Comprehensive Medical Terminology *for* Health Professions

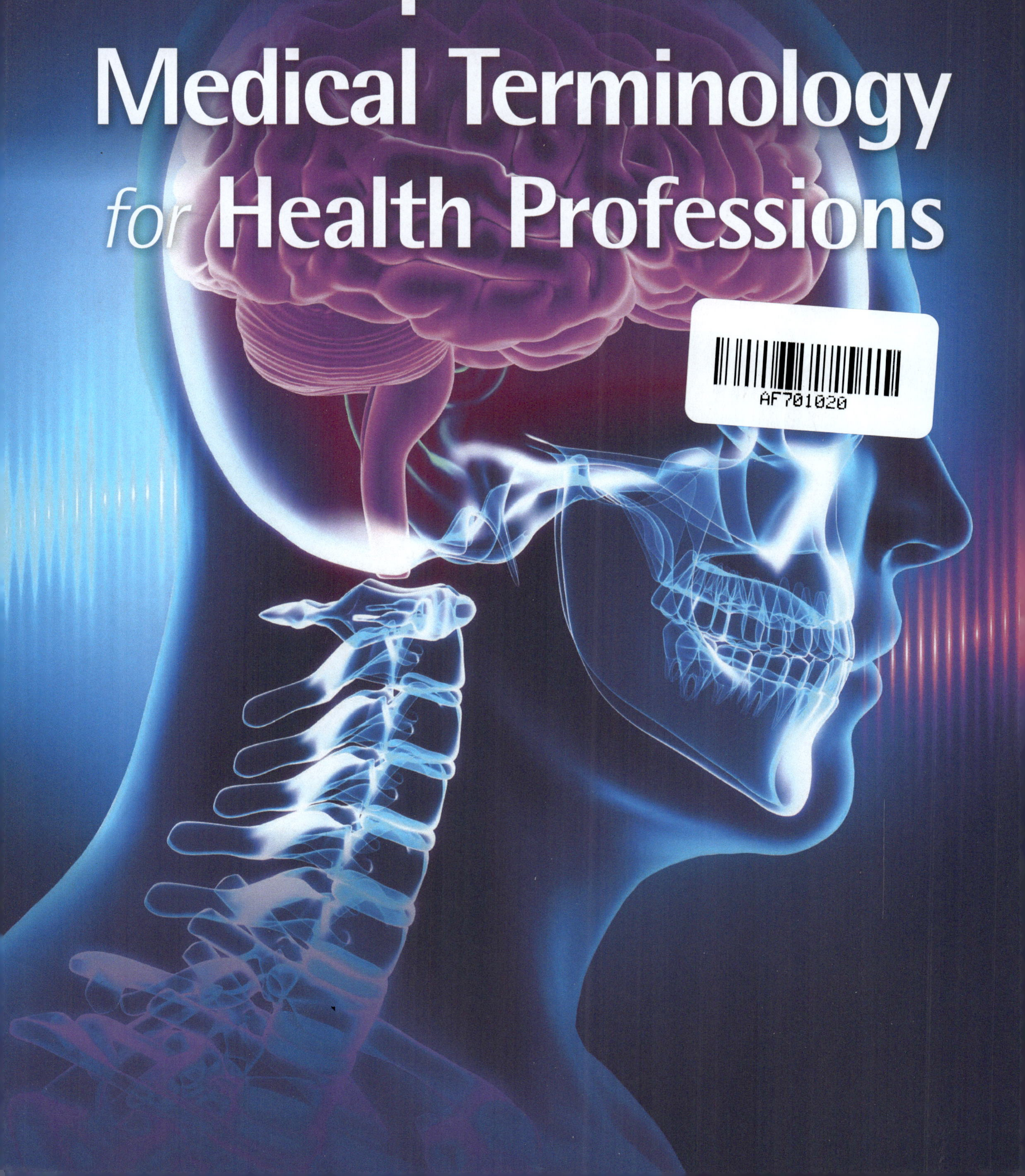

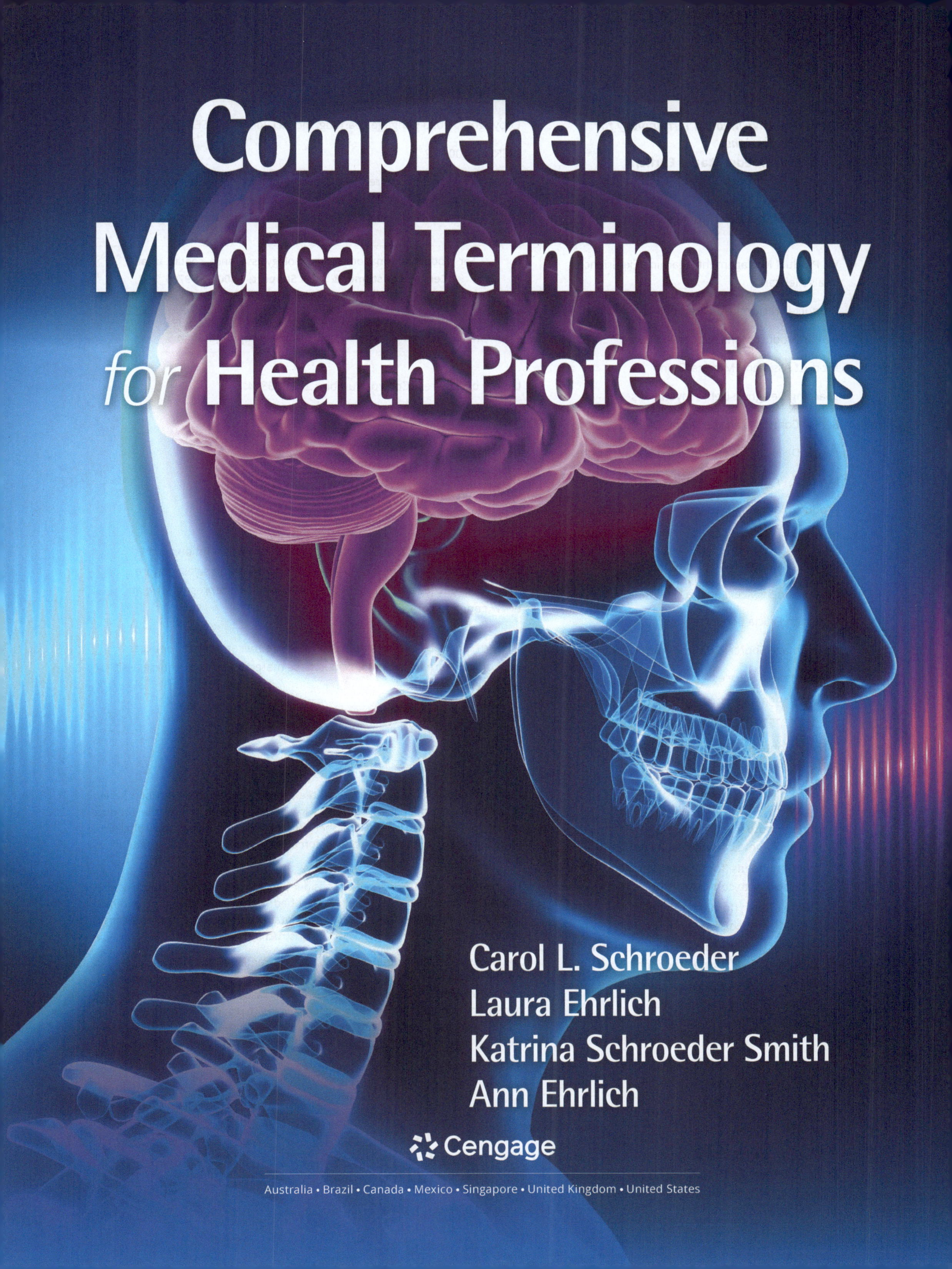

Comprehensive Medical Terminology *for* Health Professions

Carol L. Schroeder
Laura Ehrlich
Katrina Schroeder Smith
Ann Ehrlich

Cengage

Australia • Brazil • Canada • Mexico • Singapore • United Kingdom • United States

Cengage

Comprehensive Medical Terminology for Health Professions
Carol L. Schroeder, Laura Ehrlich, Katrina Schroeder Smith, Ann Ehrlich

SVP, Higher Education Product Management: Erin Joyner

VP, Product Management, Learning Experiences: Thais Alencar

Product Director: Jason Fremder

Senior Product Manager: Laura Stewart

Product Assistant: Martina Grant

Learning Designer: Debra Myette-Flis

Senior Content Manager: Anne Orgren

Digital Delivery Quality Partner: Lisa Christopher

Director, Product Marketing: Neena Bali

Product Marketing Manager: Courtney Cozzy

IP Analyst: Ashley Maynard

IP Project Manager: Anjali Kambli

Production Service: Lumina Datamatics Ltd.

Designer: Felicia Bennett

Cover Image Source: SciePro/ShutterStock.com

Interior Image Sources:

- 672719506: © MDGRPHCS/ShutterStock.com
- 178172570: © SkillUp/ShutterStock.com

Table of Contents Image Sources:
All © Cengage Learning, Inc. EXCEPT:

- Centrifuge photo (for Chapter 6): © Maxx-Studio/Shutterstock.com
- Infant photo (for Chapter 18): © iStockPhoto.com/jacobmoisan
- Photo of hands (for Chapter 19): © iStockPhoto.com/HAYKIRDI
- Photo of scan (for Chapter 20): © Mark_Kostich/Shutterstock.com
- Photo of doctor and patient (for Chapter 21): © Serhii Bobyk/Shutterstock.com
- Photo of pharmacologist (for Chapter 22): © iStockPhoto.com/Ridofranz

Library of Congress Control Number: 2021915344

ISBN: 978-0-357-51263-0

Cengage
200 Pier 4 Boulevard
Boston, MA 02210
USA

NOTICE TO THE READER

Publisher does not warrant or guarantee any of the products described herein or perform any independent analysis in connection with any of the product information contained herein. Publisher does not assume, and expressly disclaims, any obligation to obtain and include information other than that provided to it by the manufacturer.

The reader is expressly warned to consider and adopt all safety precautions that might be indicated by the activities described herein and to avoid all potential hazards. By following the instructions contained herein, the reader willingly assumes all risks in connection with such instructions.

The publisher makes no representations or warranties of any kind, including but not limited to, the warranties of fitness for particular purpose or merchantability, nor are any such representations implied with respect to the material set forth herein, and the publisher takes no responsibility with respect to such material. The publisher shall not be liable for any special, consequential, or exemplary damages resulting, in whole or part, from the readers' use of, or reliance upon, this material.

Printed in the United Kingdom by CPI Antony Rowe
Print Number: 19 Print Year: 2026

MIX Paper | Supporting responsible forestry FSC® C013604

CONTENTS

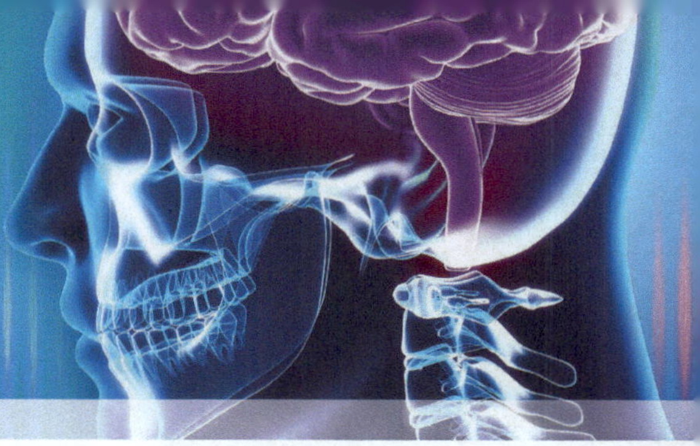

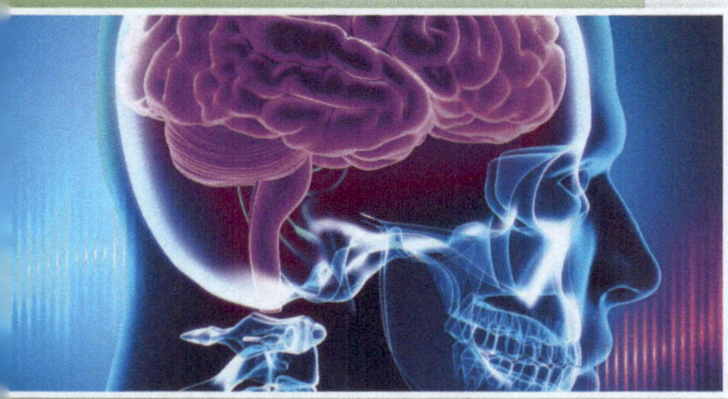

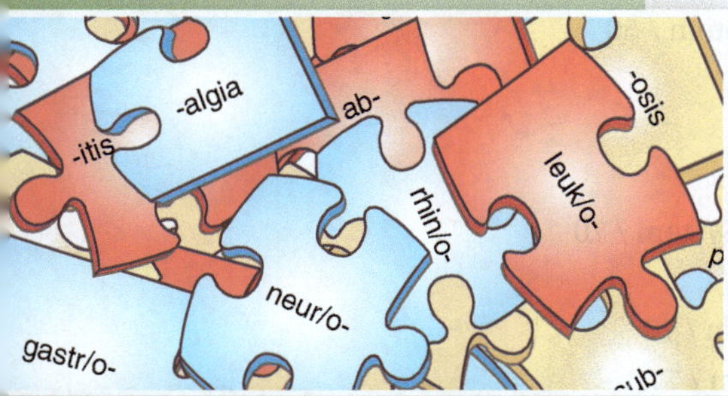

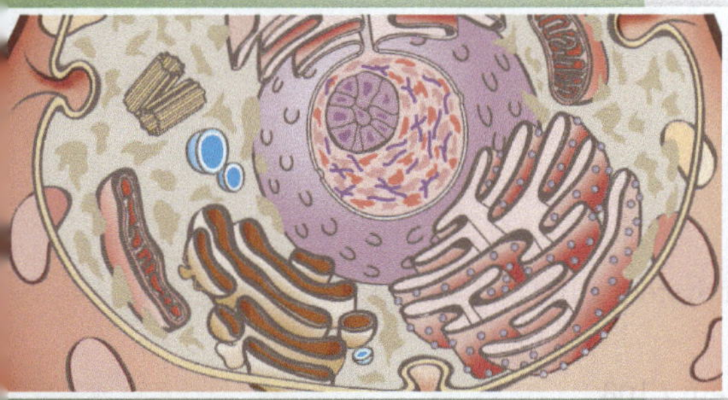

Word Part Review WPR1

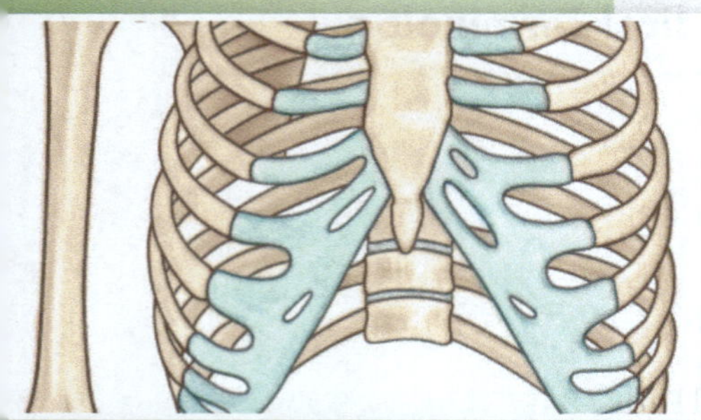

Chapter 3: The Skeletal System 56

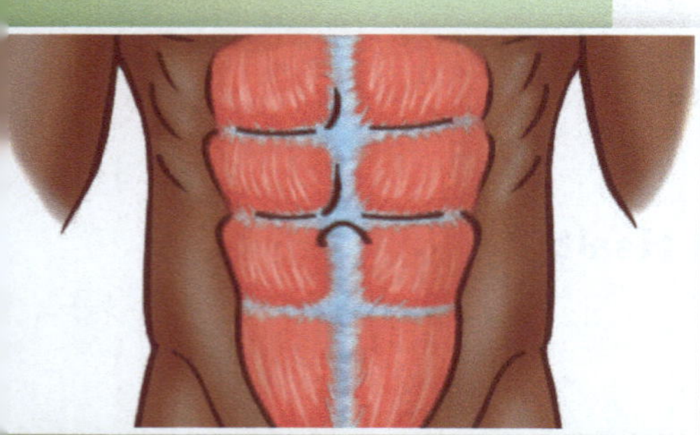

Chapter 4: The Muscular System 92

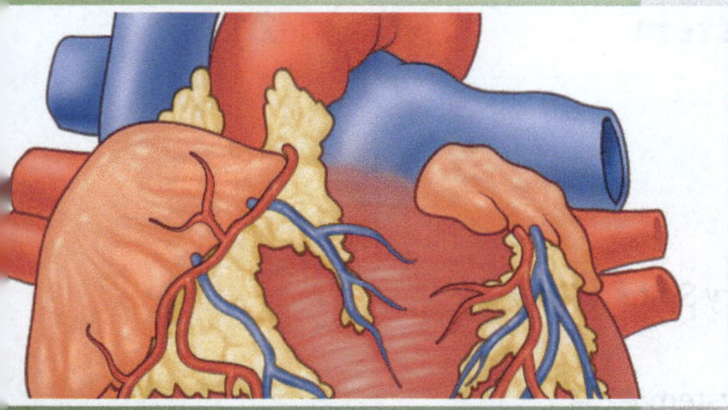

Chapter 5: The Cardiovascular System 122

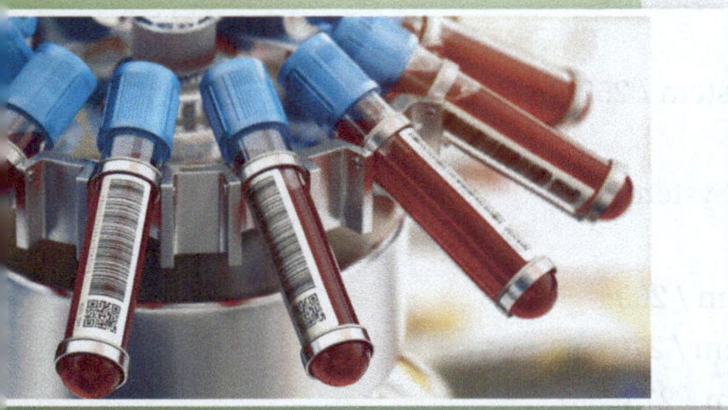

Chapter 6: The Blood System 160

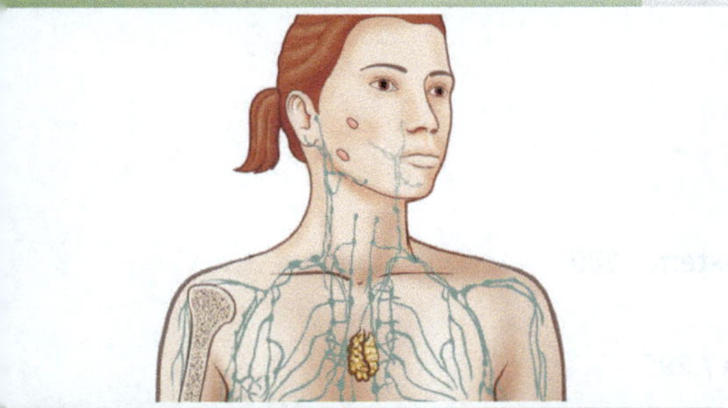

Chapter 7: The Lymphatic and Immune Systems 187

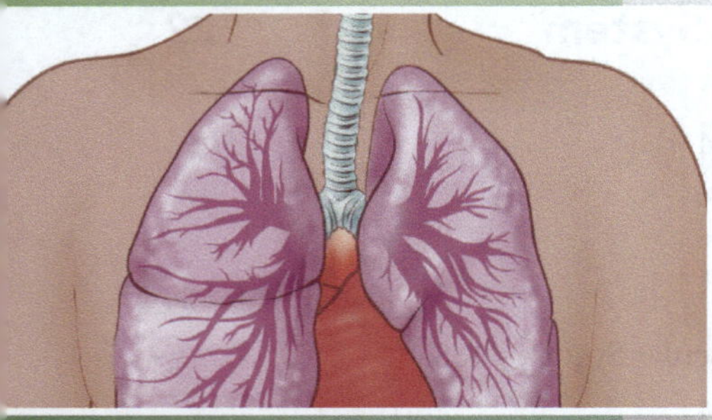

Chapter 8: The Respiratory System 217

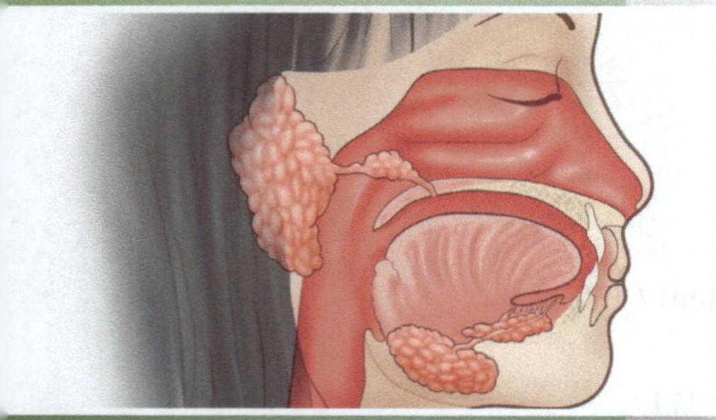

Chapter 9: The Digestive System 248

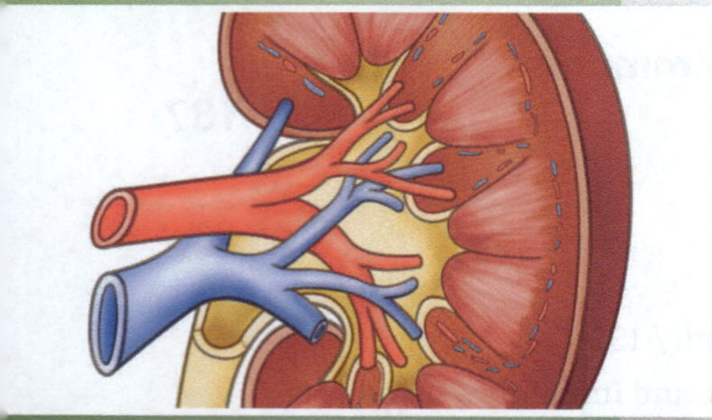

Chapter 10: The Urinary System 283

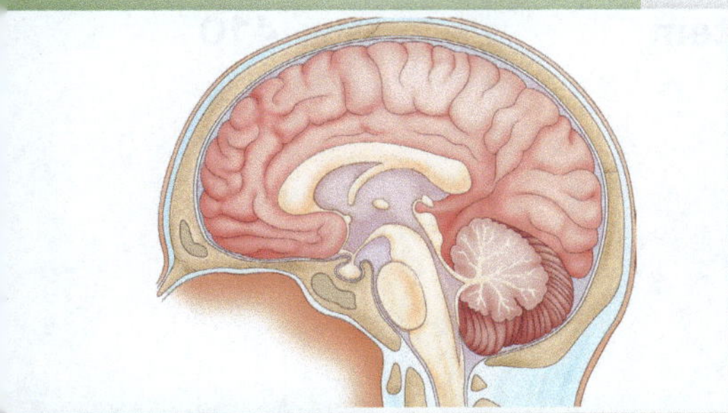

Chapter 11: The Nervous System 314

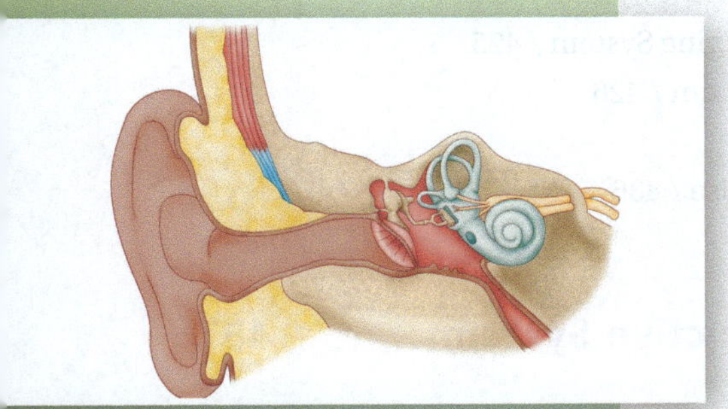

Chapter 12: Special Senses: The Eyes and Ears 347

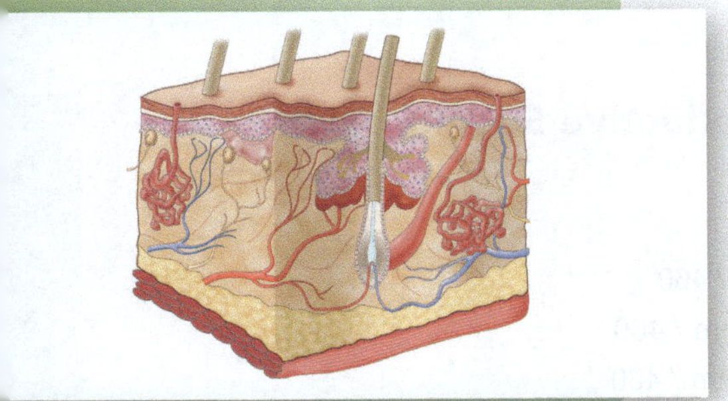

Chapter 13: Skin: The Integumentary System 379

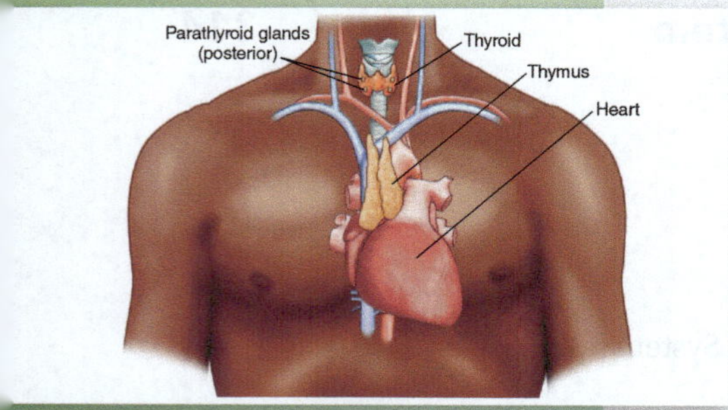

Chapter 14: The Endocrine System 410

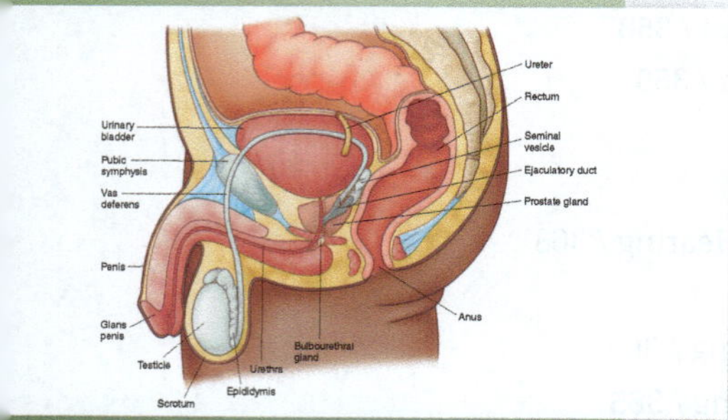

Chapter 15: The Male Reproductive System 437

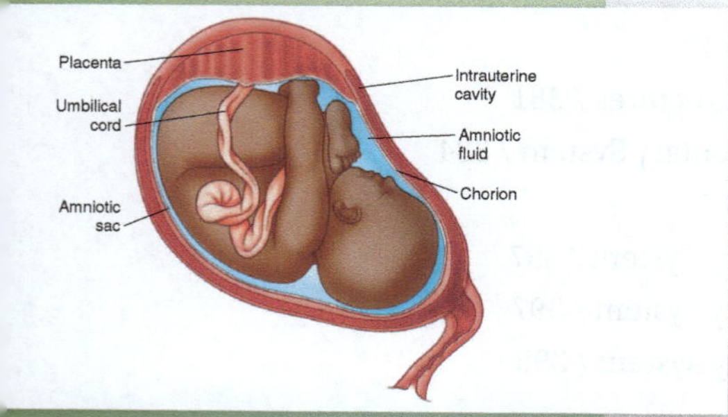

Chapter 16: The Female Reproductive System and Obstetrics 458

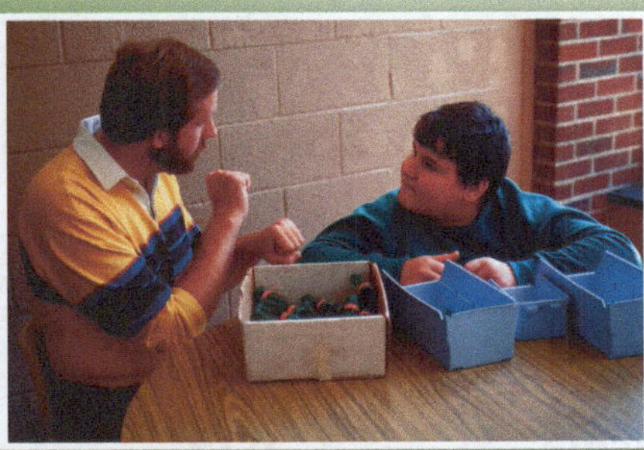

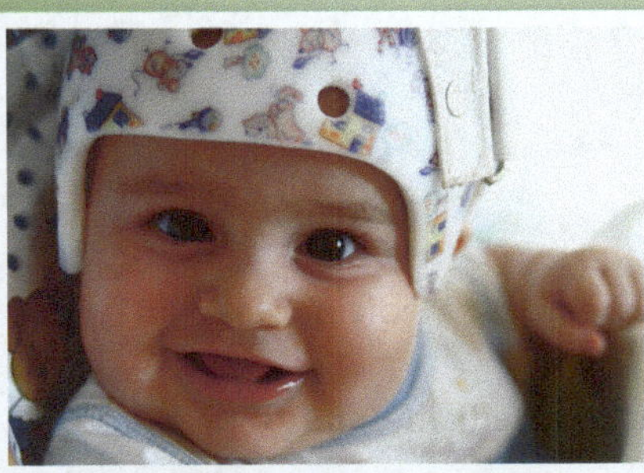

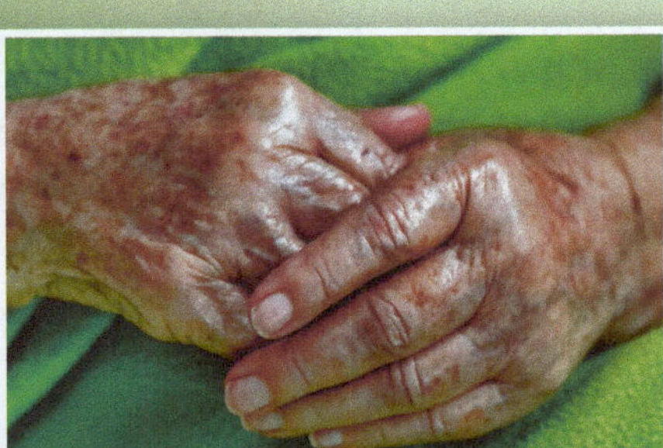

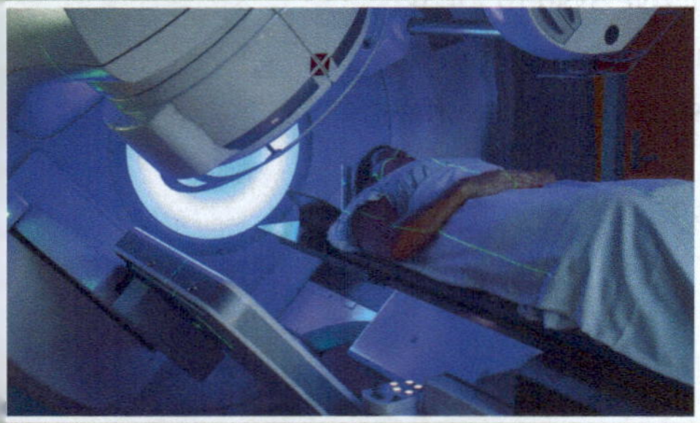

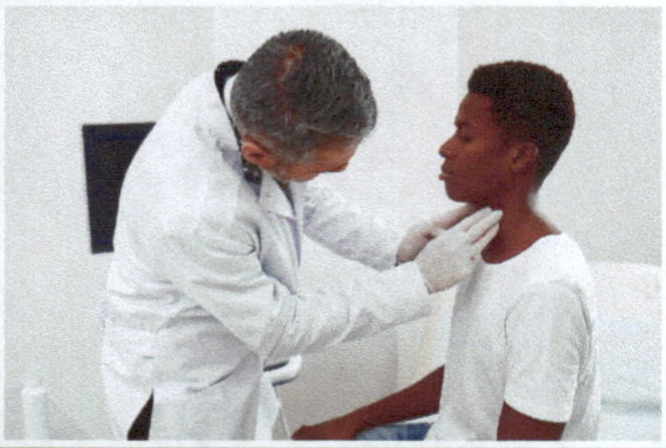

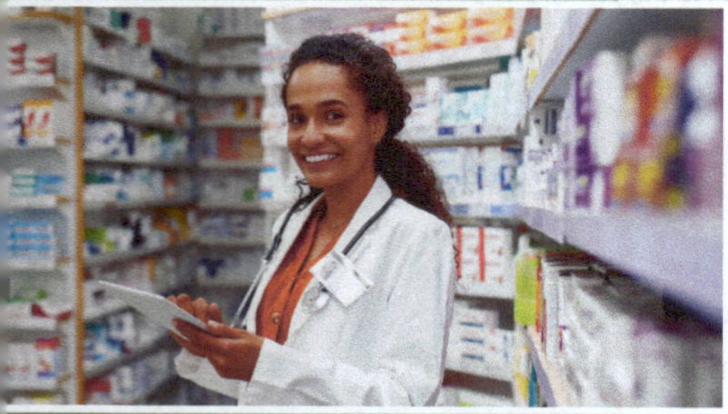

Comprehensive Medical Terminology Review 681

RS.3. The suffix ____________________ means surgical fixation.

a. -desis
b. -lysis
c. -pexy
d. -ptosis

A

a-	no, not, without, away from, negative
-a	noun ending
ab-	away from, negative, absent
abdomin/o	abdomen
-able	capable of, able to
abort/o	premature expulsion of a nonviable

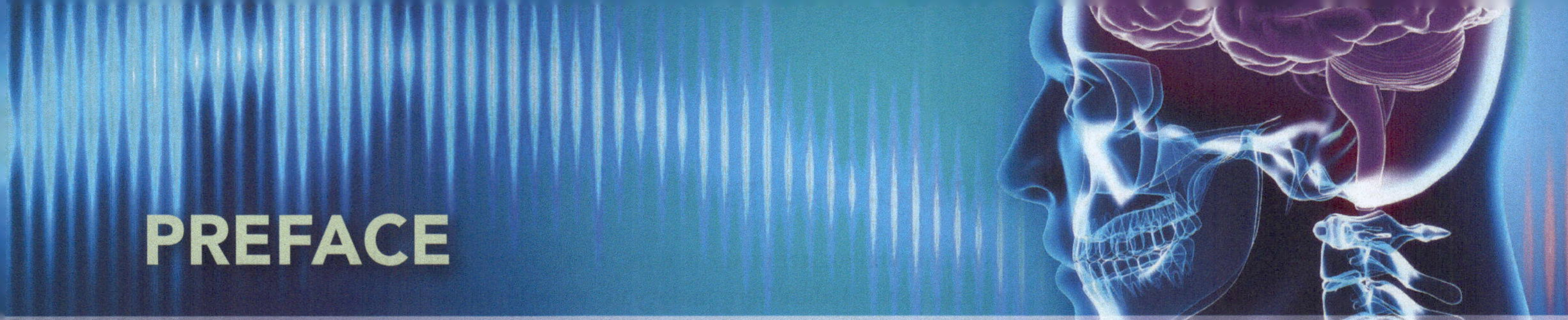

PREFACE

TO THE LEARNER

Welcome to the world of medical terminology! Learning this special language is an important step in preparing for your career as a health care professional. Here's the good news: Learning medical terms is much easier than learning a foreign language because you are already familiar with quite a few of the words, such as *appendicitis* and *tonsillectomy*. Understanding new words becomes easier with the discovery that many of these terms are made up of interchangeable word parts that are used in different combinations. Once you understand this, you'll be well on your way to translating even the most difficult medical terms, including words you have never seen before. You'll be amazed to see how quickly your vocabulary will grow!

This book and the accompanying learning materials are designed to make the process as simple as possible. Review the section "How to Use This Book" so you can find your way around easily. Once you become comfortable with the format, you'll discover you are learning more quickly than you ever imagined possible.

CONCEPTUAL APPROACH

Comprehensive Medical Terminology for Health Professions is specifically designed for students in health care programs who require in-depth competence in the terminology used in today's health care careers. This text integrates key content from the best-selling *Medical Terminology for Health Professions* text and utilizes the time-tested chapter and learning exercise structure that has made this text a leader in teaching medical terminology for over 30 years.

Intensive one-on-one conversations with instructors and in-depth research surveys helped inform and confirm the learning objectives that guided the development of each chapter. These learning objectives were key to developing the narrative content for each chapter, as well as activities and assignments for assessing students' learning. The body system and medical specialty chapter organization provides instructors with flexibility to use this text in an introductory, intermediate, or advanced medical terminology course.

Application-based activities in MindTap allow students to practice critical medical terminology concepts such as term dissection and word-building in a real-world context with exposure to a variety of medical reports used in actual practice. Audio message translation and video-based scenario activities provide students with an opportunity to apply medical terminology through simulated real-world situations that mirror those that students may encounter in actual practice.

ORGANIZATION OF THE TEXT

The text is designed to help you master medical terminology. It includes 22 chapters; a Word Part Review; a Comprehensive Medical Terminology Review with two review sessions and two simulated final tests, one each for the body system and medical specialty chapters; and three appendices. To gain the most benefit from your use of this text, take advantage of the many features, including the *Learning Exercises* plus *The Human Touch* stories and discussion questions that are included at the end of each chapter.

Primary terms are the most important terms in a chapter. When first introduced, the term appears in boldface and, if appropriate, is followed by a "sounds-like" pronunciation. Only primary terms are used as correct answers in the learning exercises and tests.

Secondary terms appear in ***orange*** italics. These terms, which are included to clarify the meaning of primary terms, are sometimes used as distracters, but not as correct answers, in the learning exercises or tests.

Each chapter begins with a **vocabulary list** consisting of 15 essential word parts and 60 medical terms selected from among the primary terms in the chapter. This list will help you focus on some of the most important terms and word parts.

Introductory Chapters and Word Part Review

Chapters 1 and 2 create the foundation that enables you to master the rest of the book. Chapter 1 introduces key word parts—the building blocks of most medical terms.

Chapter 2 introduces more word parts and provides an overview of basic terms used throughout the medical field, as well as some of the many career options open to you in health care.

After studying these chapters, complete the **Word Part Review** that follows Chapter 2. These practice activities and the accompanying test will help you determine whether you've mastered the concept of these all-important building blocks. If you are having trouble here, it is important to put more effort into learning these basics.

Body System Chapters

Chapters 3 through 16 are organized by body system. Because each body system stands alone, you can study these chapters in any sequence. Each chapter begins with an overview of the structures and functions of that system so you can relate these to the medical specialists, pathology, diagnostics, and treatment procedures that follow.

MEDICAL SPECIALTY CHAPTERS

Chapters 17 through 22 are organized by medical specialty area. Because each medical specialty area stands alone, you can study these chapters in any sequence. Each chapter begins with an overview of the specialty area, then introduces the medical terms and technical information that will help you correctly use the terminology related to this specialty during your health care career.

Chapter 17 focuses on medical terminology related to mental health including characteristics of disorders, diagnostic tools, and treatment options.

Chapter 18 provides an overview of infant and child health from birth through adolescence including growth charts, immunization schedule, and pathology specific to childhood.

Chapter 19 focuses on the medical terminology and health care considerations related to medical care of the older adult, including age-related medical problems by body system, complications related to chronic medical conditions, assisted living facilities, and death and dying.

Chapter 20 is devoted to the study of cancer, including its risk factors, different methods of classification, medical specialists, diagnostics, and treatment procedures.

Chapter 21 introduces basic diagnostic procedures, examination positions, imaging techniques, laboratory tests, and nuclear medicine. It also includes a section on alternative and complementary medicine.

Chapter 22 provides an overview of the medical terminology related to pharmacology, including the regulation, naming, and classification of drugs; common drug classes and medications; and frequently used drug administration abbreviations and symbols.

Comprehensive Medical Terminology Review

This section, which follows Chapter 22, is designed to help you prepare for your final examination. It includes study tips, a review session with practice exercises covering Chapters 1 and 2 and the body system chapters, a second review session with practice exercises covering the medical specialty chapters, a simulated final test covering Chapters 1 and 2 and the body system chapters, and a second simulated final test covering the medical specialty chapters; however, be aware that none of these questions are from the actual final test.

Appendices

Appendix A: Prefixes, Combining Forms, and Suffixes is a convenient alphabetic reference for the medical word parts. When you don't recognize a word part, you can look it up here.

Appendix B: Abbreviations and Their Meanings is an extensive list of commonly used abbreviations and their meanings. Abbreviations are important in medicine, and using them *accurately* is essential!

Appendix C: Terms Related to Diagnosis, Pathology, and Procedures gives the definitions of all the primary terms in the text relating to diagnosis, pathology, and medical procedures.

FEATURES

The focus of *Comprehensive Medical Terminology for Health Professions* is to make medical terminology relevant to students so that they will acquire the skills necessary to succeed in their health care career. Every chapter reinforces and activates students' learning and pronunciation of medical terms through engaging activities, real-life medical scenarios, and critical thinking exercises.

- The Overview introduces students to the body system structures and primary functions, related combining forms, or medical specialty area and related word parts.
- The Vocabulary list in each chapter focuses on 15 essential word parts and 60 important primary terms that help to build a working knowledge that students can build on in future health care courses. A "sounds-like" pronunciation for select primary terms assists students in correctly pronouncing the terms.
- Word parts are key to learning medical terminology. A word part breakdown included for terms made up of word parts reinforces learning these critical building blocks of medical language.

- **Primary terms**, in bold, focus students on the most important terms in the chapter. ***Secondary terms***, in orange italics, help clarify the meaning of primary terms. These terms may be used as distracters in the learning exercises, but they are never used as correct answers in learning exercises or tests.
- Learning exercises at the end of each chapter provide students with a variety of question formats that require written answers to help reinforce learning and provide practice in spelling terms. The exercises allow students to assess achievement of what the learning objectives asked them to do.
- The Human Touch: Critical Thinking Exercise and questions help students make the connection from content knowledge to application through a real-life story.
- Application-based activities in the MindTap allow students to practice critical medical terminology concepts such as term dissection and word-building in a real-world context with exposure to a variety of medical reports used in health care. Audio message translation activities and video-based scenarios provide students with an opportunity to apply medical terminology through simulated real-world situations that mirror those that students may encounter in actual practice.

INSTRUCTOR AND STUDENT RESOURCES

Additional instructor and student resources for this product are available online. Instructor assets include an Instructor Manual, Educator's Guide, PowerPoint® slides, Solution and Answer Guide, and a test bank powered by Cognero®. Student assets include PowerPoint® slides. Sign up or sign in at **www.cengage.com** to search for and access this product and its online resources.

MINDTAP

MindTap is a fully online, interactive learning experience built upon authoritative Cengage Learning content. By combining readings, multimedia activities, and assessments into a singular learning path, MindTap elevates learning by providing real-world application to better engage students. Instructors customize the learning path by selecting Cengage Learning resources and adding their own content via apps that integrate into the MindTap framework seamlessly with many learning management systems.

To learn more, visit www.cengage.com/training/mindtap.

ABOUT THE AUTHORS

CAROL L. SCHROEDER, UNIVERSITY OF WISCONSIN

Carol L. Schroeder has over 20 years of experience in finding innovative ways to present medical terminology at a level appropriate for this text's readers. Her background in technical writing, translating, and research is invaluable in continuously updating the content and in creating innovative activities and approaches—such as *The Human Touch* stories—that enable instructors to present engaging courses that help all students succeed.

LAURA EHRLICH, UNIVERSITY OF ROCHESTER SCHOOL OF NURSING

Laura Ehrlich, a registered nurse, enjoys the fast-paced, challenging environment of the emergency department as well as the knowledge that her skills save lives. She excels at explaining medical terminology to patients and training other nurses on new procedures, equipment, and technology. She is also a board-certified emergency nurse (CEN) and has been nominated for the DAISY® Award for Extraordinary Nurses.

KATRINA SCHROEDER SMITH, BOSTON CHILDREN'S HOSPITAL

Katrina Schroeder Smith is a registered dietitian who trained and works at Boston Children's Hospital, a Harvard Teaching Hospital. After finishing her dietetic internship at Simmons College, she completed the prestigious LEAH (Leadership Education in Adolescent Health) Fellowship in the adolescent department at Boston Children's Hospital. Currently she is a clinical dietitian in the adolescent clinic there, specializing in the nutritional care of young adults with HIV, eating disorders, elevated body weight, and polycystic ovarian syndrome (PCOS). She also writes guides and blogs for the Center for Young Women's Health and runs a small private practice in Brookline, Massachusetts.

ANN EHRLICH, GODDARD COLLEGE

Ann Ehrlich, who founded this series in 1988, was an experienced teacher, professional author, and lifelong student. Considered one of the leading experts in the field of medical terminology, she wrote numerous books on such health topics as dental assisting, practice management, speech therapy, and lymphedema.

ACKNOWLEDGMENTS

This new book is based on the highly successful ***Medical Terminology for Health Professions***, which recently celebrated 30 years as one of the leading texts in the health care field. We are privileged to carry on the legacy of our mother and grandmother Ann Ehrlich, whose commitment to excellence in the text and accompanying instructional materials continues to inspire us.

We are very grateful for the input of the many reviewers and instructors who provided feedback for *Comprehensive Medical Terminology for Health Professions*. Their insights, comments, suggestions, and attention to detail are very important in making the text, and its many resources, up-to-date and accurate. Special thanks to Ben Ehrlich and Elise Anderson for their input. We would each especially like to thank our families for their support throughout the research, writing, and editing processes.

Thanks also to the editorial and production staff of Cengage Learning for their very professional and extremely helpful assistance in making this new work possible, especially our editors, Deb Myette-Flis and Laura Stewart. Additionally, Anne Orgren and MT Cozzola were invaluable during the production process.

Please note that a portion of the royalties for this textbook provide scholarships for lymphedema therapists, helping to address a nationwide shortage in this field.

Carol L. Schroeder,
Laura Ehrlich, and
Katrina Schroeder Smith

REVIEWERS

Anne Russo-Ladd, MS
Instructor for Allied Health

Justin Thomas Rousse, DHSc, RHIA
Visiting Professor

Melanie Shearer, MS, MT(ASCP)PBT^{CM}, CMA(AAMA)
Associate Professor, Medical Assisting

TECHNICAL REVIEWERS—BOOK

Gratitude is extended to the technical reviewers for their expertise and feedback for the Blood System chapter, Female Reproductive System and Obstetrics chapter, and the new medical specialty chapters.

Timothy Freund, PA-C
Physician Assistant
Neonatal Associates of CNY

Robyn Kaminski, RN, MSN
Nurse Manager Electrophysiology Lab
Albany Med

Sarah M. Lawrence, PharmD, MA, BCGP
Pharmacist and Independent Educational Consultant

Dawna Martich, MSN, RN
Nursing Education Consultant-Freelance SME

Elizabeth McMahon, PhD
Licensed Psychologist in Independent Practice

Dr. Eric Phillippi
Medical Procedures of Wisconsin

Meredith Robison MSN, RN, CNML
Service Line Director, Cancer Care and Neurosciences
St. Peters Health Partners

Julia Shafer RNC, MSN
Director of Women's Services
St. Mary's Healthcare

SUBJECT MATTER EXPERTS—MINDTAP APPLY IT ACTIVITIES

Apply It Activities Lead Subject Matter Expert

A special thank you is extended to Emily Noel, BCSC, CCA, MSM for bringing her instructor and curriculum development experience, 15 years of teaching experience and guiding students in learning and mastering medical terminology, and in-depth knowledge of medical terminology and the health care arena to this project. Emily served as Lead Subject Matter Expert during the various stages of design, creation, authoring, reviewing, and technical accuracy of the Apply It activities developed for MindTap and was an integral part of the Cengage team, ensuring the content accuracy, consistency, and authenticity of all Apply It activities in the MindTap to create engaging, application-based learning experiences of the highest quality and value for students, and detailed reporting metrics for instructors.

Apply It: Medical Terminology at Work Activities Subject Matter Expert

A special thank you is extended to Cheryl J. Young, CMA (AAMA), MSHE for assisting in the development of the Medical Terminology at Work video-based Apply It activities in the MindTap.

Cheryl served as the Subject Matter Expert during the various stages in the creation, authoring, and filming of the Apply It: Medical Terminology at Work activities. Her years of clinical medical assisting and instructor experience, and expert knowledge in the use of medical terminology in actual practice, brought the highest level of authenticity to the simulated health care scenario activities. Cheryl's commitment to quality, accuracy, and the creation of authentic and realistic health care situations that represent a variety of health care professionals and settings is very much appreciated.

Apply It Activities Medical Term Mapping Subject Matter Expert

A special thank you is extended to Gregory Zaleski, MBA, RHIA for serving as the Subject Matter Expert in the selection of primary terms for the Apply It activities. Gregory's years of teaching health science undergraduate courses and curriculum development experience more than qualified him to select terms from each chapter that best aligned with each type of Apply It activity and would be the most valuable for students to experience in the real-world context of those activities, including medical reports, audio messages, and videos of medical terminology being used in actual practice.

HOW TO USE THIS BOOK

Comprehensive Medical Terminology for Health Professions is designed to help you learn and remember medical terms with surprising ease. The key lies in the following features.

OVERVIEW

The first page of each body system chapter is a chart giving an overview of the structures, related combining forms, and functions most important to that system. The first page of each medical specialty chapter introduces learners to the specialty area and related word parts.

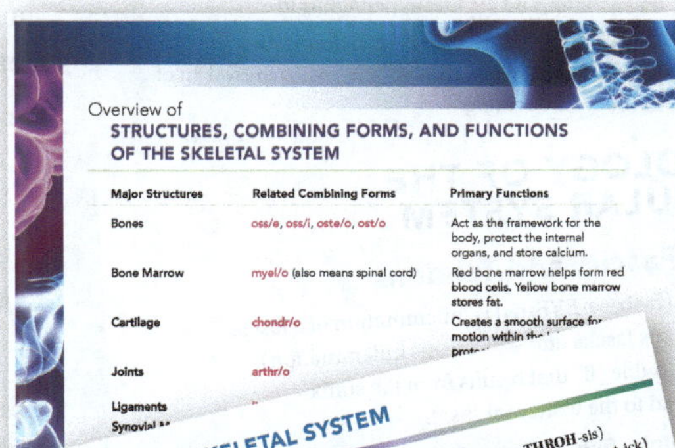
Overview of
STRUCTURES, COMBINING FORMS, AND FUNCTIONS OF THE SKELETAL SYSTEM

Major Structures	Related Combining Forms	Primary Functions
Bones	oss/e, oss/i, oste/o, ost/o	Act as the framework for the body, protect the internal organs, and store calcium.
Bone Marrow	myel/o (also means spinal cord)	Red bone marrow helps form red blood cells. Yellow bone marrow stores fat.
Cartilage	chondr/o	Creates a smooth surface for motion within the ...
Joints	arthr/o	

VOCABULARY LIST

The second page of each chapter is a 75-item vocabulary list. This list includes 15 essential word parts with their meanings and 60 primary terms from the chapter with their pronunciations. This immediately alerts you to the most important terms in the chapter and acts as a review guide. Next to each term is a box so you can check off each term when you've learned it.

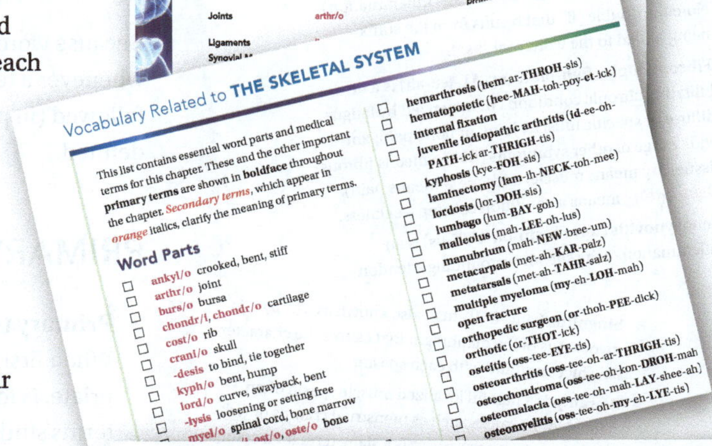
Vocabulary Related to THE SKELETAL SYSTEM

This list contains essential word parts and medical terms for this chapter. These and the other important **primary terms** are shown in **boldface** throughout the chapter. *Secondary terms*, which appear in *orange* italics, clarify the meaning of primary terms.

Word Parts
- ☐ **ankyl/o** crooked, bent, stiff
- ☐ **arthr/o** joint
- ☐ **burs/o** bursa
- ☐ **chondr/i, chondr/o** cartilage
- ☐ **cost/o** rib
- ☐ **crani/o** skull
- ☐ **-desis** to bind, tie together
- ☐ **kyph/o** bent, hump
- ☐ **lord/o** curve, swayback, bent
- ☐ **-lysis** loosening or setting free
- ☐ **myel/o** spinal cord, bone marrow
- ☐ **oss/e, oss/i, ost/o, oste/o** bone

- ☐ **hemarthrosis** (hem-ar-THROH-sis)
- ☐ **hematopoietic** (hee-MAH-toh-poy-et-ick)
- ☐ **internal fixation**
- ☐ **juvenile idiopathic arthritis** (id-ee-oh-PATH-ick ar-THRIGH-tis)
- ☐ **kyphosis** (kye-FOH-sis)
- ☐ **laminectomy** (lam-ih-NECK-toh-mee)
- ☐ **lordosis** (lor-DOH-sis)
- ☐ **lumbago** (lum-BAY-goh)
- ☐ **malleolus** (mah-LEE-oh-lus)
- ☐ **manubrium** (mah-NEW-bree-um)
- ☐ **metacarpals** (met-ah-KAR-palz)
- ☐ **metatarsals** (met-ah-TAHR-salz)
- ☐ **multiple myeloma** (my-eh-LOH-mah)
- ☐ **open fracture**
- ☐ **orthopedic surgeon** (or-thoh-PEE-dick)
- ☐ **orthotic** (or-THOT-ick)
- ☐ **ostealgia** (oss-tee-AL-jee-ah)
- ☐ **osteitis** (oss-tee-EYE-tis)
- ☐ **osteoarthritis** (oss-tee-oh-ar-THRIGH-tis)
- ☐ **osteochondroma** (oss-tee-oh-kon-DROH-mah)
- ☐ **osteomalacia** (oss-tee-oh-mah-LAY-shee-ah)
- ☐ **osteomyelitis** (oss-tee-oh-my-eh-LYE-tis)

LEARNING OBJECTIVES

The beginning of each chapter lists learning objectives to help you understand what is expected of you as you read the text and complete the learning exercises. These objectives are set off with a colored bar for easy identification.

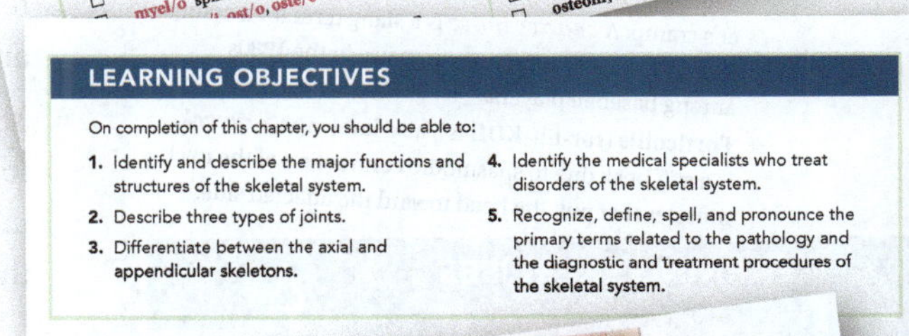
LEARNING OBJECTIVES

On completion of this chapter, you should be able to:

1. Identify and describe the major functions and structures of the skeletal system.
2. Describe three types of joints.
3. Differentiate between the axial and appendicular skeletons.
4. Identify the medical specialists who treat disorders of the skeletal system.
5. Recognize, define, spell, and pronounce the primary terms related to the pathology and the diagnostic and treatment procedures of the skeletal system.

ART PROGRAM

Our art program includes hundreds of photos and full-color illustrations that help clarify the text and contain important additional information. Review each illustration and read its caption carefully for easy and effective learning.

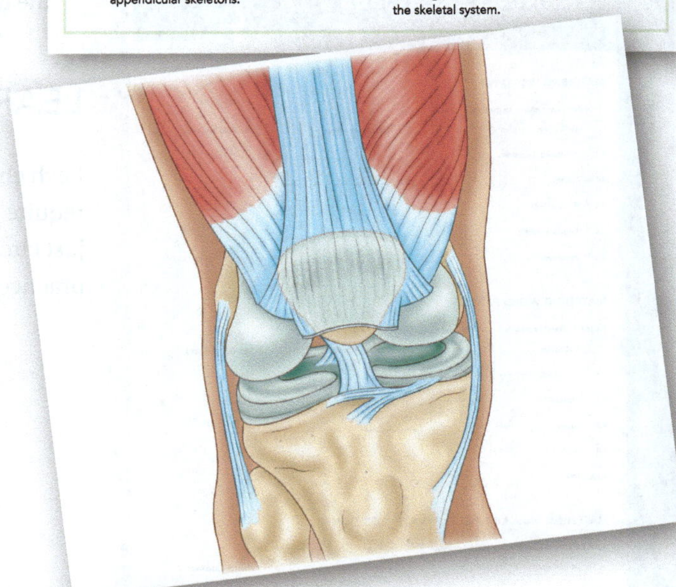

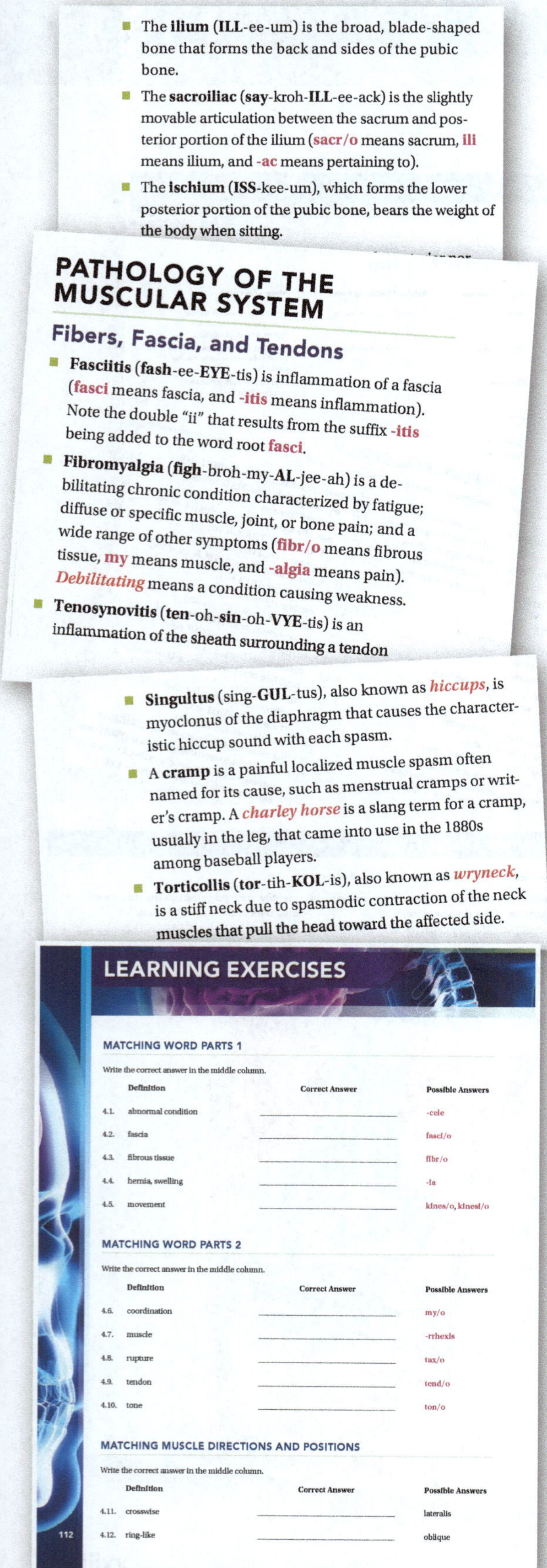

- The **ilium** (**ILL**-ee-um) is the broad, blade-shaped bone that forms the back and sides of the pubic bone.
- The **sacroiliac** (**say**-kroh-**ILL**-ee-ack) is the slightly movable articulation between the sacrum and posterior portion of the ilium (**sacr/o** means sacrum, **ili** means ilium, and **-ac** means pertaining to).
- The **ischium** (**ISS**-kee-um), which forms the lower posterior portion of the pubic bone, bears the weight of the body when sitting.

PATHOLOGY OF THE MUSCULAR SYSTEM

Fibers, Fascia, and Tendons

- **Fasciitis** (**fash**-ee-**EYE**-tis) is inflammation of a fascia (**fasci** means fascia, and **-itis** means inflammation). Note the double "ii" that results from the suffix **-itis** being added to the word root **fasci**.
- **Fibromyalgia** (**figh**-broh-my-**AL**-jee-ah) is a debilitating chronic condition characterized by fatigue; diffuse or specific muscle, joint, or bone pain; and a wide range of other symptoms (**fibr/o** means fibrous tissue, **my** means muscle, and **-algia** means pain). *Debilitating* means a condition causing weakness.
- **Tenosynovitis** (**ten**-oh-**sin**-oh-**VYE**-tis) is an inflammation of the sheath surrounding a tendon

- **Singultus** (sing-**GUL**-tus), also known as *hiccups*, is myoclonus of the diaphragm that causes the characteristic hiccup sound with each spasm.
- A **cramp** is a painful localized muscle spasm often named for its cause, such as menstrual cramps or writer's cramp. A *charley horse* is a slang term for a cramp, usually in the leg, that came into use in the 1880s among baseball players.
- **Torticollis** (**tor**-tih-**KOL**-is), also known as *wryneck*, is a stiff neck due to spasmodic contraction of the neck muscles that pull the head toward the affected side.

LEARNING EXERCISES

MATCHING WORD PARTS 1

Write the correct answer in the middle column.

	Definition	Correct Answer	Possible Answers
4.1.	abnormal condition	___	-cele
4.2.	fascia	___	fasci/o
4.3.	fibrous tissue	___	fibr/o
4.4.	hernia, swelling	___	-ia
4.5.	movement	___	kines/o, kinesi/o

MATCHING WORD PARTS 2

Write the correct answer in the middle column.

	Definition	Correct Answer	Possible Answers
4.6.	coordination	___	my/o
4.7.	muscle	___	-rrhexis
4.8.	rupture	___	tax/o
4.9.	tendon	___	tend/o
4.10.	tone	___	ton/o

MATCHING MUSCLE DIRECTIONS AND POSITIONS

Write the correct answer in the middle column.

	Definition	Correct Answer	Possible Answers
4.11.	crosswise	___	lateralis
4.12.	ring-like	___	oblique

112

"SOUNDS-LIKE" PRONUNCIATION SYSTEM

The "sounds-like" pronunciation system makes pronunciation easy by respelling the medical term with syllables you can understand—and say—at a glance. Simply pronounce the term just as it appears in parentheses, accenting the syllables as follows:

- **Primary** (strongest) **accent:** capital letters and bold type
- **Secondary accent:** lowercase letters and bold type

WORD PARTS

Because word parts are so important to learning medical terminology, whenever a term made up of word parts is introduced, the definition is followed (in parentheses) by the word parts highlighted in **magenta** and defined.

PRIMARY AND SECONDARY TERMS

- **Primary terms** are the most important medical terms in a chapter. When first introduced, the term appears in **boldface** and, if appropriate, is followed by the "sounds-like" pronunciation. These are the terms students need to concentrate on learning. Only primary terms are used as correct answers in the learning exercises and tests.
- *Secondary terms* appear in *orange* italics. These terms are included to clarify the meaning of primary terms. Although used as distracters in exercises, the secondary terms are not used as correct answers in the learning exercises or tests.

LEARNING EXERCISES

Each chapter includes 100 Learning Exercises in a variety of formats that require a one- or two-word written answer. Writing terms, rather than just circling a multiple-choice option, reinforces learning and provides practice in writing and spelling the terms.

THE HUMAN TOUCH: CRITICAL THINKING EXERCISE

A real-life short story that involves patients and pathology, along with related critical thinking questions, at the end of each chapter helps you apply what you are learning to the real world. There are no right or wrong answers, just questions to get you started thinking about and using the new medical terms you have learned.

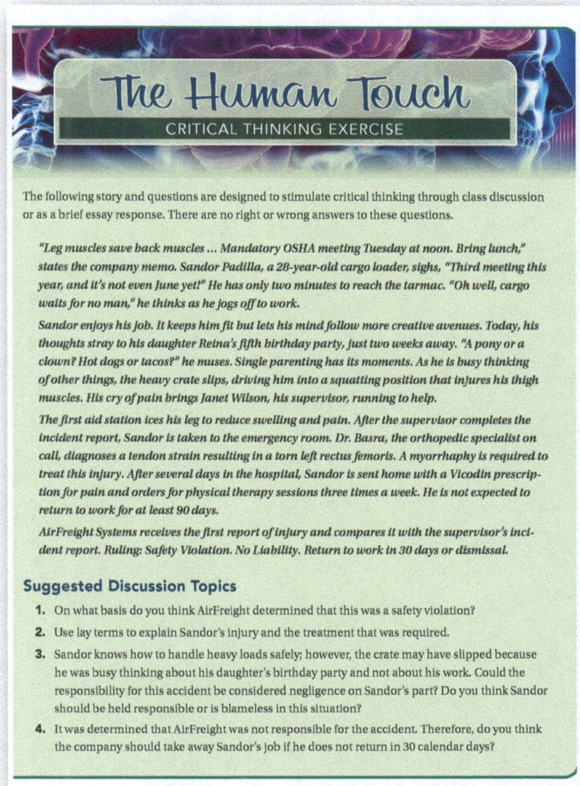

The Human Touch

CRITICAL THINKING EXERCISE

The following story and questions are designed to stimulate critical thinking through class discussion or as a brief essay response. There are no right or wrong answers to these questions.

"Leg muscles save back muscles ... Mandatory OSHA meeting Tuesday at noon. Bring lunch," states the company memo. Sandor Padilla, a 28-year-old cargo loader, sighs, "Third meeting this year, and it's not even June yet!" He has only two minutes to reach the tarmac. "Oh well, cargo waits for no man," he thinks as he jogs off to work.

Sandor enjoys his job. It keeps him fit but lets his mind follow more creative avenues. Today, his thoughts stray to his daughter Reina's fifth birthday party, just two weeks away. "A pony or a clown? Hot dogs or tacos?" he muses. Single parenting has its moments. As he is busy thinking of other things, the heavy crate slips, driving him into a squatting position that injures his thigh muscles. His cry of pain brings Janet Wilson, his supervisor, running to help.

The first aid station ices his leg to reduce swelling and pain. After the supervisor completes the incident report, Sandor is taken to the emergency room. Dr. Basra, the orthopedic specialist on call, diagnoses a tendon strain resulting in a torn left rectus femoris. A myorrhaphy is required to treat this injury. After several days in the hospital, Sandor is sent home with a Vicodin prescription for pain and orders for physical therapy sessions three times a week. He is not expected to return to work for at least 90 days.

AirFreight Systems receives the first report of injury and compares it with the supervisor's incident report. Ruling: Safety Violation. No Liability. Return to work in 30 days or dismissal.

Suggested Discussion Topics

1. On what basis do you think AirFreight determined that this was a safety violation?
2. Use lay terms to explain Sandor's injury and the treatment that was required.
3. Sandor knows how to handle heavy loads safely; however, the crate may have slipped because he was busy thinking about his daughter's birthday party and not about his work. Could the responsibility for this accident be considered negligence on Sandor's part? Do you think Sandor should be held responsible or is blameless in this situation?
4. It was determined that AirFreight was not responsible for the accident. Therefore, do you think the company should take away Sandor's job if he does not return in 30 calendar days?

CHAPTER 1

INTRODUCTION TO MEDICAL TERMINOLOGY

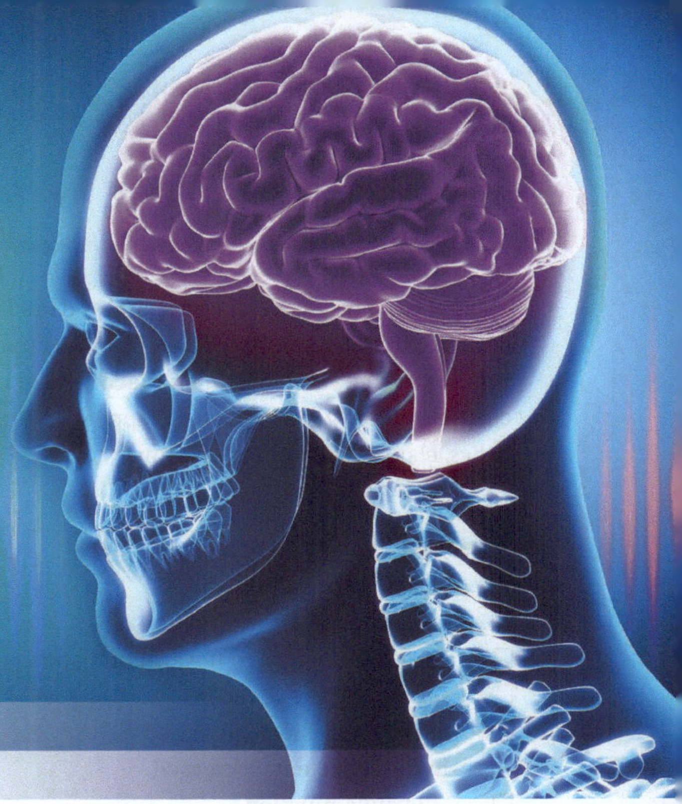

Overview of INTRODUCTION TO MEDICAL TERMINOLOGY

Primary Medical Terms	Primary terms enable you to give priority to the most important words in your study of medical terminology. These terms are shown in **black boldface**.
Word Parts Are the Key	An introduction to word parts and how they are used to create complex medical terms.
Word Roots	The word parts that usually, but not always, indicate the part of the body involved.
Combining Forms	A word root that has a vowel, usually the letter *o*, put on the end before the addition of another word root or suffix.
Combining Vowels	Letters added to a word root to create a combining form.
Suffixes	The word part attached at the end of word that usually, but not always, indicates the procedure, condition, disorder, or disease.
Prefixes	The word part attached at the beginning of word that usually, but not always, indicates location, time, number, or status.
Determining Meanings on the Basis of Word Parts	Knowledge of word parts helps decipher medical terms.
Using a Medical Dictionary or Online Resource	Guidelines to help make looking up terms online or in a medical dictionary easier.
Pronunciation	Learn how to pronounce words correctly using the "sounds-like" pronunciation system.
Spelling Is Always Important	A single spelling error can change the entire meaning of term.
Singular and Plural Endings	Unusual singular and plural endings used in medical terms.
Basic Medical Terms	Terms used to describe disease conditions.
Look-Alike, Sound-Alike Terms and Word Parts	Clarification of confusing terms and word parts that look or sound similar.
Using Abbreviations	Caution is always important when using abbreviations.

Vocabulary Related to **THE INTRODUCTION TO MEDICAL TERMINOLOGY**

This list contains essential word parts and medical terms for this chapter. These and the other important **primary terms** are shown in **boldface** throughout the chapter. *Secondary terms*, which appear in *orange* italics, clarify the meaning of primary terms.

Word Parts

- ☐ **-algia** pain, suffering
- ☐ **-dynia** pain
- ☐ **-ectomy** surgical removal, cutting out
- ☐ **-gram** picture or record
- ☐ **hyper-** excessive, increased
- ☐ **hypo-** deficient, decreased
- ☐ **-itis** inflammation
- ☐ **-osis** abnormal condition, disease
- ☐ **-ostomy** the surgical creation of an artificial opening to the body surface
- ☐ **pre-** before, in front of
- ☐ **-plasty** surgical repair
- ☐ **-rrhage** bleeding, abnormal excessive fluid discharge
- ☐ **-rrhaphy** surgical suturing
- ☐ **-rrhea** flow or discharge
- ☐ **-sclerosis** abnormal hardening

Medical Terms

- ☐ **abdominocentesis** (ab-**dom**-ih-noh-sen-**TEE**-sis)
- ☐ **acronym** (**ACK**-roh-nim)
- ☐ **acute**
- ☐ **angiography** (**an**-jee-**OG**-rah-fee)
- ☐ **appendectomy** (**ap**-en-**DECK**-toh-mee)
- ☐ **arteriosclerosis** (ar-**tee**-ree-oh-skleh-**ROH**-sis)
- ☐ **arthralgia** (ar-**THRAL**-jee-ah)
- ☐ **colostomy** (koh-**LAHS**-toh-mee)
- ☐ **cyanosis** (**sigh**-ah-**NOH**-sis)
- ☐ **dermatologist** (**der**-mah-**TOL**-oh-jist)
- ☐ **diagnosis** (**dye**-ag-**NOH**-sis)
- ☐ **diarrhea** (**dye**-ah-**REE**-ah)
- ☐ **edema** (eh-**DEE**-mah)
- ☐ **endarterial** (**end**-ar-**TEE**-ree-al)
- ☐ **eponym** (**EP**-oh-nim)
- ☐ **erythrocyte** (eh-**RITH**-roh-**sight**)
- ☐ **fissure** (**FISH**-ur)
- ☐ **fistula** (**FIS**-chuh-lah)
- ☐ **gastralgia** (gas-**TRAL**-jee-ah)
- ☐ **gastritis** (gas-**TRY**-tis)
- ☐ **gastroenteritis** (**gas**-troh-en-ter-**EYE**-tis)
- ☐ **gastrosis** (gas-**TROH**-sis)
- ☐ **hemorrhage** (**HEM**-or-idj)
- ☐ **hepatomegaly** (**hep**-ah-toh-**MEG**-ah-lee)
- ☐ **hypertension** (**high**-per-**TEN**-shun)
- ☐ **hypotension** (**high**-poh-**TEN**-shun)
- ☐ **infection** (in-**FECK**-shun)
- ☐ **inflammation** (**in**-flah-**MAY**-shun)
- ☐ **interstitial** (**in**-ter-**STISH**-al)
- ☐ **intramuscular** (**in**-trah-**MUS**-kyou-lar)
- ☐ **laceration** (**lass**-er-**AY**-shun)
- ☐ **lesion** (**LEE**-zhun)
- ☐ **malaise** (mah-**LAYZ**)
- ☐ **mycosis** (my-**KOH**-sis)
- ☐ **myelopathy** (my-eh-**LOP**-ah-thee)
- ☐ **myopathy** (my-**OP**-ah-thee)
- ☐ **natal** (**NAY**-tal)
- ☐ **neonatology** (**nee**-oh-nay-**TOL**-oh-jee)
- ☐ **neurorrhaphy** (new-**ROR**-ah-fee)
- ☐ **otorhinolaryngology** (**oh**-toh-**rye**-noh-**lar**-in-**GOL**-oh-jee)
- ☐ **palpation** (pal-**PAY**-shun)
- ☐ **palpitation** (**pal**-pih-**TAY**-shun)
- ☐ **pathology** (pah-**THOL**-oh-jee)
- ☐ **phalanges** (fah-**LAN**-jeez)
- ☐ **poliomyelitis** (**poh**-lee-oh-**my**-eh-**LYE**-tis)
- ☐ **prognosis** (prog-**NOH**-sis)
- ☐ **pyoderma** (**pye**-oh-**DER**-mah)
- ☐ **pyrosis** (pye-**ROH**-sis)
- ☐ **remission**
- ☐ **sign**
- ☐ **supination** (**soo**-pih-**NAY**-shun)
- ☐ **suppuration** (**sup**-you-**RAY**-shun)
- ☐ **supracostal** (**sue**-prah-**KOS**-tal)
- ☐ **symptom** (**SIMP**-tum)
- ☐ **syndrome** (**SIN**-drohm)
- ☐ **tenorrhaphy** (ten-**OR**-ah-fee)
- ☐ **tonsillitis** (**ton**-sih-**LYE**-tis)
- ☐ **trauma** (**TRAW**-mah)
- ☐ **triage** (tree-**AHZH**)
- ☐ **viral** (**VYE**-ral)

LEARNING OBJECTIVES

On completion of this chapter, you should be able to:

1. Define *word root, combining form, combining vowel, suffix,* and *prefix* as they are used in medical word building.
2. Use your knowledge of word parts to analyze unfamiliar medical terms.
3. Describe the steps in locating a term in a medical dictionary or online resource.
4. State the importance of spelling medical terms correctly.
5. Define *eponym*.
6. Define *acronym*.
7. Explain how to determine which medical abbreviations are not safe to use.
8. Identify the medical word parts introduced in this chapter.
9. Define the primary terms introduced in this chapter.
10. Spell the primary terms introduced in this chapter.
11. Use the "sounds-like" pronunciation system to correctly pronounce the primary terms introduced in this chapter.

PRIMARY MEDICAL TERMS

In this textbook, you will be introduced to many medical terms; however, mastering them may be easier than you anticipate because Medical Terminology for Health Professions has many features to help you learn.

- **Primary terms** appear in **boldface**. Learning these terms should be your highest priority as only primary terms are used as correct answers in the Learning Exercises and tests.
- A **vocabulary list** with 15 essential word parts and 60 key primary terms (and their pronunciations) is at the beginning of each chapter.
- *Secondary terms* appear in *orange* italics. Some of these terms are the "also known as" names for conditions or procedures. Other secondary terms clarify words used in the definitions of primary terms.

WORD PARTS ARE THE KEY

Learning medical terminology is much easier once you understand how word parts work together to form medical terms (Figure 1.1). A **compound word** is a term made up of more than one word part. This textbook includes many aids to help you reinforce your word-building skills.

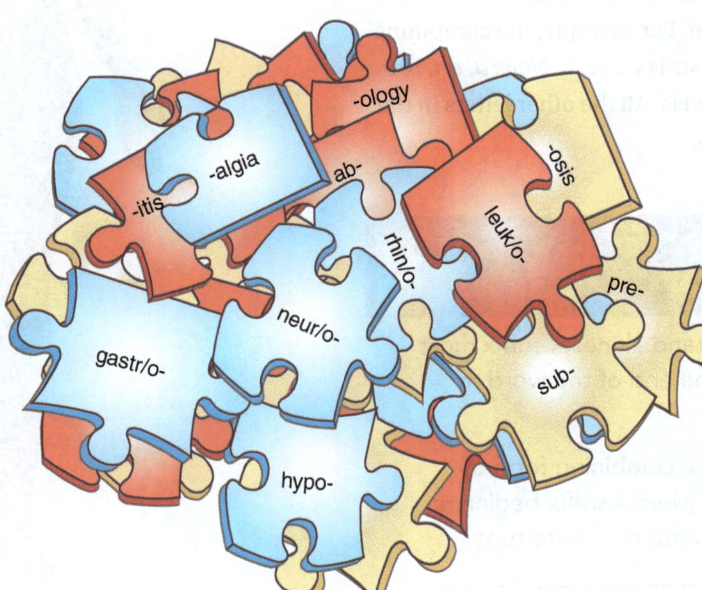

FIGURE 1.1 Word parts (word roots, combining forms, suffixes, and prefixes) make up most medical terms.

- The types of word parts and the rules for their use are explained in this chapter. Learn these rules and follow them.
- When a term is made up of recognizable word parts, these word parts and their meanings are included with the definition of that term. These word parts appear in **magenta**.
- The majority of the word parts used in medical terminology are of Latin origin, some are derived from Greek, and a few are from other languages.
- The Learning Exercises for each chapter include a "Challenge Word Building" section to help develop your skills in working with word parts.
- A **Word Part Review** follows Chapter 2. This section provides additional word part practice and enables you to evaluate your progress toward mastering the meaning of these word parts.

The Four Types of Word Parts

The four types of word parts used to create many medical terms are word roots, combining forms, suffixes, and prefixes. Guidelines for their use are shown in Table 1.1.

1. A **word root** contains the basic meaning of the term. In medical terminology, this word part usually, *but not always*, indicates the involved body part. For example, the word root meaning stomach is **gastr**.
2. A **combining form** is a word root with a combining vowel added at the end. It is used when two word roots are combined or when a suffix beginning with a consonant is added. When a combining form appears alone, it is shown with a back slash (/) between the word root and the combining vowel. For example, the combining form of the word root **gastr** is **gastr/o**. *Note: a, e, i, o, u,* and sometimes *y* are vowels. All the other letters in the alphabet are consonants.

TABLE 1.1

Word Part Guidelines

1. A word root cannot stand alone. A suffix must always be added at the end of the word to complete the term.
2. The rules for creating a combining form by adding a vowel apply when a suffix beginning with a consonant is added to a word root.
3. If a prefix is added, it is *always* placed at the beginning of the word.

3. A suffix usually, *but not always*, indicates the procedure, condition, disorder, or disease.
    - A suffix always comes at the end of the word.
    - You'll know a word part is a suffix when it is shown with a hyphen (-) in front of it. For example, the suffix **-itis** means inflammation.
4. A prefix usually, *but not always*, indicates location, time, number, or status.
    - A prefix always comes at the beginning of a word.
    - You'll know a word part is a prefix when it is shown with a hyphen (-) after it. For example, **hyper-** means excessive or increased.

WORD ROOTS

Word roots act as the foundation for most medical terms. They usually, *but not always*, describe the part of the body that is involved (Figure 1.2). As shown in Table 1.2, some word roots indicate color.

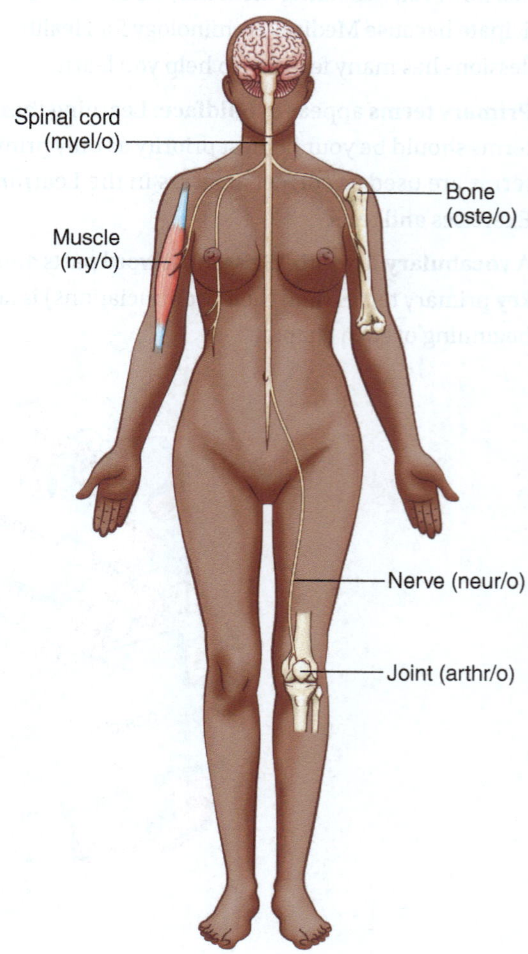

FIGURE 1.2 Word roots, shown here as combining forms, usually indicate the involved body part.

TABLE 1.2

Word Roots and Combining Forms Indicating Color

cyan/o means blue	**Cyanosis** (**sigh**-ah-**NOH**-sis) is blue discoloration of the skin caused by lack of adequate oxygen in the blood (**cyan** means blue, and **-osis** means abnormal condition or disease).
erythr/o means red	An **erythrocyte** (eh-**RITH**-roh-**sight**) is a mature red blood cell (**erythr/o** means red, and **-cyte** means cell).
leuk/o means white	A **leukocyte** (**LOO**-koh-sight) is a white blood cell (**leuk/o** means white, and **-cyte** means cell).
melan/o means black	**Melanoma** (mel-ah-**NOH**-mah) is a type of skin cancer (**melan** means black, and **-oma** means a tumor).
poli/o means gray	**Poliomyelitis** (**poh**-lee-oh-**my**-eh-**LYE**-tis) is a viral infection of the gray nerve tissue of the spinal cord (**poli/o** means gray, **myel** means spinal cord, and **-itis** means inflammation).

Combining Forms and Vowels

A combining form includes a vowel, usually the letter ***o***, added to the end of a word root. It is usually added to make the resulting medical term easier to pronounce. The rules for the use of a **combining vowel** are as follows:

- When two word roots are joined, a combining vowel is always added to the first word root. A combining vowel is used at the end of the second word root *only if the suffix begins with a consonant.*
- For example, the term **gastroenteritis** combines two word roots with a suffix: when **gastr** (stomach) is joined with the word root **enter** (small intestine), a vowel is used to make the combining form **gastr/o**.
- The word root **enter** is joined to **-itis** *without a combining vowel* because this suffix begins with a vowel. **Gastroenteritis** (**gas**-troh-en-ter-**EYE**-tis) is an inflammation of the stomach and small intestine.

SUFFIXES

A suffix is *always* added at the end of a word to complete that term. In medical terminology, suffixes usually, *but not always,* indicate a procedure, condition, disorder, or disease.

A combining vowel is used when the suffix begins with a consonant. For example, when **neur/o** (nerve) is joined with the suffix **-plasty** (surgical repair) or **-rrhaphy** (surgical suturing), the combining vowel ***o*** is used because **-plasty** and **-rrhaphy** both begin with a consonant.

- **Neuroplasty** (**NEW**-roh-**plas**-tee) is the surgical repair of a nerve.
- **Neurorrhaphy** (new-**ROR**-ah-fee) is suturing together the ends of a severed nerve.

A combining vowel is *not* used when the suffix begins with a vowel. For example, the word root **tonsill** means tonsils. No combining vowel is needed when adding either **-itis** (inflammation) or **-ectomy** (surgical removal) to **tonsill**, because they both start with a vowel (Figure 1.3). These suffixes complete the term and tell us what is happening to the tonsils.

- **Tonsillitis** (**ton**-sih-**LYE**-tis) is an inflammation of the tonsils.
- A **tonsillectomy** (**ton**-sih-**LECK**-toh-mee) is the surgical removal of the tonsils.

Suffixes as Noun Endings

A ***noun*** is a word that is the name of a person, place, or thing. In medical terminology, some suffixes change the word root into a noun. For example, the **cranium** (**KRAY**-nee-um) is the portion of the skull that encloses the brain (**crani** means skull, and **-um** is a noun ending). Suffixes that are commonly used as noun endings are shown in Table 1.3.

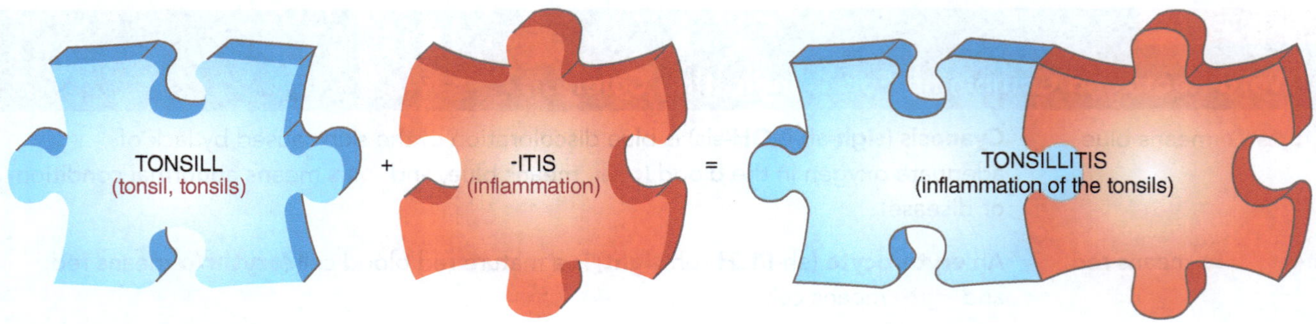

FIGURE 1.3 The term *tonsillitis* is created by adding the suffix **-itis** to the word root **tonsill**.

Suffixes Meaning "Pertaining To"

An *adjective* is a word that defines or describes. In medical terminology, many suffixes meaning "pertaining to" are used to change the meaning of a word root into an adjective. For example, the word root **cardi** means heart, and the suffix **-ac** means pertaining to. Once combined, they form the term **cardiac** (**KAR**-dee-ack), an adjective that means pertaining to the heart. Commonly used suffixes meaning pertaining to are shown in Table 1.4.

Suffixes Meaning "Abnormal Condition or Disease"

In medical terminology, many suffixes, such as **-osis**, mean "abnormal condition or disease." For example, **gastrosis** (gas-**TROH**-sis) means any disease of the stomach (**gastr** means stomach, and **-osis** means abnormal condition or disease). Commonly used suffixes meaning abnormal condition or disease are shown in Table 1.5.

TABLE 1.3

Suffixes as Noun Endings

-a	-um	-y
-e	-us	

TABLE 1.4

Suffixes Meaning "Pertaining To"

-ac	-eal	-ior
-al	-ical	-ory
-an	-ial	-ous
-ar	-ic	-tic
-ary	-ine	

Suffixes Related to Pathology

Pathology (pah-**THOL**-oh-jee) is the study of all aspects of diseases (**path** means disease, and **-ology** means study of). Suffixes related to pathology describe specific disease conditions.

- **-algia** means pain and suffering. **Gastralgia** (gas-**TRAL**-jee-ah), also known as a *stomachache*, means pain in the stomach (**gastr** means stomach, and **-algia** means pain).
- **-dynia** is another suffix meaning pain. **Gastrodynia** (**gas**-troh-**DIN**-ee-ah) also means pain in the stomach (**gastr/o** means stomach, and **-dynia** means pain). Although **gastrodynia** has the same meaning as **gastralgia**, it is not used as commonly (Figure 1.4).
- **-itis** means inflammation. **Gastritis** (gas-**TRY**-tis) is an inflammation of the stomach (**gastr** means stomach, and **-itis** means inflammation).
- **-megaly** means enlargement. **Hepatomegaly** (**hep**-ah-toh-**MEG**-ah-lee) is abnormal enlargement of

TABLE 1.5

Suffixes Meaning "Abnormal Condition or Disease"

-ago	-iasis	-osis
-esis	-ion	-pathy
-ia	-ism	

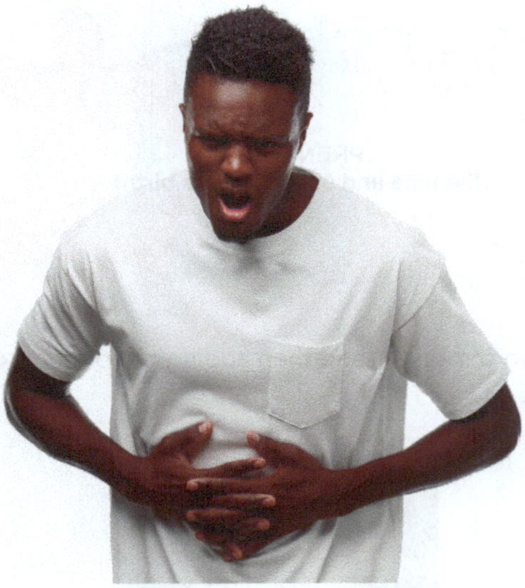

Krakenimages.com/Shutterstock.com

FIGURE 1.4 *Gastralgia* and *gastrodynia* are both terms meaning stomach pain.

the liver (**hepat/o** means liver, and **-megaly** means enlargement).

- **-malacia** means abnormal softening. **Arteriomalacia** (ar-**tee**-ree-oh-mah-**LAY**-shee-ah) is the abnormal softening of the walls of an artery or arteries (**arteri/o** means artery, and **-malacia** means abnormal softening). Notice that **-malacia** is the opposite of **-sclerosis**.
- **-necrosis** means tissue death. **Arterionecrosis** (ar-**tee**-ree-oh-neh-**KROH**-sis) is the tissue death of an artery or arteries (**arteri/o** means artery, and **-necrosis** means tissue death).
- **-sclerosis** means abnormal hardening. **Arteriosclerosis** (ar-**tee**-ree-oh-skleh-**ROH**-sis) is the abnormal hardening of the walls of an artery or arteries (**arteri/o** means artery, and **-sclerosis** means abnormal hardening). Notice that **-sclerosis** is the opposite of **-malacia**.
- **-stenosis** means abnormal narrowing. **Arteriostenosis** (ar-**tee**-ree-oh-steh-**NOH**-sis) is the abnormal narrowing of an artery or arteries (**arteri/o** means artery, and **-stenosis** means abnormal narrowing).

Suffixes Related to Procedures

Some suffixes identify the procedure that is performed on the body part indicated by the word root.

- **-centesis** is a surgical puncture to remove fluid for diagnostic purposes or to remove excess fluid. **Abdominocentesis** (ab-**dom**-ih-noh-sen-**TEE**-sis) is the surgical puncture of the abdominal cavity to remove fluid (**abdomin/o** means abdomen, and **-centesis** means a surgical puncture to remove fluid).
- **-graphy** means the process of producing a picture or record. **Angiography** (**an**-jee-**OG**-rah-fee) is the process of producing an x-ray, or radiographic study, of blood vessels after the injection of a contrast medium to make these blood vessels visible (**angi/o** means blood vessel, and **-graphy** means the process of recording).
- **-gram** means a picture or record. An **angiogram** (**AN**-jee-oh-**gram**) is the resulting film that is produced by angiography (**angi/o** means blood vessel, and **-gram** means a picture or record).
- **-plasty** means surgical repair. **Myoplasty** (**MY**-oh-**plas**-tee) is the surgical repair of a muscle (**my/o** means muscle, and **-plasty** means surgical repair).
- **-scopy** means visual examination. **Arthroscopy** (ar-**THROS**-koh-pee) is the visual examination of the internal structure of a joint (**arthr/o** means joint, and **-scopy** means visual examination).

The "Double R" Suffixes

Medical terminology suffixes beginning with two of the letter *r*, often referred to as the *double Rs*, can be particularly confusing. These word parts are of Greek rather than Latin origin. They are grouped together here to help you understand them and to remember the differences.

- **-rrhage** and **-rrhagia** mean bleeding; however, they are most often used to describe sudden, severe bleeding. A **hemorrhage** (**HEM**-or-idj) is the loss of a large amount of blood in a short time (**hem/o** means blood, and **-rrhage** means bleeding or abnormal excessive fluid discharge).
- **-rrhaphy** means surgical suturing to close a wound and includes the use of sutures, staples, or surgical glue. **Tenorrhaphy** (ten-**OR**-ah-fee) is the surgical suturing of a tendon (**ten/o** means tendon, and **-rrhaphy** means surgical suturing).
- **-rrhea** means flow or discharge and refers to the flow of most body fluids. **Diarrhea** (**dye**-ah-**REE**-ah) is the frequent flow of loose or watery stools (**dia-** means through, and **-rrhea** means flow or discharge).

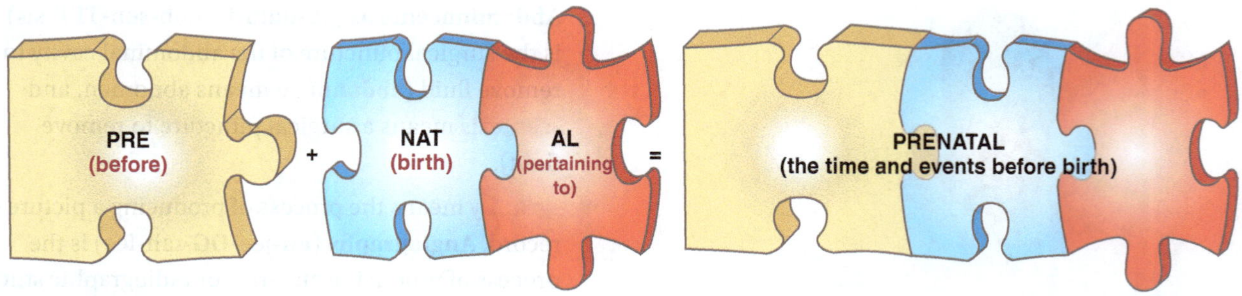

FIGURE 1.5 The term *prenatal* is created by joining the suffix **-al** to the word root **nat** and then adding the prefix **pre-**.

PREFIXES

A prefix is sometimes added to the beginning of a word to influence the meaning of that term. Prefixes usually, *but not always*, indicate location, time, or number. See Table 1.6 for a list of prefixes describing direction, quantity, size, and amount. The term **natal** (**NAY**-tal) means pertaining to birth (**nat** means birth, and **-al** means pertaining to). The following examples show how prefixes change the meaning of this term (Figures 1.5–1.8).

- **Prenatal** (pre-**NAY**-tal) means the time and events before birth (**pre-** means before, **nat** means birth, and **-al** means pertaining to).
- **Perinatal** (**pehr**-ih-**NAY**-tal) refers to the time and events surrounding birth (**peri-** means surrounding, **nat** means birth, and **-al** means pertaining to). This is the time just before, during, and just after birth.

TABLE 1.6

Prefixes Describing Direction, Quantity, Size, and Amount

ab- away from, negative, absent	**ad-** toward, to, in the direction of
dextro- right side	**sinistro-** left side
ex- out of, outside, away from	**in-** in, into, not, without
macro- large, abnormal size, long	**micro-** small
mega-, **megalo-** large, great	**oligo-** scanty, few
pre- before	**post-** after, behind

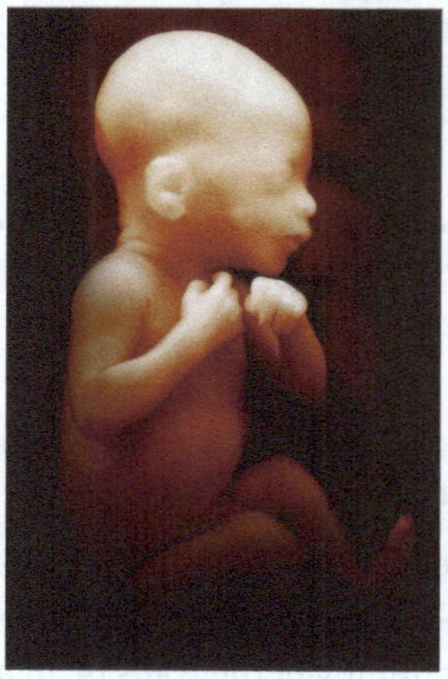

iStock.com/Chris Downie

FIGURE 1.6 The *prenatal* development of a fetus (baby).

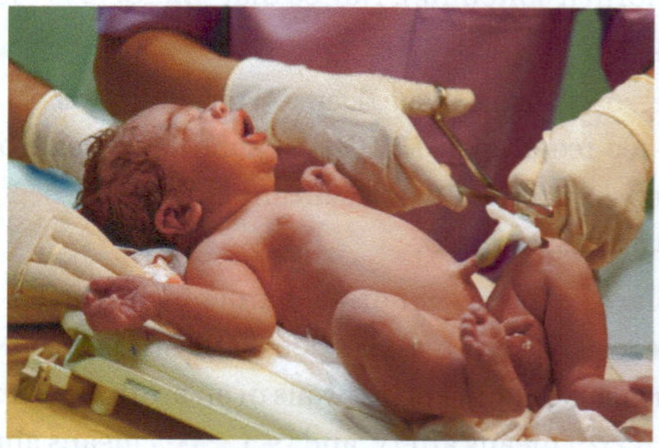

Szasz-Fabian Jozsef/Shutterstock.com

FIGURE 1.7 A *perinatal* event of the umbilical cord being cut immediately after the baby is born.

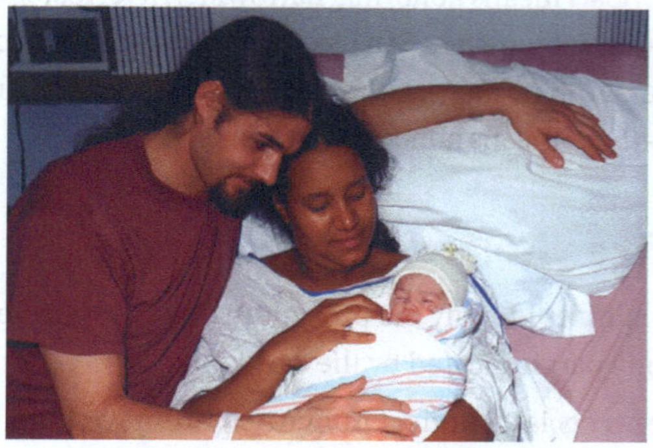

FIGURE 1.8 A happy *postnatal* moment as the parents bond with their new baby.

- **Postnatal** (pohst-**NAY**-tal) refers to the time and events after birth (**post-** means after, **nat** means birth, and **-al** means pertaining to).

Memory aid: You may know some prefixes already by using your prior knowledge and experiences. For example, a postgame press conference happens *after* a game, and a preshow reception happens *before* a performance.

Contrasting and Confusing Prefixes

Some prefixes are confusing because they are similar in spelling but opposite in meaning. The more common prefixes of this type are summarized in Table 1.7.

DETERMINING MEANINGS ON THE BASIS OF WORD PARTS

Knowing the meaning of the word parts often makes it possible to figure out the definition of an unfamiliar medical term.

Taking Terms Apart

To determine a word's meaning by looking at the component pieces, you must first separate it into word parts.

- Always start at the end of the word, with the suffix, and work toward the beginning.
- As you separate the word parts, identify the meaning of each. Identifying the meaning of each part should give you a definition of the term.
- Because some word parts have more than one meaning, it also is necessary to determine the context in which the term is being used. As used here, ***context*** means to determine which body system this term is referring to.
- If you have any doubt, use your medical dictionary or a trusted online resource to double-check your definition.
- Be aware that not all medical terms are made up of word parts.

An Example to Take Apart

Look at the term **otorhinolaryngology** (**oh**-toh-**rye**-noh-**lar**-in-**GOL**-oh-**jee**) as shown in Figure 1.9. It is made up of two combining forms, a word root, and a suffix. This is how it looks when the word parts have been separated by working from the end to the beginning.

- The suffix **-ology** means the study of.
- The word root **laryng** means larynx or throat. The combining vowel *is not used* here because the word root is joining a suffix that begins with a vowel.
- The combining form **rhin/o** means nose. The combining vowel *is used* here because the word root **rhin** is joining another word root beginning with a consonant.

TABLE 1.7

Contrasting Prefixes: Opposites

ab- means away from. **Abnormal** means not normal or away from normal.	**ad-** means toward or in the direction of. **Addiction** means being drawn toward or having a strong dependence on a drug or substance.
dys- means bad, difficult, or painful. **Dysfunctional** means an organ or body part that is not working properly.	**eu-** means good, normal, well, or easy. **Eupnea** means easy or normal breathing.
hyper- means excessive or increased. **Hypertension** is higher-than-normal blood pressure.	**hypo-** means deficient or decreased. **Hypotension** is lower-than-normal blood pressure.
inter- means between or among. **Interstitial** means between, but not within, the parts of a tissue.	**intra-** means within or inside. **Intramuscular** means within the muscle.
sub- means under, less, or below. **Subcostal** means below a rib or ribs.	**super-**, **supra-** mean above or excessive. **Supracostal** means above or outside the ribs.

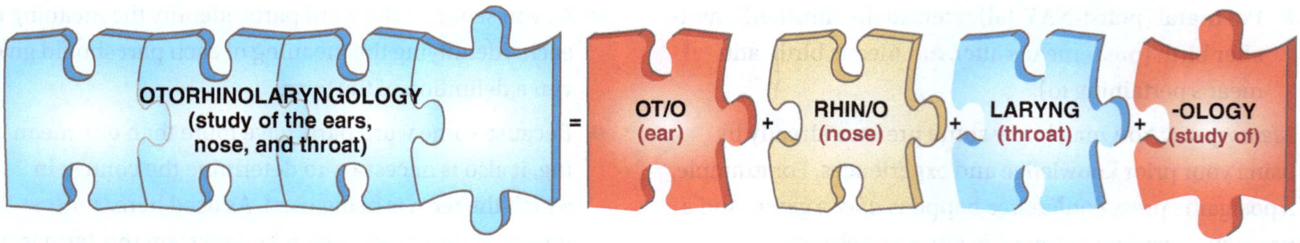

FIGURE 1.9 To determine the meaning of a medical term, the word parts are separated working from the end of the word toward the beginning.

- The combining form **ot/o** means ear. The combining vowel *is used* here because the word root **ot** is joining another word root beginning with a consonant.
- Together they form *otorhinolaryngology,* which is the study of the ears, nose, and throat (**ot/o** means ear, **rhin/o** means nose, **laryng** means throat, and **-ology** means study of). *Note:* **laryng/o** also means larynx and is discussed in Chapter 8.
- Because this is such a long term, this specialty is frequently referred to as *ENT* (ears, nose, and throat).
- A shortened version of this term is **otolaryngology** (**oh**-toh-**lar**-in-**GOL**-oh-jee), which is the study of the ears and larynx or throat (**ot/o** means ears, **laryng** means larynx, and **-ology** means study of).

Guessing at Meanings

When you are able to guess at the meaning of a term on the basis of its word parts, you must always double-check for accuracy because some terms have more than one meaning. For example, look at the term **lithotomy** (lih-**THOT**-oh-mee):

- On the basis of word parts, a **lithotomy** is a surgical incision for the removal of a stone (**lith** means stone, and **-otomy** means a surgical incision). This meaning is discussed further in Chapter 10.
- However, **lithotomy** is also the name of an examination position in which a female patient is lying on her back with her feet and legs raised and supported in stirrups. The term is used to describe this position because in the early days, this was the preferred position for lithotomy surgery. This term is discussed further in Chapter 21.
- This type of possible confusion is one of the many reasons why a medical dictionary or trusted online resource is an important medical terminology tool.

MEDICAL DICTIONARY USE

Learning to use a medical dictionary and other resources to find the definition of a term is an important part of mastering the correct use of medical terms. The following tips for dictionary use apply whether you are working with a traditional book-form dictionary or with electronic dictionary software, websites, or applications on your computer or handheld device.

If You Know How to Spell the Word

When starting to work with a printed dictionary, spend a few minutes reviewing its user guide, table of contents, and appendices. The time you spend reviewing now will be saved later when you are looking up unfamiliar terms.

- On the basis of the first letter of the word, start in the appropriate section of the dictionary. Look at the top of the page for clues. The top left word is the first term on the page. The top right word is the last term on that page.
- Next, look alphabetically for words that start with the first and second letters of the word you are researching. Continue looking through each letter until you find the term you are looking for.
- When you think you have found it, check the spelling very carefully, letter by letter, working from left to right. Terms with similar spellings have very different meanings.
- When you find the term, carefully check *all* of the definitions.

If You Do Not Know How to Spell the Word

Listen carefully to the term, and write it down. If you cannot find the word on the basis of your spelling, start looking for alternative spellings based on the beginning sound as shown in Table 1.8. *Note:* All of these examples are in

TABLE 1.8

Guidelines to Looking Up the Spelling of Unfamiliar Terms

If it sounds like	It may begin with	Example
F	F	**flatus** (**FLAY**-tus), see Chapter 9
	PH	**phlegm** (**FLEM**), see Chapter 8
J	G	**gingivitis** (**jin**-jih-**VYE**-tis), see Chapter 9
	J	**jaundice** (**JAWN**-dis), see Chapter 9
K	C	**crepitus** (**KREP**-ih-tus), see Chapter 3
	CH	**cheilitis** (kye-**LITE**-is), see Chapter 9
	K	**kyphosis** (kye-**FOH**-sis), see Chapter 3
	QU	**quadriplegia** (**kwad**-rih-**PLEE**-jee-ah), see Chapter 4
S	C	**cytology** (sigh-**TOL**-oh-jee), see Chapter 2
	PS	**psychologist** (sigh-**KOL**-oh-jist), see Chapter 17
	S	**serum** (**SEER**-um), see Chapter 5
Z	X	**xeroderma** (zee-roh-**DER**-mah), see Chapter 13
	Z	**zygote** (**ZYE**-goht), see Chapter 16

this textbook. However, you could practice looking them up in the dictionary!

Look Under Categories

Most printed dictionaries use categories such as *Diseases* and *Syndromes* to group disorders with these terms in their titles. For example:

- *Sexually transmitted disease* would be found under *Disease, sexually transmitted.*
- *Fetal alcohol syndrome* would be found under *Syndrome, fetal alcohol.*
- When you come across such a term and cannot find it listed by the first word, the next step is to look under the appropriate category.

Multiple-Word Terms

When you are looking for a term that includes more than one word, begin your search with the last term. If you do not find it there, move forward to the next word.

- For example, *congestive heart failure* is sometimes listed under *Heart failure, congestive.*

Searching for Definitions on the Internet

Online search engines such as Google are valuable resources in finding definitions and details about medical conditions and terms; however, it is important that you rely on websites, such as the National Institutes of Health (NIH) website (http://www.nih.gov), which are known to be reputable information sources.

- For better results, an Internet search should include visits to at least two reputable sites. If there is a major difference in the definitions, go on to a third site. Sometimes search engine results will include a site that is not necessarily trustworthy but has paid for good placement.
- Beware of suggested search terms. If you do not spell a term correctly, a website may guess what you were searching for. Make sure to double-check that the term you are defining is the intended term.

The same caution applies to medical dictionary applications on handheld devices. Make sure that the application comes from a reputable source, and always double-check that this definition is for the term that you intended to look up.

PRONUNCIATION

A medical term is easier to understand and remember when you know how to pronounce it properly. To help you master the pronunciation of new terms, a commonly accepted pronunciation of that word appears in parentheses next to the term.

The sounds-like pronunciation system is used in this textbook. Here the word is respelled using normal English letters to create sounds that are familiar. To pronounce a new word, just say it as it is spelled in the parentheses.

- The part of the word that receives the primary (most) emphasis when you say it is shown in uppercase boldface letters. For example, **edema** (eh-**DEE**-mah) is swelling caused by an abnormal accumulation of fluid in cells, tissues, or cavities of the body.
- A part of the word that receives secondary (less) emphasis when you say it is shown in boldface lowercase letters. For example, **appendicitis** (ah-**pen**-dih-**SIGH**-tis) means an inflammation of the appendix (**appendic** means appendix, and **-itis** means inflammation).

A Word of Caution

Frequently, there is more than one correct way to pronounce a medical term.

- The pronunciation of many medical terms is based on their Greek, Latin, or other foreign origin. However, there is a trend toward pronouncing terms as they would sound in English.
- The result is more than one "correct" pronunciation for a term. The text shows the most commonly accepted pronunciation.
- If your instructor prefers an alternative pronunciation, follow their instructions.

SPELLING IS ALWAYS IMPORTANT

Accuracy in spelling medical terms is extremely important!

- Changing just one or two letters can completely change the meaning of a word—and this difference literally could be a matter of life or death for the patient.
- The section "Look-Alike, Sound-Alike Terms and Word Parts" later in this chapter will help you become aware of some terms and word parts that are frequently confused.
- The spelling shown in this text is commonly accepted in the United States. You may encounter alternative spellings used in other English-speaking countries such as England, Australia, and Canada.

SINGULAR AND PLURAL ENDINGS

Many medical terms have Greek or Latin origins. As a result of these different origins, there are unusual rules for changing a singular word into a plural form. In addition, English endings have been adopted for some commonly used terms.

- Table 1.9 provides guidelines to help you better understand how these plurals are formed.
- Also, throughout the text, when a term with an unusual singular or plural form is introduced, both forms are included. For example, the **phalanges** (fah-**LAN**-jeez) are the bones of the fingers and toes (singular, *phalanx*) (Figure 1.10).

BASIC MEDICAL TERMS TO DESCRIBE DISEASES

Some of the medical terms that are used to describe diseases and disease conditions can be confusing. Some of the most commonly confused terms are described in Table 1.10. You will find that studying the groups of three as they are shown in the table makes it easier to master these terms.

LOOK-ALIKE, SOUND-ALIKE TERMS AND WORD PARTS

This section highlights some frequently used terms and word parts that are confusing because they look and sound alike. However, their meanings are very different. It is important that you pay close attention to these terms and word parts as you encounter them in the text.

arteri/o, ather/o, and arthr/o

- **arteri/o** means artery. **Endarterial** (**end**-ar-**TEE**-ree-al) means pertaining to the interior or lining of an artery (**end-** means within, **arteri** means artery, and **-al** means pertaining to).
- **ather/o** means plaque or fatty substance. An **atheroma** (**ath**-er-**OH**-mah) is a fatty deposit within the wall of an

TABLE 1.9

Guidelines to Unusual Plural Forms

Guideline	Singular	Plural
If the singular term ends in the suffix **-a**, the plural is usually formed by changing the ending to **-ae**.	bursa vertebra	bursae vertebrae
If the singular term ends in the suffix **-ex** or **-ix**, the plural is usually formed by changing these endings to **-ices**.	appendix index	appendices indices
If the singular term ends in the suffix **-is**, the plural is usually formed by changing the ending to **-es**.	diagnosis metastasis	diagnoses metastases
If the singular term ends in the suffix **-itis**, the plural is usually formed by changing the **-is** ending to **-ides**.	arthritis meningitis	arthritides meningitides
If the singular term ends in the suffix **-nx**, the plural is usually formed by changing the **-x** ending to **-ges**.	phalanx meninx	phalanges meninges
If the singular term ends in the suffix **-on**, the plural is usually formed by changing the ending to **-a**.	criterion ganglion	criteria ganglia
If the singular term ends in the suffix **-um**, the plural usually is formed by changing the ending to **-a**.	diverticulum ovum	diverticula ova
If the singular term ends in the suffix **-us**, the plural is usually formed by changing the ending to **-i**.	alveolus malleolus	alveoli malleoli

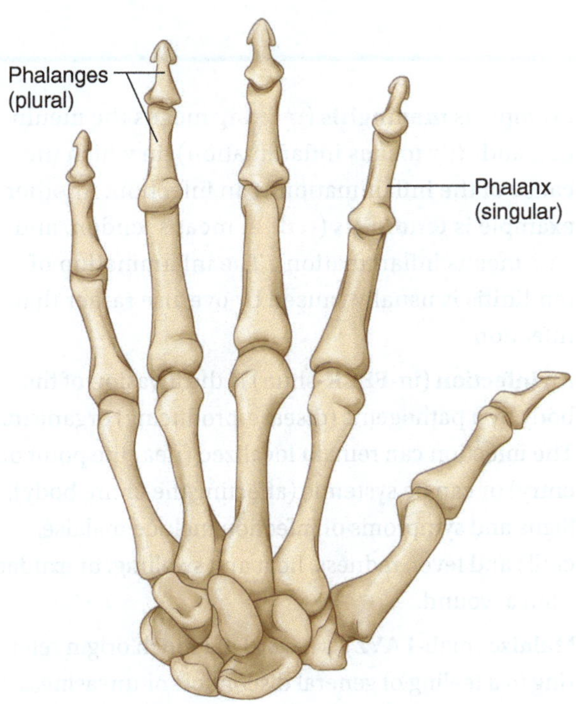

FIGURE 1.10 Singular and plural endings. A phalanx is one finger or toe bone. Phalanges are more than one finger or toe bones.

artery (**ather** means fatty substance, and **-oma** means tumor).

- **arthr/o** means joint. **Arthralgia** (ar-**THRAL**-jee-ah) means pain in a joint or joints (**arthr** means joint, and **-algia** means pain).

-ectomy, -ostomy, and -otomy

- **-ectomy** means surgical removal. An **appendectomy** (**ap**-en-**DECK**-toh-mee) is the surgical removal of the appendix (**append** means appendix, and **-ectomy** means surgical removal).
- **-ostomy** means the surgical creation of an artificial opening to the body surface. A **colostomy** (koh-**LAHS**-toh-mee) is the surgical creation of an artificial excretory opening between the colon and the body surface (**col** means colon, and **-ostomy** means the surgical creation of an artificial opening).
- **-otomy** means cutting or a surgical incision. **Pyelotomy** (**pye**-eh-**LOT**-oh-mee) is a surgical incision into the renal pelvis to remove obstructions such as a kidney stone (**pyel** means the renal pelvis, and **-otomy** means surgical incision).

TABLE 1.10

Basic Medical Terms to Describe Disease Conditions

A **sign** is objective evidence of disease, such as a fever. ***Objective*** means the sign can be evaluated or measured by the patient or others.	A **symptom** (**SIMP**-tum) is subjective evidence of a disease, such as pain or a headache. ***Subjective*** means that it can be evaluated or measured only by the patient.	A **syndrome** (**SIN**-drohm) is a set of signs and symptoms that occur together as part of a specific disease process.
A **diagnosis** (**dye**-ag-**NOH**-sis) (DX) is the identification of a disease (plural, *diagnoses*). To ***diagnose*** is the process of reaching a diagnosis.	A **differential diagnosis** (D/DX), also known as a ***rule out*** (R/O), is an attempt to determine which one of several possible diseases is causing the signs and symptoms that are present.	A **prognosis** (prog-**NOH**-sis) is a prediction of the probable course and outcome of a disease (plural, *prognoses*).
An **acute** condition has a rapid onset, a severe course, and a relatively short duration.	A **chronic** condition is of long duration. Although such diseases can be controlled, they are rarely cured.	A **remission** is the temporary, partial, or complete disappearance of the symptoms of a disease without having achieved a cure.
A **disease** is a condition in which one or more body parts are not functioning normally. Some diseases are named for their signs and symptoms. For example, ***chronic fatigue syndrome*** is a persistent, overwhelming fatigue of unknown origin (see Chapter 4).	An **eponym** (**EP**-oh-nim) is a disease, structure, operation, or procedure named for the person who discovered or described it first. For example, ***Alzheimer's disease*** is named for German neurologist Alois Alzheimer (see Chapter 11).	An **acronym** (**ACK**-roh-nim) is a word formed from the initial letter of the major parts of a compound term. For example, the acronym **laser** stands for *light amplification by stimulated emission of radiation* (see Chapter 13).

Fissure and Fistula

- A **fissure** (**FISH**-ur) is a groove or crack-like sore of the skin (see Chapter 13). This term also describes normal folds in the contours of the brain.
- A **fistula** (**FIS**-chuh-lah) is an abnormal passage, usually between two internal organs or leading from an organ to the surface of the body. A fistula may be due to surgery, injury, or the draining of an abscess.

Ileum and Ilium

- The **ileum** (**ILL**-ee-um) is the last and longest portion of the small intestine. *Memory aid: Ileum is spelled with an **e** as in intestine.*
- The **ilium** (**ILL**-ee-um) is part of the hip bone. *Memory aid: Ilium is spelled with an **i** as in hip* (Figure 1.11).

Infection and Inflammation

- Although the suffix **-itis** means inflammation, it also is commonly used to indicate infection. An example is **meningitis** (**mening** means the meninges, and **-itis** means inflammation), in which the cause of the inflammation is an infection. Another example is **tendinitis** (**tendin** means tendon, and **-itis** means inflammation). The inflammation of tendinitis is usually caused by overuse rather than infection.
- An **infection** (in-**FECK**-shun) is the invasion of the body by a pathogenic (disease-producing) organism. The infection can remain localized (near the point of entry) or can be systemic (affecting the entire body). Signs and symptoms of infection include malaise, chills and fever, redness, heat and swelling, or exudate from a wound.
- **Malaise** (mah-**LAYZ**) is a word of French origin referring to a feeling of general discomfort or uneasiness that is often the first indication of an infection or other disease.
- **Exudate** (**ECKS**-you-dayt) is any fluid, such as pus, that leaks out of an infected wound.

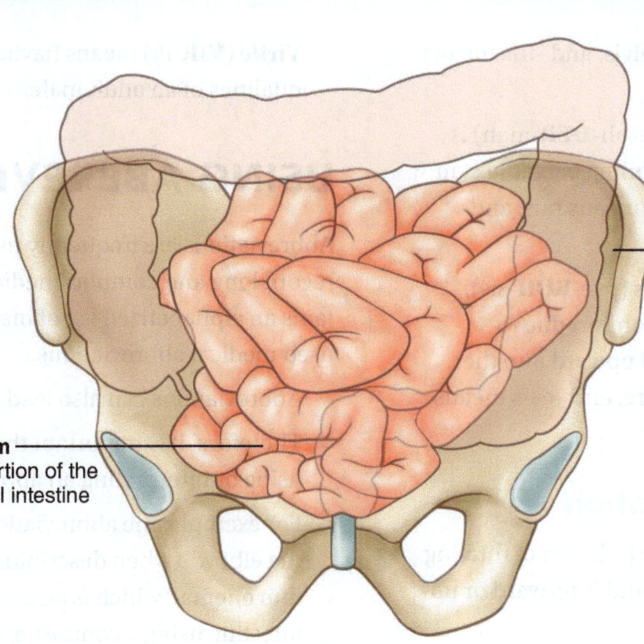

FIGURE 1.11 There is only one letter difference between *ileum* and *ilium*, but they are very different parts of the body.

- **Inflammation** (in-flah-**MAY**-shun) is a localized response to an injury or to the destruction of tissues. The key indicators of inflammation are (1) *erythema* (redness), (2) *hyperthermia* (heat), (3) *edema* (swelling), and (4) *pain*. These are caused by extra blood flowing into the area as part of the healing process.

Laceration and Lesion

- A **laceration** (**lass**-er-**AY**-shun) is a torn or jagged wound or an accidental cut.
- A **lesion** (**LEE**-zhun) is a pathologic change of the tissues due to disease or injury.

Mucous and Mucus

- The adjective **mucous** (**MYOU**-kus) describes the specialized membranes that line the body cavities.
- The noun **mucus** (**MYOU**-kus), which is pronounced the same way, refers to the fluid secreted by these mucous membranes.

myc/o, myel/o, and my/o

- **myc/o** means fungus. **Mycosis** (my-**KOH**-sis) describes any abnormal condition or disease caused by a fungus (**myc** means fungus, and **-osis** means abnormal condition or disease).
- **myel/o** means bone marrow *or* spinal cord. The term **myelopathy** (my-eh-**LOP**-ah-thee) describes any injury, degeneration or disease in the spinal cord (**myel/o** means spinal cord or bone marrow, and **-pathy** means disease).
- **my/o** means muscle. The term **myopathy** (my-**OP**-ah-thee) describes any pathologic change or disease of muscle tissue (**my/o** means muscle, and **-pathy** means disease).

-ologist and -ology

- **-ologist** means specialist. A **dermatologist** (**der**-mah-**TOL**-oh-jist) is a physician who specializes in diagnosing and treating disorders of the skin (**dermat** means skin, and **-ologist** means specialist).
- **-ology** means the study of. **Neonatology** (**nee**-oh-nay-**TOL**-oh-jee) is the study of disorders of the newborn (**neo-** means new, **nat** means birth, and **-ology** means study of).

Palpation and Palpitation

- **Palpation** (pal-**PAY**-shun) is an examination technique in which the examiner's hands are used to feel the texture, size, consistency, and location of certain body parts.
- **Palpitation** (**pal**-pih-**TAY**-shun) is a pounding or racing heart.

pyel/o, py/o, and pyr/o

- **pyel/o** means renal pelvis, which is part of the kidney. **Pyelitis** (**pye**-eh-**LYE**-tis) is an inflammation of the renal pelvis (**pyel** means renal pelvis, and **-itis** means inflammation).

- **py/o** means pus. **Pyoderma** (**pye**-oh-**DER**-mah) is any acute, inflammatory, pus-forming bacterial skin infection such as impetigo (**py/o** means pus, and **-derma** means skin).
- **pyr/o** means fever or fire. **Pyrosis** (pye-**ROH**-sis), also known as ***heartburn***, is discomfort due to the regurgitation of stomach acid upward into the esophagus (**pyr** means fever or fire, and **-osis** means abnormal condition or disease).

Supination and Suppuration

- **Supination** (**soo**-pih-**NAY**-shun) is the act of rotating the arm so that the palm of the hand is forward or upward.
- **Suppuration** (**sup**-you-**RAY**-shun) is the formation of pus.

Triage and Trauma

- **Triage** (tree-**AHZH**) is the medical screening of patients to determine their relative priority of need and the proper place of treatment (Figure 1.12).
- **Trauma** (**TRAW**-mah) means wound or injury. These are the types of injuries that might occur in an accident, shooting, natural disaster, or fire.

Viral and Virile

- **Viral** (**VYE**-ral) means pertaining to a virus (**vir** means virus or poison, and **-al** means pertaining to).

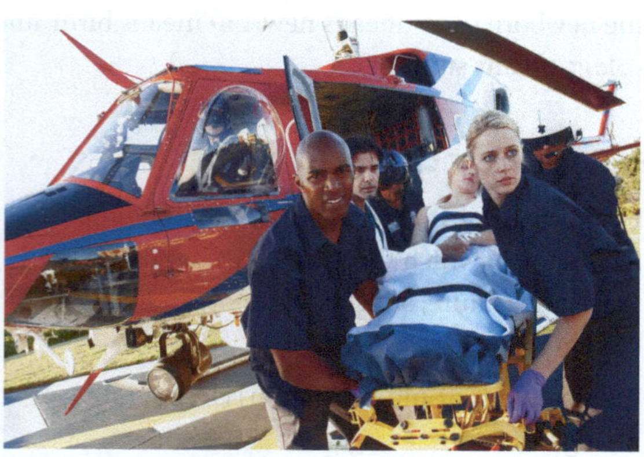

FIGURE 1.12 Triage describes the process through which emergency personnel arriving on an accident scene identify which of the injured require care first and where they can be treated most effectively.

- **Virile** (**VIR**-ill) means having the nature, properties, or qualities of an adult male.

USING ABBREVIATIONS

Abbreviations are frequently used as a shorthand way to record long and complex medical terms; Appendix B contains an alphabetized list of many of the more commonly used medical abbreviations.

- Abbreviations can also lead to confusion and errors!
- Therefore, it is important that you use caution when using or interpreting an abbreviation.
- For example, the abbreviation *BE* means both "below the elbow" (when describing an amputation) and "barium enema," which is an x-ray examination of the large intestine using a contrast medium injected into the rectum. Just imagine what a difference a mix-up would make for the patient!
- Most clinical agencies have policies for accepted abbreviations. It is important to follow this list for the facility where you are working.
- If there is any question in your mind about which abbreviation to use, always follow this rule: *When in doubt, spell it out.*

The Joint Commission, an organization founded in 1910 to standardize medical practices, publishes an official list of commonly confused "Do Not Use" abbreviations to prevent potentially fatal medical errors. The full list is available at www.jointcommission.org (see Table 1.11 for examples). Many medical facilities have their own suggested "Do Not Use" abbreviation list.

TABLE 1.11

Examples of "Do Not Use" Abbreviations

Abbreviation	Potential Problem
MS	can mean either morphine sulfate *or* magnesium sulfate
QD and QOD	mean daily and every other day, respectively; sometimes mistaken for each other
U	means unit, sometimes mistaken for 0 or 4

LEARNING EXERCISES

Matching Word Parts 1

Write the correct answer in the middle column.

	Definition	Correct Answer	Possible Answers
1.1.	bad, difficult, painful	______________	-algia
1.2.	excessive, increased	______________	dys-
1.3.	enlargement	______________	-ectomy
1.4.	pain, suffering	______________	-megaly
1.5.	surgical removal	______________	hyper-

Matching Word Parts 2

Write the correct answer in the middle column.

	Definition	Correct Answer	Possible Answers
1.6.	abnormal condition or disease	______________	hypo-
1.7.	abnormal softening	______________	-itis
1.8.	deficient, decreased	______________	-malacia
1.9.	inflammation	______________	-necrosis
1.10.	tissue death	______________	-osis

Matching Word Parts 3

Write the correct answer in the middle column.

	Definition	Correct Answer	Possible Answers
1.11.	bleeding, abnormal excessive fluid discharge	________________	**-ostomy**
1.12.	surgical creation of an artificial opening to the body surface	________________	**-otomy**
1.13.	surgical incision	________________	**-plasty**
1.14.	surgical repair	________________	**-rrhage**
1.15.	surgical suturing	________________	**-rrhaphy**

Matching Word Parts 4

Write the correct answer in the middle column.

	Definition	Correct Answer	Possible Answers
1.16.	visual examination	________________	**-ac**
1.17.	pertaining to	________________	**-rrhea**
1.18.	abnormal narrowing	________________	**-sclerosis**
1.19.	abnormal hardening	________________	**-scopy**
1.20.	flow or discharge	________________	**-stenosis**

Definitions

Select the correct answer, and write it on the line provided.

1.21. The term ________________ describes any pathologic change or disease in the spinal cord.

myelopathy   myopathy   pyelitis   pyrosis

1.22. The medical term for higher-than-normal blood pressure is ________________.

hepatomegaly   hypertension   hypotension   supination

1.23. The term *laser* is called a/an ________________ because it is made up of the initial letters of several words.

eponym   sign   acronym   combining form

1.24. Pain is classified as a ______________________.

diagnosis sign symptom syndrome

1.25. In the term *myopathy*, the suffix **-pathy** means ______________________.

abnormal condition disease inflammation swelling

Matching Terms and Definitions 1

Write the correct answer in the middle column.

	Definition	Correct Answer	Possible Answers
1.26.	white blood cell	______________	acute
1.27.	prediction of the probable course and outcome of a disorder	______________	edema
1.28.	swelling caused by an abnormal accumulation of fluid in cells, tissues, or cavities of the body	______________	leukocyte
1.29.	rapid onset	______________	prognosis
1.30.	turning the palm of the hand upward	______________	supination

Matching Terms and Definitions 2

Write the correct answer in the middle column.

	Definition	Correct Answer	Possible Answers
1.31.	examination procedure	______________	laceration
1.32.	fluid, such as pus, that leaks out of an infected wound	______________	lesion
1.33.	pathologic tissue change	______________	palpitation
1.34.	pounding heart	______________	palpation
1.35.	torn or jagged wound, or an accidental cut wound	______________	exudate

Which Word?

Select the correct answer, and write it on the line provided. *Note:* Some of the options given are similar, but have very different meanings.

1.36. The medical term ____________________ describes an inflammation of the stomach.

gastritis gastrosis

1.37. The formation of pus is called ____________________.

supination suppuration

1.38. The term meaning wound or injury is ____________________.

trauma triage

1.39. The term ____________________ means pertaining to a virus.

viral virile

1.40. An ____________________ is the surgical removal of the appendix.

appendectomy appendicitis

Spelling Counts

Find the misspelled word in each sentence. Then write that word, spelled correctly, on the line provided.

1.41. A disease named for the person who discovered it is known as an enaponym.

____

1.42. A localized response to injury or tissue destruction is called inflimmation.

____

1.43. A fisure of the skin is a groove or crack-like sore of the skin. ____________________

1.44. The medical term meaning suturing together the ends of a severed nerve is neurorraphy.

____

1.45. The medical term meaning inflammation of the tonsils is tonsilitis. ____________________

Matching Terms

Write the correct answer in the middle column.

	Definition	Correct Answer	Possible Answers
1.46.	inflammation of a tendon	______________	syndrome
1.47.	a set of signs and symptoms	______________	gastralgia
1.48.	the surgical suturing of a tendon	______________	tendinitis
1.49.	stomach pain	______________	pyoderma
1.50.	any acute, inflammatory, pus-forming bacterial skin infection	______________	tenorrhaphy

Term Selection

Select the correct answer, and write it on the line provided.

1.51. The abnormal hardening of the walls of an artery or arteries is called ______________.

arteriosclerosis   arteriostenosis   arthrostenosis   atherosclerosis

1.52. A fever is considered to be a ______________.

prognosis   sign   symptom   syndrome

1.53. An inflammation of the stomach and small intestine is known as ______________.

gastralgia   gastroenteritis   gastritis   gastrosis

1.54. The term meaning pain in a joint or joints is ______________.

arthralgia   arthritis   arthrocentesis   atherosclerosis

1.55. A ______________ is a physician who specializes in diagnosing and treating diseases and disorders of the skin.

dermatologist   dermatology   neurologist   neurology

Sentence Completion

Write the correct term on the line provided.

1.56. A word ______________________ is a word part that usually indicates the part of the body involved.

1.57. A/An ______________________ word is a term made up of more than one word part.

1.58. The word part attached at the end of word is called a/an ______________________.

1.59. A combining ______________________ is added to the end of a word root to make the resulting term easier to pronounce.

1.60. The word part attached at the beginning of word is called a/an ______________________.

True/False

If the statement is true, write **True** on the line. If the statement is false, write **False** on the line.

1.61. ________ An erythrocyte is commonly known as a red blood cell.

1.62. ________ The Joint Commission publishes an official list of common medical abbreviations it recommends be used routinely.

1.63. ________ A colostomy is the surgical creation of an artificial opening between the colon and the body surface.

1.64. ________ Malaise is often the first symptom of inflammation.

1.65. ________ An infection is the invasion of the body by a disease-producing organism.

Word Surgery

Divide each term into its component word parts. Write these word parts, in sequence, on the lines provided. When necessary, use a slash (/) to indicate a combining vowel. (You may not need all of the lines provided.)

1.66. **Otorhinolaryngology** is the study of the ears, nose, and throat.

__________ __________ __________ __________

1.67. The term **mycosis** means any abnormal condition or disease caused by a fungus.

__________ __________ __________ __________

1.68. **Poliomyelitis** is a viral infection of the gray matter of the spinal cord.

__________ __________ __________ __________

1.69. **Neonatology** is the study of disorders of the newborn.

__________ __________ __________

1.70. The term **endarterial** means pertaining to the interior or lining of an artery.

__________ __________ __________ __________

Clinical Conditions

Write the correct answer on the line provided.

1.71. Miguel required a/an ________________ injection. This term means that the medication was placed directly within the muscle.

1.72. Mrs. Tillson underwent ________________ to remove excess fluid from her abdomen.

1.73. The term *laser* is a/an ________________. This means that it is a word formed from the initial letters of the major parts of a compound term.

1.74. In an accident, Felipe Valladares broke several bones in his fingers. The medical term for these injuries is fractured ________________.

1.75. In case of a major disaster Cheng Lee, who is a trained paramedic, helps perform ________________. This is the screening of patients to determine their relative priority of need and the proper place of treatment.

1.76. Gina's physician ordered laboratory tests that would enable him to establish a differential ________________ to identify the cause of her signs and symptoms.

1.77. Jennifer plans to go to graduate school so she can specialize in ________________. This specialty is concerned with the study of all aspects of diseases.

1.78. John Randolph's cancer went into ________________. Although this is not a cure, his symptoms disappeared and he felt much better.

1.79. Mr. Jankowski describes that uncomfortable feeling as heartburn. The medical term for this condition is ________________.

1.80. Phyllis was having great fun traveling until she ate some contaminated food and developed ________________. She felt miserable and needed to stay in her hotel because of the frequent flow of loose or watery stools.

Which Is the Correct Medical Term?

Select the correct answer, and write it on the line provided.

1.81. The term ______________________ describes the surgical repair of a nerve.

neuralgia | neurorrhaphy | neurology | neuroplasty

1.82. The term ______________________ means loss of a large amount of blood in a short time.

diarrhea | hemorrhage | hepatorrhagia | otorrhagia

1.83. The term ______________________ means the tissue death of an artery or arteries.

arteriomalacia | arterionecrosis | arteriosclerosis | arteriostenosis

1.84. The term ______________________ means between, but not within, the parts of a tissue.

interstitial | intrastitial | intermuscular | intramuscular

1.85. The term ______________________ means enlargement of the liver.

hepatitis | hepatomegaly | nephromegaly | nephritis

Challenge Word Building

These terms are *not* primary terms in the chapter; however, they are made up of the following familiar word parts. For help in creating them, refer to a medical dictionary or trusted online resource.

neo- = new	**arteri/o** = artery	**-algia** = pain and suffering
	arthr/o = joint	**-itis** = inflammation
	cardi/o = heart	**-ologist** = specialist
	nat/o = birth	**-otomy** = a surgical incision
	neur/o = nerve	**-rrhea** = flow or discharge
	rhin/o = nose	**-scopy** = visual examination

1.86. A medical specialist concerned with the diagnosis and treatment of heart disease is a/an ______________________.

1.87. The term meaning a runny nose is ______________________.

1.88. The term meaning the inflammation of a joint or joints is ______________________.

1.89. A medical specialist in disorders of the newborn is a/an ______________________.

1.90. The term meaning a surgical incision into a nerve is a/an ______________________.

1.91. The term meaning inflammation of the heart is ______________________.

1.92. The term meaning pain in the nose is ______________________.

1.93. The term meaning pain in a nerve or nerves is ______________________.

1.94. The term meaning a surgical incision into the heart is a/an ______________________.

1.95. The term meaning an inflammation of the nose is ______________________.

Labeling Exercises

1.96. The combining form meaning spinal cord is

______________________.

1.97. The combining form meaning muscle is

______________________.

1.98. The combining form meaning bone is

______________________.

1.99. The combining form meaning nerve is

______________________.

1.100. The combining form meaning joint is

______________________.

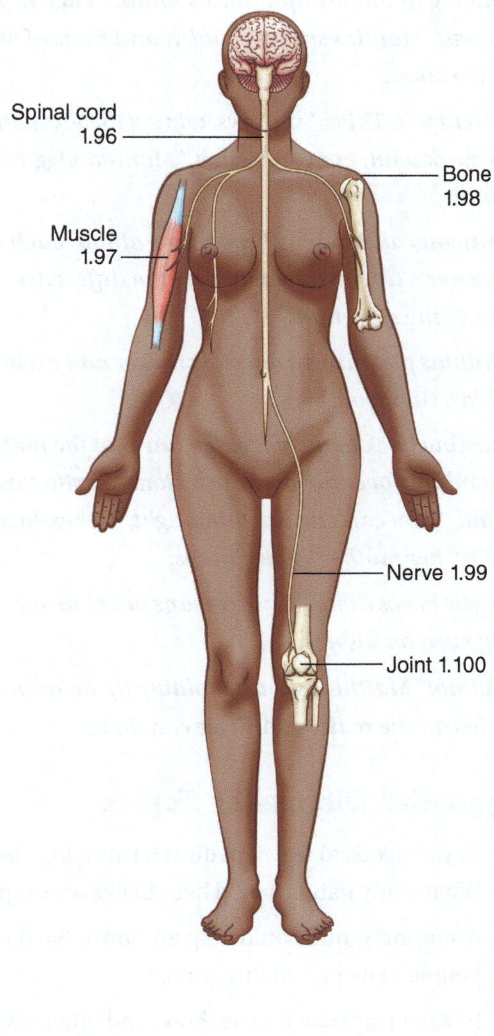

The Human Touch

CRITICAL THINKING EXERCISE

The following story and questions are designed to stimulate critical thinking through class discussion or as a brief essay response. There are no right or wrong answers to these questions.

*Baylie Hutchins sits at her kitchen table, highlighter in hand, with her medical terminology book opened to the first chapter. Her 2-year-old son, Mathias, plays with a box of animal crackers in his high chair, some even finding his mouth. "**Arteri/o**, **ather/o**, and **arthr/o**," she mutters, lips moving to shape unfamiliar sounds. "They're too much alike, and they mean totally different things." Mathias sneezes loudly, and spots of animal cracker rain on the page, punctuating her frustration.*

"Great job, Thias," she says, wiping the text with her finger. "I planned on using the highlighter to mark with, not your lunch." Mathias giggles and peeks through the tunnel made by one small hand.

"Mucous and mucus," she reads aloud, each sounding the same. Then she remembers her teacher's tip for remembering the difference, "The long word is the membrane, and the short one is the secretion."

Mathias picks up an animal cracker and excitedly shouts, "Tiger, Mommy! Tiger!" "That's right, Thias. Good job!"

*Turning back to the page, she stares at the pink word parts **-rrhagia**, **-rrhaphy**, and **-rrhea**. Stumbling over the pronunciations, Baylie closes her eyes and tries to silence the voices in her head. "You can't do anything right," her ex-husband says. "Couldn't finish if your life depended on it," her mother's voice snaps.*

*Baylie keeps at it, "**rhin/o** means nose," as she highlights that word part, "and a rhinoceros has a big horn on his nose."*

"Rhino!" Matthias shouts, holding up an animal cracker. Baylie laughs. We both have new things to learn, she realizes. And we can do it!

Suggested Discussion Topics

1. Baylie needs to learn medical terminology because she wants a career in the medical field. What study habits would help Baylie accomplish this task?
2. A support group could help empower Baylie to accomplish her goals. How could she find people to be part of this group?
3. In what ways can this textbook and other resource materials help her, and you, learn medical terminology?
4. Baylie figured out a way to remember the term for nose by using her prior knowledge of the word *rhinoceros*. Can you think of other examples of ways in which your prior knowledge and experiences help you understand the meaning of medical terms?

CHAPTER 2

THE HUMAN BODY IN HEALTH AND DISEASE

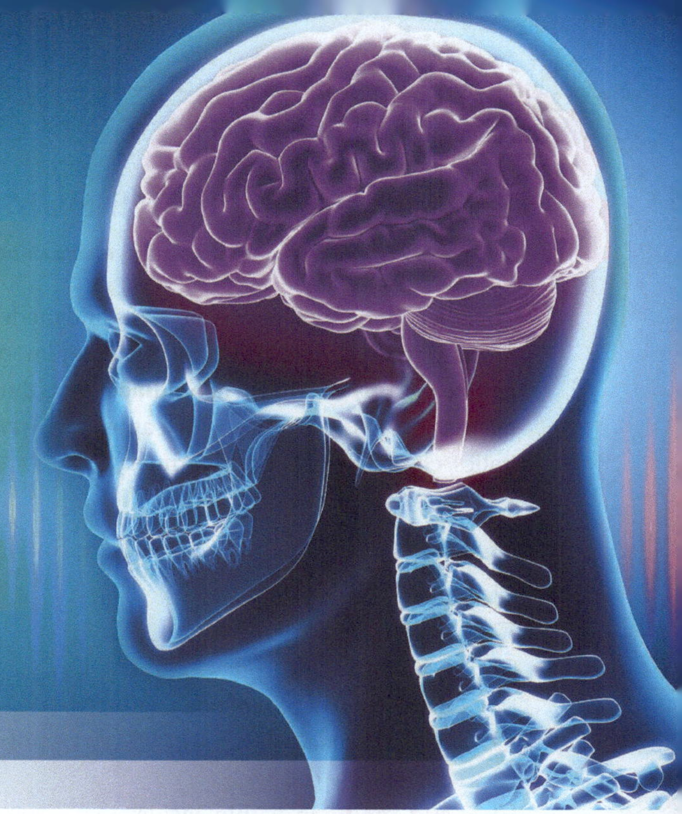

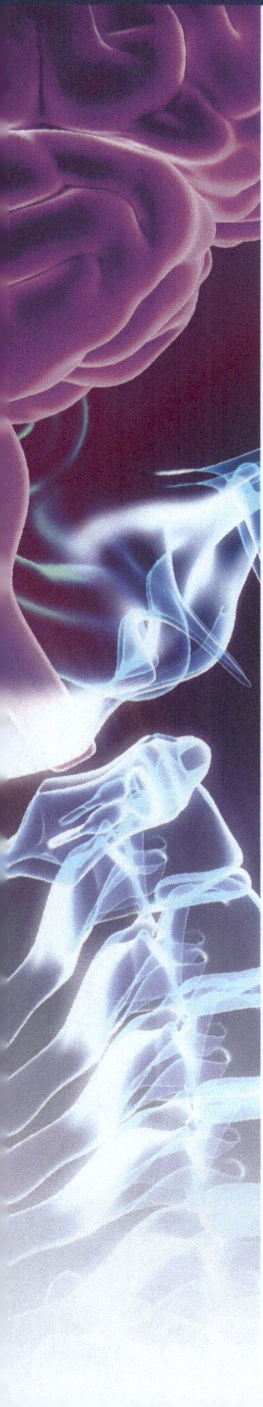

Overview of THE HUMAN BODY IN HEALTH AND DISEASE

Anatomical Reference Systems	Terms used to describe the location of body planes, directions, and cavities.
Structures of the Body	The cells, tissues, and glands that form the body systems that work together to enable the body to function properly.
Genetics	The genetic components that transfer characteristics from parents to their child.
Tissues	A group of similarly specialized cells that work together to perform specific functions.
Glands	A group of specialized cells that is capable of producing secretions.
Body Systems and Related Organs	Organs are somewhat independent parts of the body that perform specific functions. Organs with related functions are organized into body systems.
Pathology	The study of the nature and cause of disease that involve changes in structure and function.

Vocabulary Related to **THE HUMAN BODY IN HEALTH AND DISEASE**

This list contains essential word parts and medical terms for this chapter. These and the other important **primary terms** are shown in **boldface** throughout the chapter. ***Secondary terms***, which appear in ***orange*** italics, clarify the meaning of primary terms.

Word Parts

- ☐ **aden/o** gland
- ☐ **adip/o** fat
- ☐ **anter/o** before, front
- ☐ **caud/o** lower part of body, tail
- ☐ **cephal/o** head
- ☐ **cyt/o**, **-cyte** cell
- ☐ **end-**, **endo-** in, within, inside
- ☐ **exo-** out of, outside, away from
- ☐ **hist/o** tissue
- ☐ **-ologist** specialist
- ☐ **-ology** the science or study of
- ☐ **path/o**, **-pathy** disease, suffering, feeling, emotion
- ☐ **plas/i**, **plas/o**, **-plasia** development, growth, formation
- ☐ **poster/o** behind, toward the back
- ☐ **-stasis**, **-static** control, maintenance of a constant level

Medical Terms

- ☐ **abdominal cavity** (ab-**DOM**-ih-nal)
- ☐ **adenocarcinoma** (**ad**-eh-noh-**kar**-sih-**NOH**-mah)
- ☐ **adenoma** (**ad**-eh-**NOH**-mah)
- ☐ **anaplasia** (**an**-ah-**PLAY**-zhee-ah)
- ☐ **anatomy** (ah-**NAT**-oh-mee)
- ☐ **anomaly** (ah-**NOM**-ah-lee)
- ☐ **anterior** (an-**TEER**-ee-or)
- ☐ **aplasia** (ah-**PLAY**-zhee-ah)
- ☐ **atresia** (ah-**TREE**-zee-ah)
- ☐ **bloodborne transmission**
- ☐ **caudal** (**KAW**-dal)
- ☐ **cephalic** (seh-**FAL**-ick)
- ☐ **chromosome** (**KROH**-moh-sohme)
- ☐ **communicable disease** (kuh-**MEW**-nih-kuh-bul)
- ☐ **congenital disorder** (kon-**JEN**-ih-tahl)
- ☐ **cytoplasm** (**SIGH**-toh-plazm)
- ☐ **distal** (**DIS**-tal)
- ☐ **dorsal** (**DOR**-sal)
- ☐ **dysplasia** (dis-**PLAY**-zhee-ah)
- ☐ **endemic** (en-**DEM**-ick)
- ☐ **endocrine glands** (**EN**-doh-krin)
- ☐ **epidemic** (**ep**-ih-**DEM**-ick)
- ☐ **epigastric region** (**ep**-ih-**GAS**-trick)
- ☐ **etiology** (**ee**-tee-**OL**-oh-jee)
- ☐ **exocrine glands** (**ECK**-soh-krin)
- ☐ **functional disorder**
- ☐ **genetic disorder**
- ☐ **genome** (**JEE**-nohm)
- ☐ **hemophilia** (**hee**-moh-**FILL**-ee-ah)
- ☐ **histology** (hiss-**TOL**-oh-jee)
- ☐ **homeostasis** (**hoh**-mee-oh-**STAY**-sis)
- ☐ **hyperplasia** (**high**-per-**PLAY**-zhee-ah)
- ☐ **hypertrophy** (high-**PER**-troh-fee)
- ☐ **hypogastric region** (**high**-poh-**GAS**-trick)
- ☐ **hypoplasia** (**high**-poh-**PLAY**-zhee-ah)
- ☐ **iatrogenic illness** (eye-**at**-roh-**JEN**-ick)
- ☐ **idiopathic disease** (**id**-ee-oh-**PATH**-ick)
- ☐ **infectious disease** (in-**FECK**-shus)
- ☐ **inguinal** (**ING**-gwih-nal)
- ☐ **intensivist** (in-**TEN**-siv-ist)
- ☐ **medial** (**MEE**-dee-al)
- ☐ **mesentery** (**MESS**-en-**terr**-ee)
- ☐ **midsagittal plane** (mid-**SADJ**-ih-tal)
- ☐ **nosocomial infection** (**nahs**-oh-**KOH**-mee-al)
- ☐ **pandemic** (pan-**DEM**-ick)
- ☐ **pathology** (pah-**THOL**-oh-jee)
- ☐ **pelvic cavity** (**PEL**-vick)
- ☐ **peritoneum** (**pehr**-ih-toh-**NEE**-um)
- ☐ **peritonitis** (**pehr**-ih-toh-**NIGH**-tis)
- ☐ **physiology** (**fiz**-ee-**OL**-oh-jee)
- ☐ **posterior** (pos-**TEER**-ee-or)
- ☐ **proximal** (**PROCK**-sih-mal)
- ☐ **retroperitoneal** (**ret**-roh-**pehr**-ih-toh-**NEE**-al)
- ☐ **stem cells**
- ☐ **syndrome** (**SIN**-drohm)
- ☐ **thoracic cavity** (thoh-**RAS**-ick)
- ☐ **transverse plane** (trans-**VERSE**)
- ☐ **umbilicus** (um-**BILL**-ih-kus)
- ☐ **vector-borne transmission**
- ☐ **ventral** (**VEN**-tral)

LEARNING OBJECTIVES

On completion of this chapter, you should be able to:

1. Define medical terms related to body planes.
2. Define the terms describing body directions.
3. Name the body cavities.
4. List the nine regions of the thorax and abdomen.
5. Explain how the abdominal quadrants are divided and labeled.
6. Describe the four levels of structural organization of the body.
7. Define the primary terms related to cells, genetics, and genetic disorders.
8. Define the primary terms related to tissues and glands.
9. Identify the major organs and functions of the body systems.
10. Define the primary terms used to describe pathology, the modes of transmission, and the types of diseases.
11. Define the primary terms related to syndromes and congenital disorders.
12. Identify the roles of health care professionals in the various health care settings.
13. Identify medical word parts related to the human body in health and disease.
14. Spell the primary terms introduced in this chapter.
15. Pronounce the primary terms introduced in this chapter.
16. Identify common abbreviations related to the human body in health and disease.

ANATOMICAL REFERENCE SYSTEMS

Anatomical reference systems are used to describe the locations of the structural units of the body. The simplest anatomical reference is the one we learn in childhood: our right hand is on the right, and our left hand on the left.

In medical terminology, there are several additional ways to describe the location of different body parts. These anatomical reference systems include:

- Body planes
- Body directions
- Body cavities
- Structural units

When body parts work together to perform a related function, they are grouped together and are known as a body system. The digestive system, for example, is made up of the organs related to ingesting and processing of food.

Anatomy and Physiology Defined

- **Anatomy** (ah-**NAT**-oh-mee) is the study of the structures of the body. The adjective **anatomical** (ah-nah-**TOM**-ih-kal) means referring to anatomy.
- **Physiology** (**fiz**-ee-**OL**-oh-jee) is the study of the functions of the structures of the body (**physi** means nature or physical, and **-ology** means study of).

The Anatomical Position

The **anatomical position** describes the body standing in the standard position. This includes:

- Standing up straight so that the body is erect and facing forward.
- Holding the arms at the sides with the hands turned so that the palms face toward the front.

The Body Planes

Body planes are imaginary vertical and horizontal lines used to divide the body into sections for descriptive purposes (Figure 2.1). These planes are aligned to a body standing in the anatomical position.

The Vertical Planes

A **vertical plane** is an up-and-down plane that is at a right angle to the horizon.

- A **sagittal plane** (**SADJ**-ih-tal) is a vertical plane that divides the body into *unequal* left and right portions.
- The **midsagittal plane** (mid-**SADJ**-ih-tal), also known as the ***midline***, is the sagittal plane that divides the body into *equal* left and right halves (Figure 2.1).

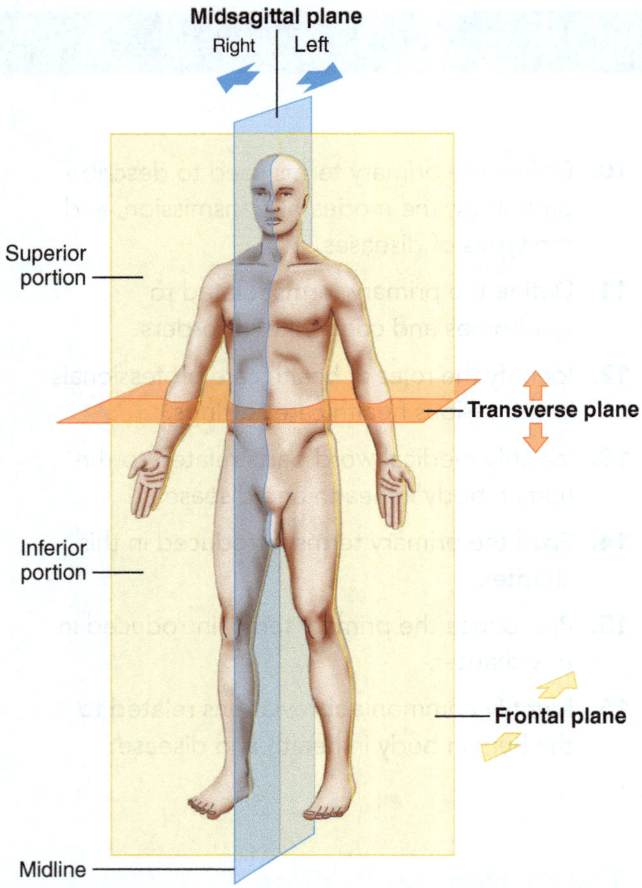

FIGURE 2.1 Body planes: the midsagittal plane divides the body into equal left and right halves. The transverse plane divides the body into superior (upper) and inferior (lower) portions. The frontal plane divides the body into anterior or ventral (front) and posterior or dorsal (back) portions.

- A **frontal plane** is a vertical plane that divides the body into anterior (front) and posterior (back) portions. Also known as the ***coronal plane***, it is located at right angles to the sagittal plane (Figure 2.1).

The Horizontal Plane

A **horizontal plane** is a flat, crosswise plane, such as the horizon.

- A **transverse plane** (trans-**VERSE**) is a horizontal plane that divides the body into superior (upper) and inferior (lower) portions. A transverse plane can be at the waist or at any other level across the body (Figure 2.1).

Body Direction Terms

The relative location of sections of the body or of an organ can be described through the use of pairs of contrasting body direction terms. These terms are illustrated in Figures 2.2 and 2.3.

- **Ventral** (**VEN**-tral) refers to the front, or belly side, of the organ or body (**ventr** means belly side of the body, and **-al** means pertaining to). *Ventral* is the opposite of *dorsal.*
- **Dorsal** (**DOR**-sal) refers to the back of the organ or body (**dors** means back of the body, and **-al** means pertaining to). *Dorsal* is the opposite of *ventral.*
- **Anterior** (an-**TEER**-ee-or) means situated in the front. It also means on the front or forward part of an organ (**anter** means front or before, and **-ior** means pertaining to). For example, the stomach is located anterior to (in front of) the pancreas. *Anterior* is also used in reference to the ventral surface of the body. *Anterior* is the opposite of *posterior.*
- **Posterior** (pos-**TEER**-ee-or) means situated in the back. It also means on the back part of an organ (**poster** means back or toward the back, and **-ior** means pertaining to). For example, the pancreas is located posterior to (behind) the stomach. The term *posterior* is also used in reference to the dorsal surface of the body. *Posterior* is the opposite of *anterior.*
- **Superior** means uppermost, above, or toward the head. For example, the lungs are located superior to (above) the diaphragm. *Superior* is the opposite of *inferior.*
- **Inferior** means lowermost, below, or toward the feet. For example, the stomach is located inferior to (below) the diaphragm. *Inferior* is the opposite of *superior.*
- **Cephalic** (seh-**FAL**-ick) means toward the head (**cephal** means head, and **-ic** means pertaining to). *Cephalic* is the opposite of *caudal.*
- **Caudal** (**KAW**-dal) means toward the lower part of the body (**caud** means tail or lower part of the body, and **-al** means pertaining to). *Caudal* is the opposite of *cephalic.*
- **Proximal** (**PROCK**-sih-mal) means situated nearest the midline or beginning of a body structure. For example, the proximal end of the humerus (bone of the upper arm) forms part of the shoulder. *Proximal* is the opposite of *distal.*
- **Distal** (**DIS**-tal) means situated farthest from the midline or beginning of a body structure. For example, the distal end of the humerus forms part of the elbow (Figure 2.3). *Distal* is the opposite of *proximal.*

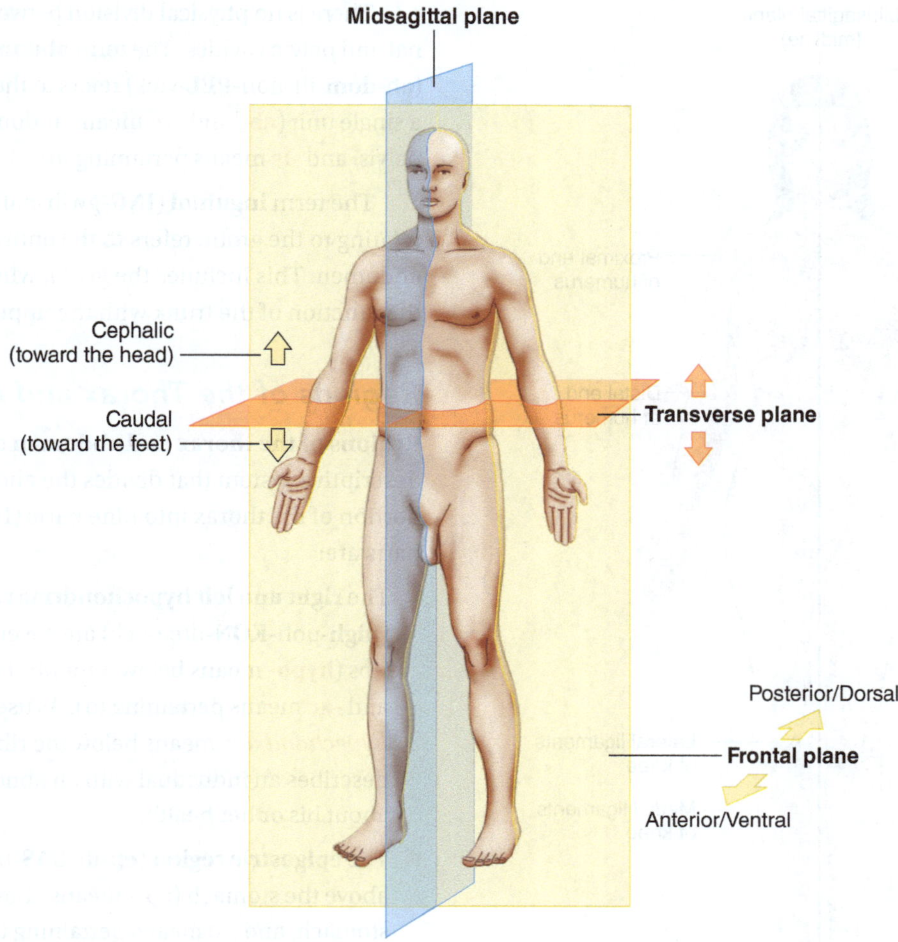

FIGURE 2.2 Body directions: *Cephalic* means toward the head, and *caudal* means toward the feet. *Anterior* means toward the front, and the front of the body is known as the ventral surface. *Posterior* means toward the back, and the back of the body is known as the dorsal surface.

- **Medial** (MEE-dee-al) means the direction toward, or nearer, the midline. For example, the medial ligament of the knee is near the inner surface of the leg (Figure 2.3). *Medial* is the opposite of *lateral*.
- **Lateral** means the direction toward, or nearer, the side of the body, away from the midline. For example, the lateral ligament of the knee is near the side of the leg. *Lateral* is the opposite of *medial*. ***Bilateral*** means relating to, or having, two sides.

Major Body Cavities

The two major **body cavities**, which are the dorsal (back) and the ventral (front) cavities, are spaces within the body that contain and protect internal organs (Figure 2.4).

The Dorsal Cavity

The **dorsal cavity**, which is located along the back of the body and head, contains organs of the nervous system that coordinate body functions and is divided into two portions:

- The **cranial cavity**, which is located within the skull, surrounds and protects the brain. ***Cranial*** means pertaining to the skull.
- The **spinal cavity**, which is located within the spinal column, surrounds and protects the spinal cord.

The Ventral Cavity

The **ventral cavity**, which is located along the front of the body, contains the organs that sustain homeostasis. **Homeostasis** (**hoh**-mee-oh-**STAY**-sis) is the processes

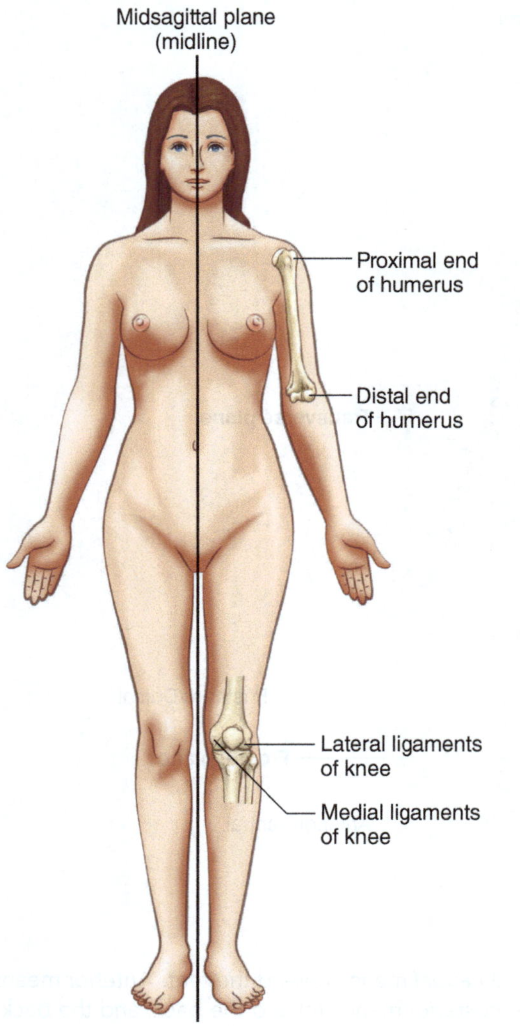

FIGURE 2.3 Body directions: *Proximal* means situated nearest the midline, and *distal* means situated farthest from the midline. *Medial* means toward or nearer the midline, and *lateral* means toward the side and away from the midline.

through which the body maintains a constant internal environment (**home/o** means constant, and **-stasis** means control). The ventral cavity is divided into the following portions:

- The **thoracic cavity** (thoh-**RAS**-ick), also known as the ***chest cavity*** or ***thorax***, surrounds and protects the heart and the lungs. The ***diaphragm*** is a muscle that separates the thoracic and abdominal cavities.
- The **abdominal cavity** (ab-**DOM**-ih-nal) contains the major organs of digestion. This cavity is frequently referred to simply as the **abdomen** (**AB**-doh-men).
- The **pelvic cavity** (**PEL**-vick) is the space formed by the hip bones and contains the organs of the reproductive and excretory systems.

There is no physical division between the abdominal and pelvic cavities. The term **abdominopelvic cavity** (ab-**dom**-ih-noh-**PEL**-vick) refers to these two cavities as a single unit (**abdomin/o** means abdomen, **pelv** means pelvis, and **-ic** means pertaining to).

The term **inguinal** (**ING**-gwih-nal), which means relating to the groin, refers to the entire lower area of the abdomen. This includes the ***groin***, which is the crease at the junction of the trunk with the upper end of the thigh.

Regions of the Thorax and Abdomen

Regions of the thorax and abdomen comprise a descriptive system that divides the abdomen and lower portion of the thorax into nine parts (Figure 2.5). These parts are:

- The **right and left hypochondriac regions** (**high**-poh-**KON**-dree-ack) are covered by the lower ribs (**hypo-** means below, **chondr/i** means cartilage, and **-ac** means pertaining to). As used here, the term ***hypochondriac*** means below the ribs. This term also describes an individual with an abnormal concern about his or her health.
- The **epigastric region** (**ep**-ih-**GAS**-trick) is located above the stomach (**epi-** means above, **gastr** means stomach, and **-ic** means pertaining to).
- The **right and left lumbar regions** (**LUM**-bar) are located near the inward curve of the spine (**lumb** means lower back, and **-ar** means pertaining to). The term ***lumbar*** describes the part of the back between the ribs and the pelvis.
- The **umbilical region** (um-**BILL**-ih-kal) surrounds the **umbilicus** (um-**BILL**-ih-kus), which is commonly known as the ***belly button*** or ***navel***. This pit in the center of the abdominal wall marks the point where the umbilical cord was attached before birth.
- The **right and left iliac regions** (**ILL**-ee-ack) are located near the hip bones (**ili** means hip bone, and **-ac** means pertaining to).
- The **hypogastric region** (**high**-poh-**GAS**-trick) is located below the stomach (**hypo-** means below, **gastr** means stomach, and **-ic** means pertaining to).

Quadrants of the Abdomen

Describing where an abdominal organ or pain is located is made easier by dividing the abdomen into four imaginary quadrants. The term **quadrant** means divided into four. As shown in Figure 2.6, the quadrants of the abdomen are as follows:

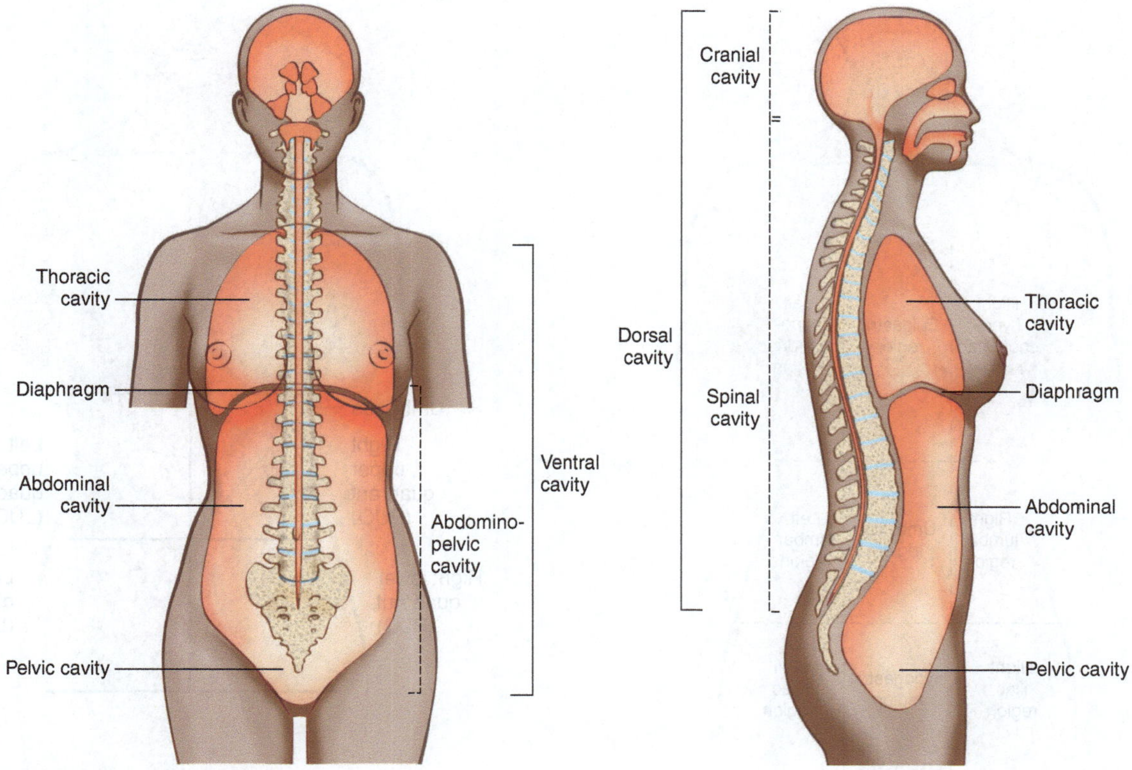

FIGURE 2.4 The major body cavities.

- Right upper quadrant (RUQ)
- Left upper quadrant (LUQ)
- Right lower quadrant (RLQ)
- Left lower quadrant (LLQ)

The Peritoneum

The **peritoneum** (**pehr**-ih-toh-**NEE**-um) is a multilayered membrane that protects and holds the organs in place within the abdominal cavity. A ***membrane*** is a thin layer of tissue that covers a surface, lines a cavity, or divides a space or organ.

- The **parietal peritoneum** (pah-**RYE**-eh-tal **pehr**-ih-toh-**NEE**-um) is the outer layer of the peritoneum that lines the interior of the abdominal wall. ***Parietal*** means cavity wall.
- The **mesentery** (**MESS**-en-**terr**-ee) is a fused double layer of the parietal peritoneum that attaches parts of the intestine to the interior abdominal wall.
- The **visceral peritoneum** (**VIS**-er-al **pehr**-ih-toh-**NEE**-um) is the inner layer of the peritoneum that surrounds the organs of the abdominal cavity. ***Visceral*** means relating to the internal organs.
- **Retroperitoneal** (**ret**-roh-**pehr**-ih-toh-**NEE**-al) means located behind the peritoneum (**retro-** means behind, **periton** means peritoneum, and **-eal** means pertaining to). For example, the location of the kidneys is retroperitoneal with one on each side of the spinal column.
- **Peritonitis** (**pehr**-ih-toh-**NIGH**-tis) is inflammation of the peritoneum.

STRUCTURES OF THE BODY

The body is made up of increasingly larger and more complex structural units. These four structural levels are the **cells**, **tissues**, **organs**, and **body systems** (Figure 2.7). Working together, these structures form the complete body and enable it to function properly.

CELLS

Cells are the basic structural and functional units of the body. Cells are specialized and grouped together to form tissues and organs.

- **Cytology** (sigh-**TOL**-oh-jee) is the study of the anatomy, physiology, pathology, and chemistry of the cell (**cyt** means cell, and **-ology** means study of).
- A **cytologist** (sigh-**TOL**-oh-jist) is a specialist in the study and analysis of cells (**cyt** means cell, and **-ologist** means specialist).

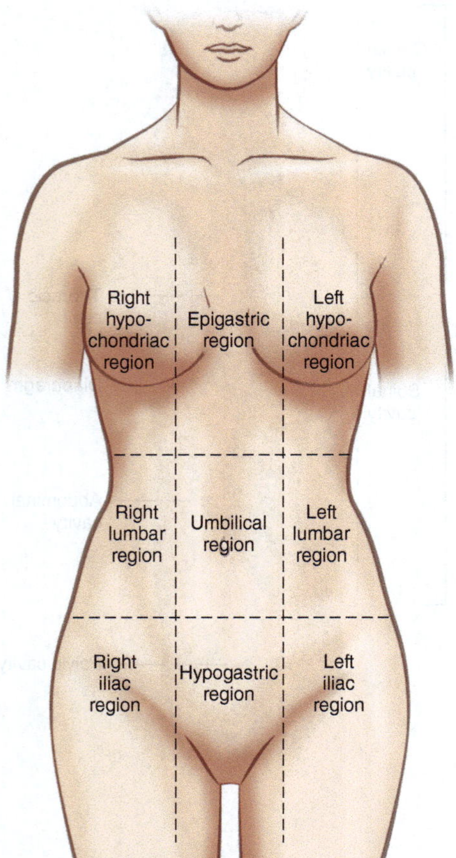

FIGURE 2.5 Regions of the thorax and abdomen.

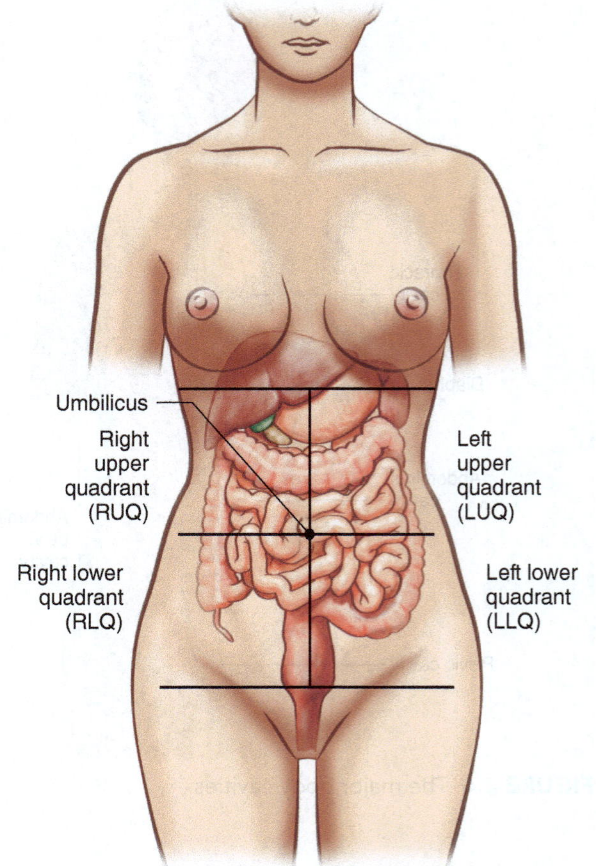

FIGURE 2.6 Division of the abdomen into quadrants.

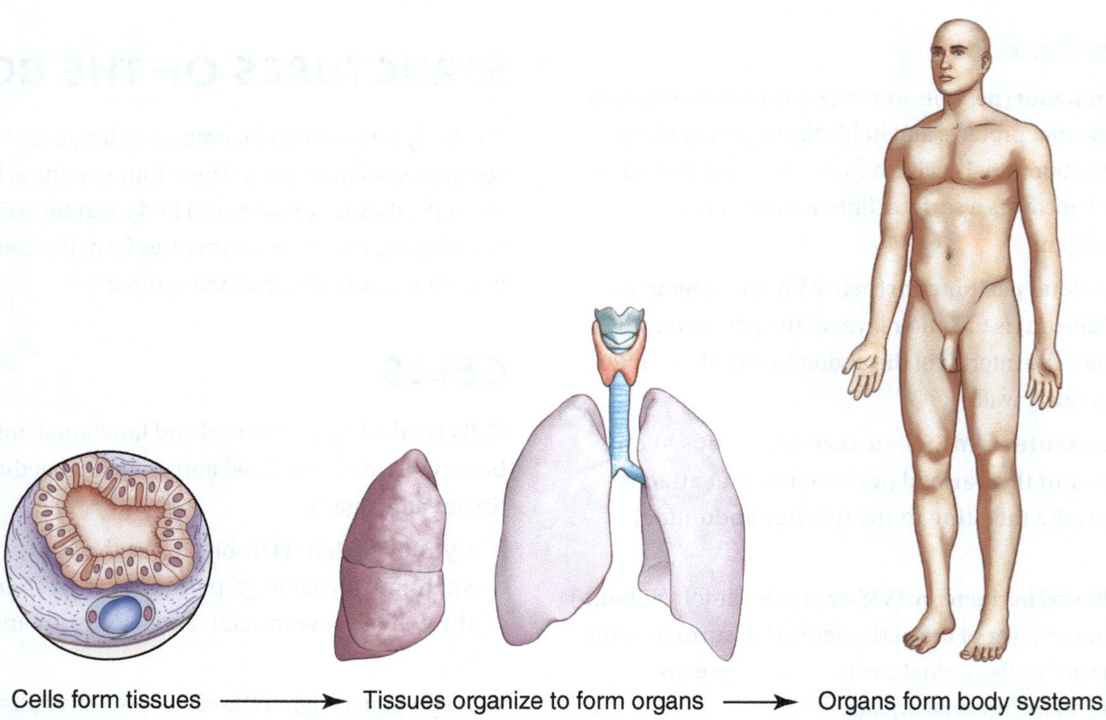

FIGURE 2.7 The human body is highly organized, from the single cell to the total organism.

The Structure of Cells

- The **cell membrane** (**MEM**-brain) is the tissue that surrounds and protects the contents of a cell from the external environment (Figure 2.8).
- **Cytoplasm** (**SIGH**-toh-plazm) is the material within the cell membrane that is *not* part of the nucleus (**cyt/o** means cell, and **-plasm** means formative material of cells).
- The **nucleus** (**NEW**-klee-us), which is surrounded by the nuclear membrane, is a structure within the cell. It has two important functions: it controls the activities of the cell, and it helps the cell divide.

Stem Cells

Stem cells differ from other kinds of cells in the body because of two characteristics:

- **Stem cells** are unspecialized cells that are able to renew themselves for long periods of time by cell division. This is in contrast to other types of cells that have a specialized role and die after a determined life span.
- Under certain conditions, stem cells can be transformed into cells with special functions, such as the cells of the heart muscle that make the heartbeat possible or the specialized cells of the pancreas that are capable of producing insulin.

Adult Stem Cells

Adult stem cells, also known as ***somatic stem cells***, are undifferentiated cells found among differentiated cells in a tissue or organ. Normally the primary role of these cells is to maintain and repair the tissue in which they are found. The term ***undifferentiated*** means not having a specialized function or structure. In contrast, the term ***differentiated*** means having a specialized function or structure.

Embryonic Stem Cells

Embryonic stem cells (em-bree-**ON**-ik) are undifferentiated cells that are unlike any specific adult cell; however, they have the important ability to form *any* adult cell. Embryonic means referring to an *embryo*, a developing fetus during its first eight weeks in the womb (**embry/o** means fertilized ovum, and **-nic** means pertaining to).

- These cells can proliferate (grow rapidly) indefinitely in a laboratory and could therefore potentially provide a source for adult muscle, liver, bone, or blood cells.

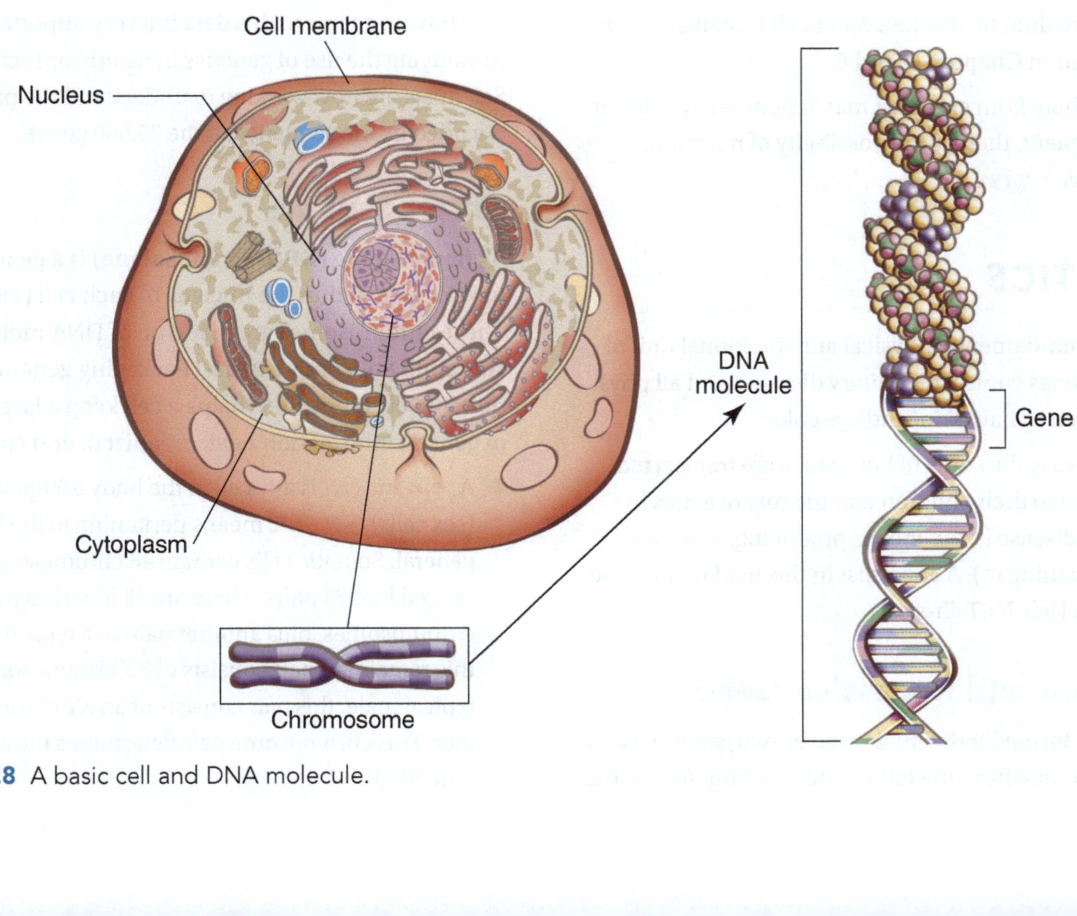

FIGURE 2.8 A basic cell and DNA molecule.

- Because these cells are more primitive than adult stem cells, an embryonic stem cell transplant does not require as perfect a match between the patient and donor as the transplantation of adult stem cells.
- Embryonic stem cells come from the *cord blood* found in the umbilical cord and placenta of a newborn infant. Embryonic stem cells from cord blood can be harvested at the time of birth without danger to mother or child. These cells are kept frozen until needed for treatment purposes (see Chapter 16).
- Embryonic stem cells can also be obtained from surplus embryos produced by in vitro (test tube) fertilization. With the informed consent of the donor couple, stem cells obtained in this manner can be used for medical treatments or scientific research. *Informed consent* means that those involved have been given information about what is involved before granting permission.

Stem Cell Therapy

Stem cell therapy, also known as *regenerative medicine*, has many potential uses to heal injuries and treat diseases.

- Cells for this purpose are usually harvested from the *hematopoietic* (blood forming) tissue of the bone marrow. They can either be harvested from the patient's own bone marrow, or transplanted from one individual to another. Stem cell transplants are discussed in Chapters 3 and 6.
- Unless there is an excellent match between the donor and recipient, there is the possibility of rejection, known as *graft versus host disease*.

GENETICS

A **gene** is a fundamental physical and functional unit of heredity. Genes control hereditary diseases and all physical traits such as hair, skin, and eye color.

Genetics is the study of how genes are transferred from parents to their children and the role of genes in health and disease (**gene** means producing, and **-tics** means pertaining to). A specialist in this field is known as a **geneticist** (jeh-**NET**-ih-sist).

Dominant and Recessive Genes

Each newly formed individual receives two genes of each genetic trait: one from the father and one from the mother.

- When a **dominant gene** is inherited from either parent, the offspring *will* inherit that genetic condition or characteristic. For example, freckles are a physical trait that is transmitted by a dominant gene. So, too, is the hereditary disease *Huntington's disease*.
- When the same **recessive gene** is inherited from both parents, the offspring *will have* that condition. For example, *sickle cell anemia* is a group of inherited red blood cell disorders that are transmitted by a recessive gene. When this gene is transmitted by both parents, the child *will have* sickle cell anemia.
- When a **recessive gene** is inherited from only one parent, and a normal gene is inherited from the other parent, the offspring *will not have* the condition. Although this child will not develop sickle cell anemia, he or she will have the *sickle cell anemia trait*. People with this trait can transmit the sickle cell gene to their offspring.

The Human Genome

A **genome** (**JEE**-nohm) is the complete set of genetic information of an organism. The Human Genome Project studied this genetic code for individual people and found that it is more than 99% identical among humans throughout the world. The first complete mapping of the *human genome*, which took 13 years to complete, was published in 2003.

Having access to this data is a very important step in studying the use of genetics in health and science. Scientists are now working to understand the proteins encoded by the sequence of the 25,000 genes.

Chromosomes

A **chromosome** (**KROH**-moh-sohme) is a genetic structure located within the nucleus of each cell (Figure 2.8). These chromosomes are made up of DNA molecules containing the body's genes. Packaging genetic information into chromosomes helps a cell keep a large amount of genetic information neat, organized, and compact.

- A *somatic cell* is any cell in the body except the gametes (sex cells). *Somatic* means pertaining to the body in general. Somatic cells contain 46 chromosomes arranged into 23 pairs. There are 22 identical pairs of chromosomes, plus another pair. In a typical female, this remaining pair consists of XX chromosomes. In a typical male, this pair consists of an XY chromosome pair. This chromosome pair determines the sex of the individual.

- A ***gamete*** (sperm or egg), also known as a ***sex cell***, is the only type of cell that *does not* contain 46 chromosomes. Instead, each ovum (egg) or sperm has 23 single chromosomes. In a female, one of these will be an X chromosome. In a male, one of these will be either an X or a Y chromosome. When a sperm and ovum join, the newly formed offspring receives 23 chromosomes from each parent, for a total of 46.
- It is the X or Y chromosome from the father that determines the sex of the child.
- A defect in chromosomes can lead to birth defects. For example, individuals with Down syndrome have 47 chromosomes instead of the usual 46.

DNA

The basic structure of the DNA molecule, which is located on the pairs of chromosomes in the nucleus of each cell, is the same for all living organisms. Human DNA contains thousands of genes that provide the information essential for heredity, determining physical appearance, disease risks, and other traits (Figure 2.8).

- **DNA**, which is an abbreviation for ***deoxyribonucleic acid***, is the main component of chromosomes, and is the material that carries the body's genetic information. It is found in the nucleus of all types of cells except erythrocytes (red blood cells). The difference here is due to the fact that erythrocytes do not have a nucleus.
- DNA is packaged in a chromosome as two spiraling strands that twist together to form a double helix. A ***helix*** is a shape twisted like a spiral staircase. A ***double helix*** consists of two of these strands twisted together.
- The DNA for each individual is different, and no two DNA patterns are exactly the same. The only exception to this rule is identical twins, which are formed from one fertilized egg that divides. Although their DNA is identical, these twins do develop characteristics that make each of them unique, such as fingerprints.
- A very small sample of DNA, such as from human hair or tissue, can be used to identify individuals in instances such as criminal investigations, paternity suits, or genealogical research. Genetic testing is discussed in Chapter 21.

Genetic Mutation

A **genetic mutation** is a change of the sequence of a DNA molecule. Potential causes of genetic mutation include exposure to radiation or environmental pollution.

- A ***somatic cell mutation*** is a change within the cells of the body. These changes affect the individual but *cannot* be transmitted to the next generation.
- A ***gametic cell mutation*** is a change within the genes in a gamete (sex cell) that *can* be transmitted by a parent to his or her children.
- ***Genetic engineering*** is the manipulating or splicing of genes for scientific or medical purposes. The production of human insulin from modified bacteria is an example of one result of genetic engineering.

Genetic Disorders

A **genetic disorder**, also known as a ***hereditary disease***, is a pathological condition caused by an absent or defective gene. Some genetic disorders are obvious at birth. Others may manifest (become evident) at any time in life. The following are examples of genetic disorders:

- **Cystic fibrosis** (CF) is a genetic disorder that is present at birth and affects both the respiratory and digestive systems (see Chapter 8).
- **Down syndrome** (DS), also known as ***trisomy 21***, is a genetic variation that is associated with a characteristic facial appearance, learning disabilities, developmental delays, and physical abnormalities such as heart valve disease (Figure 2.9). The name Down syndrome comes from English physician John Langdon Down.

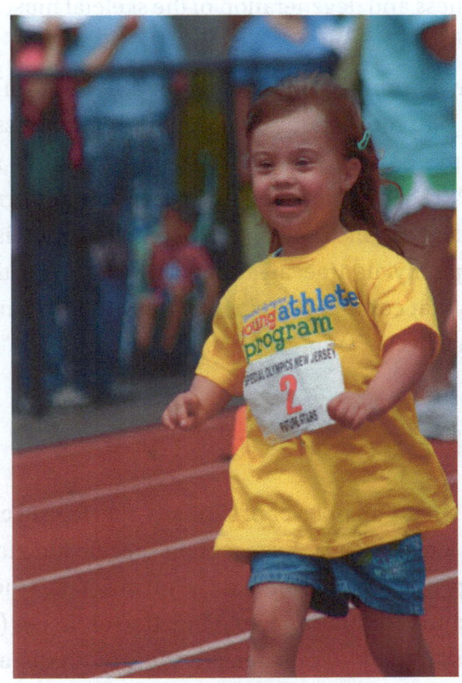

Used with permission from Special Olympics New Jersey.

FIGURE 2.9 Down syndrome is a genetic disorder usually caused by the presence of a third copy of the 21st chromosome. For this reason it is also known as *trisomy 21*.

- **Fragile X syndrome** is caused by changes in the MR1 gene that usually makes a protein needed for normal brain development. The condition is characterized by developmental delays, learning disabilities, and social and behavior problems.
- **Hemophilia** (**hee**-moh-**FILL**-ee-ah) is a hereditary bleeding disorder in which a blood-clotting factor is missing. This blood coagulation disorder, which mostly affects males, is characterized by spontaneous hemorrhages or severe bleeding following an injury.
- **Huntington's disease** (HD) is a genetic disorder that is passed from parent to child. Each child of a parent with the gene for Huntington's disease has a 50–50 chance of inheriting this single defective gene. This condition causes nerve degeneration with symptoms that most often appear in midlife. (***Degeneration*** means worsening condition.) This damage eventually results in uncontrolled movements, the loss of some mental abilities, and psychiatric disorders such as depression.
- **Marfan syndrome** is a disorder affecting the connective tissue throughout the body, including the heart, eyes, blood vessels and musculoskeletal system. People with this inherited condition often have a tall, slender build and disproportionately long arms, legs, and fingers.
- **Muscular dystrophy** (**DIS**-troh-fee) is a group of genetic diseases that are characterized by progressive weakness and degeneration of the skeletal muscles that control movement (see Chapter 4).
- **Phenylketonuria** (**fen**-il-**kee**-toh-**NEW**-ree-ah) (PKU) is a rare genetic disorder in which the essential digestive enzyme *phenylalanine hydroxylase* is missing. PKU can be detected by a blood test performed on infants at birth. With careful dietary supervision to limit phenylalanine, an amino acid found mostly in foods that contain protein, people with PKU can lead normal lives.

TISSUES

A **tissue** is a group or layer of similarly specialized cells that join together to perform certain specific functions. **Histology** (hiss-**TOL**-oh-jee) is the microscopic study of the structure, composition, and function of tissues (**hist** means tissue, and **-ology** means a study of). A **histologist** (hiss-**TOL**-oh-jist) is a non-physician specialist who studies the microscopic structure of tissues (**hist** means tissue, and **-ologist** means specialist).

The four main types of tissue are as follows:

- Epithelial tissue
- Connective tissue
- Muscle tissue
- Nerve tissue

Epithelial Tissue

Epithelial tissue (**ep**-ih-**THEE**-lee-al) forms a protective covering for all of the internal and external surfaces of the body. These tissues also form glands.

- **Epithelium** (**ep**-ih-**THEE**-lee-um) is the specialized epithelial tissue that forms the epidermis of the skin and the surface layer of mucous membranes (see Chapter 14).
- **Endothelium** (**en**-doh-**THEE**-lee-um) is the specialized epithelial tissue that lines the blood and lymph vessels, body cavities, glands, and organs.

Connective Tissue

Connective tissues support and connect organs and other body tissues. The four kinds of connective tissue are as follows:

- **Dense connective tissues**, such as bone and cartilage, form the joints and framework of the body.
- **Adipose tissue** (**AH**-deh-**pos**), also known as ***fat***, provides protective padding, insulation, and support (**adip** means fat, and **-ose** means pertaining to).
- **Loose connective tissue** holds organs in place and binds tissue together.
- **Fluid connective tissues**, which are blood and lymph, transport nutrients and waste products throughout the body.

Muscle Tissue

Muscle tissue contains cells with the specialized ability to contract and relax.

Nerve Tissue

Nerve tissue contains cells with the specialized ability to react to stimuli and to conduct electrical impulses.

Pathology of Tissue Formation

Disorders of the tissues, which are frequently due to unknown causes, can occur as the tissues form before birth or appear later in life.

Incomplete Tissue Formation

- **Aplasia** (ah-**PLAY**-zhee-ah) is the defective development, or the congenital absence, of an organ or tissue (**a-** means without, and **-plasia** means formation). An example is ***aplastic anemia***, caused by the body not producing enough new blood cells (see Chapter 6). Compare aplasia with *hypoplasia*.
- **Hypoplasia** (**high**-poh-**PLAY**-zhee-ah) is the underdevelopment of an organ or tissue, usually due to a deficiency in the number of cells (**hypo-** means deficient, and **-plasia** means formation). In ***enamel hypoplasia***, for example, the protective outer layer of developing teeth is deficient. Compare hypoplasia with *aplasia*.

Abnormal Tissue Formation

- **Anaplasia** (**an**-ah-**PLAY**-zhee-ah) is a change in the structure of cells and in their orientation to each other (**ana-** means backward, and **-plasia** means formation). This abnormal cell development is characteristic of most cancerous tumor formation. Contrast anaplasia with *hypertrophy*.
- **Dysplasia** (dis-**PLAY**-zhee-ah) is the abnormal development or growth of cells, or the presence of abnormal cells within a type of tissue (**dys-** means bad, and **-plasia** means formation). ***Cervical dysplasia***, for example, refers to abnormal cells being found on the cervix (see Chapter 16).
- **Hyperplasia** (**high**-per-**PLAY**-zhee-ah) is an increase in the number of cells in a tissue or organ (**hyper-** means excessive, and **-plasia** means formation). Some hyperplasia, such as the increase in breast tissue caused by the hormones released during pregnancy, is normal. In other types of hyperplasia the cells may be precancerous. Contrast hyperplasia with *hypertrophy*.
- **Hypertrophy** (high-**PER**-troh-fee) is a general increase in the bulk of a body part or organ that is due to an increase in the size, but not in the number, of cells in the tissues (**hyper-** means excessive, and **-trophy** means development). This enlargement is not due to tumor formation; in fact, muscle hypertrophy is the desired response to weight lifting. Contrast hypertrophy with *anaplasia* and *hyperplasia*.

GLANDS

A **gland** is a group of specialized epithelial cells that are capable of producing secretions. A ***secretion*** is the substance produced by a gland. The two major types of glands are as follows (Figure 2.10):

- **Exocrine glands** (**ECK**-soh-krin) secrete chemical substances into ducts that lead either to other organs or out of the body. Examples include the salivary, mammary and sweat glands (**exo-** means out of, and **-crine** means to secrete) (see Chapter 13).
- **Endocrine glands** (**EN**-doh-krin), which produce hormones, do not have ducts (**endo-** means within, and **-crine** means to secrete). These hormones are secreted directly into the bloodstream and are then transported

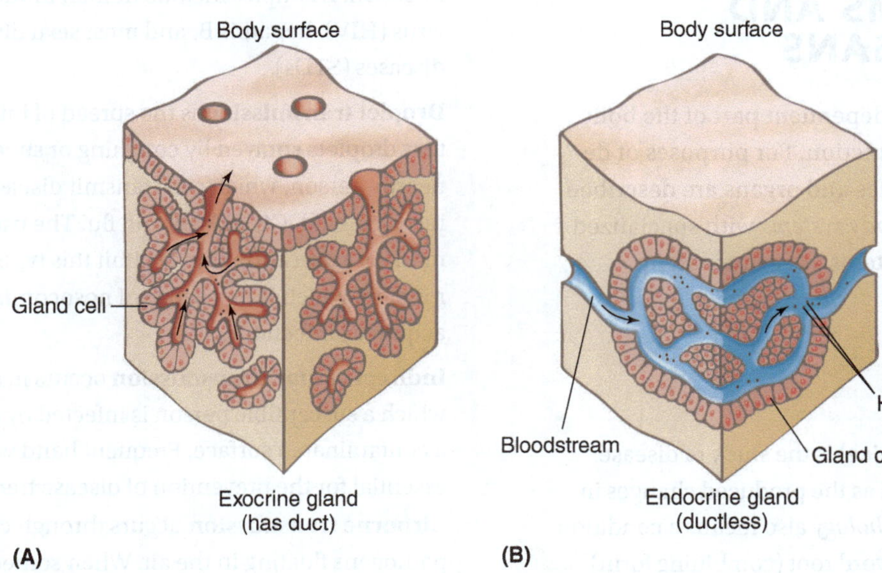

FIGURE 2.10 (A) Exocrine glands secrete their chemical substances into ducts that lead either to other organs or out of the body. (B) Endocrine glands pour their secretions directly into the bloodstream.

to organs and structures throughout the body (see Chapter 14).

Pathology and Procedures of the Glands

The word root **aden** means gland. Note that the term **adenoids**, however, refers to a mass of gland-like lymphoid tissue at the back of the upper pharynx (see Chapter 7).

- **Adenitis** (**ad**-eh-**NIGH**-tis) is the inflammation of a gland (**aden** means gland, and **-itis** means inflammation). ***Mesenteric adenitis*** is an inflammation of the lymph nodes in the abdomen that has symptoms similar to appendicitis.
- An **adenocarcinoma** (**ad**-eh-noh-**kar**-sih-**NOH**-mah) is a malignant tumor that originates in the glands and may spread to other parts of the body (**aden/o** means gland, **carcin** means cancerous, and **-oma** means tumor). ***Malignant*** means harmful, capable of spreading, and potentially life-threatening.
- An **adenoma** (**ad**-eh-**NOH**-mah) is a benign tumor that starts in the epithelial tissue of a gland or gland-like structure (**aden** means gland, and **-oma** means tumor). A ***polyp*** in the colon is a common type of adenoma (see Chapter 9). ***Benign*** means not life-threatening.
- **Adenosis** (**ad**-eh-**NOH**-sis) is any disease or condition of a gland (**aden** means gland, and **-osis** means an abnormal condition or disease).

BODY SYSTEMS AND RELATED ORGANS

A **organ** is a somewhat independent part of the body that performs a specific function. For purposes of description, the related tissues and organs are described as being organized into *body systems* with specialized functions. These body systems are explained in Table 2.1.

PATHOLOGY

Pathology (pah-**THOL**-oh-jee) is the study of disease: its nature and cause as well as the produced changes in structure and function. *Pathology* also means a condition produced by disease. The word root (combining form) **path/o** and the suffix **-pathy** mean disease; however, they also mean suffering, feeling, and emotion.

- A **pathologist** (pah-**THOL**-oh-jist) is a physician who specializes in the laboratory analysis of diseased tissue samples to confirm or establish a diagnosis (**path** means disease, and **-ologist** means specialist). These tissue specimens can be removed in biopsies, during operations, or in postmortem examinations.
- **Etiology** (**ee**-tee-**OL**-oh-jee) is the study of the causes of diseases or abnormal conditions (**eti-** means cause, and **-ology** means study of).

Disease Transmission

- A **pathogen** is a disease-producing microorganism such as a virus. ***Transmission*** is the spread of a disease. ***Contamination*** means that a pathogen is possibly present. Contamination occurs through a lack of proper hygiene standards or by failure to take appropriate infection control precautions.
- A **communicable disease** (kuh-**MEW**-nih-kuh-bul), also known as a ***contagious disease***, is any condition that is transmitted from one person to another either directly or by indirect contact with contaminated objects. ***Communicable*** means capable of being transmitted. Some diseases, such as measles, are capable of being transmitted through multiple methods.
- **Direct transmission** occurs when there is human-to-human contact in the form of touch or the exchange of bodily fluids.
- **Bloodborne transmission** is the spread of pathogens through infected blood or other body fluids. These infected fluids must enter the bloodstream to cause infection. Examples include human immunodeficiency virus (HIV), hepatitis B, and most sexually transmitted diseases (STDs).
- **Droplet transmission** is the spread of infected respiratory droplets sprayed by coughing or sneezing onto a nearby person, which can transmit diseases such as measles, cold, COVID-19, and flu. The use of a face mask as a precaution helps limit this type of transmission, which is one cause of nosocomial (hospital-acquired) infections.
- **Indirect contact transmission** occurs in situations in which a susceptible person is infected by contact with a contaminated surface. Frequent hand washing is essential for the prevention of disease transmission.
- **Airborne transmission** occurs through contact with pathogens floating in the air. When someone coughs or sneezes, certain microparticles can remain airborne for a long period of time, traveling up to 1 meter and

TABLE 2.1

Major Body Systems

Body System	Major Structures	Major Functions
Skeletal system (Chapter 3)	Bones, joints, and cartilage	Supports and shapes the body. Protects the internal organs. Forms some blood cells and stores minerals.
Muscular system (Chapter 4)	Muscles, fascia, and tendons	Holds the body erect. Makes movement possible. Moves body fluids and generates body heat.
Cardiovascular system (Chapter 5)	Heart, arteries, veins, capillaries, and blood	The heart pumps blood throughout the body to transport oxygen and nutrients to cells, and to carry waste products to the kidneys where waste is removed by filtration.
Blood system (Chapter 6)	Blood	Delivers oxygen and nutrients to the tissues and carries away waste.
Lymphatic system (Chapter 7)	Lymph, lymphatic vessels, and lymph nodes	Removes and transports waste products from the fluid between the cells. Destroys harmful substances such as pathogens and cancer cells in the lymph nodes. Returns the filtered lymph to the bloodstream where it becomes plasma again.
Immune system (Chapter 7)	Tonsils, spleen, thymus, skin, and specialized blood cells	Defends the body against invading pathogens and allergens.
Respiratory system (Chapter 8)	Nose, pharynx, trachea, larynx, and lungs	Brings oxygen into the body for transportation to the cells. Removes carbon dioxide and some water waste from the body.
Digestive system (Chapter 9)	Mouth, teeth, esophagus, stomach, small intestine, large intestine, liver, and pancreas	Digests ingested food so it can be absorbed into the bloodstream. Eliminates solid waste.
Urinary system (Chapter 10)	Kidneys, ureters, urinary bladder, and urethra	Filters blood to remove waste. Maintains the electrolyte and fluid balance within the body.
Nervous system (Chapter 11)	Nerves, brain, and spinal cord	Coordinates the reception of stimuli. Transmits messages throughout the body.
Special senses (Chapter 12)	Eyes and ears	Receive visual and auditory information and transmit it to the brain.
Integumentary system (Chapter 13)	Skin, sebaceous glands, and sweat glands	Protects the body against invasion by bacteria. Aids in regulating the body temperature and water content.
Endocrine system (Chapter 14)	Adrenal glands, gonads, pancreas, parathyroids, pineal, pituitary, thymus, and thyroid	Integrates all body functions.
Male Reproductive system (Chapter 15)	Penis and testicles	Provides the sperm necessary to fertilize an ovum.
Female Reproductive system (Chapter 16)	Ovaries, uterus, and vagina	Produces new life through the process of conception and birth.

exposing someone even after the infected person is gone. Examples include tuberculosis, measles, COVID-19, and chicken pox. The spread of pathogens via aerosol particles is especially concerning in health care settings during ***aerosol-generating procedures*** such as endotracheal intubation or open suctioning. An ***aerosol*** is a fine liquid particle suspended in air or another gas.

- **Food-borne and waterborne transmission**, also known as ***fecal-oral transmission***, is caused by eating or drinking contaminated food or water that has not been properly treated to remove contamination or kill any pathogens present.
- **Vector-borne transmission**, or an ***insect bite***, is the spread of certain disease through blood-sucking vectors. As used here, the term ***vector*** describes insects such as flies, mites, fleas, and ticks that carry or transmit such disease. Mosquitoes are the most common vectors, and the diseases they transmit include malaria and West Nile virus.

Outbreaks of Diseases

- An **epidemiologist** (**ep**-ih-**dee**-mee-**OL**-oh-jist) is a specialist in the study of outbreaks of disease within a population group (**epi-** means above, **dem/i** means population, and **-ologist** means specialist). The ***Centers for Disease Control and Prevention*** (CDC) is the national health protection agency in the United States. The CDC tracks outbreaks of diseases across the country and works to help prevent their spread.
- **Endemic** (en-**DEM**-ick) refers to the ongoing presence of a disease within a population, group, or area (**en-** means within, **dem** means population, and **-ic** means pertaining to). For example, the common cold is endemic because it is always present within the general population.
- An **epidemic** (**ep**-ih-**DEM**-ick) is a sudden and widespread outbreak of a disease within a specific population group or area (**epi-** means above, **dem** means population, and **-ic** means pertaining to). For example, a sudden widespread outbreak of whooping cough is an epidemic.
- **Pandemic** (pan-**DEM**-ick) refers to an outbreak of a disease occurring over a large geographic area, possibly worldwide (**pan-** means entire, **dem** means population, and **-ic** means pertaining to). For example, the worldwide spread of HIV and COVID-19 are pandemics (see Chapter 7).

Types of Diseases

- An **organic disorder** (or-**GAN**-ick) produces symptoms that are detectable physical changes in the body. For example, varicella (chickenpox), characterized by a rash consisting of hundreds of small blisters, is an organic disorder caused by a virus (see Chapter 7).
- A **functional disorder**, also known as a ***non-organic disorder***, produces physical symptoms for which no disease or other organic cause can be identified. Chronic fatigue syndrome is an example of a functional disorder (see Chapter 4).
- An **iatrogenic illness** (eye-**at**-roh-**JEN**-ick) is an unfavorable response due to prescribed medical treatment. For example, severe burns resulting from radiation therapy are iatrogenic. *Iatrogenic* comes from the Greek word for "caused by a healer".
- An **idiopathic disease** (**id**-ee-oh-**PATH**-ick) is any disease without a known cause (**idi/o** means peculiar to the individual, **path** means disease, and **-ic** means pertaining to). ***Idiopathic*** means without a known cause.
- An **infectious disease** (in-**FECK**-shus) is an illness caused by living pathogenic organisms such as bacteria and viruses (see Chapter 7).
- A **nosocomial infection** (**nahs**-oh-**KOH**-mee-al in-**FECK**-shun), also known as a ***hospital-acquired infection*** (HAI), is a disease acquired in a hospital or clinical setting. For example, multidrug-resistant *Staphylococcus aureus* (MRSA) infections are often spread in hospitals (see Chapter 7). *Nosocomial* comes from the Greek word for hospital.

Syndromes

A **syndrome** (**SIN**-drohm) is a set of signs and symptoms that occur together as part of a specific disease process. Some conditions, such as Down syndrome and fetal alcohol syndrome, include this term in their name.

- **Metabolic syndrome** is a common medical condition characterized by risk factors for developing heart disease, stroke, and type 2 diabetes. These factors may include elevated blood pressure, central adiposity (excessive fat in the abdomen), high insulin levels in the blood, and high cholesterol and triglyceride levels.

Congenital Disorders

- A **congenital disorder** (kon-**JEN**-ih-tahl) is an abnormal condition that exists at the time of birth.

Congenital means existing at birth. These conditions can be caused by a developmental disorder before birth, prenatal risk factors, premature birth, or injuries during the birth process.

Developmental Disorders

A **developmental disorder**, also known as a *birth defect*, can result in an anomaly or malformation such as the absence of a limb or the presence of an extra toe. An **anomaly** (ah-**NOM**-ah-lee) is a deviation from what is regarded as normal.

- The term **atresia** (ah-**TREE**-zee-ah) describes the congenital absence or narrowing of a normal body opening or passage. For example, anal atresia is the congenital absence of the opening at the bottom end of the anus; pulmonary atresia is the absence of a pulmonary valve.

Prenatal Risk Factors

Prenatal risk factors include the mother's health, her behavior, and the prenatal medical care she does or does not receive before delivery.

- An example of a problem with the mother's health is a *rubella* infection (see Chapter 7). Birth defects often develop if a pregnant woman contracts this viral infection early in her pregnancy.
- An example of a problem caused by the mother's behavior is **fetal alcohol syndrome** (FAS), which is the result of the mother's consumption of alcohol during the pregnancy (see Chapter 18).
- Examples of problems caused by lack of adequate prenatal medical care are premature delivery or a low birth-weight baby.

Premature Birth and Birth Injuries

- **Premature birth**, which is a birth that occurs earlier than the 37th week of development, can cause serious health problems because the baby's body systems have not had time to form completely.
- **Birth injuries** are disorders that occur as a result of trauma during labor or delivery.

HEALTH CARE PROFESSIONALS

Health care professionals caring for the wellbeing of patients during their lifetime include doctors, nurses, administrative staff, and allied health professionals.

Allied health professions include roles outside of medicine, nursing, and pharmacy. Allied health professionals are an essential part of health care teams, and include dental hygienists, emergency medical technicians (EMTs), medical interpreters, nutritionists, physical therapists, mental health practitioners, phlebotomists, x-ray technicians, and respiratory therapists.

In many medical office or clinic settings, the following health care specialists work as a **primary care specialists** (PCP):

- A **general practitioner** (GP), or *family practice physician*, provides ongoing care for patients of all ages.
- An **internist** is a physician who specializes in diagnosing and treating diseases and disorders of the internal organs and related body systems.
- A **pediatrician** (**pee**-dee-ah-**TRISH**-un) is a physician who specializes in diagnosing, treating, and preventing disorders and diseases of infants and children. This specialty is known as **pediatrics** (**ped** means child, and **-iatrics** means a field of medicine).
- A **geriatrician** (**jer**-ee-ah-**TRISH**-un), or *gerontologist*, is a physician who specializes in the care of older people (Figure 2.11). **Geriatrics** is the branch of medicine relating to the health of older adults (**ger** means old age, and **-iatrics** means field of medicine).
- A **nurse practitioner** (NP) is a nurse with graduate training who often works as a primary care provider.
- A **physician assistant** (PA) is a licensed professional who works under the supervision of a physician. NPs and PAs also work in hospitals and other health care settings and usually have a master's degree.

Other health care professionals in a clinic or medical office setting include:

- A **medical receptionist** schedules and registers patients for appointments and may also work as a medical assistant.
- A **medical assistant** or *clinical medical assistant* performs administrative and clinical tasks in a doctor's office, such as coding patients' medical information, measuring a patient's vital signs, administering injections, and drawing blood. Medical assistants also work in long-term care facilities caring for the elderly.
- A **certified medical assistant** (CMA) is a medical assistant certified through the American Association of Medical Assistants.

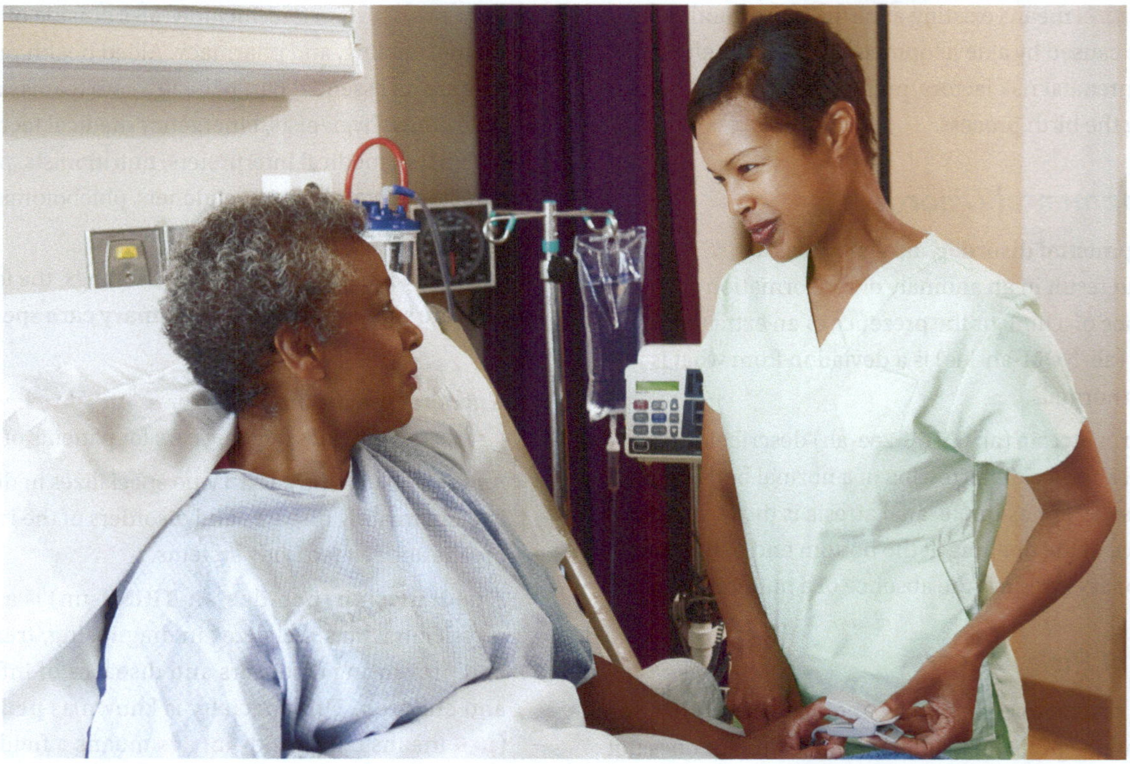

Monkey Business Images/Shutterstock.com

FIGURE 2.11 A CNA taking a pulse oximetry reading.

- A **medical coder** reviews patients' medical records for insurance purposes, assigning codes for treatment and services based on universal alphanumeric codes for medical diagnoses, equipment, and procedures. ***Alphanumeric*** means consisting of both letters and numbers.

In a hospital setting, different departments and specialists care for patients.

- The **emergency room** (ER), also called an ***emergency department***, focuses on diagnosing and treating life-threatening emergency medical conditions. Patients are triaged (see Chapter 1) by nursing staff before receiving additional care. Critically ill patients are treated first.
    - An **emergency physician** is a doctor who specializes in high-acuity medicine in the ER. ***Acuity*** refers to the level of severity of an illness.
    - An **emergency medical technician** (EMT) is a licensed health care professional who works in a pre-hospital setting on an ambulance, or in an emergency room.
- A **registered nurse** (RN) is a licensed health care professional who works in a variety of health care settings. RNs assess patients and provide care following a doctor's orders.
- A **licensed vocational nurse** (LVN), also known as a ***licensed practical nurse*** (LPN) in certain states, works under the supervision of a doctor or an RN to provide basic patient care.
- A **certified nursing assistant** (CNA) works under the supervision of an RN to provide basic patient care.
- A **pharmacist** is a licensed medical professional who dispenses prescribed medication to patients (see Chapter 22).
- The **intensive care unit** (ICU), or ***critical care unit***, provides continuously monitored care for critically ill patients. Some hospitals have specialized ICUs for burn and trauma patients, cardiac patients, or neurological patients.
- An **intensivist** (in-TEN-siv-ist) is a physician specializing in the care of critically ill patients hospitalized in the ICU.
- A **hospitalist** is a physician focusing on the general medical care of hospitalized patients.

- A **telemetry** (teh-**LEM**-eh-tree) unit provides continuous cardiac monitoring for patients with heart problems not requiring intensive care (**tele** means distant, and **-metry** means to measure). The term *telemetry* refers to the electronic transmission of data about the patient's heart rhythm.
- A **medical/surgical** unit (med/surg) provides nursing care for lower-acuity patients who are recovering from surgery or require continued drug therapy or monitoring.

ABBREVIATIONS RELATED TO THE HUMAN BODY IN HEALTH AND DISEASE

Table 2.2 presents an overview of the abbreviations related to the terms introduced in this chapter. *Note:* To avoid errors or confusion, always be cautious when using abbreviations.

TABLE 2.2

Abbreviations Related to the Human Body in Health and Disease

anatomy and physiology = A & P	**A & P** = anatomy and physiology
deoxyribonucleic acid = DNA	**DNA** = deoxyribonucleic acid
general practitioner = GP	**GP** = general practitioner
Huntington's disease = HD	**HD** = Huntington's disease
left lower quadrant = LLQ	**LLQ** = left lower quadrant
left upper quadrant = LUQ	**LUQ** = left upper quadrant
physician assistant = PA	**PA** = physician assistant
right lower quadrant = RLQ	**RLQ** = right lower quadrant
right upper quadrant = RUQ	**RUQ** = right upper quadrant

LEARNING EXERCISES

Matching Word Parts 1

Write the correct answer in the middle column.

	Definition	Correct Answer	Possible Answers
2.1.	fat	______________	**aden/o**
2.2.	front	______________	**adip/o**
2.3.	gland	______________	**anter/o**
2.4.	specialist	______________	**-ologist**
2.5.	study of	______________	**-ology**

Matching Word Parts 2

Write the correct answer in the middle column.

	Definition	Correct Answer	Possible Answers
2.6.	cell	______________	**caud/o**
2.7.	head	______________	**cephal/o**
2.8.	lower part of the body	______________	**cyt/o**
2.9.	out of	______________	**endo-**
2.10.	within	______________	**exo-**

Matching Word Parts 3

Write the correct answer in the middle column.

	Definition	Correct Answer	Possible Answers
2.11.	back	______________	**hist/o**
2.12.	control	______________	**path/o**
2.13.	disease, suffering, emotion	______________	**-plasia**

2.14. formation ______________________ **poster/o**

2.15. tissue ______________________ **-stasis**

Definitions

Select the correct answer, and write it on the line provided.

2.16. A/An ______________________ is acquired in a hospital setting.

iatrogenic illness | idiopathic disease | nosocomial infection | organic disorder

2.17. When a ______________________ is inherited from only one parent, the offspring will have that genetic condition or characteristic.

dominant gene | genome | recessive gene | recessive trait

2.18. The tonsils, spleen, and thymus are part of the ______________________ body system.

immune | endocrine | lymphatic | digestive

2.19. The term ______________________ means the direction toward or nearer the midline.

distal | lateral | medial | proximal

2.20. The primary role of the ______________________ is to maintain and repair in which they are found.

adult stem cells | cord blood | embryonic stem cells | hematopoietic stem cells

2.21. The body system that integrates all body functions is the ______________________ system.

nervous | lymphatic | endocrine | integumentary

2.22. The inflammation of a gland is known as ______________________.

atresia | adenitis | adenoma | adenosis

2.23. The ______________________ tissues support and connect organs and other body tissues.

epithelia | connective | muscle | adipose

2.24. A ______________________ is a fundamental physical and functional unit of heredity.

cell | gamete | gene | genome

2.25. A physician focusing on the general medical care of hospitalized patients is known as a/an

________________________.

intensivist emergency physician hospitalist general practitioner

Matching Regions of the Thorax and Abdomen

Write the correct answer in the middle column.

	Definition	Correct Answer	Possible Answers
2.26.	above the stomach	____________________	epigastric region
2.27.	belly button area	____________________	hypochondriac region
2.28.	below the ribs	____________________	hypogastric region
2.29.	below the stomach	____________________	iliac region
2.30.	hip bone area	____________________	umbilical region

Which Word?

Select the correct answer, and write it on the line provided.

2.31. The term ________________________ refers to the entire lower area of the abdomen.

inguinal umbilicus

2.32. The study of how genes are transferred from parents to their children and the role of genes in health and disease is known as ________________________.

cytology genetics

2.33. A specialist in the study of the outbreaks of disease is a/an ________________________.

epidemiologist pathologist

2.34. A/An ________________________ is the smallest structural level of the human body.

cell organ

2.35. The location of the stomach is ________________________ to the diaphragm.

inferior superior

Spelling Counts

Find the misspelled word in each sentence. Then write that word, spelled correctly, on the line provided.

2.36. The mesantry is a fused double layer of the parietal peritoneum. ____________________

2.37. Hemaphilia is a group of hereditary bleeding disorders in which a blood-clotting factor is missing.

____

2.38. Hypretrophy is a general increase in the bulk of a body part or organ due to an increase in the size, but not in the number, of cells in the tissues. ____________________

2.39. The protective covering for all of the internal and external surfaces of the body is formed by epithealial tissues. ____________________

2.40. An abnomolly is any deviation from what is regarded as normal. ____________________

Abbreviation Identification

Write the correct terms for the abbreviations on the lines provided.

2.41. **HD** ____________________

2.42. **CMA** ____________________

2.43. **GP** ____________________

2.44. **LUQ** ____________________

2.45. **ICU** ____________________

Term Selection

Select the correct answer, and write it on the line provided.

2.46. The term meaning situated nearest the midline or beginning of a body structure is ____________________.

distal lateral medial proximal

2.47. The term meaning situated in the back is ____________________.

anterior superior posterior ventral

2.48. The body is divided into anterior and posterior portions by the ______________________ plane.

frontal horizontal sagittal transverse

2.49. The body is divided into equal vertical left and right halves by the ______________________ plane.

coronal midsagittal sagittal transverse

2.50. Part of the elbow is formed by the ______________________ end of the humerus.

distal lateral medial proximal

Sentence Completion

Write the correct term or terms on the lines provided.

2.51. ______________________ is a genetic variation that is associated with characteristic facial appearance, learning disabilities, and physical abnormalities such as heart valve disease.

2.52. Diseases such as measles, cold, COVID-19, and flu are spread by ______________________ transmission.

2.53. The heart and the lungs are surrounded and protected by the ______________________ cavity.

2.54. An unfavorable response to prescribed medical treatment, such as severe burns resulting from radiation therapy, is known as a/an ______________________ illness.

2.55. The genetic structures located within the nucleus of each cell are known as ______________________. These structures are made up of the DNA molecules containing the body's genes.

Word Surgery

Divide each term into its component word parts. Write these word parts, in sequence, on the lines provided. When necessary use a slash (/) to indicate a combining vowel. (You may not need all of the lines provided.)

2.56. **Embryonic** stem cells are undifferentiated cells that are unlike any specific adult cell.

__________ __________ __________ __________

2.57. Hormones are secreted directly into the bloodstream by the **endocrine** glands.

__________ __________ __________ __________

2.58. A **histologist** is a specialist in the study of the organization of tissues at all levels.

__________ __________ __________ __________

2.59. The term **retroperitoneal** means located behind the peritoneum.

_______ _______ _______ _______

2.60. An **epidemiologist** is a specialist in the study of outbreaks of disease within a population group.

_______ _______ _______ _______

2.61. The study of the causes of diseases is known as **etiology**.

_______ _______ _______ _______

2.62. The term **homeostasis** refers to the processes through which the body maintains a constant internal environment.

_______ _______ _______ _______

2.63. A **pandemic** is an outbreak of a disease occurring over a large geographic area, possibly worldwide.

_______ _______ _______ _______

2.64. The **epigastric** region is located above the stomach.

_______ _______ _______ _______

2.65. An **idiopathic** disease is an illness without known cause.

_______ _______ _______ _______

Clinical Conditions

Write the correct answer on the line provided.

2.66. Mr. Tseng died of cholera during a sudden and widespread outbreak of this disease in his village. Such an outbreak is described as being a/an _______________.

2.67. Brenda Farmer's doctor could not find any physical changes to explain her symptoms. The doctor refers to this as a/an _______________ disorder.

2.68. Gerald Carlson was infected with hepatitis B through _______________ transmission.

2.69. To become a specialist in the study and analysis of cells, Lee Wong signed up for courses in _______________.

2.70. Malaria and West Nile virus are spread by mosquitoes. This is known as _______________ transmission.

2.71. Jose Ortega complained of pain in the lower right area of his abdomen. Using the system that divides the abdomen into four sections, his doctor recorded the pain as being in the lower right ______________.

2.72. Ralph Jenkins was very sick after drinking contaminated water during a camping trip. His doctor says that he contracted the illness through ______________ transmission.

2.73. Tracy Ames has a bladder inflammation. This organ of the urinary system is located in the ______________ cavity.

2.74. Mrs. Reynolds was referred by her GP to a doctor specializing in the ______________ system, which includes the skin, as well as the sebaceous and sweat glands.

2.75. Ashley Goldberg is fascinated by genetics. She wants to specialize in this field and is studying to become a/an ______________.

Which Is the Correct Medical Term?

Select the correct answer, and write it on the line provided.

2.76. Debbie Sanchez fell against a rock and injured her left hip and upper leg. This area is known as the left ______________ region.

hypochondriac   iliac   lumbar   umbilical

2.77. A ______________ is the complete set of genetic information of an organism.

cell   gamete   gene   genome

2.78. An ______________ is a malignant tumor that originates in glandular tissue.

adenocarcinoma   adenitis   adenoma   adenosis

2.79. Nerve cells and blood vessels are surrounded and supported by ______________ connective tissue.

adipose   epithelial   liquid   loose

2.80. A mother's consumption of alcohol during pregnancy can lead to fetal alcohol syndrome, which is a /an ______________ disorder.

developmental   congenital   organic   genetic

Challenge Word Building

These terms are *not* primary terms in the chapter; however, they are made up of the following familiar word parts. If you need help in creating the term, refer to your medical dictionary.

gastr/o	**-algia**
laryng/o	**-ectomy**
my/o	**-itis**
nephr/o	**-osis**
neur/o	**-plasty**

2.81. The term meaning the surgical repair of a muscle is ____________________.

2.82. The term meaning muscle pain is ____________________.

2.83. The term meaning an abnormal condition of the stomach is ____________________.

2.84. The term meaning inflammation of the larynx is ____________________.

2.85. The term meaning the surgical removal of part of a muscle is ____________________.

2.86. The term meaning pain in the stomach is ____________________.

2.87. The term meaning surgical removal of the larynx is ____________________.

2.88. The term meaning an abnormal condition of the kidney is ____________________.

2.89. The medical term meaning surgical repair of a nerve is ____________________.

2.90. The term meaning inflammation of the kidney is ____________________.

Labeling Exercises

Identify the numbered items in the accompanying figures.

2.91. This is the right ______________________________ region.

2.92. This is the ______________________________ region.

2.93. This is the ______________________________ region.

2.94. This is the left ______________________________ region.

2.95. This is the left ______________________________ region.

2.96. This is the ______________________________ plane, which is also known as the midline.

2.97. This is the ______________________________ surface, which is also known as the ventral surface.

2.98. This arrow is pointing in a/an ______________________________ direction.

2.99. This is the ______________________________ surface, which is also known as the dorsal surface.

2.100. This is the ______________________________ plane, which is a horizontal plane.

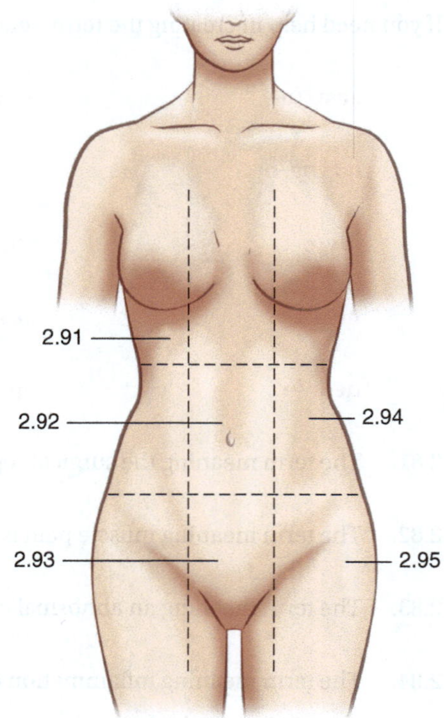

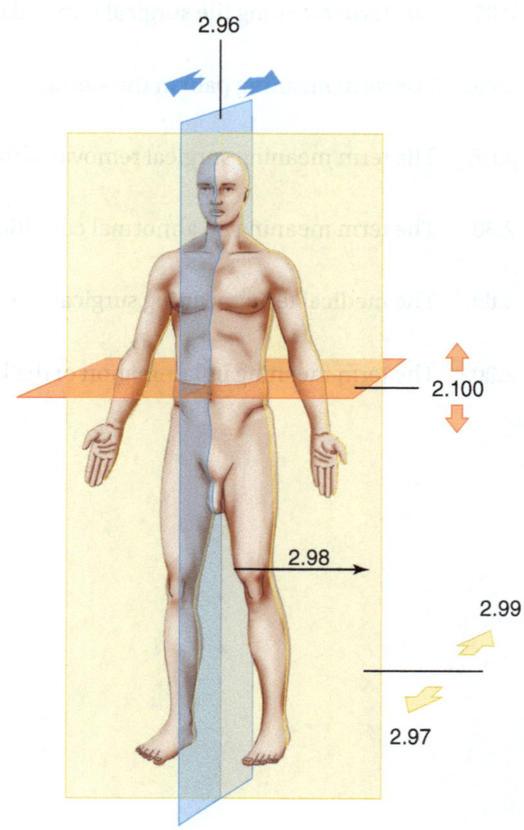

The Human Touch

CRITICAL THINKING EXERCISE

The following story and questions are designed to stimulate critical thinking through class discussion or as a brief essay response. There are no right or wrong answers to these questions.

The sign in the fifth-floor restroom read, "Dirty hands spread disease. Always use soap." Dave rinsed his hands with water, quickly ran his fingers through his hair, and then rushed into the hallway, already late for biology class.

There was an overwhelming smell as he entered the classroom, and he could immediately tell why: On each counter was sitting the day's project, a fetal pig. "Do these things have to stink?" he asked his teacher. "Well, Dave, if they didn't 'stink' of the formaldehyde, they would be rotting and could be spreading diseases. Now let's get started," the teacher said. At the end of class period, they were told, "Be sure to wash your hands thoroughly before leaving this classroom."

This reminded Dave of the lectures they had earlier in the semester about diseases caused by pathogens and how these diseases are spread. As he looked around the classroom, Dave was aware of the other students. Most were gathering up their books to go directly to lunch without washing their hands, Gail and Susan were sharing a bottle of water, Beth was rubbing her eyes, and Jim was coughing without covering his mouth. Suddenly, Dave had a mental image of pathogens everywhere: lying on hands and countertops, floating in the air—and all of these pathogens were looking for someone to infect! Dave shook his head to get rid of the mental image of **E. coli*****, tuberculosis, and COVID-19 lurking all around him. Then he went to the sink and carefully washed his hands again—this time with soap.***

Suggested Discussion Topics

1. Identify and discuss the examples of the potential disease transmission methods that are included in Dave's story, and describe what should have been done to eliminate these risks.
2. Describe how bloodborne, airborne, and food-borne diseases are transmitted, and give an example of each type of transmission.
3. Discuss what might happen in a school if a cafeteria worker has a food-borne disease and after a trip to the lavatory does not wash his or her hands. Instead, the worker goes right back to work without putting on gloves—preparing salads and cutting up fresh fruit for lunch.
4. When treating a bloody wound, the caregiver is required to wear protective gloves. Discuss the possible reasons for this. Is this step taken to protect the patient against diseases on the caregiver's hands? Is this step required to protect the caregiver from a bloodborne disease that the patient might have?

WORD PART REVIEW

The first two chapters introduced you to many word parts. In the next 15 chapters, you will learn about the body systems. You will find that mastering this information is much easier if you have already learned at least some of the word parts you met in the first two chapters.

This special **Word Part Review** is designed to reinforce your knowledge of these word parts and to confirm your mastery of them. To assist you with learning these word parts, this section is divided into two parts:

- The first part is **Word Part Practice**. It consists of 50 questions to provide practice in the use of the word parts you were introduced to in Chapters 1 and 2. It also provides opportunities to work with the use of combining vowels and word parts. If you are not certain of an answer, look it up in Chapters 1 and 2.
- The second part is a **Post-Test**. It includes 50 questions designed to enable you to evaluate your mastery of these word parts. Try to answer these questions without looking up the answers in Chapters 1 and 2.

If you are having problems in this section, ask your instructor for help *now*!

WORD PART PRACTICE SESSION

This is a practice session, and you can go back into Chapters 1 and 2 to find the answers. This is a good idea because it gives you more experience in working with the terms and word parts found in these chapters.

Matching Word Roots and Their Meanings

Enter the correct **word root** in the middle column.

	Definition	Correct Answer	Possible Answers
WP.1.	joint	______________	melan
WP.2.	skull	______________	gastr
WP.3.	red	______________	erythr
WP.4.	stomach	______________	crani
WP.5.	black	______________	arthr

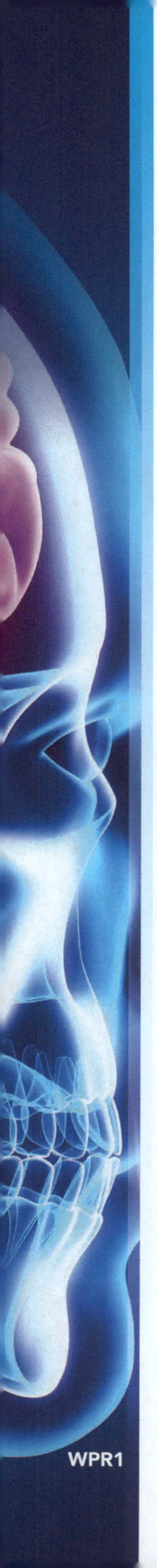

Matching Combining Forms and Their Meanings

Enter the correct **combining forms** in the middle column.

	Definition	Correct Answer	Possible Answers
WP.6.	nose	____________________	**aden/o**
WP.7.	liver	____________________	**cardi/o**
WP.8.	gland	____________________	**hepat/o**
WP.9.	heart	____________________	**ot/o**
WP.10.	ear	____________________	**rhin/o**

Matching Prefixes and Their Meanings

Enter the correct **prefix** in the middle column.

	Definition	Correct Answer	Possible Answers
WP.11.	bad, difficult	____________________	**intra-**
WP.12.	between, among	____________________	**hypo-**
WP.13.	excessive, increased	____________________	**hyper-**
WP.14.	within, inside	____________________	**inter-**
WP.15.	deficient, decreased	____________________	**dys-**

Matching Suffixes and Their Meanings

Enter the correct **suffix** in the middle column.

	Definition	Correct Answer	Possible Answers
WP.16.	abnormal condition	____________________	**-megaly**
WP.17.	bleeding	____________________	**-ologist**
WP.18.	enlargement	____________________	**-osis**
WP.19.	surgical repair	____________________	**-plasty**
WP.20.	specialist	____________________	**-rrhagia**

Matching Suffixes and Their Meanings

Enter the correct **suffix** in the middle column.

	Definition	Correct Answer	Possible Answers
WP.21.	inflammation	________________	**-algia**
WP.22.	pain, suffering	________________	**-centesis**
WP.23.	process of producing a picture or record	________________	**-ectomy**
WP.24.	surgical puncture to remove fluid	________________	**-itis**
WP.25.	surgical removal	________________	**-graphy**

Matching Suffixes and Their Meanings

Enter the correct **suffix** in the middle column.

	Definition	Correct Answer	Possible Answers
WP.26.	abnormal flow, discharge	________________	**-oma**
WP.27.	abnormal narrowing	________________	**-rrhaphy**
WP.28.	tumor	________________	**-rrhea**
WP.29.	control	________________	**-stasis**
WP.30.	to suture	________________	**-stenosis**

Word Building

Write the word you create on the line provided.

WP.31. The term ________________ means the surgical repair of the nose (**rhin/o** means nose).

WP.32. The term ________________ means the surgical removal of a kidney (**nephr/o** means kidney).

WP.33. The term ________________ means inflammation of the ear (**ot/o** means ear).

WP.34. The term __________________ means the study of disorders of the blood (**hemat/o** means blood).

WP.35. The term __________________ means inflammation of the liver (**hepat/o** means liver).

WP.36. The term __________________ means the visual examination of the interior of a joint (**arthr/o** means joint).

WP.37. The term __________________ means an inflammation of the appendix (**appendic** means appendix).

WP.38. The term __________________ means a surgical incision into the colon (**col/o** means colon).

WP.39. The term __________________ means the study of the functions of the structures of the body (**physi** means nature or physical).

WP.40. The term __________________ (ECG) means a record or picture of the electrical activity of the heart (**electr/o** means electric, and **cardi/o** means heart).

True/False

If the word part definition is accurate, write **True** on the line. If the definition is not accurate, write **False** on the line.

WP.41. __________ **myc/o** means mucous.

WP.42. __________ **peri-** means surrounding.

WP.43. __________ **hypo-** means increased.

WP.44. __________ **ather/o** means plaque or fatty substance.

WP.45. __________ **-graphy** means the process of producing a picture or record.

WP.46. __________ **pyel/o** means pus.

WP.47. __________ **-ostomy** means the surgical creation of an artificial opening to the body surface.

WP.48. __________ **hist** means tissue.

WP.49. __________ **-centesis** means to see or a visual examination.

WP.50. __________ **-cyte** means cell.

WORD PART POST-TEST

Answer these questions without looking them up in Chapters 1 and 2. If you have trouble, you should arrange to get extra help or practice more in working with word parts. Write the word part on the line provided.

PT.1. The **suffix** meaning surgical removal is ________________________.

PT.2. The **prefix** meaning under, less, or below is ________________________.

PT.3. The **suffix** meaning surgical repair is ________________________.

PT.4. The **combining form** meaning fungus is ________________________.

PT.5. The **combining form** meaning joint is ________________________.

PT.6. The **combining form** meaning muscle is ________________________.

PT.7. The **prefix** meaning between or among is ________________________.

PT.8. The **combining form** meaning bone marrow or spinal cord is ________________________.

PT.9. The **suffix** meaning a visual examination is ________________________.

PT.10. The **suffix** meaning the study of is ________________________.

Matching Word Parts 1

Matching Suffixes and Prefixes with Their Meanings.

Enter the correct **word part** in the middle column.

Definition	Correct Answer	Possible Answers
PT.11. tumor	________________________	**pre-**
PT.12. surgical suturing	________________________	**-oma**
PT.13. surrounding	________________________	**peri-**
PT.14. visual examination	________________________	**-rrhaphy**
PT.15. before	________________________	**-scopy**

Matching Word Parts 2

Matching Suffixes and Prefixes with Their Meanings.

Enter the correct **word part** in the middle column.

	Definition	Correct Answer	Possible Answers
PT.16.	abnormal hardening	____________	dys-
PT.17.	bad, difficult, painful	____________	-itis
PT.18.	inflammation	____________	-ostomy
PT.19.	surgical creation of an artificial opening	____________	-osis
PT.20.	abnormal condition or disease	____________	-sclerosis

True/False

If the statement is accurate, write **True** on the line. If the statement is not correct, write **False** on the line.

PT.21. ________ The combining form **hem/o** means blood.

PT.22. ________ The suffix **-algia** means pain.

PT.23. ________ The combining form **oste/o** means bone.

PT.24. ________ The prefix **hyper-** means deficient or decreased.

PT.25. ________ The combining form **rhin/o** means nose.

Word Surgery

Use your knowledge of word parts to identify the parts of these terms. Write the word parts, in sequence, on the lines provided. When necessary, use a slash (/) to indicate a combining vowel.

PT.26. The term meaning the surgical repair of a nerve is **neuroplasty**. This word is made up of the word parts

____________________ and ____________________.

PT.27. The term describing any pathological change or disease in the spinal cord is **myelopathy.** This term is made up of the word parts ____________________ and ____________________.

PT.28. The medical condition **pyrosis** is commonly known as heartburn. This term is made up of the word parts ____________ and ____________.

PT.29. The **endocrine** glands produce hormones but do not have ducts. This term is made up of the word parts ____________ and ____________.

PT.30. The term meaning a mature red blood cell is **erythrocyte**. This term is made up of the word parts ____________ and ____________.

Word Building

Write the word you create on the line provided.

Regarding Nerves (neur/o means nerve)

PT.31. A surgical incision into a nerve is a/an ____________.

PT.32. The study of the nervous system is known as ____________.

PT.33. The surgical repair of a nerve or nerves is a/an ____________.

PT.34. The term meaning to suture the ends of a severed nerve is ____________.

PT.35. Abnormal softening of the nerves is called ____________.

PT.36. A specialist in diagnosing and treating disorders of the nervous system is a/an ____________.

PT.37. The term meaning inflammation of a nerve or nerves is ____________.

Relating to Blood Vessels (angi/o means relating to blood vessels)

PT.38. The death of the walls of blood vessels is ____________.

PT.39. The abnormal hardening of the walls of blood vessels is ____________.

PT.40. The abnormal narrowing of a blood vessel is ____________.

PT.41. The surgical removal of a blood vessel is a/an ____________.

PT.42. The process of recording a picture of blood vessels is called ____________.

Missing Words

Write the missing word on the line provided.

PT.43. The surgical repair of an artery is a/an ______________________ (**arteri/o** means artery).

PT.44. The medical term meaning inflammation of the larynx is ______________________ (**laryng/o** means larynx).

PT.45. The surgical removal of all or part of the colon is a/an ______________________ (**col/o** means colon).

PT.46. The abnormal softening of muscle tissue is ______________________ (**my/o** means muscle).

PT.47. The term meaning any abnormal condition of the stomach is ______________________ (**gastr/o** means stomach).

PT.48. The term meaning the study of the heart is ______________________ (**cardi/o** means heart).

PT.49. The term meaning inflammation of the colon is ______________________ (**col/o** means colon).

PT.50. The term meaning a surgical incision into a vein is ______________________ (**phleb/o** means vein).

CHAPTER 3

THE SKELETAL SYSTEM

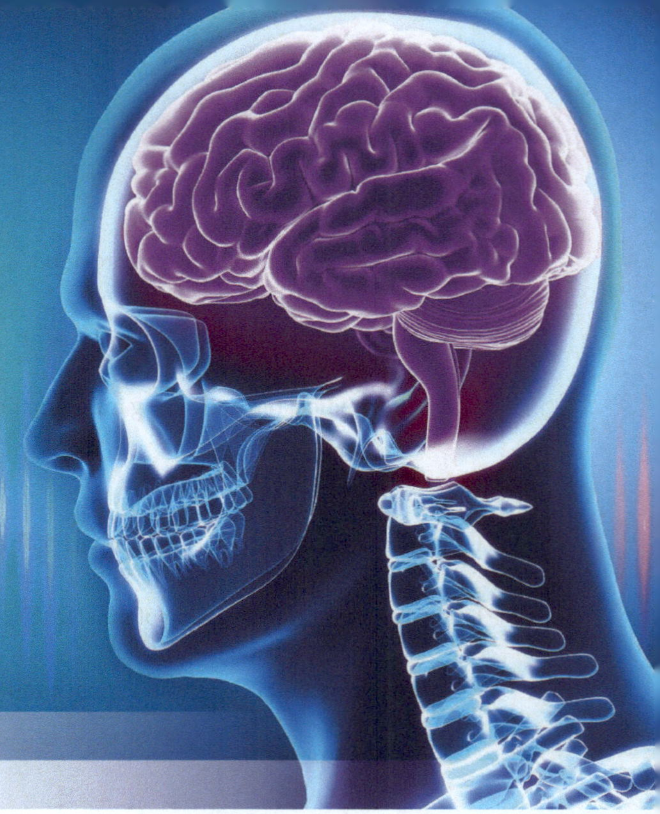

Overview of

STRUCTURES, COMBINING FORMS, AND FUNCTIONS OF THE SKELETAL SYSTEM

Major Structures	Related Combining Forms	Primary Functions
Bones	oss/e, oss/i, oste/o, ost/o	Act as the framework for the body, protect the internal organs, and store calcium.
Bone Marrow	myel/o (also means spinal cord)	Red bone marrow helps form red blood cells. Yellow bone marrow stores fat.
Cartilage	chondr/o	Creates a smooth surface for motion within the joints and protects the ends of the bones.
Joints	arthr/o	Work with the muscles to make a variety of motions possible.
Ligaments	ligament/o	Connect one bone to another.
Synovial Membrane	synovi/o, synov/o	Forms the lining of synovial joints and secretes synovial fluid.
Synovial Fluid	synovi/o, synov/o	Lubricant that makes smooth joint movements possible.
Bursa	burs/o	Cushions areas subject to friction during movement.

Vocabulary Related to **THE SKELETAL SYSTEM**

This list contains essential word parts and medical terms for this chapter. These and the other important **primary terms** are shown in **boldface** throughout the chapter. *Secondary terms*, which appear in *orange* italics, clarify the meaning of primary terms.

Word Parts

- ☐ **ankyl/o** crooked, bent, stiff
- ☐ **arthr/o** joint
- ☐ **burs/o** bursa
- ☐ **chondr/i**, **chondr/o** cartilage
- ☐ **cost/o** rib
- ☐ **crani/o** skull
- ☐ **-desis** to bind, tie together
- ☐ **kyph/o** bent, hump
- ☐ **lord/o** curve, swayback, bent
- ☐ **lumb/o** lumbar, lower back
- ☐ **myel/o** spinal cord, bone marrow
- ☐ **oss/e**, **oss/i**, **ost/o**, **oste/o** bone
- ☐ **scoli/o** curved, bent
- ☐ **spondyl/o** vertebrae, vertebral column, backbone
- ☐ **synovi/o**, **synov/o** synovial membrane, synovial fluid

Medical Terms

- ☐ **acetabulum** (**ass**-eh-**TAB**-you-lum)
- ☐ **allogeneic** (**al**-loh-jen-**EEH**-ick)
- ☐ **ankylosing spondylitis** (**ang**-kih-**LOH**-sing **spon**-dih-**LYE**-tis)
- ☐ **arthrodesis** (**ar**-throh-**DEE**-sis)
- ☐ **arthroscopy** (ar-**THROS**-koh-pee)
- ☐ **autologous** (aw-**TOL**-uh-guss)
- ☐ **avascular necrosis** (ay-**VAS**-cue-ler neh-**KROH**-sis)
- ☐ **callus** (**KAL**-us)
- ☐ **chondromalacia** (**kon**-droh-mah-**LAY**-shee-ah)
- ☐ **comminuted fracture** (**KOM**-ih-**newt**-ed)
- ☐ **compression fracture**
- ☐ **costochondritis** (**kos**-toh-kon-**DRIGH**-tis)
- ☐ **crepitation** (**krep**-ih-**TAY**-shun)
- ☐ **dual x-ray absorptiometry** (ab-**sorp**-shee-**OM**-eh-tree)
- ☐ **fat embolus** (**EM**-boh-lus)
- ☐ **gout** (**GOWT**)
- ☐ **hallux valgus** (**HAL**-ucks **VAL**-guss)
- ☐ **hemarthrosis** (**hem**-ar-**THROH**-sis)
- ☐ **hematopoietic** (**hee**-**MAH**-toh-poy-**et**-ick)
- ☐ **internal fixation**
- ☐ **juvenile idiodiopathic arthritis** (**id**-ee-oh-**PATH**-ick ar-**THRIGH**-tis)
- ☐ **kyphosis** (kye-**FOH**-sis)
- ☐ **laminectomy** (**lam**-ih-**NECK**-toh-mee)
- ☐ **lordosis** (lor-**DOH**-sis)
- ☐ **lumbago** (lum-**BAY**-goh)
- ☐ **malleolus** (mah-**LEE**-oh-lus)
- ☐ **manubrium** (mah-**NEW**-bree-um)
- ☐ **metacarpals** (met-ah-**KAR**-palz)
- ☐ **metatarsals** (met-ah-**TAHR**-salz)
- ☐ **multiple myeloma** (**my**-eh-**LOH**-mah)
- ☐ **open fracture**
- ☐ **orthopedic surgeon** (**or**-thoh-**PEE**-dick)
- ☐ **orthotic** (or-**THOT**-ick)
- ☐ **osteitis** (**oss**-tee-**EYE**-tis)
- ☐ **osteoarthritis** (**oss**-tee-oh-ar-**THRIGH**-tis)
- ☐ **osteochondroma** (**oss**-tee-oh-kon-**DROH**-mah)
- ☐ **osteomalacia** (**oss**-tee-oh-mah-**LAY**-shee-ah)
- ☐ **osteomyelitis** (**oss**-tee-oh-**my**-eh-**LYE**-tis)
- ☐ **osteopenia** (**oss**-tee-oh-**PEE**-nee-ah)
- ☐ **osteoporosis** (**oss**-tee-oh-poh-**ROH**-sis)
- ☐ **osteoporotic hip fracture** (**oss**-tee-oh-pah-**ROT**-ick)
- ☐ **Paget's disease** (**PAJ**-its)
- ☐ **pathologic fracture**
- ☐ **percutaneous vertebroplasty** (**per**-kyou-**TAY**-nee-us **VER**-tee-broh-**plas**-tee)
- ☐ **podiatrist** (poh-**DYE**-ah-trist)
- ☐ **polymyalgia rheumatica** (**pol**-ee-my-**AL**-jee-ah roo-**MA**-tih-kah)
- ☐ **prosthesis** (pros-**THEE**-sis)
- ☐ **radiculopathy** (rah-**dick**-you-**LOH**-path-ee)
- ☐ **rheumatoid arthritis** (**ROO**-mah-toyd ar-**THRIGH**-tis)
- ☐ **rickets** (**RICK**-ets)
- ☐ **scoliosis** (**skoh**-lee-**OH**-sis)
- ☐ **spina bifida** (**SPY**-nah **BIF**-ih-dah)
- ☐ **spinal stenosis** (steh-**NOH**-sis)
- ☐ **spiral fracture**
- ☐ **spondylolisthesis** (**spon**-dih-loh-liss-**THEE**-sis)
- ☐ **spondylosis** (**spon**-dih-**LOH**-sis)
- ☐ **stem cell transplant**
- ☐ **subluxation** (**sub**-luck-**SAY**-shun)
- ☐ **synovectomy** (sin-oh-**VECK**-toh-mee)
- ☐ **vertebrae** (**VER**-teh-bray)

LEARNING OBJECTIVES

On completion of this chapter, you should be able to:

1. Identify the major functions and structures of the skeletal system.
2. Describe three types of joints.
3. Differentiate between the axial and appendicular skeletons.
4. Identify the major bones in the body.
5. Identify the medical specialists who treat disorders of the skeletal system.
6. Identify medical word parts of the skeletal system.
7. Define the primary terms related to the pathology and the diagnostic and treatment procedures of the skeletal system.
8. Spell the primary terms related to the skeletal system.
9. Pronounce the primary terms related to the skeletal system.
10. Identify common abbreviations related to the skeletal system.

STRUCTURES AND FUNCTIONS OF THE SKELETAL SYSTEM

The skeletal system consists of the bones, bone marrow, cartilage, joints, ligaments, synovial membranes, synovial fluid, and bursae. This body system has many important functions:

- Bones act as the framework of the body.
- Bones support and protect the internal organs.
- Joints work in conjunction with muscles, ligaments, and tendons, making possible the wide variety of body movements. (Muscles and tendons are discussed in Chapter 4.)
- Calcium, a mineral required for normal nerve and muscle function, is stored in bones.
- Red bone marrow, which plays an important role in the formation of blood cells, is located within spongy bone.

The Formation of Bones

A newborn's skeleton begins as fragile membranes and cartilage, but after three months it starts turning into bone in a process called **ossification** (**oss**-uh-fih-**KAY**-shun), which continues through adolescence.

Even after growth is completed, this process of new bone formation continues as *osteoclast* cells break down old or damaged bone and *osteoblast* cells help rebuild the bone. Ossification repairs the minor damage to the skeletal system that occurs during normal activity and also repairs bones after injuries such as fractures.

THE STRUCTURE OF BONES

Bone is the form of connective tissue that is the second hardest tissue in the human body. Only dental enamel is harder than bone.

The Tissues of Bone

Although it is a dense and rigid tissue, bone is also capable of growth, healing, and reshaping itself (Figure 3.1).

- **Periosteum** (**pehr**-ee-**OSS**-tee-um) is the tough, fibrous tissue that forms the outermost covering of bone (**peri-** means surrounding, **oste** means bone, and **-um** is a noun ending).
- **Compact bone**, also known as ***cortical bone***, is the dense, hard, and very strong bone that forms the protective outer layer of bones. When measured by weight, compact bone accounts for more than 75% of the body's bone matter.
- **Spongy bone**, also known as ***cancellous bone***, is porous ("sponge-like"), which makes it lighter and weaker than compact bone.
  - Red bone marrow is often located within this spongy bone, which is commonly found in the ends and inner portions of long bones as well as in the pelvic bones, the ribs, and the vertebrae of the spinal column.
  - The major bones of the arms and legs, including the femur and humerus, are examples of *long bones*.

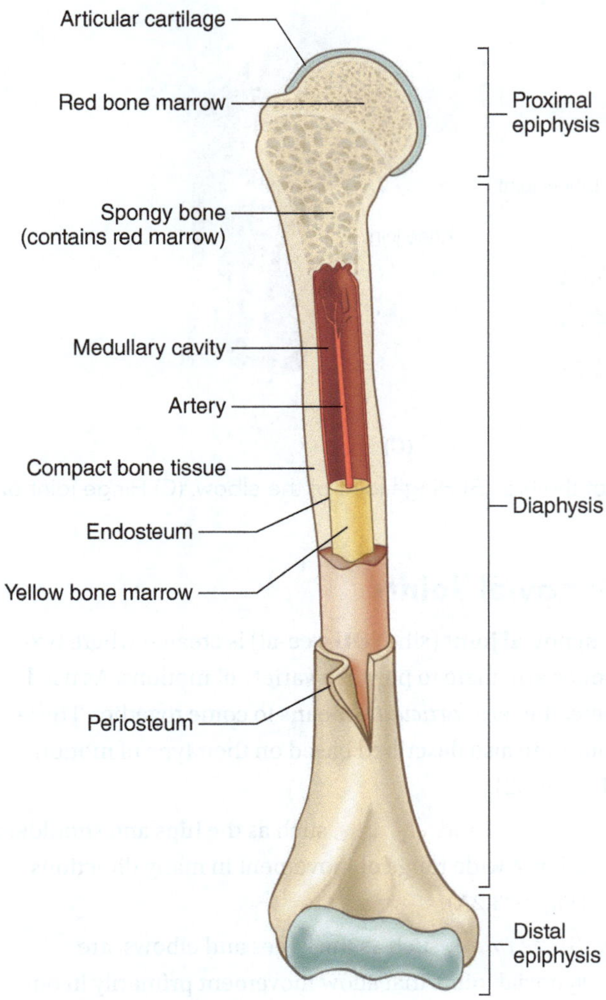

FIGURE 3.1 Anatomic features of a typical long bone.

- *Short bones* include the bones of the wrist and ankle. They are roughly cube-shaped, and are made up of spongy bone covered with a layer of compact bone.
- Bones with a large percentage of spongy bone are weaker and more susceptible to fractures.

- The **medullary cavity** (**MED**-you-**lehr**-ee) is the central cavity located in the shaft of long bones, where it is surrounded by compact bone. It is here that red and yellow bone marrow are stored. *Medullary* means pertaining to the inner section.
- The **endosteum** (en-**DOS**-tee-um) is the tissue that lines the medullary cavity (**end-** means within, **oste** means bone, and **-um** is a noun ending).

Bone Marrow

- *Red bone marrow*, which is located within the spongy bone, is a hematopoietic tissue that manufactures red blood cells, hemoglobin, white blood cells, and thrombocytes. These types of cells are discussed in Chapter 6.
- **Hematopoietic** (**hee-MAH**-toh-poy-**et**-ick) means pertaining to the formation of blood cells (**hemat/o** means blood, and **-poietic** means pertaining to formation). This term is also spelled *hemopoietic*.
- *Yellow bone marrow* functions as a fat storage area. It is composed chiefly of fat cells and is located in the medullary cavity of long bones. Most bone marrow is red from birth through early adolescence, after which about half of it is gradually replaced by yellow bone marrow.

Cartilage

- **Cartilage** (**KAR**-tih-lidj) is the smooth, rubbery, blue-white connective tissue that acts as a shock absorber between bones. Cartilage, which is more elastic than bone, also makes up the flexible parts of the skeleton such as the outer ear and the tip of the nose.
- **Articular cartilage** (ar-**TICK**-you-lar **KAR**-tih-lidj) covers the surfaces of bones where they *articulate*, or come together, to form joints. This cartilage makes smooth joint movement possible and protects the bones from rubbing against each other (Figures 3.1 and 3.3).
- The **meniscus** (meh-**NIS**-kus) is the curved, fibrous cartilage found in some joints, such as the knee and the temporomandibular joint of the jaw (Figure 3.3).

Anatomic Landmarks of Bones

- The **diaphysis** (dye-**AF**-ih-sis) is the shaft of a long bone (Figure 3.1).
- The **epiphyses** (ep-**PIF**-ih-seez) are the wider ends of long bones such as the femurs of the legs (singular *epiphysis*). Each epiphysis is covered with articular cartilage to protect it. The *proximal epiphysis* is the end of the bone located nearest to the midline of the body. The *distal epiphysis* is the end of the bone located farthest away from the midline of the body.
- A **foramen** (foh-**RAY**-men) is an opening in a bone through which blood vessels, nerves, and ligaments pass (plural, *foramina*). For example, the spinal cord passes through the *foramen magnum* of the occipital bone at the base of the skull.
- A **process** is a normal projection on the surface of a bone that most commonly serves as an attachment for a muscle or tendon. For example, the *mastoid process* is the bony projection located on the temporal bones just behind the ears (Figure 3.6).

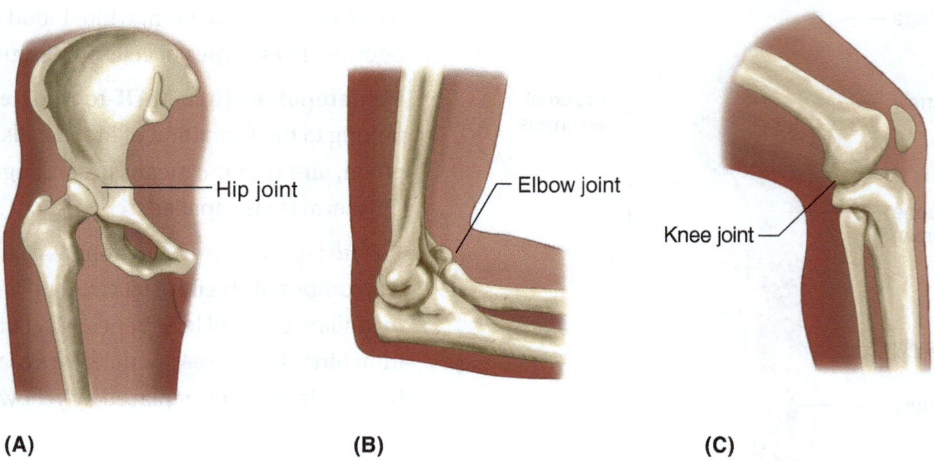

FIGURE 3.2 Examples of *synovial joints.* (A) Ball-and-socket joint of the hip. (B) Hinge joint of the elbow. (C) Hinge joint of the knee.

JOINTS

Joints, which are also known as ***articulations***, are the place of union between two or more bones. There are three main types of joints: fibrous, cartilaginous, and synovial. Joints are classified either according to their construction or based on the degree of movement they allow.

Fibrous Joints

Fibrous joints, consisting of inflexible layers of dense connective tissue, hold the bones tightly together. In adults these joints, which are also known as ***sutures***, allow little or no movement. In newborns and very young children, some fibrous joints are movable before they have solidified.

- The **fontanelles** (**fon**-tah-**NELLS**), also known as the ***soft spots***, are normally present on the skull of a newborn. These flexible soft spots facilitate the passage of the infant through the birth canal. They also allow for the growth of the skull during the first year. As the child matures, and the sutures close, the fontanelles gradually harden.

Cartilaginous Joints

Cartilaginous joints (**kar**-tih-**LADJ**-ih-nus) allow only slight movement and consist of bones connected entirely by cartilage. For example:

- Where the ribs connect to the sternum (breast bone), shown in Figure 3.8, these joints allow movement during breathing.
- The **pubic symphysis** (**PEW**-bick **SIM**-fih-sis) allows some movement to facilitate childbirth. This joint is located between the pubic bones in the anterior (front) of the pelvis as shown in Figure 3.12.

Synovial Joints

A **synovial joint** (sih-**NOH**-vee-al) is created where two bones articulate to permit a variety of motions. As used here, the term *articulate* means to come together. These joints are also described based on their type of motion (Figure 3.2).

- ***Ball-and-socket joints***, such as the hips and shoulders, allow a wide range of movement in many directions (Figure 3.2A).
- ***Hinge joints***, such as the knees and elbows, are synovial joints that allow movement primarily in one direction or plane (Figures 3.2B and 3.2C).

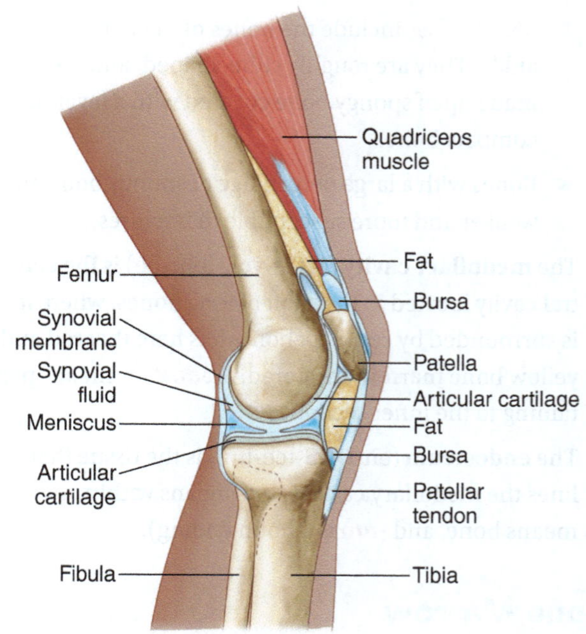

FIGURE 3.3 A lateral view of the knee showing the structures of a *synovial joint* and *bursa*.

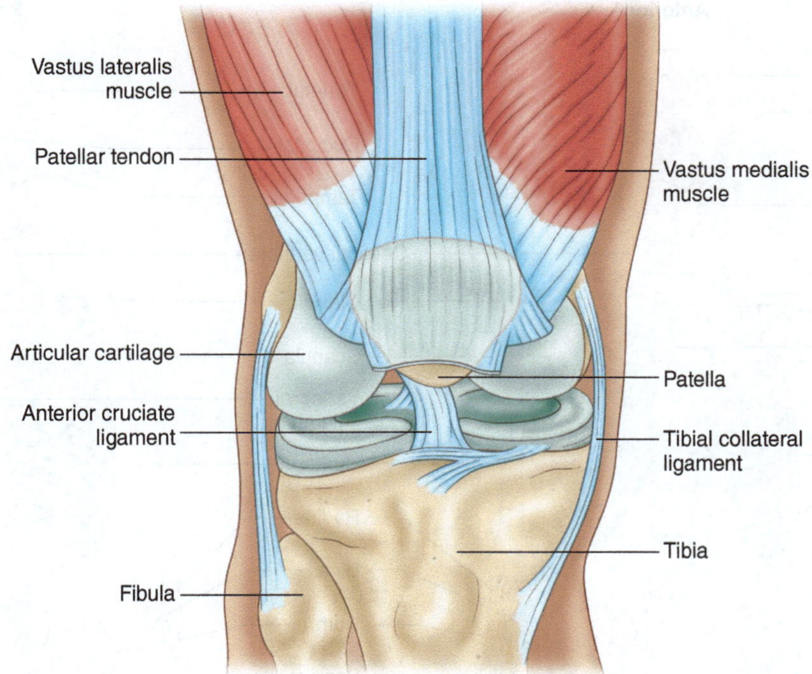

FIGURE 3.4 Major ligaments of the knee. This anterior view of the knee shows the complex system of ligaments that make its movements possible.

Components of Synovial Joints

Synovial joints consist of several components that make complex movements possible (Figure 3.3).

- The **synovial capsule** is the outermost layer of strong fibrous tissue that resembles a sleeve as it surrounds the joint.
- The **synovial membrane** lines the capsule and secretes synovial fluid.
- **Synovial fluid**, which flows within the synovial cavity, acts as a lubricant to make the smooth movement of the joint possible.
- **Ligaments** (**LIG**-ah-mentz) are bands of fibrous tissue that form joints by connecting one bone to another bone or by joining a bone to cartilage. Complex hinge joints, such as the knee shown in Figures 3.3 and 3.4, are made up of a series of ligaments that permit movement in different directions.
- A **bursa** (**BER**-sah) is a fibrous sac that acts as a cushion to ease movement in areas that are subject to friction, such as in the shoulder, elbow, and knee joints where a tendon passes over a bone (plural, *bursae*).

THE SKELETON

The typical adult human skeleton consists of approximately 206 bones, as shown in Figure 3.5. Depending upon the age of the individual, the exact number of bones ranges from 206 to 350. For descriptive purposes, the skeleton is divided into the axial and appendicular skeletal systems.

Axial Skeleton

The **axial skeleton** protects the major organs of the nervous, respiratory, and circulatory systems. In the human, the axial skeleton consists of the 80 bones of the head and body that are organized into five parts. These are (1) the bones of the skull; (2) the ossicles (bones) of the middle ear; (3) the hyoid bone, located on the throat between the chin and the thyroid; (4) the rib cage; and (5) the vertebral column.

Appendicular Skeleton

The **appendicular skeleton** makes body movement possible and also protects the organs of digestion, excretion, and reproduction. In the human, the appendicular skeleton consists of 126 bones that are organized into (1) the ***upper extremities*** (shoulders, arms, forearms, wrists, and hands) and (2) the ***lower extremities*** (hips, thighs, legs, ankles, and feet).

An ***appendage*** is anything that is attached to a major part of the body and the term ***appendicular*** means referring to an appendage. An ***extremity*** is the terminal end of a body part such as an arm or leg.

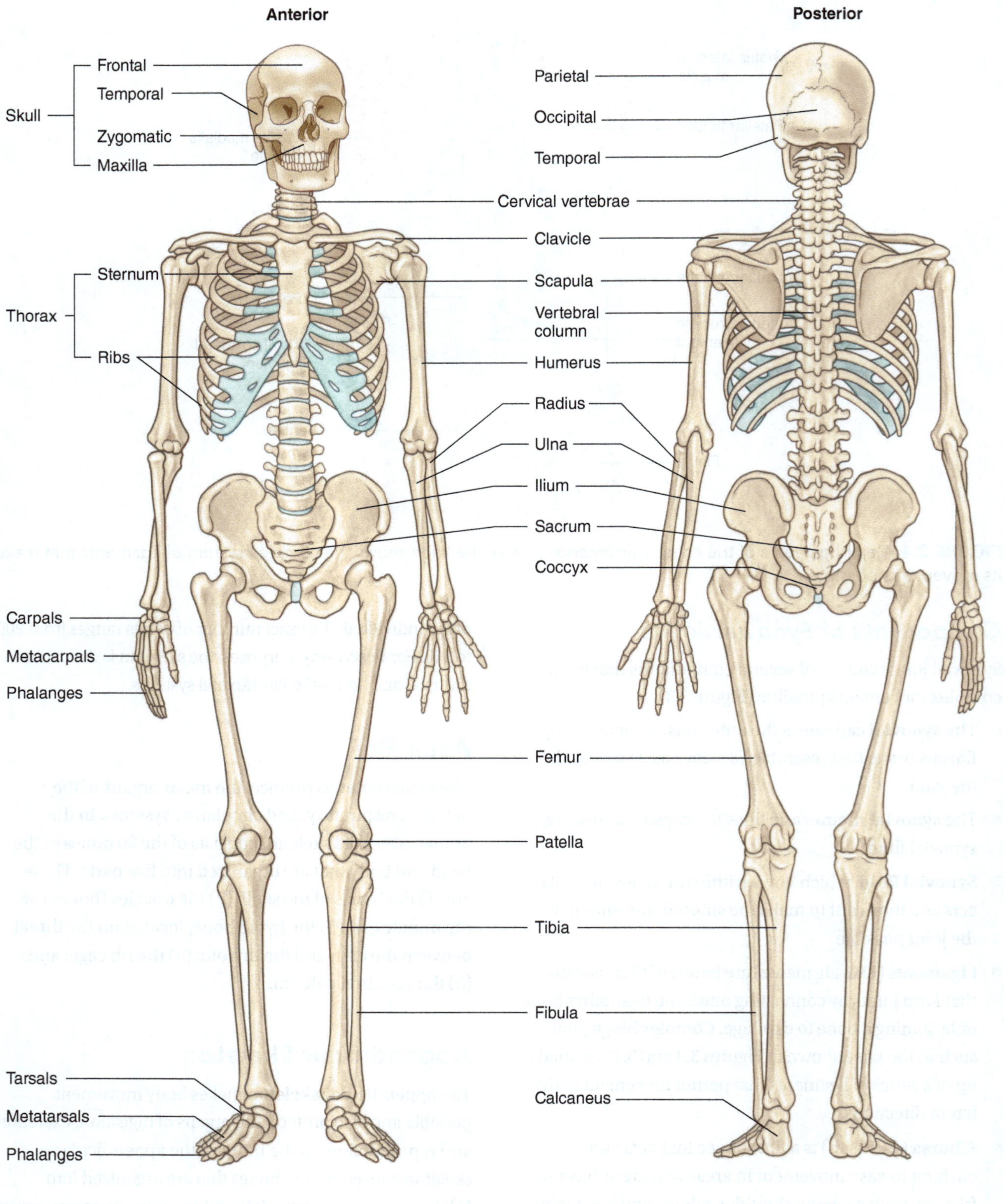

FIGURE 3.5 Anterior and posterior views of the human skeleton.

Bones of the Skull

The **skull** consists of the 8 bones that form the cranium, 14 bones that form the face, and 6 bones in the middle ear. As you study the following bones of the skull, refer to Figures 3.6 and 3.7.

The Bones of the Cranium

The **cranium** (**KRAY**-nee-um), which is made up of the following eight bones, is the portion of the skull that encloses and protects the brain (**crani** means skull, and **-um** is a noun ending). The cranial bones are joined

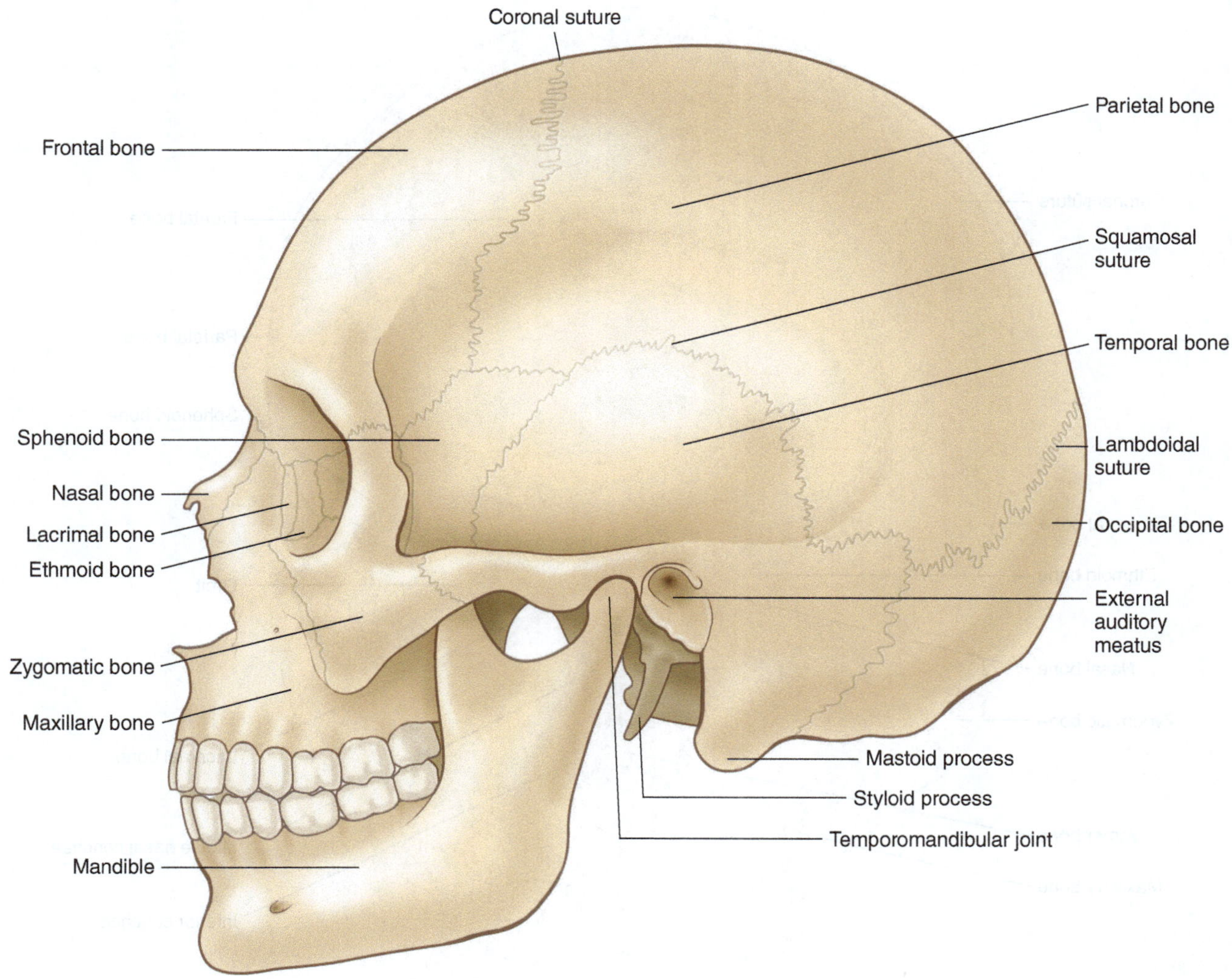

FIGURE 3.6 Lateral view of the adult human skull.

by jagged fibrous joints that are often referred to as sutures.

- The **frontal bone** is the anterior portion of the cranium that forms the forehead. This bone houses the frontal sinuses and forms the roof of the ethmoid sinuses, the nose and part of the socket that protects the eyeball.
- The **parietal bones** (pah-**RYE**-eh-tal) are two of the largest bones of the skull. Together they form most of the roof and upper sides of the cranium.
- The **occipital bone** (ock-**SIP**-ih-tal) forms the back part of the skull and the base of the cranium.
- The two **temporal bones** form the sides and base of the cranium.
- The **external auditory meatus** (mee-**AY**-tus) is the opening of the external auditory canal of the outer ear. This canal is located within the temporal bone on each side of the skull. A *meatus* is the external opening of a canal.
- The **sphenoid bone** (**SFEE**-noid) is an irregular, wedge-shaped bone at the base of the skull. This bone makes contact with all of the other cranial bones and helps form the base of the cranium, the sides of the skull, and the floors and sides of the eye sockets.
- The **ethmoid bone** (**ETH**-moid) is light, spongy bone located at the roof and sides of the nose. Here it separates the nasal cavity from the brain, and it also forms a portion of each orbit. An *orbit* is the bony socket that surrounds and protects each eyeball.

The Auditory Ossicles

The **auditory ossicles** (**OSS**-ih-kulz) are the three tiny bones located in each middle ear. These bones, known as the *malleus*, *incus*, and *stapes*, are discussed in Chapter 13.

The Bones of the Face

- The face is made up of the following 14 bones. Some of these bones contain air-filled cavities known as sinuses. Among the purposes of these sinuses is to lighten the weight of the skull. These sinuses are discussed in Chapter 8.

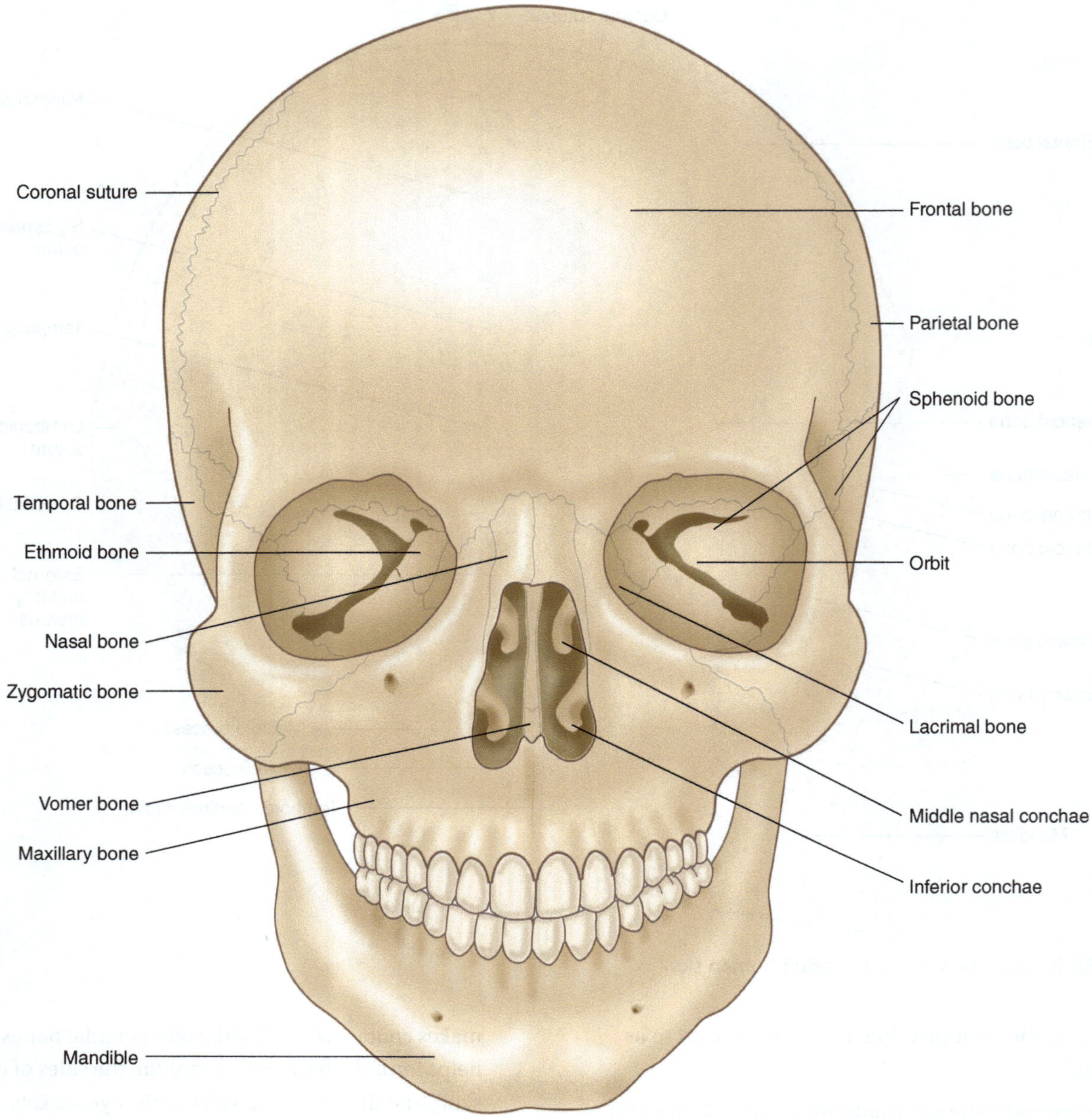

FIGURE 3.7 Anterior view of the adult human skull.

- The two **nasal bones** form the upper part of the bridge of the nose.
- The two **zygomatic bones** (**zye**-goh-**MAT**-ick), also known as the *cheekbones*, articulate with the frontal bone that makes up the forehead.
- The two **maxillary bones** (**MACK**-sih-**ler**-ee) form most of the upper jaw (singular, *maxilla*). These bones are also known as the *maxillae*.
- The two **palatine bones** (**PAL**-ah-tine) form the anterior (front) part of the hard palate of the mouth and the floor of the nose.
- The two **lacrimal bones** (**LACK**-rih-mal) make up part of the orbit (socket of the eye) at the inner angle.
- The two **inferior conchae** (**KONG**-kee *or* **KONG**-kay) are the thin, scroll-like bones that form part of the interior of the nose (singular, *concha*).
- The **vomer bone** (**VOH**-mer) forms the base for the nasal septum. The *nasal septum* is the cartilage wall that divides the two nasal cavities.
- The **mandible** (**MAN**-dih-bul), also known as the *jawbone*, is the only movable bone of the skull. The mandible is attached to the skull at the **temporomandibular joint** (**tem**-poh-roh-man-**DIB**-you-lar), which is commonly known by its abbreviation, *TMJ* (Figure 3.6).

Thoracic Cavity

The **thoracic cavity** (thoh-**RAS**-ick), also known as the ***rib cage***, is the bony structure that protects the heart and lungs. It consists of the ribs, sternum, and upper portion of the spinal column extending from the neck to the diaphragm, but not including the arms.

The Ribs

The 12 pairs of **ribs**, which are also known as ***costals***, attach posteriorly to the thoracic vertebrae (**cost** means rib, and **-al** means pertaining to) (Figure 3.8).

- The first seven pairs of ribs are called ***true ribs***, and they attach anteriorly to the sternum.
- The next three pairs of ribs are called ***false ribs***, and they attach anteriorly to cartilage that connects them to the sternum.
- The last two pairs of ribs are called ***floating ribs***, because they are only attached posteriorly to the vertebrae but are not attached anteriorly.

The Sternum

The **sternum** (**STER**-num), which is also known as the ***breast bone***, is a flat, dagger-shaped bone located in the middle of the chest. By joining with the ribs, it forms the front of the rib cage. This is divided into three parts (Figure 3.8).

- The **manubrium** (mah-**NEW**-bree-um) is the bony structure that forms the upper portion of the sternum.
- The **body of the sternum**, also known as the ***gladiolus***, is the bony structure that forms the middle portion of the sternum.
- The **xiphoid process** (**ZIF**-oid) is the structure made of cartilage that forms the lower portion of the sternum. *Xiphoid* comes from the Greek word for a straight sword.

The Shoulders

The shoulders form the **pectoral girdle** (**PECK**-toh-rahl), which supports the arms and hands. This is also known as the ***shoulder girdle***. As used here, the term *girdle* refers to a structure that encircles the body. As you study the bones of the shoulder, refer to Figures 3.5 and 3.8.

- The **clavicle** (**KLAV**-ih-kul), also known as the ***collarbone***, is a slender bone that connects the manubrium of the sternum to the scapula.
- The **scapula** (**SKAP**-you-lah) is also known as the ***shoulder blade*** (plural, *scapulae*).
- The **acromion** (ah-**KROH**-mee-on) is an extension of the scapula that forms the high point of the shoulder.

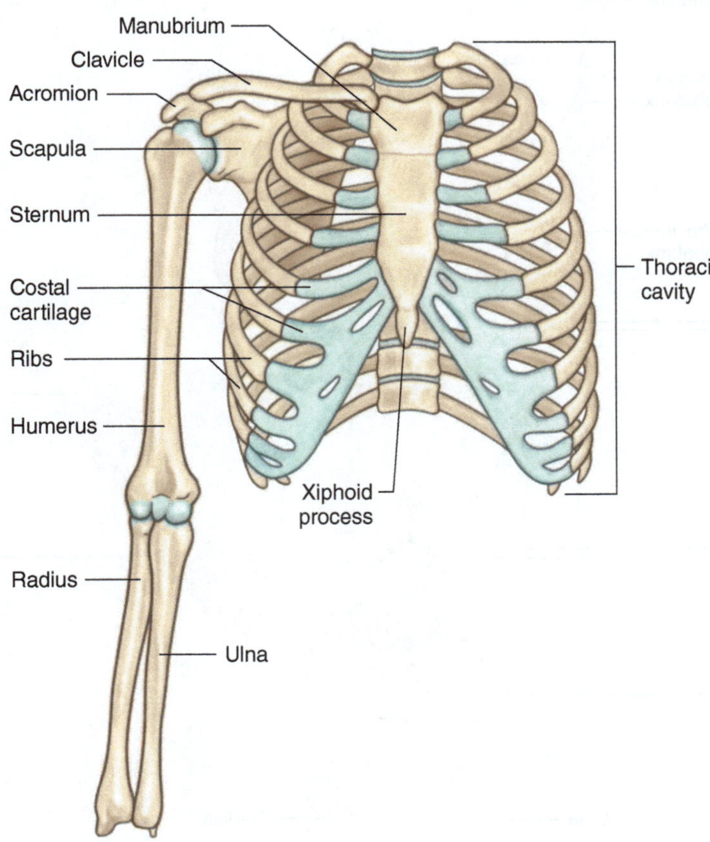

FIGURE 3.8 Anterior view of the ribs, shoulder, and arm. (Cartilaginous structures are shown in blue.)

The Arms

- As you study the bones of the arms, refer to Figures 3.5 and 3.8.
- The **humerus** (**HEW**-mer-us) is the bone of the upper arm (plural, *humeri*).
- The **radius** (**RAY**-dee-us) is the smaller and shorter bone in the forearm. The radius runs up the thumb side of the forearm (plural, *radii*).
- The **ulna** (**ULL**-nah) is the larger and longer bone of the forearm (plural, *ulnae*). The proximal end of the ulna articulates with the distal end of the humerus to form the elbow joint.
- The **olecranon** (oh-**LEK**-rah-non), commonly known as the *funny bone*, is the large, proximal tip of the ulna. This forms the point of the elbow and exposes a nerve that tingles when struck.

The Wrists, Hands, and Fingers

As you study these bones, refer to Figure 3.9.

- The eight **carpals** (**KAR**-palz) are the bones that form the wrist (singular, *carpal*). These bones form a narrow bony passage known as the *carpal tunnel*. The median nerve and the tendons of the fingers pass through this tunnel to reach the hand. *Carpal tunnel syndrome* is described in Chapter 4.
- The **metacarpals** (met-ah-**KAR**-palz) are the five bones that form the palms of the hand.
- The **phalanges** (fah-**LAN**-jeez) are the 14 bones of the fingers (singular, *phalanx*). The bones of the toes are also known as phalanges.
- Each of the four fingers has three bones. These are the distal (outermost), middle, and proximal (nearest the hand) phalanges.
- The thumb has two bones. These are the distal and proximal phalanges.

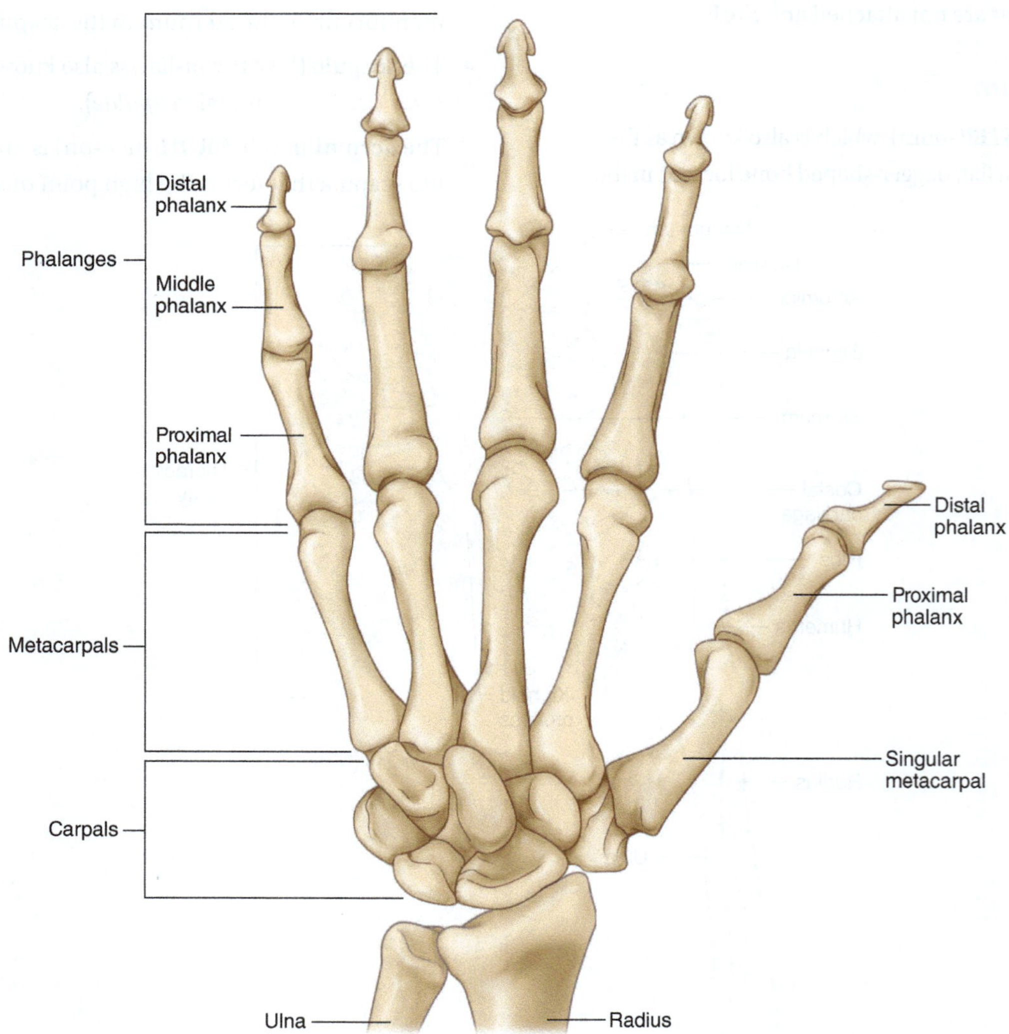

FIGURE 3.9 Superior view of the bones of the lower left arm, wrist, and hand.

The Spinal Column

The **spinal column**, which is also known as the ***vertebral column***, protects the spinal cord and supports the head and body. The spinal column consists of 26 **vertebrae** (**VER**-teh-bray). Each of these bony units is known as a **vertebra** (**VER**-teh-bruh), and the term ***vertebral*** means pertaining to the vertebrae.

The Structures of Vertebrae

As you study the structures of a vertebra, refer to Figure 3.10.

- The anterior portion of the vertebra is solid to provide strength and is known as the ***body of the vertebra***.
- The posterior portion of a vertebra is known as the **lamina** (**LAM**-ih-nah) (plural, *laminae*). The transverse and spinous processes extend from this area and serve as attachments for muscles and tendons.
- The ***vertebral foramen*** is the opening in the middle of the vertebra. This opening allows the spinal cord to pass through and to protect the spinal cord.

Intervertebral Disks

Intervertebral disks (**in**-ter-**VER**-teh-bral), which are made of cartilage and pads of tissue, separate and cushion the vertebrae from each other and allow for movement of the spinal column. Their inner core is the ***nucleus pulposus***, which is made up of a soft, gelatinous material that allows the intervertebral disks to act as shock absorbers (Figure 3.18A).

The Types of Vertebrae

As you study the types of vertebrae, refer to Figures 3.11A and 3.11B.

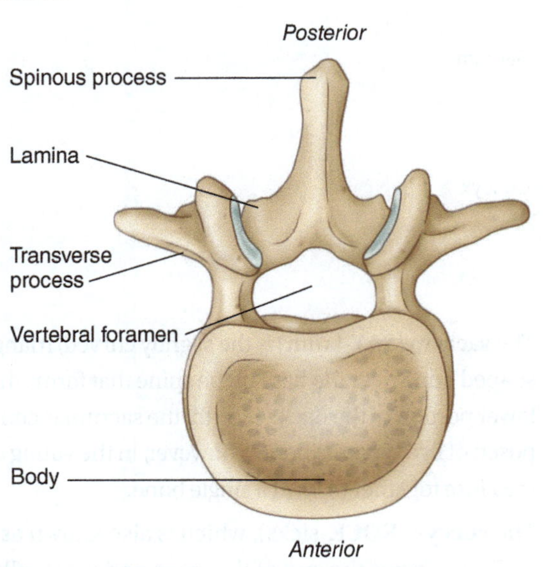

FIGURE 3.10 Characteristics of a typical vertebra.

- The **cervical vertebrae** (**SER**-vih-kal) are the first set of seven vertebrae, and they form the neck. The term ***cervical*** means pertaining to the neck, and these vertebrae are also known as **C1–C7**.
- The **thoracic vertebrae** (thoh-**RASS**-ick), known as **T1–T12**, are the second set of 12 vertebrae. Each of these vertebrae has a pair of ribs attached to it, and together they form the outward curve of the spine. ***Thoracic*** means pertaining to the thoracic cavity.

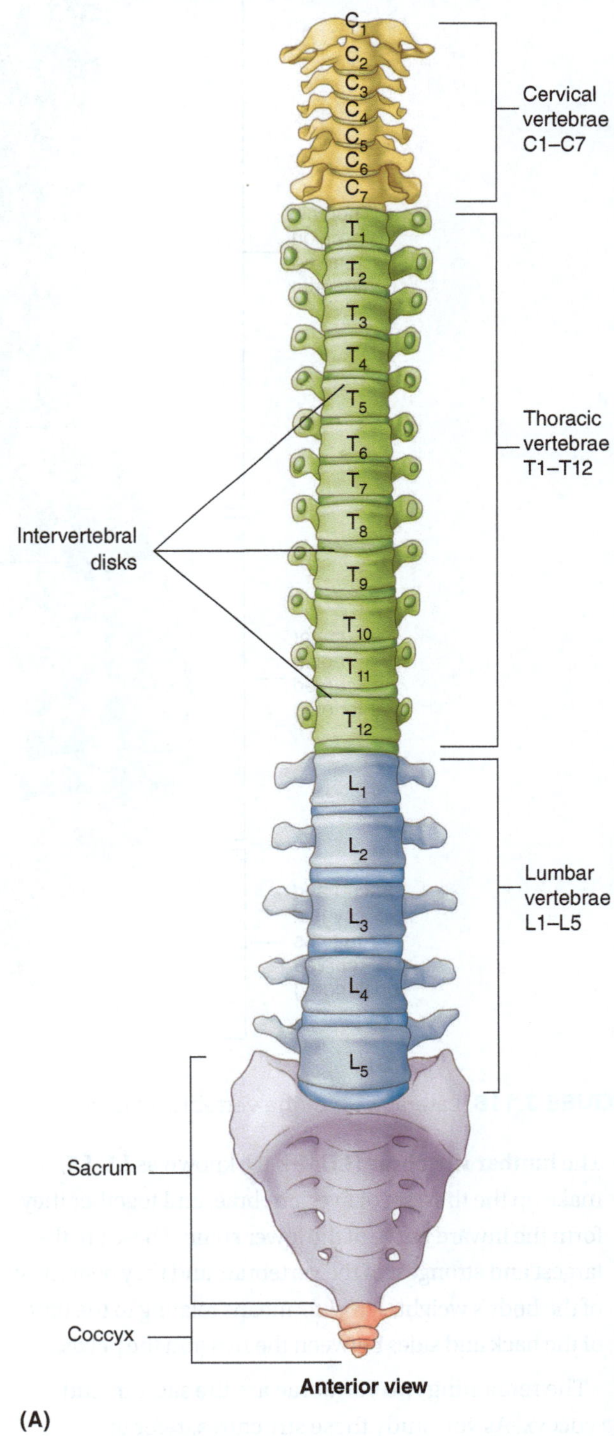

FIGURE 3.11A Anterior view of the vertebral column.

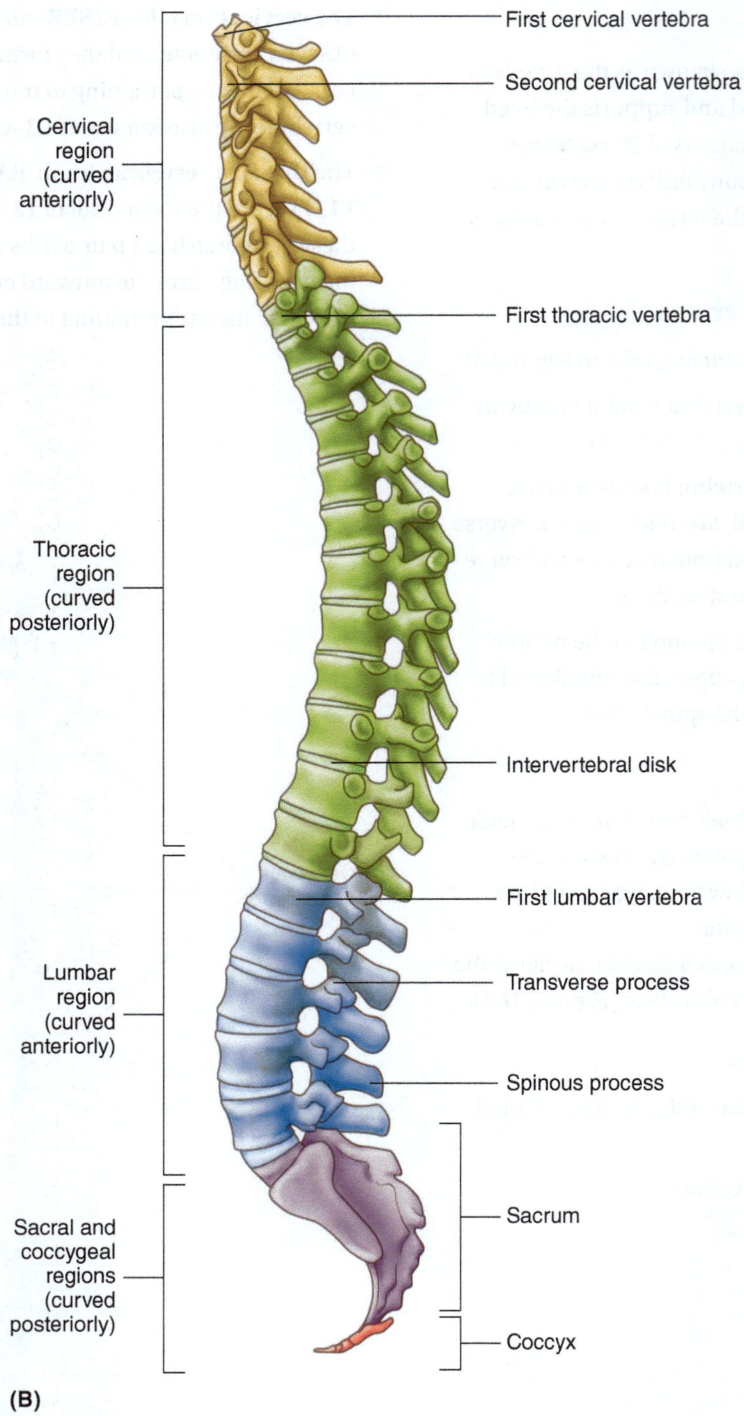

FIGURE 3.11B Lateral view of the vertebral column.

- The **lumbar vertebrae** (**LUM**-bar), known as **L1–L5**, make up the third set of five vertebrae, and together they form the inward curve of the lower spine. These are the largest and strongest of the vertebrae, and they bear most of the body's weight. ***Lumbar*** means relating to the part of the back and sides between the ribs and the pelvis.

The remaining two vertebrae are the sacrum and the coccyx. As you study these structures, refer to Figures 3.11A and 3.11B.

- The **sacrum** (**SAY**-krum) is the slightly curved, triangular-shaped bone near the base of the spine that forms the lower portion of the back. At birth, the sacrum is composed of five separate bones; however, in the young child, they fuse together to form a single bone.
- The **coccyx** (**KOCK**-sicks), which is also known as the ***tailbone***, forms the end of the spine and is actually made up of four small vertebrae that are entirely or partially fused together. The term *coccyx* comes from

the Greek for word for cuckoo, because it was thought that its shape resembled a cuckoo's beak.

The Pelvis

The **pelvis**, also known as the ***bony pelvis***, protects internal organs and supports the lower extremities. In addition to the sacrum and coccyx, it includes the ***pelvic girdle***, a cup-shaped ring of bone at the lower end of the trunk consisting of the *ilium*, *ischium*, and *pubis* (Figures 3.12–3.14).

- The **ilium** (**ILL**-ee-um) is the broad, blade-shaped bone that forms the back and sides of the pubic bone.
- The **sacroiliac** (**say**-kroh-**ILL**-ee-ack) is the slightly movable articulation between the sacrum and posterior portion of the ilium (**sacr/o** means sacrum, **ili** means ilium, and **-ac** means pertaining to).
- The **ischium** (**ISS**-kee-um), which forms the lower posterior portion of the pubic bone, bears the weight of the body when sitting.
- The **pubis** (**PEW**-bis), which forms the anterior portion of the pubic bone, is located just below the urinary bladder.
- At birth, the *ilium*, *ischium*, and *pubis* are three separate bones. As the child matures, these bones fuse to form the left and right **pubic bones**, which are held securely together by the pubic symphysis. A ***symphysis*** is a place where two bones are closely joined.
- The **pubic symphysis** (**PEW**-bik **SIM**-fih-sis) is the cartilaginous joint that unites the left and right pubic bones.

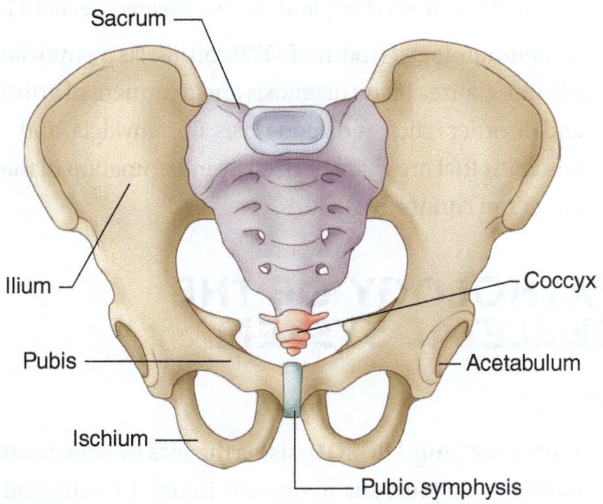

FIGURE 3.12 Anterior view of the pelvis.

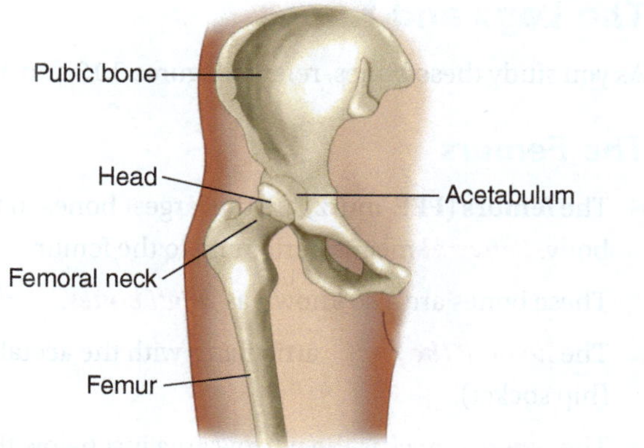

FIGURE 3.13 Structures of the proximal end of the femur and the acetabulum (hip socket).

- The **acetabulum** (**ass**-eh-**TAB**-you-lum), also known as the ***hip socket***, is the large circular cavity in each side of the pelvis that articulates with the head of the femur to form the hip joint (Figures 3.12–3.14).

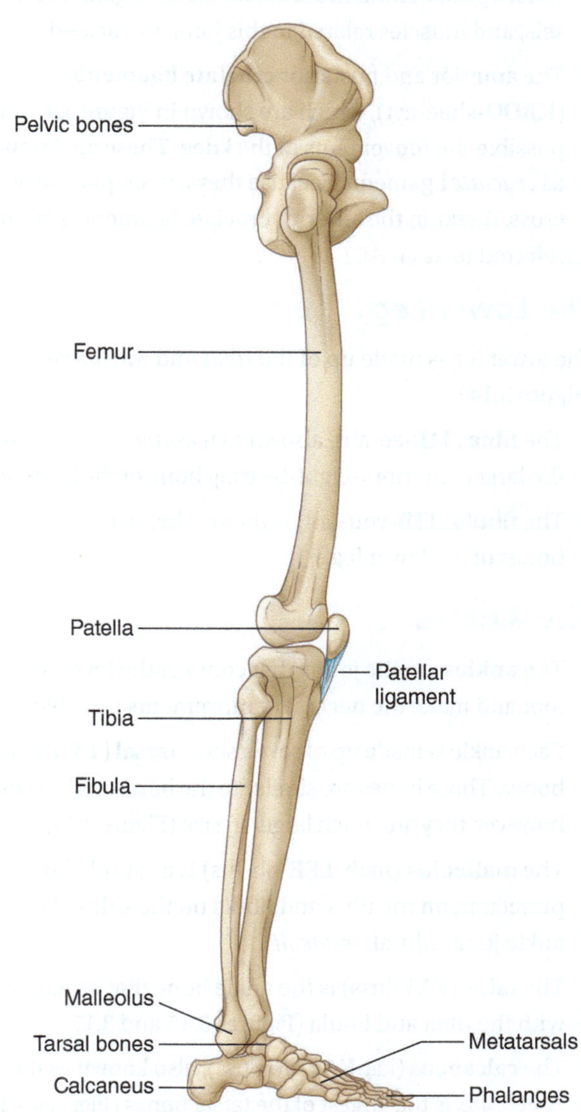

FIGURE 3.14 Lateral view of bones of the lower extremity.

The Legs and Knees

As you study these bones, refer to Figures 3.13 and 3.14.

The Femurs

- The **femurs** (**FEE**-murz) are the largest bones in the body. *Femoral* means pertaining to the femur.
- These bones are also known as *thigh bones*.
- The *head of the femur* articulates with the acetabulum (hip socket).
- The *femoral neck* is the narrow area just below the head of the femur.

The Knees

- The **patella** (pah-**TEL**-ah), also known as the *kneecap*, is the bony anterior portion of the knee.
- The term **popliteal** (pop-**LIT**-ee-al) describes the posterior space behind the knee where the ligaments, vessels, and muscles related to this joint are located.
- The anterior and posterior **cruciate ligaments** (**KROO**-shee-ayt), which are shown in Figure 3.4, make possible the movements of the knee. These are known as *cruciate* ligaments because they are shaped like a cross. A tear in the anterior cruciate ligament is often referred to as an *ACL injury*.

The Lower Legs

The lower leg is made up of the *tibia* and the *fibula* (Figure 3.14).

- The **tibia** (**TIB**-ee-ah), also known as the *shinbone*, is the larger anterior weight-bearing bone of the lower leg.
- The **fibula** (**FIB**-you-lah) is the smaller of the two bones of the lower leg.

The Ankles

- The **ankles** are the joints that connect the lower leg and foot and make the necessary movements possible.
- Each ankle is made up of seven short **tarsal** (**TAHR**-sal) bones. These bones are similar to the bones of the wrists; however, they are much larger in size (Figure 3.15).
- The **malleolus** (mah-**LEE**-oh-lus) is a rounded bony projection on the tibia and fibula on the sides of each ankle joint (plural, *malleoli*).
- The **talus** (**TAY**-luss) is the ankle bone that articulates with the tibia and fibula (Figures 3.15 and 3.17).
- The **calcaneus** (kal-**KAY**-nee-uss), also known as the *heel bone*, is the largest of the tarsal bones (Figures 3.14 and 3.15).

The Feet and Toes

The feet and toes are made up of the following bones as shown in Figure 3.15.

- The five **metatarsals** (met-ah-**TAHR**-salz) form that part of the foot to which the toes are attached.
- The **phalanges** are the bones of the toes. The great toe has two phalanges. Each of the other toes has three phalanges. The bones of the fingers are also called phalanges.

MEDICAL SPECIALTIES RELATED TO THE SKELETAL SYSTEM

- A **chiropractor** (**KYE**-roh-**prack**-tor) holds a Doctor of Chiropractic (DC) degree and specializes in the manipulative treatment of disorders originating from misalignment of the spine. *Manipulative treatment* involves manually adjusting the positions of the bones.
- An **orthopedic surgeon** (**or**-thoh-**PEE**-dick), also known as an *orthopedist*, is a physician who specializes in diagnosing and treating diseases and disorders involving the bones, joints, and muscles.
- An **osteopath** (**oss**-tee-oh-**PATH**) holds a Doctor of Osteopathy (DO) degree and uses traditional forms of medical treatment in addition to specializing in treating health problems by spinal manipulation (**oste/o** means bone, and **-path** means disease). This type of medical practice is known as *osteopathy*; however, that term is also used to mean any bone disease.
- A **podiatrist** (poh-**DYE**-ah-trist) holds a Doctor of Podiatry (DP) or Doctor of Podiatric Medicine (DPM) degree and specializes in diagnosing and treating disorders of the foot (**pod** mean foot, and **-iatrist** means specialist).
- A **rheumatologist** (roo-mah-**TOL**-oh-jist) is a physician who specializes in the diagnosis and treatment of arthritis and disorders such as osteoporosis, fibromyalgia, and tendinitis that are characterized by inflammation in the joints and connective tissues.

PATHOLOGY OF THE SKELETAL SYSTEM

Joints

- **Ankylosis** (**ang**-kih-**LOH**-sis) is the loss or absence of mobility in a joint due to disease, injury, or a surgical procedure (**ankyl** means crooked, bent, or stiff, and

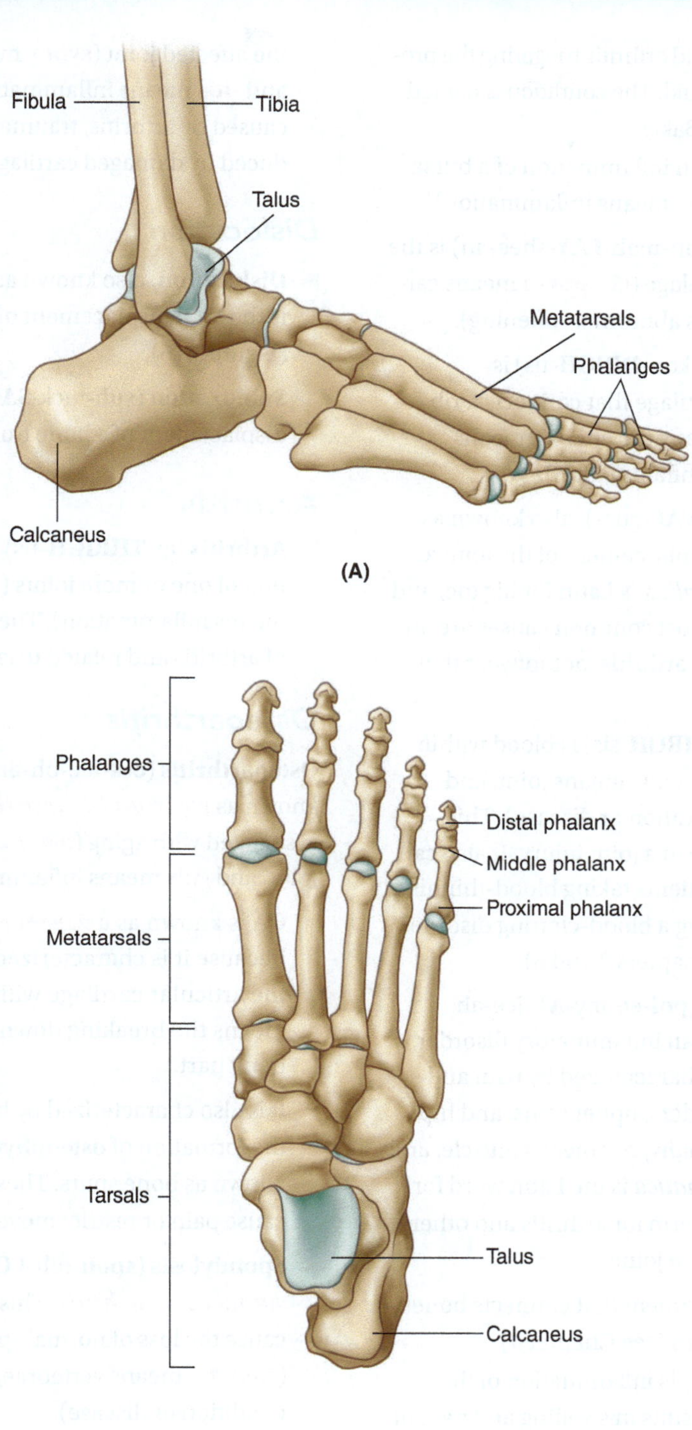

FIGURE 3.15 Bones of the right ankle and foot. (A) Lateral view. (B) Superior view.

-osis means abnormal condition or disease). ***Mobility*** means being capable of movement.

- **Adhesive capsulitis** (ad-**HEE**-siv **kap**-suh-**LIE**-tis), also known as ***frozen shoulder***, is painful ankylosis of the shoulder (**capsul** means little box, and **-itis** means inflammation). It is caused by ***adhesions*** (see Chapter 4) forming in the synovial capsule surrounding the shoulder, making the joint become thicker and tighter.
- **Arthrosclerosis** (**ar**-throh-skleh-**ROH**-sis) is stiffness of the joints, especially in the elderly (**arthr/o** means joint, and **-sclerosis** means abnormal hardening).
- A **Baker's cyst**, also known as a ***popliteal cyst***, is a fluid-filled sac behind the knee. This usually results from a

condition such as rheumatoid arthritis triggering the production of excess synovial fluid. The condition is named for British surgeon William Baker.

- **Bursitis** (ber-**SIGH**-tis) is an inflammation of a bursa (**burs** means bursa, and **-itis** means inflammation).
- **Chondromalacia** (**kon**-droh-mah-**LAY**-shee-ah) is the abnormal softening of cartilage (**chondr/o** means cartilage, and **-malacia** means abnormal softening).
- **Costochondritis** (**kos**-toh-kon-**DRIGH**-tis) is an inflammation of the cartilage that connects a rib to the sternum (**cost/o** means rib, **chondr** means cartilage, and **-itis** means inflammation).
- **Hallux valgus** (**HAL**-ucks **VAL**-guss), also known as a ***bunion***, is an abnormal enlargement of the joint at the base of the great toe (*hallux* is Latin for big toe, and *valgus* means bent). The most common causes are an inherited structural defect, arthritis, or footwear that causes stress on the joint.
- **Hemarthrosis** (**hem**-ar-**THROH**-sis) is blood within a joint (**hem** means blood, **arthr** means joint, and **-osis** means abnormal condition or disease). This condition is frequently due to a joint injury. It also can occur spontaneously in patients taking blood-thinning medications or those having a blood-clotting disorder such as hemophilia (see Chapters 2 and 6).
- **Polymyalgia rheumatica** (**pol**-ee-my-**AL**-jee-ah roo-**MA**-tih-kah) (PMR) is an inflammatory disorder of the muscles and joints characterized by pain and stiffness in the neck, shoulders, upper arms, and hips and thighs (**poly-** means many, **my** means muscle, and **-algia** means pain). *Rheumatica* is the Latin word for ***rheumatism***, an obsolete term for arthritis and other disorders causing pain in the joints.
- A ***sprain*** occurs when a ligament that connects bones to a joint is wrenched or torn (see Chapter 4).
- **Synovitis** (sin-oh-**VYE**-tiss) is inflammation of the synovial membrane that results in swelling and pain of the affected joint (**synov** means synovial membrane, and **-itis** means inflammation). This condition can be caused by arthritis, trauma, infection, or irritation produced by damaged cartilage.

Dislocation

- **Dislocation**, also known as ***luxation*** (luck-**SAY**-shun), is the total displacement of a bone from its joint (Figure 3.16).
- **Subluxation** (**sub**-luck-**SAY**-shun) is the partial displacement of a bone from its joint (Figure 3.16).

Arthritis

- **Arthritis** (ar-**THRIGH**-tis) is an inflammatory condition of one or more joints (**arthr** means joint, and **-itis** means inflammation). There are more than 100 types of arthritis and related diseases.

Osteoarthritis

Osteoarthritis (**oss**-tee-oh-ar-**THRIGH**-tis) (OA), also known as ***wear-and-tear arthritis***, is most commonly associated with aging (**oste/o** means bone, **arthr** means joint, and **-itis** means inflammation) (Figure 3.17).

- OA is known as a ***degenerative joint disease*** because it is characterized by the wearing away of the articular cartilage within the joints. ***Degenerative*** means the breaking down or impairment of a body part.
- It is also characterized by hypertrophy of bone and the formation of **osteophytes** (**OSS**-tee-oh-**fites**), also known as bone spurs. These bony projections can cause pain or restrict movement in a joint.
- **Spondylosis** (**spon**-dih-**LOH**-sis) is also known as ***spinal osteoarthritis***. This degenerative disorder can cause the loss of normal spinal structure and function (**spondyl** means vertebrae, and **-osis** means abnormal condition or disease).

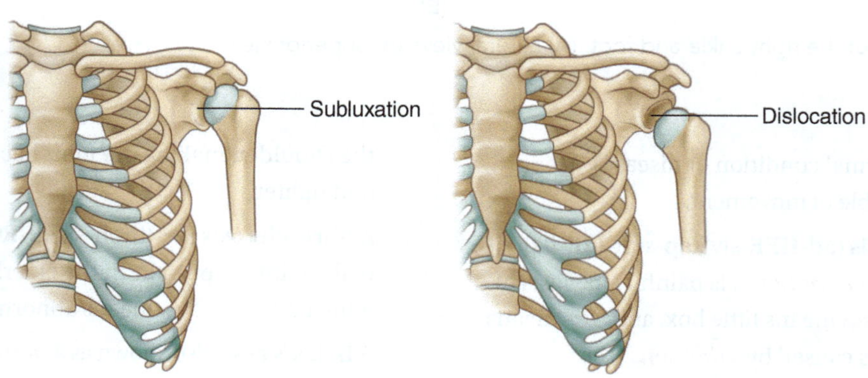

FIGURE 3.16 *Subluxation* and *dislocation* shown on an anterior view of the left shoulder.

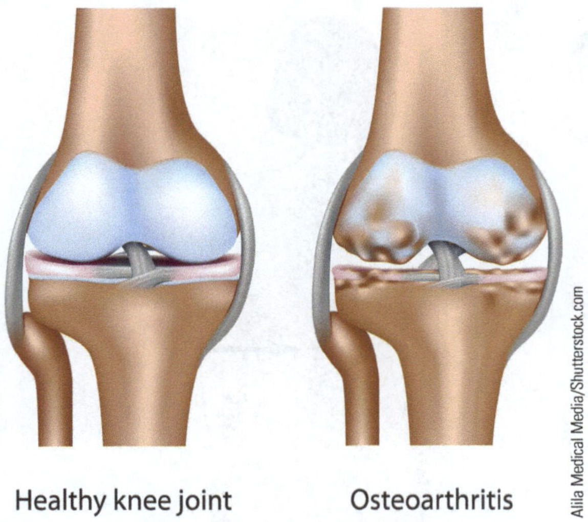

FIGURE 3.17 Damage to the knee joint caused by *osteoarthritis*.

Gout

Gout (**GOWT**), also known as ***gouty arthritis***, is a type of inflammatory arthritis characterized by deposits of urate crystals in the joints; often the big toe. Joints affected by gout are typically hot, red, and excruciatingly sensitive. High levels of uric acid in the blood, caused by medications, alcohol consumption, diet, and/or disease, can lead to the formation of urate crystals.

- ***Pseudogout*** is a form of arthritis that most commonly affects the knees or wrists. Like gout, it is caused by deposits in the joint; however, the cause of pseudogout is a buildup of calcium pyrophosphate crystals.

Rheumatoid Arthritis

Rheumatoid arthritis (**ROO**-mah-toyd ar-**THRIGH**-tis) (RA) is a chronic autoimmune disorder in which the joints and some organs of other body systems are attacked. ***Autoimmune disorders*** are described in Chapter 7.

- As RA progressively attacks the synovial membranes, they become inflamed and thickened so that the joints are increasingly swollen, painful, and immobile.

Ankylosing Spondylitis

Ankylosing spondylitis (**ang**-kih-**LOH**-sing **spon**-dih-**LYE**-tis) (AS) is a type of arthritis that primarily causes inflammation of the joints between the vertebrae (**spondyl** means vertebrae, and **-itis** means inflammation). ***Ankylosing*** refers to progressive stiffening leading to ankylosis, which is the loss or absence of mobility in a joint. This inflammatory disease can cause the vertebrae in the spine to fuse, limiting mobility and restricting lung capacity.

Juvenile Idiopathic Arthritis

Juvenile idiopathic arthritis (**id**-ee-oh-**PATH**-ick ar-**THRIGH**-tis) (JIA), formerly called ***juvenile rheumatoid arthritis***, is an autoimmune disorder that affects children ages 16 years or younger, with symptoms that include stiffness, pain, joint swelling, skin rash, fever, slowed growth, and fatigue. Many children with JIA outgrow it.

Psoriatic Arthritis

Psoriatic arthritis (PsA) is an inflammatory form of arthritis developed by about 20% of all people with the autoimmune skin disease psoriasis (see Chapter 13).

The Spinal Column

- A **herniated disk** (**HER**-nee-**ayt**-ed), also known as a ***slipped*** or ***ruptured disk***, is the breaking apart of an intervertebral disk resulting in a bulge that can put pressure on spinal nerve roots (Figure 3.18B).

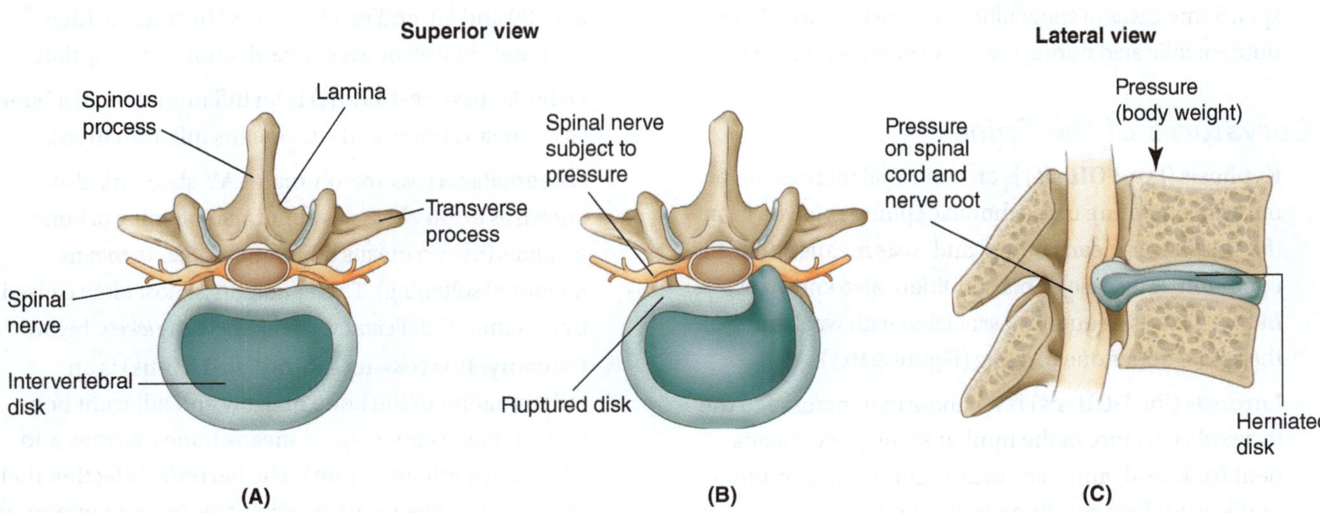

FIGURE 3.18 (A) Superior view of a normal intervertebral disk. (B) Superior and (C) lateral views of a ruptured disk causing pressure on a spinal nerve. The portion of the disk pressing on the nerve roots usually shrinks over time.

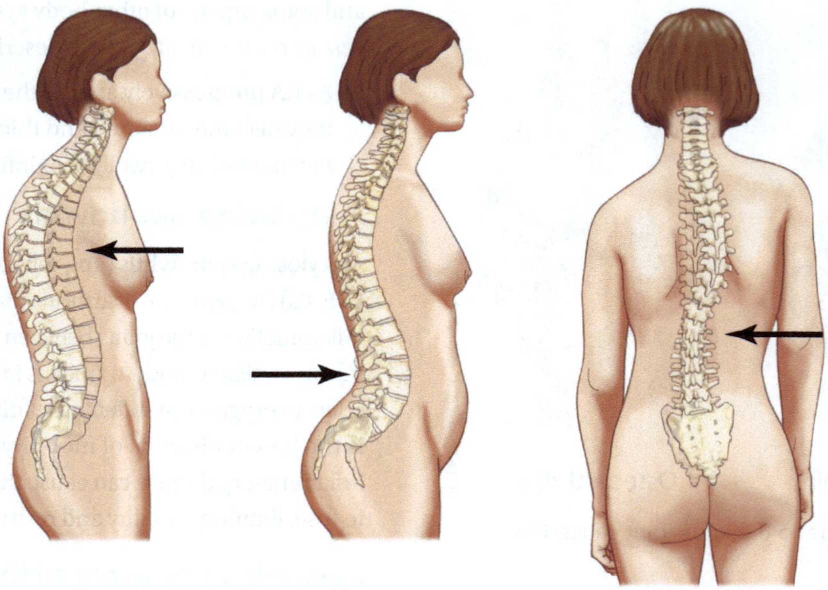

FIGURE 3.19 Abnormal curvatures of the spine. (A) Kyphosis. (B) Lordosis. (C) Scoliosis. (Normal curvatures are shown in shadow.)

- **Lumbago** (lum-**BAY**-goh), also known as ***low back pain*** (LBP), is the general term for pain in the lumbar region of the spine (**lumb** means lumbar, and **-ago** means diseased condition).
- **Spondylolisthesis** (**spon**-dih-loh-liss-**THEE**-sis) is the forward slipping movement of the body of one of the lower lumbar vertebrae on the vertebra or sacrum below it (**spondyl/o** means vertebrae, and **-listhesis** means slipping).
- **Spina bifida** (**SPY**-nah **BIF**-ih-dah) is a congenital defect that occurs during early pregnancy when the spinal canal fails to close completely around the spinal cord to protect it. ***Spina*** means pertaining to the spine. ***Bifida*** means split. Some cases of spina bifida are due to a lack of the nutrient folic acid during the early stages of pregnancy.

Curvatures of the Spine

- **Kyphosis** (kye-**FOH**-sis) is an abnormal increase in the outward curvature of the thoracic spine as viewed from the side (**kyph** means hump, and **-osis** means abnormal condition or disease). This condition, also known as ***hunchback***, is frequently associated with weakening of the spinal bones due to aging (Figure 3.19A).
- **Lordosis** (lor-**DOH**-sis) is an abnormal increase in the forward curvature of the lumbar spine (**lord** means bent backward, and **-osis** means abnormal condition or disease). This condition is also known as ***swayback*** (Figure 3.19B).
- **Scoliosis** (**skoh**-lee-**OH**-sis) is an abnormal lateral (sideways) curvature of the spine (**scoli** means curved, and **-osis** means abnormal condition or disease). Scoliosis most often occurs during the pre-puberty growth spurt around ages 10–12 (Figure 3.19C).

Bones

- **Avascular necrosis** (ay-**VAS**-cue-ler neh-**KROH**-sis), also known as ***osteonecrosis***, is an area of bone tissue death caused by insufficient blood flow, often to the hip (**a-** means without, **vascul** means blood vessels, and **-ar** means pertaining to; and **necrosis** means tissue death). It most commonly occurs in patients between ages 30 and 50, and can be caused by trauma, high-dose steroid use, or excessive alcohol consumption.
- **Osteitis** (**oss**-tee-**EYE**-tis) is an inflammation of a bone (**oste** means bone, and **-itis** means inflammation).
- **Osteomalacia** (**oss**-tee-oh-mah-**LAY**-shee-ah), also known as ***adult rickets***, is abnormal softening of bones in adults (**oste/o** means bone, and **-malacia** means abnormal softening). This condition is most often caused by a vitamin D deficiency. Compare with *rickets*, below.
- **Osteomyelitis** (**oss**-tee-oh-**my**-eh-**LYE**-tis) is an inflammation of the bone marrow and adjacent bone (**oste/o** means bone, **myel** means bone marrow, and **-itis** means inflammation). The bacterial infection that causes osteomyelitis often originates in another part of the body and spreads to the bone via the bloodstream.

- **Paget's disease** (**PAJ**-its) is a chronic bone disease of unknown cause named for Sir James Paget. The condition is characterized by the abnormal breakdown of bone, usually in the pelvis, skull, spine, and legs, followed by abnormal bone formation. The new bone is often structurally enlarged, misshapen, and weak.
- **Periostitis** (**pehr**-ee-oss-**TYE**-tis) is an inflammation of the periosteum (**peri-** means surrounding, **ost** means bone, and **-itis** means inflammation). This condition is often associated with shin splints, which are discussed in Chapter 4.
- **Radiculopathy** (rah-**dick**-you-**LOH**-path-ee) is a condition caused by the compression of a nerve in the spine, sometimes referred to as a ***pinched nerve*** (**radicul/o** means root or nerve, and **-pathy** means disease). This may cause pain, numbness, or weakness along the path of the nerve (see Chapter 11).
- **Rickets** (**RICK**-ets) is a deficiency disease occurring in children. This condition is characterized by defective bone growth resulting from a lack of vitamin D necessary for the body to maintain calcium and phosphorus levels in the bones. The incidence of rickets in the U.S. has decreased due to the fortification of milk with vitamin D.
- **Spinal stenosis** (steh-**NOH**-sis) is a narrowing of the spaces within the spine, potentially putting pressure on the nerves and spinal cord that may cause pain.
- **Short stature**, formerly known as ***dwarfism***, is a condition resulting from the failure of the bones of the limbs to grow to an appropriate length compared to the size of the head and trunk. More than 200 different conditions can cause short stature, which is defined as an average adult height of no more than 4 feet 10 inches. Some adults of short stature prefer to be referred to as ***little people***.
- **Clubfoot**, also known as ***talipes***, describes any congenital deformity of the foot involving the talus (ankle bones).

Bone Tumors

- **Primary bone cancer** is a relatively rare malignant tumor that originates in a bone. *Malignant* means becoming progressively worse and life-threatening.
- **Secondary bone cancer**, or ***bone metastasis***, occurs when cancer cells metastasize (spread) to the bones from other organs such as the breasts, prostate, or lungs. Malignancies, sarcomas, and tumors are further discussed in Chapter 20.
- **Multiple myeloma** (**my**-eh-**LOH**-mah) is a type of cancer that occurs in blood-making plasma cells found in the red bone marrow (**myel** means bone marrow, and **-oma** means tumor). This condition, which is more common in African Americans, weakens the bones and can impact other body systems such as the kidneys.
- An **osteochondroma** (**oss**-tee-oh-kon-**DROH**-mah) is a benign bony projection covered with cartilage (**oste/o** means bone, **chondr** means cartilage, and **-oma** means tumor). ***Benign*** means something that is not life-threatening and does not recur. This type of outgrowth of tissue is also known as an ***exostosis*** (plural, *exostoses*).

Osteoporosis and Osteopenia Compared

Osteoporosis (**oss**-tee-oh-poh-**ROH**-sis) (OP) is a marked loss of bone density and an increase in bone porosity frequently associated with aging (**oste/o** means bone, **por** means small opening, and **-osis** means abnormal condition or disease). It is most common in women over 50 years old due to the decrease in estrogen after menopause.

Osteopenia (**oss**-tee-oh-**PEE**-nee-ah) is thinner-than-average bone density (**oste/o** means bone, and **-penia** means deficiency). This term is used to describe the condition of someone who does not yet have osteoporosis but has a greater-than-average chance of developing it. Risk factors for osteopenia include aging, smoking, drinking, long-term use of steroid medication, and a lack of calcium in the diet. Young people with eating disorders who do not consume enough calories may also develop the condition.

Osteoporosis-Related Fractures

Osteoporosis is primarily responsible for three types of fractures:

- A **compression fracture** occurs when the bone is pressed together (compressed) on itself. These fractures are sometimes caused by the spontaneous collapse of weakened vertebrae or can be due to an injury. This results in pain and loss of height, and it can lead to the development of the spinal curvature known as kyphosis.
- A **Colles fracture** (**KAHL**-es), which is named for the Irish surgeon Abraham Colles, is also known as a ***broken wrist***. This fracture occurs at the lower end of the radius, often when a person tries to stop a fall by landing on his or her hands. The impact of the fall

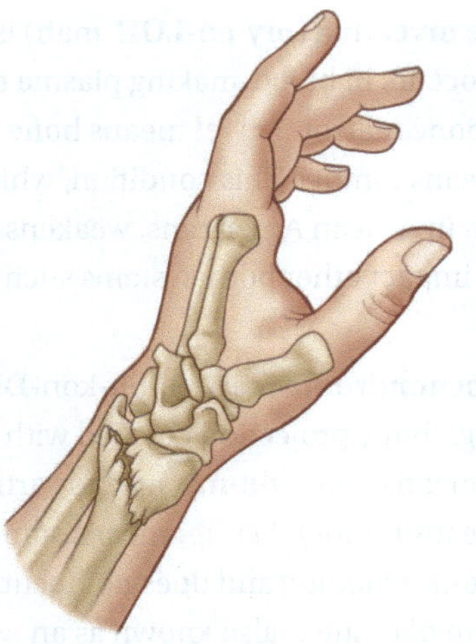

FIGURE 3.20 A Colles fracture of the left wrist.

causes the bone weakened by osteoporosis to break (Figure 3.20).

- An **osteoporotic hip fracture** (oss-tee-oh-pah-**ROT**-ick), also known as a ***broken hip***, is usually caused by weakening of the bones due to osteoporosis and can occur either spontaneously or as the result of a fall. Complications from these fractures can result in the loss of function, mobility, and independence, or death. *Osteoporotic* means pertaining to or caused by the porous condition of bones.

Fractures

A **fracture**, which is a ***broken bone***, is described in terms of its complexity. As you study this section, follow Figure 3.21.

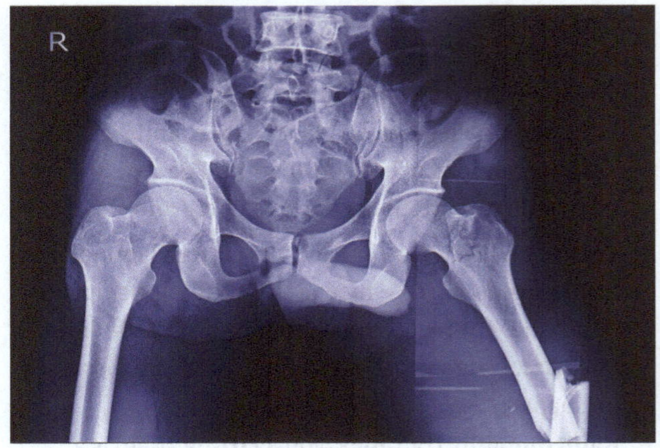

FIGURE 3.22 An x-ray showing an anteroposterior (AP) view of a closed fracture of the femur.

- A **closed fracture**, also known as a ***simple fracture*** or a ***complete fracture***, is one in which the bone is broken, but there is no open wound in the skin (see also Figure 3.22).
- An **open fracture**, also known as a ***compound fracture***, is one in which the bone is broken and there is an open wound in the skin.
- In a **comminuted fracture** (**KOM**-ih-**newt**-ed), the bone is splintered or crushed. Comminuted means crushed into small pieces.
- An **incomplete fracture**, in which the bone does not break into two separate pieces, occurs primarily in children.
- In a **greenstick fracture**, one side of the bone is broken and the other side is only bent.
- In a **buckle fracture**, also called a ***torus fracture***, the affected side of the bone is compressed and buckles but does not break.

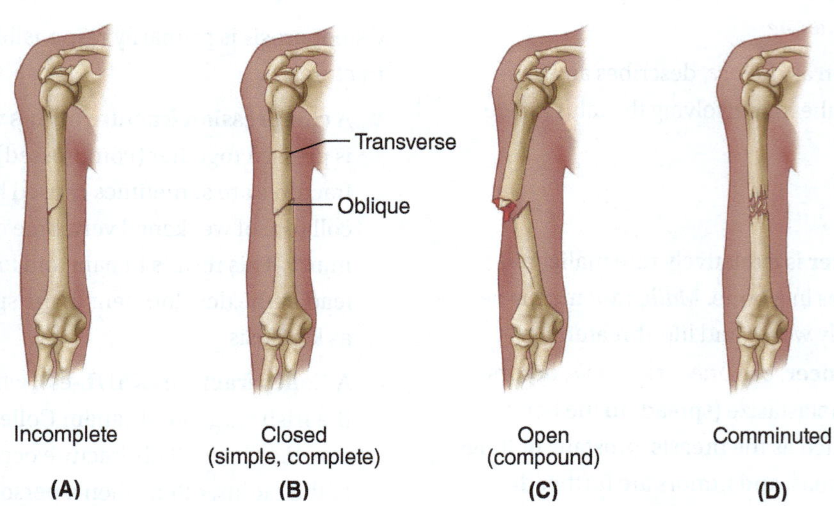

FIGURE 3.21 Types of bone fractures. (A) Incomplete. (B) Closed (simple, complete). (C) Open (compound). (D) Comminuted.

- An **oblique fracture** occurs at an angle across the bone.
- A **pathologic fracture** occurs when a bone breaks under normal strain. This is due to bones being weakened by osteoporosis or a disease process such as cancer.
- A **spiral fracture** is a complete fracture in which the bone has been twisted apart. This type of fracture occurs as the result of a severe twisting motion such as in a sports injury or automobile accident.
- A **stress fracture**, which is an overuse injury, is a small crack in the bone that often develops from chronic, excessive impact. Additional overuse and sports injuries are discussed in Chapter 4.
- A **transverse fracture** occurs straight across, perpendicular to the shaft of the bone.

Additional Terms Associated with Fractures

- A **fat embolus** (**EM**-boh-lus) can form when a long bone is fractured due to an accident or surgery, and fat cells from yellow bone marrow are released into the blood. An ***embolus*** is any foreign matter circulating in the blood that can become lodged and block the blood vessel. This is blockage is called an ***embolism*** (see Chapter 5).
- **Crepitation** (**krep**-ih-**TAY**-shun), also known as ***crepitus***, is the grating sound heard when the ends of a broken bone move together. This term refers to any unusual crackling sound or sensation within the body. It is frequently used to describe the popping or clicking sound heard in the movements of some joints.
- As the bone heals, a **callus** (**KAL**-us) forms as a bulging deposit around the area of the break. This tissue eventually becomes bone. A *callus* is also a thickening of the skin caused by repeated rubbing.

DIAGNOSTIC PROCEDURES OF THE SKELETAL SYSTEM

- **X-ray imaging**, also known as ***radiography***, uses a form of electromagnetic radiation to create ***x-rays***. These images help visualize bone fractures and other abnormalities of hard-tissue internal structures (Figure 3.22).
- **Arthroscopy** (ar-**THROS**-koh-pee) is the visual examination of the internal structure of a joint (**arthr/o** means joint, and **-scopy** means visual examination) using an instrument called an ***arthroscope***. The terms ***knee*** and ***shoulder arthroscopy*** are also used to refer to minimally invasive surgery performed using an arthroscope.
- A **bone marrow biopsy** is a diagnostic test that may be necessary after abnormal types or numbers of red or white blood cells are found in a complete blood count test.
- ***Bone marrow aspiration*** is the use of a syringe to withdraw tissue from the red bone marrow. This procedure is used to obtain tissue for diagnostic purposes or to collect bone marrow for medical procedures such as stem cell transplantation.
- **Magnetic resonance imaging** (MRI) is used to image soft tissue structures such as the interior of complex joints. It is not the most effective method of imaging hard tissues such as bone.
- ***Bone scans***, ***computed tomography*** *(CT)*, and ***arthrocentesis***, which are additional diagnostic procedures, are discussed in Chapter 21.

Bone Density Testing

Bone density testing (BDT) is used to determine losses or changes in bone density. These tests are used to diagnose conditions such as osteoporosis, osteomalacia, osteopenia, and Paget's disease. ***Bone density*** measures the amount of mineral in the bones, usually in the hip and spine, and compares the results with an established norm.

- **Ultrasonic bone density testing** is a screening test for osteoporosis or other conditions that cause a loss of bone mass. In this procedure, sound waves are used to take measurements of the calcaneus (heel) bone. If the results indicate risks, more definitive testing is indicated.
- **Dual x-ray absorptiometry** (ab-**sorp**-shee-**OM**-eh-tree) (DXA) is a low-exposure radiographic measurement of the spine and hips to measure bone density. This test produces more accurate results than ultrasonic bone density testing.

TREATMENT PROCEDURES OF THE SKELETAL SYSTEM

Medications

Bisphosphonates are a class of drugs used to slow the loss of bone density due to osteoporosis, reducing the risk of broken bones.

Low dose *hormone replacement therapy* is sometime used in the short term to maintain bone density in women at high risk for bone loss after menopause.

Stem Cell Transplants

A **stem cell transplant**, also known as a *bone marrow transplant* (BMT), is used to treat certain types of cancers, such as leukemia and lymphomas. Leukemia is discussed in Chapter 6, and lymphomas are discussed in Chapter 20.

- In this treatment, initially both the cancer cells and the patient's bone marrow are destroyed with high-intensity radiation and chemotherapy.
- Next, healthy bone marrow stem cells are infused into the recipient's blood. These cells migrate to the spongy bone, where they multiply to form cancer-free red bone marrow. *Stem cells* produced by the bone marrow eventually develop into blood cells. See Chapter 2 for more information on stem cells.

Types of Bone Marrow Transplants

An **allogeneic stem cell transplant**, also known as an *allogeneic bone marrow transplant*, uses healthy stem cells from a compatible donor, often a sibling. However, unless this is a perfect match, there is the danger that the recipient's body will reject the transplant. Umbilical cord blood frozen immediately after birth is another source of allogeneic stem cells. **Allogeneic** (**al**-loh-jen-**EEH**-ick) means originating within another.

In an **autologous stem cell transplant**, also known as an *autologous bone marrow transplant*, the patient receives his or her own bone marrow cells, which have been harvested (usually from the hip), cleansed, treated, and stored before the remaining bone marrow in the patient's body undergoes treatment. **Autologous** (aw-**TOL**-uh-guss) means originating within an individual.

A *peripheral blood stem cell transplant* utilizes blood-forming stem cells from the bloodstream of the patient or donor. After the cells are removed and stored, the blood is returned to the donor.

Medical Devices

- An **orthotic** (or-**THOT**-ick) is a mechanical appliance, such as a shoe insert, leg brace, or a splint, which is specially designed to support, control, correct, or compensate for impaired limb function.
- A **prosthesis** (pros-**THEE**-sis) is a substitute for a diseased or missing body part, such as a leg that has been amputated (plural, *prostheses*).

Joints

- *ACL reconstruction* is a surgery to replace a torn anterior cruciate ligament (ACL) in the knee.
- **Arthrodesis** (**ar**-throh-**DEE**-sis), also known as *surgical ankylosis*, is the surgical fusion (joining together) of two bones to stiffen a joint, such as an ankle, elbow, or shoulder (**arthr/o** means joint, and **-desis** means to bind, tie together). This procedure is performed to treat severe arthritis or a damaged joint by immobilizing it.
- **Arthroscopic surgery** (**ar**-throh-**SKOP**-ick) is a minimally invasive procedure for the treatment of the interior of a joint. For example, torn cartilage can be removed with the use of an arthroscope and instruments inserted through small incisions (Figure 3.23).
- **Bone grafting** is a surgical procedure using transplanted bone, often from a hip, leg, or rib, to repair and rebuild bones damaged by injury or disease. Bone grafts in dentistry often use a synthetic bone grafting material instead of actual bone, or combine allograft bone with other materials. *Allograft* means the bone or tissue comes from a donor or cadaver. The opposite is *autograft*, meaning that the patient's own bone or tissue is used.
- A **synovectomy** (sin-oh-**VECK**-toh-mee) is the surgical removal of a synovial membrane from a joint, usually the knee (**synov** means synovial membrane, and **-ectomy** means surgical removal). This procedure, which can be performed endoscopically, is used to repair joint damage caused by rheumatoid arthritis or other inflammatory processes.

Joint Replacements

Arthroplasty (**AR**-throh-**plas**-tee) means the surgical repair of a damaged joint (**arthr/o** means joint, and **-plasty** means surgical repair). The term now usually refers to the resurfacing of the bones, or the surgical placement of an artificial joint. These procedures are named for the involved joint and the amount of the joint that is replaced (Figures 3.24 and 3.25).

- The joint replacement part is a prosthesis that is commonly referred to as an *implant*.
- A **total knee replacement** (TKR) means that all of the parts of the knee are replaced. This procedure, also known as a *total knee arthroplasty* (Figure 3.24), is usually necessitated by damage to the joint from arthritis.

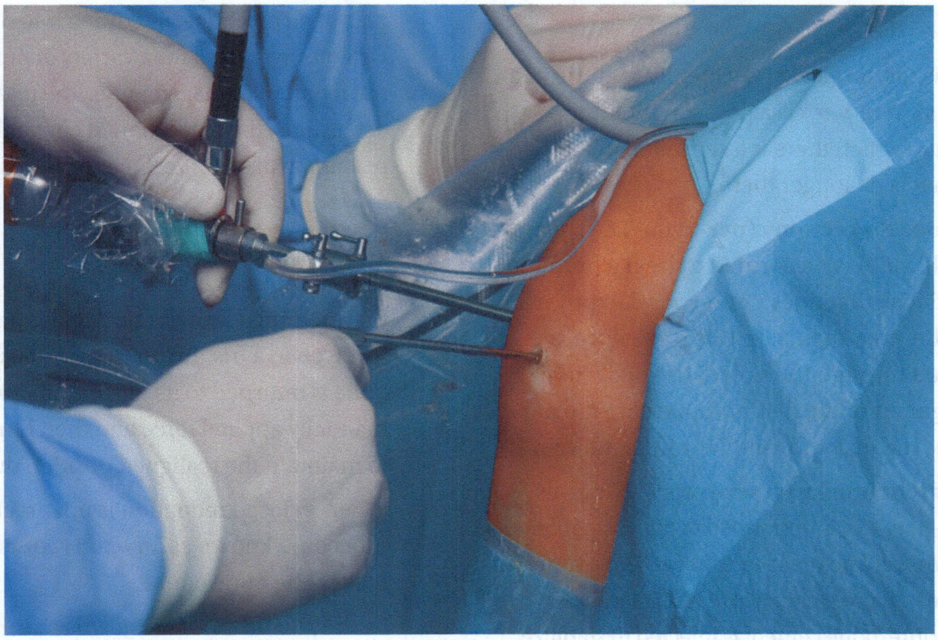

FIGURE 3.23 During arthroscopic surgery, the physician is able to view the interior of the knee on a monitor.

- A **partial knee replacement** (PKR) is a procedure in which only part of the knee is replaced. This can be the medial (inner) or lateral (outer) part of the joint, or the front patella (kneecap). The anterior and posterior cruciate ligaments are preserved.
- A **total hip replacement** (THR), also known as a ***total hip arthroplasty***, is performed to restore a damaged hip to full function. During the surgery, a plastic liner with a metal shell is fitted into the acetabulum to restore a smooth surface. The head of the femur is removed and replaced with a metal or ceramic ball attached to a metal shaft that is fitted into the femur (see Figure 3.25). These smooth surfaces restore the function of the hip joint.
- ***Hip resurfacing arthroplasty*** is an alternative to removing the head of the femur. Function is restored to the hip by placing a metal cap over the head of the femur to allow it to move smoothly over a metal lining in the acetabulum. This technique is sometimes used in younger, more active patients.
- ***Shoulder replacement surgery*** repairs injuries to this joint by replacing the top of the humerus with a metal ball, and the damaged portion of the socket with a plastic prosthesis.
- **Revision surgery** is the replacement of a worn or failed implant.

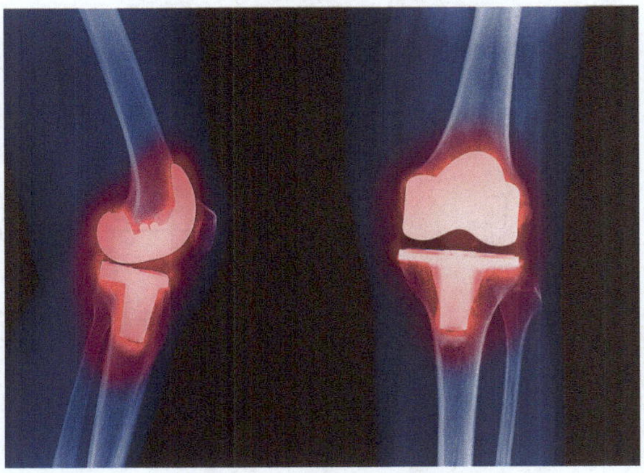

FIGURE 3.24 X-ray (radiograph) of a total knee replacement. On the film the metallic components appear lighter than the bone.

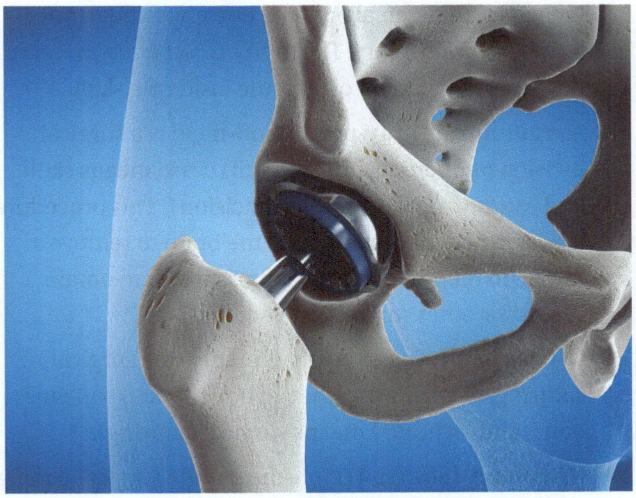

FIGURE 3.25 Total hip replacement (THR).

Spinal Column

- **Amputation** is the surgical or accidental removal of a limb. ***Phantom limb pain*** is a post-amputation phenomenon in which there is a sensation of pain from a body part that is no longer there.
- A **percutaneous diskectomy** (**per**-kyou-**TAY**-nee-us dis-**KECK**-toh-mee) is performed to treat a herniated intervertebral disk that does not respond to physical therapy or other treatments. In this procedure, a thin tube is inserted through the skin of the back to remove the fragment of the disk compressing the nerve. ***Percutaneous*** means performed through the skin.
- **Percutaneous vertebroplasty** (**per**-kyou-**TAY**-nee-us **VER**-tee-broh-**plas**-tee) is performed to treat osteoporosis-related compression fractures (**vertebr/o** means vertebra, and **-plasty** means surgical repair). In this minimally invasive procedure, bone cement is injected to stabilize compression fractures within the spinal column.
- A **laminectomy** (**lam**-ih-**NECK**-toh-mee) is the surgical removal of the lamina, or posterior portion, of a vertebra (**lamin** means lamina, and **-ectomy** means surgical removal). This procedure, also known as ***decompression surgery***, relieves pressure on the spinal cord by enlarging the spinal canal.
- **Spinal fusion** is a technique to immobilize part of the spine by joining together (fusing) two or more vertebrae. ***Fusion*** means to join together.

Bones

- A **decompressive craniectomy** (**kray**-nee-**ECK**-toh-mee) is the surgical removal of a portion of the skull (**crani** means skull, and **-ectomy** means surgical removal). This procedure is performed to relieve increased intracranial pressure due to swelling from a traumatic brain injury. The term ***intracranial pressure*** describes the amount of pressure inside the skull.
- A **craniotomy** (**kray**-nee-**OT**-oh-mee) is a surgical incision or opening into the skull (**crani** means skull, and **-otomy** means a surgical incision). This procedure is performed to gain access to the brain to remove a tumor, to relieve intracranial pressure, or to obtain access for other surgical procedures.
- **Osteorrhaphy** (**oss**-tee-**OR**-ah-fee) is the surgical suturing, or wiring together, of bones (**oste/o** means bone, and **-rrhaphy** means surgical suturing).
- **Osteotomy** (**oss**-tee-**OT**-oh-mee) is the surgical cutting and reshaping of a bone (**oste** means bone, and **-otomy** means a surgical incision). This may include removing part or all of a bone, or cutting into or through a bone. Osteotomy is used for a variety of purposes, including the repair of damaged joints, the realignment of dental occlusions, the correction of congenital defects, and the reshaping of arthritic knees and hips.

Treatment of Fractures

- **Closed reduction**, also known as ***manipulation***, is the attempted non-surgical realignment of the bone involved in a fracture or joint dislocation. The affected bone is returned to its normal anatomic alignment by manually applied force and then is usually immobilized to maintain the realigned position during healing.
- When a closed reduction is not practical, a surgical procedure known as an ***open reduction*** is required to realign the bone parts.
- **Immobilization**, also known as ***stabilization***, is the act of holding, suturing, or fastening the bone in a fixed position with strapping or a cast.
- **Traction** is a pulling force exerted on a limb in a distal direction in an effort to return the bone or joint to normal alignment.

External and Internal Fixation

- **External fixation** is a fracture treatment procedure in which pins are placed through the soft tissues and bone so that an external appliance can be used to hold the pieces of bone firmly in place during healing. When healing is complete, the appliance is removed (Figure 3.26).

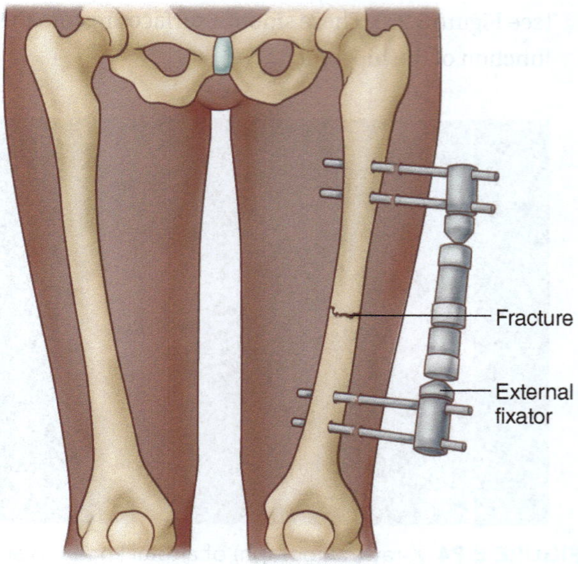

FIGURE 3.26 *External fixation* of the femur stabilizes the bone and is removed after the bone has healed.

- **Internal fixation**, also known as ***open reduction internal fixation*** (ORIF), is a fracture treatment in which a plate or pins are placed directly into the bone to hold the broken pieces in place. This form of fixation is *not* usually removed after the fracture has healed (Figure 3.27).

ABBREVIATIONS RELATED TO THE SKELETAL SYSTEM

Table 3.1 presents an overview of the abbreviations related to the terms introduced in this chapter. *Note:* To avoid errors or confusion, always be cautious when using abbreviations.

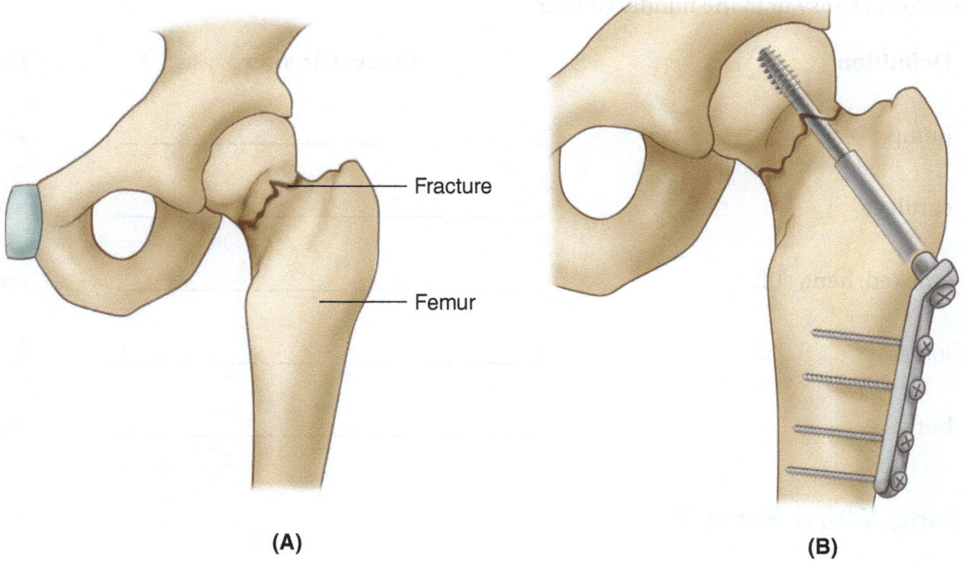

FIGURE 3.27 *Internal fixation* of a fractured hip. (A) Fracture of the femoral neck. (B) *Internal fixation* pins are placed to stabilize the bone. These pins are not usually removed after the bone has healed.

TABLE 3.1

Abbreviations Related to the Skeletal System

bone density testing = BDT	**BDT** = bone density testing
osteoarthritis = OA	**OA** = osteoarthritis
osteoporosis = OP	**OP** = osteoporosis
partial knee replacement = PKR	**PKR** = partial knee replacement
polymyalgia rheumatica = PMR	**PMR** = polymyalgia rheumatica
rheumatoid arthritis = RA	**RA** = rheumatoid arthritis
total hip replacement = THR	**THR** = total hip replacement
total knee replacement = TKR	**TKR** = total knee replacement

LEARNING EXERCISES

Matching Word Parts 1

Write the correct answer in the middle column.

	Definition	Correct Answer	Possible Answers
3.1.	hump	______________	**ankyl/o**
3.2.	cartilage	______________	**arthr/o**
3.3.	crooked, bent, stiff	______________	**burs/o**
3.4.	joint	______________	**kyph/o**
3.5.	bursa	______________	**chondr/i, chondr/o**

Matching Word Parts 2

Write the correct answer in the middle column.

	Definition	Correct Answer	Possible Answers
3.6.	cranium, skull	______________	**cost/o**
3.7.	rib	______________	**crani/o**
3.8.	setting free, loosening	______________	**-desis**
3.9.	spinal cord, bone marrow	______________	**-lysis**
3.10.	to bind, tie together	______________	**myel/o**

Matching Word Parts 3

Write the correct answer in the middle column.

	Definition	Correct Answer	Possible Answers
3.11.	vertebrae	______________	**oste/o**
3.12.	curved	______________	**spondyl/o**

3.13. swayback bent ______________________ **lord/o**

3.14. synovial membrane ______________________ **synovi/o**, **synov/o**

3.15. bone ______________________ **scoli/o**

Definitions

Select the correct answer, and write it on the line provided.

3.16. The shaft of a long bone is known as the ______________________.

distal epiphysis endosteum proximal diaphysis epiphysis

3.17. Seven short ______________________ bones make up each ankle.

carpal metatarsal phalanx tarsal

3.18. The upper portion of the sternum is the ______________________.

clavicle mandible manubrium xiphoid process

3.19. A ______________________ is movable.

cartilaginous joint fibrous joint suture joint synovial joint

3.20. The ______________________ bone is located just below the urinary bladder.

ilium ischium pubis sacrum

3.21. The opening in a bone through which blood vessels, nerves, and ligaments pass is a

______________________.

foramen foramina process symphysis

3.22. A/An ______________________ connects one bone to another bone.

articular cartilage ligament synovial membrane phalange

3.23. The hip socket is known as the ______________________.

acetabulum malleolus patella trochanter

3.24. The bones of the fingers and toes are known as the ______________________.

carpals metatarsals tarsals phalanges

3.25. A normal projection on the surface of a bone that serves as an attachment for muscles and tendons is

known as a/an ______________________.

cruciate exostosis popliteal process

Matching Structures

Write the correct answer in the middle column.

	Definition	Correct Answer	Possible Answers
3.26.	breast bone	____________	clavicle
3.27.	cheekbones	____________	olecranon
3.28.	collar bone	____________	sternum
3.29.	kneecap	____________	patella
3.30.	point of the elbow	____________	zygomatic

Which Word?

Select the correct answer, and write it on the line provided.

3.31. The attempted non-surgical realignment of the bone involved in a fracture or joint dislocation is known as ____________.

closed reduction   external fixation

3.32. A chronic bone disease that is characterized by the abnormal breakdown of bone followed by abnormal bone formation is known as ____________.

osteomalacia   Paget's disease

3.33. An ____________ bone marrow transplant uses bone marrow cells from a donor.

allogeneic   autologous

3.34. A percutaneous ____________ is performed to treat osteoporosis-related compression fractures.

diskectomy   vertebroplasty

3.35. The ____________ skeleton makes body movement possible and also protects the organs of digestion, excretion, and reproduction.

axial   appendicular

Spelling Counts

Find the misspelled word in each sentence. Then write that word, spelled correctly, on the line provided.

3.36. The medical term for the condition commonly known as low back pain is lumbaego.

____

3.37. A condition caused by the compression of a nerve in the spine is called radicalopathy.

____

3.38. Ankylosing spondilitis is a form of rheumatoid arthritis that primarily causes inflammation of the joints between the vertebrae. ________________________

3.39. Bisphosfonates are a class of drugs used to slow the loss of bone density due to osteoporosis.

____

3.40. An orthepedic surgeon specializes in diagnosing and treating disorders involving the bones.

____

Abbreviation Identification

Write the correct answer on the line provided.

3.41. **BMT** ________________________

3.42. **OP** ________________________

3.43. **DXA** ________________________

3.44. **RA** ________________________

3.45. **TMJ** ________________________

Term Selection

Select the correct answer, and write it on the line provided.

3.46. The term meaning the death of bone tissue due to lack of blood flow is ________________________.

osteitis deformans osteomyelitis avascular necrosis osteoporosis

3.47. An abnormal increase in the forward curvature of the lumbar spine is known as

________________________.

kyphosis lordosis scoliosis spondylosis

3.48. The condition known as ____________________ is a congenital defect.

juvenile idiopathic arthritis adhesive capsulitis rheumatoid arthritis spina bifida

3.49. A type of cancer that occurs in blood-making cells found in the red bone marrow is known as a/an ____________________.

primary bone cancer Ewing's sarcoma multiple myeloma osteochondroma

3.50. The bulging deposit that forms around the area of the break during the healing of a fractured bone is a ____________________.

callus crepitation crepitus luxation

Sentence Completion

Write the correct term or terms on the lines provided.

3.51. A/An ____________________ is performed to gain access to the brain or to relieve intracranial pressure.

3.52. The partial displacement of a bone from its joint is known as ____________________.

3.53. The procedure that stiffens a joint by joining two bones is ____________________. This is also known as surgical ankylosis.

3.54. The surgical placement of an artificial joint is known as ____________________.

3.55. A medical term for the condition commonly known as a bunion is ____________________.

Word Surgery

Divide each term into its component word parts. Write these word parts, in sequence, on the lines provided. When necessary, use a slash (/) to indicate a combining vowel. (You may not need all of the lines provided.)

3.56. **Hemarthrosis** is blood within a joint.

__________ __________ __________ __________

3.57. An **osteochondroma** is a benign bony projection covered with cartilage.

__________ __________ __________ __________

3.58. **Osteomalacia**, also known as adult rickets, is abnormal softening of bones in adults.

__________ __________ __________ __________

3.59. **Periostitis** is an inflammation of the periosteum.

_______ _______ _______ _______

3.60. **Spondylolisthesis** is the forward slipping movement of the body of one of the lower lumbar vertebrae on the vertebra or sacrum below it.

_______ _______ _______ _______

True/False

If the statement is true, write **True** on the line. If the statement is false, write **False** on the line.

3.61. ________ Osteopenia is thinner-than-average bone density. This term is used to describe the condition of someone who does not yet have osteoporosis, but is at risk for developing it.

3.62. ________ One of the functions of bones is the support and protection of the internal organs.

3.63. ________ Costochondritis is an inflammation of the cartilage that connects a rib to the sternum.

3.64. ________ Dislocation is the partial displacement of a bone from its joint.

3.65. ________ Arthroscopic surgery is a minimally invasive procedure for the treatment of the interior of a joint.

Clinical Conditions

Write the correct answer on the line provided.

3.66. When Bobby Kuhn fell out of a tree, the bone in his arm was partially broken. Dr. Grafton described this as a/an ________________ fracture and told the family that this type of fracture occurs primarily in children.

3.67. Eduardo Sanchez was treated for an inflammation of the bone and bone marrow. The medical term for this condition is ________________.

3.68. Beth Hubert's breast cancer spread to her bones. These new sites are referred to as ________________.

3.69. As she got older, the increased curvature of Mrs. Morton's upper spine, sometimes referred to as hunchback, got worse. The medical term for this condition is ________________.

3.70. Henry Turner wears a brace to compensate for the impaired function of his leg. The medical term for this orthopedic appliance is a/an ______________________.

3.71. As the result of a head injury in an auto accident, Sam Cheng required a/an ______________________ to relieve the rapidly increasing intracranial pressure.

3.72. Mrs. Gilmer has leukemia and requires a bone marrow transplant. Part of the treatment was the harvesting of her bone marrow so she could receive it later as a/an ______________________ bone marrow transplant.

3.73. Betty Greene has been running for several years; however, now her knees hurt. Dr. Morita diagnosed her condition as ______________________, which is an abnormal softening of the cartilage in these joints.

3.74. Patty Turner (age 7) has symptoms that include a skin rash, fever, slowed growth, fatigue, and swelling in the joints. She was diagnosed as having juvenile ______________________ arthritis.

3.75. Heather Lewis has a very sore shoulder. Dr. Plunkett diagnosed this as an inflammation of the bursa and said that Heather's condition is ______________________.

Which Is the Correct Medical Term?

Select the correct answer, and write it on the line provided.

3.76. Rodney Horner is being treated for a ______________________ fracture in which the ends of the bones were crushed together.

Colles comminuted compound spiral

3.77. Alex Jordan's herniated disk did not respond to physical therapy or other treatment, so her orthopedic surgeon performed a/an ______________________ to remove a fragment of the disk.

arthroplasty laminectomy percutaneous vertebroplasty percutaneous discectomy

3.78. Mrs. Palmer is at high risk for osteoporosis. To obtain a definitive evaluation of the status of her bone density, Mrs. Palmer's physician ordered a/an ______________________ test.

dual x-ray absorptiometry x-ray ultrasonic bone density MRI

3.79. In an effort to return a fractured bone to normal alignment, Dr. Wong ordered ______________________.

This procedure exerts a pulling force on the distal end of the affected limb.

external fixation immobilization internal fixation traction

3.80. Baby Juanita was treated for talipes, a congenital deformity of the foot involving the talus (ankle bones).

The physician referred to this condition as ______________________.

osteomalacia rickets scoliosis clubfoot

Challenge Word Building

These terms are *not* primary terms in the chapter; however, they are made up of the following familiar word parts. If you need help in creating the term, refer to your medical dictionary.

poly-	**arthr/o**	**-ectomy**
	chondr/o	**-itis**
	cost/o	**-malacia**
	crani/o	**-otomy**
	oste/o	**-pathy**
		-sclerosis

3.81. Abnormal hardening of bone is known as ______________________.

3.82. The surgical removal of a rib or ribs is a/an ______________________.

3.83. Any disease of cartilage is known as ______________________.

3.84. A surgical incision into a joint is a/an ______________________.

3.85. Inflammation of cartilage is known as ______________________.

3.86. The surgical removal of a joint is a/an ______________________.

3.87. Inflammation of more than one joint is known as ______________________.

3.88. Any disease involving the bones and joints is known as ______________________.

3.89. A surgical incision or division of a rib or ribs is a/an ______________________.

3.90. Abnormal softening of the skull is known as ______________________.

Labeling Exercises

Identify the numbered items on the accompanying figures.

3.91. ____________________ vertebrae

3.92. ____________________

3.93. ____________________

3.94. ____________________

3.95. ____________________

3.96. ____________________

3.97. ____________________ bone

3.98. ____________________ bone

3.99. ____________________

3.100. ____________________

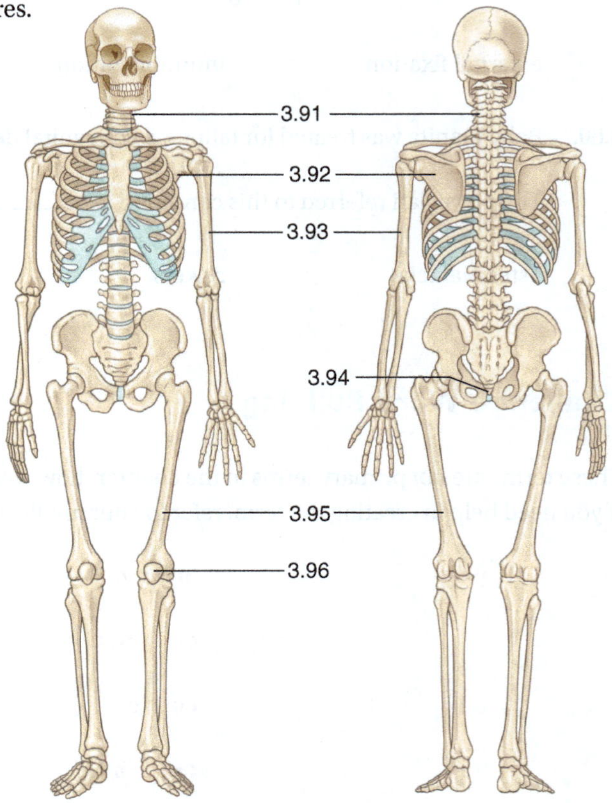

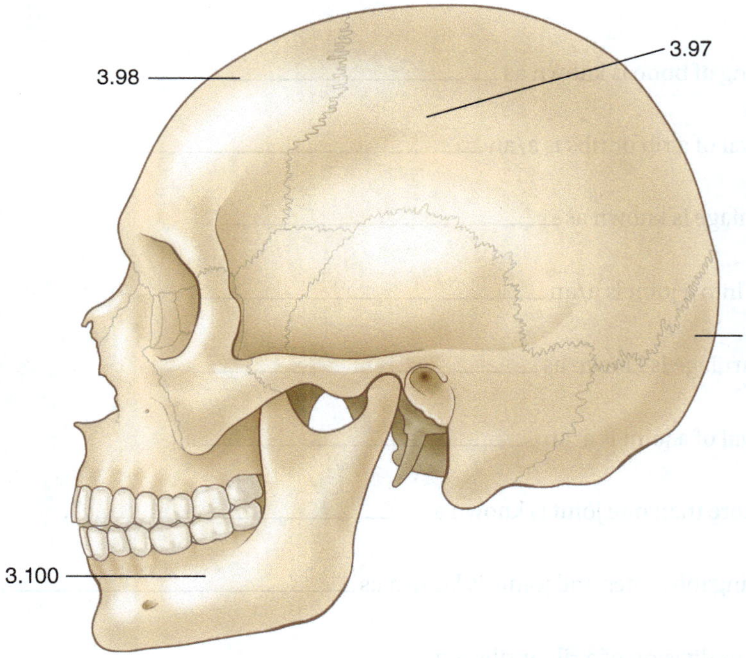

The Human Touch

CRITICAL THINKING EXERCISE

The following story and questions are designed to stimulate critical thinking through class discussion or as a brief essay response. There are no right or wrong answers to these questions.

Dr. Johnstone didn't like what he saw. The x-rays of Gladys Gwynn's hip showed a fracture of the femoral neck and severe osteoporosis of the hip. Mrs. Gwynn had been admitted to the orthopedic ward of Hamilton Hospital after a fall that morning at Sunny Meadows, an assisted-living facility. The accident had occurred when Sheri Smith, a new aide, lost her grip while helping Mrs. Gwynn in the shower.

A frail but alert and cheerful woman of 85, Mrs. Gwynn has osteoarthritis and osteoporosis that have forced her to rely on a walker. Although her finances are limited, she has been living at Sunny Meadows since her husband's death four years ago. Dr. Johnstone knew that she didn't have any close relatives, and he did not think that she had signed a health care proxy designating someone to help with medical decisions like this.

A total hip replacement would be the logical treatment for a younger patient because it could restore some of her lost mobility. However, for a frail patient like Mrs. Gwynn, internal fixation of the fracture might be the treatment of choice. This would repair the break but not improve her mobility.

Dr. Johnstone needs to make a decision soon, but he knows that Mrs. Gwynn is groggy from pain medication. With one more look at the x-ray, Dr. Johnstone sighs and walks toward Mrs. Gwynn's room.

Suggested Discussion Topics

1. Because of the pain medication, Gladys Gwynn may not be able to speak for herself. Since she has no relatives to help, is it appropriate for Dr. Johnstone to make the decision about surgery for her? Given these circumstances, is it possible that when Gladys moved into Sunny Meadows they had her sign a Health Care Power of Attorney to someone at the facility?
2. Because the accident happened when Sheri Smith was helping Mrs. Gwynn, do you think Sheri should be held responsible for the accident? Since Sheri is an employee of Sunny Meadows, should that facility be held responsible?
3. The recovery time for internal fixation surgery is shorter than that following a total hip replacement. The surgery is also less expensive and has a less strenuous recovery period; however, Mrs. Gwynn probably will not be able to walk again. Given the patient's condition, and the limited resources available for health care, which procedure should be performed?
4. Would you have answered Question 3 differently if Mrs. Gwynn were your mother?

CHAPTER **4**

THE MUSCULAR SYSTEM

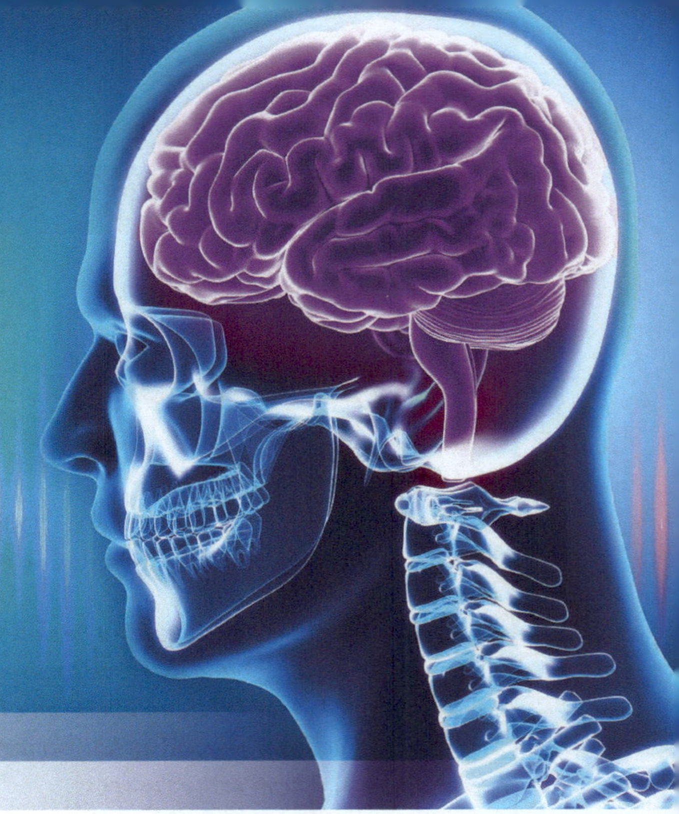

Overview of

STRUCTURES, COMBINING FORMS, AND FUNCTIONS OF THE MUSCULAR SYSTEM

Major Structures	Related Combining Forms	Primary Functions
Muscles	musculo/o, my/o, myos/o	Make body movement possible, hold body erect, move body fluids, and produce body heat.
Fascia	fasci/o	Cover, support, and separate muscles.
Tendons	ten/o, tend/o, tendin/o	Attach muscles to bones.

Vocabulary Related to **THE MUSCULAR SYSTEM**

This list contains essential word parts and medical terms for this chapter. These and the other important **primary terms** are shown in **boldface** throughout the chapter. *Secondary terms*, which appear in *orange* italics, clarify the meaning of primary terms.

Word Parts

- ☐ **bi-** twice, double, two
- ☐ **clon/o** violent action
- ☐ **dys-** bad, difficult, or painful
- ☐ **fasci/o** fascia, fibrous band
- ☐ **fibr/o** fibrous tissue, fiber
- ☐ **-ia** abnormal condition, disease, plural of **-ium**
- ☐ **-ic** pertaining to
- ☐ **kines/o**, **kinesi/o** movement
- ☐ **my/o** muscle
- ☐ **-plegia** paralysis, stroke
- ☐ **-rrhexis** rupture
- ☐ **tax/o** coordination, order
- ☐ **ten/o**, **tend/o**, **tendin/o** tendon, stretch out, extend, strain
- ☐ **ton/o** tone, stretching, tension
- ☐ **tri-** three

Medical Terms

- ☐ **abduction** (ab-**DUCK**-shun)
- ☐ **adduction** (ah-**DUCK**-shun)
- ☐ **adhesion** (ad-**HEE**-zhun)
- ☐ **ataxia** (ah-**TACK**-see-ah)
- ☐ **atonic** (ah-**TON**-ick)
- ☐ **atrophy** (**AT**-roh-fee)
- ☐ **bradykinesia** (**brad**-ee-kih-**NEE**-zee-ah)
- ☐ **carpal tunnel syndrome** (**KAR**-pul)
- ☐ **chronic fatigue syndrome**
- ☐ **circumduction** (ser-kum-**DUCK**-shun)
- ☐ **compartment syndrome**
- ☐ **contracture** (kon-**TRACK**-chur)
- ☐ **dorsiflexion** (**dor**-sih-**FLECK**-shun)
- ☐ **dyskinesia** (**dis**-kih-**NEE**-zee-ah)
- ☐ **dystonia** (dis-**TOH**-nee-ah)
- ☐ **electromyography** (ee-**leck**-troh-my-**OG**-rah-fee)
- ☐ **epicondylitis** (**ep**-ih-**kon**-dih-**LYE**-tis)
- ☐ **ergonomics** (er-goh-**NOM**-icks)
- ☐ **exercise physiologist** (**fiz**-ee-**OL**-oh-jist)
- ☐ **fasciitis** (**fas**-ee-**EYE**-tis)
- ☐ **fibromyalgia** (**figh**-broh-my-**AL**-jee-ah)
- ☐ **ganglion cyst** (**GANG**-glee-on **SIST**)
- ☐ **heel spur**
- ☐ **hemiparesis** (**hem**-ee-pah-**REE**-sis)
- ☐ **hemiplegia** (**hem**-ee-**PLEE**-jee-ah)
- ☐ **hernia** (**HER**-nee-ah)
- ☐ **hyperkinesia** (**high**-per-kye-**NEE**-zee-ah)
- ☐ **hypotonia** (**high**-poh-**TOH**-nee-ah)
- ☐ **impingement syndrome** (im-**PINJ**-ment **SIN**-drohm)
- ☐ **innervation** (**in**-err-**VAY**-shun)
- ☐ **insertion**
- ☐ **intermittent claudication** (**klaw**-dih-**KAY**-shun)
- ☐ **muscular dystrophy** (**DIS**-troh-fee)
- ☐ **myasthenia gravis** (**my**-as-**THEE**-nee-ah **GRAH**-vis)
- ☐ **myoclonus** (my-**OK**-luh-nus)
- ☐ **myofascial release** (my-oh-**FASH**-ee-ahl)
- ☐ **myoparesis** (**my**-oh-pah-**REE**-sis)
- ☐ **myorrhaphy** (my-**OR**-ah-fee)
- ☐ **neuromuscular** (**new**-roh-**MUS**-kyou-lar)
- ☐ **oblique** (oh-**BLEEK**)
- ☐ **origin**
- ☐ **paralysis** (pah-**RAL**-ih-sis)
- ☐ **paraplegia** (**pahr**-ah-**PLEE**-jee-ah)
- ☐ **physiatrist** (**fiz**-ee-**AT**-rist)
- ☐ **plantar fasciitis** (**PLAN**-tar **fas**-ee-**EYE**-tis)
- ☐ **polymyositis** (**pol**-ee-**my**-oh-**SIGH**-tis)
- ☐ **pronation** (proh-**NAY**-shun)
- ☐ **quadriplegia** (**kwad**-rih-**PLEE**-jee-ah)
- ☐ **sarcopenia** (**sar**-koh-**PEE**-nee-ah)
- ☐ **shin splint**
- ☐ **singultus** (sing-**GUL**-tus)
- ☐ **sphincter** (**SFINK**-ter)
- ☐ **sprain**
- ☐ **tendinopathy** (**ten**-din-**OP**-ah-thee)
- ☐ **tenodesis** (ten-**ODD**-eh-sis)
- ☐ **tenolysis** (ten-**OL**-ih-sis)
- ☐ **tenosynovitis** (**ten**-oh-sin-oh-**VYE**-tis)
- ☐ **tenotomy** (ten-**OT**-ah-mee)
- ☐ **torticollis** (**tor**-tih-**KOL**-is)
- ☐ **transverse** (trans-**VERSE**)

LEARNING OBJECTIVES

On completion of this chapter, you should be able to:

1. Describe the functions and structures of the muscular system.
2. Identify the types of muscles.
3. Define the primary terms related to muscle movements.
4. Explain how the muscles are named.
5. Identify the medical specialists who treat disorders of the muscular system.
6. Identify medical word parts of the muscular system.
7. Define the primary terms related to the pathology and the diagnostic and treatment procedures of the muscular system.
8. Spell the primary terms related to the muscular system.
9. Pronounce the primary terms related to the muscular system.
10. Identify common abbreviations related to the muscular system.

FUNCTIONS OF THE MUSCULAR SYSTEM

- Muscles hold the body erect and make movement possible.
- Muscle movement generates nearly 85% of the heat that keeps the body warm.
- Muscles move food through the digestive system.
- Muscle movements, such as walking, aid the flow of blood through veins as it returns to the heart.
- Muscle action moves fluids through the ducts and tubes associated with other body systems.

STRUCTURES OF THE MUSCULAR SYSTEM

The muscular and skeletal systems are sometimes referred to jointly as the *musculoskeletal* system. Because of the interactions of these two systems, they provide the body with form, support, stability, and the ability to move.

The body has more than 600 muscles, which make up about 40–45% of the body's weight. Skeletal muscles are made up of fibers that are covered with fascia and are attached to bones by tendons.

Muscle Fibers

Muscle fibers are the long, slender cells that make up muscles. Each muscle consists of a group of fibers that are bound together by connective tissue.

Fascia

Fascia (**FASH**-ee-ah) is a band of connective tissue that envelops, separates, or binds together muscles or groups of muscles (plural, *fasciae* or *fascias*). Fascia is flexible to allow muscle movements.

The term **myofascial** (**my**-oh-**FASH**-ee-ahl) means pertaining to muscle tissue and fascia (**my/o** means muscle, **fasci** means fascia, and **-al** means pertaining to).

Tendons

- A **tendon** is a narrow band of nonelastic, dense, fibrous connective tissue that attaches a muscle to a bone. Do not confuse tendons with *ligaments*, which are bands of fibrous tissue that form joints by connecting one bone to another bone (Figure 4.1). See Chapter 3 for more information on ligaments.
- For example, the ***patellar tendon*** attaches muscles to the bottom of the patella (kneecap), and the ***Achilles tendon*** attaches the gastrocnemius muscle (the major

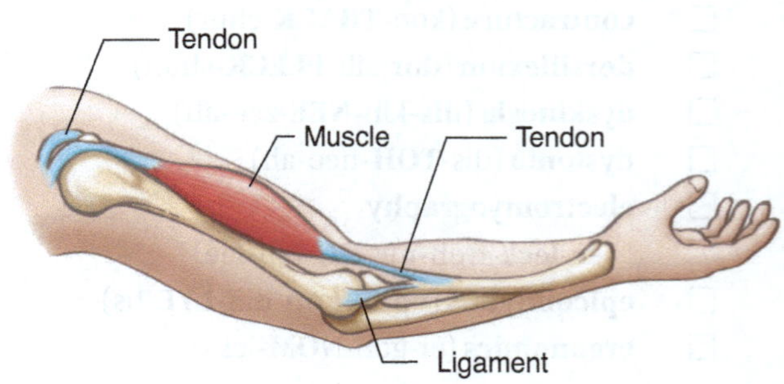

FIGURE 4.1 *Tendons* attach muscle to bone. *Ligaments* join bone to bone.

muscle of the calf of the leg) to the heel bone (Figure 4.10).

- An ***aponeurosis*** is a sheet-like fibrous connective tissue resembling a flattened tendon that connects muscles together or to a bone (plural, *aponeuroses*). As an example, the abdominal aponeurosis can be seen in Figure 4.9.

TYPES OF MUSCLE TISSUE

The three types of muscle tissue are *skeletal*, *smooth*, and *myocardial* (Figure 4.2). These muscle types are described according to their appearance and function.

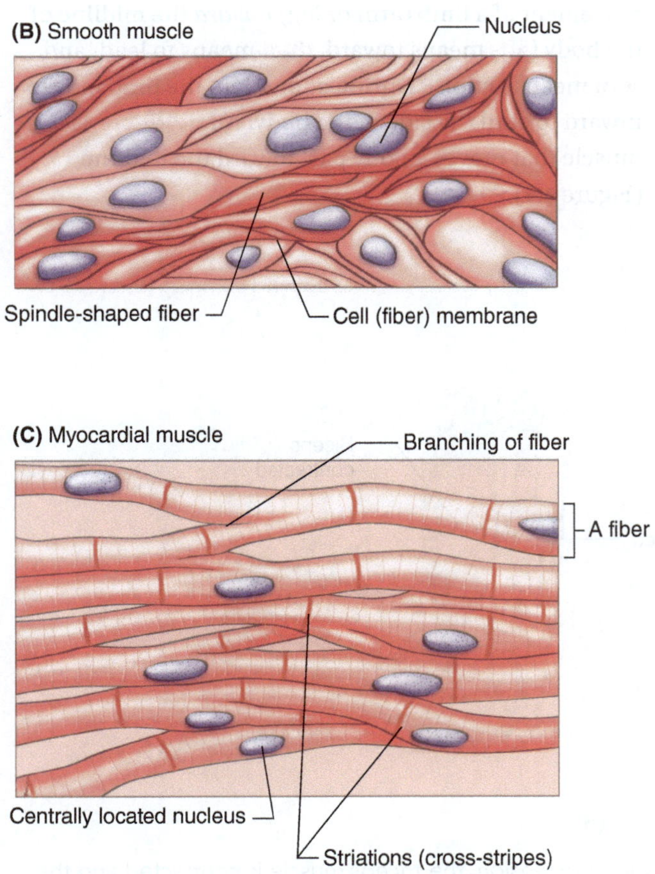

FIGURE 4.2 Types of muscle tissue. (A) Skeletal muscle. (B) Smooth muscle. (C) Myocardial muscle.

Skeletal Muscles

- **Skeletal muscles** are attached to the bones of the skeleton and make body motions possible (Figure 4.2A).
- Skeletal muscles are also known as ***voluntary muscles*** because we have conscious (voluntary) control over these muscles.
- Skeletal muscles are also known as ***striated muscles*** because, under a microscope, the dark and light bands in the muscle fibers create a striped appearance. ***Striated*** means striped.

Smooth Muscles

Smooth muscles are located in the walls of internal organs such as the digestive tract, blood vessels, and ducts leading from glands (Figure 4.2B). Their function is to move and control the flow of fluids through these structures.

- Smooth muscles are also known as ***involuntary muscles*** because they are under the control of the autonomic nervous system and are *not* under voluntary control. The autonomic nervous system is discussed in Chapter 11.
- Smooth muscles are also known as ***unstriated muscles***. This is because they do *not* have the dark and light bands that produce the striped appearance seen in striated muscles.
- Smooth muscles are also known as ***visceral muscles*** because they are found in hollow structures such as those of the digestive and urinary systems. *Visceral* means relating to the internal organs. These muscles are found in large internal organs, with the exception of the heart.

Myocardial Muscle

Myocardial muscles (**my**-oh-**KAR**-dee-al), also known as ***myocardium*** or ***cardiac muscle***, form the muscular walls of the heart (**my/o** means muscle, **cardi** means heart, and **-al** means pertaining to) (Figure 4.2C).

Myocardial muscle is like striated skeletal muscle in appearance but is similar to smooth muscle in that its action is involuntary. It is the constant contraction and relaxation of the myocardial muscle that causes the heartbeat. This topic is discussed in Chapter 5.

MUSCLE CONTRACTION AND RELAXATION

A wide range of muscle movements are made possible by the combination of specialized muscle types, muscle innervation, and the organization of muscles into antagonistic muscle pairs.

Muscle Innervation

Muscle **innervation** (**in**-err-**VAY**-shun) is the stimulation of a muscle by an impulse transmitted by a motor nerve. Motor nerves enable the brain to stimulate a muscle to contract. When the stimulation stops, the muscle relaxes. Motor nerves control the body's voluntary muscular contractions.

If the nerve impulse is disrupted due to an injury or disease, the muscle is unable to function properly. For example, it can be paralyzed or unable to contract properly. These conditions are described later in this chapter.

Neuromuscular (**new**-roh-**MUS**-kyou-lar) means pertaining to the relationship between a nerve and muscle (**neur/o** means nerve, **muscul** means muscle, and **-ar** means pertaining to). Nerves are further described in Chapter 11.

Antagonistic Muscle Pairs

All muscles are arranged in antagonistic pairs. The term ***antagonistic*** refers to working in opposition to each other. Muscles within each pair are made up of specialized cells that can change length or shape by contracting and relaxing. When one muscle of the pair contracts, the opposite muscle of the pair relaxes. It is these contrasting motions that make contraction and relaxation possible.

- **Contraction** is the tightening of a muscle. As the muscle contracts, it becomes shorter and thicker, causing the ***belly*** (center) of the muscle to enlarge.
- **Relaxation** occurs when a muscle returns to its original form. As the muscle relaxes, it becomes longer and thinner, and the belly is no longer enlarged.

As an example, the triceps and biceps work as a pair to make movement of the arm possible (Figure 4.3).

CONTRASTING MUSCLE MOTION

These muscle motions, which occur as pairs of opposites, are described in the following text and illustrated in Figures 4.4–4.8.

Abduction and Adduction

Abduction (ab-**DUCK**-shun) is the movement of a limb (arm or leg) *away from* the midline of the body (**ab-** means away from, **duct** means to lead, and **-ion** means action). During abduction, the limb moves outward away from the side of the body. An ***abductor*** is a muscle that moves a body part away from the midline.

In contrast, **adduction** (ah-**DUCK**-shun) is the movement of a limb (arm or leg) *toward* the midline of the body (**ad-** means toward, **duct** means to lead, and **-ion** means action). During adduction, the limb moves inward toward the side of the body. An ***adductor*** is a muscle that moves a body part toward the midline (Figure 4.4).

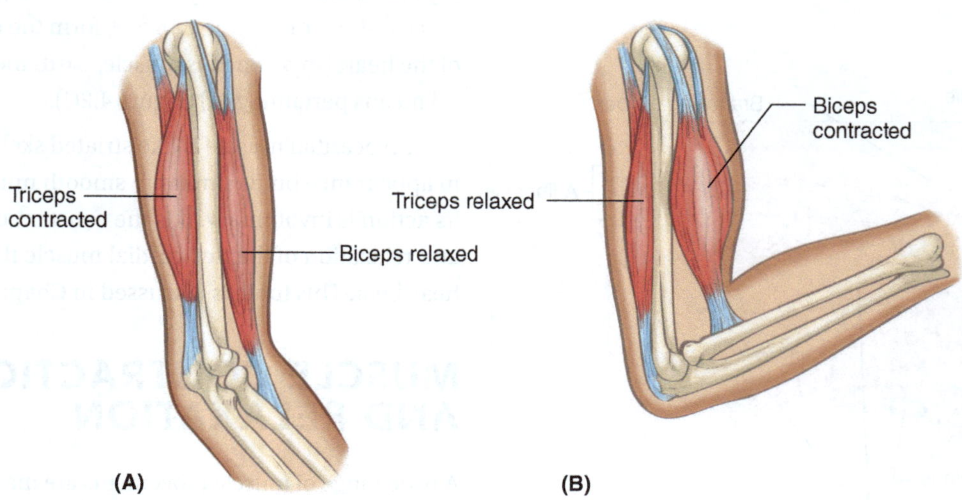

FIGURE 4.3 An antagonistic muscle pair of the upper arm. (A) During *extension*, the *triceps* muscle is contracted and the *biceps* muscle is relaxed. (B) During *flexion*, the *triceps* muscle is relaxed and the *biceps* muscle is contracted.

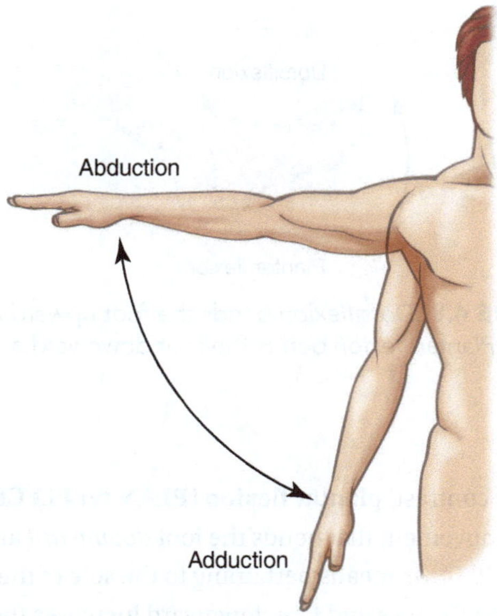

FIGURE 4.4 *Abduction* moves the arm away from the body. *Adduction* moves the arm toward the body.

Flexion and Extension

Flexion (**FLECK**-shun) means decreasing the angle between two bones by bending a limb at a joint (**flex** means to bend, and **-ion** means action). During flexion, the knee or elbow is bent. A ***flexor muscle*** bends a limb at a joint.

In contrast, **extension** means increasing the angle between two bones or the straightening out of a limb (**ex-** means away from, **tens** means to stretch out, and **-ion** means action). During extension, the knee or elbow is straightened. An ***extensor muscle*** straightens a limb at a joint (Figure 4.5).

- **Hyperextension** is the extreme extension or overextension of a limb or body part beyond its normal limit. For example, movement of the head far backward or far forward beyond the normal range of motion causes hyperextension of the muscles of the neck.

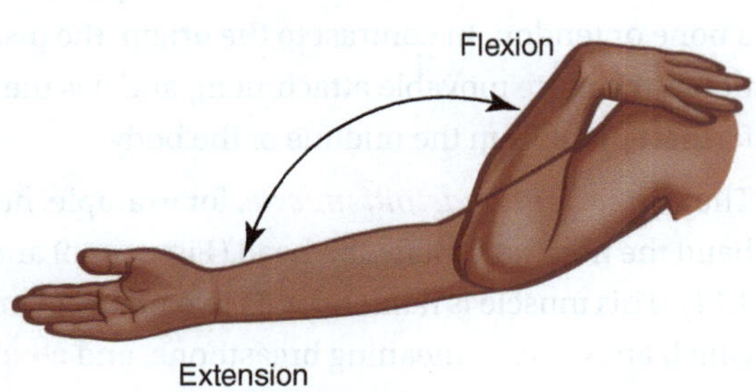

FIGURE 4.5 *Extension* increases the angle of the elbow and moves the hand away from the body. *Flexion* decreases the angle of the elbow and moves the hand toward the body.

Elevation and Depression

Elevation is the act of raising or lifting a body part. For example, the elevation of the ***levator anguli oris*** muscles of the face raises the corners of the mouth into a smile. A ***levator*** is a muscle that raises a body part.

In contrast, **depression** is the act of lowering a body part. The ***depressor anguli oris***, for example, lowers the corner of the mouth into a frown. A ***depressor*** muscle lowers a body part. See Figure 4.9 for illustrations of some of the muscles of the face.

Rotation and Circumduction

Rotation is a circular movement around an axis such as the shoulder joint. An ***axis*** is an imaginary line that runs lengthwise through the center of the body, and rotation turns a bone on its own axis.

In contrast, **circumduction** (**ser**-kum-**DUCK**-shun) is the circular movement at the far end of a limb. An example of circumduction is the swinging motion of the far end of the arm (Figure 4.6).

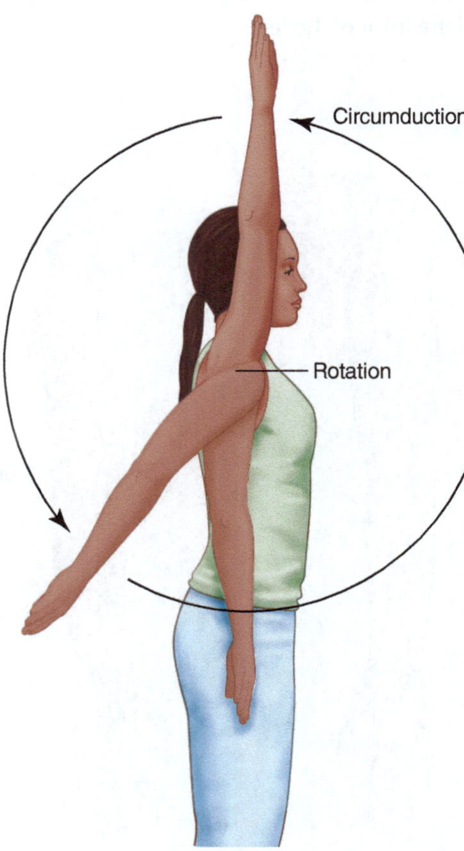

FIGURE 4.6 *Rotation* is a circular movement around an axis such as the shoulder joint. *Circumduction* is the circular movement at the far end of a limb.

- A *rotator muscle* turns a body part on its axis. For example, the head of the **humerus** (**HYUM**-er-us), which is the bone of the upper arm, rotates within the shoulder joint.
- The *rotator cuff* is the group of muscles and their tendons that hold the head of the humerus securely in place as it rotates within the shoulder joint (Figure 4.13).

Supination and Pronation

Supination (**soo**-pih-**NAY**-shun) is the act of rotating the arm or the leg so that the palm of the hand or sole of the foot is turned forward or upward. An easy way to remember this is to think of carrying a bowl of *soup*, which sounds like the beginning of the term.

In contrast, **pronation** (proh-**NAY**-shun) is the act of rotating the arm or leg so that the palm of the hand or sole of the foot is turned downward or backward (Figure 4.7).

Dorsiflexion and Plantar Flexion

Dorsiflexion (**dor**-sih-**FLECK**-shun) is the movement that bends the foot *upward* at the ankle. Pointing the toes and foot upward decreases the angle between the top of the foot and the front of the leg.

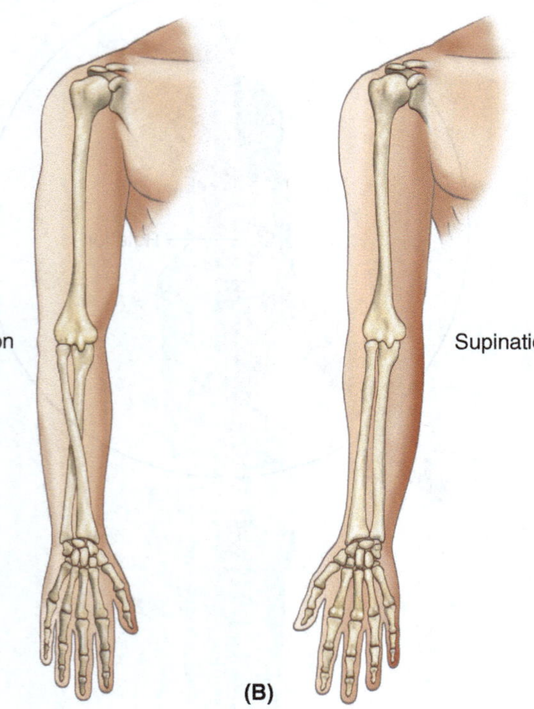

FIGURE 4.7 (A) *Pronation* is turning the arm so the palm of the hand is turned downward. (B) *Supination* is turning the arm so that the palm of the hand is turned upward.

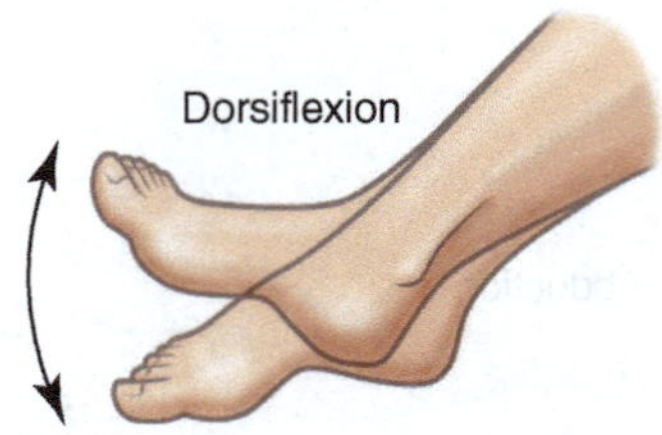

FIGURE 4.8 *Dorsiflexion* bends the foot upward at the ankle. *Plantar flexion* bends the foot downward at the ankle.

In contrast, **plantar flexion** (**PLAN**-tar **FLECK**-shun) is the movement that bends the foot *downward* at the ankle. *Plantar* means pertaining to the sole of the foot. Pointing the toes and foot downward increases the angle between the top of the foot and the front of the leg (Figure 4.8).

HOW MUSCLES ARE NAMED

As you study this section, refer to Figures 4.9–4.12. In Figures 4.9 and 4.10, many of the *superficial* muscles are labeled. These muscles are so called because they are located near the surface, just under the skin.

Muscles Named for Their Origin and Insertion

The movements of skeletal muscles are made possible by two points of attachment. These are known as the origin and insertion, and some muscles are also named for these points.

- The **origin** is where the muscle begins, and it is located nearest the midline of the body or on a less movable part of the skeleton. The origin is the less movable attachment.
- The **insertion** is where the muscle ends by attaching to a bone or tendon. In contrast to the origin, the insertion is the more movable attachment, and it is the farthest point from the midline of the body.
- The *sternocleidomastoid muscle*, for example, helps bend the neck and rotate the head (Figures 4.9 and 4.11). This muscle is named for its two points of origin, which are **stern/o**, meaning breastbone, and **cleid/o**, meaning collar bone. The **mastoid** muscle inserts at one point of insertion into the mastoid process. (This is part of the temporal bone that is located just behind the ear.)

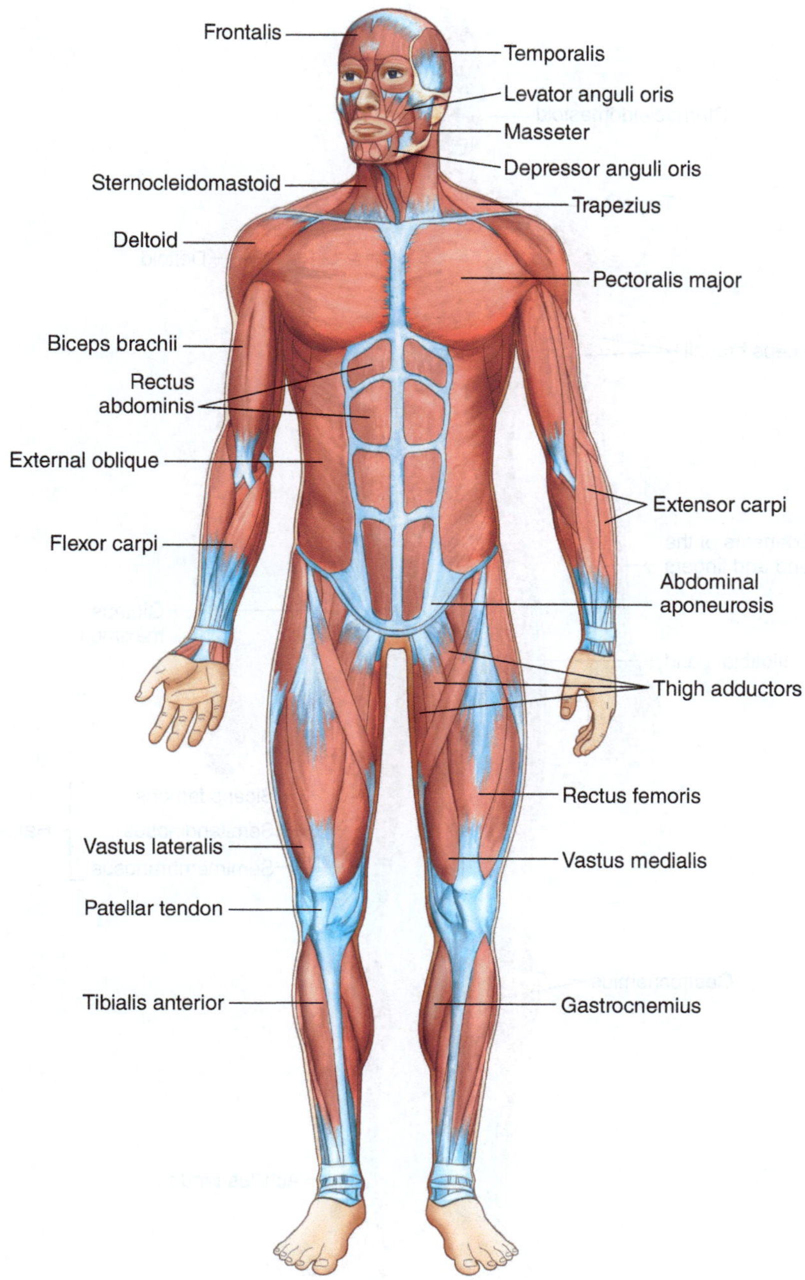

FIGURE 4.9 Superficial muscles of the body (anterior view).

Muscles Named for Their Action

Some muscles are named for their action, such as flexion or extension.

- For example, the ***flexor carpi muscles*** and the ***extensor carpi muscles*** are the pair of muscles that make flexion (bending) and extension (straightening) of the wrist possible (Figure 4.9). *Carpi* means wrist or wrist bones.

Muscles Named for Their Location

Some muscles are named for their location on the body or the organ they are near.

- The **pectoralis major** (**peck**-toh-**RAY**-lis), for example, is a thick, fan-shaped muscle situated on the anterior chest wall (Figure 4.9). ***Pectoral*** means relating to the chest.
- **Lateralis** (lat-er-**AY**-lis) means toward the side. For example, the ***vastus lateralis*** is a large muscle toward the outer side of the leg. *Vastus* is a Latin word for huge.
- **Medialis** (mee-dee-**AY**-lis) means toward the midline. The ***vastus medialis*** is a muscle toward the midline of the leg. These muscles are part of the quadriceps that flex and extend the leg at the knee (Figure 4.9).

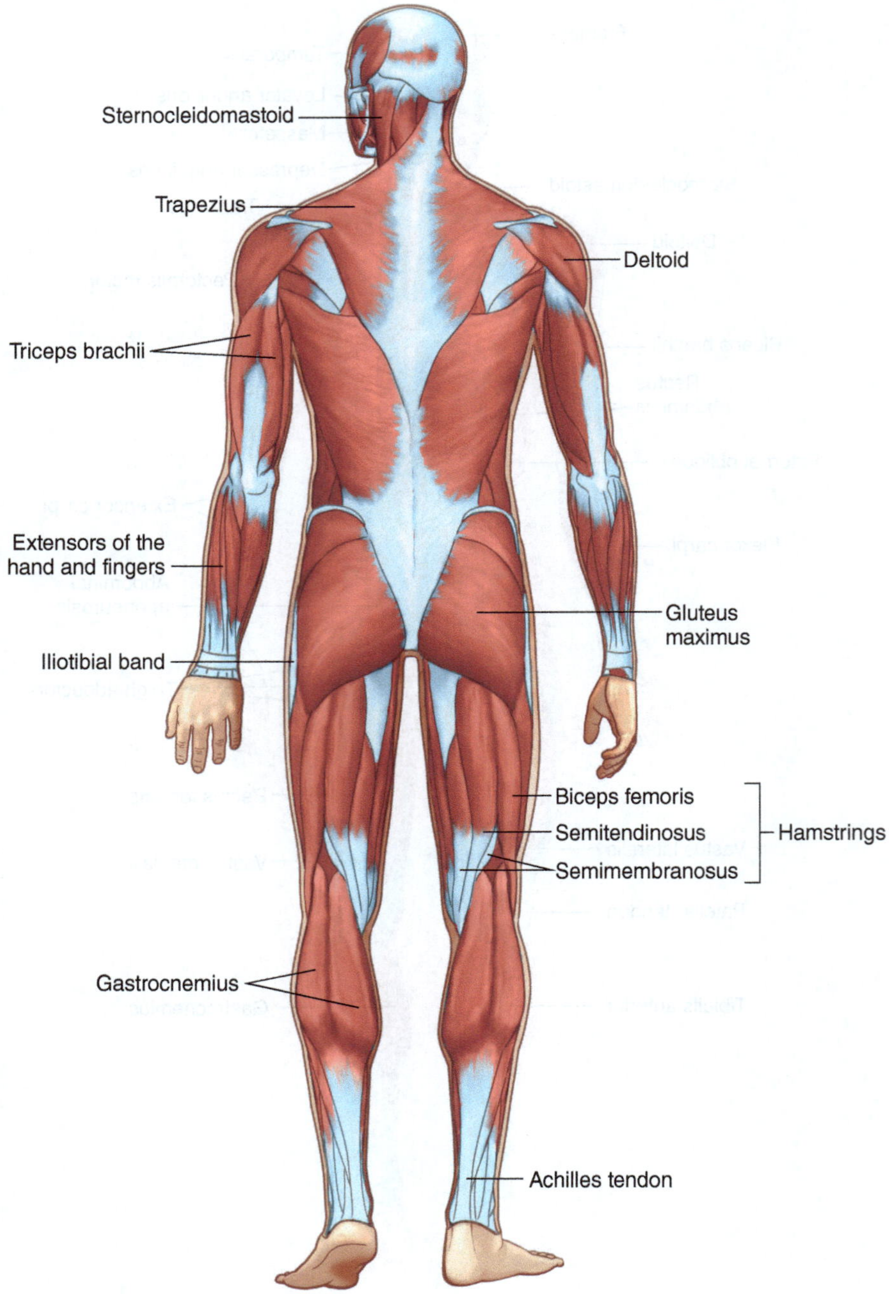

FIGURE 4.10 Superficial muscles of the body (posterior view).

Muscles Named for Fiber Direction

Some muscles are named for the direction in which their fibers run (Figure 4.12).

- **Oblique** (oh-**BLEEK**) means slanted or at an angle. As an example, the ***external oblique*** and ***internal oblique*** muscles have a slanted alignment.
- **Rectus** (**RECK**-tus) means in straight alignment with the vertical axis of the body. As an example, the *rectus abdominis* and *rectus femoris* (discussed under "Select Muscles and Their Functions") have straight alignment.
- A **sphincter** (**SFINK**-ter) is a ring-like muscle that tightly constricts the opening of a passageway. A sphincter is named for the passage involved. As an example, the ***anal sphincter*** closes the anus.
- **Transverse** (trans-**VERSE**) means in a crosswise direction. An example is the *transverse abdominis* muscle in the abdomen, which has a crosswise alignment.

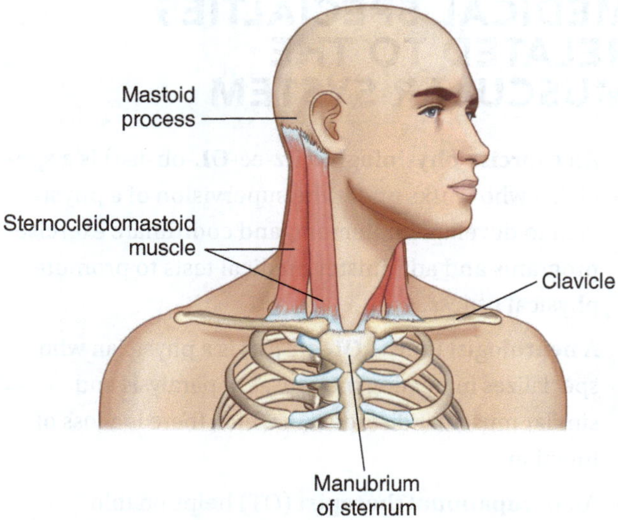

FIGURE 4.11 The *sternocleidomastoid muscle* is named for its *origins* and *insertion*.

Muscles Named for Number of Divisions

Muscles may be named according to the number of divisions forming them. See the muscles of the arm in Figure 4.3 as examples of this.

- The **biceps brachii** (**BYE**-seps **BRAY**-kee-eye), also known as the ***biceps***, is formed from two divisions (**bi-** means two, and **-ceps** means head).
- The **triceps brachii** (**TRY**-seps **BRAY**-kee-eye), also known as the ***triceps***, is formed from three divisions (**tri-** means three, and **-ceps** means head).
- These muscles flex and extend the upper arm. *Note:* The singular and plural of the terms *biceps* and *triceps* are the same.

Muscles Named for Their Size or Shape

Some muscles are named because they are broad or narrow, or large or small.

- The **gluteus maximus** (**GLOO**-tee-us **MAX**-ih-mus) is the largest muscle of the buttock (Figure 4.10). *Maximus* means great or large.
- Other muscles are named because they are shaped like a familiar object. For example, the **deltoid muscle** (**DEL**-toyd), located on the shoulder, is shaped like an inverted triangle, which is the Greek letter *delta*.

Muscles Named for Strange Reasons

Some muscles, such as the hamstrings, have seemingly strange names. The reason this group of muscles is so named is because these are the muscles by which a butcher hangs a slaughtered pig.

- The **hamstring group**, located at the back of the upper leg, consists of three separate muscles: the *biceps femoris*, *semitendinosus*, and *semimembranosus* muscles. The primary functions of the hamstrings are knee flexion and hip extension (Figure 4.10).

SELECT MUSCLES AND THEIR FUNCTIONS

Each of the body's 650 muscles has a specific role. Here are just a few listed with their function.

Muscles of the Head

- The **frontalis** (fron-**TAY**-lis), or ***occipitofrontalis***, muscle is in the forehead. It raises and lowers the eyebrows.

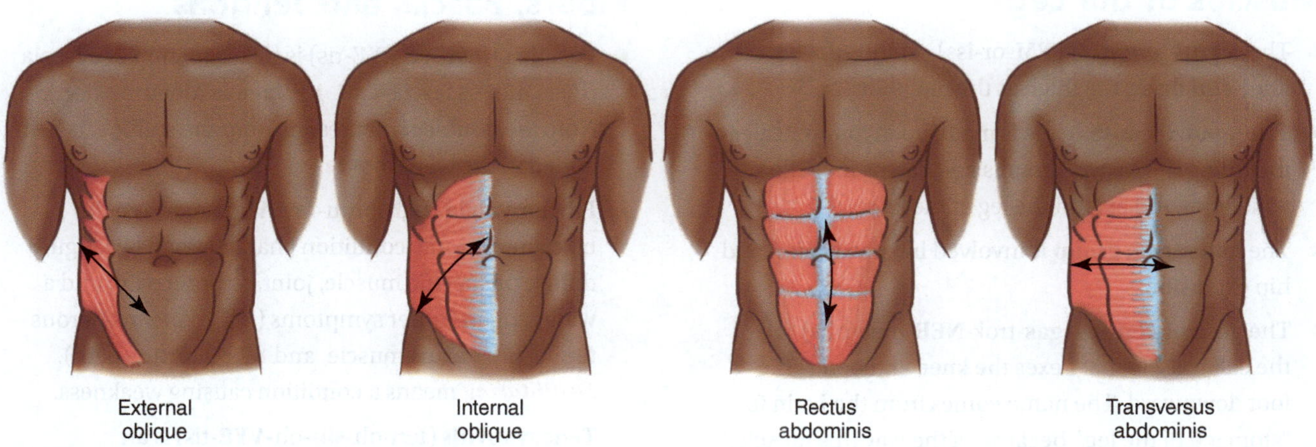

FIGURE 4.12 Many of the muscles of the trunk are named for their direction.

- The **temporalis** (**tem**-poh-**RAY**-lis) muscle moves the lower jaw up and back to close the mouth.
- The **masseter** (mah-**SEE**-ter) muscle, which is one of the strongest in the body, moves the lower jaw up to close the mouth when chewing.

Muscles of the Trunk

- In the male, the **pectoralis major** makes up the bulk of the chest muscles. In the female, this muscle lies under the breasts.
- The **external oblique** and **internal oblique muscles** are found in the abdomen. The external oblique muscles flex and rotate the vertebral column. They also flex the torso and compress the abdomen. The internal oblique muscles flex the spine, support the abdominal contents, help us breathe, and rotate the spine.
- The **rectus abdominis** (ab-**DOM**-ih-nus) helps flex the trunk, assists in breathing, and supports the spine.
- The **transverse abdominis** is located on the side of the abdomen. This *core* muscle is engaged when a person laughs or coughs.

Muscles of the Shoulders and Arms

- The **deltoid** forms the muscular cap of the shoulder (Figures 4.9 and 4.10).
- The **trapezius** (trah-**PEE**-zee-us) muscle moves the head and shoulder blade.
- The **biceps brachii**, located in the anterior upper arm, flexes the elbow.
- The **triceps brachii**, located in the posterior upper arm, extends the elbow.

Muscles of the Legs

- The **rectus femoris** (**FEM**-or-iss) extends the leg at the knee and flexes the thigh at the hip joint.
- The **quadriceps femoris** is made up of four muscles, including the vastus lateralis and vastus medialis, which flex and extend the leg at the knee.
- The **hamstring group** is involved in knee flexion and hip extension.
- The **gastrocnemius** (**gas**-trok-**NEE**-mee-uhs) is the calf muscle that flexes the knee and bends the foot downward. The name comes from the Latin for "stomach of the leg," because of the way this muscle bulges out.

MEDICAL SPECIALTIES RELATED TO THE MUSCULAR SYSTEM

- An **exercise physiologist** (**fiz**-ee-**OL**-oh-jist) is a specialist who works under the supervision of a physician to develop, implement, and coordinate exercise programs and administer medical tests to promote physical fitness.
- A **neurologist** (new-**ROL**-oh-jist) is a physician who specializes in treating the causes of paralysis and similar muscular disorders in which there is a loss of function.
- An **occupational therapist** (OT) helps enable patients to participate in the activities of daily life, including self-care, education, work, or social interaction.
- A **physiatrist** (**fiz**-ee-**AT**-rist) is a physician who specializes in physical medicine and rehabilitation with the focus on restoring function. ***Rehabilitation*** is restoration, following disease, illness, or injury, of the ability to function in a normal or near-normal manner.
- A **physical therapist** (PT) provides treatment to prevent disability or restore function through the use of exercise, heat, massage, or other techniques.
- A **sports medicine physician** specializes in the prevention and treatment of injuries of the bones, joints, and muscles for athletes and other active individuals.

PATHOLOGY OF THE MUSCULAR SYSTEM

Fibers, Fascia, and Tendons

- **Fasciitis** (**fash**-ee-**EYE**-tis) is inflammation of a fascia (**fasci** means fascia, and **-itis** means inflammation). Note the double *ii* that results from the suffix **-itis** being added to the word root **fasci**.
- **Fibromyalgia** (**figh**-broh-my-**AL**-jee-ah) is a debilitating chronic condition characterized by fatigue; diffuse or specific muscle, joint, or bone pain; and a wide range of other symptoms (**fibr/o** means fibrous tissue, **my** means muscle, and **-algia** means pain). *Debilitating* means a condition causing weakness.
- **Tenosynovitis** (**ten**-oh-**sin**-oh-**VYE**-tis) is an inflammation of the sheath surrounding a tendon

(**ten/o** means tendon, **synov** means synovial membrane, and **-itis** means inflammation).

- **Tendinitis** (**ten**-dih-**NIGH**-tis), sometimes spelled *tendonitis*, is an acute inflammation or irritation of the tendons caused by excessive or unusual use of the joint (**tendin** means tendon, and **-itis** means inflammation).
- **Tendinosis** (**ten**-dih-**NOH**-sis) is a chronic condition characterized by pain due to repetitive overuse or an injury that has not healed (**tendin** means tendon, and **-osis** means abnormal condition).

Chronic Fatigue Syndrome

Chronic fatigue syndrome (CFS) is a disorder of unknown cause that affects many body systems.

- CFS is a debilitating and complex disorder characterized by profound fatigue that is not improved by bed rest and may be made worse by physical or mental activity.
- The symptoms of CFS are similar to those of fibromyalgia, and in fact the two diseases may be related.

Muscle Disorders

- An **adhesion** (ad-**HEE**-zhun) is a band of fibrous tissue that holds structures together abnormally. Adhesions can form in muscles or in internal organs, as the result of an injury or surgery.
- **Atrophy** (AT-roh-fee) means weakness or wearing away of body tissues and structures. Atrophy of a muscle or muscles can be caused by pathology or by disuse of the muscle over a long period of time.
- **Cachexia** (kah-**KEKS**-ee-ah) is a condition of physically wasting away due to the loss of weight and muscle mass that occurs in patients with diseases such as advanced cancer or AIDS (see Chapter 9). *Muscle wasting*, or shrinking, can also result from a lack of physical activity.
- A **hernia** (**HER**-nee-ah) occurs when tissue, such as part of an internal organ, protrudes through a weak area in the muscle normally containing it. An *inguinal hernia*, the most common type (see Chapter 15).
- **Myalgia** (my-**AL**-jee-ah) is tenderness or pain in the muscles (**my** means muscle, and **-algia** means pain).
- **Polymyositis** (**pol**-ee-**my**-oh-**SIGH**-tis) (PM) is a muscle disease characterized by the simultaneous inflammation and weakening of voluntary muscles in many parts of the body (**poly-** means many, **myos** means muscle, and **-itis** means inflammation). The affected muscles are typically those closest to the trunk or torso.
- **Rhabdomyolysis** (**rab**-doh-my-**AHL**-eh-sis) is a serious syndrome that can result from a direct or indirect muscle injury (**rhabdomy/o** means striated muscle, and **-lysis** means breakdown). The death of muscle fibers releases their contents into the bloodstream, where they can lead to complications such as renal failure.
- **Sarcopenia** (**sar**-koh-**PEE**-nee-ah) is the loss of muscle mass, strength, and function that comes with aging (**sarc/o** means flesh, and **-penia** means deficiency). A weight or resistance training program can significantly improve muscle mass and slow, but not stop, this process.

Muscle Tone

Muscle tone is the state of balanced muscle tension (contraction and relaxation) that makes normal posture, coordination, and movement possible.

- **Atonic** (ah-**TON**-ick) means lacking normal muscle tone or strength (**a-** means without, **ton** means tone, and **-ic** means pertaining to).
- **Dystonia** (dis-**TOH**-nee-ah) is a movement disorder characterized by the involuntary and sometimes repetitive contraction of certain muscles (**dys-** means bad, **ton** means tone, and **-ia** means condition). Although the word parts imply that muscle tone is the cause of dystonia, it is often a symptom of Parkinson's disease, strokes, brain injuries, and other conditions (see Chapter 11).
- **Hypotonia** (**high**-poh-**TOH**-nee-ah) is a condition in which there is diminished tone of the skeletal muscles (**hypo-** means deficient, **ton** means tone, and **-ia** means condition). Infants with hypotonia are sometimes described as having *floppy baby syndrome*.

Muscle Movement

- **Ataxia** (ah-**TACK**-see-ah) is the lack of muscle coordination during voluntary movement (**a-** means without, **tax** means coordination, and **-ia** means condition). These movements, which are often shaky and unsteady, are most frequently caused by abnormal activity in the cerebellum (see Chapter 11).
- A **contracture** (kon-**TRACK**-chur) is the permanent tightening of fascia, muscles, tendons, ligaments, or skin that occurs when normally elastic connective

tissues are replaced with nonelastic fibrous tissues. The most common causes of contractures are scarring or the lack of use due to immobilization or inactivity.

- **Intermittent claudication** (**klaw**-dih-**KAY**-shun) (IC) is pain in the leg muscles that occurs during exercise and is relieved by rest. ***Intermittent*** means coming and going at intervals, and ***claudication*** means limping. This condition, which is due to poor circulation, is associated with peripheral vascular disease (see Chapter 5).
- A **spasm** is any sudden, involuntary contraction of one or more muscles. A ***tic*** is a repeated spasm, often involving the eyelids or face. These movements are difficult or impossible to control.
- **Myoclonus** (my-**OK**-luh-nus) is the quick, involuntary jerking of a muscle or group of muscles (**my/o** means muscle, **clon** means violent action, and **-us** is a singular noun ending). Myoclonus may occur normally as a person is falling asleep or as the jerks, shakes, or spasms resulting from a neurological disorder such as epilepsy, a metabolic condition, or a response to medication. ***Clonus*** is a repetitive contraction of the muscles of the knees or ankles associated with cerebral palsy, stroke, multiple sclerosis, and other neurological conditions.
- **Singultus** (sing-**GUL**-tus), also known as ***hiccups***, is myoclonus of the diaphragm that causes the characteristic hiccup sound with each spasm.
- A **cramp** is a painful localized muscle spasm often named for its cause, such as menstrual cramps or writer's cramp. A ***charley horse*** is a slang term for a cramp, usually in the leg, that came into use in the 1880s among baseball players.
- **Torticollis** (**tor**-tih-**KOL**-is), also known as ***wryneck***, is a stiff neck due to spasmodic contraction of the neck muscles that pull the head toward the affected side.

Muscle Function

- **Bradykinesia** (**brad**-ee-kih-**NEE**-zee-ah) is extreme slowness in movement (**brady-** means slow, **kines** means movement, and **-ia** means condition). This is one of the symptoms of Parkinson's disease, which is discussed in Chapter 11.
- **Dyskinesia** (**dis**-kih-**NEE**-zee-ah) is the distortion or impairment of voluntary movement resulting in fragmented or jerky motions (**dys-** means bad, **kines** means movement, and **-ia** means condition).
- **Hyperkinesia** (**high**-per-kye-**NEE**-zee-ah), also known as ***hyperactivity***, is abnormally increased muscle function or activity (**hyper-** means excessive, **kines** means movement, and **-ia** means condition).

Myasthenia Gravis

Myasthenia gravis (**my**-as-**THEE**-nee-ah **GRAH**-vis) (MG) is a chronic autoimmune disease that affects the neuromuscular junction (where the neuron activates the muscle to contract) and produces weakness and rapid fatigue of voluntary muscles, especially in the eye, face, and throat. Eye and eyelid movement, facial expression, chewing, talking, and swallowing are often affected by this condition. ***Myasthenia*** means muscle weakness (**my** means muscle, and **-asthenia** means weakness or lack of strength). ***Gravis*** comes from the Latin word meaning grave or serious.

Muscular Dystrophy

The condition commonly known as **muscular dystrophy** (**DIS**-troh-fee) (MD) is properly referred to in the plural, which is *muscular dystrophies*. This general term describes a group of more than 30 genetic diseases that are characterized by progressive weakness and degeneration of the skeletal muscles that control movement, without affecting the nervous system. There is no specific treatment to stop or reverse muscular dystrophy. Two of the most common forms are:

- ***Duchenne muscular dystrophy*** (DMD) is the most common form of muscular dystrophy in children. This condition affects primarily boys with onset between the ages of 3 and 5 years. The disorder progresses rapidly so that most of these children are unable to walk by age 12 and later develop breathing difficulties and heart disease.
- ***Becker muscular dystrophy*** (BMD) is very similar to, but less severe than, Duchenne muscular dystrophy.

Repetitive Stress Disorders

Repetitive stress disorders (RSD), also known as ***repetitive motion disorders***, are a variety of muscular conditions that result from repeated motions performed in the course of normal work, daily activities, or recreation such as sports. The symptoms caused by these frequently repeated motions involve muscles, tendons, nerves, and joints.

- **Compartment syndrome** involves the compression of nerves and blood vessels due to swelling within the *compartment*, an enclosed space created by the fascia that separates groups of muscles in the arm or leg. This syndrome can be caused by trauma, tight bandages or casts, or repetitive activities such as running.

- **Overuse injuries** are minor tissue injuries that have not been given time to heal. These injuries can be caused by spending hours at the computer keyboard or by lengthy athletic training sessions.
- **Overuse tendinitis** (**ten**-dih-**NIGH**-tis) is an inflammation of tendons caused by excessive or unusual use of a joint (**tendin** means tendon, and **-itis** means inflammation).
- **Stress fractures**, which are usually overuse injuries, are discussed in Chapter 3.
- **Trigger finger** is the painful and progressive restriction of movement caused by an inflammation of a tendon's synovial sheath. The name comes from the snapping sound sometimes made when the finger moves, not from the trigger points mentioned below.

Myofascial Pain Syndrome

Myofascial pain syndrome (**my**-oh-**FASH**-ee-ahl) is a chronic pain disorder that affects muscles and fascia throughout the body. This condition, which is caused by a muscle being contracted repetitively, is characterized by the development of trigger points, producing local and referred muscle pain. ***Trigger points*** are tender areas that most commonly develop where the fascia comes into contact with a muscle. ***Referred pain*** describes pain that originates in one area of the body but is felt in another.

Rotator Cuff Injuries

- **Tendinopathy** (**ten**-din-**OP**-ah-thee) is the general term for irritation or degeneration of a tendon in any joint, for example in the rotator cuff (**tendin/o** means tendon, and **-pathy** means disease).
- **Impingement syndrome** (im-**PINJ**-ment), also known as ***rotator cuff tendinitis***, occurs when inflamed and swollen tendons are caught in the narrow space between the bones within the shoulder joint (Figure 4.13). This painful condition is sometimes named for the repetitive overhead movements causing it, i.e. *tennis shoulder* or *swimmer's shoulder*.
- A **rotator cuff tear** can occur as the irritated tendon weakens, or as the result of a fall or injury (Figure 4.13). A partial tear refers to a tendon that is frayed or damaged. In a complete tear, the tendon has detached from the head of the humerus.

Carpal Tunnel Syndrome

Carpal tunnel syndrome symptoms occur when the tendons that pass through the carpal tunnel into the hand are

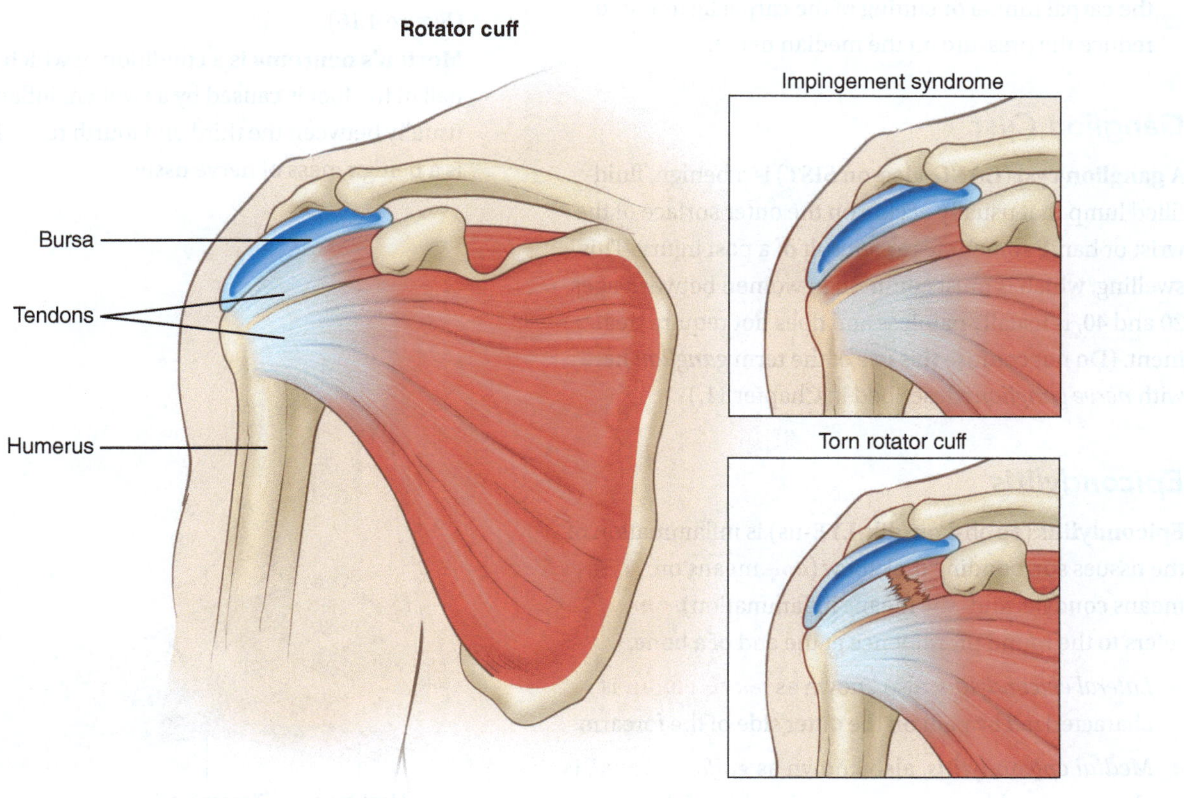

FIGURE 4.13 Views of the *rotator cuff* in health (left) and with injuries (right).

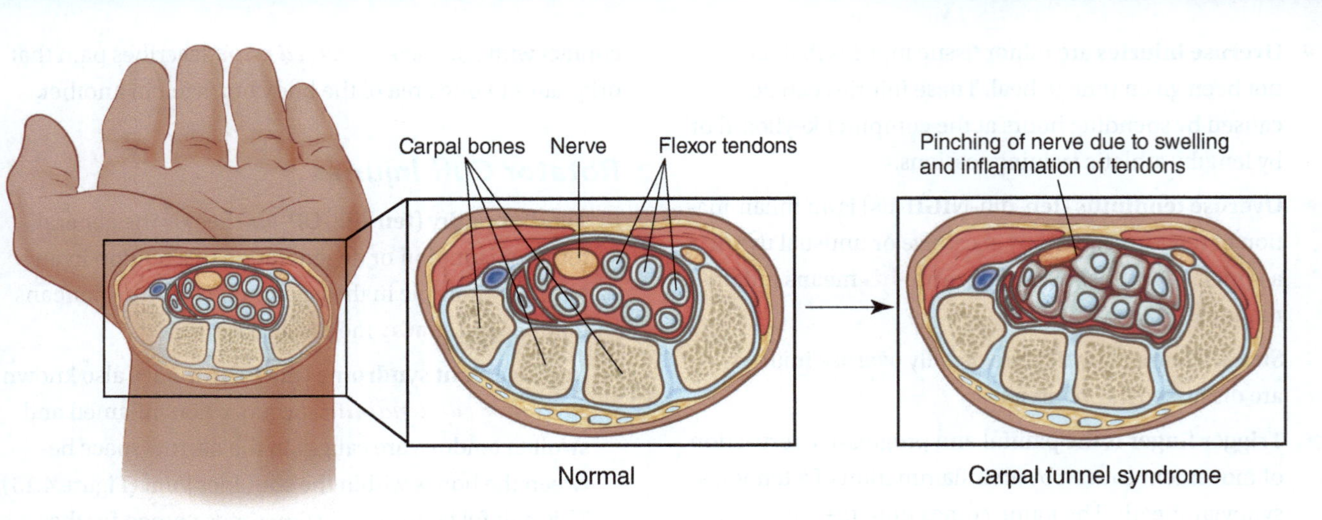

FIGURE 4.14 When the tendons that pass through the carpal tunnel become inflamed and swollen, they pinch the median nerve and cause *carpal tunnel syndrome*.

chronically overused and become inflamed and swollen. The carpal tunnel is a narrow, bony passage under the carpal ligament that is located just below the inner surface of the wrist. The median nerve and the tendons that bend the fingers pass through this tunnel (Figure 4.14). *Carpal* means pertaining to the wrist.

- This swelling creates pressure on the median nerve as it passes through the tunnel.
- **Carpal tunnel release** is the surgical enlargement of the carpal tunnel or cutting of the carpal ligament to reduce the pressure on the median nerve.

Ganglion Cyst

A **ganglion cyst** (**GANG**-glee-on **SIST**) is a benign, fluid-filled lump that usually occurs on the outer surface of the wrist or hand, sometimes as a result of a past injury. This swelling, which is most common in women between ages 20 and 40, is usually painless and does not require treatment. (Do not confuse this use of the term *ganglion* here with *nerve ganglions* described in Chapter 11.)

Epicondylitis

Epicondylitis (**ep**-ih-**kon**-dih-**LYE**-tis) is inflammation of the tissues surrounding the elbow (**epi-** means on, **condyl** means condyle, and **-itis** means inflammation). *Condyle* refers to the round prominence at the end of a bone.

- *Lateral epicondylitis*, also known as *tennis elbow*, is characterized by pain on the outer side of the forearm.
- *Medial epicondylitis*, also known as *golfer's elbow*, is characterized by pain on the palm side of the forearm.

Ankle and Foot Problems

- A **heel spur** is a calcium deposit in the plantar fascia near its attachment to the calcaneus (heel) bone, causing pain that is often mistaken for *plantar fasciitis*.
- **Plantar fasciitis** (**PLAN**-tar **fas**-ee-**EYE**-tis), also known as *plantar fasciopathy*, is an inflammation of the plantar fascia on the sole of the foot. This condition causes foot or heel pain when walking or running (Figure 4.15).
- **Morton's neuroma** is a condition in which pain on the ball of the foot is caused by a swollen, inflamed nerve, usually between the third and fourth toes. *A neuroma* is a benign mass of nerve tissue.

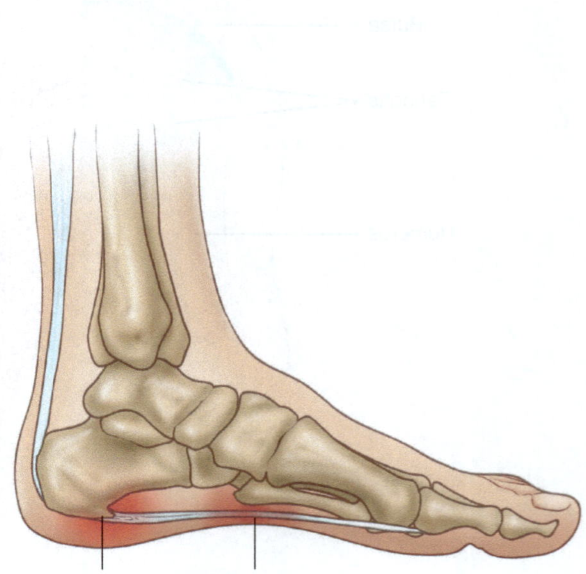

FIGURE 4.15 A *heel spur* and *plantar fasciitis*.

- **Posterior tibial tendon dysfunction** (PTTD), also known as *fallen arches*, occurs when the tendon supporting the foot's arch weakens.

Sports Injuries

In addition to some conditions already mentioned, the following injuries are frequently associated with sports overuse; however, some may also be caused by other forms of trauma (Figure 4.16).

- A *soft tissue injury* is damage to the skin, muscles, ligaments, and tendons, as opposed to the bones or internal organs. Most muscle-related sports injuries are wounds, sprains, and strains that fall into this category.
- A **sprain** is an injury to a joint, such as an ankle, knee, or wrist, which usually occurs when a ligament is wrenched or torn.
- A **strain** is an injury to the body of the muscle or to the attachment of a tendon. Strains usually are associated with overuse injuries that involve a stretched or torn muscle or tendon attachment.
- A **shin splint** is a painful condition caused by the *tibialis anterior* muscle tearing away from the tibia (shin bone). Shin splints can develop in the anterolateral (front and side) muscles or in the posteromedial (back and middle) muscles of the lower leg (Figures 4.9 and 4.10). This type of injury is usually caused by repetitive stress to the lower leg, such as running on uneven or hard surfaces.
- A **hamstring injury** can be a strain or tear on any of the three hamstring muscles that straighten the hip and bend the knee. When these muscles contract too quickly, an injury can occur that is characterized by sudden and severe pain in the back of the thigh.
- **Achilles tendinitis** (**ten**-dih-**NIGH**-tis) is a painful inflammation of the Achilles tendon caused by excessive stress being placed on that tendon.
- **Iliotibial band syndrome** (**ill**-ee-oh-**TIB**-ee-al) (ITBS) is an overuse injury causing pain, usually just above the knee joint. The iliotibial band runs diagonally from the top of the pelvis down to the tibia. ITBS is caused by this band rubbing against bone, often in the area of the knee.

Spinal Cord Injuries

As described in Chapter 3, the spinal cord is surrounded and protected by the bony vertebrae. This protection is

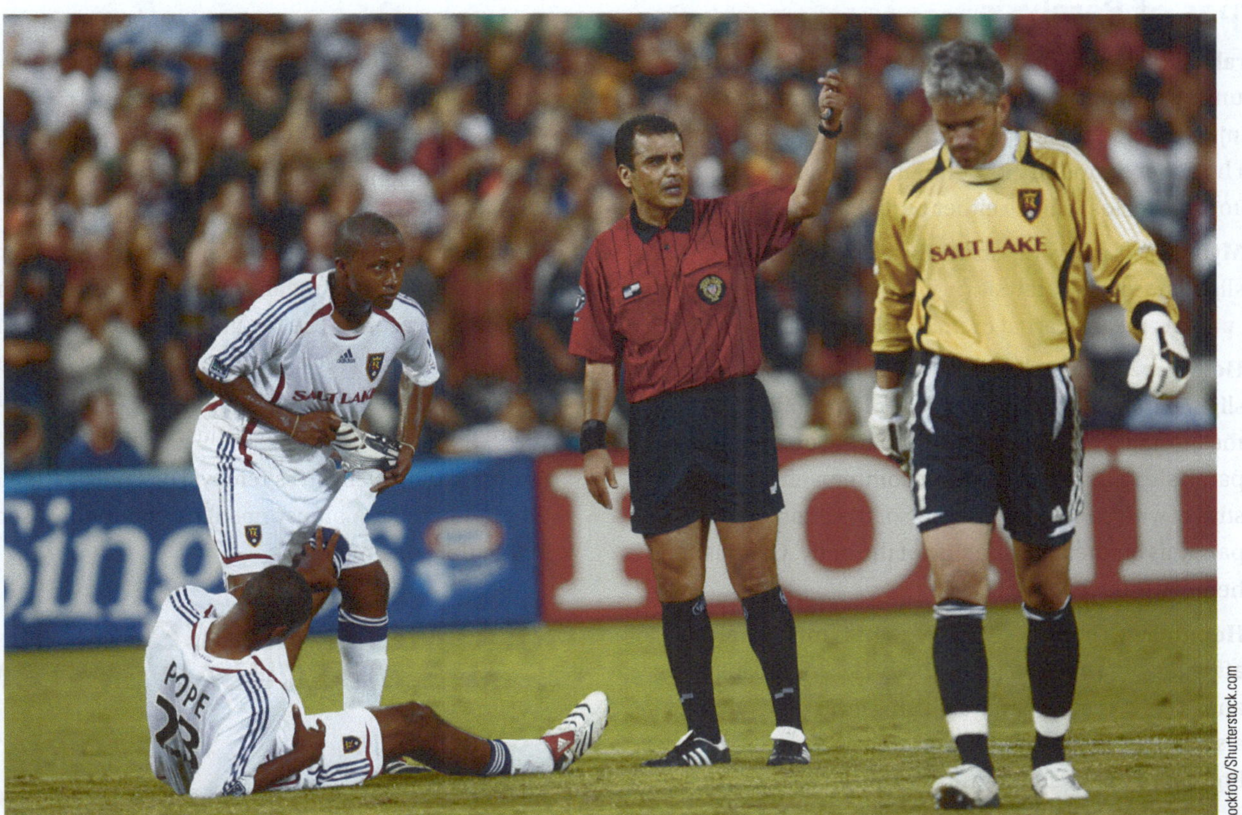

FIGURE 4.16 Sprains and strains are common sports injuries caused by wrenching, tearing, or overusing a muscle or tendon.

essential because the spinal cord is soft, with the consistency of toothpaste.

- The type of paralysis caused by a **spinal cord injury** (SCI) is determined by the level of the vertebra closest to the injury (see Chapter 11). The higher on the spinal cord the injury occurs, the greater the area of the body that may be affected.
- An injury occurs when a vertebra is broken and a piece of the broken bone is pressing into the spinal cord. The cord can also be injured if the vertebrae are pushed or pulled out of alignment.
- When the spinal cord is injured, the ability of the brain to communicate with the body below the level of the injury may be reduced or lost altogether. When that happens, the affected parts of the body will not function normally.
- An ***incomplete injury*** means that the person has some function below the level of the injury, even though that function isn't normal.
- A ***complete injury*** means that there is complete loss of sensation and muscle control below the level of the injury; however, a complete injury does not mean that there is no hope of any improvement.

Types of Paralysis

Paralysis (pah-**RAL**-ih-sis) is the loss of sensation and voluntary muscle movements in a muscle through disease or injury to its nerve supply (plural, *paralyses*). Damage can be either temporary or permanent, and sensory and motor control loss can be either partial or total.

- **Myoparesis** (**my**-oh-pah-**REE**-sis) is a weakness or slight muscular paralysis (**my/o** means muscle, and **-paresis** means partial or incomplete paralysis).
- **Hemiparesis** (**hem**-ee-pah-**REE**-sis) is a weakness or slight paralysis affecting one side of the body (**hemi-** means half, and **-paresis** means partial or incomplete paralysis). It is one of the most common effects of a stroke, with damage to one side of the brain causing paralysis on the opposite side of the body. Contrast hemiparesis with *hemiplegia*.
- **Hemiplegia** (**hem**-ee-**PLEE**-jee-ah) is total paralysis affecting only one side of the body (**hemi-** means half, and **-plegia** means paralysis). This form of paralysis is also associated with strokes, as well as other diseases or injuries of the brain. Contrast with *hemiparesis*.
- **Paraplegia** (**pahr**-ah-**PLEE**-jee-ah), also known as ***partial paralysis***, is the paralysis of both legs and the lower part of the body. An individual affected with paraplegia is known as a ***paraplegic***.
- **Quadriplegia** (**kwad**-rih-**PLEE**-jee-ah), also known as ***tetraplegia***, is paralysis of all four extremities (**quadr/i** means four, and **-plegia** means paralysis). An individual affected with quadriplegia is known as a ***quadriplegic***.

DIAGNOSTIC PROCEDURES OF THE MUSCULAR SYSTEM

Deep tendon reflexes (DTRs) are tested with a reflex hammer that is used to strike a tendon (Figure 4.17). ***Reflexes*** are involuntary responses to a stimulus. The purpose of this exam, also called a ***knee-jerk test***, is to determine whether there is homeostasis between the spinal cord and the peripheral nervous system. When the tendon is tapped, the muscle should immediately contract.

No response or an abnormal response can indicate a disruption of the nerve supply to the involved muscles. Reflexes also are lost in deep coma or because of medication such as heavy sedation.

- **Range-of-motion testing** (ROM) is a diagnostic procedure to evaluate joint mobility and muscle strength (Figure 4.18). *A* ***goniometer*** is a tool used to measure range-of-motion movements in a joint such as the elbow or knee. ROM exercises are used to increase strength, flexibility, and mobility.
- **Electromyography** (ee-**leck**-troh-my-**OG**-rah-fee) (EMG) is a diagnostic test that measures the electrical activity within muscle fibers in response to nerve stimulation (**electr/o** means electricity, **my/o** means muscle, and **-graphy** means the process of producing a picture or record). The resulting record is called an ***electromyogram***. Electromyography is most frequently used when people have symptoms of weakness and examination shows impaired muscle strength.
- A **muscle biopsy** involves removal of a plug of tissue for examination. A biopsy needle is commonly used to obtain this specimen.

TREATMENT PROCEDURES OF THE MUSCULAR SYSTEM

Medications

- An **antispasmodic**, also known as an ***anticholinergic***, is administered to suppress smooth muscle contractions of the stomach, intestine, or bladder.

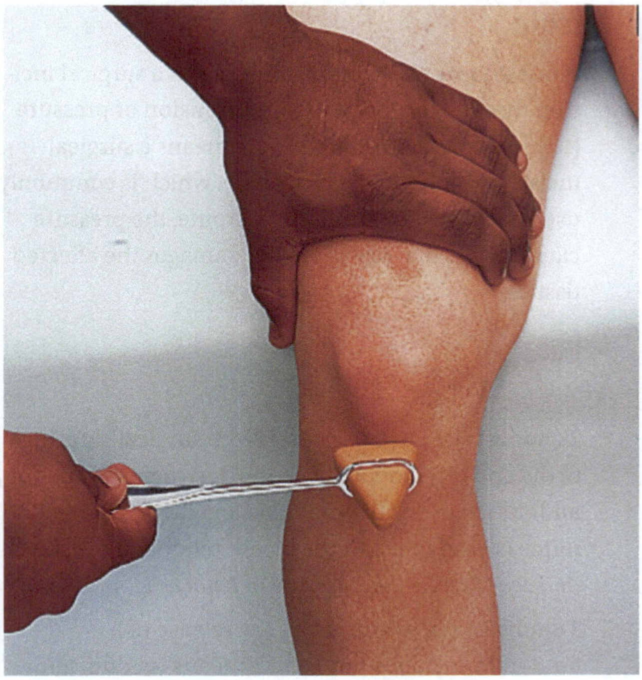

(A)

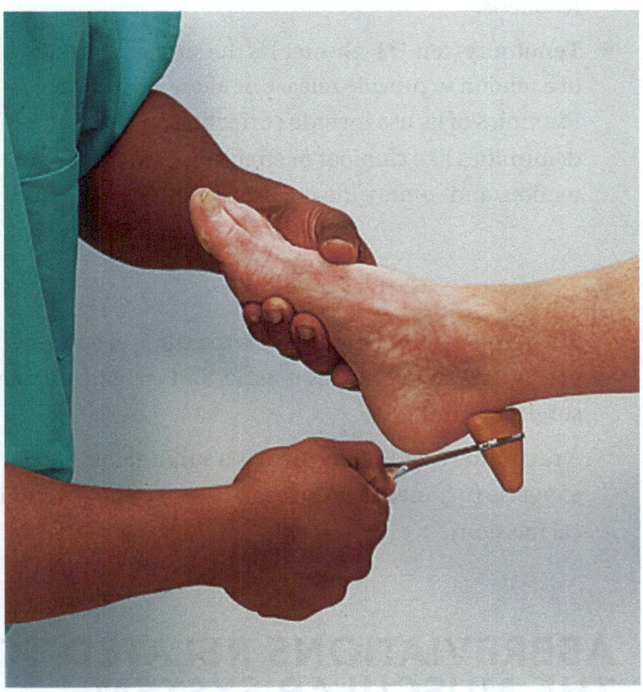

(B)

FIGURE 4.17 Assessment of *deep tendon reflexes.* (A) Testing the *patellar reflex.* (B) Testing the *Achilles tendon reflex. Note:* If gloves are not worn during assessment, hand washing must be done before and after touching the patient.

For example, ***atropine*** is an antispasmodic that can be administered preoperatively to relax smooth muscles during surgery.

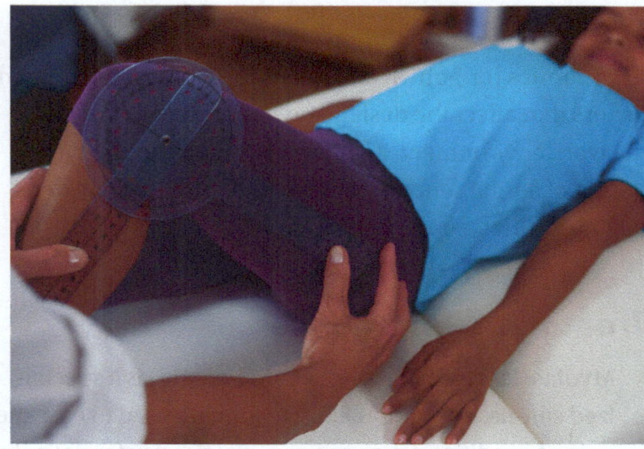

iStock.com/Wavebreakmedia

FIGURE 4.18 *Range-of-motion testing* uses a goniometer to evaluate joint mobility. The results are expressed in degrees.

- **Cortisone** (**KOR**-tih-sohn) is a **corticosteroid drug** injected to relieve pain and inflammation in a specific joint (see also Chapter 14).
- ***Anabolic steroids*** are used to replace muscle loss caused by disease and are sometimes used illegally by athletes and bodybuilders wanting to build muscle mass (see Chapter 14).
- A **muscle relaxant** is administered to relax certain muscles and to relieve the stiffness, pain, and discomfort caused by strains, sprains, or other muscle injuries. These medications act on the central nervous system and may have a negative interaction with alcohol and some antidepressants (see Chapter 11).
- **Neuromuscular-blocking drugs** cause temporary paralysis by blocking the transmission of nerve stimuli to the muscles. These drugs are used as an adjunct to anesthesia during surgery to cause skeletal muscles to relax. As used here, ***adjunct*** means in addition to.
- **Platelet-rich plasma therapy** (PRP) is a treatment in which some of the patient's own blood is separated to create a concentrated platelet-rich plasma. This is then injected into a joint such as the knee to promote healing and pain relief.
- **Viscosupplementation** uses direct injections of hyaluronic acid into the knee to increase the joint's viscous fluid, providing temporary relief from arthritis pain. They are sometimes referred to as ***chicken shots*** because the fluid is usually extracted from processed chicken or rooster combs.

Ergonomics

Ergonomics (er-goh-**NOM**-icks) is the study of the human factors that affect the design and operation of tools and the work environment. This term is usually applied to the design of equipment and workspaces, with the goal of reducing injuries, strain, and stress.

Treatment Techniques

- **Myofascial release** (**my**-oh-**FASH**-ee-ahl) is a specialized soft-tissue manipulation technique used to ease the pain of conditions such as fibromyalgia, myofascial pain syndrome, movement restrictions, temporomandibular joint (TMJ) disorders, and carpal tunnel syndrome.
- **Occupational therapy** (OT) consists of activities to promote recovery and rehabilitation to assist patients in performing **activities of daily living** (ADL). ADLs include grooming, eating, and dressing.
- **Physical therapy** (PT) is treatment to prevent disability or restore function through the use of exercise, heat, massage, or other techniques.
- **Therapeutic ultrasound** is a physical therapy technique that uses high-frequency sound waves to treat muscle injuries by generating heat deep within muscle tissue. This heat eases pain, reduces muscle spasms, and accelerates healing by increasing the flow of blood into the target tissues.
- **Transcutaneous electrical nerve stimulation** (TENS) is a method of pain control achieved by wearing a device that delivers small electrical impulses, as needed, to the nerve endings through the skin (**trans-** means across, **cutane** means skin, and **-ous** means pertaining to). These electrical impulses cause changes in muscles, such as numbness or contractions, which produce temporary pain relief. The term ***transcutaneous*** means performed through the unbroken skin.

RICE

The most common first aid treatment for soft tissue injuries is known by the acronym *RICE*. These letters stand for **R**est, **I**ce, **C**ompression, and **E**levation. Rest and ice are recommended for the first few days after the injury to ease pain. Compression, such as wrapping with a stretch bandage, and elevation help minimize swelling.

After the first few days, as the pain decreases, using heat, accompanied by stretching and light exercises, helps bring blood to the injured area to speed healing.

Fascia

- A **fasciotomy** (**fash**-ee-**OT**-oh-mee) is a surgical incision through the fascia to relieve tension or pressure (**fasci** means fascia, and **-otomy** means a surgical incision). Without this procedure, which is commonly used to treat compartment syndrome, the pressure causes a loss of circulation that damages the affected tissues.

Tendons

- **Tenodesis** (ten-**ODD**-eh-sis) is the surgical suturing of the end of a tendon to a bone (**ten/o** means tendon, and **-desis** means to bind or tie together). This technique is used to repair the biceps tendon in the shoulder. *Tenodesis* is the opposite of *tenolysis*.
- **Tenolysis** (ten-**OL**-ih-sis) is the release of a tendon from adhesions (**ten/o** means tendon, and **-lysis** means to set free). *Tenolysis* is the opposite of *tenodesis*.
- **Tenotomy** (ten-**OT**-ah-mee) is the surgical cutting of a tendon to provide release or allow lengthening. Examples of its use include correcting contraction deformities like clubfoot or strabismus (**ten** means tendon, and **-otomy** means surgical incision).

Muscles

- **Myorrhaphy** (my-**OR**-ah-fee) is the surgical suturing of a muscle (**my/o** means muscle, and **-rrhaphy** means surgical suturing).
- A **myotomy** (my-**OT**-oh-mee) is a surgical incision into a muscle (**my** means muscle, and **-otomy** means surgical incision).

ABBREVIATIONS RELATED TO THE MUSCULAR SYSTEM

Table 4.1 presents an overview of the abbreviations related to the terms introduced in this chapter. *Note:* To avoid errors or confusion, always be cautious when using abbreviations.

TABLE 4.1

Abbreviations Related to the Muscular System

activities of daily living = ADL	**ADL** = activities of daily living
carpal tunnel syndrome = CTS	**CTS** = carpal tunnel syndrome
chronic fatigue syndrome = CFS	**CFS** = chronic fatigue syndrome
electromyography = EMG	**EMG** = electromyography
intermittent claudication = IC	**IC** = intermittent claudication
muscular dystrophy = MD	**MD** = muscular dystrophy
myasthenia gravis = MG	**MG** = myasthenia gravis
occupational therapy, occupational therapist = OT	**OT** = occupational therapy, occupational therapist
polymyositis = PM	**PM** = polymyositis
repetitive stress disorder = RSD	**RSD** = repetitive stress disorder
range-of-motion testing = ROM	**ROM** = range-of-motion testing

CHAPTER 4

LEARNING EXERCISES

Matching Word Parts 1

Write the correct answer in the middle column.

	Definition	Correct Answer	Possible Answers
4.1.	abnormal condition	______________________	**-cele**
4.2.	fascia	______________________	**fasci/o**
4.3.	fibrous tissue	______________________	**fibr/o**
4.4.	hernia, swelling	______________________	**-ia**
4.5.	movement	______________________	**kines/o**, **kinesi/o**

Matching Word Parts 2

Write the correct answer in the middle column.

	Definition	Correct Answer	Possible Answers
4.6.	coordination	______________________	**my/o**
4.7.	muscle	______________________	**-rrhexis**
4.8.	rupture	______________________	**tax/o**
4.9.	tendon	______________________	**tend/o**
4.10.	tone	______________________	**ton/o**

Matching Muscle Directions and Positions

Write the correct answer in the middle column.

	Definition	Correct Answer	Possible Answers
4.11.	crosswise	______________________	lateralis
4.12.	ring-like	______________________	oblique

4.13. slanted at an angle ______________________ rectus

4.14. straight ______________________ sphincter

4.15. toward the side ______________________ transverse

Definitions

Select the correct answer, and write it on the line provided.

4.16. The ______________________ muscles are under voluntary control.

involuntary unstriated skeletal visceral

4.17. A/An ______________________ is a calcium deposit in the plantar fascia near its attachment to the calcaneus bone.

heel spur impingement syndrome overuse injury shin splint

4.18. Turning the hand so the palm is upward is called ______________________.

extension flexion pronation supination

4.19. One of the symptoms of Parkinson's disease is ______________________, which is extreme slowness of movement.

bradykinesia dyskinesia hypotonia hyperactivity

4.20. A/An ______________________ is a specialist who develops, implements, and coordinates exercise programs and administers medical tests to promote physical fitness.

neurologist physiatrist physiologist physical therapist

4.21. The term ______________________ means pertaining to muscle tissue and fascia.

aponeurosis fibrous sheath myocardium myofascial

4.22. A/An ______________________ is a narrow band of nonelastic, fibrous connective tissue that attaches a muscle to a bone.

aponeurosis fascia ligament tendon

4.23. A band of fibers that holds structures together abnormally is a/an ______________________. These bands can form as the result of an injury or surgery.

adhesion aponeurosis atrophy contracture

4.24. The paralysis of both legs and the lower part of the body is known as ______________.

hemiparesis | hemiplegia | paraplegia | quadriplegia

4.25. The surgical suturing of the end of a tendon to a bone is known as ______________.

tenodesis | tenotomy | tendinosis | tenolysis

Matching Structures

Write the correct answer in the middle column.

	Definition	Correct Answer	Possible Answers
4.26.	heart muscle	______________	gluteus maximus
4.27.	buttock muscle	______________	myocardial
4.28.	fibrous connective tissue	______________	sphincter
4.29.	muscular cap of shoulder	______________	tendon
4.30.	ring-like muscle	______________	deltoid

Which Word?

Select the correct answer, and write it on the line provided.

4.31. An injury to the body of the muscle or the attachment of a tendon is known as a ______________. These are usually associated with overuse injuries that involve a wrenched or torn muscle or tendon attachment.

sprain | strain

4.32. The ______________ muscles are named for their location toward the outer side of the body.

lateralis | medialis

4.33. The condition of abnormal muscle tone that causes the impairment of voluntary muscle movement is known as ______________.

ataxia | dystonia

4.34. Inflamed and swollen tendons caught in the narrow space between the bones within the shoulder joint cause the condition known as ______________.

impingement syndrome | intermittent claudication

4.35. The ______________ forms the muscular cap of the shoulder.

triceps brachii   deltoid

Spelling Counts

Find the misspelled word in each sentence. Then write that word, spelled correctly, on the line provided.

4.36. An antispasmydic is administered to suppress smooth muscle contractions of the stomach, intestine, or bladder. ______________

4.37. A physiaitrist is a physician who specializes in physical medicine and rehabilitation. ______________

4.38. Myasthenia gravus is a chronic autoimmune disease that affects the neuromuscular junction and produces serious weakness of voluntary muscles. ______________

4.39. A ganglian cyst is a harmless, fluid-filled swelling that occurs most commonly on the outer surface of the wrist. ______________

4.40. Pronetion is the movement that turns the palm of the hand downward or backward. ______________

Abbreviation Identification

Write the correct answer on the line provided.

4.41. **CFS** ______________

4.42. **DTRs** ______________

4.43. **ROM** ______________

4.44. **RSD** ______________

4.45. **SCI** ______________

Term Selection

Select the correct answer, and write it on the line provided.

4.46. ______________ is the stimulation of a muscle by an impulse transmitted by a motor nerve.

Abduction   Innervation   Adduction   Contracture

4.47. The term meaning a weakness or slight muscular paralysis is ______________.

myoclonus   hemiplegia   hypotonia   myoparesis

4.48. The term ________________ means abnormally increased muscle function or activity.

hyperkinesia hypertonia dyskinesia hypotonia

4.49. A/An ________________ injury can be a strain or tear on any of the three muscles that straighten the hip and bend the knee.

Achilles tendon hamstring myofascial shin splint

4.50. A ________________ muscle is named for its shape or size.

pectoralis major triceps brachii gluteus maximus sphincter

Sentence Completion

Write the correct term or terms on the lines provided.

4.51. An inflammation of the tissues surrounding the elbow is known as ________________.

4.52. The movement during which the knees or elbows are bent to decrease the angle of the joints is known as ________________.

4.53. Pain in the leg muscles that occurs during exercise and is relieved by rest is known as ________________. This condition is due to poor circulation and is associated with peripheral vascular disease.

4.54. A weakness or slight muscular paralysis is known as ________________.

4.55. A stiff neck due to spasmodic contraction of the neck muscles that pull the head toward the affected side is known as ________________, or wryneck.

Word Surgery

Divide each term into its component word parts. Write these word parts, in sequence, on the lines provided. When necessary, use a slash (/) to indicate a combining vowel. (You may not need all of the lines provided.)

4.56. **Electromyography** is a diagnostic test that measures the electrical activity within muscle fibers.

________ ________ ________ ________

4.57. **Hyperkinesia** means abnormally increased muscle function or activity.

________ ________ ________ ________

4.58. **Myoclonus** is the sudden, involuntary jerking of a muscle or group of muscles.

_____________ _____________ _____________ _____________

4.59. **Polymyositis** is a muscle disease characterized by the simultaneous inflammation and weakening of voluntary muscles in many parts of the body.

_____________ _____________ _____________ _____________

4.60. **Sarcopenia** is the loss of muscle mass, strength, and function that comes with aging.

_____________ _____________ _____________ _____________

True/False

If the statement is true, write **True** on the line. If the statement is false, write **False** on the line.

4.61. _______ Overuse tendinitis is inflammation of tendons caused by excessive or unusual use of a joint.

4.62. _______ Hemiplegia is the total paralysis of the lower half of the body.

4.63. _______ A spasm is a sudden, involuntary contraction of one or more muscles.

4.64. _______ Ataxia is the distortion of voluntary movement such as in a tic or spasm.

4.65. _______ Myocardial muscles are located in the walls of internal organs such as the digestive tract, blood vessels, and ducts leading from glands.

Clinical Conditions

Write the correct answer on the line provided.

4.66. George Quinton developed a swelling on the outer surface of his wrist. His doctor diagnosed this as being a/an ____________________ and explained that this was a harmless, fluid-filled swelling.

4.67. Raul Valladares has a protrusion of a muscle substance through a tear in the fascia surrounding it. This condition is known as a/an ____________________.

4.68. Louisa Ferraro experienced ____________________ of her leg muscles due to the disuse of these muscles over a long period of time.

4.69. Jasmine Franklin has ____________________. This is a condition in which there is diminished tone of the skeletal muscles.

4.70. Carolyn Goodwin complained of profound fatigue that is not improved by bed rest and was made worse by physical or mental activity. After ruling out other causes, her physician diagnosed her condition as being ______________________ syndrome.

4.71. Chuan Lee, who is a runner, required treatment for ______________________. This condition is a painful inflammation of the Achilles tendon caused by excessive stress being placed on that tendon.

4.72. For the first several days after his fall, Bob Hill suffered severe muscle pain. This condition is known as ______________________.

4.73. Jorge Guendulay could not play for his team because of a/an ______________________. This is a painful condition caused by the muscle tearing away from the tibia.

4.74. Due to a spinal cord injury, Marissa Giannati suffers from ______________________, which is paralysis of all four limbs.

4.75. Duncan McDougle has slight paralysis on one side of his body. This condition, which was caused by a stroke, is known as ______________________.

Which Is the Correct Medical Term?

Select the correct answer, and write it on the line provided.

4.76. The term *muscular* ______________________ describes a group of genetic diseases characterized by progressive weakness and degeneration of the skeletal muscles.

atonic | ataxia | dystonia | dystrophy

4.77. The surgical enlargement of the carpal tunnel or cutting of the carpal ligament to relieve nerve pressure is called ______________________.

carpal tunnel syndrome | compartment syndrome | carpal tunnel release | rhabdomyolysis

4.78. During ______________________, the arm moves inward and toward the side of the body.

abduction | adduction | circumduction | rotation

4.79. A surgical incision into a muscle is known as ______________________.

myoclonus | myorrhaphy | myotomy | myoparesis

4.80. The term ______________________ means bending the foot upward at the ankle.

abduction | dorsiflexion | elevation | plantar flexion

Challenge Word Building

These terms are *not* primary terms in the chapter; however, they are made up of the following familiar word parts. If you need help in creating the term, refer to your medical dictionary.

poly-	**card/o**	**-algia**
	fasci/o	**-desis**
	herni/o	**-ectomy**
	my/o	**-itis**
	sphincter/o	**-necrosis**
		-otomy
		-pathy
		-rrhaphy

4.81. Any abnormal condition of skeletal muscles is known as ______________________.

4.82. Pain in several muscle groups is known as ______________________.

4.83. The death of individual muscle fibers is known as ______________________.

4.84. Surgical suturing of torn fascia is known as ______________________.

4.85. The removal of multiple muscles is known as ______________________.

4.86. The surgical attachment of a fascia to another fascia or to a tendon is known as

______________________.

4.87. Inflammation of the muscle of the heart is known as ______________________.

4.88. The surgical removal of fascia is a/an ______________________.

4.89. The surgical suturing of a defect in a muscular wall, such as the repair of a hernia, is a/an

______________________.

4.90. An incision into a sphincter muscle is a/an ______________________.

Labeling Exercises

Identify the movements in the accompanying figures by writing the correct term on the line provided.

4.91. ____________________

4.92. ____________________

4.93. ____________________

4.94. ____________________

4.95. ____________________

4.96. ____________________

4.97. ____________________

4.98. ____________________

4.99. ____________________

4.100. ____________________

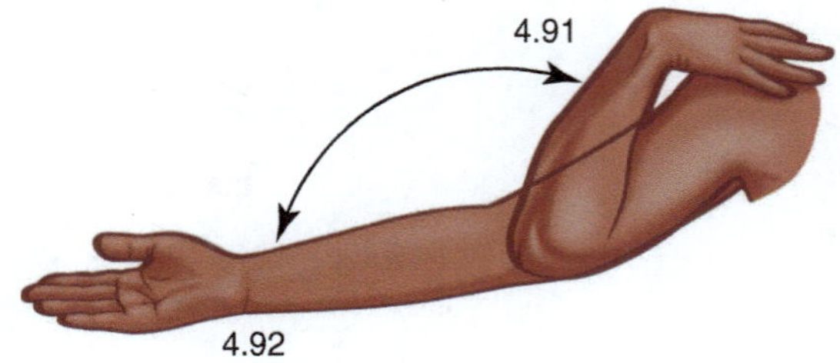

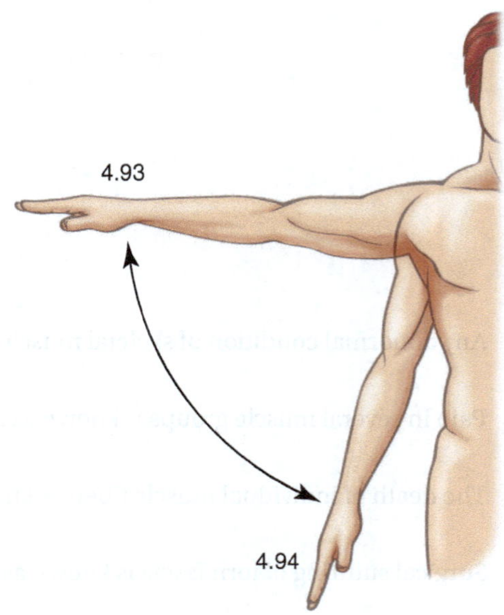

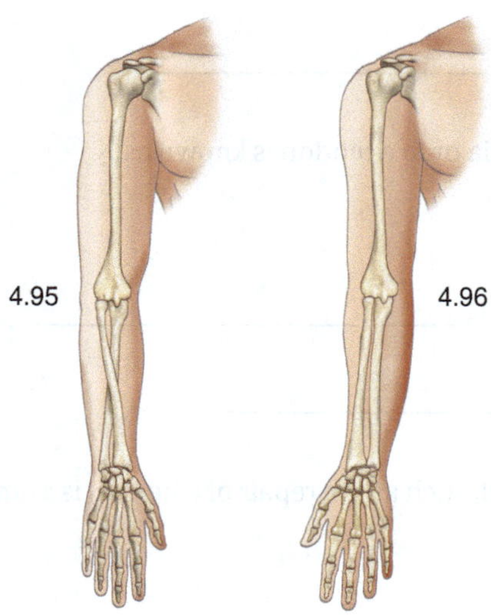

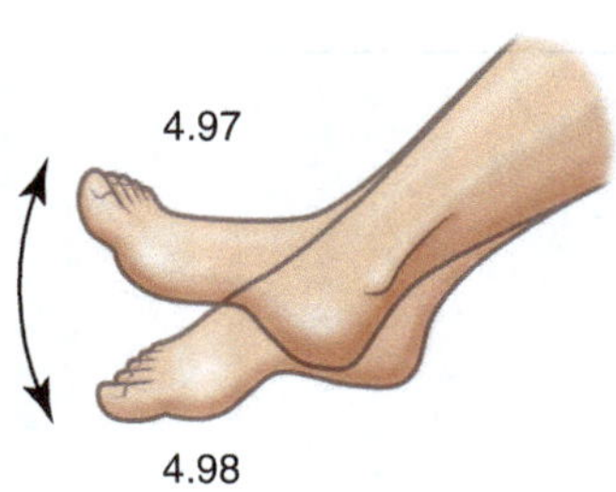

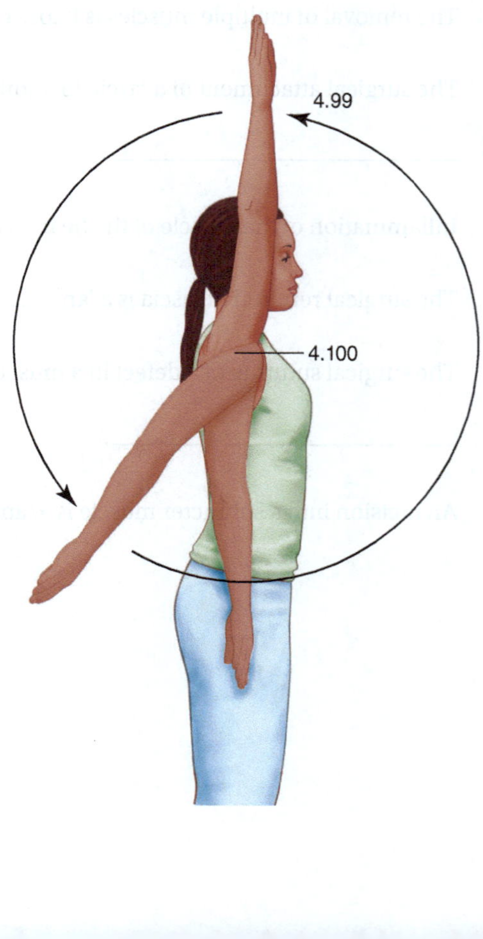

The Human Touch

CRITICAL THINKING EXERCISE

The following story and questions are designed to stimulate critical thinking through class discussion or as a brief essay response. There are no right or wrong answers to these questions.

"Leg muscles save back muscles ... Mandatory OSHA meeting Tuesday at noon. Bring lunch," states the company memo. Sandor Padilla, a 28-year-old cargo loader, sighs, "Third meeting this year, and it's not even June yet!" He has only two minutes to reach the tarmac. "Oh well, cargo waits for no man," he thinks as he jogs off to work.

Sandor enjoys his job. It keeps him fit but lets his mind follow more creative avenues. Today, his thoughts stray to his daughter Reina's fifth birthday party, just two weeks away. "A pony or a clown? Hot dogs or tacos?" he muses. Single parenting has its moments. As he is busy thinking of other things, the heavy crate slips, driving him into a squatting position that injures his thigh muscles. His cry of pain brings Janet Wilson, his supervisor, running to help.

The first aid station ices his leg to reduce swelling and pain. After the supervisor completes the incident report, Sandor is taken to the emergency room. Dr. Basra, the orthopedic specialist on call, diagnoses a tendon strain resulting in a torn left rectus femoris. A myorrhaphy is required to treat this injury. After several days in the hospital, Sandor is sent home with a Vicodin prescription for pain and orders for physical therapy sessions three times a week. He is not expected to return to work for at least 90 days.

AirFreight Systems receives the first report of injury and compares it with the supervisor's incident report. Ruling: Safety Violation. No Liability. Return to work in 30 days or dismissal.

Suggested Discussion Topics

1. On what basis do you think AirFreight determined that this was a safety violation?
2. Use lay terms to explain Sandor's injury and the treatment that was required.
3. Sandor knows how to handle heavy loads safely; however, the crate may have slipped because he was busy thinking about his daughter's birthday party and not about his work. Could the responsibility for this accident be considered negligence on Sandor's part? Do you think Sandor should be held responsible or is blameless in this situation?
4. It was determined that AirFreight was not responsible for the accident. Therefore, do you think the company should take away Sandor's job if he does not return in 30 calendar days?

CHAPTER 5

THE CARDIOVASCULAR SYSTEM

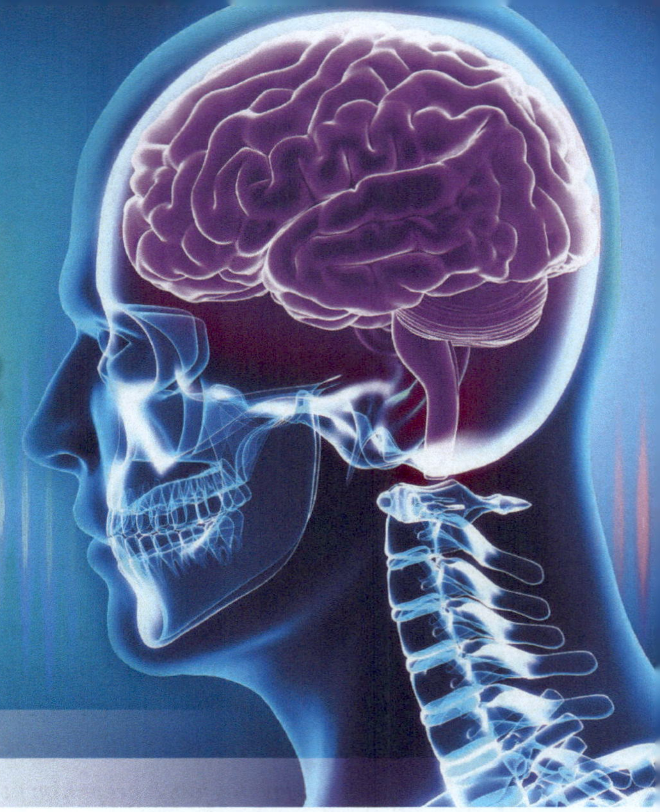

Overview of

STRUCTURES, COMBINING FORMS, AND FUNCTIONS OF THE CARDIOVASCULAR SYSTEM

Major Structures	Related Combining Forms	Primary Functions
Heart	**card/o**, **cardi/o**	Receives blood from the veins and pumps blood into the arteries.
Blood Vessels	**angi/o**, **vas/o**	Transport blood to and from all areas of the body.
Arteries	**arteri/o**	Transport blood away from the heart to all parts of the body.
Capillaries	**capill/o**	Permit the exchange of nutrients and waste products between the blood and the cells.
Veins	**phleb/o**, **ven/o**	Return blood from all body parts to the heart.
Blood	**hem/o**, **hemat/o**	Brings oxygen and nutrients to the cells and carries away waste.

Vocabulary Related to **THE CARDIOVASCULAR SYSTEM**

This list contains essential word parts and medical terms for this chapter. These and the other important **primary terms** are shown in **boldface** throughout the chapter. *Secondary terms*, which appear in *orange* italics, clarify the meaning of primary terms.

Word Parts

- ☐ **angi/o** blood or lymph vessels
- ☐ **aort/o** aorta
- ☐ **arteri/o** artery
- ☐ **ather/o** plaque, fatty substance
- ☐ **brady-** slow
- ☐ **capill/o** capillary
- ☐ **cardi/o** heart
- ☐ **end/o** within
- ☐ **hem/o**, **hemat/o** blood, relating to the blood
- ☐ **peri-** surrounding
- ☐ **phleb/o** vein
- ☐ **-sclerosis** abnormal hardening
- ☐ **tachy-** fast, rapid
- ☐ **thromb/o** clot
- ☐ **ven/o** vein

Medical Terms

- ☐ **ACE inhibitor**
- ☐ **anemia** (ah-**NEE**-mee-ah)
- ☐ **aneurysm** (**AN**-you-rizm)
- ☐ **angina** (an-**JIGH**-nuh)
- ☐ **angioplasty** (**AN**-jee-oh-**plas**-tee)
- ☐ **anticoagulant** (**an**-tih-koh-**AG**-you-lant)
- ☐ **aorta** (ay-**OR**-tah)
- ☐ **aortic stenosis** (ay-**OR**-tick steh-**NOH**-sis)
- ☐ **arrhythmia** (ah-**RITH**-mee-ah)
- ☐ **atherectomy** (**ath**-er-**ECK**-toh-mee)
- ☐ **atherosclerosis** (**ah**-theh-roh-skleh-**ROH**-sis)
- ☐ **atrial fibrillation** (**AY**-tree-al **fih**-brih-**LAY**-shun)
- ☐ **automated external defibrillator** (dee-**FIB**-rih-**lay**-ter)
- ☐ **beta-blocker** (BAY-tah-**blok**-er)
- ☐ **bradycardia** (**brad**-ee-**KAR**-dee-ah)
- ☐ **capillaries** (**KAP**-uh-**ler**-eez)
- ☐ **cardiac arrest**
- ☐ **cardiac catheterization** (**KAR**-dee-ack **kath**-eh-ter-eye-**ZAY**-shun)
- ☐ **cardiomyopathy** (**kar**-dee-oh-my-**OP**-ah-thee)
- ☐ **carotid endarterectomy** (kah-**ROT**-id **end**-ar-ter-**ECK**-toh-mee)
- ☐ **cholesterol** (koh-**LES**-ter-ol)
- ☐ **chronic venous insufficiency**
- ☐ **coronary artery disease**
- ☐ **coronary thrombosis** (**KOR**-uh-**nerr**-ee throm-**BOH**-sis)
- ☐ **defibrillation** (dee-**fih**-brih-**LAY**-shun)
- ☐ **diastole** (dye-**AS**-toh-lee)
- ☐ **diuretic** (**dye**-you-**RET**-ick)
- ☐ **electrocardiogram** (ee-**leck**-troh-**KAR**-dee-oh-**gram**)
- ☐ **electrophysiologist** (eh-**LEK**-troh-**fiz**-ee-ol-oh-jist)
- ☐ **embolism** (**EM**-boh-lizm)
- ☐ **embolus** (**EM**-boh-lus)
- ☐ **endocarditis** (**en**-doh-kar-**DYE**-tis)
- ☐ **erythrocytes** (eh-**RITH**-roh-sights)
- ☐ **heart murmur**
- ☐ **hemoglobin** (**HEE**-moh-**gloh**-bin)
- ☐ **hypertension**
- ☐ **hypoperfusion** (**high**-poh-per-**FYOU**-zhun)
- ☐ **ischemia** (iss-**KEE**-mee-ah)
- ☐ **long QT syndrome**
- ☐ **mitral valve prolapse** (**MY**-tral **VALV** proh-**LAPS**)
- ☐ **myocardial infarction** (**my**-oh-**KAR**-dee-**al** in-**FARK**-shun)
- ☐ **orthostatic hypotension** (**or**-thoh-**STAT**-ick **high**-poh-**TEN**-shun)
- ☐ **pericardium** (**pehr**-ih-**KAR**-dee-um)
- ☐ **peripheral artery disease**
- ☐ **phlebitis** (fleh-**BYE**-tis)
- ☐ **Raynaud's disease** (ray-**NOHZ**)
- ☐ **sinoatrial node** (**sigh**-noh-**AY**-tree-ahl)
- ☐ **systole** (**SIS**-toh-lee)
- ☐ **tachycardia** (**tack**-ee-**KAR**-dee-ah)
- ☐ **telemetry nurse** (teh-**LEM**-eh-tree)
- ☐ **temporal arteritis** (**TEM**-poh-**ral ar**-teh-**RYE**-tis)
- ☐ **thallium stress test** (**THAL**-ee-um)
- ☐ **thrombolytic** (**throm**-boh-**LIT**-ick)
- ☐ **thrombosis** (throm-**BOH**-sis)
- ☐ **thrombotic occlusion** (throm-**BOT**-ick ah-**KLOO**-zhun)
- ☐ **thrombus** (**THROM**-bus)
- ☐ **varicose veins** (**VAHR**-ih-**kohs VAYNS**)
- ☐ **venous thromboembolism**
- ☐ **ventricular fibrillation** (ven-**TRICK**-you-lar **fih**-brih-**LAY**-shun)
- ☐ **ventricular tachycardia** (ven-**TRICK**-you-lar **tack**-ee-**KAR**-dee-ah)

LEARNING OBJECTIVES

On completion of this chapter, you should be able to:

1. Describe the heart in terms of chambers, valves, blood flow, heartbeat, and blood supply.
2. State the difference between the systemic and pulmonary circulation.
3. Describe the cardiac cycle.
4. Differentiate among the three different types of blood vessels.
5. Describe the major functions of the three types of blood vessels.
6. Describe the basic components of blood.
7. Identify the medical specialists who treat disorders of the cardiovascular system.
8. Identify medical word parts of the cardiovascular system.
9. Define the primary terms related to the pathology and the diagnostic and treatment procedures of the cardiovascular system.
10. Describe the types of cardiac arrhythmia.
11. Spell the primary terms related to the cardiovascular system.
12. Pronounce the primary terms of the cardiovascular system.
13. Identify common abbreviations related to the cardiovascular system.

FUNCTIONS OF THE CARDIOVASCULAR SYSTEM

The cardiovascular system consists of the heart, blood vessels, and blood. **Cardiovascular** (**kar**-dee-oh-**VAS**-kyou-lar) means pertaining to the heart and blood vessels (**cardi/o** means heart, **vascul** means blood vessels, and **-ar** means pertaining to).

These structures work together to efficiently pump blood to all body tissues.

- Blood is a fluid tissue that transports oxygen and nutrients to the body tissues.
- Blood returns some waste products from these tissues to the kidneys and carries carbon dioxide back to the lungs.
- Blood cells also play important roles in the immune system (see Chapter 7), and in the endocrine system (see Chapter 14).
- See Chapter 6 for more information about the blood system.

STRUCTURES OF THE CARDIOVASCULAR SYSTEM

The major structures of the cardiovascular system are the heart, blood vessels, and blood.

The Heart

The **heart** is a hollow, muscular organ located in the thoracic cavity, between the lungs (Figure 5.1). This small organ, about the size of a fist, is a very effective pump that furnishes the power to maintain the blood flow needed throughout the entire body (Figures 5.2 and 5.3). The ***apex*** is the lower tip of the heart.

The Pericardium

The **pericardium** (**pehr**-ih-**KAR**-dee-um), also known as the ***pericardial sac***, is the double-walled membranous sac that encloses the heart (**peri-** means surrounding, **cardi** means heart, and **-um** is a singular noun ending). ***Membranous*** means pertaining to membrane, which is a thin layer of pliable tissue that covers or encloses a body part.

- The ***parietal pericardium*** is a fibrous sac that surrounds and protects the heart.
- ***Pericardial fluid*** is found between these two layers, where it acts as a lubricant to prevent friction as the heart beats.
- The ***visceral pericardium*** is the inner layer of the pericardium that also forms the outer layer of the heart. When referred to as the outer layer of the heart, it is known as the *epicardium* (Figure 5.4).

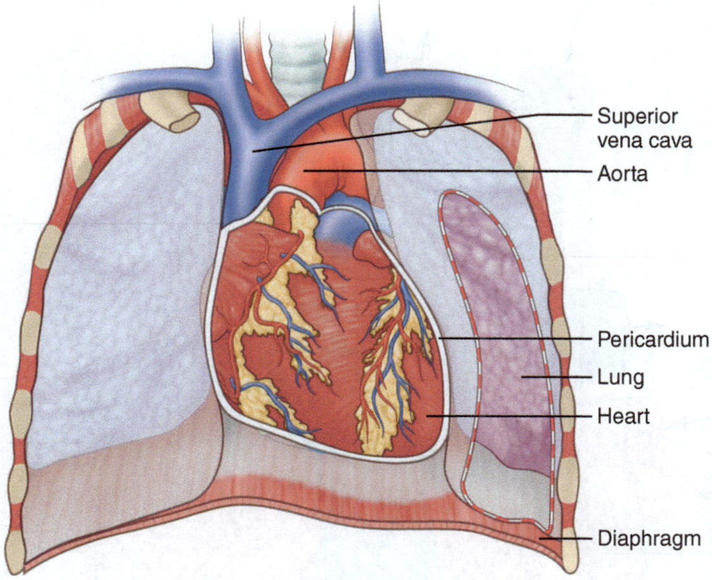

FIGURE 5.1 The heart is located in the thoracic cavity between the lungs.

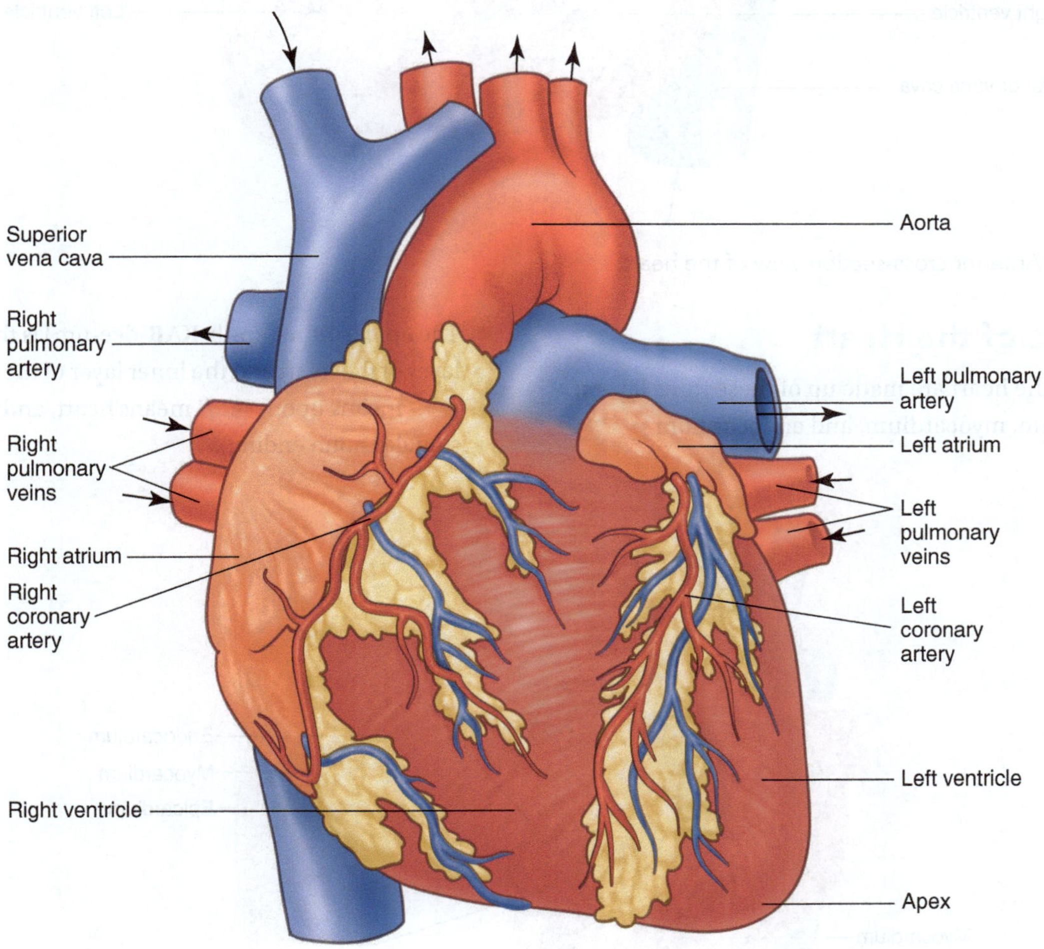

FIGURE 5.2 Anterior external view of the heart.

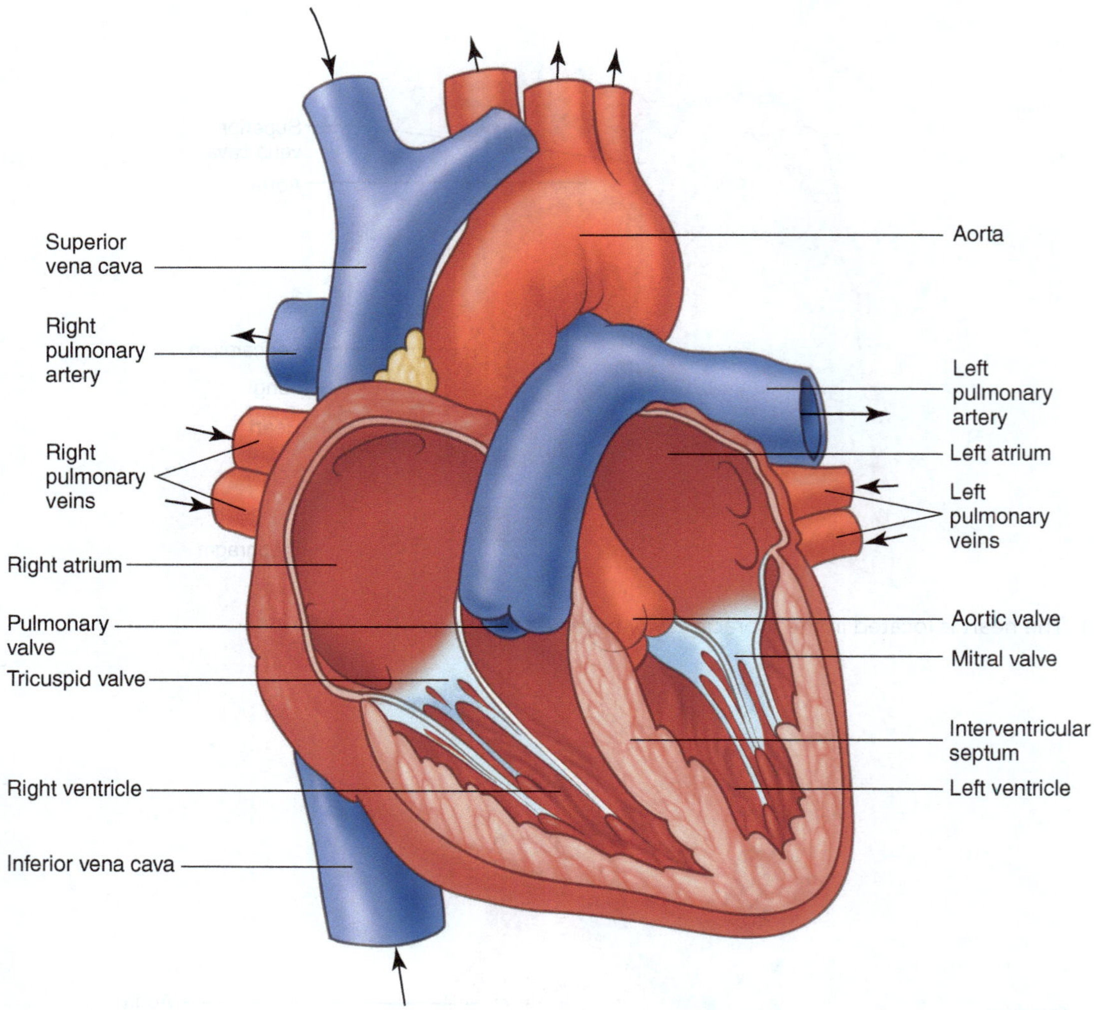

FIGURE 5.3 Anterior cross-section view of the heart.

The Walls of the Heart

The walls of the heart are made up of these three layers: the epicardium, myocardium, and endocardium (Figure 5.4).

- The **epicardium** (**ep**-ih-**KAR**-dee-um) is the external layer of the heart and the inner layer of the pericardium (**epi-** means upon, **cardi** means heart, and **-um** is a singular noun ending).

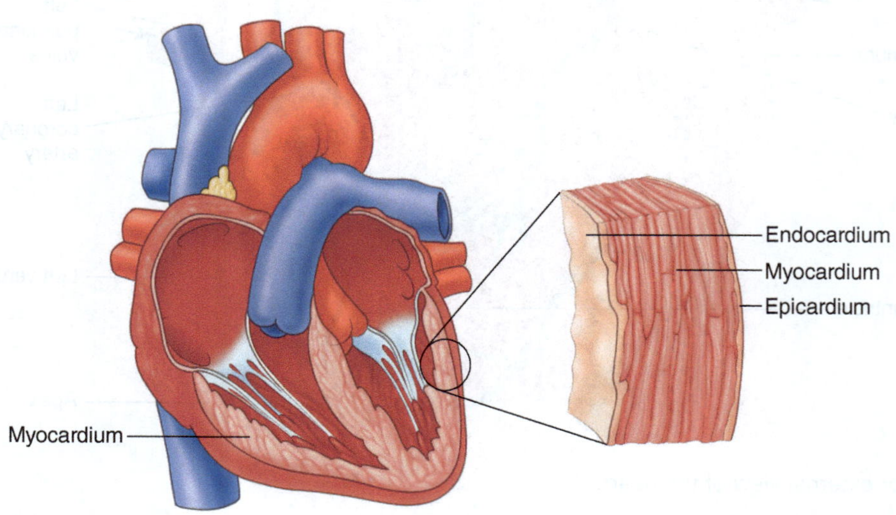

FIGURE 5.4 A simplified view of the tissues of the heart walls.

- The **myocardium** (my-oh-**KAR**-dee-um) is the middle and thickest of the heart's three layers (**my/o** means muscle, **cardi** means heart, and **-um** is a singular noun ending). Also known as ***myocardial muscle***, this consists of specialized cardiac muscle tissue that is capable of the constant contraction and relaxation that creates the pumping movement necessary to maintain the flow of blood throughout the body. Myocardial muscle is discussed in Chapter 4.
- The **endocardium** (en-doh-**KAR**-dee-um), which consists of epithelial tissue, is the inner lining of the heart (**endo-** means within, **cardi** means heart, and **-um** is a singular noun ending). This is the surface that comes into direct contact with the blood as it is being pumped through the heart.

Blood Supply to the Myocardium

The myocardium, which beats constantly, must have a continuous supply of oxygen and nutrients plus prompt waste removal to survive. If for any reason this blood supply is disrupted, the myocardium of the affected area dies.

- The **coronary arteries** (**KOR**-uh-**nerr**-ee), which supply oxygen-rich blood to the myocardium, are shown in red in Figure 5.6 (**coron** means crown, and **-ary** means pertaining to). The veins, which are shown in blue, remove waste products from the myocardium. The term ***coronary*** originates from the Latin word for crown, because these arteries encircle the heart. This is also the etymology of the name *coronavirus*, the type of virus with crown-like spikes on its surface that is the cause of COVID-19.

The Chambers of the Heart

The heart is divided into four chambers, each of which has a specialized function (Figure 5.3):

- The **atria** (**AY**-tree-ah) are the two upper chambers of the heart, and these chambers are divided by the ***interatrial septum***. A ***septum*** is a wall that separates two chambers.
- The atria are the receiving chambers, and all blood enters the heart through these chambers. The singular form of *atria* is *atrium.*
- The **ventricles** (**VEN**-trih-kuhls) are the two lower chambers of the heart, and these chambers are divided by the ***interventricular septum***.
- The walls of the ventricles are thicker than those of the atria because the ventricles must pump blood throughout the entire body.

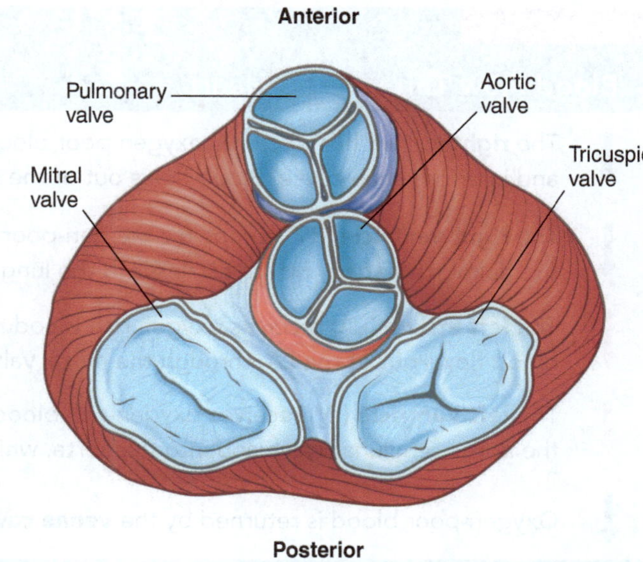

FIGURE 5.5 The valves of the heart viewed from above with the atria removed.

- The term ***ventricle*** is also defined as a normal hollow chamber of the brain (see Chapter 11).

The Valves of the Heart

The flow of blood through the heart is controlled by four valves as described in this section. If any of these valves are not working correctly, blood cannot flow properly through the heart and cannot be pumped effectively to all parts of the body (Figures 5.3 and 5.5).

- The **tricuspid valve** (try-**KUS**-pid) controls the opening between the right atrium and the right ventricle. The term ***tricuspid*** means having three cusps (points), and this describes the shape of this valve.
- The **pulmonary valve** (**PULL**-mah-**nair**-ee) is located between the right ventricle and the pulmonary artery. ***Pulmonary*** means pertaining to the lungs.
- The **mitral valve** (**MY**-tral) is located between the left atrium and left ventricle. ***Mitral*** means shaped like a bishop's mitre (hat). This valve is also known as the ***bicuspid valve*** because ***bicuspid*** means having two cusps (points), which describes the shape of this valve.
- The **aortic valve** (ay-**OR**-tick) is located between the left ventricle and the aorta (**aort** means aorta, and **-ic** means pertaining to).
- The flow of blood through the heart is summarized in Table 5.1. The red arrows indicate oxygenated blood, and blue arrows indicate deoxygenated blood. ***Oxygenated*** means oxygen rich, or containing an adequate supply of oxygen. ***Deoxygenated*** means oxygen poor, or not yet containing an adequate supply of oxygen.

TABLE 5.1

Blood Flow Through the Heart

↓ The **right atrium** (RA) receives oxygen-poor blood from all tissues, except the lungs, through the superior and inferior venae cavae. Blood flows out of the RA through the tricuspid valve into the right ventricle.
↓ The **right ventricle** (RV) pumps the oxygen-poor blood through the pulmonary semilunar valve and into the pulmonary artery, which carries it to the lungs.
↓ The **left atrium** (LA) receives oxygen-rich blood from the lungs through the four pulmonary veins. The blood flows out of the LA, through the mitral valve, and into the left ventricle.
↓ The **left ventricle** (LV) receives oxygen-rich blood from the left atrium. Blood flows out of the LV through the aortic semilunar valve and into the aorta, which carries it to all parts of the body, except the lungs.
↓ Oxygen-poor blood is returned by the **venae cavae** to the right atrium, and the cycle continues.

Systemic and Pulmonary Circulation

Blood is pumped through the systemic and pulmonary circulation systems. Together, the blood in these systems brings oxygen to the cells and removes waste products from the cells (Figure 5.6).

Pulmonary circulation is the flow of blood only between the heart and lungs.

- The **pulmonary arteries** carry deoxygenated blood out of the right ventricle and into the lungs. This is the only place in the body where deoxygenated blood is carried by arteries instead of veins.
- In the lungs, carbon dioxide from the body is exchanged for oxygen from the inhaled air.
- The **pulmonary veins** carry the oxygenated blood from the lungs into the left atrium of the heart. This is the only place in the body where veins carry oxygenated blood.

Systemic circulation includes the flow of blood to all parts of the body *except* the lungs.

- Oxygenated blood flows out of the left ventricle and into arterial circulation.
- The veins carry deoxygenated blood into the right atrium.
- From here, the blood flows into the pulmonary circulation before being pumped out of the heart into the arteries again.

The Heartbeat

The **heartbeat** is the ability to pump blood effectively throughout the body; the contraction and relaxation (beating) of the heart must occur in exactly the correct sequence.

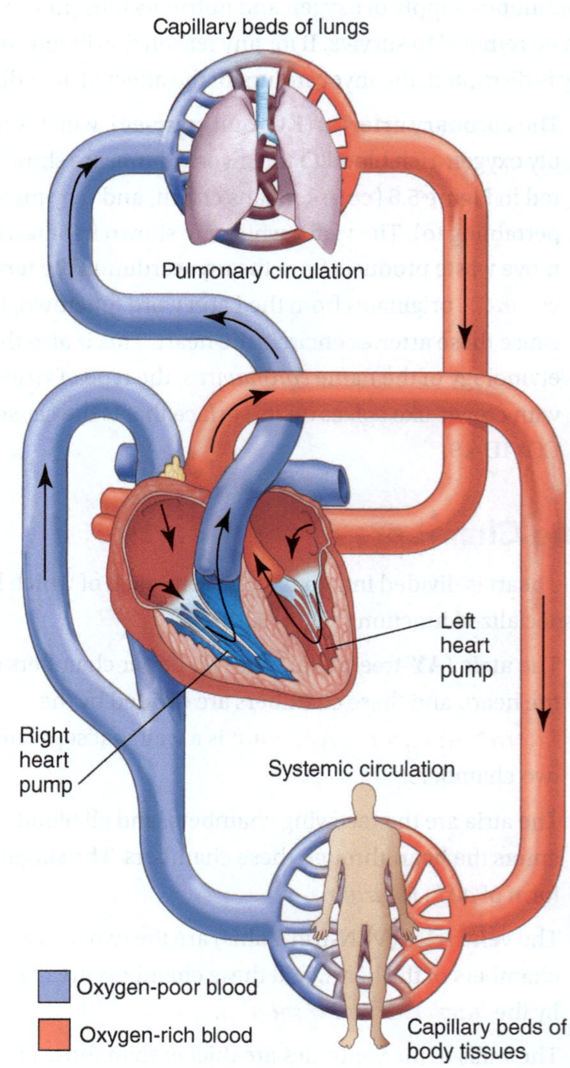

FIGURE 5.6 Systemic and pulmonary blood circulation.

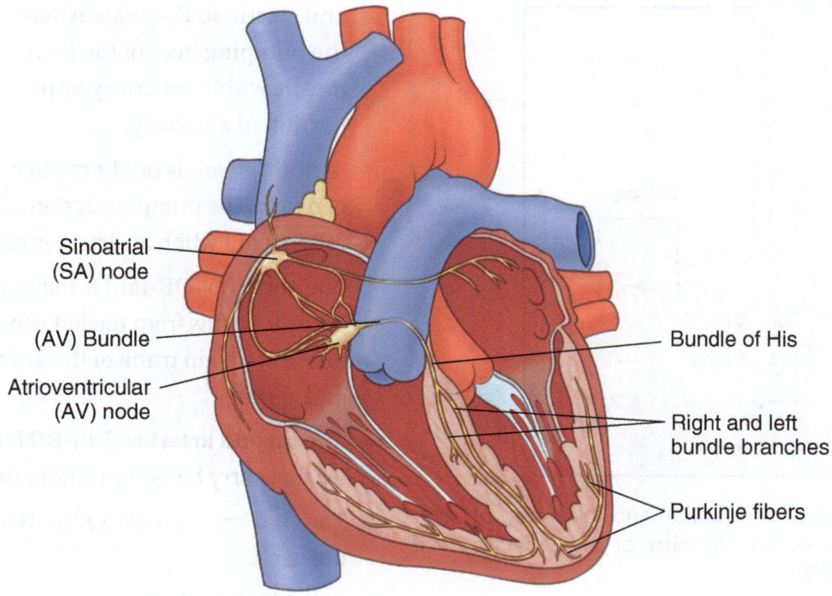

FIGURE 5.7 An electrical impulse from the SA node travels to the AV node and causes the ventricle to contract.

- The rate and regularity of the heartbeat is determined by ***electrical impulses*** from nerves that stimulate the myocardium of the chambers of the heart.
- The specialized myocardial muscles that make this pumping action possible are described in Chapter 4.
- Also known as the ***conduction system***, these electrical impulses are controlled by the sinoatrial (SA) node, atrioventricular (AV) node, and bundle of His (Figure 5.7).

The Sinoatrial Node

- The **sinoatrial** (SA) **node** (**sigh**-noh-**AY**-tree-ahl) is located in the posterior wall of the right atrium near the entrance of the superior vena cava (Figure 5.7).
- The SA node establishes the basic rhythm and rate of the heartbeat. For this reason, it is known as the ***natural pacemaker*** of the heart.
- Electrical impulses from the SA node start each wave of muscle contraction in the heart.
- The impulse in the right atrium spreads over the muscles of both atria, causing them to contract simultaneously. This contraction forces blood into the ventricles.

The Atrioventricular Node

- The impulses from the SA node also travel to the **atrioventricular** (AV) **node** (**ay-tree-oh-ven-TRICK-you-lar**).
- The AV node is located on the floor of the right atrium near the interatrial septum (Figure 5.7). From here, it transmits the electrical impulses onward to the bundle of His.

The Bundle of His

- The **bundle of His** (**HISS**) is a group of fibers located within the interventricular septum. These fibers carry an electrical impulse to ensure the sequence of the heart contractions (Figure 5.7). These electrical impulses travel onward to the right and left ventricles and the Purkinje fibers. It is named after German cardiologist Wilhelm His.
- **Purkinje fibers** (per-**KIN**-jee) are specialized conductive fibers located within the walls of the ventricles. These fibers, named for Czech physiologist Jan Purkinje, relay the electrical impulses to the cells of the ventricles, and it is this stimulation that causes the ventricles to contract. This contraction of the ventricles forces blood out of the heart and into the aorta and pulmonary arteries (Figure 5.7).

Electrical Waves

The activities of the electrical conduction system of the heart can be visualized as wave movements on a monitor or as an *electrocardiogram* (EKG or ECG). The term ***sinus rhythm*** refers to the normal beating of the heart (Figures 5.8 and 5.15A).

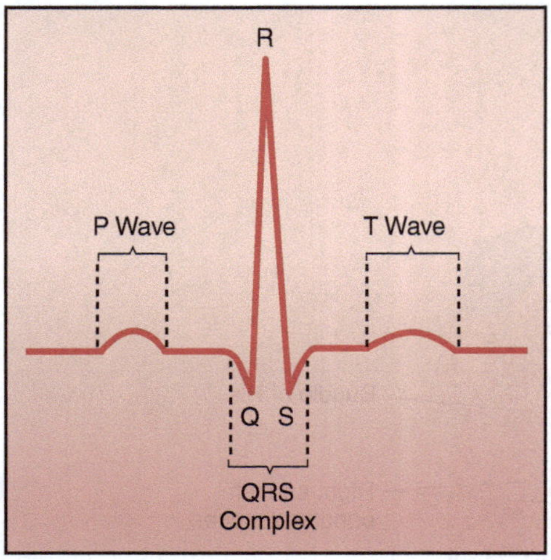

FIGURE 5.8 The waves of contraction and relaxation of the heart can be visualized on a monitor or as an electrocardiogram (EKG or ECG).

- The ***P wave*** is due to the stimulation (contraction) of the atria.
- The ***QRS complex*** shows the stimulation (contraction) of the ventricles. The atria relax as the ventricles contract.
- The ***T wave*** is the recovery (relaxation) of the ventricles.

The Cardiac Cycle

The **cardiac cycle** is one complete heartbeat, during which deoxygenated blood is converted to oxygenated blood in the lungs and pumped by the heart to the body. It is made up of two phases:

- **Systole** (**SIS**-toh-lee) is the period of contraction that the ventricles undergo while pumping blood into the aorta and the pulmonary artery. This is also referred to as the ***systolic phase***.
- **Diastole** (dye-**AS**-toh-lee) is the period of relaxation that follows as the chambers refill with blood. This is also referred to as the ***diastolic phase***.

THE BLOOD VESSELS

There are three types of blood vessels: arteries, capillaries, and veins. These vessels form the arterial and venous circulatory systems (Figures 5.9 and 5.10).

Arteries

- The **arteries** are large blood vessels that carry blood away from the heart to all regions of the body.
- The walls of the arteries are composed of three layers. This structure makes the arteries muscular and elastic so they can expand and contract with the pumping beat of the heart. The term ***endarterial*** means within an artery or pertaining to the inner portion of an artery.
- ***Arterial blood*** is bright red in color because it is oxygen rich. The pumping action of the heart causes blood to spurt out when an artery is cut.
- The **aorta** (ay-**OR**-tah) is the largest blood vessel in the body. It begins from the left ventricle of the heart and forms the main trunk of the arterial system (Figures 5.2 and 5.9).
- The **carotid arteries** (kah-**ROT**-id) are the major arteries that carry blood upward to the head.
- The ***common carotid artery*** is located on each side of the neck.
- It divides into the ***internal carotid artery***, which brings oxygen-rich blood to the brain, and the ***external carotid artery***, which brings blood to the face.
- Any disruption in this blood flow can result in a stroke or other brain damage.
- The **arterioles** (ar-**TEE**-ree-ohlz) are the smaller, thinner branches of arteries that deliver blood to the capillaries. As blood enters one end of the capillary bed, the rate of flow of arterial blood slows.

Capillaries

Capillaries (**KAP**-uh-**ler**-eez), which are only one epithelial cell in thickness, are the smallest blood vessels in the body. The capillaries form networks of expanded vascular beds that have the important role of delivering oxygen and nutrients to the cells of the tissues (Figure 5.11).

- The capillaries further slow the flow of blood to allow plasma to flow into the tissues. It is here that the exchange of oxygen, nutrients, and waste materials occur within the surrounding cells.
- After leaving the cells, 90% of this fluid, which is now oxygen-poor and contains some waste products, enters the opposite end of the capillary bed through the venules.
- The 10% of this fluid that is left behind in the tissues becomes lymph. This is explained in Chapter 7.

Veins

Veins form a low-pressure collecting system to return oxygen-poor blood to the heart (Figures 5.10–5.12).

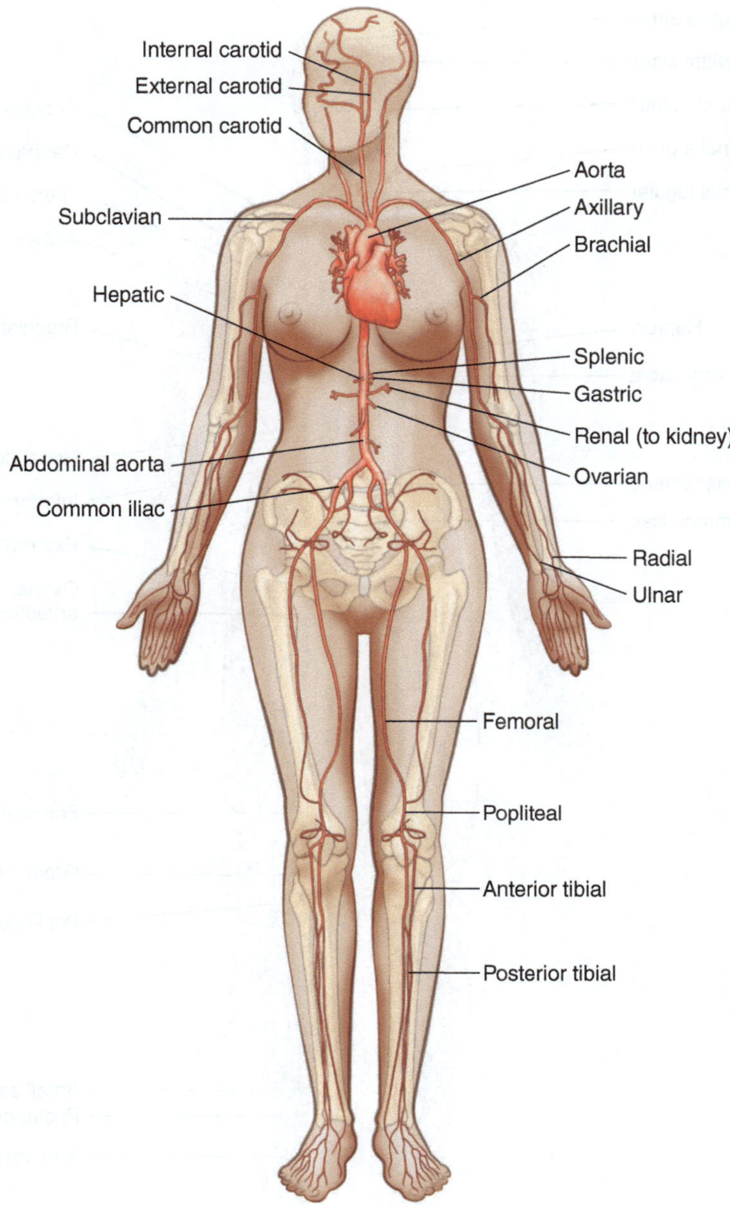

FIGURE 5.9 Anterior view of arterial circulation.

- **Venules** (**VEN**-youls) are the smallest veins that join to form the larger veins (**ven** means vein, and **-ules** means small ones).
- The walls of the veins are thinner and less elastic than those of the arteries.
- The venous blood continues its flow at an increased speed as it continues its return journey to the heart. ***Venous*** means relating to, or contained in, the veins.
- Veins have valves that enable blood to flow only toward the heart and to prevent it from flowing away from the heart (Figure 5.12).
- ***Superficial veins*** are located near the body surface.
- ***Deep veins*** are located within the tissues and away from the body surface.

The Venae Cavae

- The **venae cavae** (**VEE**-nee **KAY**-vee) are the two largest veins in the body. These are the veins that return blood into the heart (singular, *vena cava*).
- The ***superior vena cava*** transports blood from the upper portion of the body to the heart (Figures 5.2 and 5.3).

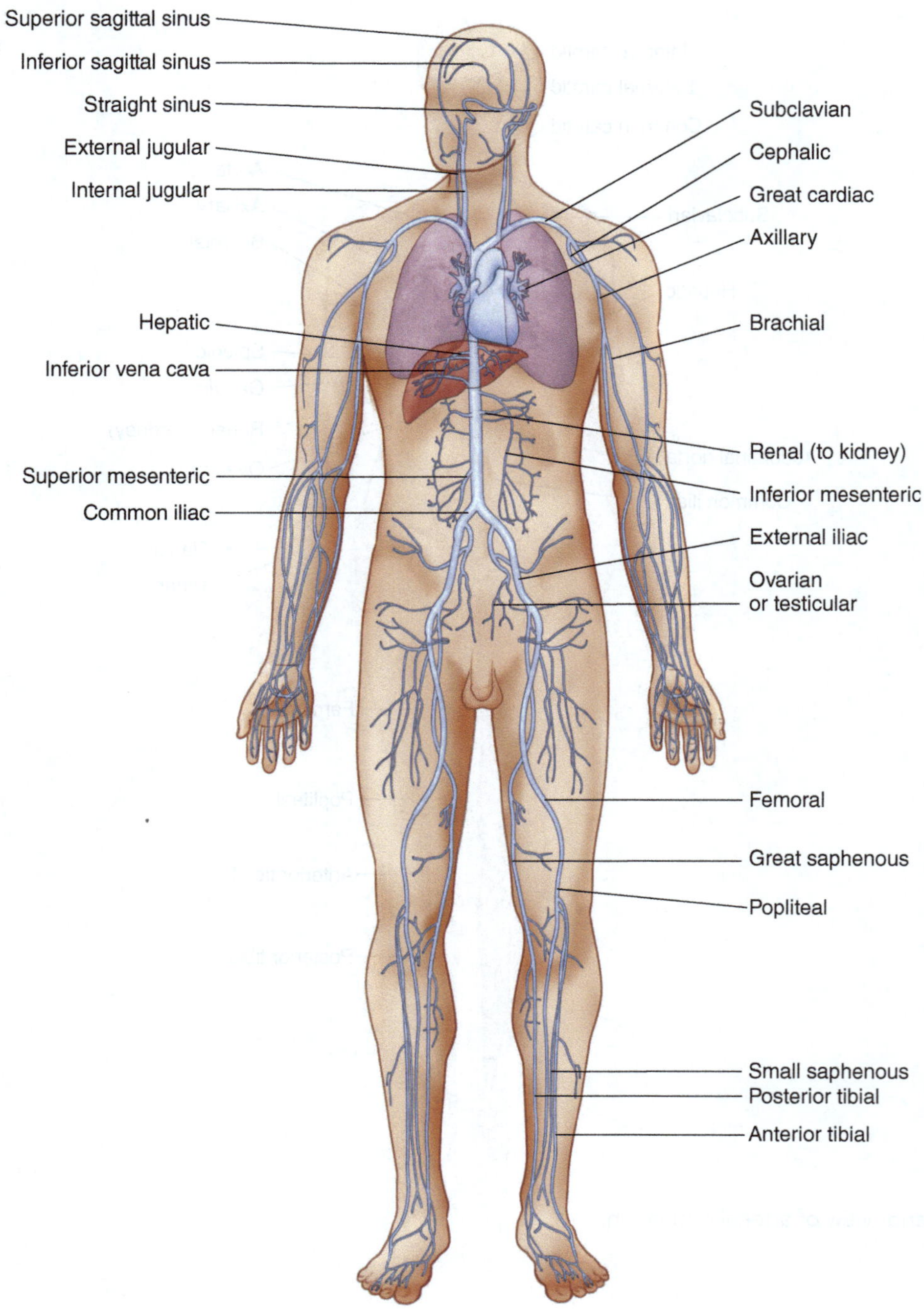

FIGURE 5.10 Anterior view of venous circulation.

- The ***inferior vena cava*** transports blood from the lower portion of the body to the heart (Figures 5.3 and 5.10).

Pulse and Blood Pressure

- The **pulse** is the rhythmic pressure against the walls of an artery caused by the contraction of the heart. The ***heart rate*** is discussed in Chapter 21.
- **Blood pressure** is the measurement of the amount of systolic and diastolic pressure exerted against the walls of the arteries. How to record blood pressure is discussed in Chapter 21. See Table 5.3 for blood pressure classifications.
- **Systolic pressure** (sis-**TOL**-ick), which occurs when the ventricles contract, is the highest pressure against the walls of an artery.
- **Diastolic pressure** (dye-ah-**STOL**-ick), which occurs when the ventricles are relaxed, is the lowest pressure against the walls of an artery.

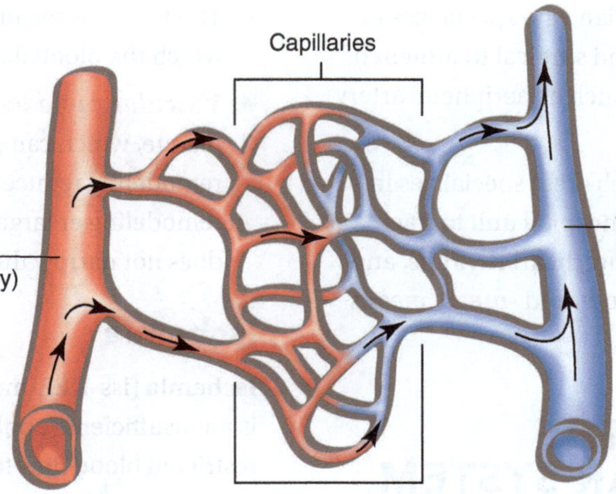

FIGURE 5.11 Oxygen-rich arterial blood is delivered by arterioles to the capillaries. After the oxygen has been extracted, the oxygen-poor blood is returned to circulation as venous blood.

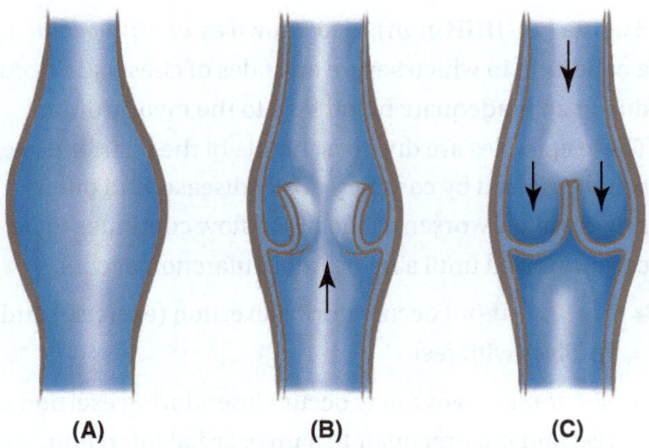

FIGURE 5.12 Veins contain valves to prevent the backward flow of blood. (A) External view of the vein shows wider area of valve. (B) Internal view with the valve open as blood flows through it toward the heart. (C) Internal view with the valve closed to prevent the backflow of blood.

BLOOD

Blood is the fluid tissue in the body. It is composed of 55% liquid plasma and 45% formed elements (red and white blood cells, and platelets). See Chapter 6 for more detailed information about the blood system.

Plasma

Plasma (**PLAZ**-mah) is a straw-colored fluid that contains nutrients, hormones, and waste products. Plasma is 92% water. The remaining 8% consists mainly of proteins, including the clotting proteins.

- **Serum** (**SEER**-um) is the clear, pale yellow plasma fluid that remains after the blood cells and the clotting proteins have been removed.
- **Fibrinogen** (figh-**BRIN**-oh-jen) and **prothrombin** (proh-**THROM**-bin) are the clotting proteins found in plasma.

Formed Elements of the Blood

The formed elements of blood include erythrocytes, leukocytes, and platelets (thrombocytes).

- **Erythrocytes** (eh-**RITH**-roh-**sights**), also known as ***red blood cells*** (RBCs), are mature red blood cells.
- **Leukocytes** (**LOO**-koh-**sights**), also known as ***white blood cells*** (WBCs), are the blood cells involved in defending the body against many infective organisms and foreign substances.
- **Platelets** (**PLAYT**-lets), also called **thrombocytes** (**THROM**-boh-sights), are the smallest formed elements of the blood. They play an important role in the clotting of blood.

MEDICAL SPECIALTIES RELATED TO THE CARDIOVASCULAR SYSTEM

- A **cardiologist** (**kar**-dee-**OL**-oh-jist) is a physician who specializes in diagnosing and treating abnormalities, diseases, and disorders of the heart (**cardi** means heart, and **-ologist** means specialist).
- An **electrophysiologist** (eh-**LEK**-troh-**fiz**-ee-ol-oh-jist) is a doctor specializing in the diagnosis and treatment of heart arrhythmias.

- A **vascular surgeon** is a physician who specializes in the diagnosis, management, and surgical treatment of disorders of the blood vessels such as peripheral artery disease and varicose veins.
- A **telemetry nurse** (teh-**LEM**-eh-tree) specializes in the use of technology within a hospital unit to track vital signs such as blood pressure, heart rhythms, and oxygen levels (**tele** means remote, and **-metry** means to measure).

PATHOLOGY OF THE CARDIOVASCULAR SYSTEM

Disorders of the heart can be congenital or can develop at any time throughout life. Heart disease is the leading cause of death in the United States.

Congenital Heart Defects

Congenital heart defects are structural abnormalities caused by the failure of the heart to develop normally before birth and are the most common type of birth defect. ***Congenital*** means present at birth. Some congenital heart defects are apparent at birth, whereas others may not be detected until later in life. The most common type is ***ventricular septal defect*** (VSD), which is characterized by a hole between the two ventricles.

Coronary Artery Disease

Coronary artery disease (CAD), also known as ***coronary heart disease*** (CHD) and ***ischemic heart disease***, is atherosclerosis of the coronary arteries that reduces the blood supply to the heart muscle. This creates an insufficient supply of oxygen that can cause angina (pain), myocardial infarction (heart attack), or death. CAD is the most common type of heart disease.

Atherosclerosis

Atherosclerosis (**ah**-theh-roh-skleh-**ROH**-sis) is hardening and narrowing of the arteries caused by a buildup of cholesterol plaque on the interior walls of the arteries (**ather/o** means plaque or fatty substance, and **-sclerosis** means abnormal hardening) (Figures 5.13 and 5.14).

- This type of **plaque** (**PLACK**), which is found within the lumen of an artery, is a fatty deposit similar to the buildup of rust inside a pipe. This substance is not the same as *dental plaque*, which is discussed in Chapter 9. The ***lumen*** is the opening within these vessels through which the blood flows.
- ***Vascular remodeling*** refers to the changes caused by plaque, which can protrude inward or outward. Inward remodeling reduces the vessel size, and outward remodeling enlarges it. Although outward remodeling does not narrow the lumen, it can lead to a rupture.

Ischemia

Ischemia (iss-**KEE**-mee-ah) is a condition in which there is an insufficient supply of oxygen in the tissues due to restricted blood flow to a part of the body (**isch** means to hold back, and **-emia** means blood). For example, ***cardiac ischemia*** is the lack of blood flow and oxygen to the heart muscle. See also *ischemic stroke* in Chapter 11.

Angina

Angina (an-**JIGH**-nuh), also known as ***angina pectoris***, is a condition in which severe episodes of chest pain occur due to an inadequate blood flow to the myocardium. These episodes are due to ischemia of the heart muscle, usually caused by coronary artery disease, and often progressively worsen as the blood flow continues to be compromised until a myocardial infarction occurs.

- ***Stable angina*** occurs during exertion (exercise) and resolves with rest.
- ***Unstable angina*** may occur either during exertion or rest and is a precursor to a myocardial infarction.

Myocardial Infarction

A **myocardial infarction** (**my**-oh-**KAR**-dee-al in-**FARK**-shun) (MI), commonly known as a ***heart attack***, is the occlusion (blockage) of one or more coronary arteries caused by plaque buildup. As used here, ***occlusion*** means total blockage.

- The term ***infarction*** means a sudden insufficiency of blood.
- An ***infarct*** is a localized area of dead tissue caused by a lack of blood. Tissue death is known as ***necrosis***, from the Greek word for death.
- This damage to the myocardium impairs the heart's ability to pump blood throughout the body (Figure 5.13).
- The most frequently recognized symptoms of a myocardial infarction include pain or pressure in the middle of the chest that may spread to the back, jaw, or left arm. Many individuals having a heart attack have mild symptoms or none at all.
- Women are more likely to have atypical symptoms, including weakness and fatigue.

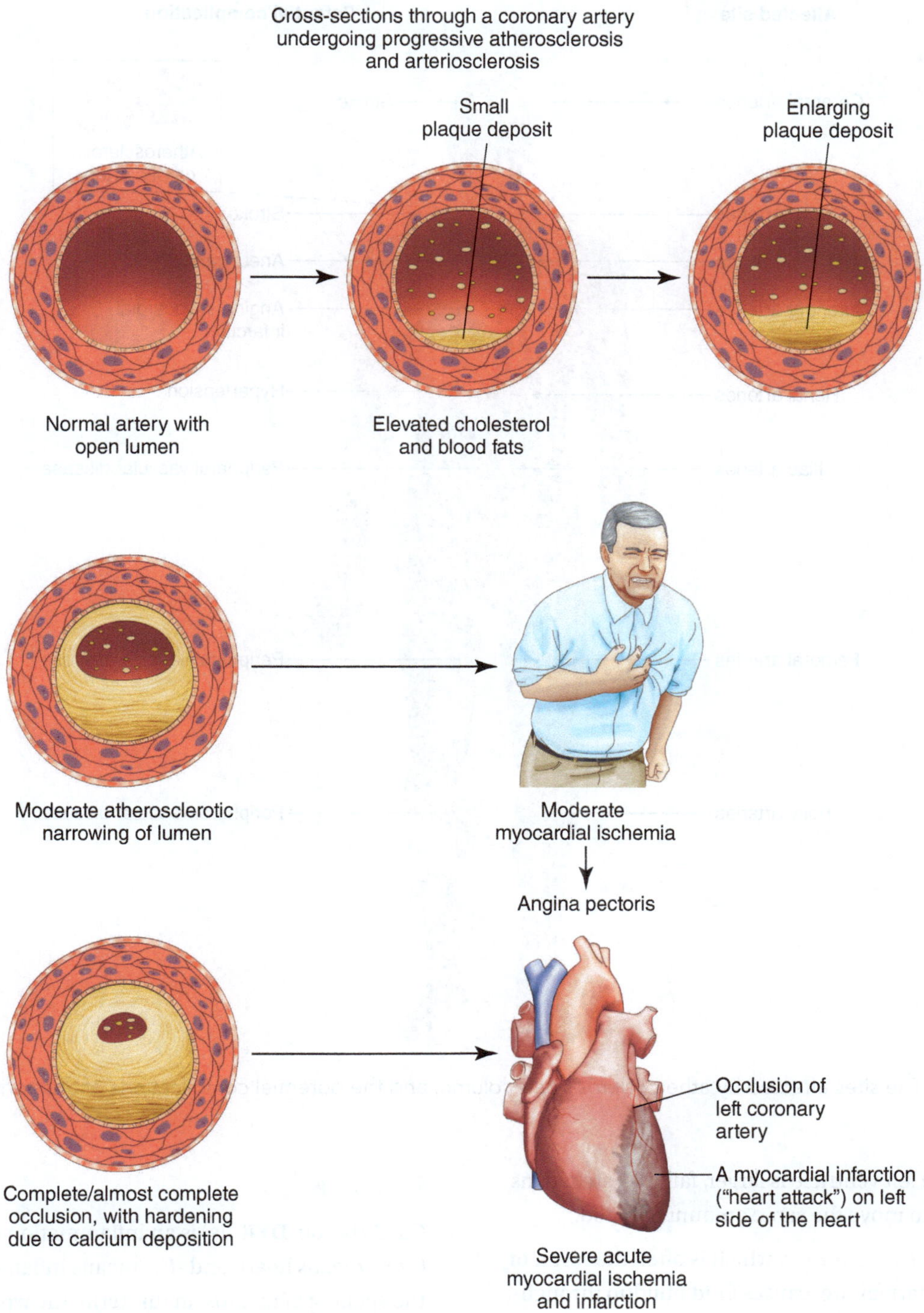

FIGURE 5.13 The progression of coronary artery disease resulting in a myocardial infarction.

Heart Failure

Heart failure occurs most commonly in the elderly, often after the heart has been weakened or damaged by other health issues. In this chronic condition, the heart is unable to pump out all of the blood that it receives. The decreased pumping action causes congestion. The term *congestion* describes a fluid buildup.

- *Congestive heart failure* (CHF) causes fluid to back up, which results in edema (swelling). This chronic condition can cause an accumulation of fluid in the lungs, which is also known as *pulmonary edema*.
- *Left-sided heart failure* is defined as systolic failure or diastolic failure depending on whether the pumping or relaxing action of the heart is affected.

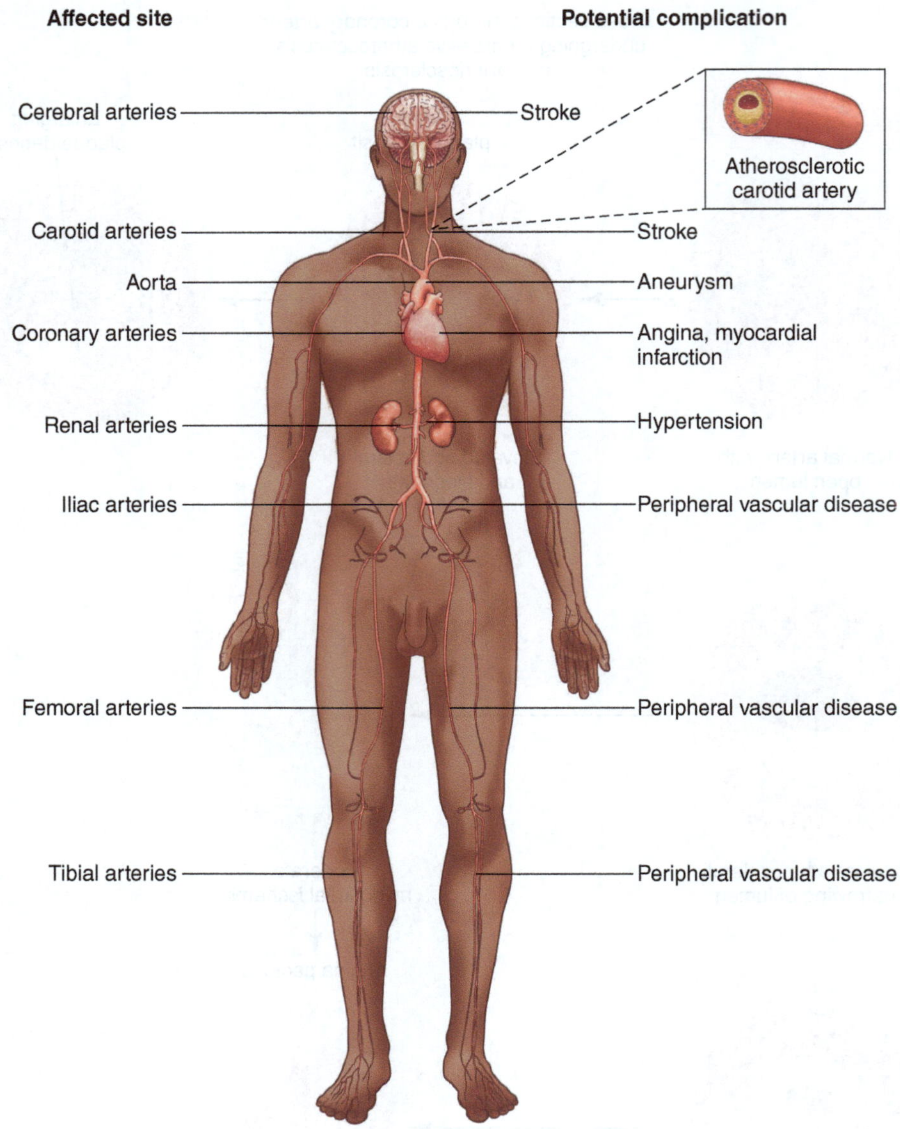

FIGURE 5.14 The sites affected by atherosclerosis (left column) and the potential complications of this condition (right column).

Because the left ventricle is larger, failure here means more work to move the same amount of blood.

- ***Right-sided heart failure***, which is often the result of left-sided heart failure, causes fluid buildup throughout the rest of the body. This occurs because the right side of the heart is unable to efficiently pump blood throughout the rest of the body. Due to the pressure of gravity, this edema, or swelling, is first noticeable in the feet and legs. As this swelling worsens, it can also affect the liver, gastrointestinal tract, or arms.
- **Cardiomegaly** (**kar**-dee-oh-**MEG**-ah-lee) is the abnormal enlargement of the heart that is frequently associated with heart failure as the heart enlarges in an effort to compensate for its decreased pumping ability (**cardi/o** means heart, and **-megaly** means enlargement).

Carditis

Carditis (kar-**DYE**-tis) is an inflammation of the heart (**card** means heart, and **-itis** means inflammation). Note the spelling of *carditis*: in this term, the word root (combining form) **card/o** is used instead of **cardi/o** to avoid having a double *i* when it is joined with the suffix **-itis**.

Endocarditis (**en**-doh-kar-**DYE**-tis) is an inflammation of the inner lining of the heart (**endo-** means within, **card** means heart, and **-itis** means inflammation).

- **Infective endocarditis** or ***bacterial endocarditis*** is an inflammation of the lining or valves of the heart caused by the presence of bacteria in the bloodstream. One cause of this condition is bleeding during dental surgery, because it allows bacteria from the mouth to enter the bloodstream.

- **Pericarditis** (**pehr**-ih-kar-**DYE**-tis) is an inflammation of the pericardium (**peri-** means surrounding, **card** means heart, and **-itis** means inflammation). This inflammation causes an accumulation of fluid within the pericardial sac, and this excess fluid restricts the movement of the heart, reducing the ability of the heart to pump blood throughout the body.
- **Myocarditis** (**my**-oh-kar-**DYE**-tis) is an inflammation of the myocardium (heart muscle) that develops as a rare complication of a viral infection (**my/o** means muscle, **card** means heart, and **-itis** means inflammation).

Diseases of the Myocardium

- **Cardiomyopathy** (**kar**-dee-oh-my-**OP**-ah-thee) is the term used to describe all diseases of the heart muscle (**cardi/o** means heart, **my/o** means muscle, and **-pathy** means disease).
- ***Dilated cardiomyopathy*** is a disease of the heart muscle that causes the heart to become enlarged and to pump less strongly. The progression of this condition is usually slow and only presents with symptoms when quite advanced. ***Dilation*** means the expansion of a hollow structure.

Heart Valves

- A **heart murmur** is an abnormal blowing or clicking sound heard when listening to the heart or a neighboring large blood vessel. Heart murmurs are most often caused by defective heart valves, but they do not usually require surgery unless they affect the patient's quality of life.
- **Mitral valve prolapse** (**MY**-tral **VALV** proh-**LAPS**) (MVP) is the abnormal protrusion of a mitral valve that results in the inability of the valve to close completely. ***Prolapse*** means the falling or dropping down of an organ or internal part.
- **Valvular stenosis** (steh-**NOH**-sis) is a condition in which there is narrowing, stiffening, thickening, or blockage of one or more valves of the heart. ***Stenosis*** is the abnormal narrowing of an opening. These conditions are named for the affected valve.
- **Heart valve disease**, also known as ***valvular heart disease***, is a degenerative disorder that prevents heart valves from opening and closing properly, leading to fatigue, shortness of breath, and lightheadedness.
- **Aortic stenosis** (ay-**OR**-tick steh-**NOH**-sis), also known as *aortic valve stenosis*, is a buildup of calcium and fat deposits in the aortic valve, a condition most prevalent in adults over age 65. This causes a narrowing that prevents the valve from opening fully.
- **Mitral valve regurgitation**, also called *insufficiency* or *incompetency*, occurs when the mitral valve does not close tightly, thus allowing blood to leak back through the opening.

Arrhythmia and Cardiac Arrest

- **Arrhythmia** (ah-**RITH**-mee-ah) is the loss of the normal rhythm of the heartbeat. This can be a minor, temporary episode, or it can be a fatal event. The severity of this episode depends on how much the heart's ability to pump blood is compromised. Rather than being an abnormality in the heart muscle, arrhythmias are usually caused by an abnormality in the electrical conduction system of the heart. These arrythmias are named for the heart rate:
    - **Bradycardia** (**brad**-ee-**KAR**-dee-ah) is an abnormally slow resting heart rate (**brady-** means slow, **card** means heart, and **-ia** means abnormal condition). The term *bradycardia* is usually applied to a heartbeat rate of less than 60 beats per minute (BPM). This condition can occur when the passage of electricity from top to bottom of the heart is partially or totally blocked. Bradycardia is the opposite of *tachycardia*.
    - **Tachycardia** (**tack**-ee-**KAR**-dee-ah) is an abnormally rapid resting heart rate (**tachy-** means rapid, **card** means heart, and **-ia** means abnormal condition). The term *tachycardia* is usually applied to a heartbeat rate of greater than 100 BPM. Tachycardia is the opposite of *bradycardia*.
- **Supraventricular tachycardia** (**soo**-prah-ven-**TRICK**-you-lar **tack**-ee-**KAR**-dee-ah) (SVT), also known as ***paroxysmal supraventricular tachycardia***, is an episode that begins and ends abruptly during which there are very rapid and regular heartbeats that originate at or above the atrioventricular (AV) node (Figure 5.15C). Compare *supraventricular tachycardia* with *ventricular tachycardia*.
- **Ventricular tachycardia** (ven-**TRICK**-you-lar **tack**-ee-**KAR**-dee-ah), also known as ***V-tach***, is a very rapid heartbeat that begins within the ventricles. This condition is potentially fatal because the heart is beating so rapidly that it is unable

to adequately pump blood through the body. For some patients, this condition can be controlled with an implantable cardioverter-defibrillator. Compare *ventricular tachycardia* with *supraventricular tachycardia*.

- **Asystole** (ay-**SIS**-toh-lee), also known as a *flat line* (**a-** means without, and **systole** means contraction), is the complete lack of electrical activity in the heart. The resulting lack of heart contractions, with no blood pumping from the heart and no blood flow through the body, is one of the conditions required for a medical practitioner to certify death.
- **Cardiac arrest** is an event in which the heart abruptly stops beating or develops an arrhythmia that prevents it from pumping blood effectively. *Sudden cardiac death* results when treatment of cardiac arrest is not provided within a few minutes.
- **Heart block** is a congenital or acquired arrhythmia caused by the electrical signal moving through the heart being partially or completely blocked from reaching the ventricles.
- **Long QT syndrome** (LQTS) is an inherited or medically acquired heart rhythm disorder that can cause fast, chaotic, and potentially dangerous arrhythmias. The name comes from the unusual pattern on the electrocardiogram of those with this disease.

Atrial and Ventricular Fibrillations

The term **fibrillation** (**fih**-brih-**LAY**-shun) describes a potentially life-threatening fast and irregular heartbeat, compared to the fast but regular rhythm of tachycardia. The addition of the term *atrial* or *ventricular* identifies which heart chambers are affected.

- **Atrial fibrillation** (**AY**-tree-al **fih**-brih-**LAY**-shun), also known as *A-fib*, is the most common type of tachycardia. It occurs when the normal rhythmic contractions of the atria are replaced by rapid, uncontrolled twitching of the muscular heart wall. This causes an irregular and quivering action of the atria (Figure 5.15B). Some of the increased electrical impulses reach the ventricles, and this makes them contract more rapidly and less efficiently than normal, producing an irregular rate of 80–180 BPM or more.
- **Ventricular fibrillation** (ven-**TRICK**-you-lar **fih**-brih-**LAY**-shun), also known as *V-fib*, consists of rapid, irregular, and useless contractions of the ventricles. Instead of pumping strongly, the heart muscle quivers ineffectively. This condition is the cause of many sudden cardiac deaths (Figure 5.15D).
- **Palpitation** (**pal**-pih-**TAY**-shun) is a pounding or racing heartbeat with or without irregularity in rhythm. This condition is associated with certain heart disorders; however, it can also occur due to imbalance of thyroid hormone, stress, anxiety, exercise, or medications. Note that this is not the same word as *palpation*, an examination technique described in Chapter 21.

Blood Vessel Abnormalities

- **Vasculitis** (**vas**-kyou-**LYE**-tis) is the inflammation of a blood vessel (**vascul** means blood vessels, and **-itis** means inflammation). There are many types of vasculitis, including *phlebitis* (described below) and *angiitis* or *arteritis* (inflammation of the arteries).
  - **Temporal arteritis** (**TEM**-poh-**ral ar**-teh-**RYE**-tis), sometimes called *giant cell arteritis*, is caused by inflammation of the temporal arteries supplying blood to the head and brain. Symptoms include headaches, double vision, and jaw pain. Temporal arteritis can cause unilateral or bilateral blindness, and more rarely, a stroke.
- A **hemangioma** (hee-**man**-jee-**OH**-mah) is a benign tumor made up of newly formed blood vessels (**hem** means blood, **angi** means blood or lymph vessel, and **-oma** means tumor) (see "Birthmarks" in Chapter 13).
- **Hypoperfusion** (**high**-poh-per-**FYOU**-zhun) is a deficiency of blood passing through an organ or body part. *Perfusion* is the circulation of blood through an organ or tissues.

Arteries

- An **aneurysm** (**AN**-you-rizm) is a localized weak spot or balloon-like enlargement of the wall of an artery. The rupture of an aneurysm can be fatal because of the rapid loss of blood. Aneurysms are named for the artery involved such as *aortic aneurysm*, *abdominal aortic aneurysm*, and *thoracic aortic aneurysm*.
- **Arteriosclerosis** (ar-**tee**-ree-oh-skleh-**ROH**-sis), also known as *hardening of the arteries*, is any of a group of diseases characterized by thickening and the loss of elasticity of arterial walls (**arteri/o** means artery, and **-sclerosis** mean abnormal hardening).
- **Carotid artery stenosis**, also known as *arteriostenosis*, is the abnormal narrowing of the carotid artery supplying blood to the brain, increasing the chance of blood clots that could cause an ischemic stroke (see Chapter 11). This condition is usually the result of atherosclerosis.

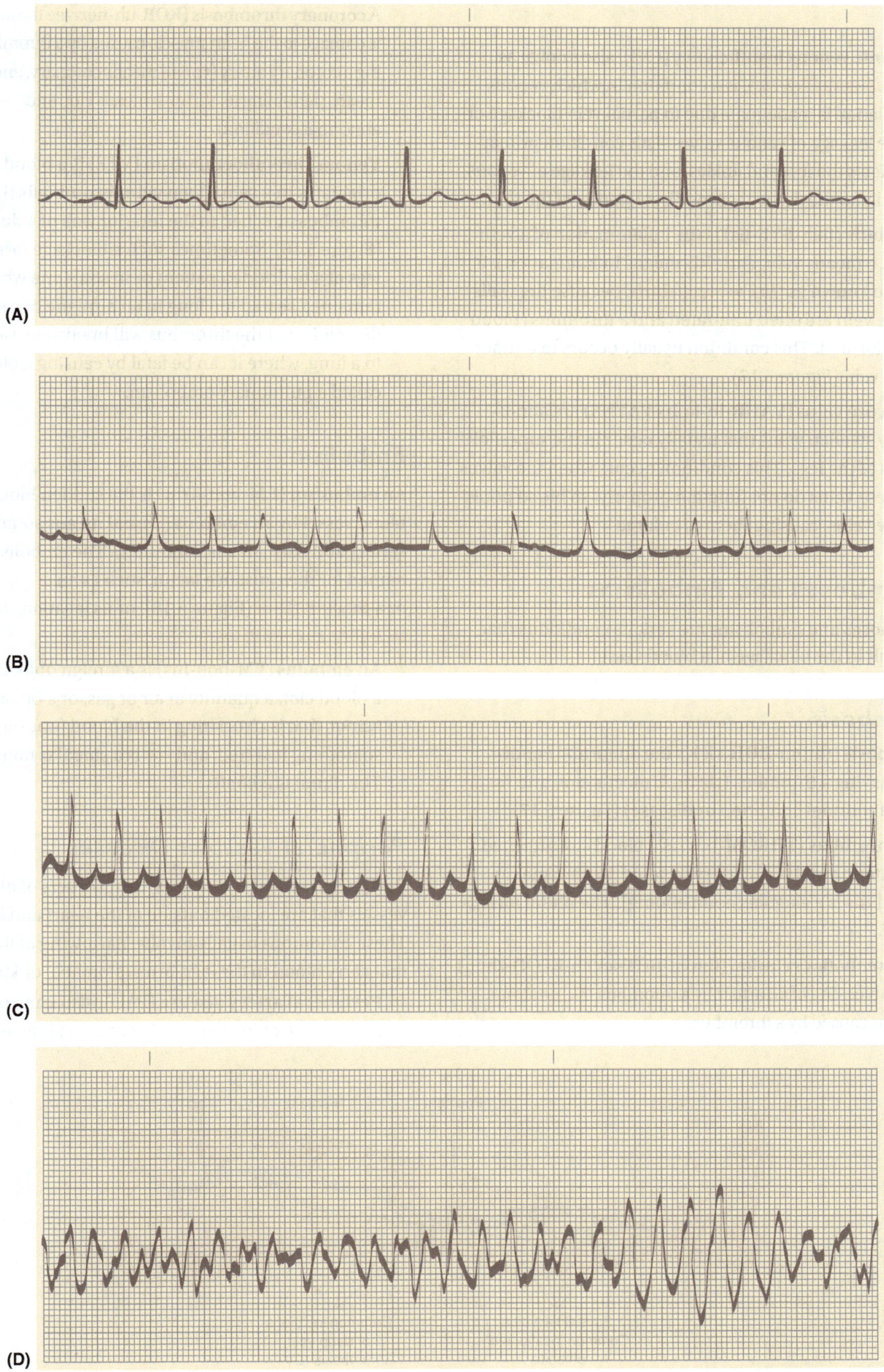

FIGURE 5.15 Electrocardiograms of heart rhythms. (A) Normal sinus rhythm. (B) Atrial fibrillation. (C) Supraventricular tachycardia. (D) Ventricular fibrillation.

Veins

- **Chronic venous insufficiency** (CVI), also known as ***venous insufficiency***, is a condition in which venous circulation is inadequate due to partial vein blockage or to the leakage of venous valves. This condition primarily affects the feet and ankles, and the leakage of venous blood into the tissues causes discoloration of the skin.
- **Phlebitis** (fleh-**BYE**-tis) is the inflammation of a vein (**phleb** means vein, and **-itis** means inflammation). It is also known as ***thrombophlebitis***, because the walls of the vein are often infiltrated and a thrombus (blood clot) formed. This condition usually occurs in a superficial vein (Figure 5.16).
- **Varicose veins** (**VAHR**-ih-**kohs VAYNS**) are abnormally swollen veins that usually occur in the superficial veins of the legs. This condition occurs when the valves in these veins do not function properly, so blood pools in the veins, causing them to enlarge.

Thromboses and Embolisms

Thromboses and embolisms are serious conditions that can result in the blockage of a blood vessel.

Thrombosis

Thrombosis (throm-**BOH**-sis) is the abnormal condition of having a thrombus (**thromb** means clot, and **-osis** means abnormal condition or disease) (Figure 5.17).

A **thrombus** (**THROM**-bus) is a blood clot attached to the interior wall of an artery or vein (**thromb** means clot, and **-us** is a singular noun ending). The plural form is *thrombi.*

- A **thrombotic occlusion** (throm-**BOT**-ick ah-**KLOO**-zhun) is the blocking of an artery by a thrombus. ***Thrombotic*** means caused by a thrombus.
- A **coronary thrombosis** (**KOR**-uh-**nerr**-ee throm-**BOH**-sis) is damage to the heart muscle caused by a thrombus blocking a coronary artery (**coron** means coronary, and **-ary** means pertaining to; **thromb** means clot, and **-osis** means abnormal condition).
- **Venous thromboembolism** (VTE) is a blood clot that originates in a vein. **Deep vein thrombosis** (DVT) is a thrombus attached to the interior wall of a deep vein (Figure 5.16). Sometimes such a blockage forms in the legs of a bedridden patient or in someone who has remained seated too long in an airplane or car. The danger is that the thrombus will break loose and travel to a lung, where it can be fatal by causing a blockage, called a pulmonary embolism.

Embolism

An **embolism** (**EM**-boh-lizm) is the sudden blockage of a blood vessel by an embolus (**embol** means something inserted, and **-ism** means condition). The embolism is often named for the causative factor, such as an ***air embolism*** or a ***fat embolism*** (Figure 5.18), or its location, such as ***pulmonary embolism***.

- An **embolus** (**EM**-boh-lus) is a foreign object, such as a blood clot, a quantity of air or gas, or a bit of tissue or tumor, that is circulating in the blood (**embol** means something inserted, and **-us** is a singular noun ending). The plural is *emboli.*

Peripheral Vascular Diseases

Peripheral vascular diseases are disorders of blood vessels that are located outside of the heart and brain. These conditions usually involve narrowing of the vessels that carry blood to the legs, arms, stomach, or kidneys.

- **Peripheral artery disease** (PAD), also known as ***peripheral arterial occlusive disease***, is an example

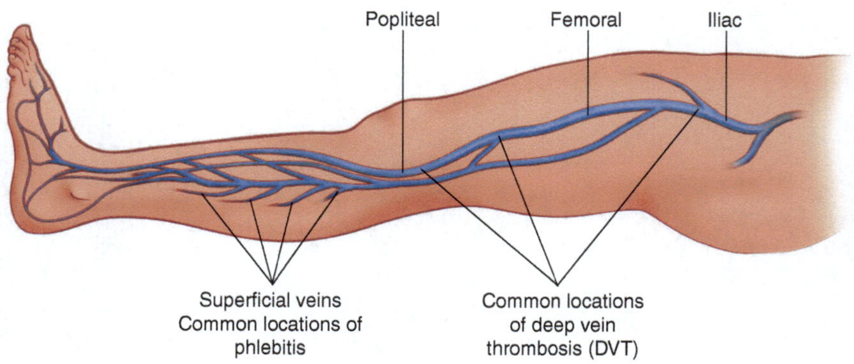

FIGURE 5.16 Common sites for the development of phlebitis and deep vein thrombosis.

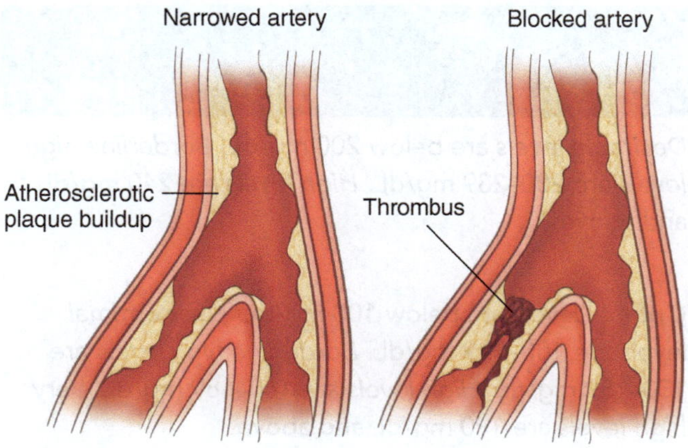

FIGURE 5.17 A thrombus is a blood clot attached to the interior wall of an artery or vein.

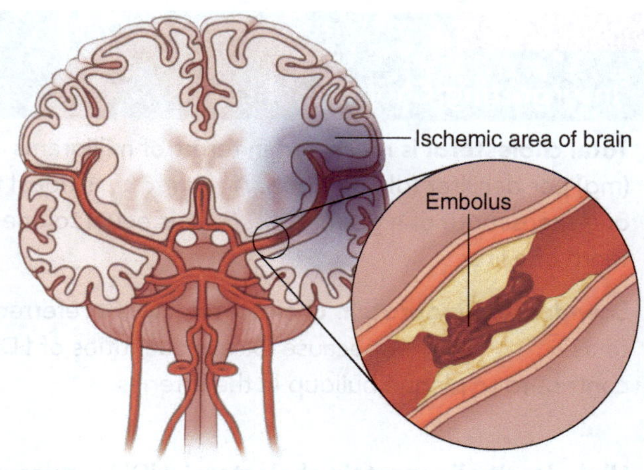

FIGURE 5.18 An embolus is a foreign object circulating in the blood.

of a peripheral vascular disease that is caused by atherosclerosis. This condition is a common and serious problem affecting 15–20% of adults over 70 years of age. Impaired circulation to the extremities and vital organs can cause changes in the skin color and temperature.

- One method of determining the severity of PAD is using the ***ankle-brachial index*** to compare the blood pressure at the ankle with the blood pressure in the arm.
- Peripheral arterial disease is also involved with *intermittent claudication*, which is discussed in Chapter 4.
- **Gangrene** is tissue death caused by a severe shortage of blood supply due to illness, injury, and/or infection. It is most common in those with peripheral artery disease. This condition usually affects fingers, toes, or limbs; untreated, it can lead to sepsis.

- **Raynaud's disease** (ray-**NOHZ**) is a peripheral arterial occlusive disease in which intermittent attacks are triggered by cold temperatures or stress. The symptoms, which are due to constricted circulation, are associated with numbness and include skin in the affected areas turning white or blue.

Cholesterol

- **Cholesterol** (koh-**LES**-ter-ol) is a fatty substance that travels through the blood and is found in all parts of the body. It aids in the production of cell membranes, some hormones, and vitamin D. Some cholesterol comes from dietary sources, and some is created by the liver. Excessively high levels of certain types of cholesterol can lead to heart disease (Table 5.2).

- **Hyperlipidemia** (**high**-per-**lip**-ih-**DEE**-mee-ah) is the general term used to describe elevated levels of cholesterol and other fatty substances in the blood (**hyper-** means excessive, **lipid** means fat, and **-emia** means blood condition).

Hypertension

Hypertension (HTN), commonly known as ***high blood pressure***, is the elevation of arterial blood pressure to a level that is likely to cause damage to the cardiovascular system. Hypertension is the opposite of *hypotension*. (One way to remember the difference between the two is to think of the *E* in *hypertension* as standing for Elevated, and the *O* in *hypotension* as standing for Low.)

- ***Essential hypertension***, also known as ***primary hypertension*** or ***idiopathic hypertension***, is consistently elevated blood pressure of unknown cause. ***Idiopathic*** means a disease of unknown cause.
- The classifications of blood pressure for adults with this condition are summarized in Table 5.3.
- ***Secondary hypertension*** is caused by a different medical problem, such as a kidney disorder or a tumor on the adrenal glands. When the other problem is resolved, the secondary hypertension usually improves.
- ***Malignant hypertension*** is characterized by very high blood pressure. This condition, which can be fatal, is usually accompanied by damage to the organs, brain, and optic nerves, or failure of the heart and kidneys.
- ***Pulmonary hypertension*** is high blood pressure in the lungs that is usually the result of chronic heart or lung

TABLE 5.2

Interpreting Cholesterol Levels

Total cholesterol is measured in terms of milligrams (mg) per deciliter (dL) of blood. A ***milligram*** is equal to one-thousandth of a gram. A ***deciliter*** is equal to one-tenth of a liter.	*Desirable levels* are below 200 mg/dL. *Borderline high levels* are 200–239 mg/dL. *High levels* are 240 mg/dL and above.
Low-density lipoprotein cholesterol (LDL) is referred to as ***bad cholesterol*** because excess quantities of LDL contribute to plaque buildup in the arteries.	*Optimal levels* are below 100 mg/dL. *Near optimal* levels are 100–129 mg/dL. *Borderline high* levels are 130–159 mg/dL. *High levels* are 160–189 mg/dL. *Very high levels* are 190 mg/dL and above.
High-density lipoprotein cholesterol (HDL) is referred to as ***good cholesterol*** because it carries unneeded cholesterol back to the liver for processing and does not contribute to plaque buildup.	*At risk levels* are below 40 mg/dL. *Desirable levels* are 60 mg/dL and above.
Triglycerides (try-**GLIS**-er-eyeds) are combinations of ***fatty acids*** attached to glycerol that are also found normally in the blood in limited quantities.	*Normal levels* are below 150 mg/dL. *Borderline high levels* are 150–199 mg/dL. *High levels* are 200–499 mg/dL. *Very high levels* are 500 mg/dL and above.

Source: National Heart, Lung, and Blood Institute of the National Institutes of Health, 2014.

TABLE 5.3

Blood Pressure Classifications for Adults

Category	Systolic (mm Hg) Top Number	Diastolic (mm Hg) Bottom Number
Normal blood pressure	less than 120	less than 80
Elevated	between 120 and 129	less than 80
Stage 1 Hypertension	between 130 and 139	between 80 and 89
Stage 2 Hypertension	140 or higher	90 or higher

disease. This condition requires the right ventricle of the heart to work harder in order to circulate blood to the lungs.

Hypotension

Hypotension (**high**-poh-**TEN**-shun) is lower-than-normal arterial blood pressure. Symptoms can include dizziness, light-headedness, or fainting. *Hypotension* is the opposite of *hypertension*.

- **Orthostatic hypotension** (**or**-thoh-**STAT**-ick **high**-poh-**TEN**-shun), also known as ***postural hypotension***, is low blood pressure that occurs upon standing up and remains lower than normal as long as the patient remains standing. ***Orthostatic*** means relating to an upright or standing position.

DIAGNOSTIC PROCEDURES OF THE CARDIOVASCULAR SYSTEM

- **Blood tests**, **computed tomography** (CT) **scans**, **MRIs**, and **ultrasonic diagnostic procedures** are discussed in Chapter 21.
- **Angiography** (**an**-jee-**OG**-rah-fee) is an x-ray of the blood vessels after the injection of a contrast medium (**angi/o** means blood vessel, and **-graphy** means the process of recording). The resulting film is an ***angiogram*** (Figure 5.19) that is used to study blood flow in the arteries, veins, and blood vessels of the heart.

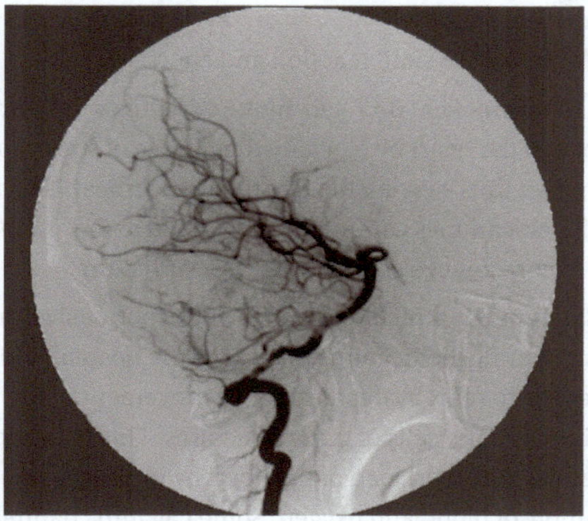

FIGURE 5.19 In angiography, the blood vessels (in black) are made visible through the use of a contrast medium.

- **Cardiac catheterization** (**KAR**-dee-ack **kath**-eh-ter-eye-**ZAY**-shun) is a diagnostic and treatment procedure in which a catheter is passed into a vein or artery and then guided into the heart (Figure 5.20). A contrast dye injected through the catheter during angiography shows any disruptions in blood flow, and angioplasty (widening a narrowed blood vessel) can then be performed via the catheter. See the section on clearing blocked arteries later in this chapter.

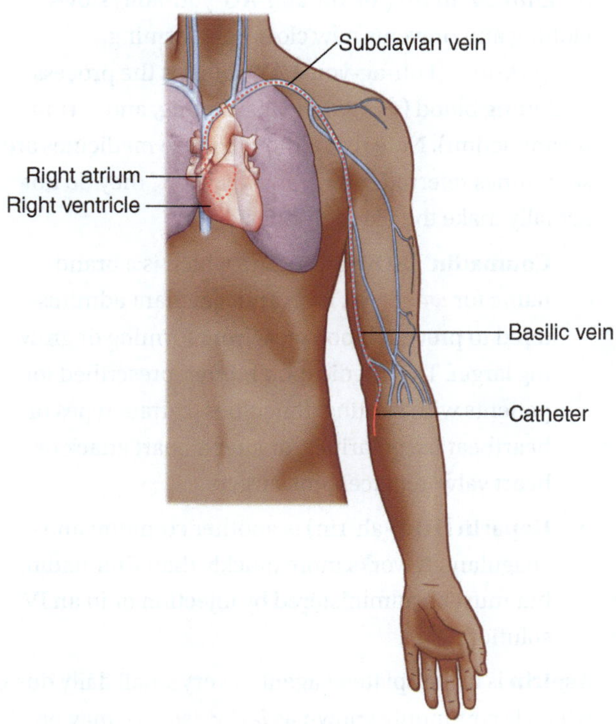

FIGURE 5.20 In *cardiac catheterization*, a catheter is passed into a vein or artery and then guided into the heart.

- ***Digital subtraction angiography*** (DSA) uses computer assistance to clarify the view of the area of interest in the cardiovascular system by "subtracting" the soft tissue and bones from the images.
- **Duplex ultrasound** is a diagnostic procedure to image the structures of the blood vessels and the flow of blood through these vessels. This is a combination of ***diagnostic ultrasound*** to show the structure of the blood vessels and ***Doppler ultrasound*** to show the movement of the red blood cells through these vessels. Diagnostic and Doppler ultrasounds are discussed in Chapter 21.
- **Venography** (vee-**NOG**-rah-fee) is a radiographic test that provides an image of specific veins after a contrast dye is injected (**ven/o** means vein, and **-graphy** means the process of recording). The resulting film is a ***venogram***.

Electrocardiography

Electrocardiography (ee-**leck**-troh-kar-dee-**OG**-rah-fee) is the noninvasive process of recording the electrical activity of the myocardium (**electr/o** means electric, **cardi/o** means heart, and **-graphy** means the process of recording a picture or record) (Figure 5.21). A ***noninvasive*** procedure does not require the insertion of an instrument or device through the skin or a body opening for diagnosis or treatment.

- An **electrocardiogram** (ee-**leck**-troh-**KAR**-dee-oh-**gram**) (EKG or ECG) is a record of the electrical activity of the myocardium (**electr/o** means electric, **cardi/o** means heart, and **-gram** means picture or record) (Figure 5.15).

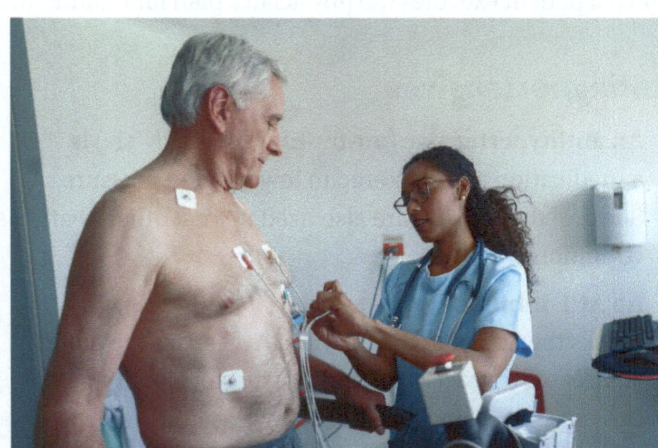

iStock.com/andresr

FIGURE 5.21 In *electrocardiography*, the electrical activity of the myocardium is captured and externally recorded by electrodes placed on the skin.

- A **Holter monitor** is a portable electrocardiograph that is worn by an ambulatory patient to continuously monitor the heart rates and rhythms over a 24- to 48-hour period, or longer. An ***implantable loop recorder*** (ILR) is a subcutaneous device implanted beneath the skin of the chest to continuously monitor heart rhythm for up to three years.
- A **stress test** is performed to assess cardiovascular health and function during and after stress. This involves recording an electrocardiogram while the patient either exercises on a treadmill or is injected with a chemical to increase the patient's heart rate if he or she is unable to use a treadmill. The test can also be performed in conjunction with an ***echocardiography***, which uses ultrasonic waves to evaluate motion of the heart (see Chapter 21).
- A **thallium stress test** (**THAL**-ee-um) (TST) is a nuclear imaging test performed by injecting a small amount of thallium into the bloodstream to evaluate how well blood flows through the coronary arteries of the heart muscle during exercise. If the thallium is not taken up equally by all heart muscle cells, the TST will show a decrease in blood flow to part of the heart.

TREATMENT PROCEDURES OF THE CARDIOVASCULAR SYSTEM

Medications

Many heart conditions are controlled with medications; however, successful treatment depends on patient adherence. ***Adherence*** is the accuracy and consistency with which a patient executes the physician's plan for treatment.

Antihypertensives

- An **antihypertensive** (**an**-tih-**high**-per-**TEN**-siv) is a medication administered to lower blood pressure. Some of these drugs are also used to treat other heart conditions.
- An **ACE inhibitor** (***angiotensin-converting enzyme***) blocks the action of the enzyme that causes the blood vessels to contract, resulting in hypertension. When this enzyme is blocked, the blood vessels are able to relax (dilate), which reduces the blood pressure. These medications are used primarily to treat hypertension and heart failure. ***Angiotensin II receptor blockers*** (ARBs) have a similar action and effect.
- A **beta-blocker** (**BAY**-tah-**blok**-er) reduces the workload of the heart by blocking the release of stress hormones, thus slowing the rate of the heartbeat. This type of medication is commonly prescribed to lower blood pressure, relieve angina, or treat heart failure.
- **Calcium channel blockers** are antihypertensive, antiarrhythmic medications that cause the heart and blood vessels to relax by decreasing the movement of calcium into the cells of these structures. This relaxation reduces the workload of the heart by increasing the supply of blood and oxygen. Some calcium channel-blocking agents are used to treat hypertension or to relieve and control angina.
- A **diuretic** (**dye**-you-**RET**-ick) is an antihypertensive medication administered to increase urine output to rid the body of excess sodium and water. These medications are administered to treat hypertension and heart failure by reducing the amount of fluid circulating in the blood.

Additional Medications

- An **anti-arrhythmic** (**an**-tih-ah-**RITH**-mick) is a medication that stops or prevents irregularities of the heartbeat.
- An **anticoagulant** (**an**-tih-koh-**AG**-you-lant) slows clotting and prevents new clots from forming. ***Coagulation*** (koh-**ag**-you-**LAY**-shun) is the process of clotting blood (**coagul** means clotting, and **-ation** means action). Note that although these medicines are sometimes referred to as ***blood thinners***, they do not actually make the blood thinner.
  - **Coumadin**® (**KOO**-mah-din), which is a brand name for ***warfarin***, is an anticoagulant administered to prevent blood clots from forming or growing larger. This medication is often prescribed for patients with clotting difficulties, certain types of heartbeat irregularities, or after a heart attack or heart valve replacement surgery.
  - **Heparin** (**HEP**-ah-rin) is another common anticoagulant. It works more quickly than Coumadin, but must be administered by injection or in an IV solution.
- **Aspirin** is an antiplatelet agent. A very small daily dose, which is commonly known as ***baby aspirin***, may be

recommended to reduce the risk of a heart attack or stroke by reducing the ability of the blood to clot.

- **Cholesterol-lowering drugs** are used to combat hyperlipidemia by reducing the undesirable cholesterol levels in the blood.
- **Digitalis** (**dij**-ih-**TAL**-is), available as the drug preparation *digoxin*, strengthens the contraction of the heart muscle, slows the heart rate, and helps eliminate fluid from body tissues. The drug, which contains extracts from the foxglove plant (which belongs the plant genus *Digitalis*), is used to treat and prevent certain types of arrhythmias, as well as for some other heart conditions.
- A **thrombolytic** (**throm**-boh-**LIT**-ick), also known as a *clot-busting drug*, dissolves or causes a thrombus to break up (**thromb/o** means clot, and **-lytic** means to destroy). The use of drugs to break up a thrombus is called *thrombolytic therapy*.
- **Tissue plasminogen activator** (plaz-**MIN**-oh-jen) (tPA) is a thrombolytic that is administered to some patients having a heart attack or stroke. If administered within a few hours after symptoms begin, this medication can dissolve the damaging blood clots. *Note:* Use caution with the abbreviation tPA, which can be confused with other drug abbreviations.
- A **vasoconstrictor** (**vas**-oh-kon-**STRICK**-tor) causes blood vessels to narrow. Examples of these medications include antihistamines and decongestants. A vasoconstrictor is the opposite of a *vasodilator*.
- A **vasodilator** (**vas**-oh-dye-**LAYT**-or) causes blood vessels to expand. A vasodilator is the opposite of a *vasoconstrictor*.
- **Nitroglycerin** (**nye**-troh-**GLIH**-seh-rin) (NTG) is a drug with antihypertensive properties that works by dilating the veins, reducing the workload of the heart. It can be administered sublingually (under the tongue), transdermally, or intravenously. Nitroglycerin is used to treat hypertension, angina, and myocardial infarction. In the event of myocardial infarction, a patient with a prescription for nitroglycerin may be instructed to take it while awaiting emergency medical assistance.

Nutritional Interventions

Patients with hypertension as well as other cardiac issues such as heart failure are often prescribed a diet with restricted sodium intake such as the *Dietary Approaches to Stop Hypertension (DASH) diet*. Snack foods as well as most fast food and processed foods tend to be high in sodium, even if they don't taste salty. Patients with high cholesterol or other cardiac disease might be prescribed a diet limited in saturated fat and cholesterol. All foods that come from animals (i.e., dairy, poultry, seafood, meat, eggs) contain cholesterol.

Cardiac Surgery

Heart surgery today ranges from the correction of congenital heart defects in children to complete heart transplantation.

Clearing Blocked Arteries and Veins

- **Angioplasty** (**AN**-jee-oh-**plas**-tee) is the technique of mechanically widening a narrowed or obstructed blood vessel (**angi/o** means blood vessel, and **-plasty** means surgical repair).
- **Balloon angioplasty**, also known as *percutaneous transluminal coronary angioplasty* (PTCA), is a procedure in which a small balloon on the end of a catheter is used to open a partially blocked coronary artery by flattening the plaque deposit and stretching the lumen (Figure 5.22).
- **Laser angioplasty** involves a laser on the end of a catheter, which uses beams of light to remove the plaque deposit. It can be used separately or prior to PTCA.
- A **stent** is a wire-mesh tube that is commonly placed after the artery has been opened. This provides support to the arterial wall, keeps the plaque from expanding again, and prevents restenosis (Figure 5.23).
- **Restenosis** describes the condition when an artery that has been opened by angioplasty gradually closes again (**re-** means again, and **-stenosis** means narrowing).
- An **atherectomy** (**ath**-er-**ECK**-toh-mee) is the surgical removal of plaque buildup from the interior of an artery (**ather** means plaque, and **-ectomy** means surgical removal). A stent may be put in place after the atherectomy to prevent the artery from becoming blocked again.
- A **carotid endarterectomy** (kah-**ROT**-id **end**-ar-ter-**ECK**-toh-mee) is the surgical removal of the lining of a portion of a clogged carotid artery leading to the brain (**end-** means within, **arter** means artery, and **-ectomy** means surgical removal).

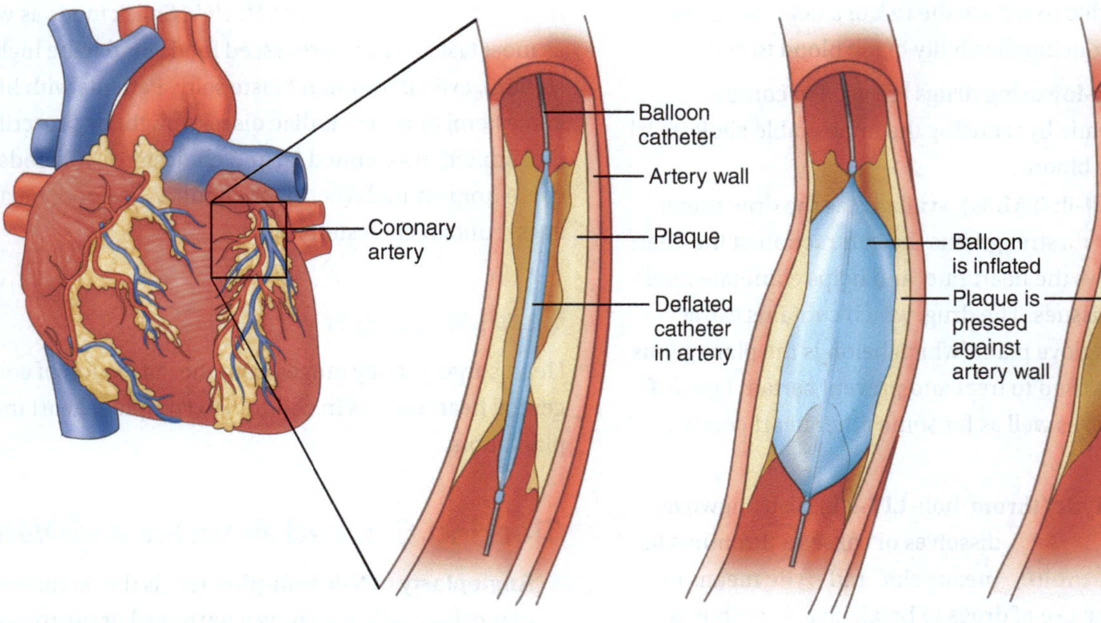

FIGURE 5.22 *Balloon angioplasty* is performed to reopen a blocked coronary artery.

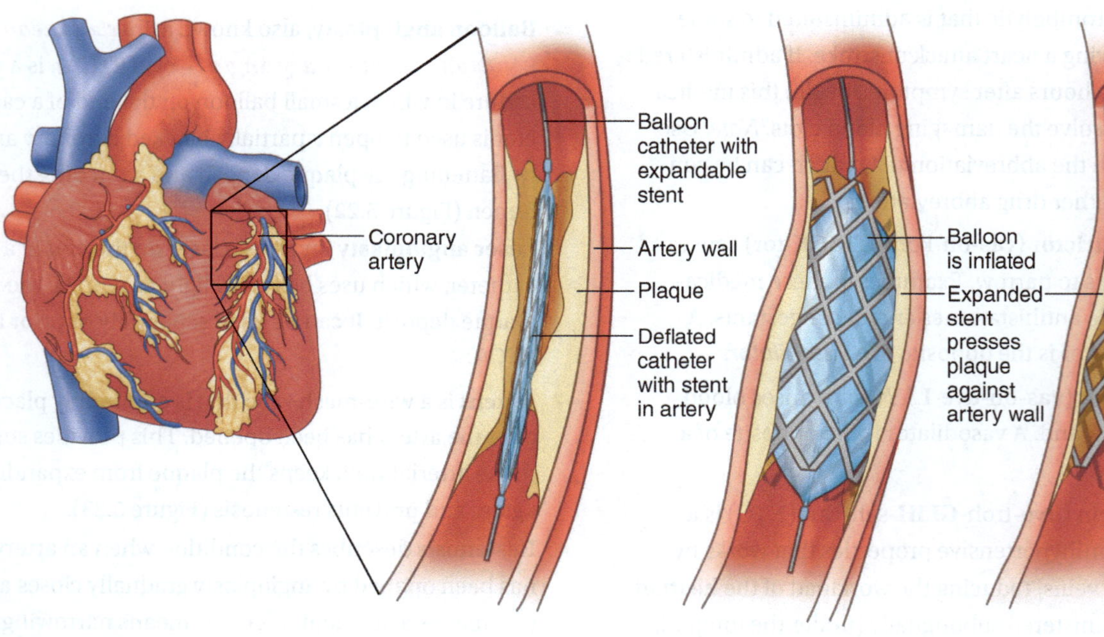

FIGURE 5.23 A *stent* is put in place to prevent *restenosis* of a treated artery.

This procedure is performed to reduce the risk of a stroke due to blood clots. Strokes are discussed in Chapter 11.

Coronary Artery Bypass Graft

Coronary artery bypass graft (CABG) is the most common type of *open-heart surgery* (Figure 5.24). In this operation, which requires opening the chest, a piece of vein from the leg or chest is implanted on the heart to replace a blocked coronary artery and to improve the flow of blood to the heart. During coronary artery bypass surgery, a *cardiopulmonary bypass* (CPB) or *heart-lung machine* is used to temporarily take over the function of the heart and lungs to maintain the circulation of blood and oxygen throughout the body. Bypassing the heart allows surgeons the opportunity to operate on the heart without it beating.

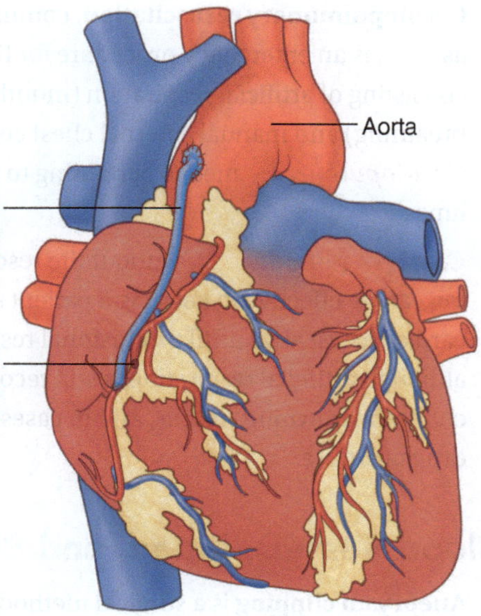

FIGURE 5.24 *Coronary artery bypass surgery* is performed to allow the flow of blood by placing vein grafts to bypass blocked arteries.

- A **minimally invasive coronary artery bypass** is an alternative technique for some bypass patients. This procedure is performed with the aid of a fiber-optic camera through small openings between the ribs.

Treatment of Cardiac Arrest, Arrhythmias, and Valves

- **Defibrillation** (dee-**fih**-brih-**LAY**-shun) is the emergency use of electrical shock to restore the heart's normal rhythm. This shock is provided by a device known as a ***defibrillator*** (Figure 5.25). **Synchronized cardioversion** is a similar procedure for restoring normal heart rhythm using a lower voltage electrical shock in a non-emergency situation.
- An **automated external defibrillator** (AED) is designed for use by nonprofessionals in emergency situations when defibrillation is required. This piece of equipment automatically samples the electrical rhythms of the heart and, if necessary, externally shocks the heart to restore a normal cardiac rhythm.
- An **implantable cardioverter-defibrillator** (**KAR**-dee-oh-**ver**-ter dee-**FIB**-rih-**lay**-ter) (ICD) is an internal double-action pacemaker. It constantly regulates the heartbeat to ensure that the heart does not beat too slowly. If a dangerous disruption of the heart's rhythm occurs, it acts as an automatic defibrillator (Figure 5.26).
- A **pacemaker** is used to treat arrhythmia. This battery-powered device can be attached externally or implanted temporarily or permanently under the skin, with connections leading into the heart to regulate the heartbeat. ***Cardiac resynchronization therapy*** is the use of a pacemaker to help the left and right heart chambers beat together and work efficiently.
- **Cardiac ablation** (ab-**LAY**-shun), also called ***catheter ablation***, is a procedure that uses radio-frequency energy (heat) or cryoablation (extreme cold) to scar or

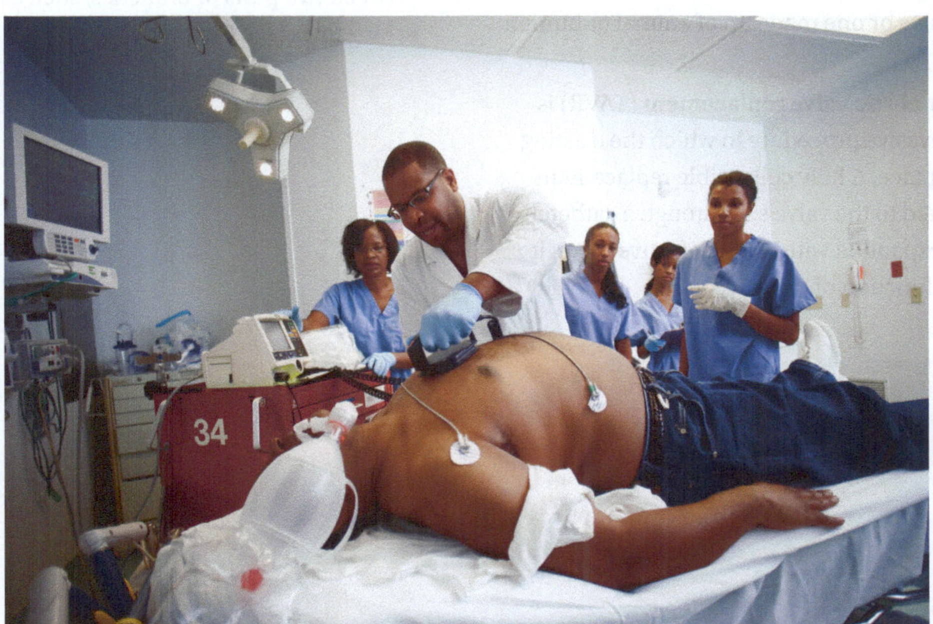

Blend Images/ERproductions Ltd/Getty Images

FIGURE 5.25 *Defibrillation* uses electrical shock to attempt to restore the heart to its usual rhythm.

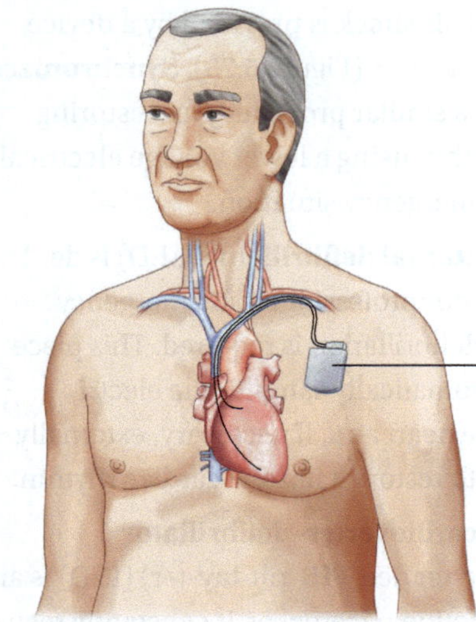

FIGURE 5.26 An *implantable cardioverter–defibrillator* constantly regulates the heartbeat and, if necessary, acts as an automatic defibrillator.

destroy the heart tissue triggering an abnormal heart rhythm. See Chapter 10 for the use of ***ablation***, which is the removal or destruction of tissue, to treat prostate cancer.

- **Valvuloplasty** (**VAL**-view-loh-**plas**-tee), or ***balloon valvuloplasty,*** is the surgical repair of a heart valve that has a narrowed opening (**valvul/o** means valve, and **-plasty** means surgical repair).
- **Heart valve replacement** is surgery to replace one of the heart's four valves, usually the aortic or mitral valve. The defective valve is replaced with either a mechanical valve or one made up of animal or human tissue.
- **Transcatheter aortic valve replacement** (TAVR) is a minimally invasive procedure in which the existing valve is left in place. A fully collapsible replacement valve is delivered to the valve site through a catheter, and after it is expanded within the defective valve, it takes over the function of the valve.
- **Cardiopulmonary resuscitation**, commonly known as ***CPR***, is an emergency procedure for life support consisting of artificial respiration (mouth-to-mouth breathing) and manual external chest compression. ***Cardiopulmonary*** means pertaining to the heart and lungs.
- ***Compression-only CPR*** without the rescue breathing can be effective in keeping a patient suffering from cardiac arrest alive until professional responders arrive, although artificial respiration is still recommended for children, drowning victims, and in cases of suspected drug overdose.

Blood Vessels, Blood, and Bleeding

- **Aneurysm clipping** is a surgical method used to isolate an aneurysm in the brain from the rest of the circulatory system by placing a small clip across its neck. This titanium clip, which remains permanently in place, prevents blood from flowing into the aneurysm.
- **Hemostasis** (**hee**-moh-**STAY**-sis) means to stop or control bleeding (**hem/o** means blood, and **-stasis** means stopping or controlling). This can be accomplished by the formation of a blood clot by the body or through the external application of pressure to block the flow of blood.
- An **anastomosis** (ah-**nas**-toh-**MOH**-sis) is a connection between blood vessels. In surgery, anastomosis is used connect two arteries, two veins, or an artery to a vein. The term also describes other connections between two parts or branches, such as two loops of the intestines (see Chapter 9).

ABBREVIATIONS RELATED TO THE CARDIOVASCULAR SYSTEM

Table 5.4 presents an overview of the abbreviations related to the terms introduced in this chapter. *Note:* To avoid errors or confusion, always be cautious when using abbreviations.

TABLE 5.4

Abbreviations Related to the Cardiovascular System

atrial fibrillation = A-fib	**A-fib** = atrial fibrillation
automated external defibrillator = AED	**AED** = automated external defibrillator
cardiac catheterization = card cath, CC	**card cath, CC** = cardiac catheterization
chronic venous insufficiency = CVI	**CVI** = chronic venous insufficiency
coronary artery bypass graft = CABG	**CABG** = coronary artery bypass graft
coronary artery disease = CAD	**CAD** = coronary artery disease
electrocardiogram = EKG, ECG	**EKG, ECG** = electrocardiogram
hypertension = HTN	**HTN** = hypertension
implantable cardioverter–defibrillator = ICD	**ICD** = implantable cardioverter–defibrillator
myocardial infarction = MI	**MI** = myocardial infarction
peripheral artery disease = PAD	**PAD** = peripheral artery disease
peripheral vascular disease = PVD	**PVD** = peripheral vascular disease
thallium stress test = TST	**TST** = thallium stress test
ventricular fibrillation = V-fib	**V-fib** = ventricular fibrillation

LEARNING EXERCISES

Matching Word Parts 1

Write the correct answer in the middle column.

	Definition	Correct Answer	Possible Answers
5.1.	aorta	______________	angi/o
5.2.	artery	______________	aort/o
5.3.	slow	______________	arteri/o
5.4.	relating to blood or lymph vessels	______________	ather/o
5.5.	plaque, fatty substance	______________	brady-

Matching Word Parts 2

Write the correct answer in the middle column.

	Definition	Correct Answer	Possible Answers
5.6.	blood or relating to the blood	______________	capill/o
5.7.	within	______________	cardi/o
5.8.	vein	______________	end/o
5.9.	heart	______________	hem/o
5.10.	capillary	______________	ven/o

Matching Word Parts 3

Write the correct answer in the middle column.

	Definition	Correct Answer	Possible Answers
5.11.	abnormal hardening	______________	phleb/o
5.12.	vein	______________	-sclerosis

5.13. fast, rapid ______________________ **tachy-**

5.14. surrounding ______________________ **thromb/o**

5.15. clot ______________________ **peri-**

Definitions

Select the correct answer, and write it on the line provided.

5.16. The ______________________ is/are located between the left ventricle and the aorta.

pulmonary valve aortic valve Purkinje fibers arterioles

5.17. Commonly known as the natural pacemaker, the medical name of the structure is the ______________________.

atrioventricular node bundle of His Purkinje fiber sinoatrial node

5.18. The myocardium receives its blood supply from the ______________________.

aorta coronary arteries inferior vena cava superior vena cava

5.19. The ______________________ return oxygen-poor blood to the heart.

veins venules capillaries arteries

5.20. The bicuspid valve is also known as the ______________________ valve.

aortic mitral pulmonary tricuspid

5.21. The ______________________ pumps blood into the pulmonary artery, which carries it to the lungs.

left atrium left ventricle right atrium right ventricle

5.22. The ______________________ are the two upper chambers of the heart.

atria ventricles venae cavae venules

5.23. A foreign object, such as a bit of tissue or air, circulating in the blood is known as a/an ______________________.

embolism embolus thrombosis thrombus

5.24. The ______________________ carries blood to all parts of the body except the lungs.

left atrium left ventricle right atrium right ventricle

5.25. The ______________ form(s) the main trunk of the arterial system.

venae cavae   arterioles   aorta   carotid artery

Matching Structures

Write the correct answer in the middle column.

	Definition	Correct Answer	Possible Answers
5.26.	clotting proteins found in plasma	______________	endocardium
5.27.	cardiac muscle	______________	epicardium
5.28.	external layer of the heart	______________	fibrinogen
5.29.	inner lining of the heart	______________	myocardium
5.30.	sac enclosing the heart	______________	pericardium

Which Word?

Select the correct answer, and write it on the line provided.

5.31. High-density ______________ is also known as good cholesterol.

lipoprotein cholesterol   total cholesterol

5.32. An abnormally slow resting heart rate is described as ______________.

bradycardia   tachycardia

5.33. In ______________ fibrillation, the heart muscle quivers ineffectively, sometimes causing sudden cardiac death.

atrial   ventricular

5.34. The highest pressure against the blood vessels is ______________ pressure, and it occurs when the ventricles contract.

diastolic   systolic

5.35. The diagnostic procedure that images the structures of the blood vessels and the flow of blood through these vessels is known as ______________.

angiography   duplex ultrasound

Spelling Counts

Find the misspelled word in each sentence. Then write that word, spelled correctly, on the line provided.

5.36. The autopsy indicated that the cause of death was a ruptured aneuryism. ______________________

5.37. A deficiency of blood passing through an organ or body part is known as hypoprefusion. ______________________

5.38. An arrhythemia is an abnormal heart rhythm in which the heartbeat is faster or slower than normal. ______________________

5.39. Reynaud's disease is a peripheral arterial occlusive disease in which symptoms are triggered by cold temperatures or stress. ______________________

5.40. An implantable cardioverter-defibrilator is a double-action pacemaker. ______________________

Abbreviation Identification

In the space provided, write the words that each abbreviation stands for.

5.41. **CAD** ______________________

5.42. **EKG, ECG** ______________________

5.43. **A-fib** ______________________

5.44. **MI** ______________________

5.45. **V-fib** ______________________

Term Selection

Select the correct answer, and write it on the line provided.

5.46. The hardening and narrowing of the arteries caused by a buildup of cholesterol plaque is called ______________________.

atherosclerosis arteriosclerosis phlebitis vasculitis

5.47. A/An ______________________ reduces the workload of the heart by slowing the rate of the heartbeat.

ACE inhibitor beta-blocker calcium blocker statin inhibitor

5.48. A/An ______________________ is a blood clot that originates in a vein.

coronary thrombosis | thrombotic occlusion | embolus | venous thromboembolism

5.49. A/An ______________________ is a class of drugs administered to lower high blood pressure.

antiarrhythmic | antihypertensive | aspirin | diuretic

5.50. A bacterial infection of the lining or valves of the heart is known as infective ______________________.

endocarditis | myocarditis | pericarditis | carditis

Sentence Completion

Write the correct term on the lines provided.

5.51. A condition in which there is an insufficient supply of oxygen in the tissues due to restricted blood flow to a part of the body is called ______________________.

5.52. When the mitral valve does not close tightly, allowing blood to leak back through the opening, the condition is called mitral valve ______________________.

5.53. The surgical removal of the lining of a portion of a clogged carotid artery leading to the brain is known as a/an ______________________.

5.54. The abnormal protrusion of a heart valve that results in the inability of the valve to close completely is known as a/an ______________________.

5.55. The medication ______________________ is prescribed to treat hypertension, angina, and myocardial infarction by dilating the veins.

Word Surgery

Divide each term into its component word parts. Write these word parts, in sequence, on the lines provided. When necessary, use a slash (/) to indicate a combining vowel. (You may not need all of the lines provided.)

5.56. **Arteriosclerosis** is a group of diseases characterized by thickening and the loss of elasticity of arterial walls.

__________ __________ __________ __________

5.57. **Hyperlipidemia** is the general term used to describe elevated levels of cholesterol and other fatty substances in the blood.

______ ______ ______ ______

5.58. **Electrocardiography** is the process of recording the electrical activity of the myocardium.

______ ______ ______ ______

5.59. **Cardiomyopathy** is the term used to describe all diseases of the heart muscle.

______ ______ ______ ______

5.60. **Valvuloplasty** is the surgical repair or replacement of a heart valve.

______ ______ ______ ______

True/False

If the statement is true, write **True** on the line. If the statement is false, write **False** on the line.

5.61. _____ A thrombus is a clot or piece of tissue circulating in the blood.

5.62. _____ An atherectomy is the surgical removal of plaque buildup from the interior of an artery.

5.63. _____ Asystole is the loss of the normal rhythm of the heartbeat.

5.64. _____ A vasoconstrictor is a drug that enlarges the blood vessels.

5.65. _____ Peripheral vascular disease is a disorder of the blood vessels located outside the heart and brain.

Clinical Conditions

Write the correct answer on the line provided.

5.66. Alberta Fleetwood has a/an ________________. This condition is a benign tumor made up of newly formed blood vessels.

5.67. After his surgery, Ramon Martinez developed a deep vein ________________ in his leg.

5.68. During her pregnancy, Polly Olson suffered from abnormally swollen veins in her legs. The medical term for this condition is ________________ veins.

5.69. Thomas Wilkerson suffers from episodes of severe chest pain due to inadequate blood flow to the myocardium. This is a condition known as ________________.

5.70. When Mr. Klein stands up too quickly, his blood pressure drops. His physician describes this as postural or ________________.

5.71. The cardiologist suspected that Wade Casper had ________________, based on his family history of this disorder that can cause fast, chaotic arrhythmias.

5.72. Dr. Lawson read her patient's ________________. This diagnostic record is also known as an ECG or EKG.

5.73. Jason Turner was referred to a specialist in heart arrythmias, known as a/an ________________.

5.74. Darlene Nolan was diagnosed as having a deep vein thrombosis. Her doctor immediately prescribed a/an ________________ to cause the thrombus to dissolve.

5.75. Hamilton Edwards Sr. suffers from ________________. This is atherosclerosis of the coronary arteries that reduces the blood supply to the heart muscle.

Which Is the Correct Medical Term?

Select the correct answer, and write it on the line provided.

5.76. A/An ________________ is characterized by the loss of elasticity of arterial walls.

vasculitis atherosclerosis arteriosclerosis carotid artery stenosis

5.77. Temporal ________________ is an inflammation of the temporal arteries supplying blood to the head and brain.

arteritis phlebitis vasculitis ischemia

5.78. Inflammation of a vein is known as ________________.

arteriostenosis endocarditis phlebitis carditis

5.79. Tissue death caused by a severe shortage of blood supply due to illness, injury, and/or infection is called ________________.

thrombotic occlusion ischemia hemangioma gangrene

5.80. The flow of blood to all parts of the body *except* the lungs is known as ________________ circulation.

pulmonary mitral systemic sinoatrial

Challenge Word Building

These terms are *not* primary terms in the chapter; however, they are made up of the following familiar word parts. If you need help in creating the term, refer to your medical dictionary.

peri-	**angi/o**	**-ectomy**
	arter/o	**-itis**
	cardi/o	**-rrhaphy**
	phleb/o	**-graphy**
	ven/o	**-sclerosis**
		-stenosis

5.81. Inflammation of an artery or arteries is known as ______________________.

5.82. The surgical removal of a portion of a blood vessel is a/an ______________________.

5.83. The abnormal narrowing of the lumen of a vein is known as ______________________.

5.84. The surgical removal of a portion of the tissue surrounding the heart is a/an ______________________.

5.85. To surgically suture the wall of the heart is a/an ______________________.

5.86. The abnormal hardening of a vein is known as ______________________.

5.87. The suture repair of any vessel, especially a blood vessel, is a/an ______________________.

5.88. The graphic study of the movements of the heart is known as ______________________.

5.89. To suture the tissue surrounding the heart is a/an ______________________.

5.90. A radiographic test that provides an image of specific veins after a contrast dye is injected is a/an ______________________.

Labeling Exercises

Identify the numbered items in the accompanying figures.

5.91. superior ______________________

5.92. right ______________________

5.93. right ____________________

5.94. left pulmonary ____________________

5.95. left pulmonary ____________________

5.96. ____________________ valve

5.97. ____________________ valve

5.98. ____________________

5.99. ____________________ valve

5.100. ____________________ valve

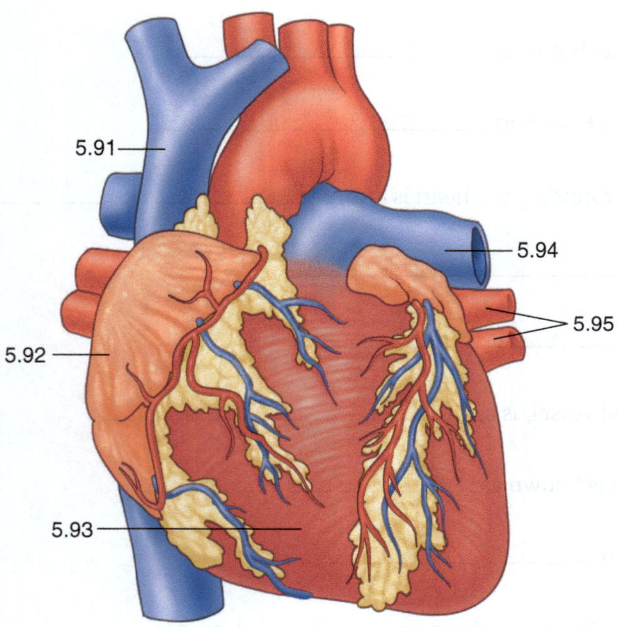

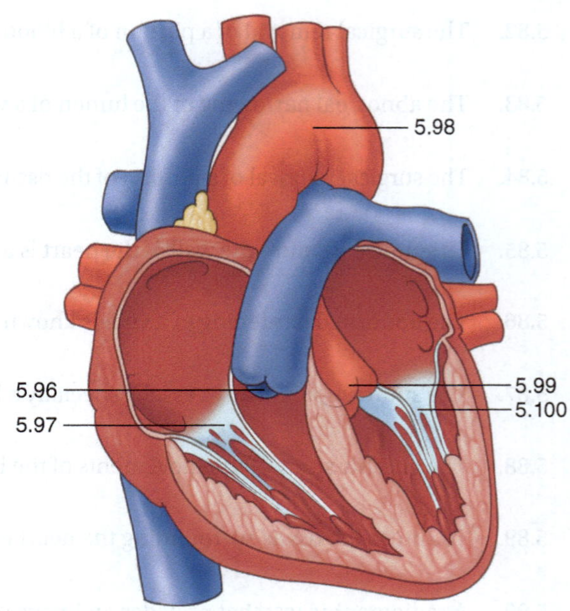

The Human Touch

CRITICAL THINKING EXERCISE

The following story and questions are designed to stimulate critical thinking through class discussion or as a brief essay response. There are no right or wrong answers to these questions.

Randi Marchant, a 42-year-old waitress, was vacuuming the family room when she felt that painful squeezing in her chest again. This was the third time today, but this one really hurt. She sat down to catch her breath and stubbed out the cigarette she had left smoldering in the half-filled ashtray by the couch. Randi's husband, Jimmy, and stepdaughter Melonie had pestered her until she finally had taken time off work to see her doctor. Dr. Harris found that her blood pressure was 158/88—probably owing to the noon rush stress at work, she rationalized. At least her cholesterol test was only 30 points above average this time. It had been slowly coming down, even though she was having a hard time following the DASH diet her doctor her doctor had recommended.

Another wave of pain tightened its icy fingers around her heart, and moved up into both sides of her jaw. Randi thought, "Probably just a little acid reflux. Since the pain doesn't radiate down my left arm, it couldn't be my heart, could it?"

"Don't think about the pain," she told herself. "Think of something else. For dinner tonight I'll make—" Randi fell to the floor, clutching her chest, just as Melonie walked in. She saw her stepmother slumped on the floor and screamed, "Help, somebody, help!"

Suggested Discussion Topics

1. What information in the story indicates that Randi might be a candidate for heart disease?
2. Discuss why Randi thought this was not a heart attack.
3. What can Melonie do immediately to try to save Randi's life?
4. Assuming that Randi is suffering a myocardial infarction, discuss why it is important that she receive appropriate treatment quickly.

CHAPTER 6

THE BLOOD SYSTEM

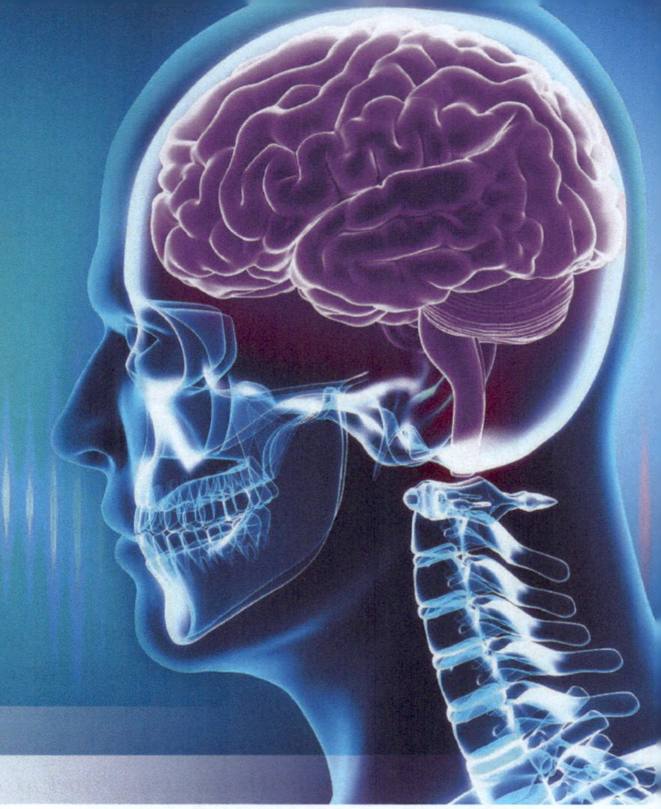

Overview of STRUCTURES, COMBINING FORMS, AND FUNCTIONS OF THE BLOOD SYSTEM

Major Structures	Related Combining Forms	Primary Functions
Blood	hem/o, hemat/o	Brings oxygen and nutrients to the cells and carries away waste.
Plasma	plasma, plasm/o	Contains nutrients, hormones, waste products, and clotting proteins.
Erythrocytes (red blood cells)	erythr/o	Transport oxygen to the tissues.
Leukocytes (white blood cells)	leuk/o	Support the immune system.
Platelets (thrombocytes)	thromb/o	Play an important role in the clotting of blood.

Vocabulary Related to **THE BLOOD SYSTEM**

This list contains essential word parts and medical terms for this chapter. These and the other important **primary terms** are shown in **boldface** throughout the chapter. *Secondary terms*, which appear in *orange* italics, clarify the meaning of primary terms.

Word Parts

- ☐ **chromat/o** color
- ☐ **coagul/o** clotting, coagulation
- ☐ **-emia** blood, blood condition
- ☐ **erythr/o** red
- ☐ **fibrin/o** fibrin, fibers, threads of a clot
- ☐ **-globin** protein
- ☐ **hem/o**, **hemat/o** blood, relating to the blood
- ☐ **leuk/o** white
- ☐ **myel/o** spinal cord, bone marrow
- ☐ **-oid** resembling
- ☐ **-penia** deficiency
- ☐ **phleb/o** vein
- ☐ **plasma**, **plasm/o** something molded or formed, plasma
- ☐ **-poiesis** to make
- ☐ **-stasis** maintenance of a constant level

Medical Terms

- ☐ **allogeneic transfusion** (**al**-loh-jen-**EEH**-ick)
- ☐ **anticoagulant** (**an**-tih-koh-**AG**-you-lant)
- ☐ **antigen** (**AN**-tih-jen)
- ☐ **aplastic anemia** (ay-**PLAS**-tick ah-**NEE**-mee-ah)
- ☐ **autologous transfusion** (aw-**TOL**-uh-guss)
- ☐ **basophils** (**BAY**-soh-fills)
- ☐ **coagulation** (koh-**ag**-you-**LAY**-shun)
- ☐ **coagulopathy** (koh-**ag**-you-**LOP**-ah-thee)
- ☐ **comprehensive metabolic panel**
- ☐ **decompression sickness**
- ☐ **direct antiglobulin test**
- ☐ **eosinophils** (**ee**-oh-**SIN**-oh-fills)
- ☐ **erythrocyte** (eh-**RITH**-roh-site)
- ☐ **erythropoietin** (eh-**rith**-roh-**POY**-eh-tin)
- ☐ **fibrin** (**FYE**-brin)
- ☐ **fibrinogen** (fye-**BRIN**-oh-jen)
- ☐ **globulins** (**GLOB**-you-lins)
- ☐ **granulocytes** (**GRAN**-you-loh-**sights**)
- ☐ **hematologist** (**hee**-mah-**TOL**-oh-jist)
- ☐ **hematopoiesis** (hee-**MAT**-oh-poh-**ee**-sis)
- ☐ **hematocrit** (hee-**MAT**-oh-krit)
- ☐ **hemoglobin** (**HEE**-moh-**gloh**-bin)
- ☐ **hemolysis** (heh-**MOL**-eh-sis)
- ☐ **hemolytic anemia** (**hee**-moh-**LIT**-ick ah-**NEE**-mee-ah)
- ☐ **hemophilia** (**hee**-moh-**FILL**-ee-ah)
- ☐ **hemostasis** (**hee**-moh-**STAY**-sis)
- ☐ **hemorrhage** (**HEM**-or-idj)
- ☐ **heparin** (**HEP**-ah-rin)
- ☐ **hereditary spherocytosis** (**sfee**-roh-sigh-**TOH**-sis)
- ☐ **immunoglobulins** (**im**-you-noh-**GLOB**-you-lins)
- ☐ **leukemia** (loo-**KEE**-mee-ah)
- ☐ **leukocytes** (**LOO**-koh-sights)
- ☐ **leukopenia** (**loo**-koh-**PEE**-nee-ah)
- ☐ **lipoprotein panel blood test**
- ☐ **lymphocytes** (**LIM**-foh-sights)
- ☐ **megakaryocytes** (**meg**-ah-**KAH**-ree-oh-sights)
- ☐ **monocytes** (**MON**-oh-sights)
- ☐ **multiple myeloma** (**my**-eh-**LOH**-mah)
- ☐ **neutropenia** (**new**-troh-**PEE**-nee-ah)
- ☐ **neutrophils** (**NEW**-troh-fills)
- ☐ **non-Hodgkin's lymphoma**
- ☐ **pancytopenia** (**pan**-sight-oh-**PEE**-nee-ah)
- ☐ **pernicious anemia** (per-**NISH**-us ah-**NEE**-mee-ah)
- ☐ **phagocytes** (**FAG**-oh-sights)
- ☐ **phlebotomist** (fleh-**BOT**-oh-mist)
- ☐ **plasma** (**PLAZ**-mah)
- ☐ **plasmapheresis** (**plaz**-mah-feh-**REE**-sis)
- ☐ **platelets** (**PLAYT**-lets)
- ☐ **prothrombin time** (proh-**THROM**-bin)
- ☐ **reticulocytes** (reh-**TIK**-you-loh-sights)
- ☐ **Rh factor**
- ☐ **sepsis** (**SEP**-sis)
- ☐ **serum**
- ☐ **sickle cell anemia**
- ☐ **thalassemia** (**thal**-ah-**SEE**-mee-ah)
- ☐ **therapeutic plasma exchange**
- ☐ **thrombocytes** (**THROM**-boh-sights)
- ☐ **thrombocytopenia** (**throm**-boh-**sigh**-toh-**PEE**-nee-ah)
- ☐ **transfusion reaction**
- ☐ **Von Willebrand disease** (von **VIL**-eh-brond)

LEARNING OBJECTIVES

On completion of this chapter, you should be able to:

1. Explain the functions of the hematologic system.
2. Identify the major components of blood and the major functions of each component.
3. Differentiate between the four blood types.
4. Identify the medical specialists who treat disorders of the blood system.
5. Identify the medical word parts of the blood system.
6. Define the primary terms related to the pathology and treatment procedures of hematologic diseases, including blood clotting disorders, blood cancers, and diseases of the bone marrow cells.
7. Describe the diagnostic test procedures of the blood system, including basic blood tests and their purpose.
8. Spell the primary terms of the blood system.
9. Pronounce the primary terms of the blood system.
10. Identify common abbreviations related to the blood system.

FUNCTIONS OF THE BLOOD SYSTEM

The blood system, also known as the **hematologic system**, consists of the blood and bone marrow. **Hematologic** (HEE-mat-oh-**lah**-jik) means pertaining to the blood (**hemat/o** means blood, **-log** means the study of, and **-ic** means pertaining to).

Blood delivers oxygen and nutrients to the tissues, and transports carbon dioxide, blood cells, immune cells, antibodies, and hormones throughout the body. Blood also removes waste products from tissues and delivers them to the liver and kidneys, and returns carbon dioxide to the lungs. The blood plays an important role in fighting inflammation, and helps regulate skin temperature as well as the pH and water balance in the body.

STRUCTURES OF THE BLOOD

Blood is the fluid tissue in the body. It is composed of 55% liquid plasma and 45% formed elements (blood cells and platelets) suspended in the plasma (Figure 6.1).

Plasma

Plasma (**PLAZ**-mah) is a straw-colored fluid that contains nutrients, hormones, and waste products. Plasma is 92% water. The remaining 8% consists mainly of the blood proteins albumin and globulins, and the clotting proteins fibrinogen and prothrombin. These proteins are all produced in the liver.

- **Albumin** (al-**BYOU**-min) is the main protein in the blood and helps prevent fluid from leaking out of the blood vessels into other tissues.
- **Globulins** (**GLOB**-you-lins) are a group of proteins in the blood that play an important role in the immune system.
- **Fibrinogen** (figh-**BRIN**-oh-jen) and **prothrombin** (proh-**THROM**-bin) are the clotting proteins found in plasma. They are important for clot formation to control bleeding.
- **Serum** (**SEER**-um) is the clear, pale yellow plasma fluid that remains after the blood cells and clotting proteins have been removed.

Formed Elements of the Blood

The **formed elements** of blood include three categories of cells: erythrocytes, leukocytes, and thrombocytes thrombocytes (platelets). They are called formed elements because they have a definite structure and shape.

Erythrocytes

Erythrocytes (eh-**RITH**-roh-**sights**), also known as ***red blood cells*** (RBCs), are mature red blood cells produced by the red bone marrow (**erythr/o** means red, and **-cytes** means cells). The primary role of these cells, which make up about 45% of the blood by volume, is to transport oxygen to the tissues.

Oxygen is transported by **hemoglobin** (**HEE**-moh-**gloh**-bin) (Hgb), which is a blood protein pigment of the erythrocytes (**hem/o** means blood, and

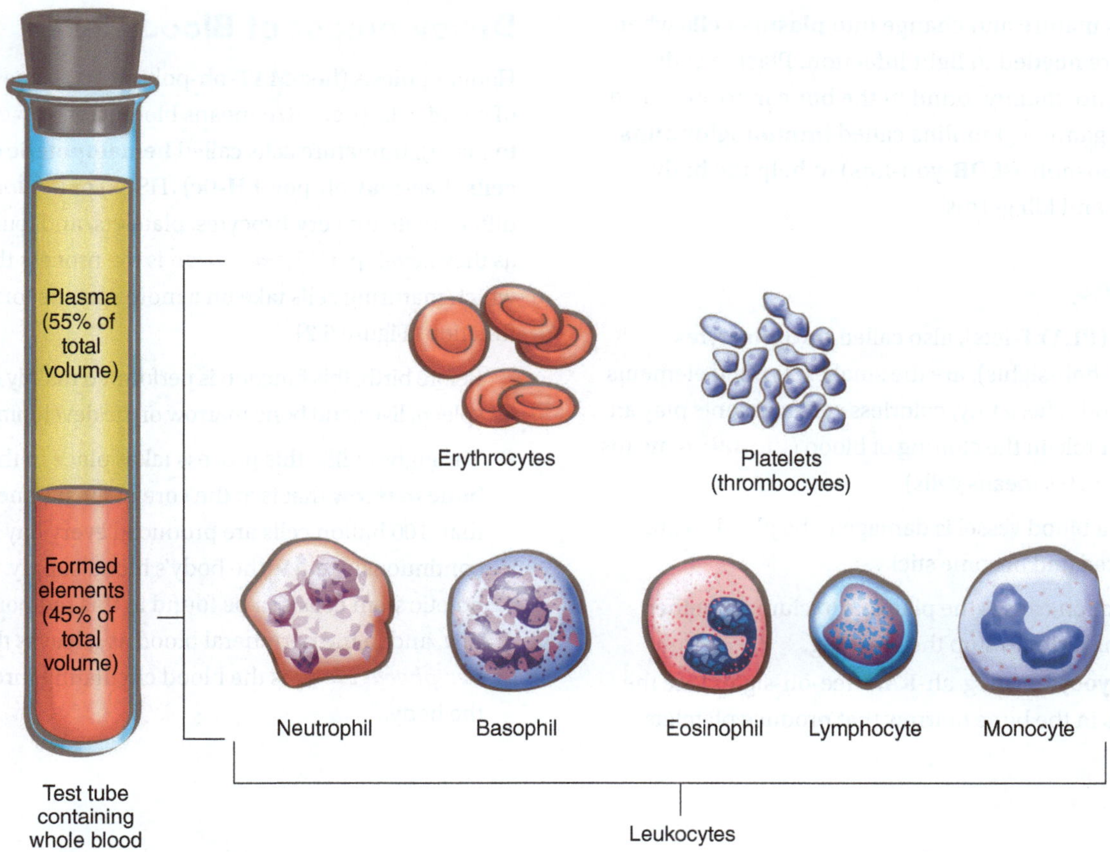

FIGURE 6.1 Components of the blood.

-globin means protein). Hemoglobin contains a red-colored compound called ***heme*** that gives blood its color.

Erythropoietin (eh-**rith**-roh-**POY**-eh-tin) (EPO) is a hormone produced in the kidneys that promotes the production of erythrocytes in the bone marrow. Measurement of the erythropoietin level in the blood is used to detect certain medical conditions.

Leukocytes

Leukocytes (**LOO**-koh-**sights**), also known as ***white blood cells*** (WBCs), are the blood cells involved in supporting the immune system in defending the body against infective organisms and foreign substances (**leuk/o** means white, and **-cytes** means cells). The following are the major groups of leukocytes:

- **Neutrophils** (**NEW**-troh-fills), which are formed in red bone marrow, are the most common type of WBCs. Neutrophils, along with macrophages, are called phagocytes. **Phagocytes** (**FAG**-oh-sights) are cells that play a major role in the immune system's defense against pathogens such as bacteria, viruses, and fungi by engulfing the pathogens and consuming them (**phag/o** means to eat or swallow, and **-cytes** means cells). Phagocytes are discussed further in Chapter 7.
- **Basophils** (**BAY**-soh-fills), which are also formed in red bone marrow, are the least common type of WBCs. Basophils are responsible for the histamines that cause the symptoms of allergic reactions.
- **Eosinophils** (**ee**-oh-**SIN**-oh-fills) are formed in red bone marrow and then migrate to tissues throughout the body. These cells destroy some parasites, and play a major role in allergic reactions.
- Neutrophils, eosinophils, and basophils are all called **granulocytes** (**GRAN**-you-loh-**sights**) because they have small granules containing proteins. When there is a serious infection, the body produces more granulocytes.
- **Lymphocytes** (**LIM**-foh-sights) include T cells and B cells. These are formed in the red bone marrow, lymph nodes, and the spleen. Lymphocytes identify foreign substances and germs (bacteria or viruses) in the body and produce antibodies that specifically target them. Lymphocytes are discussed further in Chapter 7.

Monocytes (**MON**-oh-sights) are also formed in the red bone marrow, lymph nodes, and the spleen. They are the largest type of white blood cells. Through ***phagocytosis***, which is the the ingestion of bacteria or other material by phagocytes, monocytes provide immunological defenses against many infectious organisms.

- B cells mature and change into **plasma cells** when they are needed to fight infection. Plasma cells, which are mainly found in the bone marrow, make active gamma globulins called **immunoglobulins** (**im**-you-noh-**GLOB**-you-lins) to help the body attack and kill germs.

Platelets

Platelets (**PLAYT**-lets), also called **thrombocytes** (**THROM**-boh-sights), are the smallest formed elements of the blood. These tiny, colorless cell fragments play an important role in the clotting of blood (**thromb/o** means clot, and **-cytes** means cells).

- When a blood vessel is damaged, the platelets are activated and become sticky.
- This action causes the platelets to clump together, forming a clot to stop the bleeding.

Megakaryocytes (**meg**-ah-**KAH**-ree-oh-sights) are the large cells in the bone marrow that produce platelets.

Development of Blood Cells

Hematopoiesis (hee-**MAT**-oh-poh-**ee**-sis) is the formation of blood cells (**hemat/o** means blood, and **-poiesis** means to make). Immature cells called **hematopoietic stem cells** (hee-**mat**-oh-poy-**EH**-tic) (HSCs) or ***hemocytoblasts*** differentiate into erythrocytes, platelets, and leukocytes as they develop. ***Differentiation*** is the process through which maturing cells take on a more specific form and function (Figure 6.2).

- Before birth, this function is performed mainly in the spleen, liver, and bone marrow of the developing embryo.
- Throughout life, this process takes place in the **red bone marrow** that is at the core of most bones. More than 100 billion cells are produced every day in order to continuously renew the body's blood supply. Hematopoietic stem cells can be found in this red bone marrow, and in the peripheral blood as it leaves the bone. ***Peripheral blood*** is the blood circulating throughout the body.

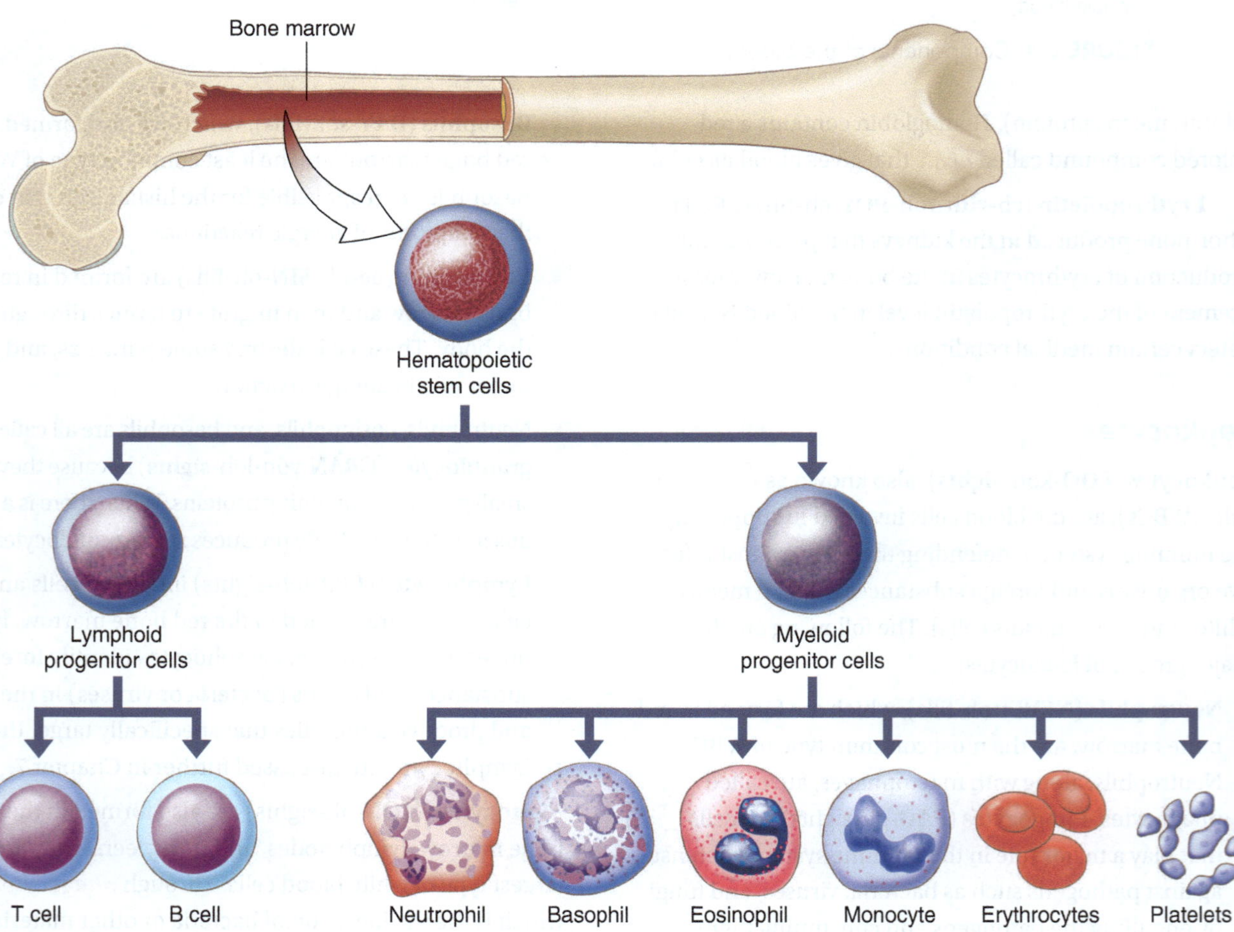

FIGURE 6.2 Blood cell formation from stem cells in bone marrow.

- **Reticulocytes** (reh-**TIK**-you-loh-sights) are red blood cells that have just been released from the bone marrow. They will mature in about a day in the bloodstream. The reticulocyte count in a blood sample is indicative of how well the bone marrow, liver, and kidneys are functioning. A high count can also indicate extensive blood loss.
- T cells and B cells are among the lymphocytes that originate in the bone marrow. B cells mature there, while T cells migrate to the **thymus**, where they are referred to as ***thymocytes***. The thymus facilitates the maturation of these cells that are an important part of the immune system's ability to provide cell-mediated immunity. See Chapter 14 for additional functions of the thymus.

ABO Blood Types

Blood types are classified according to the presence or absence of certain antigens. An **antigen** (**AN**-tih-jen) is any substance that the body regards as being foreign, thus sometimes triggering an adverse reaction. Traditionally, blood type is listed as type (represented by a letter) followed by Rh factor (represented by + or –), such as A– or O+.

The four major blood types are called **A**, **AB**, **B**, and **O**. The A, AB, and B groups are based on the presence of the A and/or B antigens on the red blood cells. In type O blood, both the A and B antigens are absent (Figure 6.3). (The O actually represents a zero, referring to the lack of either A or B antigens.)

The Rh Factor

The **Rh factor** defines the presence or absence of the Rh antigen on red blood cells. The Rh factor is so named because this antigen was first found in rhesus monkeys. It is pronounced as the letters, *R H*.

- About 85% of Americans have the Rh antigen, and these individuals are described as being ***Rh positive*** (Rh+).
- The remaining 15% of Americans *do not have* the Rh antigen, and these individuals are described as being ***Rh negative*** (Rh–).
- The Rh factor is an important consideration when cross-matching blood for transfusions.
- The Rh factor can cause difficulties when an Rh-positive infant is born to an Rh-negative mother.

Genetic Determination of Blood Type

The factors that determine blood type and the Rh factor are part of the genetic code passed on from parent to child. Each biological parent donates one ABO gene to their child, meaning that there are six different possible combinations. The A and B genes are dominant and the O gene is recessive, giving the results shown in Table 6.1

Blood type	A	B	AB	O
Erythrocytes (red blood cells)	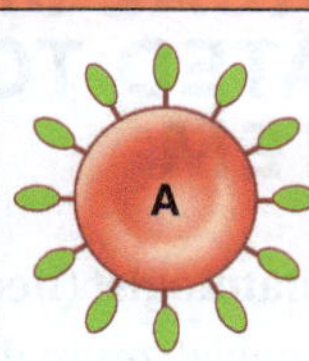	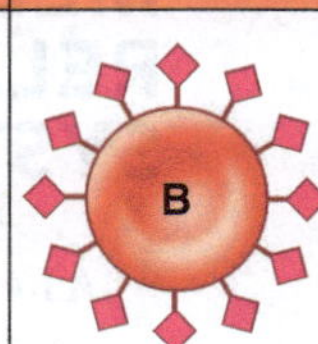	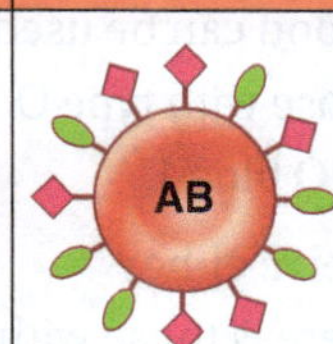	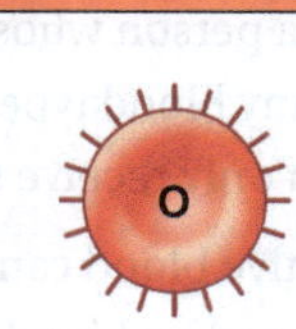
Antibodies in plasma	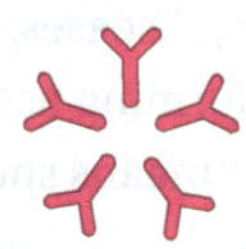 Anti-B	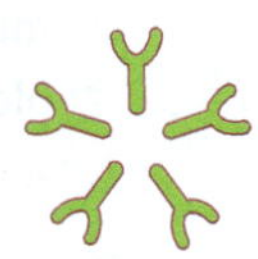 Anti-A	None	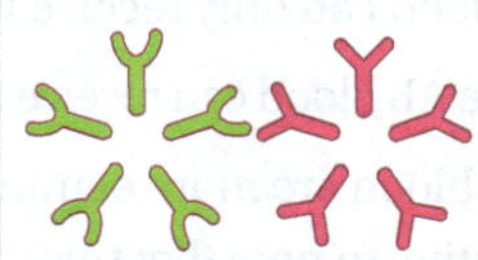 Anti-A and Anti-B
Antigens in red blood cells	A antigen	B antigen	A and B antigen	None
Can receive blood from:	**A, O**	**B, O**	**AB, A, B, O** (all types)	**O**
Can donate blood to:	**A, AB**	**B, AB**	**AB**	**AB, A, B, O** (all types)

FIGURE 6.3 Blood type classifications for transfusions.

TABLE 6.1

Parent 1's Blood Type	Parent 2's Blood Type	Child's Blood Type
A	A	A
A	O	A
B	B	B
B	O	B
O	O	O
A	B	AB

- Every individual also inherits one Rh factor gene from each biological parent, with the Rh-positive gene always dominant. During pregnancy, problems can occur if the mother is Rh negative and the fetus is Rh positive. An early prenatal blood test is used to determine whether this is the case. If it is, a medication called ***Rho(D) immune globulin*** (RhoGAM) is administered to prevent the mother's body from producing Rh antibodies that might harm the fetus.

Matching Blood Types

Blood types must be matched in specific ways for blood transfusions, to prevent antigens that are present in the recipient's blood type from being attacked by the antibodies in the blood received via transfusion.

- Type O– blood is considered a universal donor for red blood cells because it doesn't contain any antigens. A ***universal donor*** is a person whose blood can be used in transfusions for any blood type. Those with type O blood, however, can only receive type O blood.
- Those with Rh-positive blood can receive either Rh-positive or Rh-negative blood, whereas those with Rh-negative blood can only receive Rh-negative blood.
- Those with type AB blood can receive all types of blood.
- Some types of blood are more common than others, and it's interesting to note that this varies widely in different parts of the world. In the United States, O+ and A+ together account for about 70% of all people. Although AB negative is found in a very small percentage of the population, *a* ***rare blood type*** refers to when some of the 600 other known antigens beyond A and B are either present or absent.

Blood Gases

Blood gases are gases that are normally dissolved in the fluid portion of blood. The major blood gases are *oxygen* (O_2), *carbon dioxide* (CO_2), and *nitrogen* (N_2). Red blood cells transport oxygen from the lungs to all the tissues of the body, and return carbon dioxide to the lungs to be eliminated. Nitrogen is inhaled along with oxygen, but the human body is not able to absorb nitrogen in its gaseous form. Food and water are the primary sources of the nitrogen the body needs.

Hemostasis

- **Hemostasis** (**hee**-moh-**STAY**-sis) means to stop or control bleeding (**hem/o** means blood, and **-stasis** means stopping or controlling). The body attempts to do this by automatically constricting an injured blood vessel and activating factors to cause the platelets and proteins in the blood to thicken and form a clot. ***Mechanical hemostasis*** refers to the use of external means such as a tourniquet to stop the flow of blood during surgery or in an emergency.
- **Coagulation** (koh-**ag**-you-**LAY**-shun) is the process of blood clotting, or the formation of a blood clot. (**coagul** means clotting, and **-ation** means action).
- **Thrombin** and **fibrinogen** are proteins in the blood plasma that are important clotting agents. When activated by an injury, fibrinogen forms a web-like material called **fibrin** (**FYE**-brin) that aids in blood clotting and the formation of a scab to help the wound heal. As the body ages, however, increased formation of fibrin can increase the risk of dangerous blood clots.

MEDICAL SPECIALTIES RELATED TO THE BLOOD SYSTEM

- A **hematologist** (**hee**-mah-**TOL**-oh-jist) is a physician who specializes in diagnosing and treating abnormalities, diseases, and disorders of the blood and blood-forming tissues (**hemat** means blood, and **-ologist** means specialist).
- A **phlebotomist** (fleh-**BOT**-oh-mist) is a medical professional trained to draw blood from patients for laboratory tests and other procedures (Figure 6.4).

PATHOLOGY OF THE BLOOD SYSTEM

Blood Clotting Disorders

- A **hypercoagulable state** (**high**-per-koh-**AG**-you-lah-bull) occurs when the blood has an increased tendency to form clots.

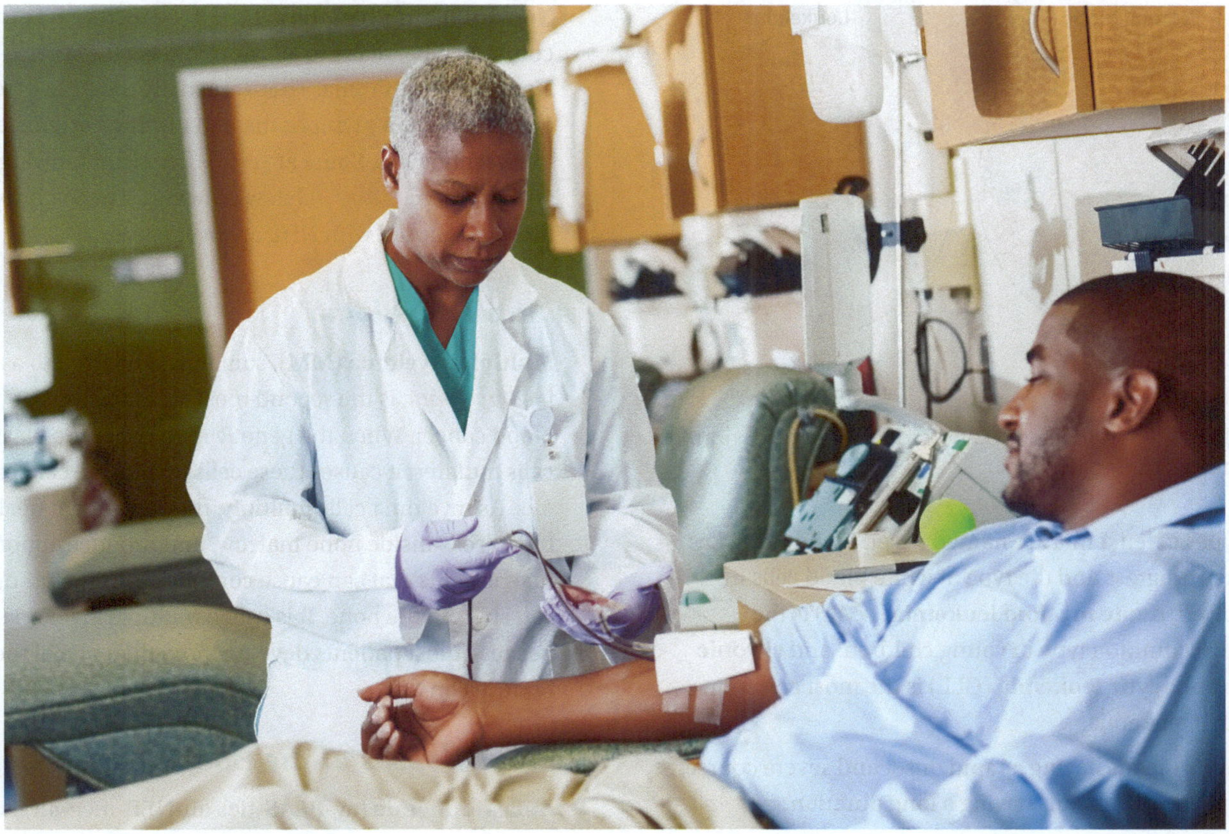

FIGURE 6.4 A phlebotomist checking a blood draw.

This condition can be genetic, with the most common cause being ***Factor V Leiden***, or acquired as a result of surgery, trauma, or medications. Individuals with this condition have an increased tendency to form blood clots, which can cause deep vein thrombosis or a pulmonary embolus. If the blood clot occurs in the arteries, it increases the risk of a stroke, a heart attack, or the loss of a limb.

- **Coagulopathy** (koh-**ag**-you-**LOP**-ah-thee), also known as a ***bleeding disorder***, occurs when the blood's ability to coagulate is impaired. Hemophilia and von Willebrand's disease are genetic disorders that can cause this reduction in clotting factors.
- **Hemophilia** (**hee**-moh-**FILL**-ee-ah) is a hereditary bleeding disorder in which a blood-clotting factor is missing, resulting in abnormal coagulation. This disorder, which mostly affects males, is characterized by spontaneous hemorrhages or severe bleeding following an injury.
- **Von Willebrand disease** (von **VIL**-eh-brond) (VWD), the most common genetic bleeding disorder, impacts women more than men. People with VWD either have a low level of the clotting protein called the ***von Willebrand factor*** in their blood, or this protein doesn't function the way it should. This can lead to heavy, hard-to-stop bleeding, and menorrhagia during menstrual periods.

Diseases of the Bone Marrow

Bone marrow diseases are caused by problems with the stem cells in the bone marrow, or with their development. The three main types of blood cancer originate in the bone marrow: leukemia, lymphoma, and multiple myeloma. Aplastic anemia, myelodysplastic syndrome, and pancytopenia are also bone marrow diseases.

Leukemia

Leukemia (loo-**KEE**-mee-ah) is a type of cancer characterized by a progressive increase in the number of abnormal leukocytes found in blood-forming tissues, other organs, and the circulating blood (**leuk** means white, and **-emia** means blood condition). These abnormal leukocytes impair the ability of the bone marrow to produce red blood cells and platelets (Figure 6.5).

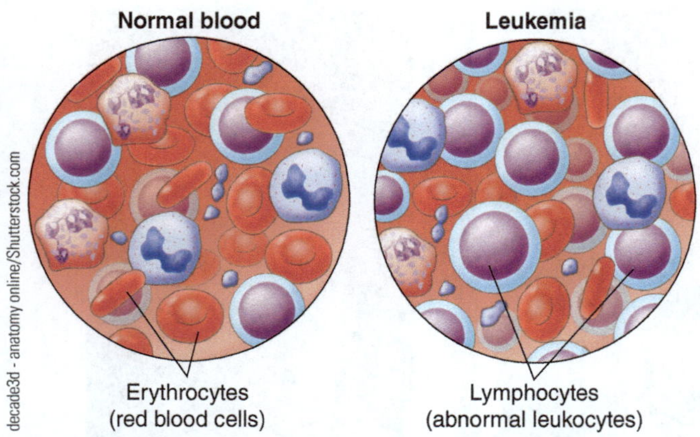

FIGURE 6.5 Normal blood and blood showing abnormal leukocytes due to leukemia.

- Types of leukemia are named based on how quickly they progress and the type of white blood cells involved. **Acute myeloid leukemia** (AML) is the most common type in young children, and **chronic lymphocytic leukemia** (CLL) is the most common adult leukemia.
- ***Acute*** means having a rapid onset and severe course, and ***chronic*** means having a long duration.
- **Myeloid** (**MY**-eh-loyd) refers to cells growing in the bone marrow. In this type of leukemia, the bone marrow produces white blood cells that develop into large numbers of leukemic cells called myeloblasts. Another term for this type of cancer is ***myelogenous***. The adjective **myeloid** means relating to the bone marrow (**myel** means bone marrow, and **-oid** means resembling).
- **Lymphocytic** (lim-foh-**SIT**-ic) means that the bone marrow is producing abnormal, ineffective lymphocytes, which are a type of leukocyte important to the immune system.

Lymphoma

Lymphoma (lim-**FOH**-mah) is a general term applied to malignancies affecting lymphoid tissues (**lymph** means lymph, and **-oma** means tumor). This includes lymph nodes, the spleen, the liver, and bone marrow. The two most common types of lymphomas are Hodgkin's lymphoma and non-Hodgkin's lymphoma.

- **Hodgkin's lymphoma** (**HODJ**-kinz) (HL), also known as ***Hodgkin's disease***, is a cancer of the immune system distinguished by the presence of large, cancerous lymphocytes known as ***Reed-Sternberg cells***. The spread of these cells compromises the body's ability to fight infection. HL is usually treatable, especially in its early stages.
- **Non-Hodgkin's lymphoma** (NHL), which is the more common type, refers to all lymphomas other than Hodgkin's lymphoma. There are many different types of non-Hodgkin's lymphomas, all of which originate in the lymphocytes. Some are ***aggressive*** (fast growing) and some are ***indolent*** (slow growing). The majority of those diagnosed with NHL are over age 65.

Multiple Myeloma

- **Multiple myeloma** (MM), sometimes referred to as just ***myeloma***, is the second most common type of blood cancer. When the genetic material in the plasma cells mutates, it causes these cells to become cancerous. As myeloma cells multiply, they crowd out healthy blood cells inside bone marrow, and produce abnormal proteins that can cause complications including soft spots in the bone. It is called multiple myeloma because most patients develop more than one of these bone lesions.

Other Diseases of the Bone Marrow Cells

- **Aplastic anemia** (ay-**PLAS**-tick ah-**NEE**-mee-ah) is a rare but serious condition characterized by an absence of *all* formed blood elements caused by the failure of blood cell production in the bone marrow (**a-** means without, **plast** means growth, and **-ic** means pertaining to). Contrast this with ***anemia***, in which there is a lower than average number of red blood cells.
- **Myelodysplastic syndrome** (**my**-eh-loh-dis-**PLAS**-tick **SIN**-drohm) (MDS) is a type of cancer in which there is insufficient production of one or more types of blood cells due to dysfunction of the bone marrow (**myel/o** means bone marrow, **dys** means bad, and **-plastic** means pertaining to formation). Some patients later develop ***acute myeloid leukemia***.
- **Pancytopenia** (**pan**-sight-oh-**PEE**-nee-ah) is a condition that is characterized by lower-than-normal quantities of erythrocytes, leukocytes, and platelets. This is usually caused by a problem in the bone marrow where the blood cells are produced as a result of cancer, lupus, or a bone marrow disorder.

Disorders of the Blood Gases

- **Decompression sickness** (DCS), also called ***the bends***, is a potentially fatal condition that can occur as a result of deep-sea diving or unpressurized air travel. During a rapid ascent from a deep-sea dive, or other compressed air environment, accumulated nitrogen can form bubbles in the blood or tissue, damaging blood vessels and tissue or triggering small blood clots. Treatment involves administering 100% oxygen, followed by recompression in a ***hyperbaric oxygen chamber*** (Figure 6.6).

- **Carbon monoxide poisoning** occurs when an abnormally high concentration of carbon monoxide builds up in the blood, resulting in **hypoxia** (deficient oxygen levels in the body's tissue and organs). Accidentally inhaling combustion fumes from improperly ventilated heaters, appliances, and engines can lead to carbon monoxide poisoning, which may cause serious tissue damage and even death.

Blood Disorders

- **Hemochromatosis** (**hee**-moh-**kroh**-mah-**TOH**-sis), also known as ***iron overload disease***, is a genetic disorder in which the intestines absorb too much iron (**hem/o** means blood, **chromat** means color, and **-osis** means abnormal condition or disease). The excess iron that is absorbed enters the bloodstream and accumulates in organs, where it causes damage.
- **Hereditary spherocytosis** (**sfee**-roh-sigh-**TOH**-sis) is a genetic disorder that causes the red blood cells to be spherical rather than flat. These malformed cells are fragile and have a shorter life span than normal erythrocytes. Their spherical shape taxes the spleen's ability to clear out the red cells and their products, possibly resulting in ***splenomegaly*** (enlargement of the spleen) and anemia.
- **Leukopenia** (**loo**-koh-**PEE**-nee-ah) is a decrease in the number of disease-fighting leukocytes circulating in the blood (**leuk/o** means white, and **-penia** means deficiency). This condition, which is also known as a ***low white blood cell count***, places the patient at an increased of risk of developing or having difficulty fighting infections.
- **Neutropenia** (**new**-troh-**PEE**-nee-ah) is the presence of abnormally few of the white blood cells called neutrophils in the blood, usually as a result of cancer treatment. This condition can lead to increased susceptibility to infection Sepsis.
- **Polycythemia** (**pol**-ee-sigh-**THEE**-mee-ah) is a condition which causes the bone marrow to produce too many erythrocytes (**poly-** means many, **cyt** means

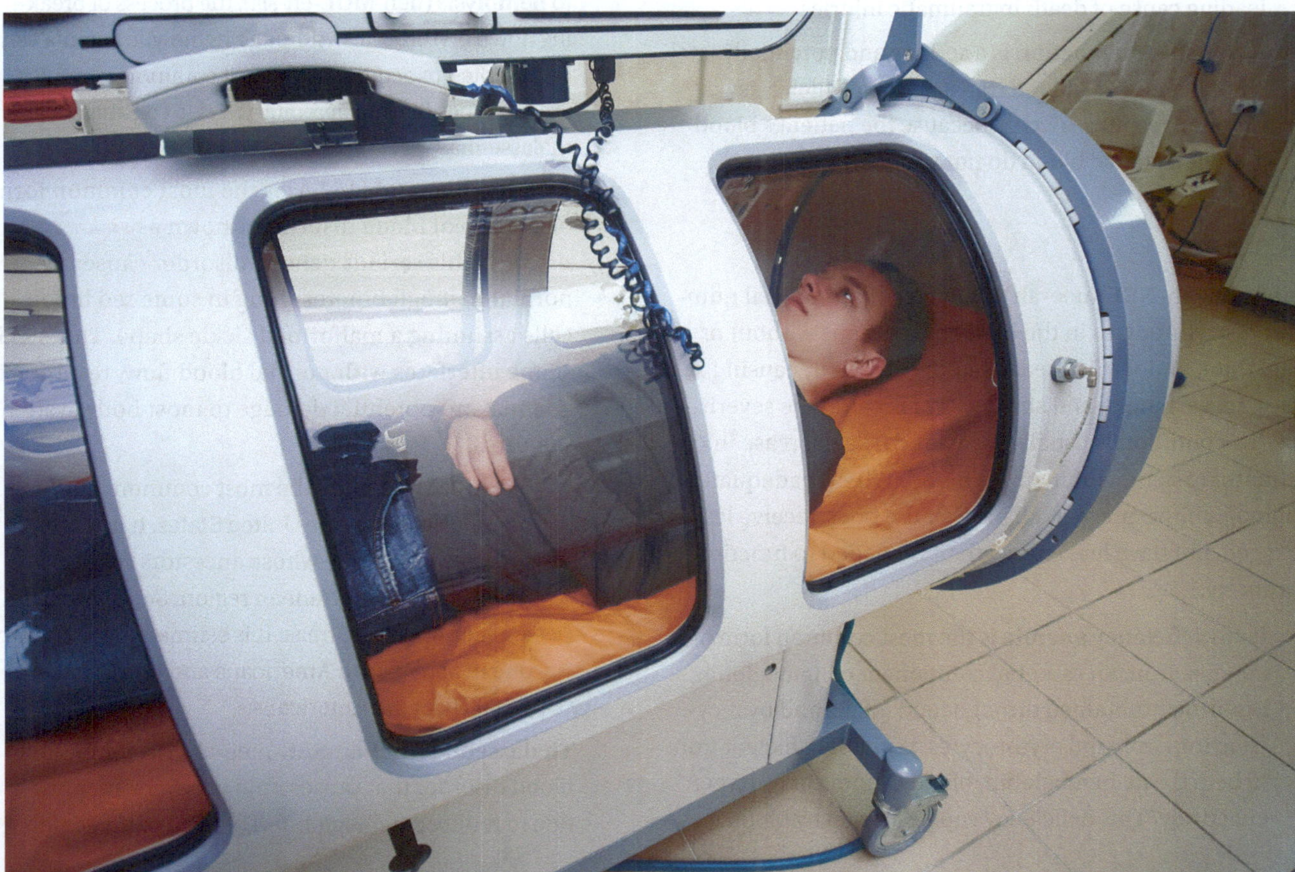

Nakleyka/Shutterstock.com

FIGURE 6.6 A patient undergoing treatment for decompression sickness.

cell, **hem** means blood, and **-ia** means abnormal condition). This abnormal increase in the number of circulating red blood cells causes the blood to thicken, increasing the risk of blood clots and other complications. A rare blood cancer called ***polycythemia vera*** is the most common cause of this condition.

- **Thrombocytopenia** (**throm**-boh-**sigh**-toh-**PEE**-nee-ah) is a condition in which there is an abnormally small number of platelets circulating in the blood (**thromb/o** means clot, **cyt/o** means cell, and **-penia** means deficiency). Because platelets help the blood to clot, this condition is sometimes associated with abnormal bleeding as a result of leukemia or infection, or as a side effect of chemotherapy or radiation treatments.
- **Thrombocytosis** (**throm**-boh-sigh-**TOH**-sis) is an abnormal increase in the number of platelets in the circulating blood (**thromb/o** means clot, **cyt** means cell, and **-osis** means abnormal condition). It is sometimes referred to as ***secondary thrombocytosis*** because the production of platelets can occur as part of the body's response to an injury.
- A **hemorrhage** (**HEM**-or-idj) is the loss of a large amount of blood in a short time (**hem/o** means blood, and **-rrhage** means bleeding). ***Hemorrhagic shock*** is a leading cause of death in traumatic injuries.
- A **transfusion reaction** is a serious and potentially fatal complication of a blood transfusion in which a severe immune response occurs because the patient's blood and the donated blood do not match.

Anemia

Anemia (ah-**NEE**-mee-ah) is a lower-than-normal number of erythrocytes in the blood (**an-** means without or less than, and **-emia** means blood condition) causing fatigue, weakness, and shortness of breath. The severity of this condition is usually measured by a decrease in the amount of hemoglobin in the blood. When inadequate hemoglobin is present, all parts of the body receive less oxygen and have less energy than is needed to function properly.

- **Iron-deficiency anemia** is the most common form of anemia. Iron, an essential component of hemoglobin, is normally obtained through food intake and by recycling iron from old erythrocytes. Without sufficient iron to help create hemoglobin, blood cannot carry oxygen effectively. This deficiency can be caused by blood loss, poor absorption of iron, or inadequate dietary intake of iron. The body's extensive iron consumption during gestation and childbirth can result in pregnancy-related anemia.
- **Megaloblastic anemia** (**MEG**-ah-loh-**blas**-tick ah-**NEE**-mee-ah) is a blood disorder characterized by anemia in which the red blood cells are larger than normal (**megalo-** means large, **blast** means immature, and **-ic** means pertaining to). This condition usually results from a deficiency of folic acid or vitamin B_{12}.
- **Pernicious anemia** (per-**NISH**-us ah-**NEE**-mee-ah) is caused by a lack of the protein ***intrinsic factor*** (IF) that helps the body absorb vitamin B_{12} from the gastrointestinal tract. Vitamin B_{12} is necessary for the formation of erythrocytes. It is called ***pernicious*** because it was once considered deadly; however, treatment is now possible by supplementing the body's vitamin B_{12}. Pernicious anemia is thought to be an autoimmune disease.
- **Hemolytic anemia** (**hee**-moh-**LIT**-ick ah-**NEE**-mee-ah) is characterized by an inadequate number of circulating red blood cells due to the premature destruction of red blood cells by the spleen (**hem/o** means relating to blood, and **-lytic** means to destroy). ***Hemolytic*** means pertaining to **hemolysis** (heh-**MOL**-eh-sis), the process of breaking down erythrocytes. Although hemolytic anemia can be inherited or acquired, the most common examples are two types that are hereditary: sickle cell anemia and thalassemia.
- **Sickle cell anemia** (SCA) is the most common form of a group of blood disorders known as ***sickle cell disease***. This serious genetic disorder causes abnormal hemoglobin, resulting in some red blood cells assuming a malformed sickle shape. This sickle shape interferes with normal blood flow, resulting in anemia and potential damage to most body systems (Figure 6.7).
  - Sickle cell anemia is the most common inherited blood disorder in the United States. It is more prevalent in people whose ancestors came from Africa, the Mediterranean region, South America, and certain other areas. It is estimated that it affects one in 500 African Americans and one in 1,000 to 1,500 Hispanic Americans.
- **Thalassemia** (**thal**-ah-**SEE**-mee-ah) is an inherited blood disorder that causes mild or severe anemia due to reduced hemoglobin. This lack of hemoglobin

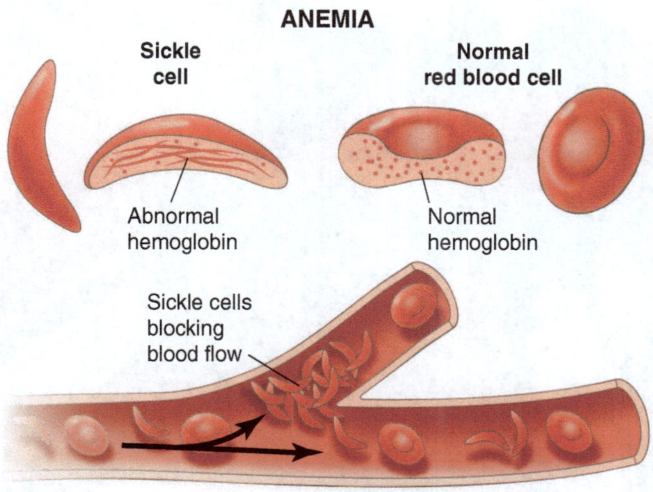

FIGURE 6.7 A sickle cell and a normal red blood cell.

results in the destruction of large numbers of erythrocytes. Thalassemia is caused by mutations of the DNA in the cells that produce hemoglobin.

Infectious Blood Diseases

- **Malaria** is a serious infectious blood disease transmitted by mosquitoes. Their bite transmits a parasite into the blood, where it travels to the liver to mature. The mature parasite multiplies in the red blood cells, causing them to rupture. People traveling to areas where malaria is prevalent should take a drug for malaria prophylaxis and avoid exposure to mosquitoes. ***Prophylaxis*** is a treatment intended to prevent a disease or stop it from spreading.
- **Sepsis** (**SEP**-sis) is a potentially life-threatening infection that results from bacteria or other infectious organisms entering the bloodstream. Sepsis can cause damage to multiple organ systems as the chemicals released into the bloodstream to fight the infection trigger inflammatory responses throughout the body. Bacteria coming into the bloodstream is ***septicemia***, sometimes incorrectly referred to as blood poisoning. Both sepsis and septicemia are derived from the Greek word for decomposition or decay.

DIAGNOSTIC PROCEDURES OF THE BLOOD SYSTEM

Blood tests are a non-invasive way to evaluate the functions of organs such as the kidneys, liver, thyroid, and heart, as well as to check for various diseases and conditions. See Chapter 21 for more information about blood tests.

Venipuncture (**VEE**-nih-punk-tyur) is the puncturing of a vein for the purpose of drawing blood. Blood specimens are often put in a **centrifuge** to separate the cellular and liquid portions of the blood for tests requiring a sample of serum or plasma (Figure 6.8).

- A **complete blood count** (CBC) measures various components of the blood in order to identify blood disorders and diseases. The test evaluates:
  - Erythrocytes
  - Leukocytes
  - Hemoglobin
  - Platelets
  - Mean corpuscular volume—the average size of the red blood cells
  - Hematocrit
- A **comprehensive metabolic panel** (CMP), also known as a ***Chem 14***, is a broad screening tool used to provide information about the state of the body's metabolism by measuring fourteen different substances in the blood. The CMP includes indicators regarding the function of the kidneys and liver, and also measures the levels of glucose, calcium, electrolytes, and proteins in the body.
- A **basic metabolic panel** (BMP), also known as a ***Profile 8***, is one of the most common lab tests. It measures seven different substances in the blood: four electrolytes (sodium, potassium, chloride, and bicarbonate), blood urea nitrogen, creatinine, and glucose. Sometimes calcium is added as an eighth substance. The BMP provides information about kidney function and electrolyte levels.

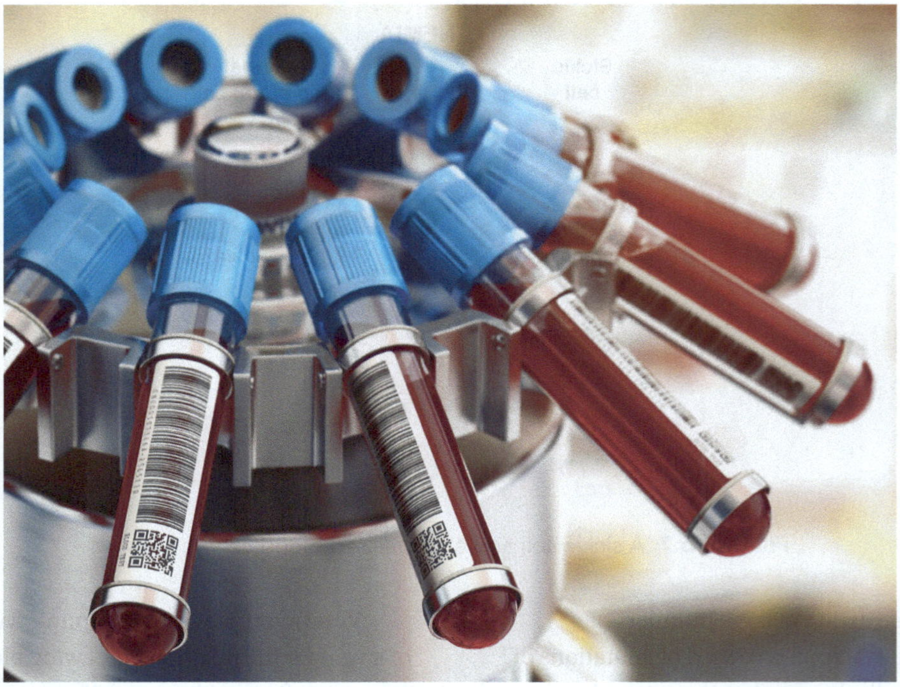

FIGURE 6.8 Centrifuging of blood specimens.

- **Blood urea nitrogen test** (you-**REE**-ah) (BUN) is a separate test used to measure the amount of urea nitrogen in the blood. Higher-than-normal levels may be indicative of problems with kidney or liver function.
- A **direct antiglobulin test** (DAT), also known as a ***direct Coombs test***, is used to investigate possible hemolytic transfusion reaction or whether a fetus or newborn has a hemolytic disease.
- A **blood clotting test**, or ***coagulation panel***, is used to test for suspected blood clotting disorders, and also to monitor patients taking blood-thinning medications.
- A **blood differential test** measures the percentage of each type of leukocyte present in the blood. This ratio is changed by the presence of infection or disease.
- **Blood enzyme tests** are used to diagnose a targeted health issue by measuring the level of specific enzymes. For example, the heart releases the cardiac enzyme ***troponin*** when it is injured, indicating a possible heart attack.
- A **blood gas analysis** or **arterial blood gas test** (ABG) measures the amount of oxygen and carbon dioxide in the blood. This can determine how well the lungs are moving oxygen into the blood and removing carbon dioxide from the blood. This test can also indicate the pH levels of the blood, or how acidic it is. These results can be indicative of lung or kidney diseases.
- A **blood glucose test** measures the level of glucose, a type of simple sugar, in the blood. Insulin is a hormone that helps the body process glucose, and the blood glucose test indicates whether enough insulin is being produced, or if it is functioning properly. These indicators are important for the diagnosis and monitoring of diabetes (see Chapter 14 for more about diabetes).
- **Erythrocyte sedimentation rate** (eh-**RITH**-roh-site) (ESR), also known as a ***sed rate***, is a test based on the speed with which the red blood cells separate from the plasma and fall to the bottom of a specialized test tube. An elevated sed rate indicates the presence of inflammation in the body.
- A ***fibrinogen activity test*** is used to determine the level of fibrinogen in the blood, which may help find the cause of abnormal bleeding.
- A ***glucose tolerance test*** is an oral test used to diagnose gestational diabetes during pregnancy, and sometimes to screen for type 2 diabetes. Two hours after drinking a syrupy glucose solution, a blood glucose test is done to see if the body has processed the glucose normally.

- **Hematocrit** (hee-**MAT**-oh-krit) (HCT) is the percentage of the blood that is made up of red blood cells (**hemat/o** means blood, and **-crit** means to separate). The ***hematocrit test*** is part of a complete blood count. A higher- or lower-than-normal hematocrit may be indicative of a disease or disorder.
- A **lipoprotein panel blood test**, or ***lipid panel***, requires that a patient fast for 8–12 hours before the blood is drawn. Laboratory tests can then detect the average levels of cholesterol and triglycerides, helping to assess the patient's risk for developing cardiovascular disease.
- **Newborn screening**, which is usually done 24 to 48 hours after birth, includes a blood test for sickle cell anemia and other genetic, hormone-related, and metabolic conditions such as cystic fibrosis and phenylketonuria (PKU). Blood is taken via a prick to the heel. See Chapter 18 for more information.
- **Prothrombin time** (proh-**THROM**-bin) (PT), also known as ***pro time***, is a blood coagulation test used to diagnose conditions associated with abnormalities of clotting time and to monitor anticoagulant therapy. A longer prothrombin time can be caused by serious liver disease, bleeding disorders, blood-thinning medicines, or a lack of vitamin K. In patients taking the anticoagulant medication warfarin, prothrombin time is expressed as an ***international normalized ratio*** (INR) in order to measure how well the medication is working.
- A **total protein test** measures the proteins albumin and globulin in the blood, and also the ratio between the two, referred to as the ***A/G ratio***.

Bone Marrow Biopsies

- A **bone marrow biopsy** is performed by inserting a small needle into a bone in order to remove a sample of the bone marrow tissue. This procedure, which is done to determine the cause of anemia or iron deficiency, and for cancer diagnosis, most commonly uses a pelvic bone such as the posterior iliac crest (Figure 6.9).
- **Bone marrow aspiration** is done to procure a sample of the ***aspirate***, or liquid portion, of the bone marrow. A syringe with a hollow needle is used to withdraw this sample, often in advance of a bone marrow biopsy.
- The **Schilling test** is a urine test used to evaluate vitamin B_{12} absorption, which is a factor in pernicious anemia.

TREATMENT PROCEDURES OF THE BLOOD SYSTEM

The treatment for blood disorders includes transfusions of blood or platelets, therapeutic plasma exchange, and stem cell transplants.

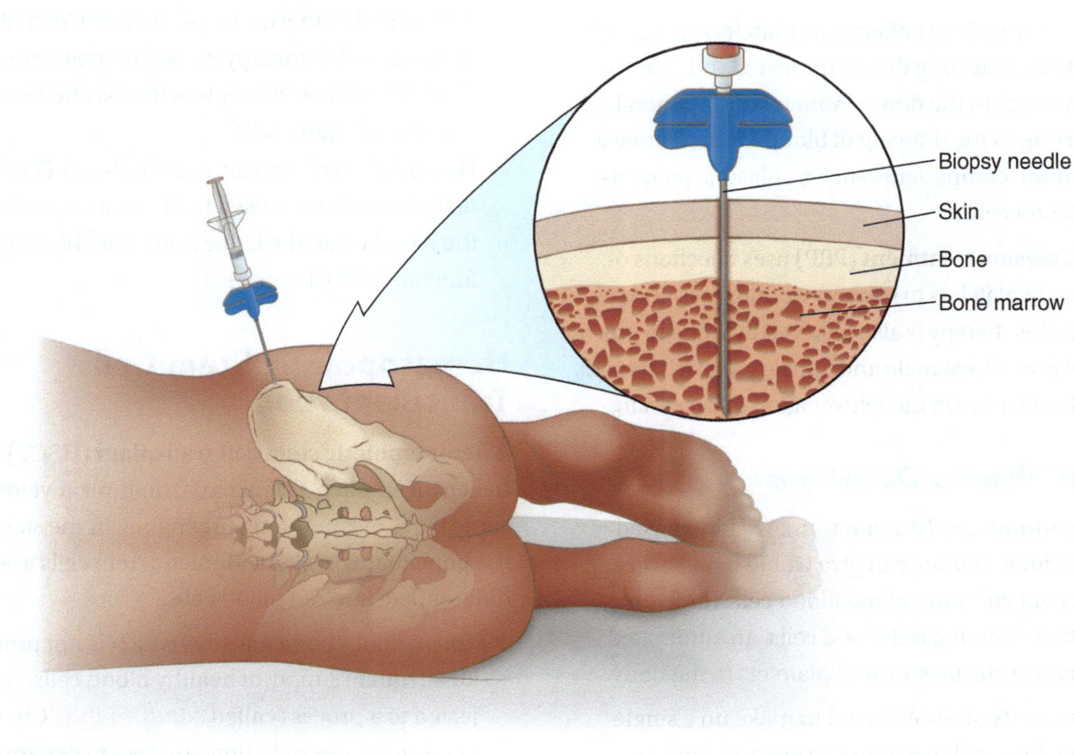

FIGURE 6.9 A bone marrow aspiration and biopsy.

Blood and Platelet Transfusions

A **blood transfusion** is a procedure in which donated blood is used to replace blood lost due to surgery, injury, or bleeding disorder. Instead of whole blood being transfused, the patient normally just receives donated red blood cells.

- An **allogeneic transfusion** (**al**-loh-jen-**EEH**-ick) uses donated blood that must be of a compatible blood type. ***Allogeneic*** means coming from a different individual, i.e., one who is genetically not the same as the recipient (**all/o** means different, **gene** means origin, and **-ic** means pertaining to).
- An **autologous transfusion** (aw-**TOL**-uh-guss) uses the patient's own blood instead of blood from a donor. This ensures a perfect match, and reduces the risk of infection. Patients will sometimes bank, or store, some of their own blood in anticipation of surgery, especially if there is a shortage of donated blood. ***Cell salvage*** is a type of autologous transfusion in which any blood lost during surgery is transfused back into the patient after filtration and washing.

Platelet transfusions are used to treat patients who have a low platelet count or poor platelet function, making them at high risk for bleeding. Cancer treatment involving radiation or chemotherapy sometimes damages cells in the red bone marrow, resulting in a decrease in their ability to generate platelets. A transfusion of platelets can help reduce the risk of infection and bleeding.

- An ***apheresis*** machine collects the platelets along with some plasma, returning the erythrocytes and most of the plasma back to the donor. Apheresis is a general term referring to the drawing of blood for the removal of one or more components such as plasma, platelets, or white blood cells.

Platelet-rich plasma treatment (PRP) uses injections of the patient's own platelets to support wound, muscle, and joint healing. This therapy is also believed by some to promote hair growth to treat male and female pattern baldness, and even to be effective in the rejuvenation of facial skin.

Blood and Plasma Donations

- **Blood donations** are the main source of blood used for transfusions. Donors can give whole blood every 56 days, or a concentration of red blood cells three times a year. When donating red blood cells, an automated process returns the plasma and platelets to the body.
- It takes five units of whole blood to make up a single unit of platelets, and they must be used within five days. Platelets can be donated every seven days.
- **Plasma donations** involves drawing the blood, separating out the plasma, and returning the red blood cells and platelets to the body. Plasma from those with blood type AB+ is collected so that it can be given to any patient in an emergency situation. It is also used to create plasma protein therapies for people with blood-clotting disorders, autoimmune diseases, and severe burns.
- **Platelet donations** can be made every seven days. It takes five units of whole blood to make up one unit of platelets, however a single platelet donation yields several transfusable units.
- **Plasmapheresis** (**plaz**-mah-feh-**REE**-sis) is the removal of blood plasma by drawing blood and then separating the blood into its cellular elements (**plasma** means plasma, and **-pheresis** means removal). The erythrocytes, leukocytes, and platelets and platelets are suspended in a solution of saline or albumin (a soluble protein) to be returned to the circulatory system, and the plasma is collected. This process makes more frequent blood donations possible.

External Treatments

- **Therapeutic plasma exchange** (TPE) is a type of plasmapheresis in which some of the patient's own blood is circulated through a device that removes the disease-causing antibodies in the plasma and replaces them with healthy donor plasma and/or a plasma substitute. This therapy is used to treat neurological disorders such as multiple sclerosis and Guillain-Barré syndrome (Figure 6.10).
- **Hemodialysis** is a treatment similar to TPE in which a dialysis machine is used to filter waste products from the blood when the kidneys are not able to perform this function (see Chapter 10).

Hematopoietic Stem Cell Transplantation

A **hematopoietic stem cell transplant** (HSCT) is used to treat cancers such as leukemia, multiple myeloma, and some types of lymphoma originating in the stem cells of the bone marrow. Hematopoietic stem cells are able to differentiate into red blood cells.

- The patient's bone marrow, which is not producing an adequate supply of healthy blood cells, is first subjected to a process called ***conditioning***. Chemotherapy and sometimes radiation are used to destroy cancerous cells and suppress the immune system. The process

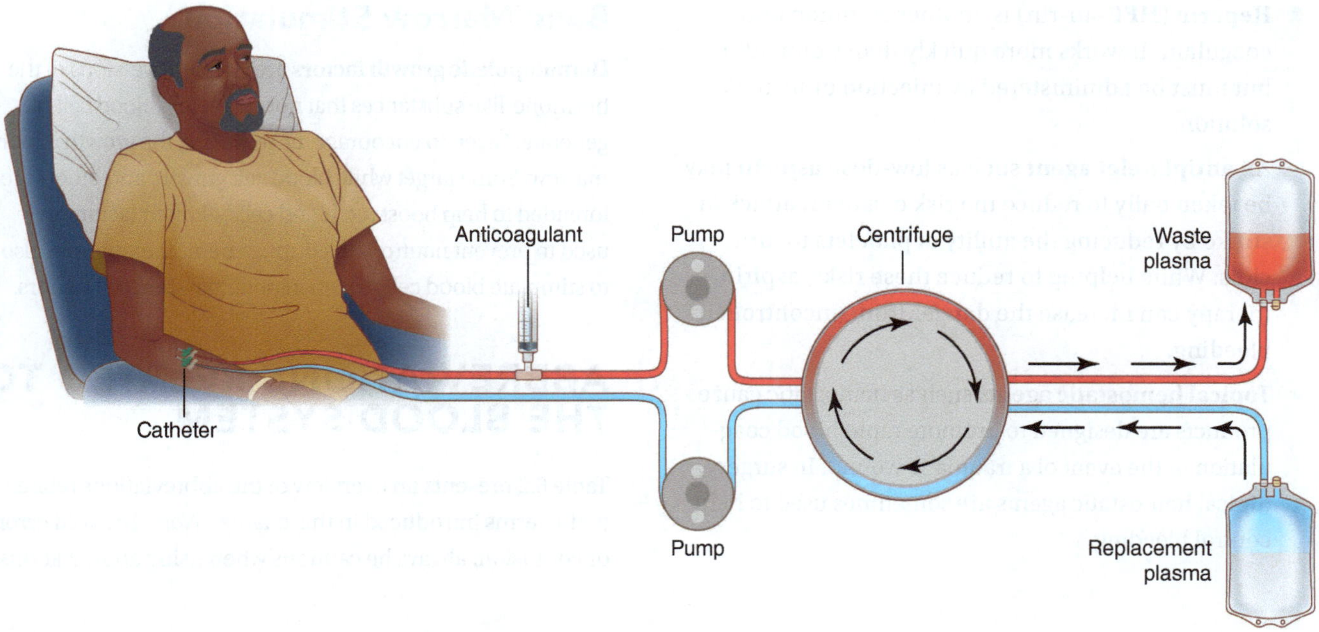

FIGURE 6.10 Therapeutic plasma exchange.

also makes room in the bone marrow for new stem cells to grow, and helps prevent the rejection of the transplanted cells.

- Once the bone marrow is ready for the transplanted stem cells, they are introduced into the bone marrow via the bloodstream. The new cells then multiply and create healthy new blood cells.
- Donor bone marrow used to be the primary source of hematopoietic stem cells, which is why this process is sometimes referred to as a ***bone marrow transplant***. Now, however, peripheral blood stem cells (PBSC) and umbilical cord blood and umbilical cord blood are the usual sources of these cells. ***Peripheral blood*** refers to blood circulating through the body, as opposed to being in the bone marrow or organs.
- **Umbilical cord blood** (UCB), sometimes referred to as ***cord blood***, is blood that remains in the umbilical cord and placenta after a baby is delivered and the umbilical cord is cut.

Types of Stem Cell Transplants

- An **autologous** (AUTO) **transplant** uses peripheral blood stem cells from the patient's own blood that are harvested and frozen prior to chemotherapy. After the treatment is completed, the thawed stem cells are administered through a catheter into the bloodstream.
- An **allogeneic** (**al**-loh-jen-**EEH**-ick) (ALLO) **transplant** requires finding a donor whose bone marrow matches the patient's. In a ***haplotype mismatched transplant***, the donor—usually a parent, child, or sibling—is only a 50% match. The term *allogeneic transplant* describes any procedure in which the recipient receives tissues, cells, or organs from a compatible donor.
- The closest match possible is necessary to avoid a serious condition called **graft-versus-host disease** (GVHD). Stem cells from umbilical cord blood are sometimes used when a close donor match cannot be found.

Medications

An **anticoagulant** (**an**-tih-koh-**AG**-you-lant) slows coagulation and prevents new clots from forming. ***Coagulation*** is the process of of blood clotting. Note that although these medicines are sometimes referred to as ***blood thinners***, they do not actually make the blood thinner.

- **Coumadin**® (**KOO**-mah-din), which is a brand name for ***warfarin***, is an anticoagulant administered to prevent blood clots from forming or growing larger. This medication is often prescribed for patients with clotting difficulties, certain types of heartbeat irregularities, or after a heart attack or heart valve replacement surgery.

- **Heparin** (**HEP**-ah-rin) is another common anticoagulant. It works more quickly than Coumadin, but must be administered by injection or in an IV solution.
- An **antiplatelet agent** such as low-dose **aspirin** may be taken daily to reduce the risk of a heart attack or stroke by reducing the ability of platelets to form clots. While helping to reduce these risks, aspirin therapy can increase the danger from uncontrolled bleeding.
- **Topical hemostatic agents** such as hemostatic gauze products are designed to promote rapid blood coagulation in the event of a traumatic wound. In surgery, topical hemostatic agents are sometimes used to help control bleeding.

Bone Marrow Stimulation

Hematopoietic growth factors are synthetic versions of the hormone-like substances that normally help blood cells regenerate. Given to encourage, or stimulate, the growth of bone marrow. Some target white blood cell growth, and others are intended to help boost red blood cells. Growth factors are used to prevent neutropenia during chemotherapy, and also to stimulate blood cell growth in potential stem cell donors.

ABBREVIATIONS RELATED TO THE BLOOD SYSTEM

Table 6.2 presents an overview of the abbreviations related to the terms introduced in this chapter. *Note:* To avoid errors or confusion, always be cautious when using abbreviations.

TABLE 6.2

Abbreviations Related to the Blood System

comprehensive metabolic panel = CMP	**CMP** = comprehensive metabolic panel
graft-versus-host disease = GVHD	**GVHD** = graft-versus-host disease
hematocrit = HCT	**HCT** = hematocrit
hemoglobin = Hgb	**Hgb** = hemoglobin
Hodgkin's lymphoma = HL	**HL** = Hodgkin's lymphoma
multiple myeloma = MM	**MM** = multiple myeloma
myelodysplastic syndrome = MDS	**MDS** = myelodysplastic syndrome
non-Hodgkin's lymphoma = NHL	**NHL** = non-Hodgkin's lymphoma
prothrombin time = PT	**PT** = prothrombin time
red blood cells = RBC	**RBC** = red blood cells
white blood cells = WBC	**WBC** = white blood cells

CHAPTER 6

LEARNING EXERCISES

Matching Word Parts 1

Write the correct answer in the middle column.

	Definition	Correct Answer	Possible Answers
6.1.	red	____________	**chromat/o**
6.2.	blood, blood condition	____________	**coagul/o**
6.3.	fibrin, fibers	____________	**-emia**
6.4.	clotting, coagulation	____________	**erythr/o**
6.5.	color	____________	**fibrin/o**

Matching Word Parts 2

Write the correct answer in the middle column.

	Definition	Correct Answer	Possible Answers
6.6.	blood, relating to the blood	____________	**-globin**
6.7.	protein	____________	**hem/o**
6.8.	spinal cord, bone marrow	____________	**leuk/o**
6.9.	resembling	____________	**myel/o**
6.10.	white	____________	**-oid**

Matching Word Parts 3

Write the correct answer in the middle column.

	Definition	Correct Answer	Possible Answers
6.11.	something molded or formed	____________	**hemat/o**
6.12.	to make	____________	**-penia**
6.13.	blood, relating to the blood	____________	**plasm/o**

6.14. maintenance of a constant level ________________ **-poiesis**

6.15. deficiency ________________ **-stasis**

Definitions

Select the correct answer, and write it on the line provided.

6.16. The term meaning white blood cells is ________________.

erythrocytes leukocytes platelets thrombocytes

6.17. The clotting protein ________________ forms a web-like material to aid in blood clotting.

hemoglobin prothrombin erythropoietin fibrinogen

6.18. A/an ________________ is any substance that the body regards as being foreign.

antigen hematopoietic stem cell thrombocyte reticulocyte

6.19. The ________________ are white blood cells that provide immunological defenses against many infectious organisms.

basophils eosinophils erythrocytes monocytes

6.20. The formation of blood cells is called ________________.

hematopoiesis plasmapheresis hemostasis erythropoietin

6.21. The ________________ are white blood cells that include T cells and B cells.

erythrocytes reticulocytes leukocytes lymphocytes

6.22. The ________________ are the smallest formed elements in the blood, and play an important role in blood clotting.

erythrocytes leukocytes monocytes platelets

6.23. Red blood cells that have just been released from the bone marrow are called ________________.

monocytes hematopoietic stem cells reticulocytes neutrophils

6.24. The process of blood clotting is called ________________.

plasmapheresis coagulation hematopoiesis coagulopathy

6.25. The ________________ are the most common type of white blood cell.

erythrocytes leukocytes neutrophils thrombocytes

Matching Structures

Write the correct answer in the middle column.

	Definition	Correct Answer	Possible Answers
6.26.	fluid containing nutrients, hormones	________________	erythrocytes
6.27.	red blood cells	________________	megakaryocytes
6.28.	cells that produce platelets	________________	plasma
6.29.	main protein in the blood	________________	albumin
6.30.	largest type of white blood cell	________________	monocytes

Which Word?

Select the correct answer, and write it on the line provided.

6.31. A ________________ is a medical professional trained to draw blood from patients.

phlebotomist hematologist

6.32. The type of cancer characterized by a progressive increase in the number of abnormal leukocytes is ________________.

leukopenia leukemia

6.33. The condition characterized by an abnormal increase in the number of circulating red blood cells is called ________________.

pancytopenia polycythemia

6.34. A ________________ test measures the percentage of each type of leukocyte present in the blood.

total protein blood differential

6.35. An ________________ transfusion uses donated blood that must be of a compatible blood type.

autologous allogeneic

Spelling Counts

Find the misspelled word in each sentence. Then write that word, spelled correctly, on the line provided.

6.36. The term *hemeostasis* means to stop or control bleeding. ________________

6.37. Plasmaphereses is the removal of blood plasma into its cellular elements. ________________

6.38. Hereditary spherosytosis is a genetic disorder that causes the red blood cells to be spherical rather than flat. ____________________

6.39. Bone marrow asperation is done to procure a sample of the aspirate, or liquid portion, of the bone marrow. ____________________

6.40. The patient lost a large amount of blood in a short time when his wound started to hemorage.

____

Abbreviation Identification

In the space provided, write the words that each abbreviation stands for.

6.41. **HGB** ____________________

6.42. **PT** ____________________

6.43. **MM** ____________________

6.44. **GVHD** ____________________

6.45. **RBC** ____________________

Term Selection

Select the correct answer, and write it on the line provided.

6.46. A potentially life-threatening infection that results from bacteria or other infectious organisms entering the bloodstream is known as ____________________.

pancytopenia leukopenia neutropenia sepsis

6.47. This blood type has no antigens on its red blood cells. ____________________

A AB B O

6.48. The blood disorder characterized by anemia in which the red blood cells are larger than normal is known as ____________________ anemia.

aplastic hemolytic megaloblastic pernicious

6.49. The term ____________ describes a condition in which the blood has an increased tendency to form blood clots.

coagulopathy hemophilia von Willebrand disease hypercoagulable state

6.50. The blood cancer ____________ occurs when the genetic material in a certain type of white blood cell mutates.

multiple myeloma non-Hodgkin's lymphoma acute myeloid leukemia myelodysplastic syndrome

Sentence Completion

Write the correct term or terms on the lines provided.

6.51. Plasma with the blood cells and the clotting proteins and removed is known as ____________.

6.52. Having an abnormally small number of platelets in the circulating blood is known as ____________.

6.53. During pregnancy, problems can occur if the mother and fetus have a difference in their blood's ____________.

6.54. A/An ____________ blood test is used to detect the average levels of cholesterol and triglycerides.

6.55. The removal of blood plasma by separating the blood into its cellular elements is called ____________.

Word Surgery

Divide each term into its component word parts. Write these word parts, in sequence, on the lines provided. When necessary, use a slash (/) to indicate a combining vowel. (You may not need all of the lines provided.)

6.56. **Thrombocytosis** is an abnormal increase in the number of platelets in the circulating blood.

____________ ____________ ____________ ____________

6.57. **Aplastic** anemia is characterized by an absence of *all* formed blood elements.

____________ ____________ ____________ ____________

6.58. **Phagocytes** are cells that play a major role in the immune system's defense against pathogens by engulfing the pathogens and consuming them

________ ________ ________ ________

6.59. **Hemochromatosis** is characterized by the overabsorption of iron in the intestine.

________ ________ ________ ________

6.60. An **allogeneic** transplant requires finding a donor whose bone marrow matches the patient's.

________ ________ ________ ________

True/False

If the statement is true, write **True** on the line. If the statement is false, write **False** on the line.

6.61. _____ Hematocrit is the percentage of the blood that is made up of white blood cells.

6.62. _____ Sickle cell anemia is a serious genetic disorder that causes abnormal hemoglobin.

6.63. _____ Blood removes waste products from tissues and delivers them to the liver and kidneys.

6.64. _____ Hemostasis is the process of clotting blood.

6.65. _____ Pernicious anemia is caused by a lack of iron.

Clinical Conditions

Write the correct answer on the line provided.

6.66. Wes Red Crow was treated in a hyperbaric oxygen chamber after developing ____________________ as a result of ascending to the ocean surface too rapidly after his dive.

6.67. When Santiago Lopes scraped his knee on the playground, the wound wouldn't stop bleeding because he suffers from the hereditary bleeding disorder known as ____________________.

6.68. Olivia Melius was found unconscious and rushed to the hospital after a malfunctioning space heater caused her to suffer from ____________________.

6.69. When Colin Weiss suffered a flare-up from multiple sclerosis, the clinic had him come in four times to have some of his plasma replaced with plasma from a donor. This treatment is called ____________________.

6.70. When Arjun Patel was brought to the ER with symptoms of a possible a heart attack, a _______________ test was performed to check for the cardiac enzyme troponin.

6.71. Juanita Gomez was diagnosed as having _______________. This condition is characterized by lower-than-normal quantities of red blood cells, white blood cells, and platelets.

6.72. Dr. Mian reviewed the results of David Barnett's _______________. This test provides information about the state of the patient's metabolism by measuring fourteen different substances in the blood.

6.73. Before his trip to Papua New Guinea, Jimbo Weatherill was advised to avoid exposure to mosquitoes in order to prevent contracting _______________.

6.74. Francesca Schmidt always had abnormally heavy bleeding during her menstrual period. The cause was diagnosed as the genetic disorder known as _______________.

6.75. Hamilton Edwards Sr. suffers from _______________. This is a genetic disorder that causes the red blood cells to be spherical rather than flat.

Which Is the Correct Medical Term?

Select the correct answer, and write it on the line provided.

6.76. Hormone-like substances given to encourage, or stimulate, the growth of bone marrow are called _______________.

hemostatic agents | heparin | anticoagulant | hematopoietic growth factors

6.77. The percentage of the blood that is made up of red blood cells is the _______________.

hematopoiesis | hematocrit | prothrombin time | erythropoietin

6.78. One group of proteins in the plasma that play an important role in the immune system are the _______________.

globulins | formed elements | neutrophils | basophils

6.79. The process of breaking down red blood cells is called _______________.

anemia | hemolysis | hemochromatosis | sepsis

6.80. An inherited blood disorder that causes mild or severe anemia due to reduced hemoglobin is called

________________________.

thalassemia   von Willebrand disease   sickle cell anemia   hemophilia

Challenge Word Building

These terms are *not* primary terms in the chapter; however, they are made up of the following familiar word parts. If you need help in creating the term, refer to your medical dictionary.

anti-
macro-

coagul/o
cyt/o
erythr/o
fibr/o
granul/o
hem/o
leuk/o
myel/o
plasm/a
platelet
thromb/o

-able
-atic
-crit
-globin
-ic
-osis
-pathy
-penia
-pheresis
-poiesis
-rrhagic
-uria

6.81. A disease such as sickle cell anemia associated with the hemoglobin in the blood is

________________________.

6.82. A substance or agent that promotes hemostasis is a ________________________.

6.83. Blood that is capable of clotting is said to be ________________________.

6.84. The formation and development of white blood cells is ________________________.

6.85. Red blood cells in the urine is called ________________________.

6.86. A shortage of platelets for normal blood clotting is called ________________________.

6.87. This term means relating to, or occurring, in blood plasma ________________________.

6.88. A blood bank procedure that removes platelets from the blood is called ________________________.

6.89. In this type of blood cancer, the bone marrow is replaced by fibrous scar tissue.

____

6.90. The condition marked by a decrease in the number of granulocytes is called

________________________.

Labeling Exercises

Identify the numbered items in the accompanying figures.

6.91. ____________________

6.92. ____________________ elements

6.93. ____________________

6.94. ____________________

6.95. ____________________

6.96. ____________________

6.97. ____________________

6.98. ____________________

6.99. ____________________

6.100. ____________________

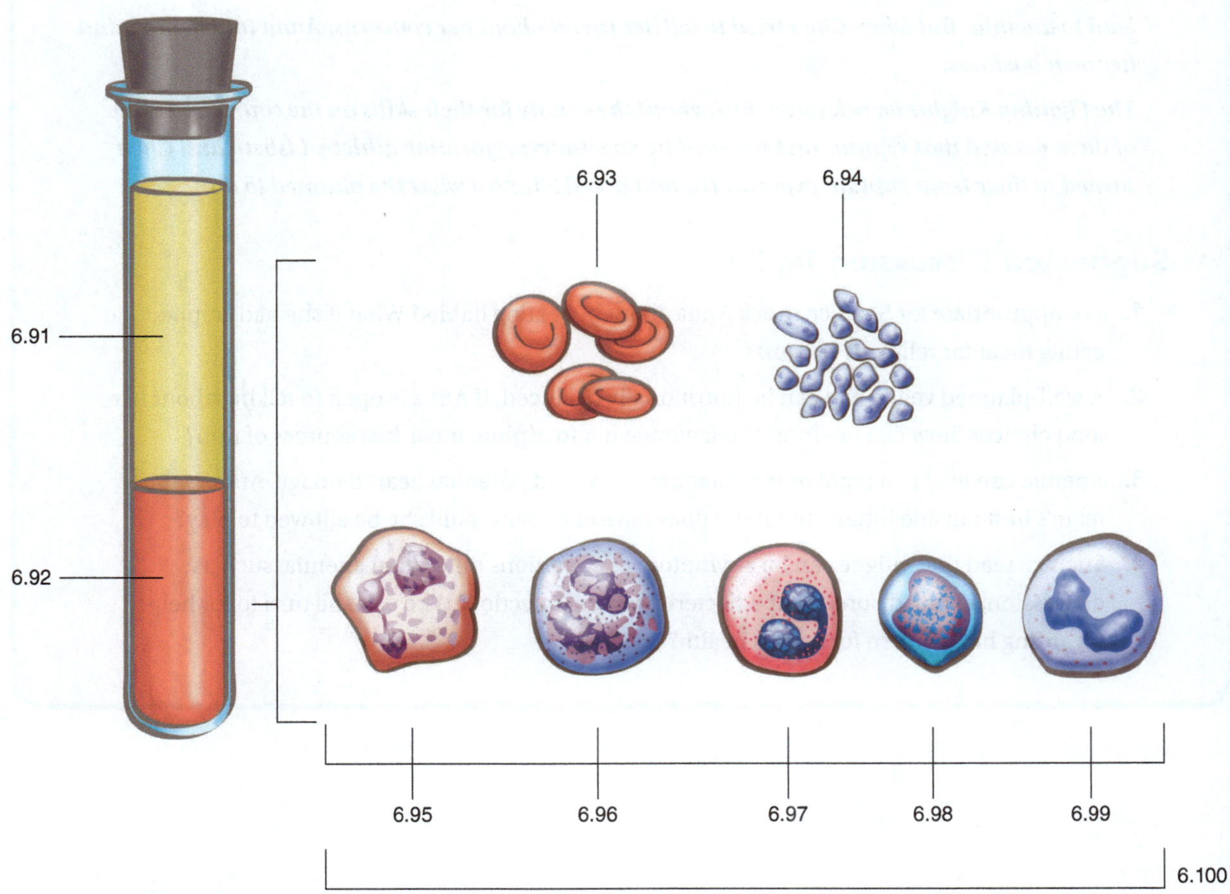

The Human Touch

CRITICAL THINKING EXERCISE

The following story and questions are designed to stimulate critical thinking through class discussion or as a brief essay response. There are no right or wrong answers to these questions.

The Fighting Knights went into the volleyball season undefeated. Team captain Shanice hoped to get a college scholarship based on her skills as a setter and her leadership ability. She was counting on Anna, a sophomore standout on last year's junior varsity team, to help carry the Fighting Knights to victory. After a crushing loss in their preview game against the Central High Bulldogs, a few players approached Shanice to express their concerns about Anna. They knew from a team social over the summer, as well as her impassioned social media posts about animal rights, that Anna had recently decided to go vegan. Fellow player Lisbeth shared that during a night out over Labor Day weekend, Anna had only picked at a salad during dinner and then dozed off during the movie. That wasn't like her, Lisbeth confided.

Another teammate, Chen, mentioned that a few days ago Anna had a hard time catching her breath and recovering between weight training sets. Anna had brushed the problem off as PMS, but Lisbeth and Chen both noticed that Anna seemed to be tired all the time. Chen wondered if it might be because Anna didn't seem to have many sources of iron in her current diet, which can lead to anemia. But when Chen tried to tell her friend about her concerns, Anna told her to mind her own business.

The Fighting Knights were known throughout the county for their skills on the court, and none of them wanted that reputation tarnished by one underperforming athlete. Lisbeth and Chen turned to their team captain expectantly, and asked Shanice what she planned to do.

Suggested Discussion Topics

1. Is it appropriate for Shanice to ask Anna about her eating habits? What if she had stopped eating meat for religious reasons?
2. A well-planned vegan diet can be nutritionally balanced. If Anna is open to talking about her food choices, how can her friends encourage her to explore meat-free sources of iron?
3. Anemia can lead to a rapid or irregular heartbeat and potential heart damage. Anna is the team's best outside hitter—but if she does have anemia, should she be allowed to play?
4. Shanice read that fatigue can be a symptom of conditions other than anemia, such as depression, eating disorders, or a bacterial or viral infection. Who can she turn to for help regarding her concern for Anna's health?

CHAPTER 7

THE LYMPHATIC AND IMMUNE SYSTEMS

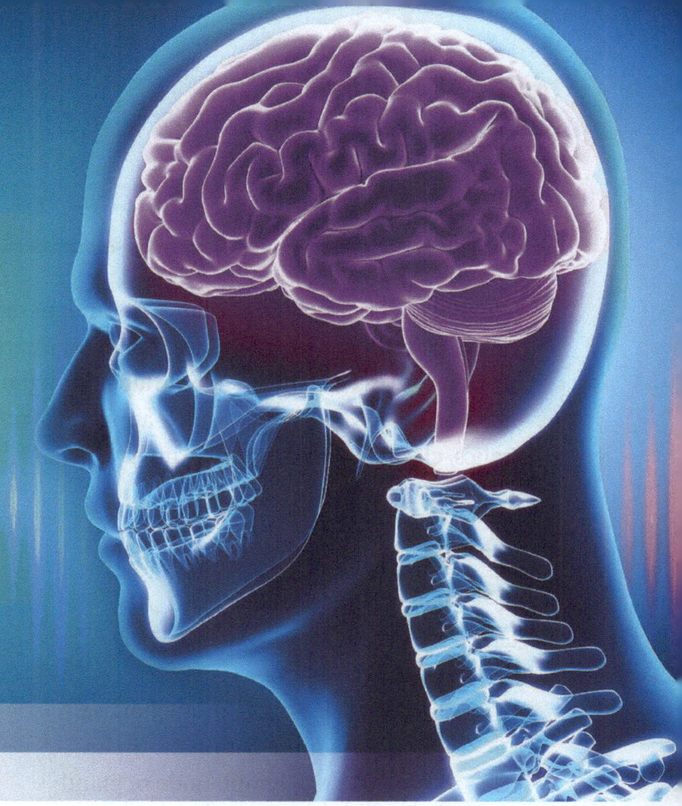

Overview of STRUCTURES, COMBINING FORMS, AND FUNCTIONS OF THE LYMPHATIC AND IMMUNE SYSTEMS

Major Structures	Related Combining Forms	Primary Functions
Lymph	lymph/o	The fluid that removes cellular waste products, pathogens, and dead blood cells from the tissues.
Lymphatic Vessels and Ducts	lymphangi/o	The capillaries, vessels, and ducts that return lymph from the tissues to the venous bloodstream.
Lymph Nodes	lymphaden/o	Bean-shaped structures of the lymphatic system where pathogens and other harmful substances are filtered from the lymph by specialized cells of the immune system.
Tonsils and Adenoids	tonsill/o, adenoid/o	Lymphoid structures of the lymphatic system that protect the entry to the respiratory system.
Spleen	splen/o (*Note:* This combining form is spelled with only one e.)	A sac-like mass of lymphoid tissue with protective roles in both the immune and lymphatic systems.
Bone Marrow	myel/o	Produces lymphocytes, which are specialized leukocytes (white blood cells).
Lymphocytes	lymphocyt/o	Specialized leukocytes that play important roles in immune reactions.
Thymus	thym/o	A gland located in the upper chest with specialized roles in both the lymphatic and immune systems.

Vocabulary Related to **THE LYMPHATIC AND IMMUNE SYSTEMS**

This list contains essential word parts and medical terms for this chapter. These and the other important **primary terms** are shown in **boldface** throughout the chapter. ***Secondary terms***, which appear in ***orange*** italics, clarify the meaning of primary terms.

Word Parts

- ☐ **anti-** against
- ☐ **-cocci** spherical bacteria
- ☐ **-cyte** cell
- ☐ **-edema** swelling
- ☐ **immun/o** immune, protection, safe
- ☐ **lymph/o** lymph, lymphatic tissue
- ☐ **lymphaden/o** lymph node or gland
- ☐ **lymphangi/o** lymph vessel
- ☐ **-lytic** to destroy
- ☐ **macro-** large
- ☐ **-oma** tumor
- ☐ **phag/o**, **-phage** eat, swallow
- ☐ **splen/o** spleen
- ☐ **-tic** pertaining to
- ☐ **tox/o** poison, poisonous

Medical Terms

- ☐ **acquired immunity**
- ☐ **acquired immunodeficiency syndrome** (**im**-you-noh-deh-**FISH**-en-see)
- ☐ **allergen** (**AL**-er-jen)
- ☐ **allergist** (**AL**-er-jist)
- ☐ **allergy**
- ☐ **anaphylaxis** (**an**-ah-fih-**LACK**-sis)
- ☐ **antibiotic-resistant bacteria**
- ☐ **antibiotics**
- ☐ **antibody** (**AN**-tih-**bod**-ee)
- ☐ **antifungal** (**an**-tih-**FUNG**-gul)
- ☐ **antigen** (**AN**-tih-jen)
- ☐ **antigen-antibody reaction**
- ☐ **autoimmune disorder** (**aw**-toh-ih-**MYOUN**)
- ☐ **bacilli** (bah-**SILL**-eye)
- ☐ **bacteria** (back-**TEE**-ree-ah)
- ☐ **candidiasis** (kan-dih-**DYE**-ah-sis)
- ☐ **complement system** (**KOM**-pleh-ment)
- ☐ **COVID-19** (**KOH**-vid)
- ☐ **cytokines** (**SIGH**-toh-kyens)
- ☐ **cytomegalovirus** (**sigh**-toh-**meg**-ah-loh-**VYE**-rus)
- ☐ **hemolytic** (**hee**-moh-**LIT**-ick)
- ☐ **herpes zoster** (**HER**-peez **ZOS**-ter)
- ☐ **human immunodeficiency virus** (**im**-you-noh-deh-**FISH**-en-see)
- ☐ **immunodeficiency disorder** (**im**-you-noh-deh-**FISH**-en-see)
- ☐ **immunoglobulins** (**im**-you-noh-**GLOB**-you-lins)
- ☐ **immunologist** (**im**-you-**NOL**-oh-jist)
- ☐ **immunosuppressant** (**im**-you-noh-soo-**PRES**-ant)
- ☐ **immunotherapy** (**im**-you-noh-**THER**-ah-pee)
- ☐ **infectious disease specialist**
- ☐ **infectious mononucleosis** (**mon**-oh-**new**-klee-**OH**-sis)
- ☐ **influenza** (**in**-floo-**EN**-zah)
- ☐ **interferons** (**in**-ter-**FEAR**-onz)
- ☐ **Lyme disease** (**LIME**)
- ☐ **lymphadenopathy** (lim-**fad**-eh-**NOP**-ah-thee)
- ☐ **lymphangioma** (lim-**fan**-jee-**OH**-mah)
- ☐ **lymphedema** (**lim**-feh-**DEE**-mah)
- ☐ **lymphocytes** (**LIM**-foh-sights)
- ☐ **lymphologist** (lim-**FOL**-oh-jist)
- ☐ **lymphoscintigraphy** (**lim**-foh-sin-**TIH**-grah-fee)
- ☐ **macrophage** (**MACK**-roh-fayj)
- ☐ **malaria** (mah-**LAY**-ree-ah)
- ☐ **measles**
- ☐ **natural immunity**
- ☐ **opportunistic infection** (**op**-ur-too-**NIHS**-tick)
- ☐ **parasite** (**PAR**-ah-sight)
- ☐ **pathogen** (**PATH**-oh-jen)
- ☐ **rabies** (**RAY**-beez)
- ☐ **rickettsia** (rih-**KET**-see-ah)
- ☐ **rubella** (roo-**BELL**-ah)
- ☐ **spirochetes** (**SPY**-roh-keets)
- ☐ **splenomegaly** (**splee**-noh-**MEG**-ah-lee)
- ☐ **staphylococci** (**staf**-ih-loh-**KOCK**-sigh)
- ☐ **streptococci** (**strep**-toh-**KOCK**-sigh)
- ☐ **synthetic immunoglobulins**
- ☐ **synthetic interferon**
- ☐ **systemic reaction** (sis-**TEH**-mik)
- ☐ **toxoplasmosis** (**tock**-soh-plaz-**MOH**-sis)
- ☐ **varicella** (**var**-ih-**SEL**-ah)
- ☐ **West Nile virus**
- ☐ **Zika virus**

LEARNING OBJECTIVES

On completion of this chapter, you should be able to:

1. Describe the major functions and structures of the lymphatic and immune systems.
2. Describe the types of immunity.
3. Explain the process of the immune response.
4. Identify the medical specialists who treat disorders of the lymphatic and immune systems.
5. Identify the medical word parts of the lymphatic system.
6. Define the primary terms related to the pathology and the diagnostic and treatment procedures of the lymphatic and immune systems.
7. Name the types of pathogens.
8. Spell the primary terms of the lymphatic and immune systems.
9. Pronounce the primary terms of the lymphatic and immune systems.
10. Identify common abbreviations related to the lymphatic and immune systems.

FUNCTIONS OF THE LYMPHATIC SYSTEM

The three main functions of the lymphatic system are to:

1. Absorb fats and fat-soluble vitamins through the lacteals of the small intestine.
2. Remove waste products from the tissues and cooperate with the immune system in destroying invading pathogens.
3. Return filtered lymph to the veins at the base of the neck.

Absorption of Fats and Fat-Soluble Vitamins

Food is digested in the small intestine, which is lined with small finger-like projections known as ***villi***. Each *villus* (singular) contains lacteals and blood vessels.

- **Lacteals** (**LACK**-tee-ahlz) are specialized structures of the lymphatic system that absorb those fats that cannot be transported by the bloodstream. These dietary fats are transformed in the cells of the lacteals. The lymphatic vessels then return them to the venous circulation so they can be used throughout the body as nutrients.
- The blood vessels absorb the nutrients, fats, and fat-soluble vitamins from the digested food directly into the bloodstream for use throughout the body. This is discussed further in Chapter 9.

Interstitial Fluid and Lymph Creation

Interstitial fluid (**in**-ter-**STISH**-al), which is also known as ***intercellular*** or ***tissue fluid***, is plasma from arterial blood that flows out of the arterioles and into the capillaries, and then flows into the spaces between the cells of the tissues.

- This fluid delivers nutrients, oxygen, and hormones to the cells.
- When interstitial fluid leaves the cells, it brings with it waste products and protein molecules that were created within the cells. About 90% of this fluid returns to the bloodstream.

Lymph (**LIMF**) is made up of the remaining 10% of the returning interstitial fluid. Lymph is a clear, watery fluid containing electrolytes and proteins. It plays essential roles in the lymphatic system as it works in close cooperation with the immune system.

- Lymph collects the protein molecules created within the cells as it leaves. Lymph also removes dead cells, debris, and pathogens (including cancer cells) from the intercellular spaces.
- The lymph enters very small capillaries within the tissues and then flows into progressively larger vessels and ducts as it travels in a one-way trip upward toward the neck.
- At this stage, the lymph begins to play an active role in cooperation with the immune system to protect the body against invading microorganisms and diseases. These functions are described in the section "The Immune System's First Line of Defense."

STRUCTURES OF THE LYMPHATIC SYSTEM

Many of the structures of the lymphatic system cooperate and also perform roles in other body systems.

Lymphatic Circulation

The **lymphatic circulatory system** and blood circulatory system work closely together, and because of these similarities the lymphatic circulatory system is often referred to as the ***secondary circulatory system***. However, it is also very important to understand the differences in these two systems. While studying this section, compare Figure 7.1 with Figures 5.9 and 5.10 (arterial and venous circulation) in Chapter 5.

- Blood circulates throughout the entire body in a loop, pumped by the heart. The bloodstream flows in an open system in which it leaves and reenters the blood vessels through the capillaries.
- Since the lymphatic system does not have a pump-like organ, it must depend on the pumping motion of muscles to move the fluid.
- Lymph flows in only one direction. From its point of origin, lymph can move only upward until it returns to the circulatory system at the base of the neck. Once lymph enters a lymphatic capillary, it must continue this upward flow.
- Blood is filtered by the kidneys, and waste products are excreted by the urinary system. Lymph is filtered by lymph nodes, which are located along lymphatic vessels. These nodes contain specialized cells of the immune system.
- The color of blood makes the arteries and veins readily visible. Since lymph is a clear fluid, the lymphatic vessels are not readily visible.

Lymphatic Capillaries

Lymphatic capillaries are microscopic, blind-ended (sealed on one end) tubes located near the surface of the body with capillary walls that are only one cell in thickness. These cells separate briefly to allow the lymph to enter the capillary. Then the action of the cells as they close forces the lymph to flow upward and forward (Figure 7.2).

Lymphatic Vessels and Ducts

Lymph flows from the lymphatic capillaries into the progressively larger **lymphatic vessels**, which are located deeper within the tissues. Like veins, lymphatic vessels have valves to prevent the backward flow of lymph.

The larger lymphatic vessels eventually join together to form two ducts. Each duct drains a specific part of the body and returns the lymph to the venous circulation (Figure 7.1).

- The **right lymphatic duct** collects lymph from the right side of the head and neck, the upper right quadrant of the body, and the right arm. The right lymphatic duct empties into the right subclavian vein. The ***subclavian*** vein is the proximal part of the main vein of the arm.
- The **thoracic duct**, which is the largest lymphatic vessel in the body, collects lymph from the left side of the head and neck, the upper left quadrant of the trunk, the left arm, the entire lower portion of the trunk, and both legs. The thoracic duct empties into the left subclavian vein.

Lymph Nodes

Each small, bean-shaped **lymph node** contains specialized lymphocytes that are capable of destroying pathogens. Unfiltered lymph flows into the nodes, and here the lymphocytes destroy harmful substances such as bacteria, viruses, and malignant cells. Additional structures within the node filter the lymph to remove other impurities. After these processes are complete, the lymph leaves the node and continues its journey to become part of the venous circulation again.

There are between 400 and 700 lymph nodes located along the larger lymphatic vessels, and approximately half of these nodes are in the abdomen. Most of the other nodes are positioned on the branches of the larger lymphatic vessels throughout the body. In addition, there are the three major groups of lymph nodes that are named for their locations (Figure 7.1).

- **Cervical lymph nodes** (**SER**-vih-kal) are located along the sides of the neck (**cervic** means neck, and **-al** means pertaining to).
- **Axillary lymph nodes** (**AK**-sih-lar-ee) are located under the arms in the area known as the armpits (**axill** means armpit, and **-ary** means pertaining to).
- **Inguinal lymph nodes** (**ING**-gwih-nal) are located in the inguinal (groin) area of the lower abdomen (**inguin** means groin, and **-al** means pertaining to).

Lymphocytes

Lymphocytes (**LIM**-foh-sights), also known as ***lymphoid cells***, are leukocytes that are formed in bone marrow as stem cells (**lymph/o** means lymph, and **-cytes** means cells).

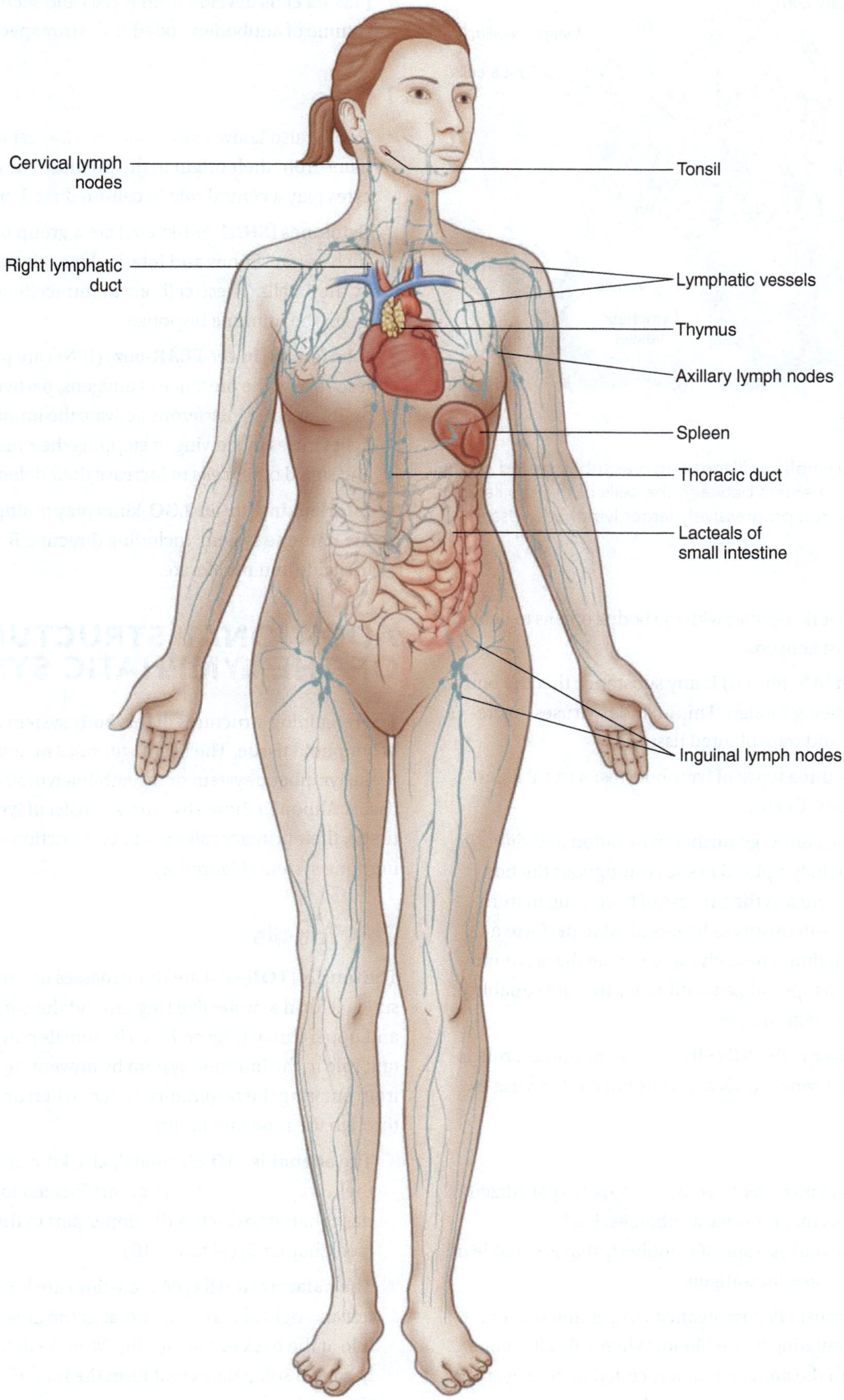

FIGURE 7.1 The vessels and organs of the lymphatic system.

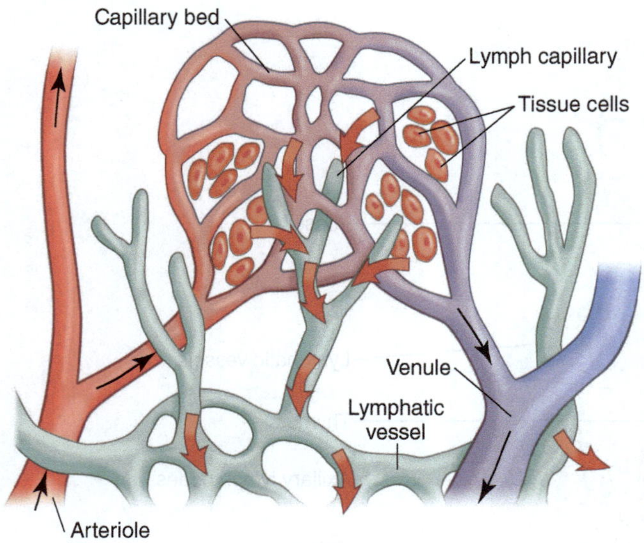

FIGURE 7.2 *Lymph capillaries* begin as tubes sealed on one end. Lymph enters between the cells of the capillary wall and flows into progressively larger lymphatic vessels.

Lymphocytes work together with the body's organs to defend the body against antigens.

- An **antigen** (**AN**-tih-jen) is any substance that the body regards as being foreign. This includes viruses, bacteria, toxins, and transplanted tissues.

  There are three types of lymphocytes: natural killer cells, B cells, and T cells.

- Lymphocytes undergo further maturation and differentiation in lymphoid tissues throughout the body. ***Maturation*** means the process of becoming mature. ***Differentiation*** means to be modified to perform a specific function. These changes enable these lymphocytes to act as specialized antibodies that are capable of attacking specific antigens.
- **Natural killer cells** (NK cells) play an important role in the killing of cancer cells and cells infected by viruses.

B Cells

- **B cells**, also known as ***B lymphocytes***, are specialized lymphocytes that produce antibodies. Each lymphocyte makes a specific antibody that is capable of destroying a specific antigen.
- B cells are most effective against viruses and bacteria that are circulating in the blood. When a B cell is confronted with the antigen that it is coded to destroy, then that B cell is transformed into a plasma cell.
- **Plasma cells** develop from B cells and secrete a large volume of antibodies coded to destroy specific antigens.

T Cells

- **T cells**, also known as ***T lymphocytes***, get the *T* in their name from their origin in the thymus. These lymphocytes play a central role in cell-mediated immunity.
- **Cytokines** (**SIGH**-toh-kyens) are a group of proteins such as interferons and interleukins released primarily by the T cells. These cells act as intracellular signals to begin the immune response.
- **Interferons** (**in**-ter-**FEAR**-onz) (IFNs) are produced in response to the presence of antigens, particularly viruses or tumor cells. Interferons activate the immune system, fight viruses by slowing or stopping their multiplication, and signal other cells to increase their defenses.
- **Interleukins** (**in**-ter-**LOO**-kinz) play multiple roles in the immune system, including directing B and T cells to divide and proliferate.

ADDITIONAL STRUCTURES OF THE LYMPHATIC SYSTEM

The remaining structures of this body system are made up of lymphoid tissue. The term ***lymphoid*** means pertaining to the lymphatic system or resembling lymph or lymphatic tissue. Although these structures consist of lymphoid tissue, their primary roles are in conjunction with the immune system (Figure 7.3).

The Tonsils

The **tonsils** (**TON**-sils) are three masses of lymphoid tissue that form a protective ring around the back of the nose and upper throat (Figure 7.4). The tonsils play an important role in the immune system by preventing pathogens from entering the respiratory system when one breathes through the nose and mouth.

- The **adenoids** (**AD**-eh-noids), also known as the ***nasopharyngeal tonsils***, are located in the nasopharynx, which is the upper part of the pharynx (see Chapter 8) (Figure 7.4B).
- The **palatine tonsils** (**PAL**-ah-tine) are located on the left and right sides of the throat in the area that is visible at the back of the mouth. ***Palatine*** describes the hard and soft palates that form the roof of the mouth (Figure 7.4A).

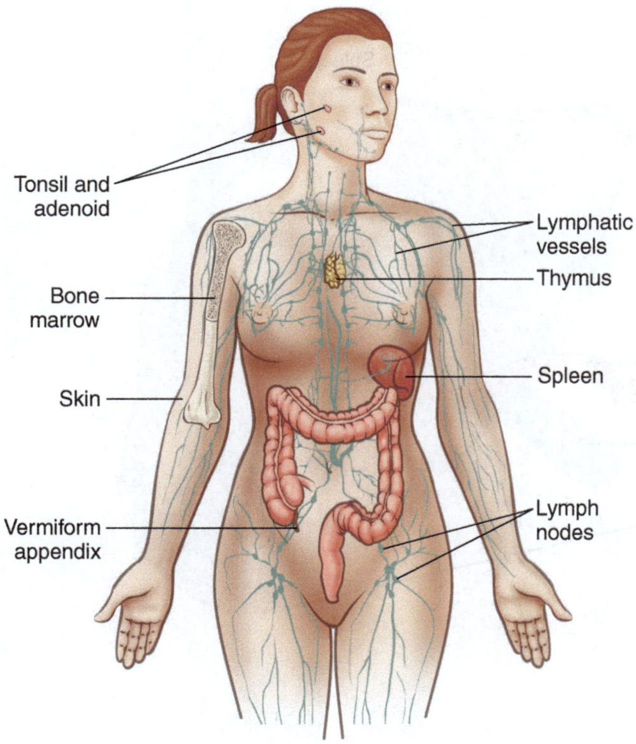

FIGURE 7.3 Structures consisting of lymphoid tissues play many important roles in the immune system.

- The **lingual tonsils** (**LING**-gwal) are located at the base of the tongue; however, they are not readily visible. ***Lingual*** means pertaining to the tongue (Figure 7.4A).

The Thymus Gland

The **thymus** (**THIGH**-mus), which is a mass of lymphoid tissue located above the heart, reaches its greatest size at puberty and becomes smaller with age (Figure 7.3).

- As part of the endocrine system, the thymus secretes a hormone that stimulates the maturation of lymphocytes into T cells (see Chapter 14).
- These T cells, which are essential to the immune system, leave the thymus through the bloodstream and the lymphatic system.

The Vermiform Appendix

The **vermiform appendix**, commonly referred to as the ***appendix***, hangs from the lower portion of the cecum, which is the first section of the large intestine. Although its purpose was unknown for many years, recent research indicates that the appendix may play an important role in the immune system.

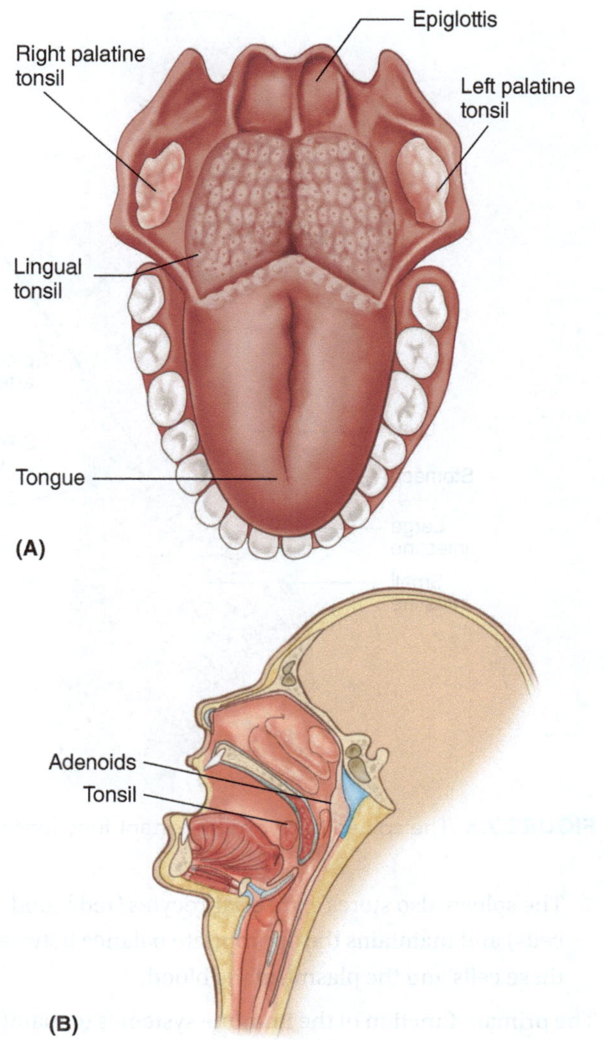

FIGURE 7.4 The *tonsils* form a protective ring around the entrance to the respiratory system.

The Spleen

The **spleen** is a sac-like mass of lymphoid tissue located in the left upper quadrant of the abdomen, just inferior to (below) the diaphragm and posterior to (behind) the stomach (Figure 7.5).

- The spleen filters microorganisms and other foreign material from the blood.
- The spleen forms lymphocytes and monocytes, which are specialized leukocytes (white blood cells) with important roles in the immune system.
- The spleen has the **hemolytic** (hee-moh-**LIT**-ick) function of destroying worn-out erythrocytes (red blood cells) and releasing their hemoglobin for reuse (**hem/o** means blood, and **-lytic** means to destroy).

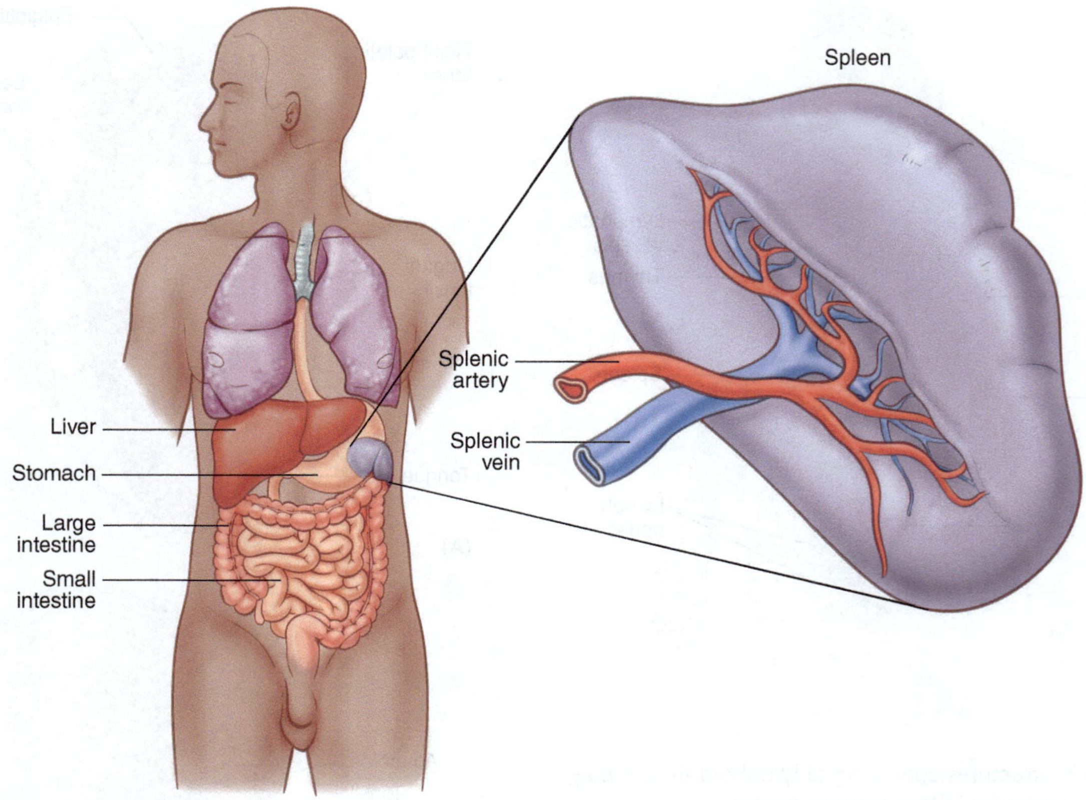

FIGURE 7.5 The spleen performs important functions related to both the immune and cardiovascular systems.

- The spleen also stores extra erythrocytes (red blood cells) and maintains the appropriate balance between these cells and the plasma of the blood.

The primary function of the immune system is to maintain good health and to protect the body from harmful substances such as:

- ***Pathogens***, which are disease-producing microorganisms.
- ***Allergens***, which are substances that produce allergic reactions.
- ***Toxins***, which are poisonous or harmful substances.
- ***Malignant cells***, which are potentially life-threatening cancer cells. *Note:* Cancer, which can attack any body system, is covered in Chapter 20.
- The immune system first attempts to prevent the entry of these harmful substances into the body. If harmful substances do gain entry into the body, the immune system immediately begins working to destroy them.
- The immune system uses a complex system of chemical signaling between specialized cells to identify, attack, and remember antigens.
- This is accomplished by coordinating a highly specific response based on the type of antigen and differentiating it from the body's own tissues to avoid attacking itself.
- After encountering an antigen once, the immune system's "memory" of the invader enables the body to mount a more efficient future defense against that antigen.

The Immune System's First Line of Defense

Unlike other body systems, the immune system is not contained within a single set of organs or vessels. Instead, its functions use structures from several other body systems. The first line of defense includes:

- **Intact skin** that wraps the body in a physical barrier to prevent invading organisms from entering the body. ***Intact*** means that there are no cuts, scrapes, open sores, or breaks in the skin. The skin is also covered with an ***acid mantle*** that makes it an inhospitable environment for most bacteria.
- The **respiratory system** traps breathed-in foreign matter with nose hairs and the moist mucous membrane lining of the respiratory system. The tonsils form a protective ring around the entrance to the throat. If foreign matter gets past these barriers, coughing and sneezing help expel it from the respiratory system.

- The **digestive system** uses the acids and enzymes produced by the stomach to destroy invaders that are swallowed or consumed with food.
- The structures of the **lymphatic system** and specialized leukocytes (white blood cells) work together in specific ways to attack and destroy pathogens that have succeeded in entering the body.

The Antigen–Antibody Reaction

The **antigen–antibody reaction**, also known as the ***immune reaction***, involves binding antigens to antibodies. This reaction labels a potentially dangerous antigen so it can be recognized and destroyed by other cells of the immune system. The immune system immediately responds to the presence of any antigen (Figure 7.6).

- **Tolerance** refers to an acquired unresponsiveness to a specific antigen. The term is also used to describe a decline in the effective response to a drug, usually due to repeated use.

An **antibody** (**AN**-tih-**bod**-ee) is a disease-fighting protein created by the immune system in response to the presence of a specific antigen (the prefix **anti-** means against). The terms ***antibody*** and ***immunoglobulin*** are often used interchangeably.

Immunoglobulins

- **Immunoglobulins** (im-you-noh-**GLOB**-you-lins) bind with specific antigens in the antigen–antibody response. The five primary types of immunoglobulins, which are secreted by plasma cells, are also known as antibodies (Table 7.1).

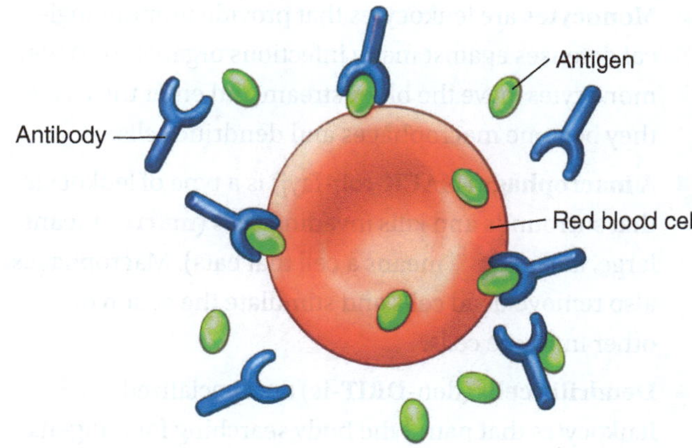

FIGURE 7.6 Antibodies bind together with foreign antigens to neutralize them and to flag them for destruction by the macrophages.

Phagocytes

Phagocytes (**FAG**-oh-sights) are specialized leukocytes that act as part of the antigen–antibody reaction by destroying substances such as cell debris, dust, pollen, and pathogens by the process of phagocytosis (**phag/o** means to eat or swallow, and **-cytes** means cells). ***Phagocytosis*** is the process of destroying pathogens by surrounding and swallowing them. Phagocytes include monocytes, macrophages, dendritic cells, and mast cells. Mast cells are discussed in Chapter 13.

TABLE 7.1

Immunoglobulins and Their Roles

Immunoglobulin G **(IgG)** is the most abundant class of antibodies, and is found in blood and lymph. These antibodies are active against bacteria, fungi, viruses, and foreign particles.
Immunoglobulin A **(IgA)** is the class of antibodies produced predominantly against ingested antigens. These antibodies are found in body secretions such as saliva, sweat, or tears, and they function to prevent the attachment of viruses and bacteria to the epithelial surfaces that line most organs.
Immunoglobulin M **(IgM)** is the class of antibodies that are found in circulating body fluids. These are the first antibodies to appear in response to an initial exposure to an antigen.
Immunoglobulin D **(IgD)** is the class of antibodies found only on the surface of B cells. These antibodies are important in B cell activation.
Immunoglobulin E **(IgE)** is the class of antibodies produced in the lungs, skin, and mucous membranes. These antibodies are responsible for allergic reactions.

Note: Synthetic immunoglobulins, which are used as medications, are discussed in the section "Antibody Therapy."

- **Monocytes** are leukocytes that provide immunological defenses against many infectious organisms. When monocytes leave the bloodstream and enter the tissue, they become macrophages and dendritic cells.
- A **macrophage** (**MACK**-roh-fayj) is a type of leukocyte that surrounds and kills invading cells (**macro-** means large, and **-phage** means a cell that eats). Macrophages also remove dead cells and stimulate the action of other immune cells.
- **Dendritic cells** (den-**DRIT**-ic) are specialized leukocytes that patrol the body searching for antigens that produce infections. When such a cell is found, the dendritic cell grabs it, swallows it, and alerts B and T cells to act against this specific antigen.

The Complement System

The **complement system** (**KOM**-pleh-ment) is a group of proteins that normally circulate in the blood in an inactive form. When needed, these cells complement the ability of antibodies to ward off pathogens by combining with them to dissolve and remove pathogenic bacteria and other foreign cells. *Complement* means to complete or make whole.

Immunity

Immunity is the state of being resistant to a specific disease. This resistance can be present naturally, or it can be acquired.

- **Natural immunity**, which is also known as *passive immunity*, is resistance to a disease present without the administration of an antigen or exposure to a disease. Natural immunity is present at birth, and can be augmented when breast milk passes from a nursing mother to her baby.
- **Acquired immunity** is obtained by having had a contagious disease. Being *vaccinated* against a contagious disease provides protection against that disease, such as measles or polio, without the risks of actually having the disease.
- A *vaccine* is a preparation containing an antigen, consisting of whole or partial disease-causing organisms, which have been killed or weakened. An *mRNA vaccine* is a form of vaccine containing genetic instructions for a surface protein from the target virus. The mRNA vaccine instructs cells to create the protein, which the body recognizes as foreign, and then builds antibodies against it.
- *Vaccination* provides protection against a disease; however, for some conditions a periodic booster is required to maintain the effectiveness of the immunization.

MEDICAL SPECIALTIES RELATED TO THE LYMPHATIC AND IMMUNE SYSTEMS

The lymphatic and immune systems work in close cooperation to protect and maintain the health of the body. Some medical specialists treat disorders that affect both of these body systems.

- An **allergist** (**AL**-er-jist) specializes in diagnosing and treating conditions of altered immunologic reactivity, such as allergic reactions.
- An **infectious disease specialist** is a physician who specializes in diagnosing and treating diseases caused by microorganisms such as viruses, bacteria, and parasites.
- An **immunologist** (**im**-you-**NOL**-oh-jist) specializes in diagnosing and treating disorders of the immune system (**immun** means protected, and **-ologist** means specialist).
- A **lymphologist** (lim-**FOL**-oh-jist) is a physician who specializes in diagnosing and treating disorders of the lymphatic system (**lymph** means lymphatic system, and **-ologist** means specialist).

PATHOLOGY AND DIAGNOSTIC PROCEDURES OF THE LYMPHATIC SYSTEM

- **Lymphadenitis** (lim-**fad**-eh-**NIGH**-tis), commonly known as *swollen glands*, is an inflammation of the lymph nodes (**lymphaden** means lymph node, and **-itis** means inflammation). The terms *lymph nodes* and *lymph glands* are sometimes used interchangeably. Swelling of the lymph nodes is frequently an indication of an infection.
- **Lymphadenopathy** (lim-**fad**-eh-**NOP**-ah-thee) is any disease process affecting a lymph node or nodes (**lymphaden/o** means lymph node, and **-pathy** means disease).
- A **lymphangioma** (lim-**fan**-jee-**OH**-mah) is a benign tumor formed by an abnormal collection of lymphatic vessels due to a congenital malformation of the

lymphatic system (**lymph** means lymph, **angi** means lymph vessel, and **-oma** means tumor).

- A **ruptured spleen** is a medical emergency that occurs when the covering of the spleen is torn, usually as the result of a blow to the abdomen.
- **Splenomegaly** (**splee**-noh-**MEG**-ah-lee) is an abnormal enlargement of the spleen (**splen/o** means spleen, and **-megaly** means enlargement). This condition can be due to bleeding caused by an injury, an infectious disease such as mononucleosis, or abnormal functioning of the immune system.
- **Tonsillitis** and **tonsillectomy** are discussed in Chapter 1.
- **Lymphoscintigraphy** (**lim**-foh-sin-**TIH**-grah-fee) is a diagnostic test that is performed to detect damage or malformations of the lymphatic vessels. A radioactive substance is injected into lymph ducts, and a scanner or probe is used to follow the movement of the substance on a computer screen.

Lymphedema

Lymphedema (**lim**-feh-**DEE**-mah) (LE) is swelling of the tissues due to an abnormal accumulation of lymph fluid within the tissues (**lymph** means lymph, and **-edema** means swelling). This is not the type of swelling that occurs due to an injury such as a sprained ankle. It is caused by damage to the lymphatic system that prevents lymph from draining properly. Because lymph is rich in protein, which is an environment that pathogens thrive in, lymphedema is often associated with infections.

- ***Primary lymphedema*** is a hereditary condition of the lymphatic system that develops with swelling beginning in the feet and progressing into the ankles and in an upward direction along the legs. The disorder occurs most frequently in females, and the symptoms begin to appear during puberty.
- ***Secondary lymphedema*** is caused by damage to lymphatic vessels that is most frequently due to cancer treatment, surgery, trauma, or burns.
- Primary and secondary lymphedema are most commonly treated with compression and exercise to control the swelling and to minimize the infections. ***Compression*** uses specialized clothing such as socks, stockings, and sleeves or bandages to exert pressure, which can be used to improve circulation and lymph flow. Although this treatment helps, at this time it is not possible to cure lymphedema.
- **Bioimpedance spectroscopy** (**BYE**-oh-im-**pee**-dens) is a noninvasive method of diagnosing lymphedema. It measures the resistance to an electrical current passed through the affected limb, with abnormally low results showing a buildup of lymph. If this condition can be diagnosed with this technique at an early stage, there is hope that it will not develop any further.

PATHOLOGY AND DIAGNOSTIC PROCEDURES OF THE IMMUNE SYSTEM

The effectiveness of the immune system depends upon the individual's:

- *General health.* If the immune system is compromised by poor health, it cannot be fully effective.
- *Age.* Older individuals usually have more acquired immunity; however, their immune system tends to respond less quickly and effectively to new challenges. Babies and very young children do not have as much acquired immunity, and their bodies sometimes have difficulty resisting challenges to the immune system.
- *Heredity.* Genes and genetic disorders affect the individual's general health and the functioning of his or her immune system.

Allergic Reactions

- An **allergic reaction** occurs when the body's immune system reacts to a harmless allergen such as pollen, food, or animal dander as if it were a dangerous invader.
- An **allergy**, also known as ***hypersensitivity***, is an overreaction by the body to a particular antigen. For *allergic rhinitis*, an allergic reaction to airborne allergens, see Chapter 8.
- An **allergen** (**AL**-er-jen) is a substance that produces an allergic reaction in an individual.
- A **localized allergic response**, also known as a ***cellular response***, includes redness, itching, and burning where the skin has come into contact with an allergen. For example, contact with poison ivy can cause a localized allergic response in the form of an itchy rash (see Chapter 13). Although the body reacts mildly the

first time it is exposed to the allergen, sensitivity is established, and future contacts can cause much more severe symptoms.

- A **systemic reaction** (sis-**TEH**-mik), which is also known as **anaphylaxis** (**an**-ah-fih-**LACK**-sis) or *anaphylactic shock*, is a severe response to an allergen. As shown in Figure 7.7, the symptoms of this response develop quickly. Without prompt medical aid, the patient can die within a few minutes.
- A *scratch test* is a diagnostic test to identify commonly troublesome allergens such as tree pollen and ragweed. Swelling and itching indicate an allergic reaction (Figure 7.8).
- The *allergen-specific immunoglobulin E* (IgE) blood test is sometimes used to determine whether a person is allergic to a particular substance.
- **Antihistamines** are medications administered to relieve or prevent the symptoms of allergy to wind-borne pollens and other types of allergies. Antihistamines work by preventing the effects of *histamine*, which is a substance produced by the body that causes the itching, sneezing, runny nose, and watery eyes of an allergic reaction.

Autoimmune Disorders

An **autoimmune disorder** (**aw**-toh-ih-**MYOUN**), also known as an *autoimmune disease*, is any of a large group of diseases characterized by a condition in which the immune system produces antibodies against its own tissues, mistaking healthy cells, tissues, or organs for antigens.

- This abnormal functioning of the immune system appears to be genetically transmitted and predominantly occurs in women during the childbearing years.

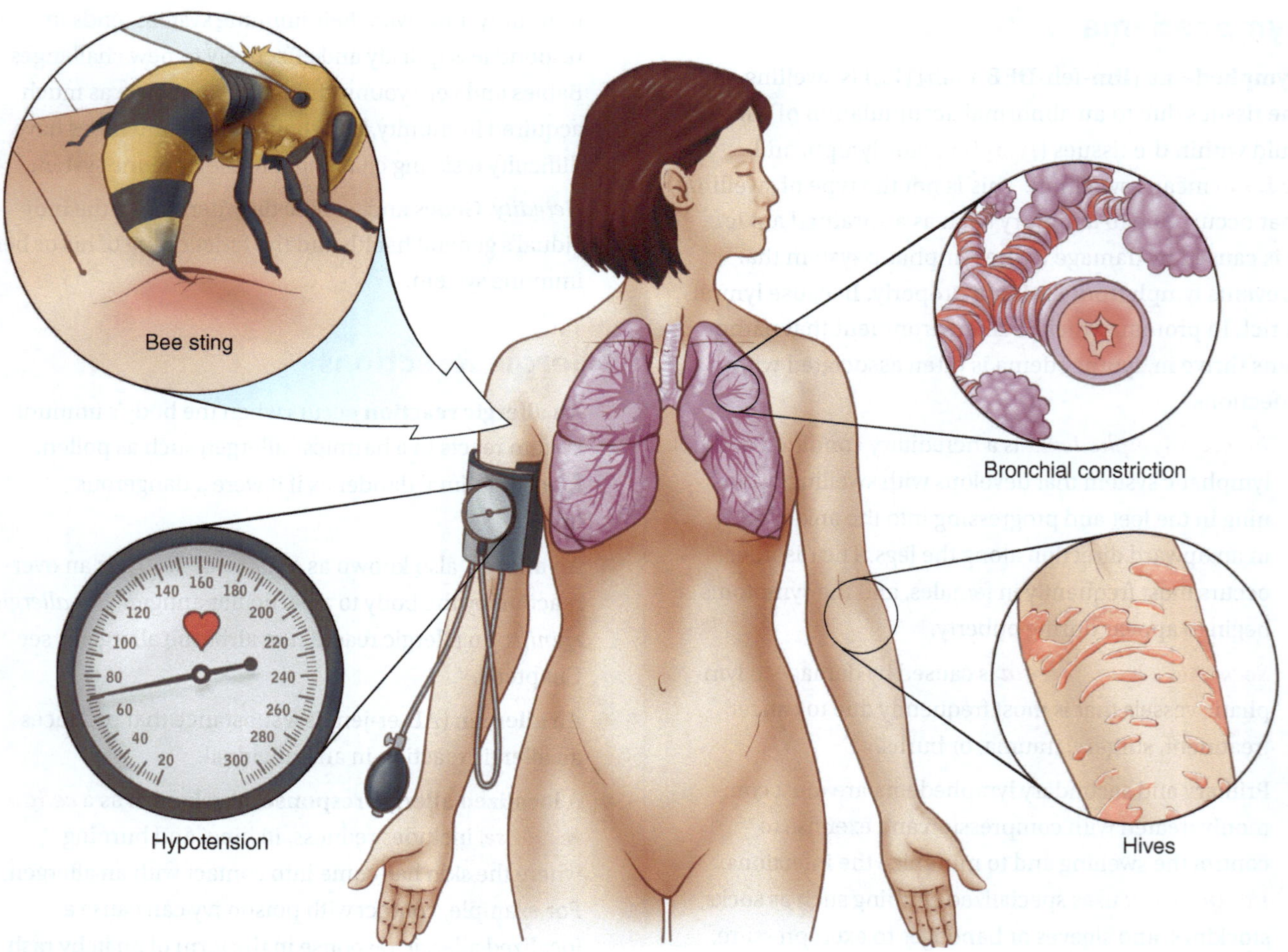

FIGURE 7.7 A severe anaphylactic allergic reaction involves several body systems and requires prompt treatment. Shown here are the many systems that may respond to a bee sting.

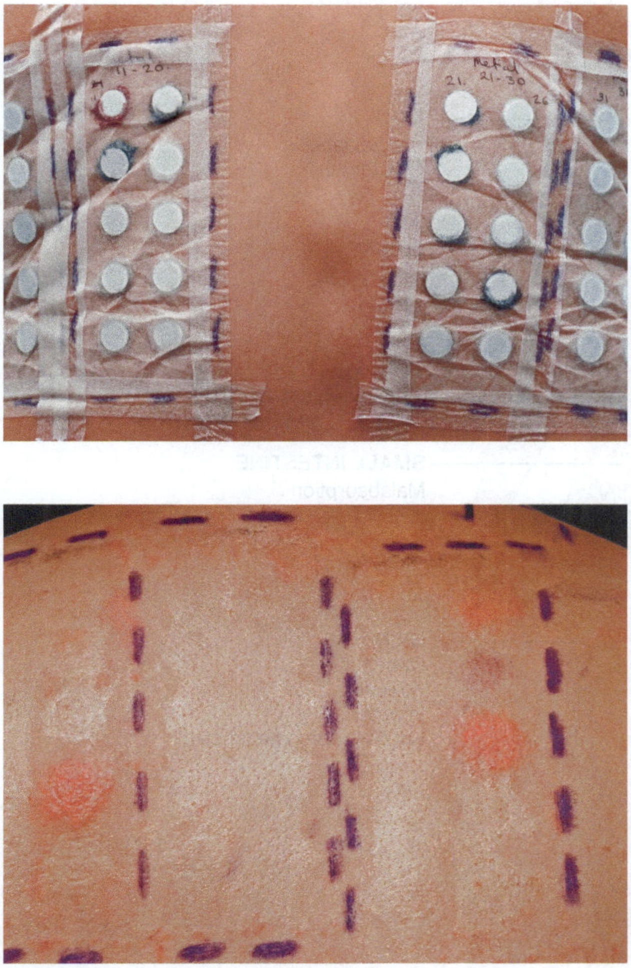

Andy Lidstone/Shutterstock.com

Andy Lidstone/Shutterstock.com

FIGURE 7.8 In scratch tests, allergens are placed on the skin, the skin is scratched, and the allergen is labeled. Reactions usually begin to occur within 20 minutes.

- It is estimated that 3% of Americans have an autoimmune disorder, with women affected 2.7 times more often than men. Autoimmune disorders affect most body systems. For examples, see Table 7.2. To learn more, see the chapters for each body system referenced in the table.

Immunodeficiency Disorders

An **immunodeficiency disorder** (**im**-you-noh-deh-**FISH**-en-see) occurs when the immune response is compromised. ***Compromised*** means weakened or not functioning properly.

- **Severe combined immunodeficiency** (SCID) is an inherited condition in which abnormalities in the immune system cause an increased susceptibility to infection and failure to thrive as a result of infections. Although the condition is rare, testing for it is now routinely included during infant newborn screening.

HIV: Human Immunodeficiency Virus

The **human immunodeficiency virus** (**im**-you-noh-deh-**FISH**-en-see), commonly known as ***HIV***, is a bloodborne infection in which the virus damages or kills the T cells of the immune system, causing it to progressively fail, thus leaving the body at risk of developing many life-threatening opportunistic infections (Figure 7.9). HIV can be ***perinatally*** acquired (transmitted from a mother who is HIV+ to her child during pregnancy, childbirth, or

TABLE 7.2

Examples of Autoimmune Disorders and the Affected Body Systems

Body System	Autoimmune Disorder	See Chapter
Skeletal System	*Rheumatoid arthritis* affects joints and connective tissue.	3
Muscular System	*Myasthenia gravis* affects nerve and muscle synapses.	4
Cardiovascular System	*Pernicious anemia* affects the red blood cells.	5
Digestive System	*Crohn's disease* affects the intestines, ileum, or the colon.	9
Nervous System	*Multiple sclerosis* affects the brain and spinal cord.	11
Integumentary System	*Scleroderma* affects the skin and connective tissues.	13
Endocrine System	*Graves' disease* affects the thyroid gland.	14

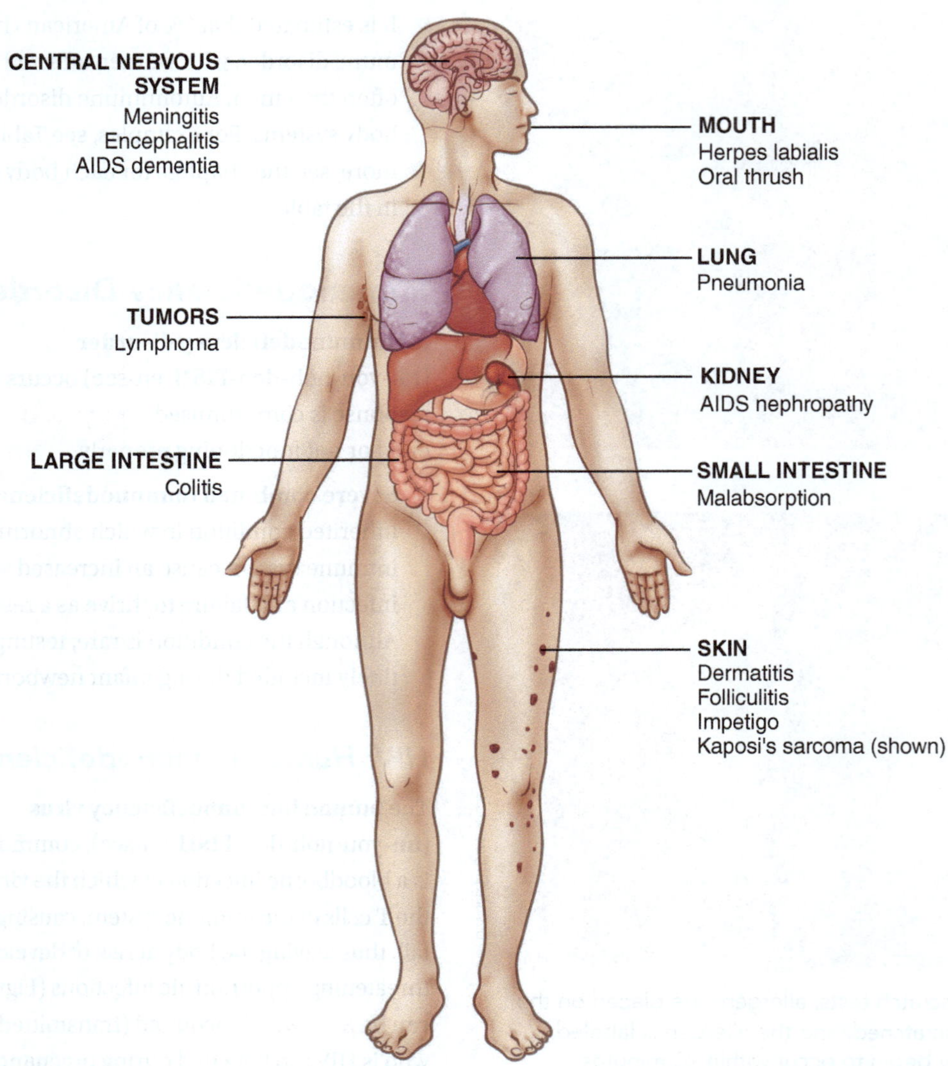

FIGURE 7.9 Pathologies associated with acquired immunodeficiency syndrome (AIDS). Each condition is discussed in the appropriate body system chapter.

breastfeeding) or ***behaviorally*** acquired (transmitted from a person who is HIV+ through unprotected sex or sharing needles). Current prevention and treatment medications make HIV transmission much more preventable than it was in the past (see the section "HIV Treatment").

- **Acquired immunodeficiency syndrome**, commonly known as ***AIDS***, is the most advanced and fatal stage of an HIV infection.
- An **opportunistic infection** (**op**-ur-too-**NIHS**-tick) is caused by a pathogen that does not normally produce an illness in healthy humans. However, when the host is debilitated, these pathogens are able to cause an infection. ***Debilitated*** means weakened by another condition.
- **Kaposi's sarcoma** (**KAP**-oh-seez sar-**KOH**-mah) is an example of an opportunistic infection that is frequently associated with HIV. This cancer causes patches of abnormal tissue to grow under the skin; in the lining of the mouth, nose, and throat; or in other organs.
- **ELISA**, which is the acronym for ***enzyme-linked immunosorbent assay***, is a blood test used to screen for the presence of HIV antibodies, as well as Lyme disease and other infectious conditions.
- An ***HIV differentiation assay*** is used to confirm a positive ELISA test.

TREATMENT OF THE IMMUNE SYSTEM

A variety of treatment procedures are used to correct or control the symptoms of disorders of the immune system.

Immunotherapy

Immunotherapy (**im**-you-noh-**THER**-ah-pee), also called ***biological therapy***, is a disease treatment that involves either stimulating or repressing the immune response (**immun/o** means immune, and **-therapy** means treatment).

- In the treatment of cancers, immunotherapy is used to stimulate the immune response to fight the malignancy. ***Stimulate*** means to cause greater activity.
- In the treatment of allergies, immunotherapy is used to repress the body's sensitivity to a particular allergen. ***Repress*** means to decrease or stop a normal response. This treatment is also known as ***allergy desensitization*** or ***allergen immunotherapy***.

Antibody Therapy

- **Synthetic immunoglobulins**, also known as ***immune serum***, are used as a post-exposure preventive measure against certain viruses, including rabies and some types of hepatitis. ***Post-exposure*** means that the patient has been exposed to the virus, for example, by being bitten by an animal with rabies. The goal of this treatment is to provide temporary immunity to prevent the disease from developing.
- **Synthetic interferon** is used in the treatment of multiple sclerosis, hepatitis C, and some cancers.
- **Monoclonal antibodies** are any of a class of antibodies produced in the laboratory by identical offspring of a clone of specific cells. These artificially produced antibodies are used to enhance the patient's immune response to certain types of cancer. See Chapter 20 for more information.

HIV Treatment

- Treatment for HIV includes ***antiretroviral therapy*** (ART), which is sometimes referred to as a ***treatment regimen*** because often it is more than one drug and they must be taken in combination with each other. Although there is no cure for HIV, these drugs help control the impact of the disease on the immune system and the ability of a person to transmit the disease.
- There are medications that can be taken to prevent HIV transmission, either after exposure or prior to exposure to the virus. ***Pre-exposure prophylaxis*** (PrEP) is a daily preventative drug for people at high risk of HIV infection such as people who use IV drugs and men who have sex with men. ***Post-exposure prophylaxis*** (PEP) is for people who have had suspected or confirmed exposure to the virus, such as in the case of a sexual assault, and is taken for 28 days.

Immunosuppression

Immunosuppression (**im**-you-noh-sup-**PRESH**-un) is treatment to repress or interfere with the ability of the immune system to respond to stimulation by antigens.

- An **immunosuppressant** (**im**-you-noh-soo-**PRES**-ant) is a substance that prevents or reduces the body's normal immune response. This medication is administered to prevent the rejection of donor tissue and to depress autoimmune disorders.
- A **corticosteroid drug** (**kor**-tih-koh-**STEHR**-oid) is a synthetic hormone that closely resembles the cortisol secreted by the adrenal glands. The natural production of corticosteroids by the endocrine system is discussed in Chapter 14.
- A **cytotoxic drug** (**sigh**-toh-**TOK**-sick) is a medication that kills or damages cells (**cyt/o** means cell, **tox** means poison, and **-ic** means pertaining to). These drugs are used as immunosuppressants or as antineoplastics. *Antineoplastics* are discussed in the "Chemotherapy" section in Chapter 20.

PATHOGENIC ORGANISMS

A **pathogen** (**PATH**-oh-jen) is a microorganism that causes a disease in humans. A ***microorganism*** is a living organism that is so small it can be seen only with the aid of a microscope. ***Pathogenic*** means capable of producing disease (Figure 7.10).

Bacteria

Bacteria (back-**TEE**-ree-ah) are one-celled microscopic organisms (singular, *bacterium*). Most bacteria are not harmful to humans. The following list shows some of the bacteria that are pathogenic.

- **Bacilli** (bah-**SILL**-eye) are rod-shaped, spore-forming bacteria (**bacilli** means rod-shaped). (The singular is *bacillus*.)

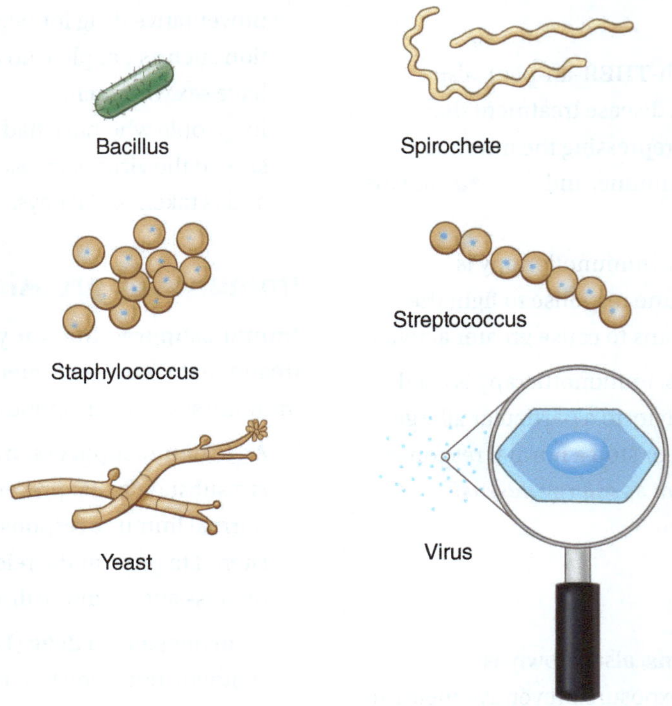

FIGURE 7.10 Shown here are examples of types of pathogens. The single virus shown at the right is magnified to illustrate details of its structure.

- **Anthrax** (AN-thraks) is a contagious disease that can be transmitted through livestock infected with *Bacillus anthracis*. Spores grown in laboratories have been used in biological warfare.
- A **rickettsia** (rih-**KET**-see-ah) is a small bacterium that lives in lice, fleas, ticks, and mites (plural, *rickettsiae*). ***Rocky Mountain spotted fever*** is caused by a rickettsia that is transmitted to humans by the bite of an infected tick.
- **Lyme disease** (**LIME**) is transmitted to humans by the bite of a tick that has had contact with a deer infected with the spirochete *Borrelia burgdorferi*. It is named for Old Lyme, Connecticut, where it was first diagnosed. Symptoms of Lyme disease include fever, headache, fatigue, and a characteristic skin rash known as *erythema migrans*. If untreated, Lyme disease can spread to the joints, heart, and nervous system. Syphilis is also caused by spirochetes (see Chapter 15).
- **Spirochetes** (**SPY**-roh-keets) are long, slender, spiral-shaped bacteria that have flexible walls and are capable of movement.
- **Shigellosis** is an infection caused by the bacteria *Shigella*, which can cause diarrhea and fever and can be prevented by hand washing and good hygiene.
- **Staphylococci** (**staf**-ih-loh-**KOCK**-sigh) are a group of about 30 species of bacteria that form irregular groups or clusters resembling grapes (**staphyl/o** means clusters or bunches of grapes, and **-cocci** means spherical bacteria). (The singular is *staphylococcus*.) Most staphylococci are harmless and reside normally on the skin and mucous membranes of humans and other organisms; however, others are capable of producing very serious infections.
- **Staphylococcus aureus** (**staf**-ih-loh-**KOCK**-us **OR**-ee-us), also known as ***staph aureus***, is a form of staphylococcus that often infects wounds and causes serious problems such as toxic shock syndrome or food poisoning.
- **Streptococci** (**strep**-toh-**KOCK**-sigh) are bacteria that form a chain (**strept/o** means twisted chain, and **-cocci** means spherical bacteria). (The singular is *streptococcus*.) Many streptococcal species are harmless; however, other members of this group are responsible for serious illnesses such as strep throat, meningitis (see Chapter 11), endocarditis (see Chapter 5), and necrotizing fasciitis (see Chapter 13).

Antibiotic-Resistant Bacteria

Antibiotic-resistant bacteria occur when antibiotics fail to kill all of the bacteria they target. When this occurs, the surviving bacteria become resistant to this particular drug. As more and more bacteria become resistant to first-line antibiotics, the consequences are severe because the illness lasts longer, and the risk of complications and death increases.

Originally these infections were nosocomial (hospital or clinic acquired), but now these antibiotic-resistant bacteria are increasingly common in the general population.

Methicillin-resistant Staphylococcus aureus, commonly known as ***MRSA***, is one of several types of bacteria that are now resistant to most antibiotics.

- The first symptom of MRSA looks like small, red bumps with a black top. These bumps soon become abscesses that require immediate care.
- MRSA infections are serious, difficult to treat, can be fatal, and often occur repeatedly as breaks in the skin allow the bacteria entry. These infections are becoming increasingly present in the general population.

Fungus and Yeast Infections

A **fungus** (**FUNG**-gus) is a simple parasitic organism (plural, *fungi*). Some of these fungi are harmless to humans; others are pathogenic. **Tinea pedis**, commonly known as ***athlete's foot***, is a fungal infection that develops between the toes (see Chapter 13). ***Aspergillosis*** is a rare infection caused by mold (a type of fungus) inhaled into the lungs.

Yeast is a type of fungus. An example is **candidiasis** (**kan**-dih-**DYE**-ah-sis), which is also known as a ***yeast infection***. (Note that the fungus involved is not related to the microscopic fungus from the *saccharomycetaceae* family used in baking.) Yeast infections occur on the skin or mucous membranes in warm, moist areas such as the vagina or mouth and are caused by the pathogenic yeast *Candida albicans*. ***Oral thrush*** is a yeast infection that occurs in the mouth, especially in infants (see Chapter 18), whereas ***vaginal candidiasis*** occurs in the vagina (see Chapter 16).

Parasites

A **parasite** (**PAR**-ah-sight) is a plant or animal that lives on or within another living organism at the expense of that organism.

- **Giardiasis** (gee-are-**DIE**-uh-sis) is a diarrheal disease caused by the parasite *Giardia*. The most common method of transmission is via water that has been contaminated with feces.
- **Malaria** (mah-**LAY**-ree-ah) is caused by a parasite that lives in certain mosquitoes and is transferred to humans by the bite of an infected mosquito. Symptoms develop from 1 to 4 weeks after being infected and include fever, shaking, chills, headache, muscle aches, and fatigue.
- **Toxoplasmosis** (**tock**-soh-plaz-**MOH**-sis) is a disease caused by a parasite that is most commonly transmitted from pets to humans by contact with contaminated animal feces. A pregnant woman should avoid such contact because it can cause diseases in the developing fetus.
- ***Trichomoniasis*** is a common sexually transmitted disease caused by the parasite *Trichomonas vaginalis* (see Chapter 16).

Viral Infections

Viruses (**VYE**-rus-ez) are very small infectious agents that live only by invading other cells. After invading the cell, the virus reproduces and then breaks the wall of the infected cell to release the newly formed viruses. These viruses spread to other cells and repeat the process.

- **COVID-19** (**KOH**-vid) is a highly contagious viral infection caused by the *SARS-CoV-2* virus. This coronavirus, discovered in 2019, became a global pandemic starting in 2020 (Figure 7.11). COVID-19 spreads via droplet, airborne, and contact transmission, with an incubation period of up to 14 days. Symptoms are wide-ranging and can include fever, body aches, pneumonia, hypoxia, abdominal pain, diarrhea, and loss of taste and smell. The disease is named for **CO**rona**VI**rus **D**isease 2019. ***Coronavirus*** is a type of virus that has crown-like structures on the surface (**corona** means crown).

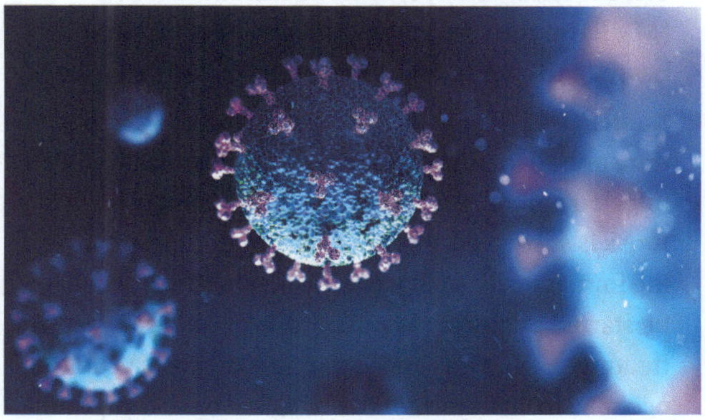

Andrii Vodolazhskyi/Shutterstock.com

FIGURE 7.11 Coronavirus, illustrated here as it appears under a microscope, is a type of virus that has crown-like structures on the surface.

- **Ebola** (ee-**BOH**-lah) is a rare and generally fatal disease transmitted by contact with any bodily fluids infected with the *Ebola* virus. Ebola can only be transmitted when symptoms are present. Early symptoms, which usually appear within 21 days of exposure, include high fever, vomiting, and diarrhea. Late symptoms include massive internal bleeding and organ failure.
- **Influenza** (**in**-floo-**EN**-zah), commonly known as the ***flu***, is a highly contagious viral respiratory infection that usually occurs in seasonal epidemics. Flu symptoms include fever, sore throat, muscle aches, cough, runny nose, and fatigue. Complications can include pneumonia. A vaccine is available annually to protect against the most common strains of influenza.
- **Measles** is an acute, highly contagious infection that is transmitted by respiratory droplets of the *rubeola* virus. Symptoms include a red, itchy rash over the entire body, a high fever, runny nose, and coughing. Measles can be dangerous, especially for babies and young children, and complications may include bronchitis and permanent hearing loss. The incidence of measles in the United States is on the rise due to an increase in unvaccinated children.
- **Mumps** is an acute viral infection that is characterized by the swelling of the parotid glands, which are the salivary glands located just in front of the ears. In adults, mumps can also cause painful swelling of the ovaries or testicles.
- **Rubella** (roo-**BELL**-ah), also known as ***German measles***, is a viral infection characterized by a low-grade fever, swollen glands, inflamed eyes, and a fine, pink rash. Although not usually severe or long-lasting, rubella is serious in a woman during early pregnancy because it can cause defects in a developing fetus.
- The **measles, mumps, and rubella vaccination** (MMR) immunization can prevent these three viral illnesses and should be administered in early childhood.
- **Rabies** (**RAY**-beez) is an acute viral infection that is transmitted to humans through the bite or saliva of an infected animal. An infected animal is said to be ***rabid***. If risk is suspected, it is necessary to undergo testing immediately so that post-exposure treatment can be started as quickly as possible. Without testing and treatment, the signs and symptoms of rabies usually occur 30 to 90 days after the bite, and once symptoms have developed, rabies is almost always fatal.
- **West Nile virus** is spread to humans by the bite of an infected mosquito. A mild form of this condition has flu-like symptoms. A more severe variety spreads to the spinal cord and brain. West Nile virus is a member of the *Flavivirus* genus, which also includes the viruses that cause the mosquito-borne tropical disease dengue fever.
- **Zika virus** is spread to humans by the bite of an infected mosquito, by a woman to her fetus, or through sexual intercourse. People do not normally get sick enough to go to the hospital, but it can cause fever, rash, and birth defects.

Herpesviruses

The group of herpesviruses, which includes *varicella zoster*, *Epstein-Barr*, *cytomegalovirus*, and *herpes simplex*, causes a variety of diseases in humans.

- **Cytomegalovirus** (**sigh**-toh-**meg**-ah-loh-**VYE**-rus) (CMV) is found in most body fluids (**cyt/o** means cell, **megal/o** means large, **vir** means virus, and **-us** is a singular noun ending). It is most often present as a ***silent infection*** in which the individual has no signs or symptoms of the infection, although it can potentially cause a serious illness when the individual has a weakened immune system, or when it is transmitted from a mother to her unborn child. This transmission can cause serious congenital disabilities to the child.
- **Varicella** (**var**-ih-**SEL**-ah), also known as ***chickenpox***, is caused by the herpesvirus *Varicella zoster* and is highly contagious. The condition is characterized by a fever and a rash consisting of hundreds of itchy, fluid-filled blisters that burst and form crusts (Figure 7.12A).
- **Herpes zoster** (**HER**-peez **ZOS**-ter) (HZ), commonly known as ***shingles***, is an acute viral infection characterized by painful skin eruptions that follow the underlying route of an inflamed nerve (Figure 7.12B). This inflammation occurs when the dormant varicella (chickenpox) virus is reactivated later in life. A vaccine is available to help prevent shingles and is recommended for adults age 60 years and older.
- ***Postherpetic neuralgia*** is a complication that may follow herpes zoster if nerve fibers have been damaged during the outbreak. The resulting pain can be severe and persistent.
- **Infectious mononucleosis** (**mon**-oh-**new**-klee-**OH**-sis), also known as ***mono***, is caused by the *Epstein-Barr* virus, and is most common in adolescents and young adults. This condition is characterized by fever, a sore throat, and enlarged lymph nodes. Swelling of the spleen or liver involvement can also develop.

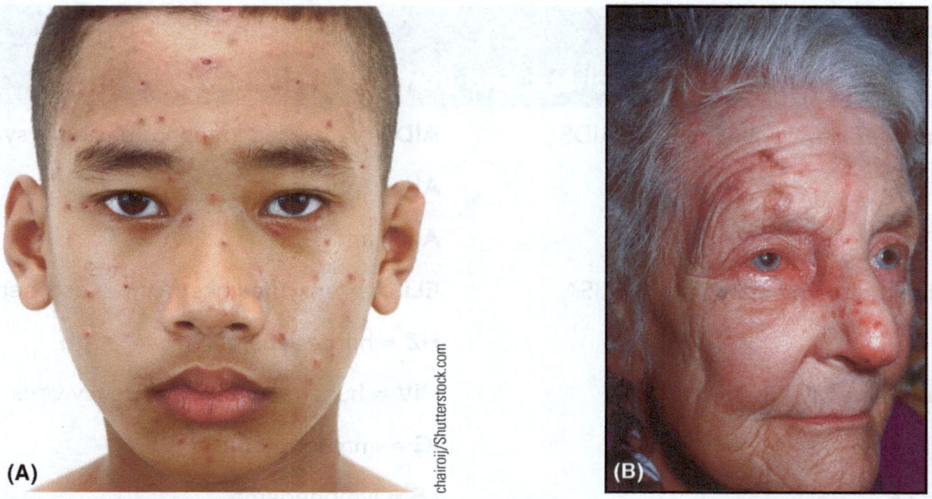

FIGURE 7.12 Varicella, or chickenpox (A), is caused by the varicella zoster virus, which can remain dormant until later in life when it erupts as herpes zoster, or shingles (B).

- **Roseola** (**row**-zee-**OH**-la), also called ***sixth disease***, is common in infants ages 6 months to 2 years and is characterized by a high fever followed by a rash.

Medications to Control Infections

- **Antibiotics** are medications capable of inhibiting growth or killing pathogenic bacterial microorganisms (**anti-** means against, **bi/o** means life, and **-tic** means pertaining to). ***Inhibit*** means to slow the growth or development. Antibiotics are effective against most bacterial infections; however, they are not effective against viral infections.
- A **bactericide** (back-**TEER**-ih-side) is a substance that causes the death of bacteria (**bacteri** means bacteria, and **-cide** means causing death). This group of antibiotics includes penicillins and cephalosporins.
- A **bacteriostatic** agent slows or stops the growth of bacteria (**bacteri/o** means bacteria, and **-static** means causing control). This group of antibiotics includes tetracycline, sulfonamide, and erythromycin.
- An **antifungal** (**an**-tih-**FUNG**-gul) is an agent that destroys or inhibits the growth of fungi (**anti-** means against, **fung** means fungus, and **-al** means pertaining to). Lotrimin is an example of a topical antifungal that is applied to treat or prevent athlete's foot. This type of medication is also known as an ***antimycotic***.
- An **antiviral drug** (**an**-tih-**VYE**-ral) is used to treat viral infections or to provide temporary immunity (**anti-** means against, **vir** means virus, and **-al** means pertaining to).

ABBREVIATIONS RELATED TO THE LYMPHATIC AND IMMUNE SYSTEMS

Table 7.3 presents an overview of the abbreviations related to the terms introduced in this chapter. *Note:* To avoid errors or confusion, always be cautious when using abbreviations.

TABLE 7.3

Abbreviations Related to the Lymphatic and Immune Systems

acquired immunodeficiency syndrome = AIDS	**AIDS** = acquired immunodeficiency syndrome
antibody = Ab	**Ab** = antibody
antigen = Ag	**Ag** = antigen
enzyme-linked immunosorbent assay = ELISA	**ELISA** = enzyme-linked immunosorbent assay
herpes zoster = HZ	**HZ** = herpes zoster
human immunodeficiency virus = HIV	**HIV** = human immunodeficiency virus
immunoglobulin = IG	**IG** = immunoglobulin
lymphedema = LE	**LE** = lymphedema
measles, mumps, and rubella vaccination = MMR	**MMR** = measles, mumps, and rubella vaccination
methicillin-resistant staph aureus = MRSA	**MRSA** = methicillin-resistant staph aureus
severe combined immunodeficiency = SCID	**SCID** = severe combined immunodeficiency
varicella = VZV	**VZV** = varicella

CHAPTER 7

LEARNING EXERCISES

Matching Word Parts 1

Write the correct answer in the middle column.

	Definition	Correct Answer	Possible Answers
7.1.	against	____________	anti-
7.2.	eat, swallow	____________	lymphaden/o
7.3.	lymph node	____________	lymphangi/o
7.4.	lymph vessel	____________	phag/o
7.5.	poison	____________	tox/o

Matching Word Parts 2

Write the correct answer in the middle column.

	Definition	Correct Answer	Possible Answers
7.6.	swelling	____________	immun/o
7.7.	to destroy	____________	-cyte
7.8.	protection, safe	____________	-lytic
7.9.	spleen	____________	-edema
7.10.	cell	____________	splen/o

Matching Types of Pathogens

Write the correct answer in the middle column.

	Definition	Correct Answer	Possible Answers
7.11.	bacteria capable of movement	________________	parasites
7.12.	chain-forming bacteria	________________	spirochetes
7.13.	cluster-forming bacteria	________________	staphylococci
7.14.	live only by invading cells	________________	streptococci
7.15.	live within other organisms	________________	viruses

Definitions

Select the correct answer, and write it on the line provided.

7.16. The ________________ has/have a hemolytic function.

appendix   lymph nodes   spleen   tonsils

7.17. The term ________________ means slowing or stopping the growth of bacteria.

bactericidal   bacteriostatic   antibiotic   antimycotic

7.18. The medical term for the condition commonly known as shingles is ________________.

cytomegalovirus   herpes zoster   rubella   varicella

7.19. Proteins that activate the immune system, fight viruses by slowing or stopping their multiplication, and signal other cells to increase their defenses are known as ________________.

T cells   immunoglobulins   interferons   synthetic immunoglobulins

7.20. The ________________ plays specialized roles in both the lymphatic and immune systems.

bone marrow   liver   spleen   thymus

7.21. The protective ring of lymphoid tissue around the back of the nose and upper throat is formed by the ________________.

lacteals   lymph nodes   tonsils   villi

7.22. Secondary ________________ can be caused by cancer treatments, burns, or injuries.

lymphadenitis   lymphangioma   lymphadenopathy   lymphedema

7.23. Fats that cannot be transported by the bloodstream are absorbed by the ________________ that are located in the villi that line the small intestine.

lacteals | lymph nodes | B cells | spleen

7.24. The parasite ________________ is most commonly transmitted from pets to humans by contact with contaminated animal feces.

herpes zoster | malaria | rabies | toxoplasmosis

7.25. A/An ________________ is a type of leukocyte that surrounds and kills invading cells. This type of cell also removes dead cells and stimulates the action of other immune cells.

B lymphocyte | macrophage | platelet | T lymphocyte

Matching Structures

Write the correct answer in the middle column.

	Definition	Correct Answer	Possible Answers
7.26.	filter harmful substances from lymph	________________	complement system
7.27.	lymphoid tissue hanging from the lower portion of the cecum	________________	intact skin
7.28.	cells combine with antibodies to ward off pathogens	________________	lymph nodes
7.29.	stores extra erythrocytes	________________	spleen
7.30.	wraps the body in a physical barrier	________________	vermiform appendix

Which Word?

Select the correct answer, and write it on the line provided.

7.31. The ________________ act as intracellular signals to begin the immune response.

cytokines | macrophages

7.32. A ________________ drug is a medication that kills or damages cells.

corticosteroid | cytotoxic

7.33. The ______________________ develop from B cells and secrete large bodies of antibodies coded to destroy specific antigens.

interleukins plasma cells

7.34. The antibody therapy known as ______________________ is used to treat multiple sclerosis, hepatitis C, and some cancers.

monoclonal antibodies synthetic interferon

7.35. Infectious mononucleosis is caused by a ______________________.

spirochete virus

Spelling Counts

Find the misspelled word in each sentence. Then write that word, spelled correctly, on the line provided.

7.36. Raybees is an acute viral infection that is transmitted to humans through the bite or saliva of an infected animal. ______________________

7.37. The adanoids, which are also known as the nasopharyngeal tonsils, are located in the nasopharynx. ______________________

7.38. Lymphiscintigraphy is a diagnostic test that is performed to detect damage or malformations of the lymphatic vessels. ______________________

7.39. A bactirecide is a substance that causes the death of bacteria. ______________________

7.40. Varichella is commonly known as chickenpox. ______________________

Abbreviation Identification

In the space provided, write the words that each abbreviation stands for.

7.41. **IG** ______________________

7.42. **SCID** ______________________

7.43. **LE** ______________________

7.44. **MMR** ______________________

7.45. **Ag** ______________________

Term Selection

Select the correct answer, and write it on the line provided.

7.46. ______________ immunity is the state of being resistant to a specific disease obtained by having had a contagious disease.

Passive | Acquired | Natural | Partial

7.47. An opportunistic infection that is frequently associated with HIV is ______________.

COVID-19 | Kaposi's sarcoma | myasthenia gravis | tinea pedis

7.48. Malaria is caused by a ______________ that is transferred to humans by the bite of an infected mosquito.

parasite | rickettsia | spirochete | virus

7.49. Bacilli, which are rod-shaped, spore-forming bacteria, cause ______________.

Lyme disease | measles | rubella | anthrax

7.50. Swelling of the parotid glands is a symptom of ______________.

measles | mumps | shingles | rubella

Sentence Completion

Write the correct term on the line provided.

7.51. A severe systemic reaction to an allergen causing serious symptoms that develop very quickly is known as ______________.

7.52. A ______________ is a physician who specializes in diagnosing and treating disorders of the lymphatic system.

7.53. An HIV differentiation assay is used for confirmation if a/an ______________ test, which stands for enzyme-linked immunosorbent assay, is positive.

7.54. A/An ______________ is a benign tumor formed by an abnormal collection of lymphatic vessels.

7.55. An ______________ specializes in diagnosing and treating disorders of the immune system.

Word Surgery

Divide each term into its component word parts. Write these word parts, in sequence, on the lines provided. When necessary, use a slash (/) to indicate a combining vowel. (You may not need all of the lines provided.)

7.56. **Lymphocytes** are leukocytes that are formed in bone marrow as stem cells.

________ ________ ________ ________

7.57. An **antibiotic** is a medication capable of inhibiting growth or killing pathogenic bacterial microorganisms.

________ ________ ________ ________

7.58. A **lymphangioma** is a benign tumor formed by an abnormal collection of lymphatic vessels.

________ ________ ________ ________

7.59. **Cytomegalovirus** is a member of the *herpesvirus* family that causes a variety of diseases.

________ ________ ________ ________

7.60. The spleen has the **hemolytic** function of destroying worn-out erythrocytes and releasing their hemoglobin for reuse.

________ ________ ________ ________

True/False

If the statement is true, write **True** on the line. If the statement is false, write **False** on the line.

7.61. ________ An antigen is any substance that the body regards as being foreign.

7.62. ________ Lymph carries nutrients and oxygen to the cells.

7.63. ________ Phagocytes are a group of proteins that circulate in the blood in inactive form.

7.64. ________ Roseola is characterized by a high fever followed by a rash.

7.65. ________ Ebola is a common disease transmitted by parasites.

Clinical Conditions

Write the correct answer on the line provided.

7.66. Dr. Wei diagnosed her patient as having an enlarged spleen due to damage caused by his injuries. The medical term for this condition is ________________.

7.67. The newborn screening for Juanita Phillips's baby showed that the infant has ________________. This is an inherited condition in which abnormalities in the immune system cause an increased susceptibility to infection and failure to thrive as a result of infections.

7.68. Mr. Grossman described his serious illness as being caused by a "superbug infection." His doctor describes these bacteria as being ________________.

7.69. Dorothy Peterson was diagnosed with a ________________ after her car accident. This is a medical emergency that occurs when the covering of the spleen is torn, usually as the result of a blow to the abdomen.

7.70. Every day since his kidney transplant, Mr. Lanning must take a/an ________________ to prevent rejection of the donor organ.

7.71. Rosita Sanchez is 2 months pregnant, and she and her doctor are worried because her rash was diagnosed as ________________. They are concerned because this condition can produce defects in Rosita's developing child.

7.72. Tarana Inglis took ________________ to relieve the symptoms of her allergies.

7.73. The ________________ virus is spread to humans through the bite of an infected mosquito. The more severe variety spreads to the spinal cord and brain.

7.74. John Fogelman was diagnosed with having lymphedema after undergoing ________________. This is a noninvasive method of diagnosing lymphedema by passing an electrical current through the affected limb.

7.75. Jane Bell is infected with HIV. Her doctor prescribed her a/an ________________ drug used to treat viral infections or to provide temporary immunity.

Which Is the Correct Medical Term?

Select the correct answer, and write it on the line provided.

7.76. The ____________ are specialized lymphocytes that produce antibodies. Each lymphocyte makes a specific antibody that is capable of destroying a specific antigen.

B cells bacilli immunoglobulins T cells

7.77. Any of a large group of diseases characterized by a condition in which the immune system produces antibodies against its own tissues is known as a/an ______________ disorder.

autoimmune allergy rubella immunodeficiency

7.78. The ______________ lymph nodes are located in the groin.

axillary cervical inguinal subcutaneous

7.79. ______________ is a highly contagious viral infection caused by the SARS-CoV-2 virus.

COVID-19 Zika Toxoplasmosis AIDS

7.80. A/An ______________ drug is used either as an immunosuppressant or as an antineoplastic.

corticosteroid cytotoxic immunoglobulin monoclonal

Challenge Word Building

These terms are *not* primary terms in the chapter; however, they are made up of the following familiar word parts. If you need help in creating the term, refer to your medical dictionary.

adenoid/o	**-ectomy**
immun/o	**-ic**
lymphaden/o	**-itis**
lymphangi/o	**-ology**
splen/o	**-oma**
tox/o	**-rrhaphy**
thym/o	

7.81. The study of the immune system is known as ______________________________.

7.82. Surgical removal of the spleen is a/an ______________________________.

7.83. Inflammation of the thymus is known as ______________________________.

7.84. Inflammation of the lymph vessels is known as ______________________________.

7.85. The term meaning to suture the spleen is ______________________________.

7.86. The surgical removal of the adenoids is a/an ______________________________.

7.87. The surgical removal of a lymph node is a/an ______________________________.

7.88. A tumor originating in the thymus is known as ______________________.

7.89. Another word for poisonous is ______________________.

7.90. Inflammation of the spleen is known as ______________________.

Labeling Exercises

Identify the numbered items on the accompanying figures.

7.91. tonsils and ______________________

7.92. Lymphocytes are formed in bone ______________________.

7.93. large intestine and ______________________

7.94. ______________________

7.95. ______________________

7.96. ______________________ lymph nodes

7.97. Right ______________________ empties into the right subclavian vein.

7.98. ______________________ duct

7.99. ______________________ lymph nodes

7.100. ______________________ lymph nodes

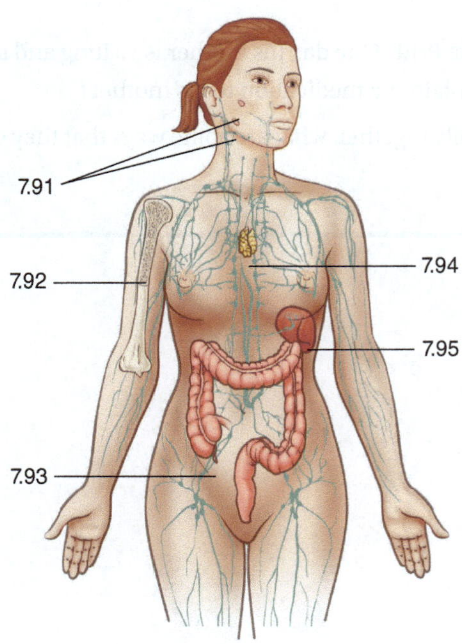

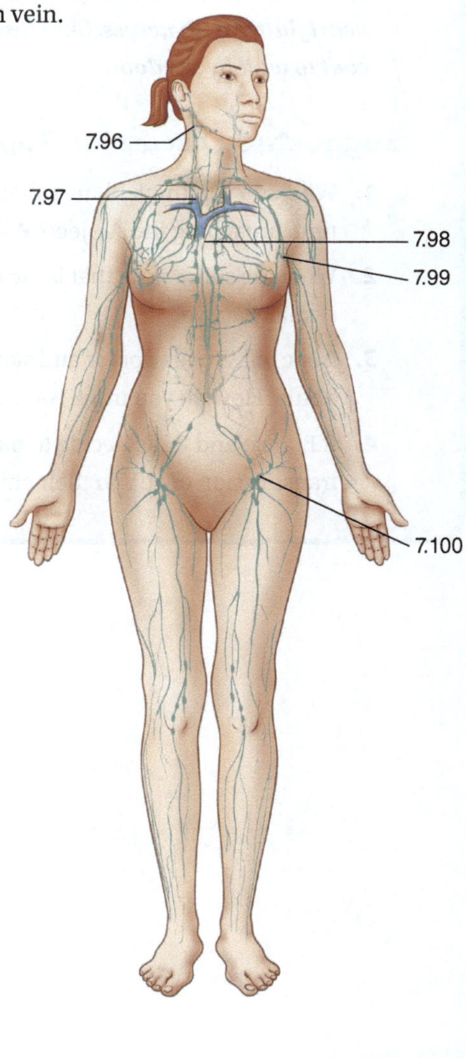

The Human Touch

CRITICAL THINKING EXERCISE

The following story and questions are designed to stimulate critical thinking through class discussion or as a brief essay response. There are no right or wrong answers to these questions.

Blanca Cortez applies her lipstick and smiles into the mirror. She's got a second date tonight with a friend's cousin who just moved to town. Isaac is everything she's been looking for in a partner: taller than her, with a sarcastic personality and great taste in music. She's excited but also nervous about where the relationship could go. Blanca has perinatally acquired HIV and when she disclosed her status to her last boyfriend prior to being sexually active he turned into a different person. She would be crushed if the same thing happened with Isaac.

It's hard for Blanca to be vulnerable with new people, maybe in part because she was adopted as a young child and has had trust issues. She has worked hard to overcome these feelings in therapy but sometimes her depression and anxiety have become too much to bear, causing her to become non-adherent to her ART medications.

She checks her phone, sees that Isaac has texted that he's on his way to pick her up, and feels her heart flutter with nerves. She closes her eyes, takes several cleansing breaths, then zips up her coat to wait by the door.

Suggested Discussion Topics

1. When do you think Blanca should disclose her HIV status to Isaac? Why might she have a hard time broaching the subject? What would the consequences be if she decided not to tell him?
2. What are some ways that Isaac can protect himself from acquiring HIV if he and Blanca become sexually active?
3. Isaac talks to his doctor and starts to take PrEP. One day his mother is visiting and sees the pill bottle. How do you think Isaac could explain the medication to his mother?
4. If Blanca and Isaac decide to have a family together, what are some ways that they can prevent transmission of HIV to their child?

CHAPTER 8

THE RESPIRATORY SYSTEM

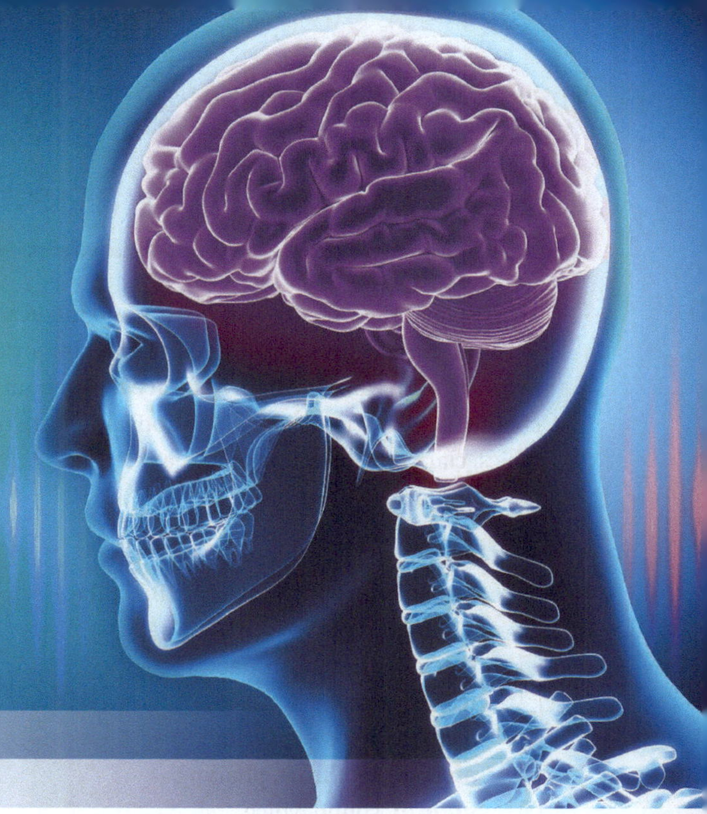

Overview of

STRUCTURES, COMBINING FORMS, AND FUNCTIONS OF THE RESPIRATORY SYSTEM

Major Structures	Related Combining Forms	Primary Functions
Nose	nas/o	Exchanges air during inhaling and exhaling; warms, moisturizes, and filters inhaled air.
Sinuses	sinus/o	Produce mucus for the nasal cavities, make bones of the skull lighter, aid in sound production.
Pharynx	pharyng/o	Transports air back and forth between the nose and the trachea.
Larynx	laryng/o	Makes speech possible.
Epiglottis	epiglott/o	Closes off the trachea during swallowing.
Trachea	trache/o	Transports air back and forth between the pharynx and the bronchi.
Bronchi	bronch/o, bronchi/o	Transports air from the trachea into the lungs.
Alveoli	alveol/o	Air sacs that exchange gases with the pulmonary capillary blood.
Lungs	pneum/o, pneumon/o, pulmon/o	Bring oxygen into the body, and remove carbon dioxide and some water waste from the body.

Vocabulary Related to **THE RESPIRATORY SYSTEM**

This list contains essential word parts and medical terms for this chapter. These and the other important **primary terms** are shown in **boldface** throughout the chapter. *Secondary terms*, which appear in *orange* italics, clarify the meaning of primary terms.

Word Parts

- ☐ **bronch/o**, **bronchi/o** bronchial tube, bronchus
- ☐ **laryng/o** larynx, throat
- ☐ **nas/o** nose
- ☐ **ox/i**, **ox/o**, **ox/y** oxygen
- ☐ **pharyng/o** throat, pharynx
- ☐ **phon/o** sound, voice
- ☐ **pleur/o** pleura, side of the body
- ☐ **-pnea** breathing
- ☐ **pneum/o**, **pneumon/o** lung, air
- ☐ **pulm/o**, **pulmon/o** lung
- ☐ **sinus/o** sinus
- ☐ **somn/o** sleep
- ☐ **spir/o** to breathe
- ☐ **thorac/o**, **-thorax** chest, pleural cavity
- ☐ **trache/o** windpipe, trachea

Medical Terms

- ☐ **anoxia** (ah-**NOCK**-see-ah)
- ☐ **antitussive** (**an**-tih-**TUSS**-iv)
- ☐ **aphonia** (ah-**FOH**-nee-ah)
- ☐ **asbestosis** (**ass**-beh-**STOH**-sis)
- ☐ **asphyxia** (ass-**FICK**-see-ah)
- ☐ **asthma** (**AZ**-mah)
- ☐ **atelectasis** (**at**-ee-**LEK**-tah-sis)
- ☐ **bradypnea** (**brad**-ihp-**NEE**-ah)
- ☐ **bronchiectasis** (**brong**-kee-**ECK**-tah-sis)
- ☐ **bronchodilator** (**brong**-koh-**DYE**-lay-tor)
- ☐ **bronchorrhea** (**brong**-koh-**REE**-ah)
- ☐ **bronchoscopy** (brong-**KOS**-koh-pee)
- ☐ **bronchospasm** (**BRONG**-koh-spazm)
- ☐ **Cheyne–Stokes respiration** (**CHAYN STOHKS**)
- ☐ **chronic obstructive pulmonary disease**
- ☐ **croup** (**KROOP**)
- ☐ **cyanosis** (**sigh**-ah-**NOH**-sis)
- ☐ **cystic fibrosis** (**SIS**-tick figh-**BROH**-sis)
- ☐ **dysphonia** (dis-**FOH**-nee-ah)
- ☐ **dyspnea** (**DISP**-nee-ah)
- ☐ **emphysema** (**em**-fih-**SEE**-mah)
- ☐ **empyema** (**em**-pye-**EE**-mah)
- ☐ **endotracheal intubation** (**en**-doh-**TRAY**-kee-al **in**-too-**BAY**-shun)
- ☐ **epistaxis** (**ep**-ih-**STACK**-sis)
- ☐ **hemoptysis** (hee-**MOP**-tih-sis)
- ☐ **hemothorax** (**hee**-moh-**THOH**-racks)
- ☐ **hypercapnia** (**high**-per-**KAP**-nee-ah)
- ☐ **hyperpnea** (**high**-perp-**NEE**-ah)
- ☐ **hypopnea** (**high**-poh-**NEE**-ah)
- ☐ **hypoxemia** (**high**-pock-**SEE**-mee-ah)
- ☐ **hypoxia** (high-**POCK**-see-ah)
- ☐ **laryngitis** (**lar**-in-**JIGH**-tis)
- ☐ **laryngoscopy** (**lar**-ing-**GOS**-koh-pee)
- ☐ **laryngospasm** (lah-**RING**-goh-spazm)
- ☐ **mediastinum** (**mee**-dee-as-**TYE**-num)
- ☐ **nebulizer** (**NEB**-you-lye-zer)
- ☐ **otolaryngologist** (**oh**-toh-**lar**-in-**GOL**-oh-jist)
- ☐ **pertussis** (per-**TUS**-is)
- ☐ **pharyngitis** (fah-rin-**JIGH**-tis)
- ☐ **pleural effusion** (eh-**FEW**-zhun)
- ☐ **pleurisy** (**PLOOR**-ih-see)
- ☐ **pleurodynia** (**ploor**-oh-**DIN**-ee-ah)
- ☐ **pneumoconiosis** (**new**-moh-**koh**-nee-**OH**-sis)
- ☐ **pneumonectomy** (**new**-moh-**NECK**-toh-mee)
- ☐ **pneumonia** (new-**MOH**-nee-ah)
- ☐ **pneumothorax** (**new**-moh-**THOH**-racks)
- ☐ **polysomnography** (**pol**-ee-som-**NOG**-rah-fee)
- ☐ **pulmonary edema** (eh-**DEE**-mah)
- ☐ **pulmonologist** (**pull**-mah-**NOL**-oh-jist)
- ☐ **pulse oximeter** (ock-**SIM**-eh-ter)
- ☐ **pyothorax** (**pye**-oh-**THOH**-racks)
- ☐ **sinusitis** (**sigh**-nuh-**SIGH**-tis)
- ☐ **sleep apnea** (**AP**-nee-ah)
- ☐ **spirometer** (spih-**ROM**-eh-ter)
- ☐ **tachypnea** (**tack**-ihp-**NEE**-ah)
- ☐ **thoracentesis** (**thoh**-rah-sen-**TEE**-sis)
- ☐ **thoracotomy** (**thoh**-rah-**KOT**-oh-mee)
- ☐ **tracheostomy** (**tray**-kee-**OS**-toh-mee)
- ☐ **tracheotomy** (**tray**-kee-**OT**-oh-mee)
- ☐ **tuberculosis** (too-**ber**-kew-**LOH**-sis)

LEARNING OBJECTIVES

On completion of this chapter, you should be able to:

1. Describe the major functions and structures of the respiratory system.
2. Differentiate between external respiration and internal respiration.
3. Identify the medical specialists who treat disorders of the respiratory system.
4. Identify medical word parts of the respiratory system.
5. Define the primary terms related to the pathology and the diagnostic and treatment procedures of the respiratory system.
6. Spell the primary terms of the respiratory system.
7. Pronounce the primary terms of the respiratory system.
8. Identify common abbreviations related to the respiratory system.

FUNCTIONS OF THE RESPIRATORY SYSTEM

The functions of the respiratory system are to:

- Deliver air to the lungs.
- Convey oxygen from the inhaled air to the blood for delivery to the body cells.
- Expel the waste products (carbon dioxide and a small amount of water) returned to the lungs by the blood through exhalation.
- Produce the airflow through the larynx that makes speech possible.

The **respiratory system** supplies the blood with oxygen for transportation to the cells in all parts of the body (Figure 8.1). Oxygen is vital to the survival and function of these cells. The respiratory system also removes carbon dioxide and some water waste from the body.

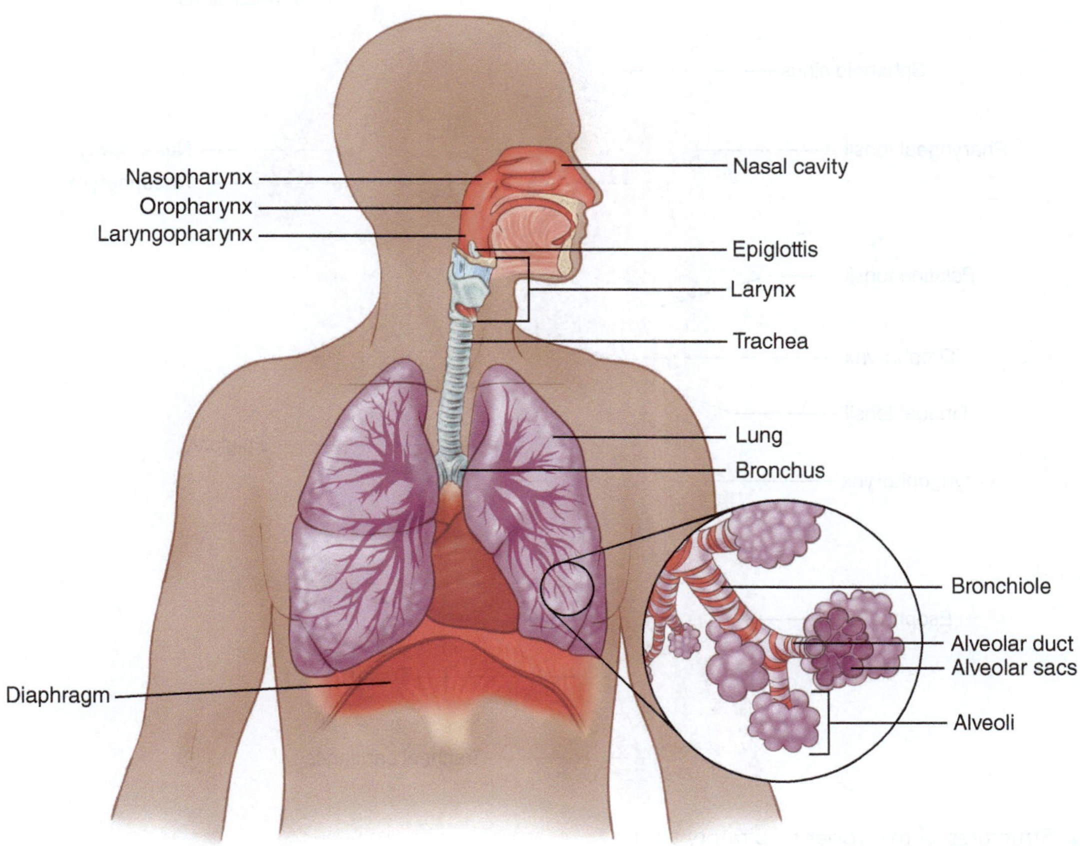

FIGURE 8.1 Structures of the respiratory system.

STRUCTURES OF THE RESPIRATORY SYSTEM

For descriptive purposes, the respiratory system is divided into upper and lower respiratory tracts (Figures 8.1 and 8.2).

- The **upper respiratory tract** consists of the nose (nostrils), mouth, pharynx, epiglottis, larynx, and trachea (Figure 8.2).
- The **lower respiratory tract** consists of the bronchial tree and lungs. These structures are located within and protected by the **thoracic cavity** (thoh-**RAS**-ick), or **thorax**, also known as the ***rib cage***.
- The upper respiratory tract and the bronchial tree of the lower respiratory tract are sometimes referred to as the ***airway***.

The Nose

Air enters the body through the **nose** and passes through the ***nasal cavity***, which is the interior portion of the nose. The ***nostrils*** are the external openings of the nose.

- The **nasal septum** (**NAY**-zal **SEP**-tum) is a wall of cartilage that divides the nose into two equal sections. A ***septum*** is a wall that separates two chambers.
- **Cilia** (**SIL**-ee-ah), the thin hairs located just inside the nostrils, filter incoming air to remove debris.
- **Mucous membranes** (**MYOU**-kus) line the nose. These specialized tissues also line the digestive, reproductive, and urinary systems as well as other parts of the respiratory system.
- **Mucus** (**MYOU**-kus) is a slippery secretion produced by the mucous membranes that protects and lubricates these tissues. In the nose, mucus helps moisten, warm, and filter the air as it enters. Notice that *mucous* and *mucus* have different spellings; however, they share the same pronunciation. Mucous is the name of the tissue (which comes first, both anatomically and alphabetically); mucus is the secretion that flows from the tissue.
- The **olfactory receptors** (ol-**FACK**-toh-ree) are nerve endings that act as the receptors for the sense of smell. They are also important to the sense of taste. These receptors are located in the mucous membrane in the upper part of the nasal cavity.

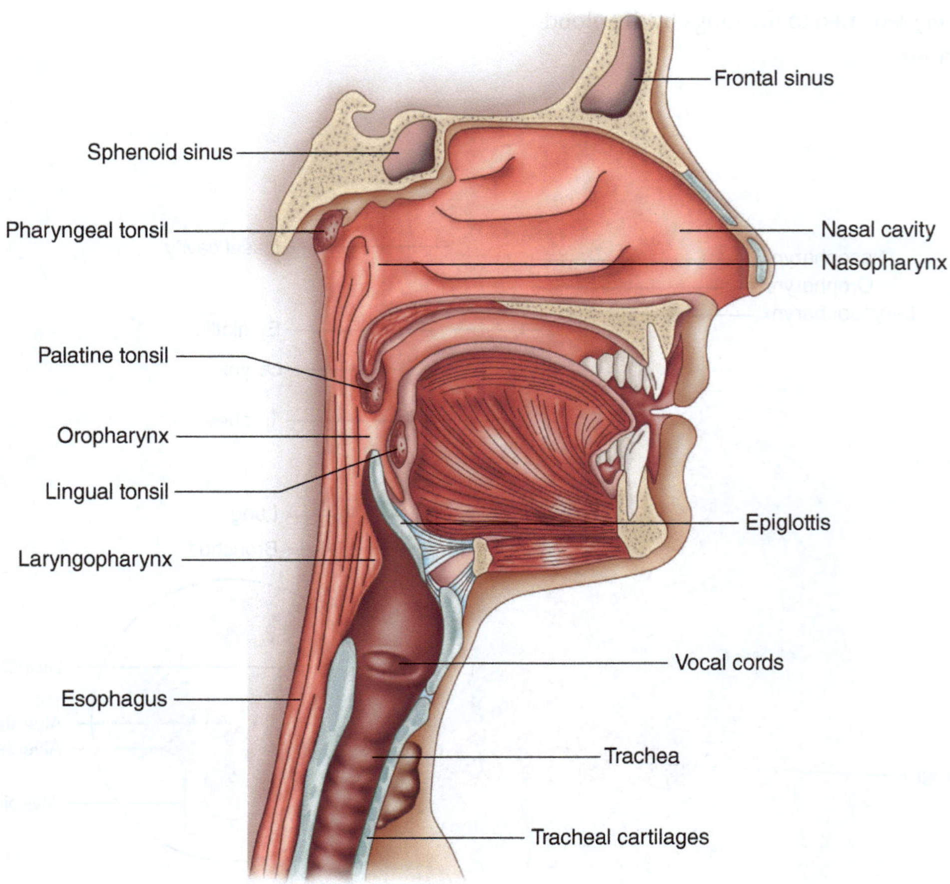

FIGURE 8.2 Structures of the upper respiratory tract.

The Tonsils

The **tonsils** and **adenoids** are part of the lymphatic system described in Chapter 7. They help protect the body from infection coming through the nose or the mouth. The tonsils, also called the ***palatine tonsils***, are located at the back of the mouth. The adenoids, also called the ***nasopharyngeal tonsils***, are higher up, behind the nose and the roof of the mouth.

The Paranasal Sinuses

The **paranasal sinuses**, which are air-filled cavities lined with mucous membrane, are located in the bones of the skull (**para-** means near, **nas** means nose, and **-al** means pertaining to). A ***sinus*** can be a sac or cavity in any organ or tissue; however, the term *sinus* most commonly refers to the paranasal sinuses.

The functions of these sinuses are (1) to make the bones of the skull lighter, (2) to help produce sound by giving resonance to the voice, and (3) to produce mucus to provide lubrication for the tissues of the nasal cavity. The sinuses are connected to the nasal cavity via short ducts. The four pairs of paranasal sinuses are located on either side of the nose and are named for the bones in which they are located.

- The **frontal sinuses** are located in the frontal bone just above the eyebrows. An infection here can cause severe pain in this area.
- The **sphenoid sinuses**, which are located in the sphenoid bone behind the eye and under the pituitary gland, are close to the optic nerves, and an infection here can damage vision.
- The **maxillary sinuses**, which are the largest of the paranasal sinuses, are located in the maxillary bones under the eyes. An infection in these sinuses can cause pain in the posterior maxillary teeth.
- The **ethmoid sinuses**, which are located in the ethmoid bones between the nose and the eyes, are irregularly shaped air cells that are separated from the orbital (eye) cavity by only a thin layer of bone.

The Pharynx

The **pharynx** (**FAR**-inks), which is commonly known as the ***throat***, receives the air after it passes through the nose or mouth, as well as food. Its role in the digestive system is discussed in Chapter 9.

The pharynx is made up of three divisions (Figure 8.2):

- The **nasopharynx** (**nay**-zoh-**FAR**-inks) is posterior to the nasal cavity and continues downward to behind the mouth (**nas/o** means nose, and **-pharynx** means throat). This portion of the pharynx is used only by the respiratory system for the transport of air and opens into the oropharynx.
- The **oropharynx** (**oh**-roh-**FAR**-inks) is the portion that is visible when looking into the mouth (**or/o** means mouth, and **-pharynx** means throat). The oropharynx is shared by the respiratory and digestive systems and transports air, food, and fluids downward to the laryngopharynx.
- The **laryngopharynx** (lah-**ring**-goh-**FAR**-inks) is also shared by both the respiratory and digestive systems (**laryng/o** means larynx, and **-pharynx** means throat). Air, food, and fluids continue downward to the openings of the esophagus and trachea where air enters the trachea and food and fluids flow into the esophagus. See the section "Protective Swallowing Mechanisms."

Larynx

The **larynx** (**LAR**-inks), also known as the ***voice box***, is a triangular chamber located between the pharynx and the trachea (Figure 8.3).

- The larynx is protected and supported by a series of nine separate cartilages. The ***thyroid cartilage*** is the largest, and when enlarged it projects from the front of the throat and is commonly known as the ***Adam's apple***.
- The larynx contains the ***vocal cords***. During breathing, the cords are separated to let air pass. During speech, they close together, and sound is produced as air is expelled from the lungs, causing the cords to vibrate against each other.

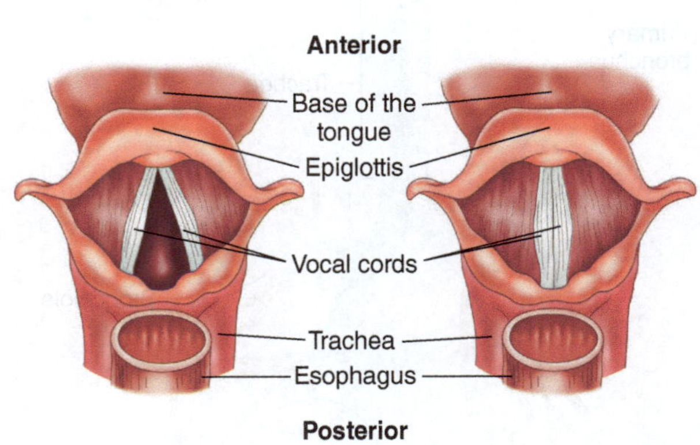

FIGURE 8.3 View of the larynx and vocal cords from above. Shown on the left, the vocal cords are open during breathing. On the right, the vocal cords vibrate together during speech.

Protective Swallowing Mechanisms

The respiratory and digestive systems share part of the pharynx. During swallowing, there is the risk of a blocked airway or aspiration pneumonia caused by food or water going into the trachea and entering the lungs instead of going into the esophagus. Two protective mechanisms act automatically during swallowing to ensure that *only* air goes into the lungs:

- The soft palate, which is the muscular posterior portion of the roof of the mouth, moves up and backward during swallowing to close off the nasopharynx. This prevents food or liquid from going up into the nose. Structures of the mouth are discussed further in Chapter 9.
- At the same time, the **epiglottis** (**ep**-ih-**GLOT**-is), a lid-like structure located at the base of the tongue, swings downward and closes off the laryngopharynx so that food does not enter the trachea and the lungs.

The Trachea

- The role of the **trachea** (**TRAY**-kee-ah) is to transport air to and from the lungs. This tube, which is commonly known as the ***windpipe***, is located directly in front of the esophagus.
- The trachea is held open by a series of flexible C-shaped cartilage rings that make it possible for the trachea to compress so that food can pass down the esophagus (Figure 8.4).

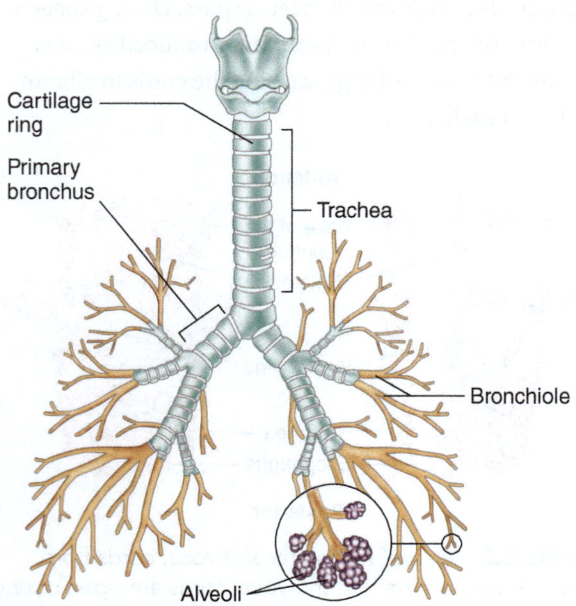

FIGURE 8.4 The trachea, bronchial tree, and alveoli.

The Bronchi

The **bronchi** (**BRONG**-kee) are two large tubes, also known as ***primary bronchi***, which branch out from the trachea and convey air into the two lungs (singular, *bronchus*). Because of the similarity of these structures to an inverted tree, this is referred to as the ***bronchial tree*** (Figures 8.1 and 8.4).

- Within the lung, each primary bronchus divides and subdivides into increasingly smaller **bronchioles** (**BRONG**-kee-ohlz), which are the smallest branches of the bronchi.

The Alveoli

Alveoli (al-**VEE**-oh-lye), also known as ***air sacs***, are very small, grapelike clusters found at the end of each bronchiole (singular, *alveolus*). The alveoli are where the exchange of oxygen and carbon dioxide takes place. Each lung contains millions of alveoli (Figures 8.1 and 8.4).

- During respiration, the alveoli are filled with air from the bronchioles.
- A network of microscopic pulmonary capillaries surrounds the alveoli. **Pulmonary** (**PULL**-mah-**nair**-ee) means relating to or affecting the lungs.
- The exchange of oxygen and carbon dioxide between the air inside the alveoli and the blood in the pulmonary capillaries occurs through the thin, elastic walls of the alveoli.
- The alveoli produce a detergent-like substance, known as a ***surfactant***, which reduces the surface tension of the fluid in the lungs. This makes the alveoli more stable so they do not collapse when an individual exhales. Premature babies often lack adequate surfactant.

The Lungs

The **lungs**, which are the essential organs of respiration, are divided into lobes (Figure 8.5). A ***lobe*** is a subdivision or part of an organ.

- The **right lung** is larger and has three lobes: the upper, middle, and lower (or superior, middle, and inferior).
- The **left lung** has only two lobes, the upper and lower, due to space restrictions because the heart is located on that side of the body.

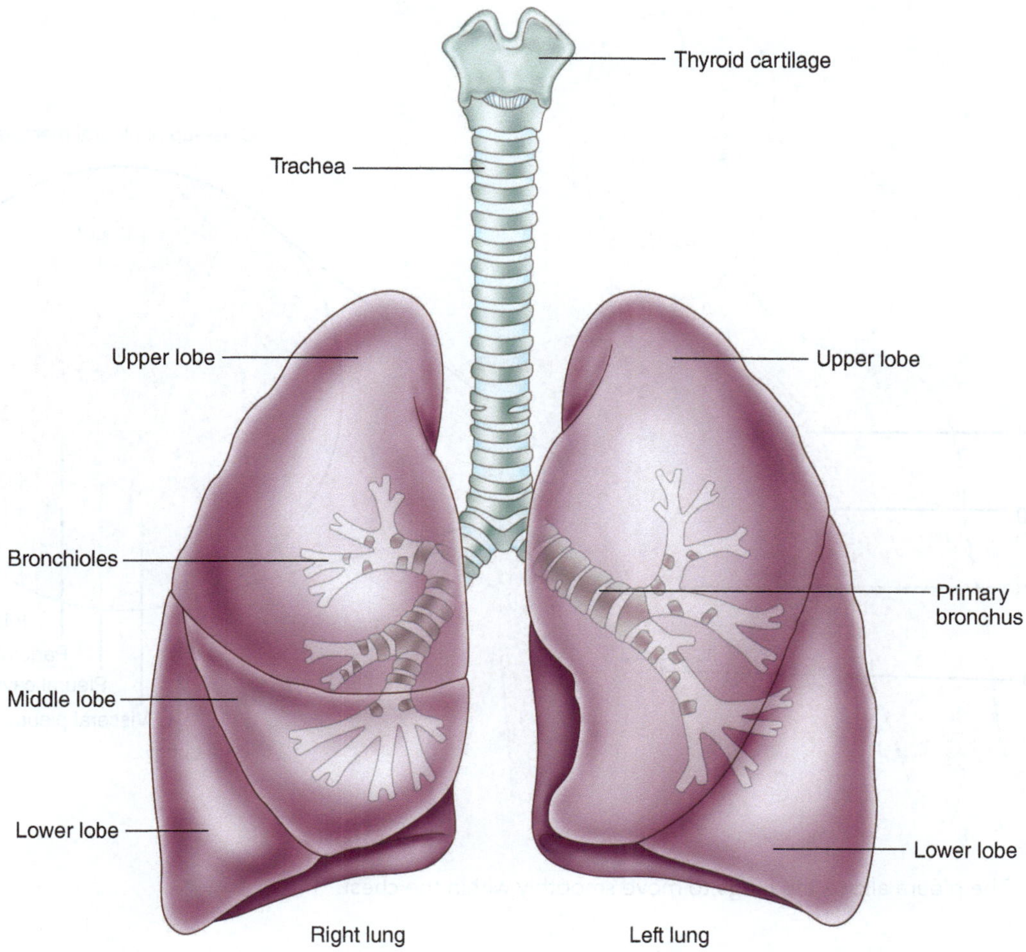

FIGURE 8.5 External view of the lungs. Note the three lobes of the right lung and the two lobes of the left lung.

The Mediastinum

The **mediastinum** (**mee**-dee-as-**TYE**-num) is the middle section of the chest cavity and is located between the lungs. This cavity contains connective tissue and organs, including the heart and its veins and arteries, the esophagus, trachea, bronchi, thymus gland, and lymph nodes (Figure 8.6).

The Pleura

The **pleura** (**PLOOR**-ah) is a thin, moist, and slippery membrane that covers the outer surface of the lungs and lines the inner surface of the thoracic cavity (Figure 8.6).

- The **parietal pleura** (pah-**RYE**-eh-tal) is the outer layer of the pleura. It lines the walls of the thoracic cavity, covers the diaphragm, and forms the sac containing each lung. The parietal pleura is attached to the chest wall. ***Parietal*** means relating to the walls of a cavity.
- The **visceral pleura** (**VIS**-er-al), which is the inner layer of pleura that covers each lung, is attached directly to the lungs. ***Visceral*** means relating to the internal organs.
- The **pleural cavity**, also known as the ***pleural space***, is the thin, fluid-filled space between the parietal and visceral pleural membranes. The fluid acts as a lubricant, allowing the membranes to slide easily over each other during respiration.

The Diaphragm

The **diaphragm** (**DYE**-ah-fram), also known as the ***thoracic diaphragm***, is a dome-shaped sheet of muscle that separates the thoracic cavity from the abdomen. It is the contraction and relaxation of this muscle that makes breathing possible.

- The **phrenic nerves** (**FREN**-ick) stimulate the diaphragm and cause it to contract (Figure 8.7).
- *Note:* The word *diaphragm* refers to a dividing structure, so the term is also used to describe a contraceptive device that separates the vagina from the cervix.

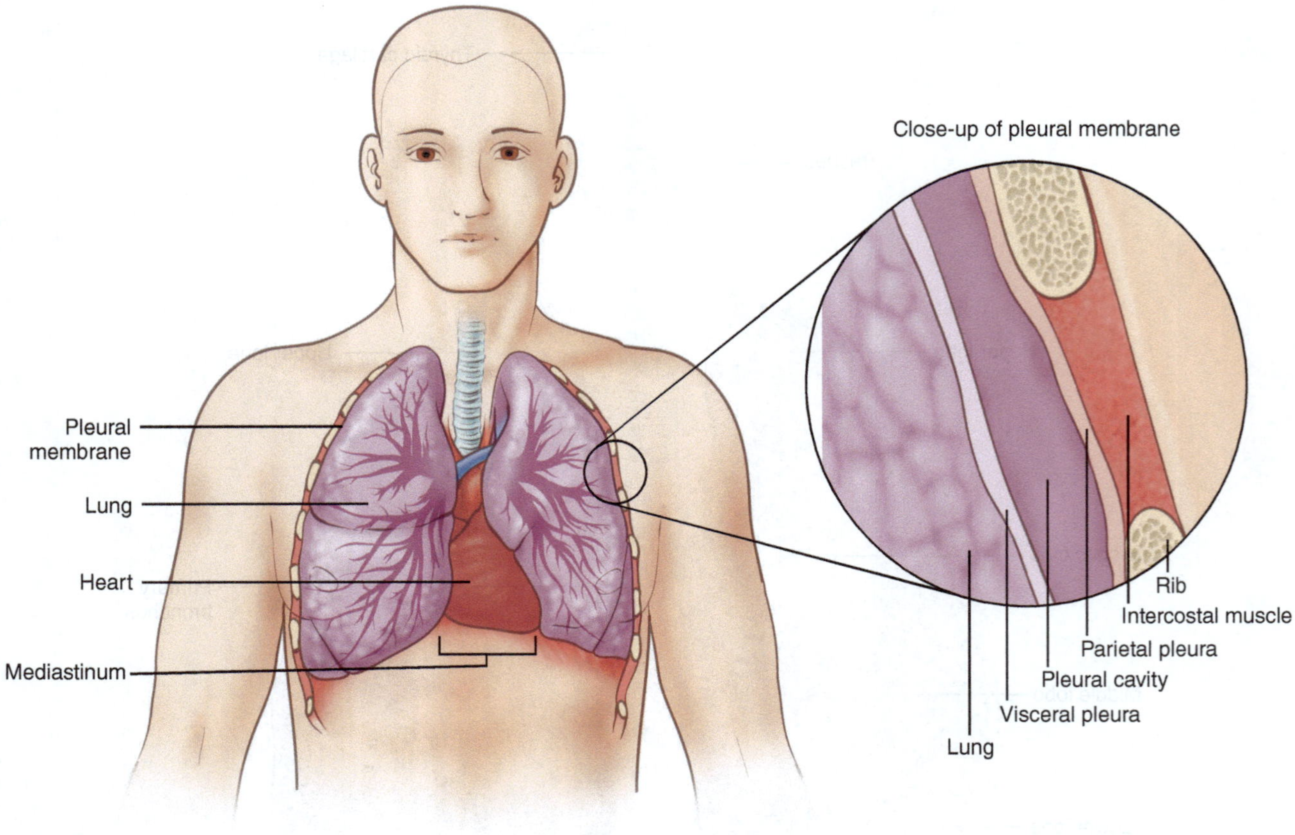

FIGURE 8.6 The pleura allows the lungs to move smoothly within the chest.

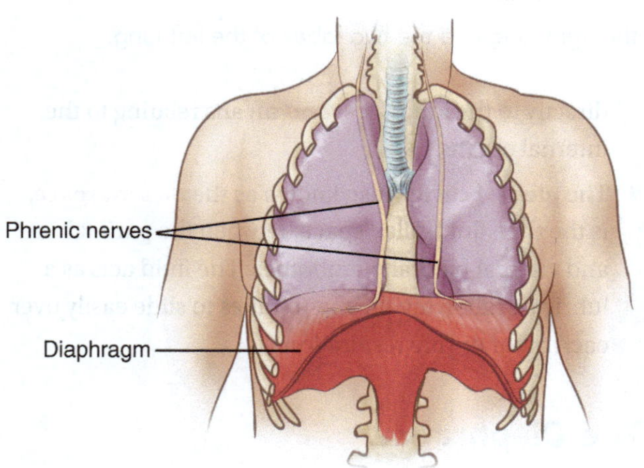

FIGURE 8.7 The diaphragm is controlled by the phrenic nerves.

RESPIRATION

Respiration, or breathing, is the exchange of oxygen for carbon dioxide that is essential to life. A single respiration, or ***breath***, consists of one inhalation and one exhalation (Figure 8.8). ***Ventilation*** is another word for moving air into and out of the lungs.

Inhalation and Exhalation

Inhalation (**in**-hah-**LAY**-shun) is the act of taking in air as the diaphragm contracts and pulls downward (Figure 8.8 left). This action causes the thoracic cavity to expand. This creates negative pressure within the thoracic cavity that draws air into the lungs.

Exhalation (**ecks**-hah-**LAY**-shun) is the act of breathing out. As the diaphragm relaxes, it moves upward, causing the thoracic cavity to become narrower. This action creates positive pressure, forcing air out of the lungs (Figure 8.8 right).

External Respiration

External respiration is the act of bringing air into and out of the lungs from the outside environment and, in the process, exchanging oxygen for carbon dioxide (Figure 8.9).

- As air is ***inhaled*** into the alveoli, oxygen immediately passes into the surrounding capillaries and is carried by the erythrocytes (red blood cells) to all body cells.
- At the same time, the waste product carbon dioxide that has passed into the bloodstream is transported into the air spaces of the lungs to be ***exhaled***.

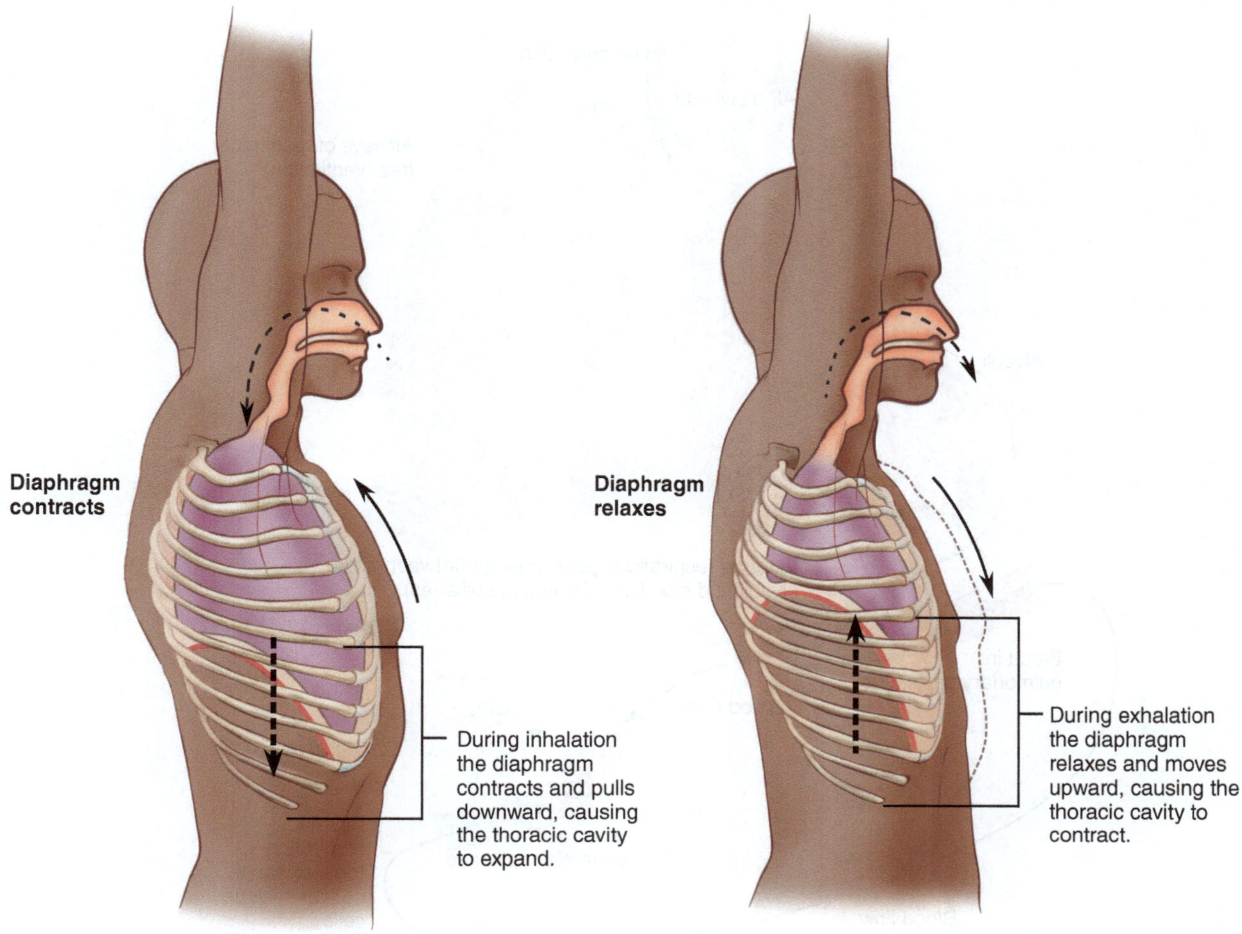

FIGURE 8.8 Movements of the diaphragm and thoracic cavity produce inhalation (left) and exhalation (right).

Internal Respiration

Internal respiration, also known as ***cellular respiration***, is the exchange of gases within the cells of the blood and tissues (Figure 8.9).

- In this process, oxygen passes from the bloodstream into the cells.
- The cells give off the waste product carbon dioxide, which passes into the bloodstream.
- The bloodstream transports the carbon dioxide to the lungs, where it is expelled during exhalation.

MEDICAL SPECIALTIES RELATED TO THE RESPIRATORY SYSTEM

- An **otolaryngologist** (**oh**-toh-**lar**-in-**GOL**-oh-jist), also known as an **ENT** (**E**ar, **N**ose, and **T**hroat), is a physician with specialized training in the diagnosis and treatment of diseases and disorders of the head and neck (**ot/o** means ear, **laryng** means larynx, and **-ologist** means specialist).
- A **pulmonologist** (**pull**-mah-**NOL**-oh-jist) is a physician who specializes in diagnosing and treating diseases and disorders of the respiratory system (**pulmon** means lung, and **-ologist** means specialist).
- A **respiratory therapist** (RT) is a licensed medical professional who specializes in treating patients who are having difficulty breathing, both in hospital and outpatient settings.
- A **thoracic surgeon** performs operations on the organs inside the thorax, or chest, including the heart, lungs, and esophagus.

PATHOLOGY OF THE RESPIRATORY SYSTEM

Chronic Obstructive Pulmonary Disease

Chronic obstructive pulmonary disease (COPD) is a group of lung diseases in which the bronchial airflow is obstructed, making it difficult to breathe out. COPD, which is most often caused by long-term smoking, is

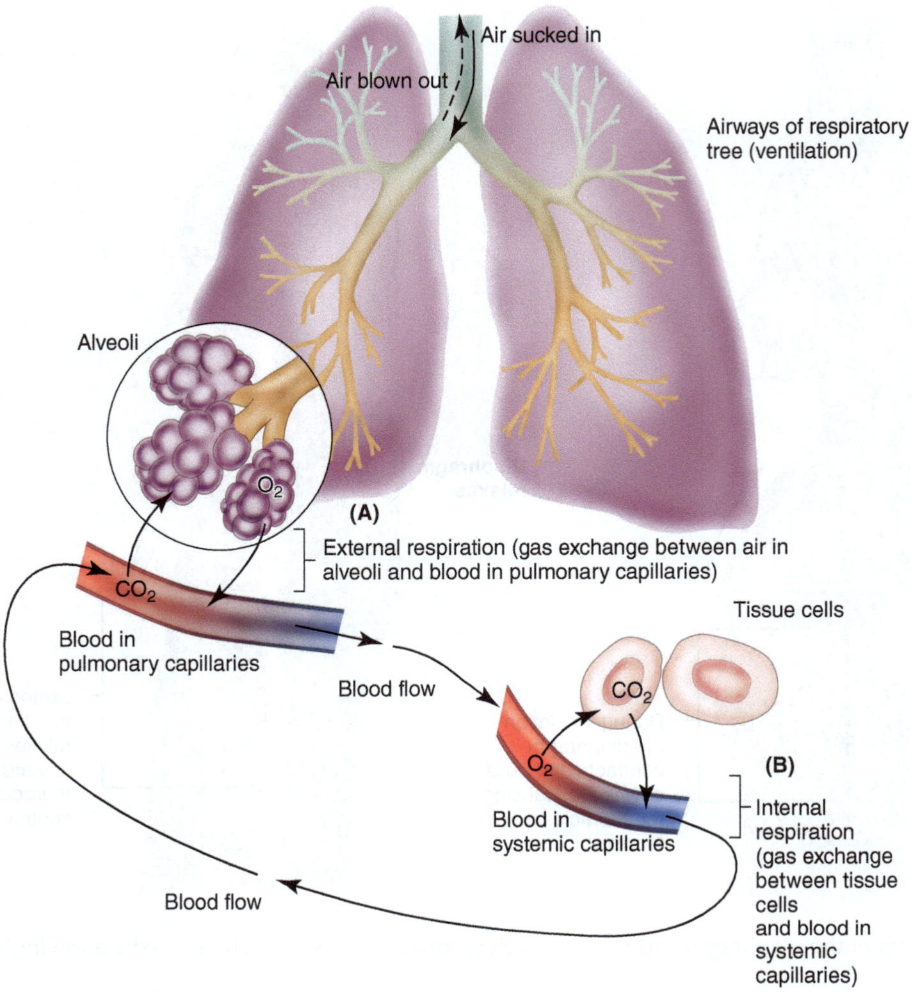

FIGURE 8.9 External and internal respiration compared. (A) External respiration occurs in the lungs. (B) Internal respiration occurs at the cellular level within the blood and tissues.

generally permanent and progressive. Most people with COPD suffer from two related conditions: chronic bronchitis and emphysema.

Chronic Bronchitis

Chronic bronchitis (brong-**KYE**-tis) is a disease in which the airways have become inflamed due to recurrent exposure to an inhaled irritant, usually cigarette smoke (**bronch** means bronchus, and **-itis** means inflammation). An increase in the number and size of mucus-producing cells results in excessive mucus production and thickening of the walls of the air passages. This causes chronic coughing, difficulty getting air into and out of the lungs, and increased risk of bacterial lung infections.

Emphysema

Emphysema (**em**-fih-**SEE**-mah) is the progressive, long-term loss of lung function, usually due to smoking. Emphysema is characterized by a decrease in the total number of alveoli, the enlargement of the remaining alveoli, and the progressive destruction of the walls of these remaining alveoli.

As the alveoli are destroyed, breathing becomes increasingly rapid, shallow, and difficult. In an effort to compensate for the loss of capacity, the lungs chronically overinflate, and the rib cage stays partially expanded all the time, resulting in a slightly rounded shape called a ***barrel chest*** (Figure 8.10).

Asthma

Asthma (**AZ**-mah) is a chronic inflammatory disease of the bronchial tubes, often triggered by an allergic reaction. An ***asthma attack*** is characterized by episodes of severe breathing difficulty, coughing, and wheezing.

Wheezing is a breath sound caused by a partially obstructed airway. The frequency and severity of

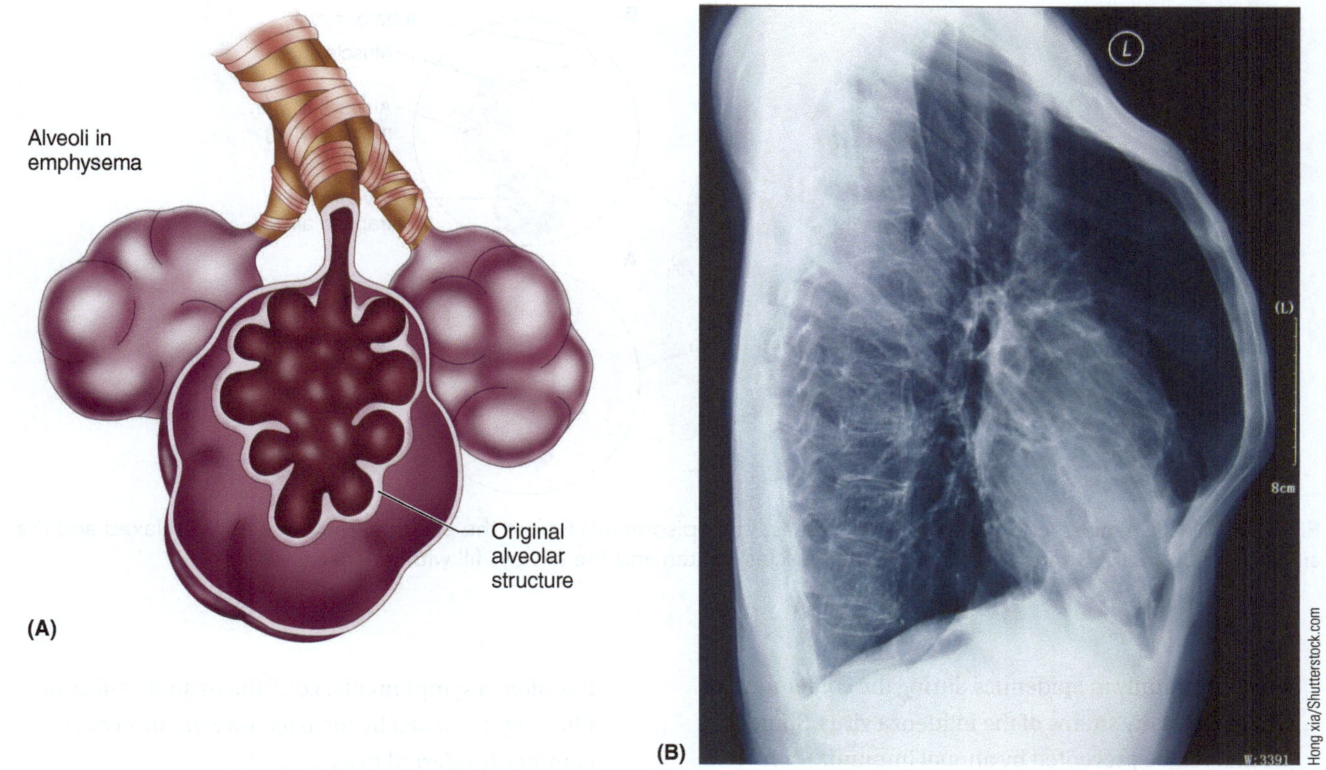

FIGURE 8.10 Emphysema. (A) Changes in the alveoli as the disease progresses. (B) Lateral x-ray showing lung enlargement and abnormal barrel chest in emphysema.

asthma attacks are influenced by a variety of factors, including allergens, environmental agents, exercise, and infection.

- Figure 8.11A shows the exterior of the airway before an attack. Figure 8.11B shows the factors within and surrounding the airway that cause breathing difficulty during an attack.
- **Airway inflammation** is the swelling and clogging of the bronchial tubes with mucus. This usually occurs after the airway has been exposed to inhaled allergens.
- A **bronchospasm** (**BRONG**-koh-spazm) is a contraction of the smooth muscle in the walls of the bronchi and bronchioles, tightening and squeezing the airway shut (**bronch/o** means bronchi, and **-spasm** means involuntary contraction).
- *Exercise-induced bronchoconstriction* is the narrowing of the airways that develops after 5 to 15 minutes of physical exertion, usually triggered by the inhalation of cold, dry air.

Upper Respiratory Diseases

- **Upper respiratory infections** (URI) and *acute nasopharyngitis* are among the terms used to describe the *common cold*. An upper respiratory infection can be caused by any one of 200 different viruses, the most common of which is the *human rhinovirus*.
- **Allergic rhinitis** (rye-**NIGH**-tis), commonly referred to as an *allergy*, is an allergic reaction to airborne allergens that causes an increased flow of mucus (**rhin** means nose, and **-itis** means inflammation). Allergies are discussed in Chapter 7. *Nonallergic rhinitis* is an inflammation of the lining of the nose caused by something other than an allergen, such as cold air, spicy food, or medication.
- **Croup** (**KROOP**) is an acute respiratory infection in children and infants characterized by obstruction of the larynx, hoarseness, and swelling around the vocal cords resulting in a barking cough and stridor. *Stridor* is a harsh, high-pitched sound caused by a blockage present when breathing in.
- **Epistaxis** (ep-ih-**STACK**-sis), also known as a *nosebleed*, is bleeding from the nose that may be caused by dry air, injury, medication to prevent blood clotting, or high blood pressure.
- **Influenza** (in-flew-**EN**-zah), also known as the *flu*, is an acute, highly contagious viral infection characterized by respiratory inflammation, fever, chills, and muscle pain. Influenza is spread by respiratory droplets and occurs

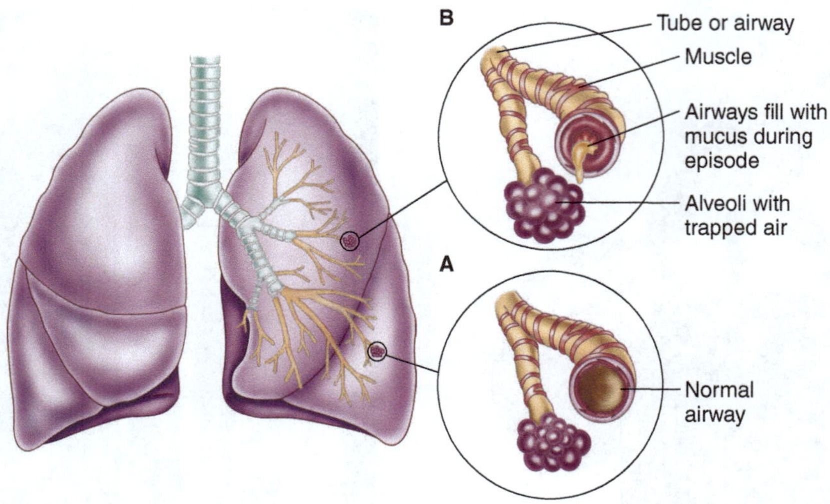

FIGURE 8.11 Changes in the airways during an asthma episode. (A) Before the episode, the muscles are relaxed and the airways are open. (B) During the episode, the muscles tighten and the airways fill with mucus.

most commonly in epidemics during the colder months. There are many strains of the influenza virus. Some strains can be prevented by annual immunization.

- **Pertussis** (per-**TUS**-is), also known as ***whooping cough***, is a contagious bacterial infection of the upper respiratory tract that is characterized by recurrent bouts of a paroxysmal cough, followed by breathlessness and a noisy inspiration. ***Paroxysmal*** means sudden or spasm-like. Childhood immunizations against diphtheria, tetanus, and acellular pertussis (DTaP or Tdap) are given together.
- **Respiratory syncytial virus** (sin-**SIH**-shul) (RSV) is a common, highly contagious viral infection spread by respiratory droplets. Most infections are mild and similar to the common cold. However, RSV can cause bronchiolitis in younger children and infants, which may require hospitalization.
- ***Bronchiolitis*** is inflammation of the bronchioles (**bronchiol** means bronchioles, and **-itis** means inflammation).
- **Rhinorrhea** (rye-noh-**REE**-ah), also known as a ***runny nose***, is the watery flow of mucus from the nose (**rhin/o** means nose, and **-rrhea** means abnormal discharge).
- **Sinusitis** (**sigh**-nuh-**SIGH**-tis) is an inflammation of the sinuses (**sinus** means sinus, and **-itis** means inflammation).

Pharynx and Larynx

- **Pharyngitis** (fah-rin-**JIGH**-tis), also known as a ***sore throat***, is an inflammation of the pharynx (**pharyng** means pharynx, and **-itis** means inflammation). It is often a symptom of a cold, flu, or sinus infection. Pharyngitis caused by the bacteria *Streptococcus* is commonly referred to as ***strep throat***.
- A **laryngospasm** (lah-**RING**-goh-spazm) is the sudden spasmodic closure of the larynx (**laryng/o** means larynx, and **-spasm** means a sudden involuntary contraction). It is sometimes associated with gastroesophageal reflux disease (GERD), which is discussed in Chapter 9.

Voice Disorders

- **Aphonia** (ah-**FOH**-nee-ah) is the loss of the ability of the larynx to produce normal speech sounds (**a-** means without, **phon** means sound or voice, and **-ia** means abnormal condition). Patients with aphonia are only able to whisper.
- **Dysphonia** (dis-**FOH**-nee-ah) is difficulty in speaking, which may include any impairment in vocal quality, including hoarseness, weakness, or the cracking of a boy's voice during puberty (**dys-** means bad, **phon** means sound or voice, and **-ia** means abnormal condition).
- **Laryngitis** (**lar**-in-**JIGH**-tis) is an inflammation of the larynx (**laryng** means larynx, and **-itis** means inflammation). This term is also commonly used to describe voice loss that is caused by this inflammation.

Trachea and Bronchi

- **Acute bronchitis**, also known as a chest cold, is inflammation of the bronchi usually caused by a viral infection. It is characterized by a productive cough, shortness of breath, and often wheezing and a low-grade fever. A *productive cough* is a cough that brings up mucus or phlegm.

- **Bronchiectasis** (**brong**-kee-**ECK**-tah-sis) is the permanent thickening of the walls of the bronchi, caused by chronic infection and inflammation (**bronch/i** means bronchus, and **-ectasis** means stretching or enlargement).
- **Bronchorrhea** (**brong**-koh-**REE**-ah) is an excessive discharge of watery mucus from the bronchi (**bronch/o** means bronchus, and **-rrhea** means abnormal flow). This is often caused by chronic bronchitis or asthma.

Pleural Cavity

- **Pleurisy** (**PLOOR**-ih-see), also known as *pleuritis*, is an inflammation of the pleura, the membranes that cover the lungs and line the pleural cavity. Pleurisy, which causes pleurodynia, may result from trauma, tuberculosis, connective tissue disease, or an infection (**pleur** means pleura, and **-isy** is a noun ending).
- **Pleurodynia** (**ploor**-oh-**DIN**-ee-ah) is a sharp chest pain that occurs when the inflamed pleural membranes rub against each other with each inhalation (**pleur/o** means pleura, and **-dynia** means pain).
- **Pleural effusion** (eh-**FEW**-zhun) is the excess accumulation of fluid in the pleural space. This produces a feeling of breathlessness because it prevents the lung from fully expanding. *Effusion* is the escape of fluid from blood or lymphatic vessels into the tissues or into a body cavity (Figure 8.12).

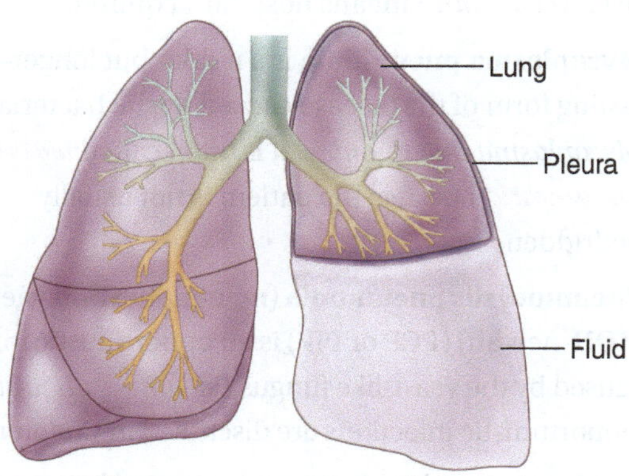

FIGURE 8.12 In pleural effusion, excess fluid in the pleural cavity prevents the lung from fully expanding.

- **Pyothorax** (**pye**-oh-**THOH**-racks), also known as *pleural empyema*, is the presence of pus in the pleural cavity between the layers of the pleural membrane resulting from a bacterial infection (**py/o** means pus, and **-thorax** means chest).
- **Empyema** (**em**-pye-**EE**-mah) refers to a collection of pus in any body cavity.
- **Hemothorax** (**hee**-moh-**THOH**-racks) is a collection of blood in the pleural cavity (**hem/o** means blood, and **-thorax** means chest). This condition often results from chest trauma, such as a stab wound, or it can be caused by disease or surgery.
- A **pneumothorax** (**new**-moh-**THOH**-racks) is the accumulation of air in the pleural space resulting in a pressure imbalance that causes the lung to fully or partially collapse (**pneum/o** means lung or air, and **-thorax** means chest). This can have an external cause, such as a stab wound through the chest wall, or it can occur when there is a lung-disease-related rupture in the pleura that allows air to leak into the pleural space (Figure 8.13).

Lungs

- **Acute respiratory distress syndrome** (ARDS) is a lung condition usually caused by trauma, pneumonia, smoke or fumes, inhaled vomit, or sepsis. *Sepsis* is a systemic bacterial infection, which is discussed in Chapter 6. ARDS is a life-threatening condition in which inflammation in the lungs and fluid in the alveoli lead to low levels of oxygen in the blood.

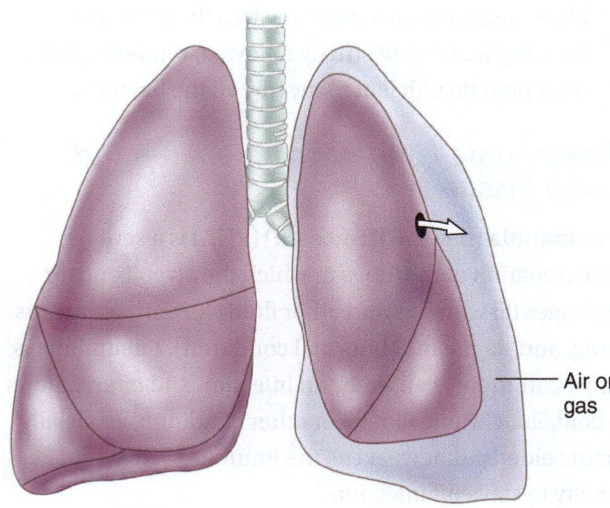

FIGURE 8.13 Pneumothorax is an accumulation of air or gas in the pleural space that causes the lung to collapse. In the left lung, a perforation in the pleura allowed air to escape into the pleural space.

- **Atelectasis** (**at**-ee-**LEK**-tah-sis), or *collapsed lung*, is the incomplete expansion of part or all of a lung due to a blockage of the air passages or pneumothorax (**atel** means incomplete, and **-ectasis** means stretching or enlargement).
- **Granuloma** (**gran**-you-**LOH**-mah) is a general term used to describe a localized area of inflammation, usually in the lungs (**granul** means granular, and **-oma** means tumor). Granulomas are most commonly caused by infections such as tuberculosis.
- **Pulmonary edema** (eh-**DEE**-mah) is an accumulation of fluid in lung tissues, especially the alveoli. *Edema* means swelling. Pulmonary edema is often a symptom of heart failure, which is discussed in Chapter 5.
- **Pulmonary embolism** (**EM**-boh-lizm) is the sudden blockage of a pulmonary artery by foreign matter or by an embolus that has formed in the leg or pelvic region.

Tuberculosis

Tuberculosis (too-**ber**-kew-**LOH**-sis) (TB), which is an infectious disease caused by *Mycobacterium tuberculosis*, usually attacks the lungs; however, it can also affect other parts of the body. Pleurisy and *hemoptysis* (coughing up blood) can be symptoms of TB in the lungs.

- TB occurs most commonly in individuals whose immune systems are weakened by another condition such as AIDS. A healthy individual can carry latent TB without showing symptoms of the disease. *Latent* means present but not active.
- *Drug-resistant tuberculosis* is a dangerous form of the disease that can occur when the prescribed drug regimen is not strictly followed, rendering the treatment insufficient to destroy all the bacteria.

Pneumonia Named for the Affected Lung Tissue

Pneumonia (new-**MOH**-nee-ah) (PNA) is a serious inflammation of the lungs in which the alveoli and air passages fill with pus and other fluids (**pneumon** means lung, and **-ia** means abnormal condition). Pneumonia is most commonly caused by an infection and often follows a cold, flu, chronic illness, or other condition, especially in the elderly, that weakens the immune system and its ability to stave off infection.

There are two types of bacterial pneumonia named for the parts of the lungs affected (Figure 8.14). These are:

- **Bronchopneumonia** (**brong**-koh-new-**MOH**-nee-ah) is a localized form of pneumonia that often affects the bronchioles (**bronch/o** means bronchial tubes, **pneumon** means lung, and **-ia** means abnormal condition). Bronchopneumonia often leads to lobar pneumonia.
- **Lobar pneumonia** affects larger areas of the lungs, often including one or more sections, or lobes, of a lung. *Double pneumonia* is lobar pneumonia involving both lungs and is usually a form of bacterial pneumonia.

Pneumonia Named for the Causative Agent

As many as 30 causes of pneumonia have been identified; however, the most common causative agents are air pollution, bacteria, fungi, viruses, and inhaled liquid or chemicals.

- **Aspiration pneumonia** (ass-pih-**RAY**-shun) can occur when a foreign substance, such as vomit, is inhaled into the lungs. As used here, *aspiration* means inhaling or drawing a foreign substance into the upper respiratory tract.
- **Community-acquired pneumonia** (CAP) is any pneumonia that results from contagious infection outside of a hospital or clinic. CAP is most commonly bacterial, but can also be caused by a virus or fungi. This is the most common form of pneumonia, and it can affect people of all ages.
- **Bacterial pneumonia** is most commonly caused by *Streptococcus pneumoniae*. *Pneumococcal pneumonia* is the only form of pneumonia that can be prevented through vaccination.
- **Hospital-acquired pneumonia**, or *nosocomial pneumonia*, is a type of pneumonia contracted during a stay in the hospital when a patient's defenses are impaired. Patients on a ventilator are particularly at risk. *Nosocomial* means hospital-acquired.
- **Mycoplasma pneumonia** is a milder but longer-lasting form of the disease caused by the bacteria *Mycoplasma pneumoniae*. It is often called *walking pneumonia* because the patient is not usually bedridden.
- **Pneumocystis pneumonia** (**new**-moh-**SIS**-tis new-**MOH**-nee-ah) (PCP or PJP) is an opportunistic infection caused by the yeast-like fungus *Pneumocystis jirovecii*. Opportunistic infections are discussed in Chapter 7.
- **Viral pneumonia**, which can be caused by several different types of viruses, accounts for approximately a third of all pneumonias.

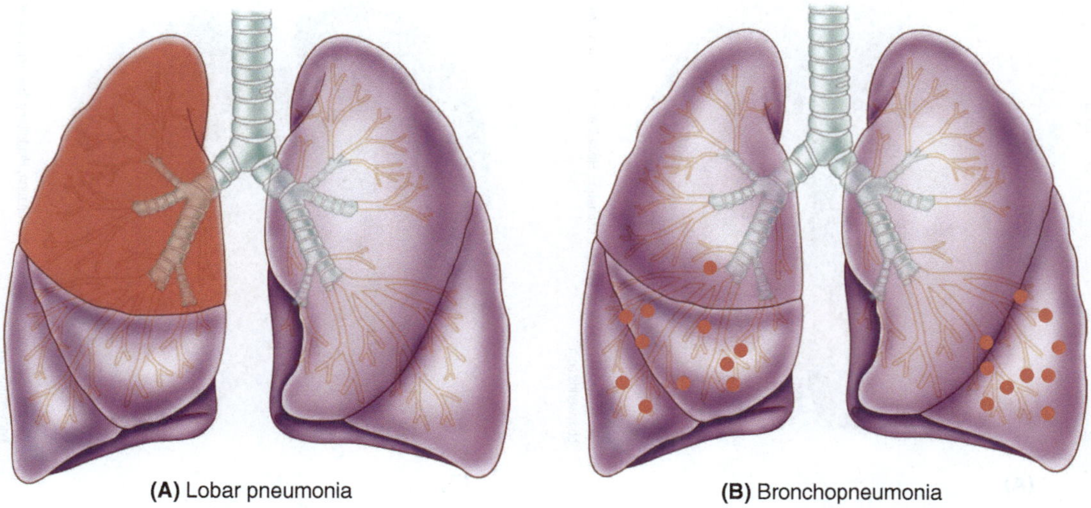

FIGURE 8.14 Types of pneumonia are usually named for the area of the lung that is involved or for the causative agent. (A) Lobar pneumonia affects larger areas of the lungs. (B) Bronchopneumonia affects the bronchioles and surrounding alveoli.

Interstitial Lung Disease

Interstitial lung disease (**in**-ter-**STISH**-al) refers to a group of almost 200 disorders that cause inflammation and scarring of the alveoli and their supporting structures. ***Interstitial*** means relating to spaces within or around a tissue or an organ. In these lung conditions the tissue around the alveoli becomes scarred or stiff, leading to a reduction of oxygen being transferred to the blood.

- **Pulmonary fibrosis** (figh-**BROH**-sis) is the progressive formation of scar tissue in the lung, resulting in decreased lung capacity and increased difficulty breathing (**fibr** means fibrous connective tissue, and **-osis** is the noun ending means abnormal condition). ***Fibrosis*** is a condition in which normal tissue is replaced by fibrotic (hardened) tissue.

Many connective tissue diseases such as rheumatoid arthritis, scleroderma, and lupus can cause pulmonary fibrosis, as can environmental toxins such as asbestos and silica. Pulmonary fibrosis can also occur without a known cause.

Environmental and Occupational Interstitial Lung Diseases

- **Pneumoconiosis** (**new**-moh-**koh**-nee-**OH**-sis) is any fibrosis of the lung tissues caused by mineral dust in the lungs after prolonged environmental or occupational contact (**pneum/o** means lung, **coni** means dust, and **-osis** means abnormal condition or disease).
  - **Asbestosis** (**ass**-beh-**STOH**-sis) is caused by asbestos particles in the lungs and usually occurs after working with asbestos (**asbest** means asbestos, and **-osis** means abnormal condition or disease).
  - **Silicosis** (**sill**-ih-**KOH**-sis) is caused by inhaling silica dust in the lungs and usually occurs after working in occupations including foundry work, quarrying, ceramics, glasswork, and sandblasting (**silic** means glass, and **-osis** means abnormal condition or disease).

Cystic Fibrosis

Cystic fibrosis (**SIS**-tick figh-**BROH**-sis) (CF) is a life-threatening genetic disorder in which the lungs and pancreas are clogged with large quantities of abnormally thick mucus. This results in damage to the lungs, poor growth, and nutritional deficiencies. Common symptoms of cystic fibrosis include wheezing and a persistent cough.

Lung Cancer

Lung cancer, which is the leading cause of cancer death in the United States, is a condition in which cancer cells form in the tissues of the lung. Important risk factors for lung cancer are smoking and inhaling secondhand smoke (Figure 8.15).

Breathing Disorders

The general term ***breathing disorders*** describes abnormal changes in the rate or depth of breathing. Specific terms

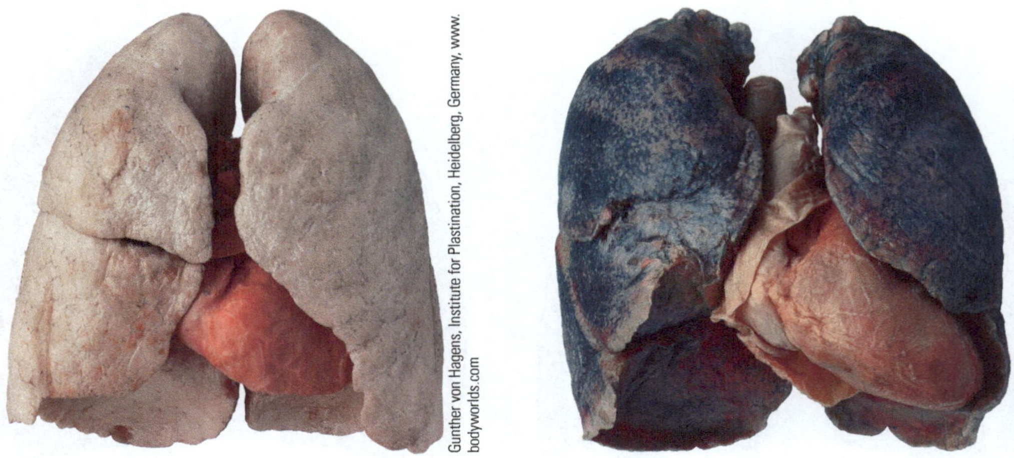

Gunther von Hagens, Institute for Plastination, Heidelberg, Germany, www.bodyworlds.com

Gunther von Hagens, Institute for Plastination, Heidelberg, Germany, www.bodyworlds.com

(A) (B)

FIGURE 8.15 Photographs of actual lung and heart specimens. (A) Healthy lungs of a nonsmoker. (B) Damaged lungs of a smoker.

describe in greater detail the changes that are occurring (Figure 8.16).

- **Eupnea** (youp-**NEE**-ah) is easy or normal breathing (**eu-** means good, and **-pnea** means breathing). This is the baseline for judging some breathing disorders (Figure 8.16A). Eupnea is the opposite *of apnea*.
- **Apnea** (**AP**-nee-ah) is the temporary absence of spontaneous respiration (**a-** means without, and **-pnea** means breathing) (Figure 8.16D). It is a common respiratory problem in premature infants. Apnea is the opposite of *eupnea*.
- **Bradypnea** (**brad**-ihp-**NEE**-ah) is an abnormally slow rate of respiration, usually of less than 10 breaths per minute (**brady-** means slow, and **-pnea** means breathing) (Figure 8.16C). Bradypnea is the opposite of *tachypnea*.
- **Cheyne–Stokes respiration** (**CHAYN STOHKS**) is an irregular pattern of breathing characterized by alternating rapid or shallow respiration followed by slower respiration or apnea (Figure 8.16E). This pattern sometimes occurs in comatose patients or those nearing death.
- **Tachypnea** (**tack**-ihp-**NEE**-ah) is an abnormally rapid rate of respiration, usually of more than 20 breaths per minute (**tachy-** means rapid, and **-pnea** means breathing) (Figure 8.16B). Tachypnea is the opposite of *bradypnea*.

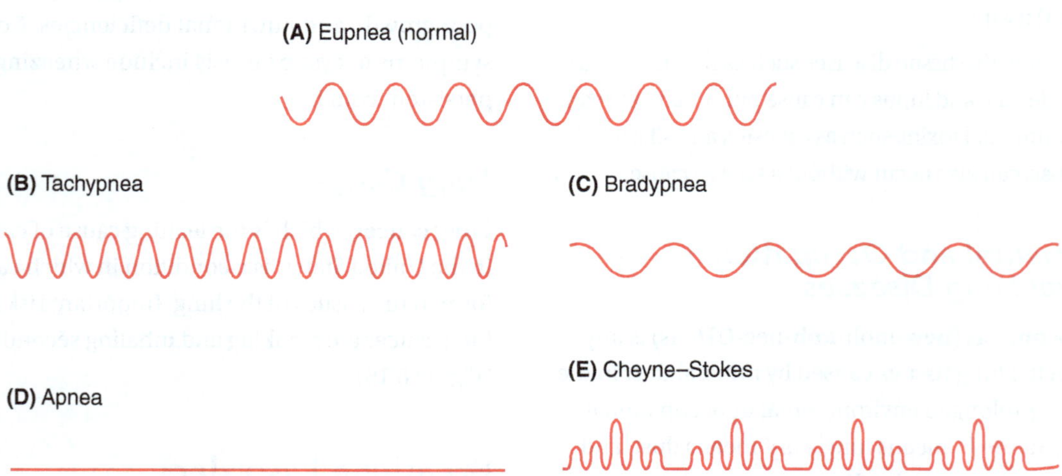

FIGURE 8.16 Respiratory patterns. (A) Eupnea is normal breathing. (B) Tachypnea is abnormally rapid breathing. (C) Bradypnea is abnormally slow breathing. (D) Apnea is the absence of breathing. (E) Cheyne–Stokes is an alternating series of abnormal patterns.

- **Dyspnea** (**DISP**-nee-ah), also known as ***shortness of breath*** (SOB), is difficult or labored breathing (**dys-** means painful, and **-pnea** means breathing). Shortness of breath can be caused by strenuous physical exertion or can be due to lung damage or heart failure.
- **Hyperpnea** (**high**-perp-**NEE**-ah), which is commonly associated with exertion, is breathing that is deeper and more rapid than is normal at rest (**hyper-** means excessive, and **-pnea** means breathing). Hyperpnea may also occur at high altitude or be caused by anemia or sepsis. Hyperpnea is the opposite of *hypopnea*.
- **Hypopnea** (**high**-poh-**NEE**-ah) is shallow or slow respiration (**hypo-** means decreased, and **-pnea** means breathing). *Note:* The second *p* is silent in the American pronunciation of this word. Hypopnea is the opposite of *hyperpnea*.
- **Hyperventilation** (**high**-per-**ven**-tih-**LAY**-shun) is an abnormally rapid rate of deep respiration that is usually associated with anxiety (**hyper-** means excessive, and **-ventilation** means breathing). This decreases the level of carbon dioxide in the blood, causing dizziness and tingling in the hands and feet.

Sleep-Related Breathing Disorders

Sleep-related breathing disorders are characterized by disruptions of normal breathing patterns that only occur during sleep and are associated with higher risks of cardiovascular disease and strokes.

- **Sleep apnea** is a potentially serious disorder in which breathing repeatedly stops and starts during sleep for periods long enough to cause a measurable decrease in blood oxygen levels. ***Obstructive sleep apnea*** (OSA) is caused by the muscles at the back of the throat relaxing and blocking the airway. It is often accompanied by periods of hypopnea, in which the airway is partially blocked.
- ***Snoring***, which can be a symptom of sleep apnea, is noisy breathing caused by vibration of the soft palate.

Coughing

- **Expectoration** (eck-**SPEK**-toh-**ray**-shun) is the act of coughing up and spitting out saliva, mucus, or other body fluid (**expector** means to cough up, and **-ation** means state or action).
- **Hemoptysis** (hee-**MOP**-tih-sis) is the expectoration of blood or blood-stained sputum derived from the lungs or bronchial tubes as the result of a pulmonary or bronchial hemorrhage (**hem/o** means blood, and **-ptysis** means spitting).

Lack of Oxygen

- **Airway obstruction**, commonly known as ***choking***, occurs when food or a foreign object partially or completely blocks the airway and prevents air from entering or leaving the lungs. This can be a life-threatening emergency requiring immediate action through the performance of ***abdominal thrusts*** on children or adults. This is also known as the ***Heimlich maneuver***. For choking infants, ***back blows*** are performed instead to try to clear the airway.
- **Anoxia** (ah-**NOCK**-see-ah) is the absence of oxygen from the body's tissues and organs even though there is an adequate flow of blood (**an-** means without, **ox** means oxygen, and **-ia** means abnormal condition). If anoxia continues for more than four to six minutes, irreversible brain damage can occur.
- **Hypoxia** (high-**POCK**-see-ah) is the condition of having deficient oxygen levels in the body's tissues and organs; however, it is less severe than anoxia (**hyp-** means deficient, **ox** means oxygen, and **-ia** means abnormal condition). This condition can be caused by a variety of factors, including trauma, lung diseases, cardiovascular problems, carbon monoxide poisoning, and high altitudes. Compare with *hypoxemia*.
- ***Altitude sickness*** is a condition that can be brought on by the lower air pressure and decreased oxygen level in the air at higher altitudes, usually above 8,000 feet. Severe altitude sickness can cause ***high-altitude pulmonary edema***, which can be life threatening.
- **Asphyxia** (ass-**FICK**-see-ah) is the loss of consciousness that occurs when the body cannot get the oxygen it needs to function. Asphyxia can be caused by choking, suffocation, drowning, or inhaling gases such as carbon monoxide.
- ***Asphyxiation*** is a state of asphyxia or suffocation. In this life-threatening condition, oxygen levels in the blood drop quickly, carbon dioxide levels rise, and unless the patient's breathing is restored within a few minutes, death or serious brain damage follows.
- **Carbon monoxide poisoning** is a potentially fatal condition in which exposure to carbon monoxide (CO) from fire or poorly vented heaters in an enclosed area causes high concentrations of CO in the bloodstream, interfering with the body's ability to utilize oxygen. Symptoms can include nausea/vomiting, dizziness, shortness of breath, headaches, lethargy, and confusion. CO poisoning is treated with oxygen therapy, including hyperbaric oxygen therapy.

- **Cyanosis** (**sigh**-ah-**NOH**-sis) is a bluish discoloration of the skin and mucous membranes caused by a lack of adequate oxygen in the blood (**cyan** means blue, and **-osis** means abnormal condition or disease).
- **Hypercapnia** (**high**-per-**KAP**-nee-ah), also known as ***CO_2 retention***, is the abnormal buildup of carbon dioxide in the blood (**hyper-** means excessive, **capn** means carbon dioxide, and **-ia** means abnormal condition). This is common in patients with respiratory disorders such as chronic obstructive pulmonary disease and sleep apnea.
- **Hypoxemia** (**high**-pock-**SEE**-mee-ah) is the condition of having low oxygen levels in the blood, usually due to respiratory disorders or heart conditions (**hyp-** means deficient, **ox** means oxygen, and **-emia** means blood). Compare with *hypoxia*.
- **Respiratory failure**, also known as ***respiratory acidosis***, is a condition in which the level of oxygen in the blood becomes dangerously low (hypoxemia) or the level of carbon dioxide becomes dangerously high (hypercapnia). It is a medical emergency that can result from a chronic condition or develop suddenly.
- **Smoke inhalation** is chemical damage and burns to the lungs caused by breathing in hot smoke containing products of combustion, including carbon monoxide.

Sudden Infant Death Syndrome

Sudden infant death syndrome (SIDS) is the sudden and unexplainable death of an apparently healthy sleeping infant between the ages of 1 month and 1 year. Although the cause of SIDS is still unknown, the Safe to Sleep® campaign recommending that infants sleep on their back instead of facedown with no blankets, pillows, or toys in the crib has significantly reduced the incidence of SIDS.

DIAGNOSTIC PROCEDURES OF THE RESPIRATORY SYSTEM

- The ***respiratory rate***, which is an important vital sign, is discussed in Chapter 21. It is a count of the number of breaths (one inhalation and one exhalation) per minute.
- ***Respiratory sounds*** such as *rales*, *rhonchi*, and *stridor* provide information about the condition of the lungs and pleura. These are described in Chapter 21.
- **Bronchoscopy** (brong-**KOS**-koh-pee) is the visual examination of the bronchi using a bronchoscope (**bronch/o** means bronchus, and **-scopy** means direct visual examination). A ***bronchoscope*** is a flexible, fiber-optic device that is passed through the nose or mouth and down the airways. It can also be used for operative procedures, such as tissue repair or the removal of a foreign object.
- A **chest x-ray** (CXR) is a valuable tool for diagnosing pneumonia, lung cancer, pneumothorax, pleural effusion, tuberculosis, and emphysema (Figure 8.10B).
- **Laryngoscopy** (**lar**-ing-**GOS**-koh-pee) is the visual examination of the larynx and vocal cords using a flexible or rigid laryngoscope inserted through the mouth (**laryng/o** means larynx, and **-scopy** means a direct visual examination). ***Indirect laryngoscopy*** is a simpler version of this test in which the larynx is viewed by shining a light on an angled mirror held at the back of the soft palate.
- A **peak flow meter** is an inexpensive handheld device used by asthma patients to measure air flow out of the lungs, revealing any narrowing of the airways in advance of an asthma attack (Figure 8.17). ***Peak expiratory flow*** (PEF) is a person's highest number on a peak flow meter.
- **Polysomnography** (**pol**-ee-som-**NOG**-rah-fee), also known as a ***sleep study***, measures physiological activity during sleep and is often performed to detect nocturnal defects in breathing associated with sleep apnea (**poly-** means many, **somn/o** means sleep, and **-graphy** means the process of recording).

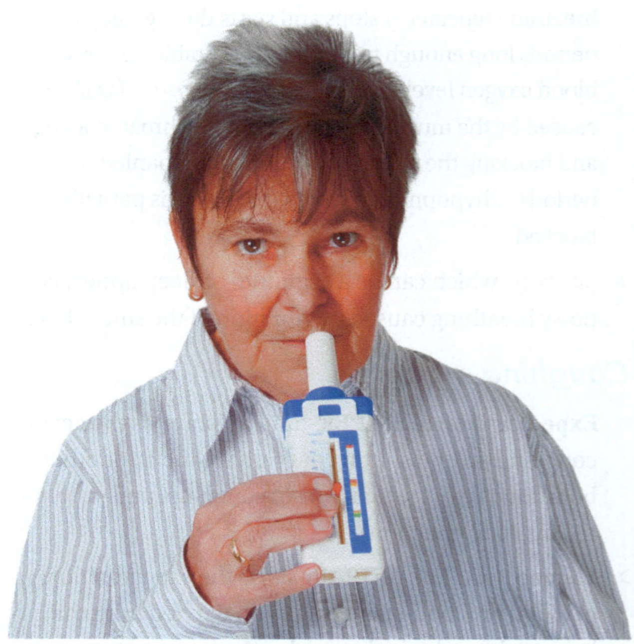

FIGURE 8.17 A peak flow meter is often used to measure how quickly a patient with asthma can expel air.

- **Pulmonary function tests** (PFTs) are a group of tests that measure volume and flow of air by using a spirometer. These tests are measured against a norm for the individual's age, height, and sex.
- A **spirometer** (spih-**ROM**-eh-ter) is a recording device that measures the amount of air inhaled or exhaled (volume) and the length of time required for each breath (**spir/o** means to breathe, and **-meter** means to measure).
- An ***incentive spirometer*** is used to help patients who have recently had surgery keep their lungs healthy during recovery.
- A **pulse oximeter** (ock-**SIM**-eh-ter) is an external monitor placed on the patient's fingertip or earlobe to measure the oxygen saturation level in the blood (**ox/i** means oxygen, and **-meter** means to measure). This is a noninvasive method of assessing basic respiratory function (Figure 8.18).
- **Sputum cytology** is a procedure in which a sample of mucus is coughed up from the lungs and then examined under a microscope to detect cancer cells.
- **Sputum culture & sensitivity** is a test in which a sample of mucus is coughed up from the lungs and monitored for bacterial growth. If bacteria grows, it is then tested for sensitivity or resistance to different antibiotics. This is used to diagnose specific types of bacterial pneumonia and determine the most effective treatment.
- **Sputum** (**SPYOU**-tum) is phlegm ejected through the mouth that can be examined for diagnostic purposes.
- **Phlegm** (**FLEM**) is thick mucus secreted by the tissues lining the respiratory passages.

Tuberculosis Testing

Two kinds of tests can be used to help detect tuberculosis infection: tuberculin skin testing and blood tests. These tests show whether the patient is infected with TB; however, they do not show whether the infection is latent or active.

- **Tuberculin skin testing**, also known as ***Mantoux PPD skin test***, is a screening test for tuberculosis in which a very small amount of tuberculin **P**urified **P**rotein **D**erivative is injected just under the top layer of the skin on the forearm. The site is checked for a reaction 48 to 72 hours later.

A positive result from either a skin or a blood test indicates the possibility of exposure to the disease, and this response warrants further testing such as a chest x-ray and sputum cytology.

TREATMENT PROCEDURES OF THE RESPIRATORY SYSTEM

Medications and Their Administration

- An **antitussive** (**an**-tih-**TUSS**-iv), commonly known as ***cough medicine***, is administered to prevent or relieve coughing (**anti-** means against, **tuss** means cough, and **-ive** means performs).
- A **decongestant**, also known as a ***nasal decongestant***, is administered orally or intranasally to relieve nasal congestion from allergies or illness.
- An **expectorant** is an oral medication that makes it easier to cough up mucus by making it thinner and less viscous. Many cold medications contain both decongestants and expectorants.

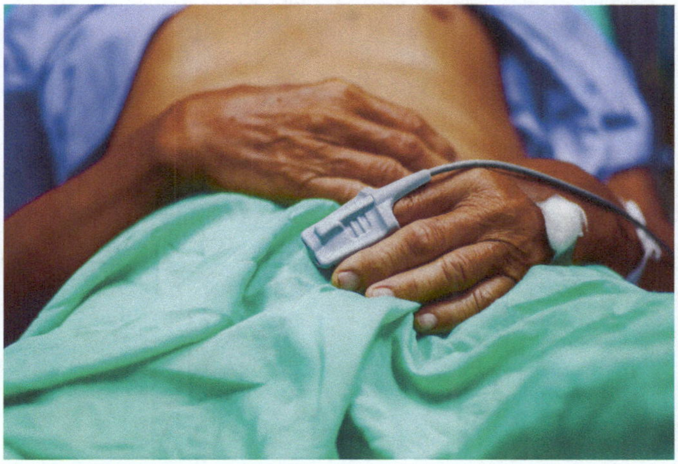

Chaikom/Shutterstock.com

FIGURE 8.18 A pulse oximeter is applied to a finger to provide continuous reassessment of the patient's levels of oxygenation.

- A **bronchodilator** (**brong**-koh-**DYE**-lay-tor) is an inhaled medication that relaxes and expands the bronchial passages into the lungs. Patients with asthma use short-acting bronchodilators as needed as *rescue medications*, while long-acting bronchodilators are used every day as controller medicines to manage the condition.
- *Controller medicines*, such as inhaled corticosteroids, are long-acting medications taken daily to prevent asthma attacks. These medications help control inflammation and stop the airways from reacting to the factors that trigger the asthma.
- A **metered-dose inhaler** (MDI) administers a specific amount of a medication such as a bronchodilator in aerosol form. A gas propellant mixes with the medicine to push it into the lungs (Figure 8.19).
- A **nebulizer** (**NEB**-you-lye-zer) is an electronic device that pumps air or oxygen through a liquid medicine to turn it into a mist, which is then inhaled by the patient via a face mask or mouthpiece.

The Nose, Throat, and Larynx

- **Endotracheal intubation** (**en**-doh-**TRAY**-kee-al **in**-too-**BAY**-shun) is the passage of a tube through the mouth into the trachea to establish or maintain an open airway, especially when a patient must be placed on a ventilator (**endo-** means within, **trache** means trachea, and **-al** means pertaining to). *Intubation* is the insertion of a tube, usually for the passage of air or fluids.
- **Functional endoscopic sinus surgery** (FESS) is a procedure performed using an endoscope in which chronic sinusitis is treated by enlarging the opening between the nose and sinus.
- A **laryngotomy** (**lar**-ing-**OT**-oh-mee) is a surgical incision into the larynx, performed when the upper part of the airway is obstructed (**laryng** means larynx, and **-otomy** means surgical incision).
- **Septoplasty** (**SEP**-toh-**plas**-tee) is the surgical repair of parts of the nasal septum (**sept/o** means septum, and **-plasty** means surgical repair), usually to correct a deviated septum. A *deviated septum* is the displacement of the nasal septum that may cause difficulty breathing through one or both nostrils. It can either be congenital or caused by an injury, and increases the likelihood of recurrent sinus infections.

The Trachea

- **Tracheostomy** (**tray**-kee-**OS**-toh-mee) is the surgical creation of a stoma into the trachea below the vocal cords to insert a temporary or permanent tube to facilitate breathing (**trache** means trachea, and **-ostomy** means surgically creating an opening). The term *tracheostomy* is used to refer to the surgical procedure and to the stoma

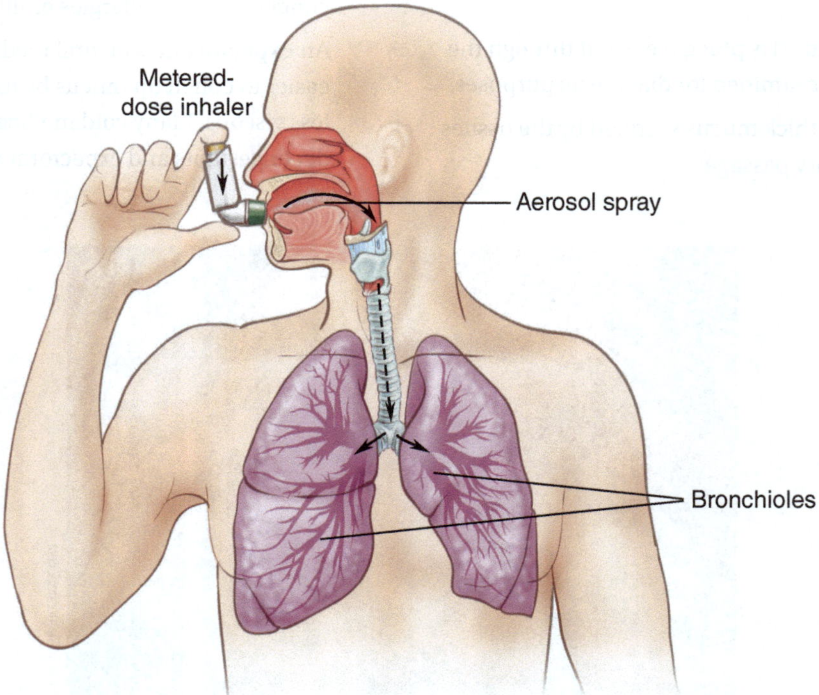

FIGURE 8.19 The metered-dose inhaler delivers medication for inhalation directly into the airways.

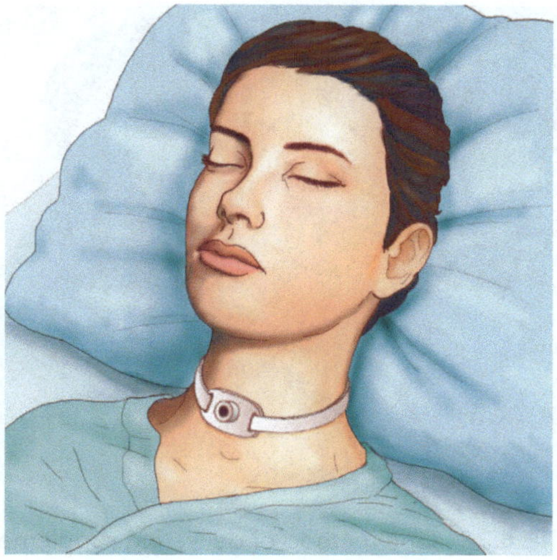

FIGURE 8.20 A tracheostomy tube creates an open airway for a patient unable to maintain his own airway.

itself. As used here, a *stoma* means a surgically created opening on a body surface (Figure 8.20).

- An emergency **tracheotomy** (**tray**-kee-**OT**-oh-mee) is a procedure in which an incision is made into the trachea to gain access to the airway below a blockage (**trache** means trachea, and **-otomy** means surgical incision).

The Lungs, Pleura, and Thorax

- A **pneumonectomy** (**new**-moh-**NECK**-toh-mee) is the surgical removal of all or part of a lung (**pneumon** means lung, and **-ectomy** means surgical removal).
- A **lobectomy** (loh-**BECK**-toh-mee) is the surgical removal of a lobe of an organ, usually the lung, brain, liver, or thyroid gland (**lob** means lobe, and **-ectomy** means surgical removal).
- **Wedge resection** is a surgery in which a small wedge-shaped piece of cancerous lung tissue is removed, along with a margin of healthy tissue around the cancer. A wedge resection removes less tissue than a lobectomy.
- **Thoracentesis** (**thoh**-rah-sen-**TEE**-sis) is the surgical puncture of the chest wall with a needle to obtain fluid from the pleural cavity (**thor/a** means thorax or chest, and **-centesis** means surgical puncture to remove fluid). This procedure is performed to remove liquid (pleural effusion, hemothorax) or air (pneumothorax) from the pleural cavity.
- A **thoracotomy** (**thoh**-rah-**KOT**-oh-mee) is a surgical incision into the chest wall to open the pleural cavity for biopsy or treatment (**thorac** means chest, and **-otomy** means surgical incision). A thoracotomy is used to gain access to the lungs, heart, esophagus, diaphragm, and other organs.
- **Video-assisted thoracic surgery** (VATS) is the use of a thoracoscope to view the inside of the pleural cavity through very small incisions. A *thoracoscope* is a specialized endoscope used for treating the thorax. This procedure is used to remove small sections of cancerous tissue and to obtain biopsy specimens to diagnose certain types of pneumonia, infections, or tumors of the chest wall. It is also used to treat repeatedly collapsing lungs.

Respiratory Therapy

- A **CPAP machine** (**C**ontinuous **P**ositive **A**irway **P**ressure) is a noninvasive ventilation device used in the treatment of sleep apnea. A face mask is connected to a pump that creates constant air pressure in the nasal passages, holding the airway open. Although this does not cure sleep apnea, it does reduce snoring and prevents dangerous apnea disturbances.
- A **BiPAP machine** (**Bi**level **P**ositive **A**irway **P**ressure) is like a CPAP machine; however, it can be set at a higher pressure for inhaling and a lower pressure for exhaling. It is used for sleep apnea in patients with neuromuscular diseases or those who find the CPAP machine uncomfortable.
- An **Ambu® bag**, or **BVM** (**B**ag **V**alve **M**ask), is an emergency resuscitator used to assist ventilation (Figure 8.21). A flexible air chamber is squeezed to force air through a face mask into the lungs of the patient, a process referred to as "bagging."
- A **ventilator** is a mechanical device for artificial respiration that is used to replace or supplement the patient's natural breathing function. The ventilator forces air into the lungs; exhalation takes place passively as the lungs contract.

Supplemental Oxygen Therapy

Supplemental oxygen is administered when the patient is unable to maintain an adequate blood oxygen saturation level from breathing normal air. Oxygen is administered by using a compressor either flowing into a hood or tent or delivered directly to the patient using one of the following devices:

- A *nasal cannula* is a small tube that divides into two nasal prongs (Figure 8.22).
- A *rebreather mask* allows the exhaled breath to be partially reused, delivering up to 60% oxygen.
- A *non-rebreather mask* allows higher levels of oxygen to be added to the air taken in by the patient.

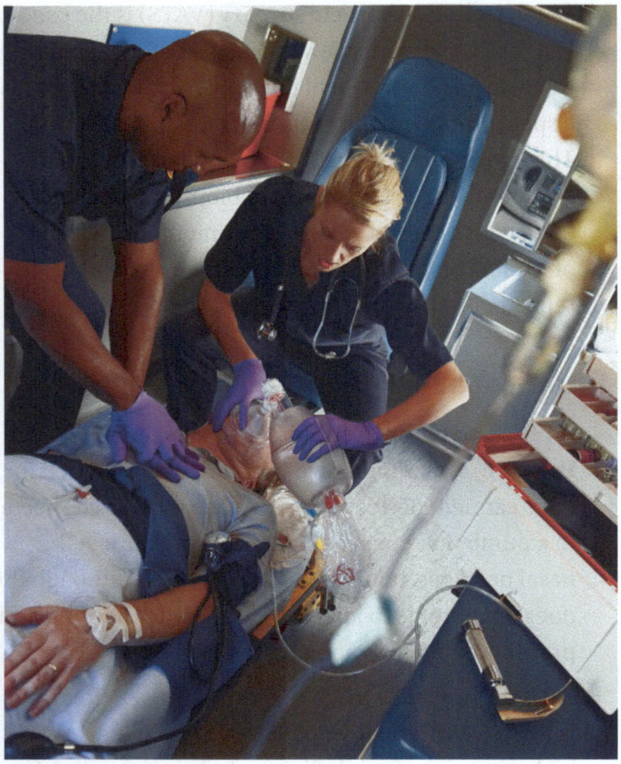

Monkey Business Images/ Shutterstock.com

FIGURE 8.21 An emergency medical technician uses an Ambu bag to assist ventilation.

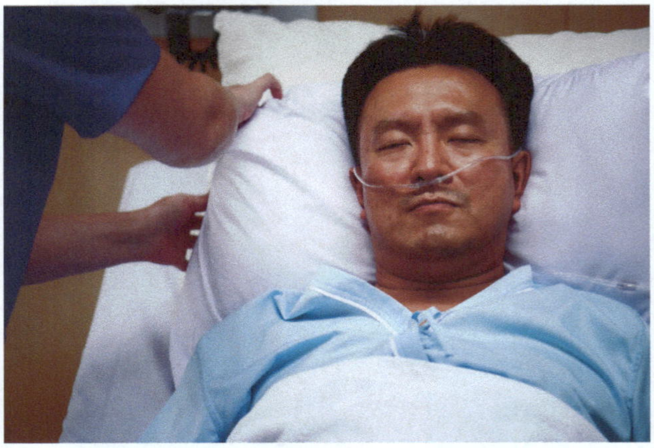

iStock.com/Rawpixel

FIGURE 8.22 One method of delivering supplemental oxygen is through a nasal cannula.

Hyperbaric oxygen therapy (**high**-per-**BARE**-ik) (HBOT) involves breathing pure oxygen in a special chamber that allows air pressure to be raised up to three times higher than normal. The lungs and the bloodstream are thus able to absorb more oxygen, which is delivered throughout the body to promote healing and fight infection. This treatment is also used for carbon monoxide poisoning.

ABBREVIATIONS RELATED TO THE RESPIRATORY SYSTEM

Table 8.1 presents an overview of the abbreviations related to the terms introduced in this chapter. *Note*: To avoid errors or confusion, always be cautious when using abbreviations.

TABLE 8.1

Abbreviations Related to the Respiratory System

acute respiratory distress syndrome = ARDS	**ARDS** = acute respiratory distress syndrome
chronic obstructive pulmonary disease = COPD	**COPD** = chronic obstructive pulmonary disease
cystic fibrosis = CF	**CF** = cystic fibrosis
functional endoscopic sinus surgery = FESS	**FESS** = functional endoscopic sinus surgery
hyperbaric oxygen therapy = HBOT	**HBOT** = hyperbaric oxygen therapy
metered-dose inhaler = MDI	**MDI** = metered-dose inhaler
pneumonia = PNA	**PNA** = pneumonia
pulmonary function tests = PFT	**PFT** = pulmonary function tests
sudden infant death syndrome = SIDS	**SIDS** = sudden infant death syndrome
tuberculosis = TB	**TB** = tuberculosis
upper respiratory infection = URI	**URI** = upper respiratory infection

LEARNING EXERCISES

Matching Word Parts 1

Write the correct answer in the middle column.

	Definition	Correct Answer	Possible Answers
8.1.	nose	______________	nas/o
8.2.	sleep	______________	laryng/o
8.3.	to breathe	______________	pharyng/o
8.4.	throat, pharynx	______________	somn/o
8.5.	larynx, throat	______________	spir/o

Matching Word Parts 2

Write the correct answer in the middle column.

	Definition	Correct Answer	Possible Answers
8.6.	lung	______________	bronch/o
8.7.	oxygen	______________	ox/o
8.8.	pleura	______________	phon/o
8.9.	bronchus	______________	pleur/o
8.10.	sound or voice	______________	pneum/o

Matching Word Parts 3

Write the correct answer in the middle column.

	Definition	Correct Answer	Possible Answers
8.11.	windpipe	______________	-pnea
8.12.	sinus	______________	pulmon/o

8.13.	lung	________________	**sinus/o**
8.14.	chest	________________	**-thorax**
8.15.	breathing	________________	**trache/o**

Definitions

Select the correct answer, and write it on the line provided.

8.16. The heart, aorta, esophagus, and trachea are located in the ________________.

dorsal cavity | manubrium | mediastinum | pleura

8.17. The ________________ acts as a lid over the entrance to the laryngopharynx.

Adam's apple | epiglottis | larynx | thyroid cartilage

8.18. The innermost layer of the pleura is known as the ________________.

parietal pleura | pleural space | pleural cavity | visceral pleura

8.19. The ________________ sinuses are located just above the eyebrows.

ethmoid | frontal | maxillary | sphenoid

8.20. The smallest divisions of the bronchial tree are the ________________.

alveoli | alveolus | bronchioles | bronchi

8.21. During respiration, the exchange of oxygen and carbon dioxide takes place through the walls of the ________________.

alveoli | arteries | capillaries | veins

8.22. The term meaning spitting blood or blood-stained sputum is ________________.

effusion | epistaxis | hemoptysis | hemothorax

8.23. Doing foundry work, quarrying, ceramics, glasswork, or sandblasting can put you at risk for ________________.

bronchopneumonia | asbestosis | pneumoconiosis | silicosis

8.24. The term ________________ means an abnormally rapid rate of respiration.

apnea | bradypnea | dyspnea | tachypnea

8.25. The term meaning any voice impairment is ________________.

aphonia | dysphonia | laryngitis | laryngospasm

Matching Structures

Write the correct answer in the middle column.

	Definition	Correct Answer	Possible Answers
8.26.	first division of the pharynx	________________	laryngopharynx
8.27.	second division of the pharynx	________________	larynx
8.28.	third division of the pharynx	________________	nasopharynx
8.29.	voice box	________________	oropharynx
8.30.	windpipe	________________	trachea

Which Word?

Select the correct answer, and write it on the line provided.

8.31. The exchange of gases within the cells of the body is known as ________________.

external respiration internal respiration

8.32. A physician who specializes in diagnosing and treating diseases and disorders of the respiratory system is a ________________.

pulmonologist respiratory therapist

8.33. The form of pneumonia that can be prevented through vaccination is ________________.

bacterial pneumonia viral pneumonia

8.34. The term commonly known as shortness of breath is ________________.

dyspnea eupnea

8.35. The emergency procedure to gain access below a blocked airway is known as a ________________.

tracheostomy tracheotomy

Spelling Counts

Find the misspelled word in each sentence. Then write the word, spelled correctly, on the line provided.

8.36. The thick mucus secreted by the tissues that line the respiratory passages is called phlem.

____

8.37. The medical term meaning an accumulation of pus in a body cavity is empiema.

____

8.38. The medical name for the disease commonly known as whooping cough is pertusis.

____

8.39. The frenic nerves stimulate the diaphragm and cause it to contract. ______________________

8.40. An antitussiff is administered to prevent or relieve coughing. ______________________

Abbreviation Identification

In the space provided, write the words that each abbreviation stands for.

8.41. **ARDS** ______________________

8.42. **CF** ______________________

8.43. **FESS** ______________________

8.44. **SIDS** ______________________

8.45. **URI** ______________________

Term Selection

Select the correct answer, and write it on the line provided.

8.46. Inhaling a foreign substance into the upper respiratory tract can cause ______________________ pneumonia.

aspiration | inhalation | inspiration | respiration

8.47. The term meaning abnormally rapid deep breathing is ______________________.

dyspnea | hyperpnea | hypopnea | hyperventilation

8.48. The term meaning the surgical creation of a stoma into the trachea to insert a breathing tube is ______________________.

bronchiectasis | thoracotomy | tracheostomy | tracheotomy

8.49. The diaphragm is relaxed during ______________________.

exhalation | inhalation | internal respiration | singultus

8.50. The chronic allergic disorder characterized by episodes of severe breathing difficulty, coughing, and wheezing is known as ______________________.

allergic rhinitis   asthma   bronchospasm   laryngospasm

Sentence Completion

Write the correct term on the line provided.

8.51. The term meaning an absence of spontaneous respiration is ______________________.

8.52. The sudden spasmodic closure of the larynx is a/an ______________________.

8.53. The term meaning the surgical puncture of the chest wall with a needle to obtain fluid from the pleural cavity is ______________________.

8.54. The term meaning pain in the pleura with each inhalation is ______________________.

8.55. A contraction of the smooth muscle in the walls of the bronchi and bronchioles that tighten and squeeze the airway shut is known as a/an ______________________.

Word Surgery

Divide each term into its component word parts. Write these word parts, in sequence, on the lines provided. When necessary, use a slash (/) to indicate a combining vowel. (You may not need all of the lines provided.)

8.56. **Bronchorrhea** means an excessive discharge of mucus from the bronchi.

__________ __________ __________ __________

8.57. The **oropharynx** is visible when looking at the back of the mouth.

__________ __________ __________ __________

8.58. **Polysomnography** measures physiological activity during sleep and is most often performed to detect nocturnal defects in breathing associated with sleep apnea.

__________ __________ __________ __________

8.59. **Pneumonectomy** is the surgical removal of all or part of a lung.

__________ __________ __________ __________

8.60. **Rhinorrhea**, also known as a runny nose, is an excessive flow of mucus from the nose.

__________ __________ __________ __________

True/False

If the statement is true, write **True** on the line. If the statement is false, write **False** on the line.

8.61. ________ A pulse oximeter is a monitor placed inside the ear to measure the oxygen saturation level in the blood.

8.62. ________ In atelectasis, the lung fails to expand because there is a blockage of the air passages or pneumothorax.

8.63. ________ Croup is an allergic reaction to airborne allergens.

8.64. ________ Hypoxemia is the condition of below-normal oxygenation of arterial blood.

8.65. ________ Emphysema is the progressive loss of lung function in which the chest sometimes assumes an enlarged barrel shape.

Clinical Conditions

Write the correct answer on the line provided.

8.66. Baby Jamison was born with ________________. This is a genetic disorder in which the lungs are clogged with large quantities of abnormally thick mucus.

8.67. Dr. Lee surgically removed a portion of the lung. This procedure is known as a/an ________________.

8.68. Wendy Barlow required a surgical incision into her larynx. This procedure is known as a/an ________________.

8.69. During his asthma attacks, Jamaal Nelson uses an inhaler containing a ________________. This medication expands the opening of the passages into his lungs.

8.70. Each year, Mr. Partin receives a flu shot to prevent ________________.

8.71. When hit during a fight, Marvin Roper's nose started to bleed. The medical term for this condition is ________________.

8.72. The doctor's examination revealed that Juanita Martinez has an accumulation of blood in the pleural cavity. This diagnosis is recorded on her chart as a/an ________________.

8.73. Duncan McClanahan had a/an ________________ performed to correct damage to the septum of his nose.

8.74. Suzanne Holderman is suffering from an inflammation of the bronchial walls. The medical term for Suzanne's condition is chronic ______________________.

8.75. Ted Coleman required the permanent placement of a breathing tube. The procedure for the placement of this tube is called a/an ______________________.

Which Is the Correct Medical Term?

Select the correct answer, and write it on the line provided.

8.76. An inflammation of the pleura that causes pleurodynia is known as ______________________.

atelectasis emphysema pleurodynia pleurisy

8.77. The substance ejected through the mouth and used for diagnostic purposes in respiratory disorders is known as ______________________.

phlegm pleural effusion saliva sputum

8.78. The term meaning a bluish discoloration of the skin caused by a lack of adequate oxygen is ______________________.

asphyxia cyanosis epistaxis hypoxia

8.79. The medical term meaning sudden spasmodic closure of the larynx is ______________________.

aphonia dysphonia laryngitis laryngospasm

8.80. The pattern of alternating periods of rapid breathing, slow breathing, and the absence of breathing is known as ______________________.

anoxia Cheyne Stokes respiration eupnea tachypnea

Challenge Word Building

These terms are *not* primary terms in the chapter; however, they are made up of the following familiar word parts. If you need help in creating the term, refer to your medical dictionary.

bronch/o	**-itis**
epiglott/o	**-ologist**
laryng/o	**-plasty**
pharyng/o	**-plegia**
pneumon/o	**-rrhagia**
trache/o	**-rrhea**
	-scopy
	-stenosis

8.81. An abnormal discharge from the pharynx is known as ______________________.

8.82. Inflammation of the lungs is known as ______________________.

8.83. A specialist in the study of the larynx is a/an ______________________.

8.84. Bleeding from the larynx is known as ______________________.

8.85. Inflammation of both the pharynx and the larynx is known as ______________________.

8.86. Abnormal narrowing of the lumen of the trachea is known as ______________________.

8.87. The surgical repair of a bronchial defect is a/an ______________________.

8.88. Inflammation of the epiglottis is known as ______________________.

8.89. The inspection of both the trachea and bronchi through a bronchoscope is a/an ______________________.

8.90. Paralysis of the walls of the bronchi is known as ______________________.

Labeling Exercises

Identify the parts of numbered items on the accompanying figure.

8.91. ______________________

8.92. ______________________

8.93. ______________________

8.94. ______________________

8.95. ______________________

8.96. ______________________ cavity

8.97. ______________________

8.98. ______________________

8.99. ______________________ lung

8.100. ______________________ sacs

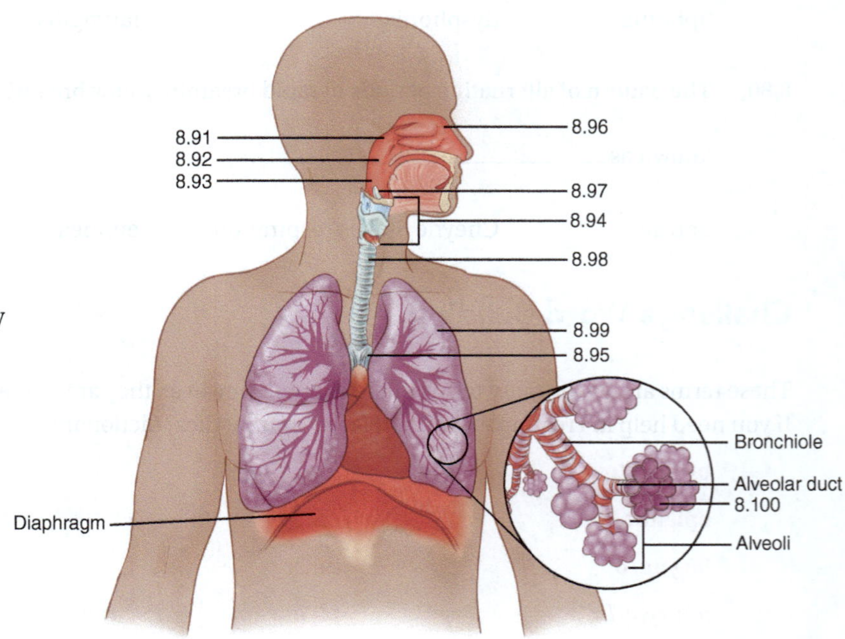

The Human Touch

CRITICAL THINKING EXERCISE

The following story and questions are designed to stimulate critical thinking through class discussion or as a brief essay response. There are no right or wrong answers to these questions.

Sylvia Gaylord works as a legal aide on the 12th floor of a tall glass-and-steel monument to modern architectural technology. On clear days, the views are spectacular. From her cubicle, Sylvia's eye catches the edge of the beautiful blue-and-white skyscraper as she reaches for her inhaler. This is the third attack since she returned from lunch four hours ago—her asthma is really bad today. But if she leaves work early again, her boss will write her up for it. Sylvia concentrates on breathing normally.

Her roommate, Kelly, is a respiratory therapist at the county hospital. Kelly says Sylvia's asthma attacks are probably triggered by the city's high level of air pollution. That can't be true. They both run in the park every morning before work, and Sylvia rarely needs to use her inhaler. The problems start when she gets to work. The wheezing and coughing were so bad today that by the time she got up the elevator and into her cubicle, she could hardly breathe.

Last night, the cable news ran a story on the unhealthy air found in some buildings. They called it "sick building syndrome" and reported that certain employees developed allergic reactions just by breathing the air. "Hmmm," she thought, "It seems like more and more people are getting sick in our office. John has had the flu twice. Sid's bronchitis turned into bronchopneumonia, and Hui complains of sinusitis. Could this building have an air quality problem?"

Suggested Discussion Topics

1. Discuss which environmental factors might cause an asthma attack.
2. Discuss what Sylvia might do to find out if her building has an air quality problem.
3. What factors did Sylvia and Kelly consider as possible triggers for Sylvia's frequent attacks?
4. If Sylvia's inhaler does not control her attack and her condition worsens, what steps should be taken promptly? Why?

CHAPTER 9

THE DIGESTIVE SYSTEM

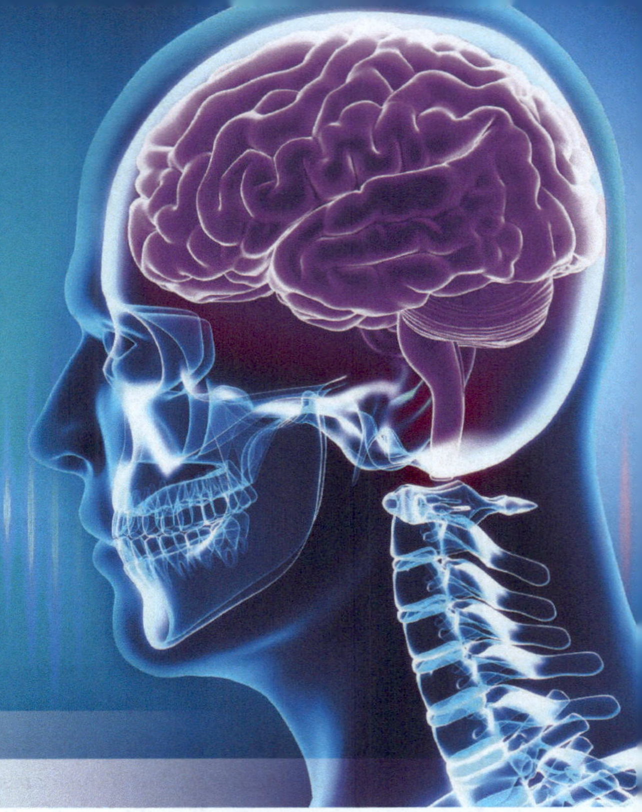

Overview of

STRUCTURES, COMBINING FORMS, AND FUNCTIONS OF THE DIGESTIVE SYSTEM

Major Structures	Related Combining Forms	Primary Functions
Mouth	or/o, stomat/o	Begins preparation of food for digestion.
Teeth	odont/i	Used for biting, tearing, and chewing in mechanical digestion.
Pharynx	pharyng/o	Transports food from the mouth to the esophagus.
Esophagus	esophag/o	Transports food from the pharynx to the stomach.
Stomach	gastr/o	Breaks down food and mixes it with gastric juices.
Small Intestine	enter/o	Mixes chyme coming from the stomach with digestive juices to complete the digestion and absorption of most nutrients.
Large Intestine	col/o, colon/o	Absorbs excess water and prepares solid waste for elimination.
Rectum and Anus	an/o, proct/o, rect/o	Control the excretion of solid waste.
Liver	hepat/o	Secretes bile and enzymes to aid in the digestion of fats.
Gallbladder	cholecyst/o	Stores bile and releases it into the small intestine as needed.
Pancreas	pancreat/o	Secretes digestive juices and enzymes into the small intestine as needed.

Vocabulary Related to **THE DIGESTIVE SYSTEM**

This list contains essential word parts and medical terms for this chapter. These and the other important **primary terms** are shown in **boldface** throughout the chapter. *Secondary terms*, which appear in *orange* italics, clarify the meaning of primary terms.

Word Parts

- ☐ **an/o** anus, ring
- ☐ **chol/e** bile, gall
- ☐ **cholecyst/o** gallbladder
- ☐ **col/o**, **colon/o** colon, large intestine
- ☐ **-emesis** vomiting
- ☐ **enter/o** small intestine
- ☐ **esophag/o** esophagus
- ☐ **gastr/o** stomach, belly
- ☐ **hepat/o** liver
- ☐ **-lithiasis** presence of stones
- ☐ **-pepsia** digest, digestion
- ☐ **-phagia** eating, swallowing
- ☐ **proct/o** anus and rectum
- ☐ **rect/o** rectum, straight
- ☐ **sigmoid/o** sigmoid colon

Medical Terms

- ☐ **aerophagia** (**ayr**-oh-**FAY**-jee-ah)
- ☐ **anastomosis** (ah-**nas**-toh-**MOH**-sis)
- ☐ **antiemetic** (**an**-tee-eh-**MET**-ick)
- ☐ **ascites** (ah-**SIGH**-teez)
- ☐ **bariatrics** (**bayr**-ee-**AT**-ricks)
- ☐ **borborygmus** (**bor**-boh-**RIG**-mus)
- ☐ **cachexia** (kah-**KEKS**-eeh-ah)
- ☐ **canker sores** (**KANE**-ker)
- ☐ **celiac disease** (**SEE**-lee-ak)
- ☐ **cheilitis** (kye-**LITE**-is)
- ☐ **cholangiography** (koh-**LAN**-jee-**og**-rah-fee)
- ☐ **cholangitis** (**koh**-lan-**JIGH**-tis)
- ☐ **cholecystectomy** (**koh**-luh-sis-**TECK**-toh-mee)
- ☐ **cholecystitis** (**koh**-luh-sis-**TYE**-tis)
- ☐ **cholelithiasis** (**koh**-luh-lih-**THIGH**-ah-sis)
- ☐ **cirrhosis** (sih-**ROH**-sis)
- ☐ **colonoscopy** (**koh**-lun-**OSS**-koh-pee)
- ☐ **colostomy** (koh-**LAHS**-toh-mee)
- ☐ **Crohn's disease** (**KROHNZ**)
- ☐ **dental prophylaxis** (**proh**-fih-**LACK**-sis)
- ☐ **diverticulitis** (**dye**-ver-tick-you-**LYE**-tis)
- ☐ **diverticulosis** (**dye**-ver-tick-you-**LOH**-sis)
- ☐ **dyspepsia** (dis-**PEP**-see-ah)
- ☐ **dysphagia** (dis-**FAY**-jee-ah)
- ☐ **endoscopy** (en-**DOS**-koh-pee)
- ☐ **enema** (**EH**-neh-ma)
- ☐ **enteritis** (**en**-ter-**EYE**-tis)
- ☐ **eructation** (eh-ruk-**TAY**-shun)
- ☐ **esophageal varices** (eh-**sof**-ah-**JEE**-al **VAYR**-ih-seez)
- ☐ **esophagogastroduodenoscopy** (eh-**sof**-ah-goh-**gas**-troh-**dew**-oh-deh-**NOS**-koh-pee)
- ☐ **gastroduodenostomy** (**gas**-troh-**dew**-oh-deh-**NOS**-toh-mee)
- ☐ **gastroesophageal reflux disease** (gas-troh-eh-**sof**-ah-**JEE**-al **REE**-flucks)
- ☐ **gastroparesis** (**gas**-troh-pah-**REE**-sis)
- ☐ **gastrostomy tube** (gas-**TROS**-toh-mee)
- ☐ **hematemesis** (**hee**-mah-**TEM**-eh-sis)
- ☐ **Hemoccult test** (**HEE**-moh-kult)
- ☐ **hepatitis** (**hep**-ah-**TYE**-tis)
- ☐ **hiatal hernia** (high-**AY**-tal **HER**-nee-ah)
- ☐ **hyperemesis** (**high**-per-**EM**-eh-sis)
- ☐ **ileus** (**ILL**-ee-us)
- ☐ **inguinal hernia** (**ING**-gwih-nal **HER**-nee-ah)
- ☐ **jaundice** (**JAWN**-dis)
- ☐ **leukoplakia** (**loo**-koh-**PLAY**-kee-ah)
- ☐ **malocclusion** (**mal**-oh-**KLOO**-zhun)
- ☐ **melena** (meh-**LEE**-nah)
- ☐ **nasogastric intubation** (**nay**-zoh-**GAS**-trick **in**-too-**BAY**-shun)
- ☐ **obesity** (oh-**BEE**-sih-tee)
- ☐ **palatoplasty** (**PAL**-ah-toh-**plas**-tee)
- ☐ **peptic ulcer disease** (**UL**-ser)
- ☐ **peristalsis** (**pehr**-ih-**STAL**-sis)
- ☐ **polyp** (**POL**-up)
- ☐ **proctologist** (prock-**TOL**-oh-jist)
- ☐ **regurgitation** (ree-**gur**-jih-**TAY**-shun)
- ☐ **salmonellosis** (**sal**-moh-nel-**LOH**-sis)
- ☐ **sigmoidoscopy** (**sig**-moi-**DOS**-koh-pee)
- ☐ **stomatitis** (**stoh**-mah-**TYE**-tis)
- ☐ **trismus** (**TRIZ**-mus)
- ☐ **ulcerative colitis** (**UL**-ser-**ay**-tiv koh-**LYE**-tis)
- ☐ **volvulus** (**VOL**-view-lus)
- ☐ **xerostomia** (**zeer**-oh-**STOH**-mee-ah)

LEARNING OBJECTIVES

On completion of this chapter, you should be able to:

1. Describe the major structures and functions of the digestive system.
2. Describe the accessory organs of the digestive system.
3. Describe the processes of digestion, absorption, and metabolism.
4. Identify the medical specialists who treat disorders of the digestive system.
5. Identify medical word parts of the digestive system.
6. Define the primary terms related to the pathology and the diagnostic and treatment procedures of the digestive system.
7. Spell the primary terms of the digestive system.
8. Pronounce the primary terms of the digestive system.
9. Identify common abbreviations related to the digestive system.

STRUCTURES AND FUNCTIONS OF THE DIGESTIVE SYSTEM

The digestive system consists primarily of the **gastrointestinal tract** (**gas**-troh-in-**TESS**-tih-nal), which is also known as the *GI tract* (**gastr/o** means stomach, **intestin** means intestine, and **-al** means pertaining to). These organs work in cooperation with *accessory organs* (Figure 9.1).

- The *upper GI tract* consists of the mouth, pharynx (throat), esophagus, and stomach. This transports food from entry into the body until digestion begins in the stomach.
- The *lower GI tract*, which is sometimes referred to as the *bowels*, is made up of the small and large intestines (sometimes called the *small and large bowels*) plus the rectum and anus. Here digestion is completed and waste material is prepared for expulsion from the body.
- The accessory organs of the digestive system are the liver, gallbladder, and pancreas.

The Oral Cavity

The major structures of the **oral cavity**, also known as the *mouth*, are the lips, hard and soft palates, salivary glands, tongue, teeth, and periodontium (Figure 9.2).

The Lips

The **lips**, which are also known as the *labia*, surround the opening to the oral cavity (singular, *labium*). The term *labia* is also used to describe parts of the female genitalia (see Chapter 16).

- During eating, the lips, tongue, and cheeks hold the food in the mouth.
- The lips also have important roles in breathing, speaking, and the expression of emotions.

The Palate

The **palate** (**PAL**-at), which forms the roof of the mouth, consists of three major parts (Figure 9.2).

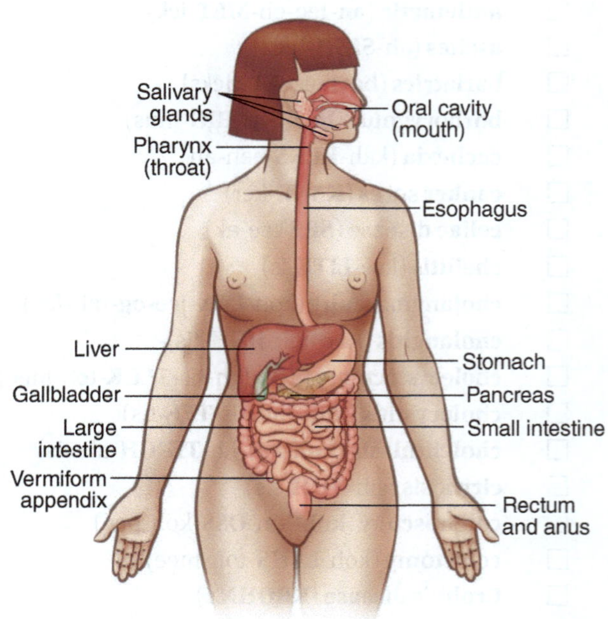

FIGURE 9.1 Major structures and accessory organs of the digestive system.

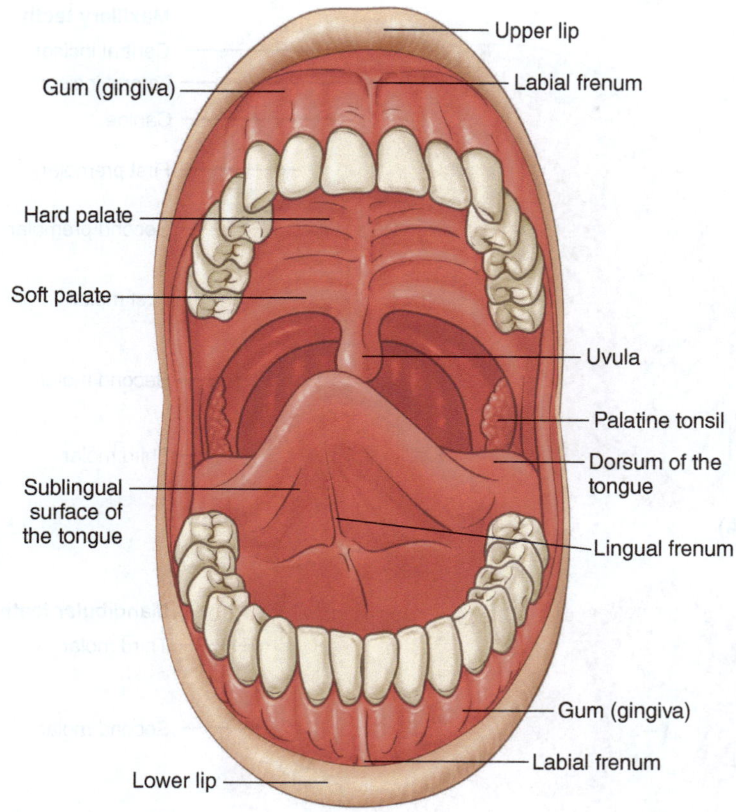

FIGURE 9.2 Structures of the tongue and oral cavity.

- The **hard palate** is the anterior portion of the palate. This area is covered with specialized mucous membrane.
- The **soft palate** is the flexible posterior portion of the palate. During swallowing, it has the important role of closing off the nasal passage to prevent food and liquid from moving upward into the nasal cavity.
- The **uvula** (**YOU**-view-lah) is the third part, and it hangs from the free edge of the soft palate. During swallowing, it moves upward with the soft palate. It also plays an important role in snoring and in the formation of some speech sounds.

The Tongue

The **tongue** is very strong, flexible, and muscular. The posterior portion of the tongue is attached. The anterior end of the tongue moves freely and is flexible. It is the structure of the tongue that makes it so important for chewing, speaking, and swallowing (Figure 9.2).

- The upper surface of the tongue is the ***dorsum***. This surface has a tough protective covering and in some areas, small bumps known as **papillae** (pah-**PILL**-ee) (singular, *papilla*). These papillae contain ***taste buds***, which are the sensory receptors for the sense of taste.
- The ***sublingual surface*** of the tongue and the tissues that lie under the tongue are covered with delicate highly vascular tissues. *Sublingual* means under the tongue. ***Highly vascular*** means containing many blood vessels.
- The presence of this rich blood supply under the tongue makes it suitable for administering certain medications sublingually by placing them under the tongue, where they are quickly absorbed into the bloodstream.
- The ***lingual frenum*** is a band of tissue that attaches the tongue to the floor of the mouth. This frenum limits the motion of the tongue.

Soft Tissues of the Oral Cavity

- The term **periodontium** (**pehr**-ee-oh-**DON**-shee-um) describes the structures that surround, support, and are attached to the teeth (**peri-** means surrounding, **odonti** means the teeth, and **-um** is a noun ending). This consists of the bone of the dental arches and the soft tissues that surround and support the teeth.
- The **gingiva** (**JIN**-jih-vah), also known as ***masticatory mucosa*** or the ***gums***, is the specialized mucous membrane that covers the bone of the dental arches and surrounds the neck of the teeth (plural *gingivae*).

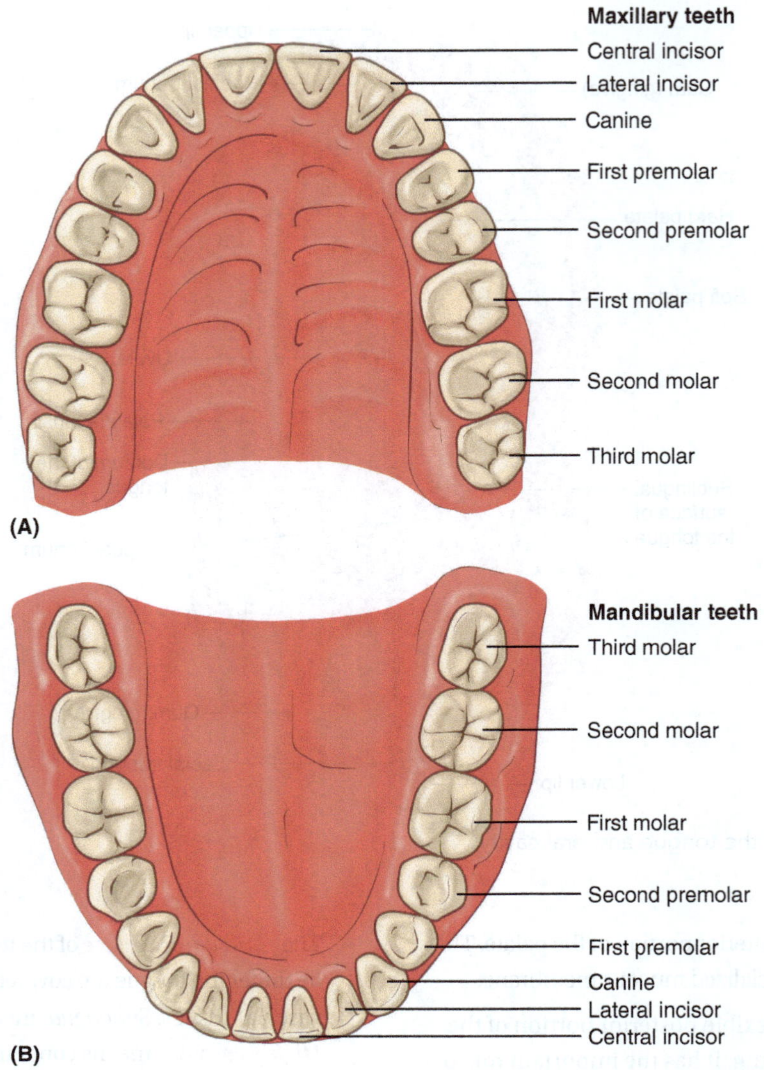

FIGURE 9.3 Four types of teeth make up adult dentition. (A) Maxillary arch. (B) Mandibular arch.

- The ***sulcus*** is an area of space between a tooth and the surrounding gingiva (plural *sulci*). A buildup of food debris and bacteria in the sulcus can lead to infection. *Sulci* is also the term for fissures in the cerebral cortex of the brain (see Chapter 11).

The Dental Arches

The **dental arches** are the bony structures of the oral cavity (Figures 9.3A and 9.3B). These arches hold the teeth firmly in position to facilitate chewing and speaking.

- The ***maxillary arch*** is commonly known as the upper jaw and consists of bones of the lower surface of the skull. This arch does not move.
- The ***mandibular arch***, commonly known as the lower jaw, is a separate bone and is the only movable component of the joint.
- The **temporomandibular joint** (**tem**-poh-roh-man-**DIB**-you-lar), commonly known as the ***TMJ***, is formed at the back of the mouth where the maxillary and mandibular arches come together.

The Teeth

The term **dentition** (den-**TISH**-un) refers to the natural teeth arranged in the upper and lower jaws. Human dentition consists of four types of teeth (Figure 9.3):

- ***Incisors*** and ***canines*** (also known as ***cuspids***). These teeth are used for biting and tearing.
- ***Premolars***, which are also known as ***bicuspids***, and ***molars***. These teeth are used for chewing and grinding.

Primary and Permanent Dentition

- The **primary dentition** is also known as the ***baby teeth***. These 20 teeth erupt during early childhood, are normally lost in late childhood, and are replaced by the permanent teeth. The primary dentition consists

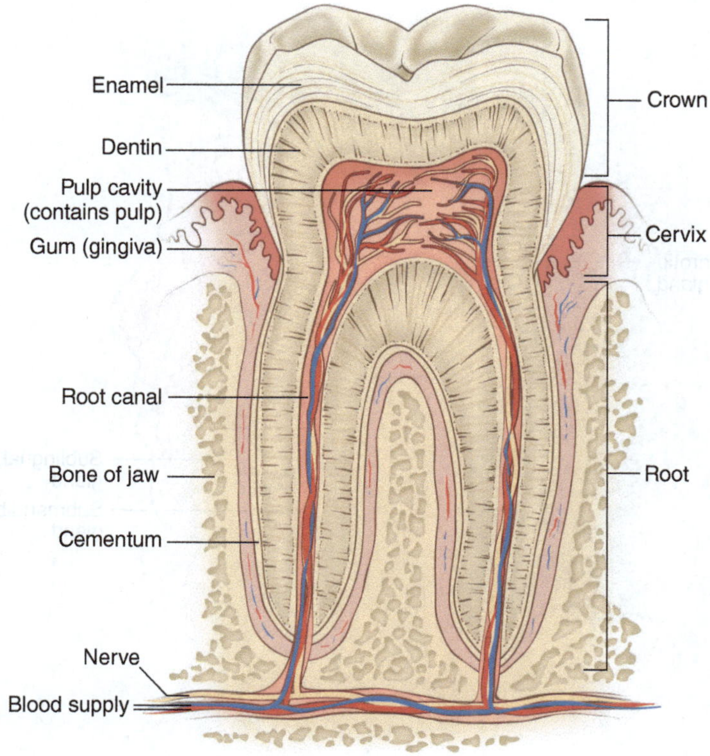

FIGURE 9.4 Structures and tissues of the tooth.

of eight incisors, four canines, and eight molars but no premolars.

- The **permanent dentition** consists of 32 teeth designed to last a lifetime. Of these teeth, 20 replace primary teeth and 12 erupt at the back of the mouth. The permanent dentition includes 8 incisors, 4 canines, 8 premolars, and 12 molars. The third molars, which are the last to erupt, are also known as ***wisdom teeth***.
- The term **occlusion**, as used in dentistry, describes any contact between the chewing surfaces of the upper and lower teeth.

Structures and Tissues of the Teeth

The **crown** is the portion of a tooth that is visible in the mouth. It is covered with ***enamel***, which is the hardest substance in the body (Figure 9.4).

- The ***roots*** of the tooth hold it securely in place within the dental arch. The roots are protected by ***cementum***. This substance is hard, but it is not as strong as enamel.
- The ***cervix***, also known as the neck of the tooth, is where the crown and root meet. The term cervix is also used in female anatomy (Chapter 16).
- ***Dentin*** makes up the bulk of the tooth. The portion that is above the gum line is covered with enamel. The root area is covered with cementum.
- The ***pulp cavity*** is the area within the crown and roots of the tooth that is surrounded by the dentin to protect the delicate pulp of the tooth. In the roots, the pulp continues in the space known as the ***root canals***.
- The ***pulp*** itself consists of a rich supply of blood vessels and nerves that provide nutrients and innervation to the tooth.

Saliva and Salivary Glands

Saliva is a colorless liquid that maintains the moisture in the mouth. It helps maintain the health of the teeth, and it begins the digestive process by lubricating food during chewing and swallowing (mechanical digestion). Saliva also contains the digestive enzyme ***amylase*** and is the first step in chemical digestion.

The three pairs of **salivary glands** (**SAL**-ih-ver-ee) secrete saliva that is carried by ducts into the mouth (Figure 9.5).

- The ***parotid glands*** are located on the face, slightly in front of each ear. The ducts for these glands are on the inside of the cheek near the upper molars.
- The ***sublingual glands*** and their ducts are located on the floor of the mouth under the tongue.
- The ***submandibular glands*** and their ducts are located on the floor of the mouth near the mandible.

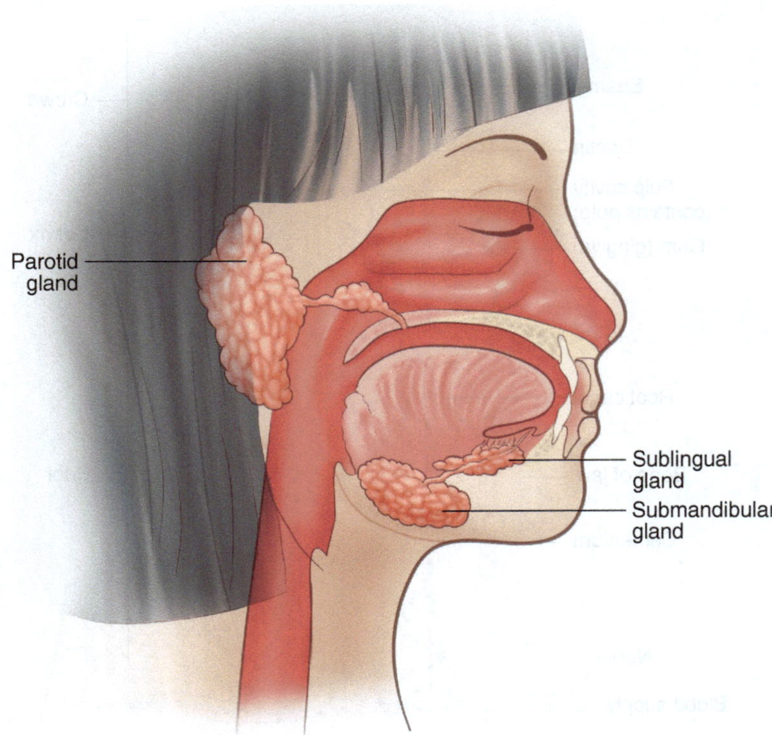

FIGURE 9.5 The salivary glands.

The Pharynx

The **pharynx** (**FAH**-rinks), which is the common passageway for both respiration and digestion, is discussed in Chapter 8.

- The pharynx plays an important role in ***deglutition***, which is commonly known as swallowing.
- The ***epiglottis*** (**ep**-ih-**GLOT**-is) is a lid-like structure that closes off the entrance to the trachea (windpipe) to prevent food and liquids from moving from the pharynx during swallowing. This is discussed further in Chapter 8.

The Esophagus

The **esophagus** (eh-**SOF**-ah-gus) is the muscular tube through which ingested food passes from the pharynx to the stomach (Figure 9.1).

- The **lower esophageal sphincter**, also known as the ***cardiac sphincter***, is a muscular ring between the esophagus and stomach. During swallowing, it relaxes to allow food to enter the stomach (Figure 9.6).
- This sphincter normally opens to allow the flow of food into the stomach and closes to prevent the stomach contents from regurgitating into the esophagus. ***Regurgitating*** means flowing backward.

The Stomach

The **stomach** is a sac-like organ composed of the ***fundus*** (upper, rounded part), ***body*** (main portion), and ***antrum*** (lower part) (Figure 9.6).

- **Rugae** (**ROO**-gay) are the folds in the mucosa lining the stomach. These folds allow the stomach to increase and decrease in size. Glands located within these folds produce gastric juices.
- **Gastric juices** made up of enzymes and hydrochloric acid aid in the beginning of food digestion. Mucus produced by glands in the stomach creates a protective coating on the lining of the stomach.
- The **pyloric sphincter** (pye-**LOR**-ick) is the ring-like muscle at the base of the stomach that controls the flow of partially digested food from the stomach to the duodenum of the small intestine.
- The **pylorus** (pye-**LOR**-us) is the narrow passage that connects the stomach with the small intestine.

The Small Intestine

The **small intestine** extends from the pyloric sphincter to the first part of the large intestine. This coiled organ is up to 20 feet in length and consists of three sections where food is digested and the nutrients are absorbed into the bloodstream (see Figure 9.1).

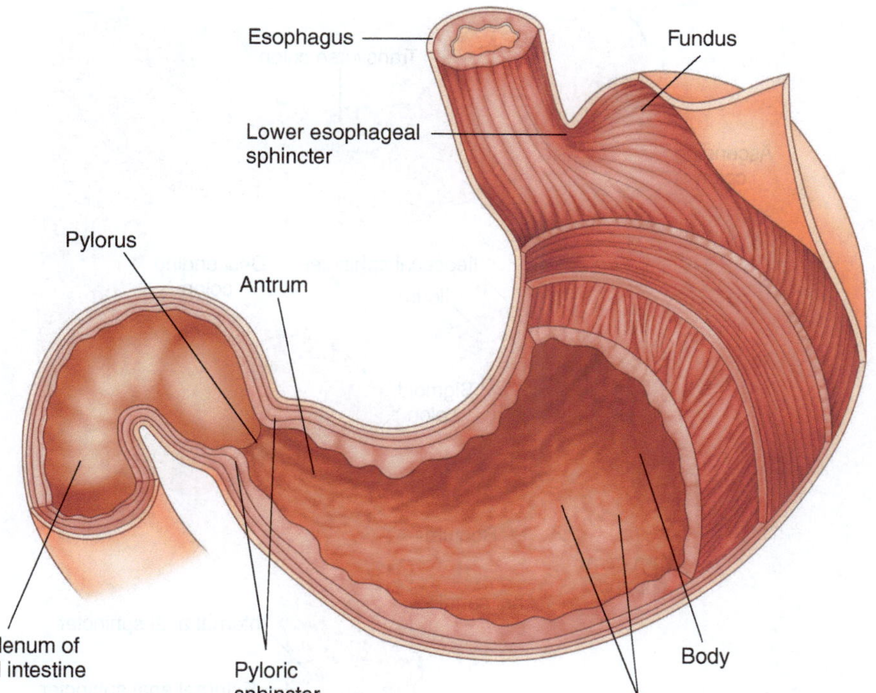

FIGURE 9.6 Structures of the stomach.

1. The **duodenum** (**dew**-oh-**DEE**-num) is the first portion of the small intestine. The duodenum extends from the pylorus of the stomach to the jejunum.
2. The **jejunum** (jeh-**JOO**-num), which is the middle portion of the small intestine, extends from the duodenum to the ileum.
3. The **ileum** (**ILL**-ee-um), which is the last and longest portion of the small intestine, extends from the jejunum to the cecum of the large intestine.

The Large Intestine

The **large intestine** extends from the end of the small intestine to the anus. It is about twice as wide as the small intestine; however, it is only one-fourth as long. It is here that the waste products of digestion are processed in preparation for excretion through the anus. The major parts of the large intestine are the cecum, colon, rectum, and anus (Figure 9.7).

The Cecum

The **cecum** (**SEE**-kum) is a pouch that lies on the right side of the abdomen. It extends from the end of the ileum to the beginning of the colon.

- The **ileocecal sphincter** (**ill**-ee-oh-**SEE**-kull) is the ring-like muscle that controls the flow from the ileum of the small intestine into the cecum of the large intestine (Figure 9.7).
- The **vermiform appendix**, commonly called the ***appendix***, hangs from the lower portion of the cecum. The term ***vermiform*** refers to a worm-like shape. The appendix, which consists of lymphoid tissue, is discussed in Chapter 7.

The Colon

The **colon**, which is the longest portion of the large intestine, is subdivided into four parts (Figure 9.7):

- The **ascending colon** travels upward from the cecum to the undersurface of the liver. ***Ascending*** means upward.
- The **transverse colon** passes horizontally across the abdominal cavity from right to left toward the spleen. ***Transverse*** means across.
- The **descending colon** travels down the left side of the abdominal cavity to the sigmoid colon. ***Descending*** means downward.
- The **sigmoid colon** (**SIG**-moid) is an S-shaped structure that continues from the descending colon above and joins the rectum below. ***Sigmoid*** means curved like the letter *S*.

The Rectum and Anus

- The **rectum** is the widest division of the large intestine. It makes up the last 4 inches of the large intestine and ends at the anus.

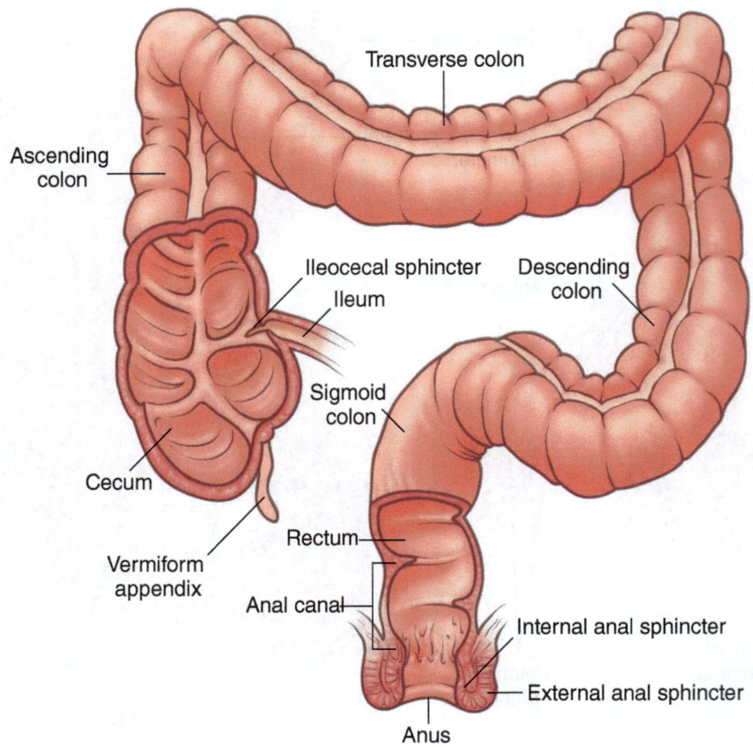

FIGURE 9.7 Structures of the large intestine.

- The **anus** is the lower opening of the digestive tract. The flow of waste through the anus is controlled by the *internal anal sphincter* and the *external anal sphincter*.
- The term **anorectal** (**ah**-noh-**RECK**-tal) refers to the anus and rectum as a single unit (**an/o** means anus, **rect** means rectum, and **-al** means pertaining to).

Accessory Digestive Organs

The **accessory organs** of the digestive system are so named because they play a key role in the digestive process but are not part of the gastrointestinal tract (Figure 9.8). The accessory digestive organs are the liver, gallbladder, and pancreas.

The Liver

The **liver** is the largest organ in the body (Figure 9.8). It has several important functions related to removing toxins from the blood and turning food into the fuel and nutrients the body needs. The term **hepatic** means pertaining to the liver (**hepat** means liver, and **-ic** means pertaining to).

- The liver removes excess glucose, which is commonly known as blood sugar, from the bloodstream and stores it as glycogen. **Glycogen** is a form of glucose that is stored in the liver and muscles. When the blood sugar level is low, the liver converts glycogen back into glucose and releases it for use by the body. Glucose and glycogen are discussed further in Chapter 14.
- **Bile**, which aids in the digestion of fats, is a digestive juice secreted by the liver that is necessary for the digestion of fat. Bile travels from the liver to the gallbladder, where it is concentrated and stored. The word part **chol/e** refers to bile.
- **Bilirubin** (bill-ih-**ROO**-bin) is a pigment formed in the liver by the breakdown of hemoglobin and excreted in bile, giving it a yellow to green color. Excessive amounts of bilirubin in the body can lead to jaundice and other diseases.

The Biliary Tree

The **biliary** tree (**BILL**-ee-air-ee) provides the channels through which bile is transported from the liver to the small intestine. Biliary means pertaining to bile.

- Small ducts in the liver join together like branches to form the biliary tree. The trunk, which is just outside the liver, is known as the *common hepatic duct*.
- The bile travels from the liver through the common hepatic duct to the gallbladder where it enters and exits through the narrow *cystic duct*.
- The cystic duct leaving the gallbladder rejoins the common hepatic duct to form the *common bile duct*.

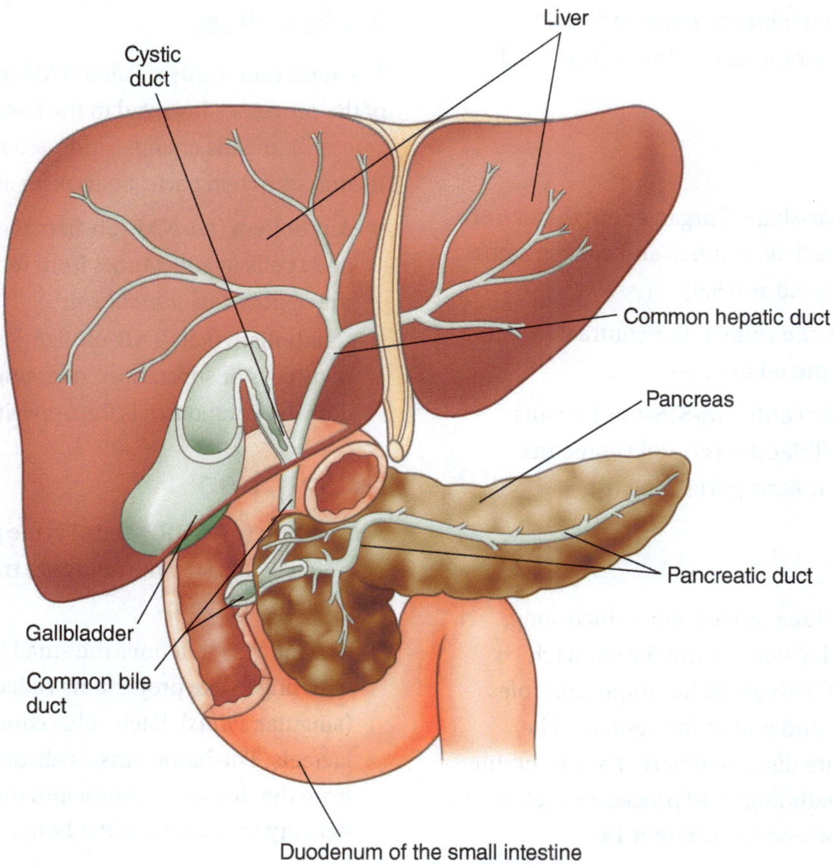

FIGURE 9.8 Accessory digestive organs: the liver, gallbladder, and pancreas.

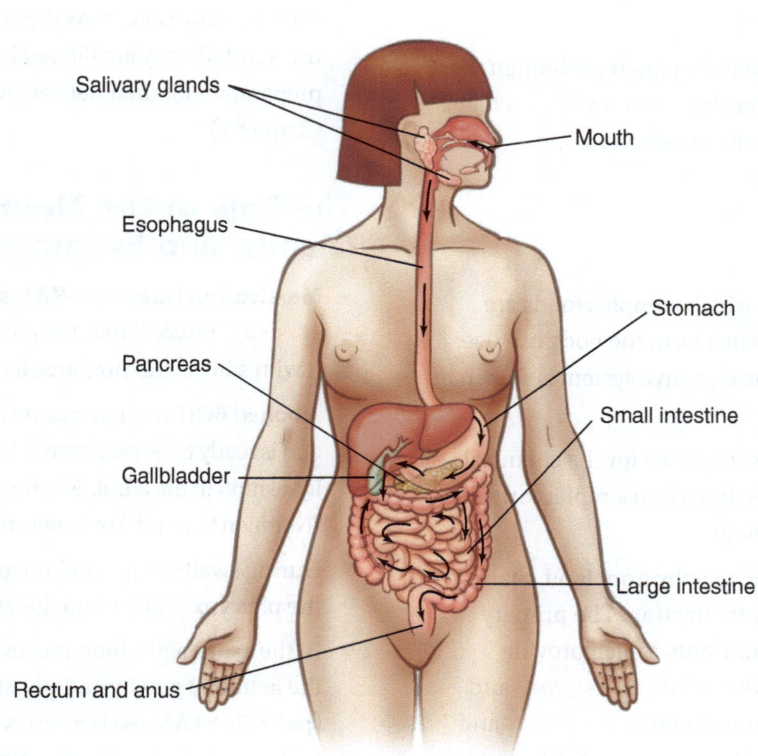

FIGURE 9.9 The pathway of food through the digestive system.

The common bile duct joins the *pancreatic duct*, and together they enter the duodenum of the small intestine.

The Gallbladder

The **gallbladder** is a pear-shaped organ about the size of an egg located under the liver. It stores and concentrates bile for later use (Figures 9.8 and 9.9).

- When bile is needed, the gallbladder contracts, forcing the bile out through the biliary tree.
- The term **cholecystic** (**koh**-luh-**SIS**-tick) means pertaining to the gallbladder (**cholecyst** means gallbladder, and **-ic** means pertaining to).

The Pancreas

- The **pancreas** (**PAN**-kree-as) is a soft, 6-inch-long, oblong gland that is located behind the stomach (Figures 9.8 and 9.9). This gland has important roles in both the digestive and endocrine systems. The digestive functions are discussed here. The endocrine functions, plus the pathology and procedures related to the pancreas, are discussed in Chapter 14.
- The pancreas produces and secretes *pancreatic juices* that aid in digestion and contain digestive enzymes and sodium bicarbonate to help neutralize stomach acids. *Pancreatic* means pertaining to the pancreas.
- The pancreatic juices leave the pancreas through the *pancreatic duct* that joins the *common bile duct* just before the entrance into the duodenum.

DIGESTION

Digestion is the process by which complex foods are broken down into nutrients in a form the body can use. The flow of food through the digestive system is shown in Figure 9.9.

- *Digestive enzymes* are responsible for the chemical changes that break foods down into simpler forms of nutrients for use by the body.
- A **nutrient** is a substance, usually from food, that is necessary for the body to function. The primary nutrients, called macronutrients, which provide the body with calories are *carbohydrates*, *fats*, and *proteins*. A **calorie** is a unit of energy. *Vitamins* and *minerals* are essential micronutrients, which means they are required only in small amounts.

Metabolism

The term **metabolism** (meh-**TAB**-oh-lizm) includes all of the processes involved in the body's use of nutrients (**metabol** means change, and **-ism** means condition). It consists of two parts: anabolism and catabolism.

- **Anabolism** (an-**NAB**-oh-lizm) is the building up of body cells or substances from nutrients. Anabolism is the opposite of *catabolism*.
- **Catabolism** (kah-**TAB**-oh-lizm) is the breaking down of body cells or substances, releasing energy and carbon dioxide. Catabolism is the opposite of *anabolism*.

Absorption

Absorption (ab-**SORP**-shun) is the process by which completely digested nutrients are transported to the cells throughout the body.

- The mucosa that lines the small intestine is covered with finger-like projections called **villi** (**VILL**-eye) (singular, *villus*). Each villus contains blood vessels and lacteals. The blood vessels absorb nutrients directly from the digestive system into the bloodstream for delivery to the cells of the body.
- The *lacteals*, which are specialized structures of the lymphatic system, absorb fats and fat-soluble vitamins that cannot be transported directly by the bloodstream. Instead they absorb these nutrients and transport them via lymphatic vessels. As these nutrients are being transported, they are filtered by the lymph nodes in preparation for their delivery to the bloodstream (see Chapter 7).

The Role of the Mouth, Salivary Glands, and Esophagus

- **Mastication** (**mass**-tih-**KAY**-shun), also known as *chewing*, breaks food down into smaller pieces, mixes it with saliva, and prepares it to be swallowed.
- A **bolus** (**BOH**-lus) is a mass of food that has been chewed and is ready to be swallowed. The term *bolus* is also used in relation to the administration of tube feeding (see "Nutrition Support") or medication, discussed in Chapter 22.
- During swallowing, food travels from the mouth into the pharynx and on into the esophagus.
- In the esophagus, food moves downward through the action of gravity and peristalsis. **Peristalsis** (**pehr**-ih-**STAL**-sis) is a series of wave-like contractions of the smooth muscles in a single direction that moves the food forward into the digestive system.

The Role of the Stomach

- The gastric juices of the stomach contain hydrochloric acid and digestive enzymes to continue the breakdown of food. Few nutrients enter the bloodstream through the walls of the stomach.
- The churning action of the stomach works with the gastric juices by converting the food into chyme. **Chyme** (**KYM**) is the semifluid mass of partly digested food that passes out of the stomach, through the pyloric sphincter, and into the small intestine.

The Role of the Small Intestine

The conversion of food into usable nutrients is completed as the chyme is moved through the small intestine by peristaltic action.

- In the duodenum, chyme is mixed with pancreatic juice and bile. The bile breaks apart large fat globules so that enzymes in the pancreatic juices can digest the fats. This action is called ***emulsification*** and must be completed before the nutrients can be absorbed into the body.
- The jejunum secretes large amounts of digestive enzymes and continues the process of digestion.
- The primary function of the ileum is to absorb nutrients from the digested food.

The Role of the Large Intestine

The role of the entire large intestine is to receive the waste products of digestion and store them until they are eliminated from the body.

- Food waste enters the large intestine where excess water is reabsorbed into the body through the walls of the large intestine, helping maintain the body's fluid balance. The remaining waste forms into feces.
- **Feces** (**FEE**-seez), also known as ***solid body waste*** or ***stool***, are expelled through the rectum and anus.
- **Defecation** (**def**-eh-**KAY**-shun), also known as a ***bowel movement*** (BM), is the evacuation or emptying of the large intestine.
- The large intestine contains gut microbiota, which help break down organic waste material. This process produces gas.
- ***Gut microbiota*** refers to the billions of bacteria present in the large intestine to protect against infection and help maintain the immune system. Studies are ongoing that show a link between gut microbiota and various physical and mental health diseases.
- **Borborygmus** (**bor**-boh-**RIG**-mus) is the rumbling noise caused by the movement of gas in the intestine.
- **Flatulence** (**FLAT**-you-lens) is the passage of gas also called ***flatus*** out of the body through the rectum.

MEDICAL SPECIALTIES RELATED TO THE DIGESTIVE SYSTEM

- **Bariatrics** (**bayr**-ee-**AT**-ricks) is the branch of medicine concerned with the prevention and management of obesity and associated diseases.
- A **dentist** holds a doctor of dental surgery (DDS) or doctor of medical dentistry (DMD) degree and specializes in diagnosing and treating diseases and disorders of teeth and tissues of the oral cavity. A ***prosthodontist*** is a dentist who specializes in the restoration and replacement of teeth.
- A **gastroenterologist** (**gas**-troh-**en**-ter-**OL**-oh-jist) is a physician who specializes in diagnosing and treating diseases and disorders of the stomach and intestines (**gastr/o** means stomach, **enter** means small intestine, and **-ologist** means specialist).
- An **oral** or **maxillofacial surgeon** (mack-**sill**-oh-**FAY**-shul) specializes in surgery of the face and jaws to correct deformities, treat diseases, and repair injuries.
- An **orthodontist** (**or**-thoh-**DON**-tist) is a dental specialist who prevents or corrects malocclusion of the teeth and related facial structures (**orth** means straight or normal, **odont** means the teeth, and **-ist** means specialist).
- A **periodontist** (**pehr**-ee-oh-**DON**-tist) is a dental specialist who prevents or treats disorders of the tissues surrounding the teeth (**peri-** means surrounding, **odont** means the teeth, and **-ist** means specialist).
- A **proctologist** (prock-**TOL**-oh-jist) is a physician who specializes in disorders of the colon, rectum, and anus (**proct** means anus and rectum, and **-ologist** means specialist).
- A **registered dietitian** (RD) or **registered dietitian nutritionist** (RDN) is a specialist in food and nutrition who practices medical nutrition therapy and counsels patients on improving their dietary intake.

PATHOLOGY OF THE DIGESTIVE SYSTEM

Tissues of the Oral Cavity

- **Canker sores**, also known as ***aphthous ulcers***, are gray-white pits with a red border in the soft tissues lining the mouth. Although the exact cause is unknown, the appearance of these very common sores is associated with stress, certain foods, or fever.
- An ***ulcer*** is an open lesion of the skin or mucous membrane resulting in tissue loss around the edges (see Chapter 13).
- **Cheilitis** (kye-**LITE**-is), also known as ***cheilosis***, is inflammation of the lips characterized by crack-like sores at the corners of the mouth (**cheil** means lips, and **-itis** means inflammation).
- **Cold sores**, also known as ***herpes labialis*** or ***fever blisters***, are blister-like sores on the lips and adjacent facial tissue that are caused by the *oral herpes simplex virus type 1* (HSV-1). Most adults have been infected by this extremely common virus, and in some, it becomes reactivated periodically, causing cold sores.
- **Leukoplakia** (loo-koh-**PLAY**-kee-ah) is an abnormal white, usually benign lesion (sore) that develops on the tongue or the inside of the cheek (**leuk/o** means white, and **-plakia** means plaque). These lesions develop in response to chronic irritation in the mouth such as smoking, chewing tobacco, or constant rubbing against a broken tooth. Occasionally, leukoplakia patches occur on the genitals, in the digestive system, or in the urinary tract.
- **Stomatitis** (**stoh**-mah-**TYE**-tis) is an inflammation of the mucosa of the mouth (**stomat** means mouth or oral cavity, and **-itis** means inflammation). *Note:* The word *stoma*, which occurs in the later section "Ostomies," refers to an artificial mouth-like opening between an organ and the body's surface.
- **Oral thrush** is a fungal infection in the mouth caused by *Candida albicans* (see Chapter 7). The symptoms are creamy white lesions on the tongue or inner cheeks. This condition occurs most often in infants, older adults with weakened immune systems, or individuals who have been taking antibiotics.
- The term **trismus** (**TRIZ**-mus), also known as ***lockjaw***, describes any restriction to the opening of the mouth caused by trauma, surgery, or radiation associated with the treatment of oral cancer. This condition causes difficulty in speaking and affects the patient's nutrition due to impaired ability to chew and swallow.
- **Xerostomia** (**zeer**-oh-**STOH**-mee-ah), also known as ***dry mouth***, is the lack of adequate saliva due to diminished secretions by the salivary glands (**xer/o** means dry, **stom** means mouth or oral cavity, and **-ia** means pertaining to). This condition can be due to medications or radiation of the salivary glands, and can cause discomfort, difficulty in swallowing, changes in the taste of food, and dental decay.

Cleft Lip and Cleft Palate

- A **cleft lip** is a birth defect in which there is a deep groove of the lip running upward to the nose as a result of the failure of this portion of the lip to close during prenatal development.
- A **cleft palate** is the failure of the palate to close during the early development of the fetus. This opening can involve the upper lip, hard palate, and/or soft palate. If not corrected, this opening between the nose and mouth makes it difficult for the child to eat and speak. Cleft lip and cleft palate can occur singly or together and usually can be corrected surgically (Figure 9.10).

Dental Diseases and Conditions

- **Bruxism** (**BRUCK**-sizm) is the involuntary grinding of the teeth that usually occurs during sleep and is associated with tension or stress. It can also occur habitually during the day. Bruxism wears away tooth structure, damages periodontal tissues, and injures the temporomandibular joint.
- **Dental caries** (**KAYR**-eez), also known as ***tooth decay*** or ***cavities***, are an infectious disease caused by bacteria that destroy the enamel and dentin of the tooth. If the decay process is not arrested, the pulp can be exposed and become infected (Figure 9.11).
- **Dental plaque** (**PLACK**), which is a major cause of dental caries and periodontal disease, forms as soft deposits in sheltered areas near the gums and between the teeth. Dental plaque consists of bacteria and bacterial by-products. In contrast, the ***plaque*** associated with heart conditions consists of deposits of cholesterol that form within blood vessels (see Chapter 5).
- **Edentulous** (ee-**DEN**-too-lus) means without teeth. This term describes the situation after the natural permanent teeth have been lost.
- **Halitosis** (hal-ih-**TOH**-sis), also known as ***bad breath***, is an unpleasant odor coming from the mouth that can be caused by dental diseases or respiratory or gastric disorders (**halit** means breath, and **-osis** means abnormal condition or disease).

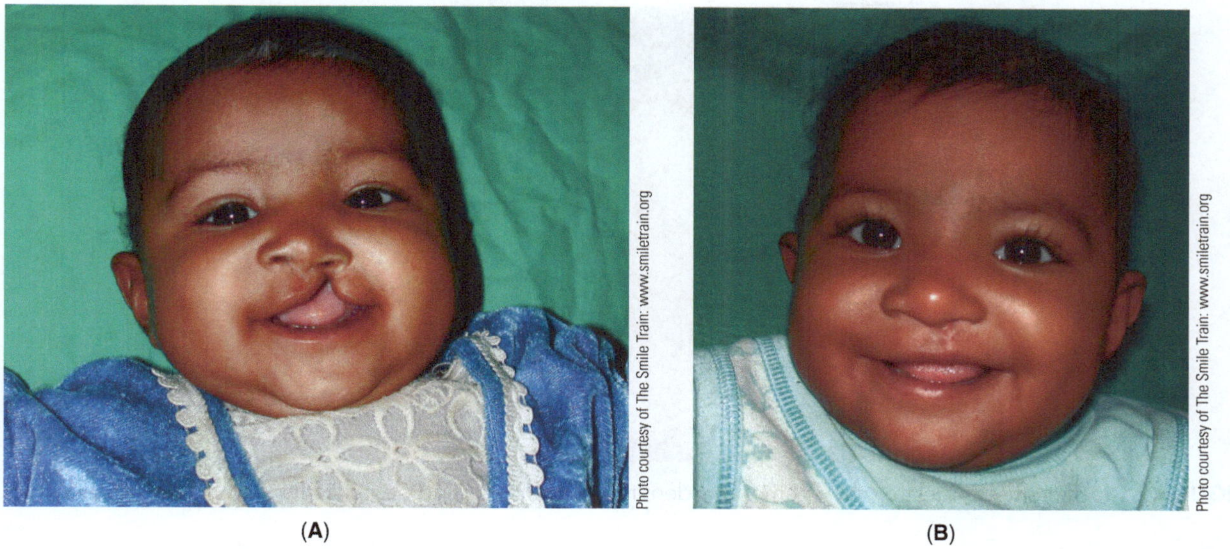

FIGURE 9.10 A child with a cleft palate (A) before and (B) after treatment.

- **Malocclusion** (**mal**-oh-**KLOO**-zhun) is any deviation from the normal positioning of the upper teeth against the lower teeth. In an ***overbite*** there is an excessive overlap of the upper and lower teeth, and in an ***underbite*** the lower teeth are in front of the upper teeth.

Periodontal Disease

Periodontal disease, also known as ***periodontitis***, is an inflammation of the tissues that surround and support the teeth (**peri-** means surrounding, **odont** means tooth or teeth, and **-al** means pertaining to). This progressive disease is classified according to the degree of tissue involvement. In severe cases, the gums and bone surrounding the teeth are involved.

- **Dental calculus** (**KAL**-kyou-luhs), also known as ***tartar***, is dental plaque that has calcified (hardened) on the teeth. These deposits irritate the surrounding tissues and cause increasingly serious periodontal diseases. The term ***calculus*** is also used to describe hard deposits, such as gallstones or kidney stones, that form in other parts of the body.
- **Gum recession** is the shrinking of gingival tissue often associated with aging.
- **Gingivitis** (**jin**-jih-**VYE**-tis) is the earliest stage of periodontal disease, and the inflammation affects only the gums (**gingiv** means gums, and **-itis** means inflammation).
- **Acute necrotizing ulcerative gingivitis** (ANUG), also known as ***trench mouth***, is caused by the abnormal growth of bacteria in the mouth. As this condition progresses, the inflammation, bleeding, deep ulceration, and death of gum tissue become more severe. ***Necrotizing*** means causing ongoing tissue death.

The Esophagus

- **Dysphagia** (dis-**FAY**-jee-ah) is difficulty in swallowing (**dys-** means difficult, and **-phagia** means swallowing).
- **Eosinophilic esophagitis** (**ee**-oh-sin-ah-**FIL**-ik eh-**sof**-ah-**JEYE**-tis) (EoE) is a chronic immune system disease in which a type of white blood cell called an ***eosinophil*** builds up in the esophagus, usually as the result of an allergy to certain foods (**esophag** means esophagus and **-itis** means inflammation). The resulting inflammation can make it difficult to swallow. This disease appears to be increasingly common in children and adults.
- **Gastroesophageal reflux disease** (**gas**-troh-eh-**sof**-ah-**JEE**-al **REE**-flucks), also known as ***GERD***, is the upward flow of acid from the stomach into the esophagus (**gastr/o** means stomach, **esophag** means esophagus, and **-eal** means pertaining to). ***Reflux*** means a backward or return flow. When this occurs, the stomach acid irritates and damages the delicate lining of the esophagus.
- **Barrett's esophagus** is a condition that occurs when the cells in the epithelial tissue of the esophagus are damaged by chronic acid exposure. Some patients with chronic GERD develop this complication, which slightly increases the risk of esophageal cancer.
- A **stricture** of the esophagus resulting from scar tissue or other damage can cause swallowing difficulties. A stricture is an abnormal narrowing of a bodily passage (see also Chapter 10).
- **Pyrosis** (pye-**ROH**-sis), also known as ***heartburn***, is a burning sensation in the chest caused by the return of acidic stomach contents into the esophagus

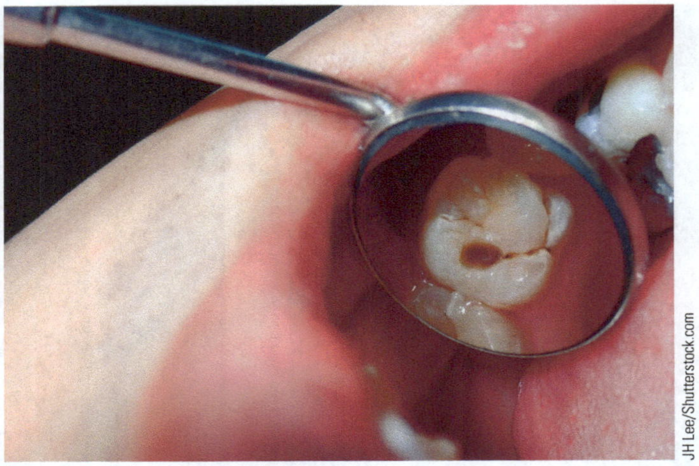

FIGURE 9.11 Bacteria can destroy the enamel and dentin of a tooth, causing dental caries.

(**pyr** means fever or fire, and **-osis** means abnormal condition or disease).

- **Esophageal varices** (eh-**sof**-ah-**JEE**-al **VAYR**-ih-seez) are enlarged and swollen veins at the lower end of the esophagus (singular, *varix*). This condition, which is associated with serious liver diseases, can cause severe bleeding if one of these veins ruptures.
- A **hiatal hernia** (high-**AY**-tal **HER**-nee-ah) is an anatomical abnormality in which a portion of the stomach protrudes upward into the chest, through an opening in the diaphragm (**hiat** means opening, and **-al** means pertaining to). A ***hernia*** is the protrusion of a part or structure through the tissues that normally contain it. This condition can cause GERD and pyrosis (Figure 9.12).

The Stomach

- **Gastritis** (gas-**TRY**-tis) is a common inflammation of the stomach lining that can cause nausea and vomiting. In chronic cases it is often caused by the bacterium *Helicobacter pylori* (**gastr** means stomach, and **-itis** means inflammation).
- **Gastroenteritis** (**gas**-troh-en-ter-**EYE**-tis) is an inflammation of the mucous membrane lining the stomach and intestines (**gastr/o** means stomach, **enter** means small intestine, and **-itis** means inflammation).
- **Gastroparesis** (**gas**-troh-pah-**REE**-sis) is a condition in which gastric motility slows down, causing delayed gastric emptying (**gastr/o** means stomach, and **-paresis** means partial paralysis).

Peptic Ulcers

Peptic ulcer disease (**UL**-ser) (PUD) is characterized by sores that affect the mucous membranes of the digestive system (**pept** means digestion, and **-ic** means pertaining to). Peptic ulcers are caused by the bacterium *Helicobacter pylori* or by medications, such as aspirin, that irritate the mucous membranes (Figure 9.13).

- ***Gastric ulcers*** are peptic ulcers that occur in the stomach.
- ***Duodenal ulcers*** are peptic ulcers that occur in the upper part of the small intestine.

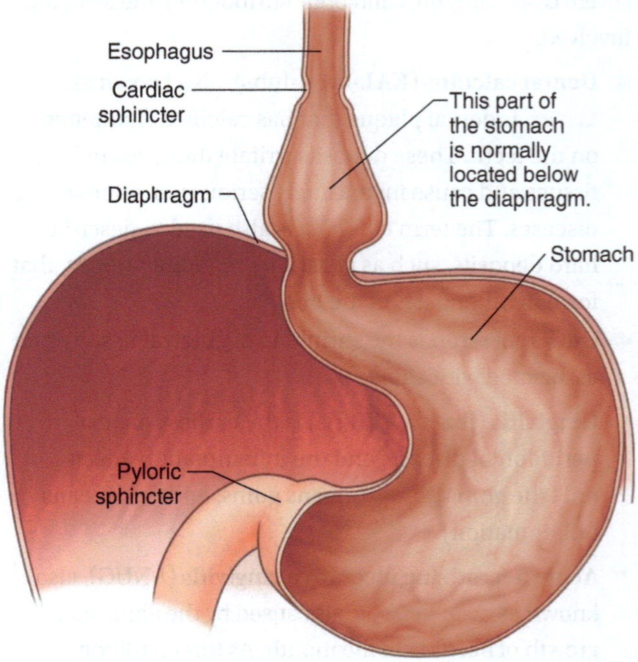

FIGURE 9.12 In a hiatal hernia, part of the stomach protrudes through the esophageal opening in the diaphragm.

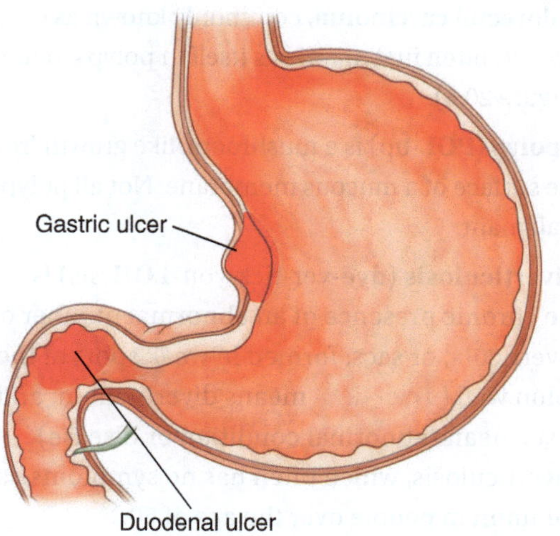

FIGURE 9.13 The locations of peptic ulcers: gastric and duodenal.

- A *perforated ulcer* is a complication of a peptic ulcer in which the ulcer erodes through the entire thickness of the organ wall.

Nutritional Disorders

- **Anorexia** (**an**-oh-**RECK**-see-ah) is the loss of appetite for food, especially when caused by disease (**an-** means without, and **-orexia** means appetite). Anorexia nervosa and other eating disorders are discussed under "Mental Health" in Chapter 17.
- **Cachexia** (kah-**KEKS**-eeh-ah) is a condition of physical wasting away due to the loss of weight and muscle mass that occurs in patients with diseases such as advanced cancer or AIDS. Although these patients might be eating enough food, their bodies are unable to absorb enough nutrients.
- **Dehydration** is a condition in which fluid loss exceeds fluid intake and disrupts the body's normal electrolyte balance (**de-** means removal, **hydra** means water, and **-tion** means the process of).
- **Failure to thrive** (FTT) is when an infant or child does not grow as expected due to any number of reasons including malabsorption or malnutrition.
- **Malabsorption** (**mal**-ab-**SORP**-shun) is a condition in which the small intestine cannot absorb nutrients from food that passes through it. **Mal-** is a prefix meaning bad or poor.
- **Malnutrition** is a lack of proper food or nutrients in the body due to a shortage of food, poor eating habits, or the inability of the body to digest, absorb, and distribute these nutrients.

Overweight and Obesity

Overweight and **obesity** (oh-**BEE**-sih-tee) are weight classifications based on BMI that are higher than a healthy weight for someone based on their height, gender, and age.

- The **body mass index** (BMI) is a ratio of weight in kilograms divided by height in meters squared. The results fall into one of these categories for adults: underweight (18.5 kg/m^2–20 kg/m^2), normal (20 kg/m^2–25 kg/m^2), overweight (25 kg/m^2–30 kg/m^2), or obese (>30 kg/m^2). A high BMI is one of many factors related to developing chronic diseases such as heart disease, cancer, or diabetes. For children under the age of 19, BMI is expressed as a percentile according to the growth chart.

Severe obesity (oh-**BEE**-sih-tee) is the condition of having a body mass index value greater than 40. BMI can indicate a high level of body fat but is not a measure of body fat.

- Obesity is frequently present as a comorbidity with conditions such as metabolic syndrome (Chapter 2), hypertension (Chapter 5), and diabetes (Chapter 14). *Comorbidity* describes the presence of more than one disease or health condition in an individual at a given time.

Indigestion and Vomiting

- **Aerophagia** (**ayr**-oh-**FAY**-jee-ah) is the excessive swallowing of air while eating or drinking and is a common cause of gas in the stomach (**aer/o** means air, and **-phagia** means swallowing).
- **Dyspepsia** (dis-**PEP**-see-ah), also known as *indigestion*, is pain or discomfort during the digestion process (**dys-** means painful, and **-pepsia** means digestion). *Functional dyspepsia* is recurring indigestion with no known cause.
- **Emesis** (**EM**-eh-sis), also known as *vomiting*, is the reflex ejection of the stomach contents outward through the mouth. Emesis is used either as a standalone term or as the suffix **-emesis**.
- **Eructation** (eh-ruk-**TAY**-shun) is the act of belching or raising gas orally from the stomach.
- **Hematemesis** (**hee**-mah-**TEM**-eh-sis) is the vomiting of coagulated blood (**hemat** means blood, and **-emesis** means vomiting). The substance that is vomited often resembles coffee grounds.
- **Hyperemesis** (**high**-per-**EM**-eh-sis) is extreme, persistent vomiting that can cause dehydration (**hyper-** means excessive, and **-emesis** means vomiting). During the early stages of pregnancy, this is known as *morning sickness*.

- **Nausea** (**NAW**-see-ah) is the urge to vomit.
- **Regurgitation** (ree-**gur**-jih-**TAY**-shun) is the return of swallowed food into the mouth.

Intestinal Disorders

- **Celiac disease** (**SEE**-lee-ak) is an autoimmune disorder characterized by a severe reaction to ingesting gluten. ***Gluten*** is a type of protein found in grains such as wheat, barley, and rye. This common disorder damages the villi of the small intestine and can cause malabsorption.
- **Gluten intolerance**, also known as ***non-celiac gluten sensitivity***, is a response to gluten involving digestive distress but not causing the intestinal tissue damage of celiac disease.
- A **food allergy** is an immune system reaction that occurs after eating a certain food (see Chapter 7).
- **Lactose intolerance** is the inability to digest dairy products due to the absence of the enzyme lactase, which is needed to process the sugar (lactose) found in milk and some other dairy products. Lactose intolerance is particularly common among African Americans and East Asians.
- **Small intestinal bacterial overgrowth** (SIBO) can cause gastrointestinal upset such as gas, bloating, diarrhea, constipation, and nausea.
- **Colorectal carcinoma**, commonly known as ***colon cancer***, often first manifests itself in polyps in the colon (Figure 20.5).
- A **polyp** (**POL**-up) is a mushroom-like growth from the surface of a mucous membrane. Not all polyps are malignant.
- **Diverticulosis** (**dye**-ver-tick-you-**LOH**-sis) is the chronic presence of an abnormal number of diverticula, or sacs, formed in weak spots of the colon wall (**diverticul** means diverticulum, and **-osis** means abnormal condition or disease). Diverticulosis, which often has no symptoms, is more common in people over the age of 50.
- A **diverticulum** (**dye**-ver-**TICK**-you-lum) is a small pouch, or sac, found in the lining or wall of a tubular organ such as the colon (plural, *diverticula*).
- **Diverticulitis** (**dye**-ver-tick-you-**LYE**-tis), which sometimes develops as a result of diverticulosis, is the inflammation or infection of one or more diverticulum in the colon (**diverticul** means diverticulum, and **-itis** means inflammation). Symptoms of this condition can include sudden abdominal pain, cramping, and nausea (Figure 9.14).
- **Enteritis** (**en**-ter-**EYE**-tis) is an inflammation of the small intestine caused by ingesting substances contaminated with viral or bacterial pathogens which causes diarrhea (**enter** means small intestine, and **-itis** means inflammation).

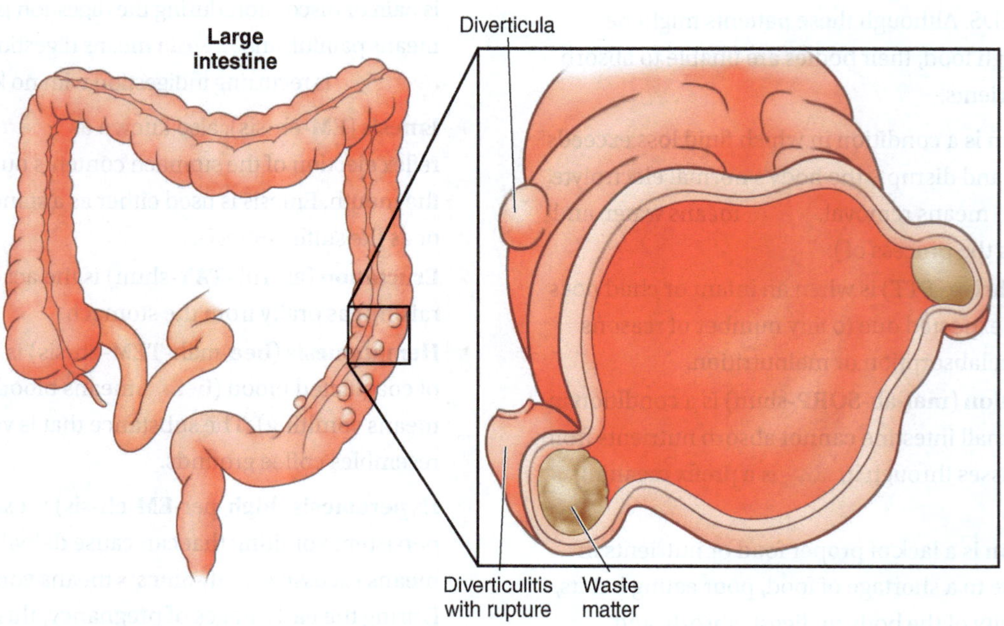

FIGURE 9.14 Diverticulitis is the inflammation of one or more diverticula in the colon.

- **Ischemic colitis** (is-**KEY**-mick koh-**LYE**-tis) occurs when part of the large intestine is partially or completely deprived of blood. If this lack of blood persists, it can lead to inflammation and permanent damage of the affected area.

Ileus

Ileus (**ILL**-ee-us) is the partial or complete blockage of the small or large intestine. This condition is also known as *paralytic ileus*, and it is caused by the stopping of the normal peristalsis of this area of the intestine. Symptoms of ileus can include severe pain, cramping, abdominal distention, vomiting, and the inability to pass gas or stools.

Postoperative ileus is a temporary impairment (stoppage) of bowel action that is considered to be a normal response to abdominal surgery. It is often present for 24 to 72 hours, depending on which part of the digestive system was treated.

Irritable Bowel Syndrome

Irritable bowel syndrome (IBS) is a common condition of unknown cause with symptoms that can include intermittent cramping and abdominal pain, accompanied by constipation or diarrhea. This condition, which is usually aggravated by stress and by eating certain foods (such as those high in fermentable short-chain carbohydrates or FODMAPs), is not believed to be caused by pathogens (bacteria or viruses).

Inflammatory Bowel Diseases

Inflammatory bowel disease (IBD) is the general name for diseases that cause inflammation and swelling in the intestines. The two most common inflammatory bowel diseases are ulcerative colitis and Crohn's disease. These conditions are becoming more common and can increase risk of colorectal cancer.

- These conditions are grouped together because both are chronic and incurable and can affect the large and small intestines. They also have similar symptoms, which can include abdominal pain, weight loss, fatigue, fever, rectal bleeding, *enteropathic arthritis*, and diarrhea.
- These conditions tend to occur at intervals of active disease known as *flares* alternating with periods of remission.

Ulcerative Colitis

Ulcerative colitis (**UL**-ser-**ay**-tiv koh-**LYE**-tis) (UC) is a chronic condition of unknown cause in which repeated episodes of inflammation in the rectum and large intestine cause ulcers (lesions in the mucous membrane) and irritation (**col** means colon, and **-itis** means inflammation) (Figure 9.15).

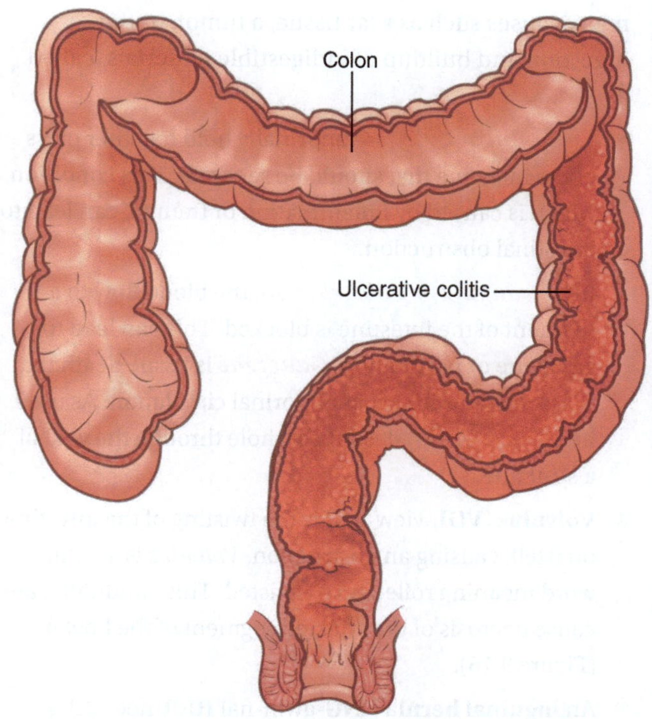

FIGURE 9.15 Ulcerative colitis causes ulcers and irritation in the rectum and large intestine.

- Ulcerative colitis usually starts in the rectum and progresses upward to the lower part of the colon; however, it can affect the entire large intestine.
- Ulcerative colitis affects only the innermost lining and not the deep tissues of the colon.

Crohn's Disease

Crohn's disease (**KROHNZ**) (CD) is a chronic autoimmune disorder that can occur anywhere in the digestive tract; however, it is most often found in the ileum and in the colon.

In contrast to ulcerative colitis, Crohn's disease generally penetrates every layer of tissue in the affected area. This can result in scarring and thickening of the walls of the affected structures. The most common complication of Crohn's disease is blockage of the intestine due to swelling and scarring.

Intestinal Obstructions

An **intestinal obstruction** is the partial or complete blockage of the small or large intestine caused by a physical obstruction. This blockage can result from many causes such as scar tissue, a tumor, or the ingestion and buildup of indigestible materials, called a *bezoar*.

- *Intestinal adhesions* abnormally hold together parts of the intestine that should be separate. This condition, which is caused by inflammation or trauma, can lead to intestinal obstruction.
- In a *strangulating obstruction*, the blood flow to a segment of the intestine is blocked. This can lead to gangrene or perforation. *Gangrene* is tissue death that is associated with a loss of normal circulation. As used here, *perforation* describes a hole through the wall of a structure.
- **Volvulus** (**VOL**-view-lus) is the twisting of the intestine on itself, causing an obstruction. *Volvulus* is a Latin word meaning rolled up or twisted. This condition can cause necrosis of the affected segment of the bowel (Figure 9.16).
- An **inguinal hernia** (**ING**-gwih-nal **HER**-nee-ah) is the protrusion of a small loop of bowel through a weak place in the lower abdominal wall or groin (**inguin** means groin, and **-al** means pertaining to). This condition can be caused by obesity, pregnancy, heavy lifting, or straining to pass a stool.
- A **strangulated hernia** occurs when a portion of the intestine is constricted inside the hernia, causing ischemia (insufficient oxygen) in this tissue by cutting off its blood supply.

Infectious Diseases of the Intestines

Infectious diseases of the intestines can be transmitted through contaminated food and water or through poor sanitation practices. The more common of these infectious diseases include the following:

- **Clostridium difficile** (klos-**TRID**-ee-um dif-us-**SEEL**), also known as *C. diff*, is a common bacterial infection, typically following the use of antibiotics that wipe out competing bacteria. This disease causes diarrhea and can lead to inflammation of the colon. Infection control measures such as hand washing and wearing gloves can help prevent its spread.
- **Dysentery** (**DIS**-en-**ter**-ee), which is a bacterial infection, occurs most frequently in tropical countries where it is spread through food or water contaminated by human feces.
- **E. coli**, which is caused by the bacterium *Escherichia coli*, is transmitted through contaminated foods that have not been adequately cooked.
- **Salmonellosis** (**sal**-muh-nel-**LOH**-sis), also referred to as *salmonella*, is transmitted by feces, either through direct contact with animals, or by eating contaminated raw or undercooked meat, poultry, seafood, and eggs or unpasteurized milk products. It is one of the most common food-borne infections in the United States.

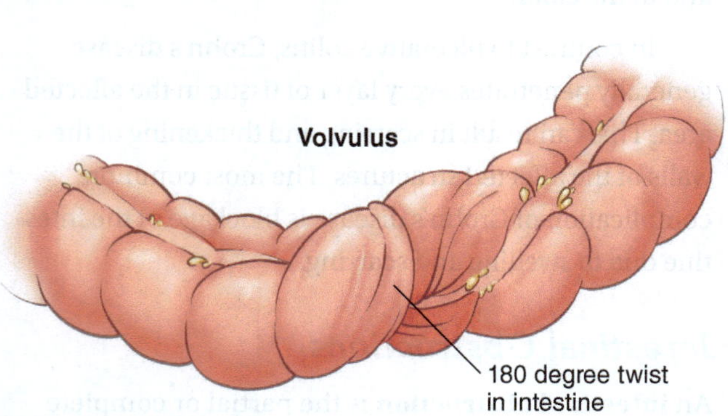

FIGURE 9.16 Volvulus is the twisting of the bowel on itself.

Anorectal and Bowel Movement Pathology

- An **anal fissure** is a small crack-like sore in the skin of the anus that can cause severe pain during a bowel movement. As used here, a *fissure* is a groove or crack-like sore of the skin.
- **Fecal incontinence** (in-**KON**-tih-nents) is the inability to control the excretion of feces. Urinary incontinence is discussed in Chapter 10.
- **Constipation** is defined as having a bowel movement fewer than three times per week. With constipation, stools are usually hard, dry, small in size, and difficult to pass. Constipation can be caused by a lack of fiber in the diet, disease, medication, and (especially in women) pelvic floor dysfunction. *Pelvic floor dysfunction* is the lack of coordination of the muscles needed for the rectum to straighten and the anal sphincter to relax.
- **Diarrhea** (**dye**-ah-**REE**-ah) is an abnormally frequent flow of loose or watery stools and can lead to dehydration (**dia-** means through, and **-rrhea** means flow or discharge).
- **Hemorrhoids** (**HEM**-oh-roids) occur when a cluster of veins, muscles, and tissues slip near or through the anal opening. These veins can become inflamed, resulting in pain, fecal leakage, itching, and bleeding.

- A **rectocele** (**RECK**-toh-seel) is a bulging of the front wall of the rectum into the vagina, usually as the result of childbirth or pregnancy (**rect/o** means rectum, and **-cele** means hernia).

Abnormal Stools

- **Hematochezia** (hee-**mat**-oh-**KEE**-zee-uh) is the presence of bright red blood in the stool. This bright red color usually indicates that the blood is coming from the lower part of the gastrointestinal tract.
- **Melena** (meh-**LEE**-nah), in contrast to *hematochezia*, is the passage of black, tarry, foul-smelling stools. This appearance of the stools is caused by the presence of digested blood and often indicates bleeding in the upper part of the gastrointestinal tract.
- **Steatorrhea** (**stee**-at-oh-**REE**-ah) is the presence of excess fat in the stool (**steat/o** means fat, and **-rrhea** means flow or discharge). This condition, which results in frothy, foul-smelling stools, is usually caused by pancreatic disease, the removal of the gallbladder, or malabsorption disorders.

The Liver

Liver disorders are a major concern because the functioning of the liver is essential to the digestive process.

- **Ascites** (ah-**SIGH**-teez) is an abnormal accumulation of serous fluid in the peritoneal cavity. This condition is usually the result of severe liver disease creating pressure on the liver's blood vessels. As used here, the term ***serous*** means a substance having a watery consistency.
- **Hepatomegaly** (**hep**-ah-toh-**MEG**-ah-lee) is the abnormal enlargement of the liver (**hepat/o** means liver, and **-megaly** means enlargement).
- **Jaundice** (**JAWN**-dis) is a yellow discoloration of the skin, mucous membranes, and eyes. This condition is caused by greater-than-normal amounts of bilirubin in the blood.
- **Hepatitis** (**hep**-ah-**TYE**-tis) is an inflammation of the liver usually caused by a viral infection (**hepat** means liver, and **-itis** means inflammation). Viral hepatitis is the leading cause of liver cancer and the most common reason for liver transplants. The three most common varieties of viral hepatitis are shown in Table 9.1.

Cirrhosis

Cirrhosis (sih-**ROH**-sis) is a chronic degenerative disease of the liver characterized by scarring (**cirrh** means yellow or orange, and **-osis** means abnormal condition or disease). ***Degenerative*** means progressive deterioration resulting in the loss of tissue or organ function.

- Cirrhosis is often caused by excessive alcohol abuse or by viral hepatitis B or C.
- The progress of cirrhosis is marked by the formation of areas of scarred liver tissue that are filled with fat. The liver damage causes abnormal conditions throughout the other body systems (Figure 9.17).

Nonalcoholic Fatty Liver Disease

The term **nonalcoholic fatty liver disease** (NAFLD) describes the accumulation of fat in the liver and is not associated with alcohol consumption. NAFLD is the leading

TABLE 9.1

The ABCs of Hepatitis

HAV	**Hepatitis A virus** is the most prevalent type of hepatitis. This highly contagious condition is transmitted mainly through contamination of food and water with infected fecal matter. A vaccine is available to provide immunity against HAV.
HBV	**Hepatitis B virus** is a bloodborne disease that is transmitted through contact with blood and other body fluids that are contaminated with this virus. A vaccine is available to provide immunity against HBV.
HCV	**Hepatitis C virus** is a bloodborne disease that is spread through contact with blood and other body fluids that are contaminated with this virus. HCV is described as a silent epidemic because it can be present in the body for years and destroy the liver before any symptoms appear. There is no vaccine available to prevent this form of hepatitis.

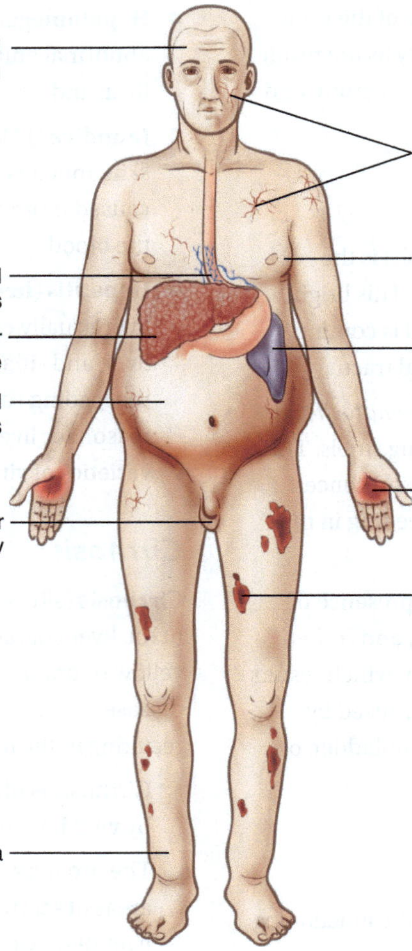

FIGURE 9.17 Clinical conditions associated with cirrhosis of the liver.

liver disorder in the United States. Patients with this disease usually have no signs or symptoms. Common comorbidities include obesity, type 2 diabetes, and high cholesterol.

Nonalcoholic steatohepatitis (**stee**-ah-toh-hep-ah-**TYE**-tis) (NASH) is a more serious form of this condition because it consists of fatty accumulations plus liver-damaging inflammation (**steat/o** means fat, **hepat** means liver, and **-itis** mean inflammation). In some cases, this will progress to cirrhosis, irreversible liver scarring, or liver cancer.

The Gallbladder

- **Cholangitis** (**koh**-lan-**JIGH**-tis) is an acute inflammation of the bile duct characterized by pain in the right upper quadrant of the abdomen, fever, and jaundice (**cholang** means bile duct, and **-itis** means inflammation). The most common cause is a bacterial infection.
- **Cholecystitis** (**koh**-luh-sis-**TYE**-tis) is inflammation of the gallbladder, usually associated with gallstones blocking the flow of bile (**cholecyst** means gallbladder, and **-itis** means inflammation).
- A **gallstone**, also known as a ***cholelith***, is a hard deposit formed in the gallbladder and bile ducts due to the concretion of bile components. The formation of stones is discussed further in Chapter 10.
- **Cholelithiasis** (**koh**-leh-lih-**THIGH**-ah-sis) is the presence of gallstones in the gallbladder or bile ducts (**chole** means bile or gall, and **-lithiasis** means presence of stones).
- Pain caused by the passage of a gallstone through the bile duct is called ***biliary colic***.

The Pancreas

Disorders of the pancreas are discussed in Chapter 14.

DIAGNOSTIC PROCEDURES OF THE DIGESTIVE SYSTEM

- **Abdominal computed tomography** (CT) is a radiographic procedure that uses x-rays to produce a detailed cross-section of the tissue structure within the abdomen, showing, for example, the presence of a tumor or obstruction. CT scans are discussed in Chapter 21.
- An **abdominal ultrasound** is a noninvasive test used to visualize internal organs by using very high-frequency sound waves. Ultrasonography is discussed in Chapter 21.
- **Cholangiography** (koh-**LAN**-jee-**og**-rah-fee) is a radiographic examination of the bile ducts with the use of a contrast medium (**cholangi/o** means bile duct, and **-graphy** means the process of recording). This test is used to identify obstructions in the liver or bile ducts that slow or block the flow of bile from the liver. The resulting record is a ***cholangiogram***.
- An **enema** (**EH**-neh-ma) is the placement of a solution into the rectum and colon to empty the lower intestine through bowel activity. An enema is sometimes part of the preparation for an endoscopic examination; however, enemas are also used to treat severe constipation and as a means of administering medication.
- **Esophagogastroduodenoscopy** (eh-**sof**-ah-goh-**gas**-troh-**dew**-oh-deh-**NOS**-koh-pee) (EGD) is an endoscopic procedure that allows direct visualization of the upper GI tract (**esophag/o** means esophagus, **gastr/o** means stomach, **duoden/o** means duodenum, and **-scopy** means visual examination). This includes the esophagus, stomach, and upper duodenum.
- A **barium swallow study** is a video fluoroscopy test using barium-coated foods or barium-containing liquids of various thicknesses to observe whether there is a danger of food being aspirated into the lungs.
- An **upper GI series** and a **lower GI series** are radiographic studies to examine the digestive system. A contrast medium called **barium** is required to make these structures visible, allowing the flow of the barium to be traced using radiography or fluoroscopy. A ***barium swallow*** is used for the upper GI series, and a ***barium enema*** is used for the lower GI series (see Chapter 21).
- **Stool tests** use a specimen of feces to examine for content and characteristics. Abnormal findings such as blood, fat, nutrients, bacteria, or parasites in the stool can help diagnose disease or malabsorption. A blood test can determine blood nutrient levels, sometimes used to test for deficiencies. For more information on stool analysis, see "Laboratory Tests" in Chapter 21.
- A **breath test** can be used to diagnose certain intestinal disorders and is named for the gas being tested. For example, the test for lactose intolerance is called a ***hydrogen breath test*** because hydrogen is found in excess levels when ingested lactose is not broken down. A breath test can also diagnose small intestine bacterial overgrowth, fructose intolerance, and *Helicobacter pylori* infection.

Endoscopic Procedures

An **endoscope** (**EN**-doh-**skope**) is an instrument used for a visual examination of internal structures (**endo-** means within, and **-scope** means an instrument for visual examination). This examination is called an **endoscopy** (en-**DOS**-koh-pee).

- An **anoscopy** (ah-**NOS**-koh-pee) is the visual examination of the anal canal and lower rectum (**an/o** means anus, and **-scopy** means visual examination).
- A ***capsule endoscopy*** is the use of a tiny video camera in a capsule that the patient swallows. For approximately eight hours, as it passes through the small intestine, this camera transmits images of the walls of the small intestine. The images are detected by sensor devices attached to the patient's abdomen and transmitted to a data recorder worn on the patient's belt.

Colon Screening

The following diagnostic tests can be used for the early detection of polyps that may cause colorectal carcinoma.

- A **colonoscopy** (**koh**-lun-**OSS**-koh-pee) is the direct visual examination of the inner surface of the entire colon from the rectum to the cecum using a colonoscope (**colon/o** means colon, and **-scopy** means visual examination).
- In a ***virtual colonoscopy***, a small, flexible tube is inserted into the rectum and an MRI or CT machine is used to produce two- and three-dimensional images of the colon. The preparation, which requires that the bowels be completely emptied, is the same for both of these types of colonoscopy and the sigmoidoscopy.
- A **sigmoidoscopy** (**sig**-moi-**DOS**-koh-pee) is the endoscopic examination of the interior of the rectum, the sigmoid colon, and possibly a portion of the descending colon (**sigmoid/o** means sigmoid colon, and **-scopy** is the visual examination).
- A **Hemoccult® test** (**HEE**-moh-kult), also known as the ***fecal occult blood test***, is a laboratory test for hidden blood

in stool (**hem** means blood, and **-occult** means hidden). The test kit is used to obtain the specimens at home, and the results are then evaluated in a laboratory.

- ***Cologuard*®** is a recently developed, noninvasive, collect-at-home stool test that uses DNA testing along with screening for hidden blood to determine the potential presence of colorectal cancer.

TREATMENT PROCEDURES OF THE DIGESTIVE SYSTEM

The Oral Cavity and Esophagus

- A **dental prophylaxis** (**proh**-fih-**LACK**-sis) is the professional examining, cleaning, and polishing of the gums and teeth to remove plaque and tartar. Often this includes x-rays to look for cavities. The term ***prophylaxis*** refers to disease prevention. Examples include vaccination to provide immunity against a specific disease.
- A **filling** is the restoration of a decaying tooth by removing the damaged area and replacing it with material to fill it in such as ***amalgam*** from metal or ***composite*** from resin to match the tooth.
- **Orthodontics** is the treatment of alignment and malocclusion of the teeth and jaw. ***Braces*** and retainers are hardware used for this purpose.
- A **dental implant** is the anchoring of a crown, bridge, or denture to the bone of the jaw. Crowns, bridges, and dentures can also be placed in the mouth without being anchored to the jaw.
  - A ***crown*** is a metal or porcelain alloy cap shaped like a tooth cemented over a damaged tooth structure. *Note*: The word *crown* also refers to the portion of the tooth visible in the mouth.
  - A ***bridge*** is a fixed dental prosthesis used to join one or more artificial teeth to the adjacent teeth.
  - A ***denture*** is a plate holding one or more replacement teeth. Conventional dentures, also known as a full or partial set of false teeth, are removable.
- An ***occlusal splint*** is a specially designed mouth guard worn at night to prevent grinding the teeth.
- ***Scaling*** and ***root planing*** is the removal of plaque and tartar below the gum line for the treatment of gum disease.
- The term **root canal** refers both to the pulp cavity in the root of the tooth and to a procedure in which diseased or damaged pulp in the root canal is removed in order to save the tooth. After it is free of infection, the cavity is filled with a protective substance and sealed.
- A **gingivectomy** (**jin**-jih-**VECK**-toh-mee) is the surgical removal of diseased gingival tissue (**gingiv** means gingival tissue, and **-ectomy** means surgical removal).
- **Maxillofacial surgery** (mack-**sill**-oh-**FAY**-shul) is specialized surgery of the face and jaws to correct deformities, treat diseases, and repair injuries.
- **Palatoplasty** (**PAL**-ah-toh-**plas**-tee) is surgical repair of a cleft palate, also used to refer to the repair of a cleft lip (**palat/o** means palate, and **-plasty** means surgical repair) (Figure 9.10).

For more detailed dental terminology, pronunciations, and images, refer to a dental dictionary or dental dictionary application on your computer, tablet, or smartphone.

Antioxidants and Probiotics

- **Antioxidants** (**an**-tee-**OCK**-sih-dantz) are chemicals such as vitamins A, C, and E; carotene; and lutein that may prevent or delay cell damage by blocking the activity of potentially harmful chemicals called *free radicals*. Antioxidants are naturally present in fruits, beans, berries, nuts, and dark chocolate.
- **Probiotics** (**pro**-bye-**AH**-tics) are living microorganisms sometimes described as "good" bacteria because of their role in aiding digestion and protecting the body from harmful bacteria (**pro-** means supporting, **biot** means life, and **-ic** means pertaining to). Probiotics are found in fermented food and beverages such as yogurt, sauerkraut, and kombucha.
- ***Prebiotics*** are the nondigestible carbohydrates that probiotics feed on and are found in fruits, vegetables, and whole grains. Some foods and supplements contain both probiotics and prebiotics.

Medications

- **Antacids**, which neutralize the acids in the stomach, are taken to relieve the discomfort of conditions such as pyrosis or to help peptic ulcers heal.
- **Proton pump inhibitors** (PPI) block the action of the enzyme in the wall of the stomach that produces acid. These medications are used to treat the symptoms of GERD.
- An **antiemetic** (**an**-tee-eh-**MET**-ick) is a medication that is administered to prevent or relieve nausea and vomiting (**anti-** means against, **emet** means vomit, and **-ic** means pertaining to).
- **Laxatives** are medications or foods given to stimulate bowel movements. ***Bulk-forming laxatives***, such as bran, treat constipation by helping fecal matter retain water and remain soft as it moves through the intestines.

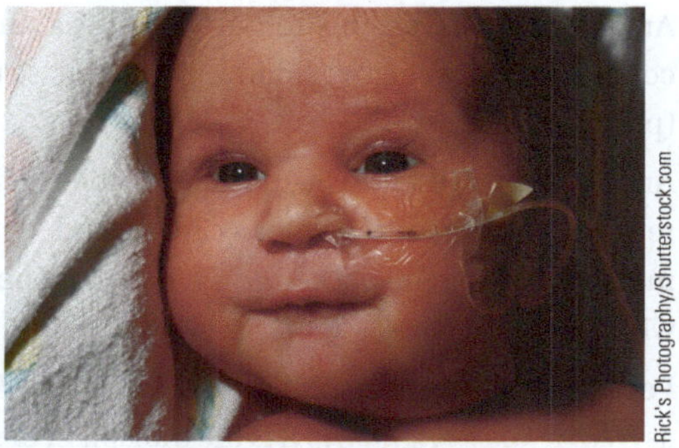

FIGURE 9.18 A baby being fed with a nasogastric tube.

- *Antimotility agents* are over-the-counter medications that reduce diarrhea symptoms by slowing digestion, allowing for more water to be reabsorbed back into the body.
- **Intravenous fluids** (**in**-trah-**VEE**-nus) (IV) are administered to combat the effects of dehydration (**intra** means within, **ven/o** means vein, and **-us** is a noun ending).
- **Oral rehydration therapy** (ORT) is a treatment in which a solution of electrolytes is administered in a liquid preparation to counteract the dehydration that can accompany diarrhea, especially in young children (**re-** means back or again, **hydra** means water, and **-tion** is the process of).

Nutrition Support

Nutrition support is helping a person get the nutrients they need through whatever means possible, such as by mouth (food), via tube (formula), or by vein (solution). This might be food- or nutrient-specific such as prescribing a gluten-free diet to someone with celiac disease. Or, it could be addressing inadequate caloric intake such as prescribing an increase in calories for someone with anorexia or failure to thrive.

- **Enteral nutrition** (EN) is feeding using the digestive system either through eating and drinking by mouth or via *tube feeding* (**enter** means small intestine and **-al** means pertaining to). Tube feedings may be given bolus, a large amount in a short period of time, or continuous, providing calories throughout the day and/or night.
- **Nasogastric intubation** (**nay**-zoh-**GAS**-trick **in**-too-**BAY**-shun) is the placement of a nasogastric feeding tube (NG tube) through the nose and into the stomach (**nas/o** means nose, **gastr** means stomach, and **-ic** means pertaining to). This temporary tube provides nutrition for patients who cannot take sufficient nutrients by mouth (Figures 9.18 and 9.19).
- A **gastrostomy tube** (gas-**TROS**-toh-mee) is a surgically placed feeding tube from the exterior of the body on the abdomen, directly into the stomach (**gastr** means stomach, and **-ostomy** means surgically creating an opening). This is also known as a *G-tube*, and it is used long term to provide nutrition for patients who cannot swallow or take sufficient nutrients by mouth (Figure 9.19). A *jejunostomy tube* is similar but placed from the abdomen into the small intestine rather than the stomach.
- **Parenteral nutrition** (pah-**REN**-ter-al) (PN) or *total parenteral nutrition* (TPN) is administered to patients who cannot or should not get their nutrition through the digestive system. Some or all of the patient's nutritional requirements are met through a specialized solution administered intravenously. *Parenteral* means not in or through the digestive system.

Bariatric Surgery

Bariatric surgery is performed to treat severe obesity by restricting the amount of food that can enter the stomach and be digested. This procedure limits food intake, decreases absorption, and forces a reduction in dietary intake in order to enable weight loss.

- *Gastric bypass surgery*, also known as Roux-en-Y gastric bypass, makes the stomach smaller by stapling a section to create a small pouch and causes food to bypass the first part of the small intestine. This procedure, which

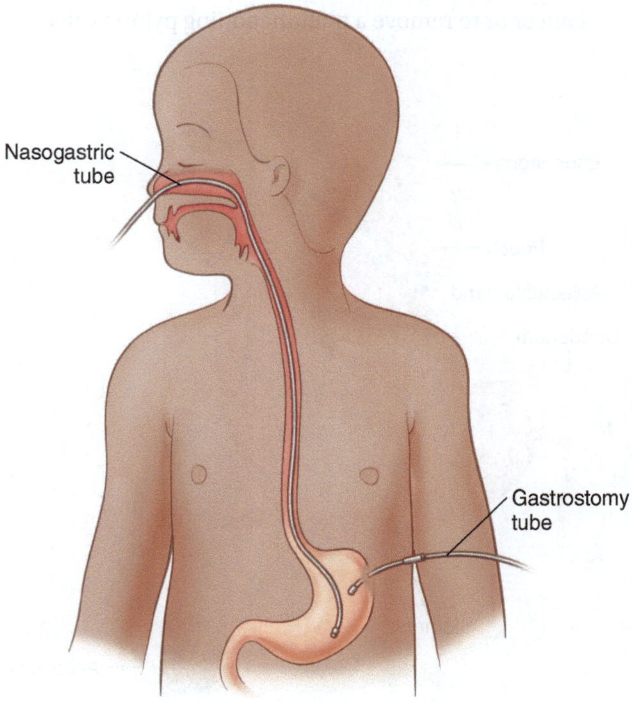

FIGURE 9.19 Nasogastric and gastrostomy tubes can be used to supply nutrition to a child or adult who cannot eat by mouth.

is the most common form of bariatric surgery, is not reversible and carries some risk of complications.

- The ***lap-band*** or ***adjustable gastric banding*** procedure involves placing an inflatable band around the exterior of the stomach to restrict the amount of food that can enter (Figure 9.20). This procedure has the advantage of being reversible through the removal of the band.
- ***Sleeve gastrectomy*** is one of several endoscopic options for bariatric surgeries requiring general anesthesia. In this procedure, the stomach is sutured to make it into a small tube, reducing its capacity by about 75%.

The Intestines

- A **colectomy** (koh-**LECK**-toh-mee) is the surgical removal of all or part of the colon (**col** means colon, and **-ectomy** means surgical removal).
- A **diverticulectomy** (**dye**-ver-**tick**-you-**LECK**-toh-mee) is the surgical removal of a diverticulum (**diverticul** means diverticulum, and **-ectomy** means surgical removal).
- A **gastroduodenostomy** (**gas**-troh-**dew**-oh-deh-**NOS**-toh-mee) is the establishment of an *anastomosis* between the upper portion of the stomach and the duodenum (**gastr/o** means stomach, **duoden** means first part of the small intestine, and **-ostomy** means surgically creating an opening). This procedure is performed to treat stomach cancer or to remove a malfunctioning pyloric valve.

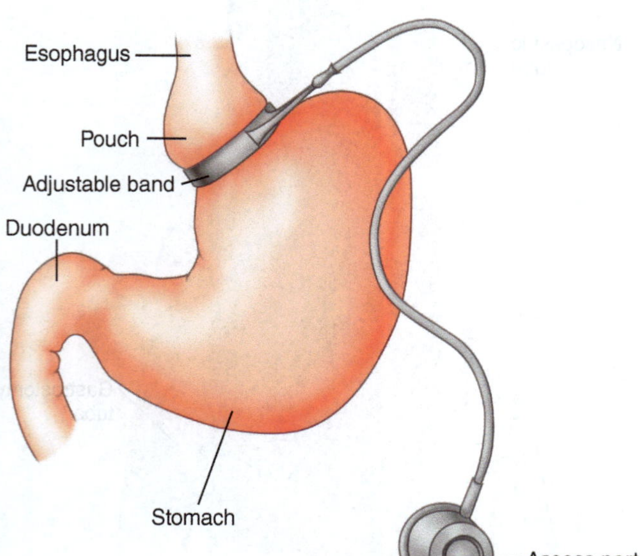

FIGURE 9.20 Lap-band adjustable gastric banding is one type of bariatric surgery.

- An **anastomosis** (ah-**nas**-toh-**MOH**-sis) is a surgical connection between two hollow, or tubular, structures (plural, *anastomoses*).
- An **ileectomy** (**ill**-ee-**ECK**-toh-mee) is the surgical removal of the ileum (**ile** means ileum, and **-ectomy** means surgical removal). *Note:* This term is spelled with a double *e*.
- **Fecal microbiota transplantation** (FMT), also known as ***fecal transplant therapy***, is the transplant of stool from a healthy donor, used to restore gut bacteria. This is used for patients whose frequent antibiotic use to treat *C. difficile* infection has wiped out good bacteria and is being studied to treat other conditions such as IBD.

Ostomies

An **ostomy** (**OSS**-toh-mee) is a surgical procedure to create an artificial opening between an organ and the body surface. This artificial opening is also known as a ***stoma***. *Ostomy* can be used alone as a noun to describe a procedure or as a suffix with the word part that describes the organ involved.

- An **ileostomy** (**ill**-ee-**OS**-toh-mee) is the surgical creation of an artificial excretory opening between the ileum, at the end of the small intestine, and the outside of the abdominal wall (**ile** means small intestine, and **-ostomy** means surgically creating an opening).
- A **colostomy** (koh-**LAHS**-toh-mee) is the surgical creation of an artificial excretory opening between the colon and the body surface (**col** means colon, and **-ostomy** means surgically creating an opening). The segment of the intestine below the ostomy is usually removed, and the fecal matter flows through the stoma

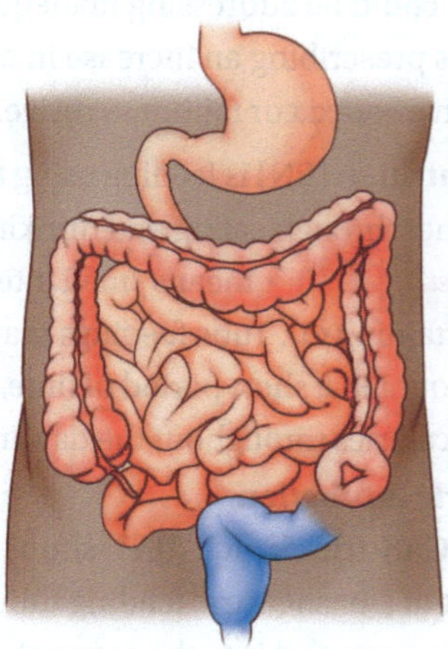

FIGURE 9.21 Colostomy sites are named for the portion of the bowel removed. Shown here is a sigmoid colostomy. The stoma is located at the end of the remaining intestine. The portion that has been removed is shown in blue.

into a disposable bag. A colostomy can be permanent or temporary to divert feces from an area that needs to heal (Figure 9.21).

The Rectum and Anus

- A **hemorrhoidectomy** (**hem**-oh-roid-**ECK**-toh-mee) is the surgical removal of hemorrhoids (**hemorrhoid** means hemorrhoid, and **-ectomy** means surgical removal). ***Rubber band ligation*** can be done instead of surgery. Rubber bands cut off the circulation at the base of an internal hemorrhoid, causing it to eventually fall off. ***Ligation*** means the tying off of blood vessels or ducts.

The Liver

- A **hepatectomy** (**hep**-ah-**TECK**-toh-mee) is the surgical removal of all or part of the liver (**hepat** means liver, and **-ectomy** means surgical removal).
- A **liver transplant** is an option for a patient whose liver has failed for a reason other than liver cancer. Because liver tissue regenerates, a ***partial liver transplant***, in which only part of the organ is donated, can be adequate. A partial liver can be donated by a living donor whose blood and tissue types match.

The Gallbladder

- A **cholecystectomy** (**koh**-luh-sis-**TECK**-toh-mee) is the surgical removal of the gallbladder (**cholecyst** means gallbladder, and **-ectomy** means surgical removal), which is not necessary for survival. An ***open cholecystectomy*** is performed through an incision in the right side of the upper abdomen. A ***laparoscopic cholecystectomy***, also known as a ***lap choley***, is the surgical removal of the gallbladder using a laparoscope and other instruments inserted through three or four small incisions in the abdominal wall. This is performed for the treatment of gallstones, which can commonly reoccur without surgical intervention.

ABBREVIATIONS RELATED TO THE DIGESTIVE SYSTEM

Table 9.2 presents an overview of the abbreviations related to the terms introduced in this chapter. *Note:* To avoid errors or confusion, always be cautious when using abbreviations.

TABLE 9.2

Abbreviations Related to the Digestive System

body mass index = BMI	**BMI** = body mass index
esophagogastroduodenoscopy = EGD	**EGD** = esophagogastroduodenoscopy
failure to thrive = FTT	**FTT** = failure to thrive
fecal microbiota transplantation = FMT	**FMT**= fecal microbiota transplantation
gastroesophageal reflux disease = GERD	**GERD** = gastroesophageal reflux disease
gastrointestinal = GI	**GI** = gastrointestinal
inguinal hernia = IH	**IH** = inguinal hernia
inflammatory bowel disease = IBD	**IBD** = inflammatory bowel disease
irritable bowel syndrome = IBS	**IBS** = irritable bowel syndrome
nasogastric tube = NG tube	**NG tube** = nasogastric tube
nonalcoholic fatty liver disease = NAFLD	**NAFLD** = nonalcoholic fatty liver disease
peptic ulcer disease = PUD	**PUD** = peptic ulcer disease
parenteral nutrition = PN	**PN** = parenteral nutrition
ulcerative colitis = UC	**UC** = ulcerative colitis

CHAPTER 9

LEARNING EXERCISES

Matching Word Parts 1

Write the correct answer in the middle column.

	Definition	Correct Answer	Possible Answers
9.1.	anus	____________	chol/e
9.2.	bile, gall	____________	an/o
9.3.	large intestine	____________	col/o
9.4.	swallowing	____________	enter/o
9.5.	small intestine	____________	-phagia

Matching Word Parts 2

Write the correct answer in the middle column.

	Definition	Correct Answer	Possible Answers
9.6.	stomach	____________	cholecyst/o
9.7.	liver	____________	esophag/o
9.8.	gallbladder	____________	gastr/o
9.9.	esophagus	____________	hepat/o
9.10.	presence of stones	____________	-lithiasis

Matching Word Parts 3

Write the correct answer in the middle column.

	Definition	Correct Answer	Possible Answers
9.11.	sigmoid colon	____________	-pepsia
9.12.	anus and rectum	____________	-emesis
9.13.	digestion	____________	proct/o
9.14.	vomiting	____________	rect/o
9.15.	rectum	____________	sigmoid/o

Definitions

Select the correct answer, and write it on the line provided.

9.16. The visual examination of the anal canal and lower rectum is known as ______________________.

anoscopy colonoscopy endoscopy sigmoidoscopy

9.17. The term ______________________ is an inflammation in the mucosa of the mouth.

salmonellosis leukoplakia stomatitis steatorrhea

9.18. The ______________________ is the last and longest portion of the small intestine.

cecum ileum jejunum pylorus

9.19. The inability to control the excretion of feces is called ______________________.

fecal incontinence constipation anal fissure hematochezia

9.20. The liver secretes ______________________, which is stored in the gallbladder for later use.

bile glycogen insulin pepsin

9.21. The ______________________ travels upward from the cecum to the undersurface of the liver.

ascending colon descending colon sigmoid colon transverse colon

9.22. The process of the building up of body cells and substances from nutrients is known as ______________________.

anabolism catabolism defecation mastication

9.23. The receptors of taste are located on the dorsum of the ______________________.

hard palate rugae tongue uvula

9.24. The bone and soft tissues that surround and support the teeth are known as the ______________________.

dentition gingiva occlusion periodontium

9.25. The condition characterized by the twisting of the intestine on itself, causing an obstruction is ______________________.

borborygmus flatus inguinal hernia volvulus

Matching Structures

Write the correct answer in the middle column.

	Definition	Correct Answer	Possible Answers
9.26.	connects the small and large intestine	______________	cecum
9.27.	S-shaped structure of the large intestine	______________	duodenum
9.28.	widest division of the large intestine	______________	jejunum
9.29.	middle portion of the small intestine	______________	rectum
9.30.	first portion of the small intestine	______________	sigmoid colon

Which Word?

Select the correct answer, and write it on the line provided.

9.31. The medical term meaning vomiting blood is ______________.

hematemesis hyperemesis

9.32. The ______________ virus is transmitted mainly through contamination of food and water with infected fecal matter.

hepatitis A hepatitis B

9.33. ______________ is characterized by a severe reaction to foods containing gluten.

Celiac disease Crohn's disease

9.34. The medical term meaning inflammation of the small intestine is ______________.

colitis enteritis

9.35. The ______________ is the accessory organ responsible for removing toxins from the blood.

gallbladder liver

Spelling Counts

Find the misspelled word in each sentence. Then write that word, spelled correctly, on the line provided.

9.36. An ilectomy is the surgical removal of the last portion of the ileum. ______________

9.37. The bacterial infection disentary occurs mostly in hot countries and is spread through food or water contaminated by human feces. ______________

9.38. The chronic degenerative disease of the liver characterized by scarring is known as serosis.

____

9.39. One example of maloclusion is an underbite where the lower teeth are in front of the upper teeth.

____

9.40. The lack of adequate saliva due to the absence of or diminished secretions by the salivary glands is known as zerostomia. ______________________

Abbreviation Identification

In the space provided, write the words that each abbreviation stands for.

9.41. **UC** ______________________

9.42. **PN** ______________________

9.43. **GERD** ______________________

9.44. **IBS** ______________________

9.45. **PUD** ______________________

Term Selection

Select the correct answer, and write it on the line provided.

9.46. Any deviation from the normal positioning of the upper teeth against the lower teeth is called ______________________.

malocclusion halitosis gingivectomy xerostomia

9.47. The medical term meaning difficulty in swallowing is ______________________.

anorexia dyspepsia dysphagia pyrosis

9.48. The involuntary grinding or clenching of the teeth is called ______________________.

bruxism edentulous malocclusion dental caries

9.49. The chronic degeneration of the liver often caused by excessive alcohol abuse is called ______________________.

cirrhosis hepatitis C hepatitis A hepatomegaly

9.50. Jaundice can be caused by an excess of the pigment ______________________.

bile bilirubin hydrochloric acid pancreatic juice

Sentence Completion

Write the correct term or terms on the lines provided.

9.51. The excessive swallowing of air while eating or drinking is known as ______________________.

9.52. The return of swallowed food to the mouth is known as ______________________.

9.53. A yellow discoloration of the skin caused by greater-than-normal amounts of bilirubin in the blood is called ______________________.

9.54. The ______________________ is the ring-like muscle that controls the flow from the stomach to the small intestine.

9.55. A medical specialist who treats issues related to the digestive system is known as a/an ______________________.

Word Surgery

Divide each term into its component word parts. Write these word parts, in sequence, on the lines provided. When necessary use a slash (/) to indicate a combining vowel. (You may not need all of the lines provided.)

9.56. An **esophagogastroduodenoscopy** is an endoscopic procedure that allows direct visualization of the upper GI tract.

__________ __________ __________ __________

9.57. A **periodontist** is a dental specialist who prevents or treats disorders of the tissues surrounding the teeth.

__________ __________ __________ __________

9.58. A **sigmoidoscopy** is the endoscopic examination of the interior of the rectum, sigmoid colon, and possibly a portion of the descending colon.

__________ __________ __________ __________

9.59. An **antiemetic** is a medication that is administered to prevent or relieve nausea and vomiting.

__________ __________ __________ __________

9.60. A **gastroduodenostomy** is the establishment of an anastomosis between the upper portion of the stomach and the duodenum.

__________ __________ __________ __________

True/False

If the statement is true, write **True** on the line. If the statement is false, write **False** on the line.

9.61. ______ Cholangitis is an acute infection of the bile duct characterized by pain in the upper right quadrant of the abdomen, fever, and jaundice.

9.62. ______ Cholangiography is an endoscopic diagnostic procedure.

9.63. ______ Acute necrotizing ulcerative gingivitis is caused by the abnormal growth of bacteria in the mouth.

9.64. ______ Bruxism means to be without natural teeth.

9.65. ______ Gastroparesis is an inflammation of the mucous membrane lining the stomach and intestines.

Clinical Conditions

Write the correct answer on the line provided.

9.66. James Ridgeview was diagnosed as having ________________, which is the partial or complete blockage of the small or large intestine.

9.67. Chang Hoon suffers from ________________. This condition is an abnormal accumulation of serous fluid in the peritoneal cavity.

9.68. Rita Martinez is a dentist. She described her patient Mr. Espinoza as being ________________, which means that he was without natural teeth.

9.69. Baby Kilgore was vomiting almost continuously. The medical term for this excessive vomiting is ________________.

9.70. A/An ________________ was performed on Mr. Schmidt to create an artificial excretory opening between his colon and body surface.

9.71. After eating, Mike Delahanty often complained about heartburn. The medical term for this condition is ________________.

9.72. After the repeated passage of black, tarry, and foul-smelling stools, Catherine Baldwin was diagnosed as having ________________. This condition is caused by the presence of digested blood in the stools.

9.73. Alberta Roberts was diagnosed as having an inflammation of one or more diverticula. The medical term for this condition is ________________.

9.74. Carlotta Hansen has blister-like sores on her lips and adjacent facial tissue. She says they are cold sores; however, the medical term for this condition is ____________________.

9.75. Lisa Wilson saw her dentist because she was concerned about bad breath. Her dentist refers to this condition as ____________________.

Which Is the Correct Medical Term?

Select the correct answer, and write it on the line provided.

9.76. The ____________________ test detects hidden blood in the stools.

anoscopy colonoscopy enema Hemoccult

9.77. A/An ____________________ is a surgical connection between two hollow or tubular structures.

anastomosis ostomy stoma sphincter

9.78. The anchoring of a crown, bridge, or denture to the bone of the jaw is called a ____________________.

root canal dental implant dental prophylaxis gingivectomy

9.79. The hardened deposit that forms on the teeth and irritates the surrounding tissues is known as ____________________.

dental calculus caries decay plaque

9.80. The surgical removal of all or part of the liver is known as ____________________.

anoplasty palatoplasty cholecystectomy hepatectomy

Challenge Word Building

These terms are *not* primary terms in the chapter; however, they are made up of the following familiar word parts. If you need help in creating the term, refer to your medical dictionary.

col/o	**-algia**
enter/o	**-ectomy**
esophag/o	**-ic**
gastr/o	**-itis**
hepat/o	**-megaly**
proct/o	**-pexy**
sigmoid/o	**-rrhaphy**

9.81. Surgical suturing of a stomach wound is known as ____________.

9.82. Pain in the esophagus is known as ____________.

9.83. The surgical removal of all or part of the sigmoid colon is a/an ____________.

9.84. Pain in and around the anus and rectum is known as ____________.

9.85. The surgical fixation of the stomach to correct displacement is a/an ____________.

9.86. Inflammation of the sigmoid colon is known as ____________.

9.87. The surgical removal of all or part of the esophagus and stomach is a/an ____________.

9.88. The term meaning relating to the liver and intestines is ____________.

9.89. Abnormal enlargement of the intestines is known as ____________.

9.90. Inflammation of the stomach, small intestine, and colon is known as ____________.

Labeling Exercises

Identify the numbered items on the accompanying figure.

9.91. ____________ glands

9.92. ____________

9.93. ____________

9.94. ____________

9.95. ____________

9.96. ____________

9.97. ____________ intestine

9.98. vermiform ____________

9.99. ____________ intestine

9.100. ____________ and anus

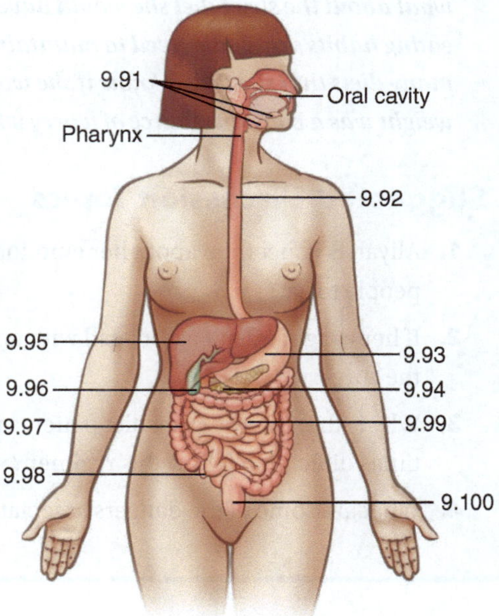

The Human Touch

CRITICAL THINKING EXERCISE

The following story and questions are designed to stimulate critical thinking through class discussion or as a brief essay response. There are no right or wrong answers to these questions.

"Bariatric Info Session: Tuesday at 7:00 PM." Aliyah looked at the flyer in her physician's waiting room, wondering if this would be the week that she would muster the courage to get more information about gastric bypass surgery. Her doctor had been telling her for two years that her elevated BMI, combined with the fact that she had type 2 diabetes, would qualify her for insurance coverage if she decided to have the operation. But surgery seemed so drastic and irreversible. She had recently been motivated by a friend's posts on social media about her weight-loss success story but then her coworker Tim told her that his cousin gained all of his weight back just a few years post-op.

Aliyah felt ashamed that she hadn't been able to lose weight on her own through diet and exercise, despite having worked with a personal trainer and a registered dietitian. Her doctor had told her that part of the bariatric evaluation consisted of meeting with a psychologist to make sure that she would be a good candidate for surgery. She didn't like the idea of talking to someone about her feelings, especially regarding the complicated role that food had always played in her life. And what about the strict diet she would have to follow in the weeks post-surgery—and the changes in eating habits she would need to maintain for the rest of her life? Aliyah had already failed at so many diets that she didn't know if she would have the willpower necessary to succeed. And yet her weight was a constant source of worry when she thought about her health.

Suggested Discussion Topics

1. Aliyah is concerned about her emotional overeating. What reasons besides hunger might cause people to eat?
2. If her weight wasn't associated with any current health problems, should she consider having the surgery?
3. Why is there a very strict diet patients must follow after bariatric surgery, and why is it sometimes difficult to follow this regimen?
4. What are some of the dangers associated with any type of surgery?

CHAPTER **10**

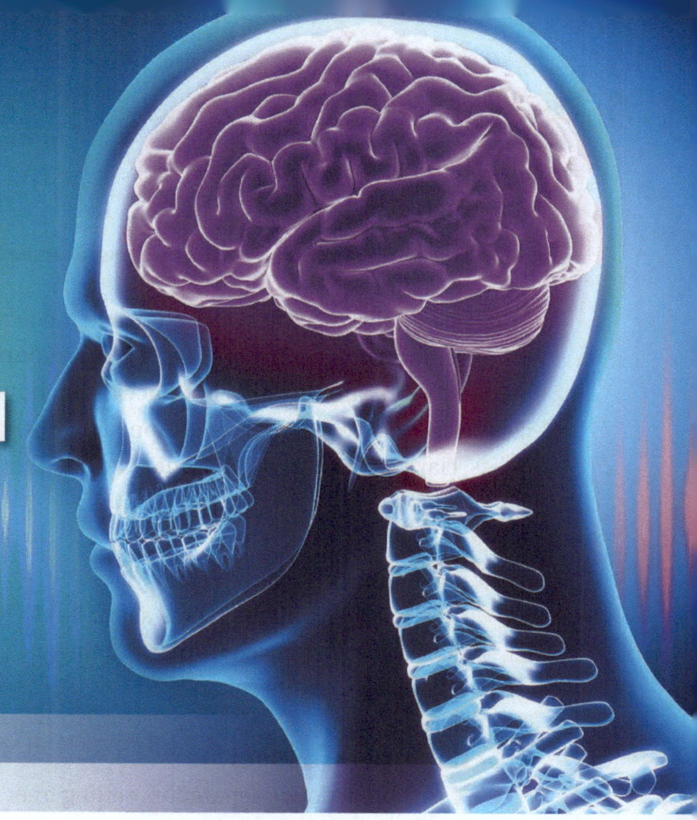

THE URINARY SYSTEM

Overview of **STRUCTURES, COMBINING FORMS, AND FUNCTIONS OF THE URINARY SYSTEM**

Major Structures	Related Combining Forms	Primary Functions
Kidneys	nephr/o, ren/o	Filter the blood to remove waste products, maintain electrolyte concentrations, and remove excess water to maintain the fluid volume within the body.
Renal Pelvis	pyel/o	Collects urine produced by the kidneys.
Urine	ur/o, urin/o	Liquid waste products to be excreted.
Ureters	ureter/o	Transport urine from the kidneys to the bladder.
Urinary Bladder	cyst/o	Stores urine until it is excreted.
Urethra	urethr/o	Transports urine from the bladder through the urethral meatus, where it is excreted.
Prostate	prostat/o	A gland of the male reproductive system that surrounds the male urethra. Disorders of this gland can disrupt the flow of urine.

Vocabulary Related to **THE URINARY SYSTEM**

This list contains essential word parts and medical terms for this chapter. These and the other important **primary terms** are shown in **boldface** throughout the chapter. ***Secondary terms***, which appear in ***orange*** italics, clarify the meaning of primary terms.

Word Parts

- ☐ **-cele** hernia, tumor, swelling
- ☐ **cyst/o** urinary bladder, cyst, sac of fluid
- ☐ **dia-** through, between, apart, complete
- ☐ **glomerul/o** glomerulus
- ☐ **hydr/o** water
- ☐ **lith/o** stone, calculus
- ☐ **-lysis** breakdown, separation, setting free, destruction, loosening
- ☐ **nephr/o** kidney
- ☐ **pyel/o** renal pelvis, bowl of kidney
- ☐ **-tripsy** to crush
- ☐ **ur/o** urine, urinary tract
- ☐ **ureter/o** ureter
- ☐ **urethr/o** urethra
- ☐ **-uria** urination, urine
- ☐ **vesic/o** urinary bladder

Medical Terms

- ☐ **ablation** (ab-**LAY**-shun)
- ☐ **acute renal failure**
- ☐ **anuria** (ah-**NEW**-ree-ah)
- ☐ **benign prostatic hyperplasia** (bee-**NINE** pros-**TAT**-ick **high**-per-**PLAY**-zee-ah)
- ☐ **chronic kidney disease**
- ☐ **cystitis** (sis-**TYE**-tis)
- ☐ **cystocele** (**SIS**-toh-seel)
- ☐ **cystolith** (**SIS**-toh-lith)
- ☐ **cystoscopy** (sis-**TOS**-koh-pee)
- ☐ **dialysis** (dye-**AL**-ih-sis)
- ☐ **diuresis** (**dye**-you-**REE**-sis)
- ☐ **dysuria** (dis-**YOU**-ree-ah)
- ☐ **ectopic kidney**
- ☐ **edema** (eh-**DEE**-mah)
- ☐ **end-stage renal disease**
- ☐ **epispadias** (**ep**-ih-**SPAY**-dee-as)
- ☐ **extracorporeal shockwave lithotripsy** (**ecks**-trah-kor-**POUR**-ee-al **shock**-wayv **LITH**-oh-**trip**-see)
- ☐ **glomerulonephritis** (gloh-**mer**-you-loh-neh-**FRY**-tis)
- ☐ **hemodialysis** (**hee**-moh-dye-**AL**-ih-sis)
- ☐ **hydronephrosis** (**high**-droh-neh-**FROH**-sis)
- ☐ **hydroureter** (**high**-droh-**YOUR**-eh-ter)
- ☐ **hyperproteinuria** (**high**-per-**proh**-tee-in-**YOU**-ree-ah)
- ☐ **hypoproteinemia**
- ☐ **hypospadias** (**high**-poh-**SPAY**-dee-as)
- ☐ **incontinence** (in-**KON**-tih-nents)
- ☐ **interstitial cystitis** (**in**-ter-**STISH**-al sis-**TYE**-tis)
- ☐ **intravenous pyelogram** (**PYE**-eh-loh-**gram**)
- ☐ **nephrolith** (**NEF**-roh-lith)
- ☐ **nephrolithiasis** (**nef**-roh-lih-**THIGH**-ah-sis)
- ☐ **nephrolysis** (neh-**FROL**-ih-sis)
- ☐ **nephrons** (**NEF**-ronz)
- ☐ **nephropathy** (neh-**FROP**-ah-thee)
- ☐ **nephrostomy** (neh-**FROS**-toh-mee)
- ☐ **nephrotic syndrome** (neh-**FROT**-ick)
- ☐ **neurogenic bladder** (new-roh-**JEN**-ick)
- ☐ **nocturia** (nock-**TOO**-ree-ah)
- ☐ **nocturnal enuresis** (**en**-you-**REE**-sis)
- ☐ **oliguria** (**ol**-ih-**GOO**-ree-ah)
- ☐ **percutaneous nephrolithotomy** (**per**-kyou-**TAY**-nee-us **nef**-roh-lih-**THOT**-oh-mee)
- ☐ **peritoneal dialysis** (**pehr**-ih-toh-**NEE**-al dye-**AL**-ih-sis)
- ☐ **polycystic kidney disease** (**pol**-ee-**SIS**-tick)
- ☐ **polyuria** (**pol**-ee-**YOU**-ree-ah)
- ☐ **prostatism** (**PROS**-tah-tizm)
- ☐ **pyelonephritis** (**pye**-eh-loh-neh-**FRY**-tis)
- ☐ **pyelotomy** (**pye**-eh-**LOT**-oh-mee)
- ☐ **renal colic**
- ☐ **suprapubic catheterization** (**soo**-prah-**PYOU**-bick **kath**-eh-ter-eye-**ZAY**-shun)
- ☐ **transurethral prostatectomy**
- ☐ **uremia** (you-**REE**-mee-ah)
- ☐ **ureterolith** (you-**REE**-ter-oh-**lith**)
- ☐ **ureterorrhagia** (you-**ree**-ter-oh-**RAY**-jee-ah)
- ☐ **urethritis** (**you**-reh-**THRIGH**-tis)
- ☐ **urethroplasty** (you-**REE**-throh-**plas**-tee)
- ☐ **urethrorrhagia** (you-**ree**-throh-**RAY**-jee-ah)
- ☐ **urethrostenosis** (you-**ree**-throh-steh-**NOH**-sis)
- ☐ **urethrotomy** (**you**-reh-**THROT**-oh-mee)
- ☐ **urinary catheterization**
- ☐ **vesicovaginal fistula** (**ves**-ih-koh-**VAJ**-ih-nahl **FIS**-tyou-lah)
- ☐ **voiding cystourethrography** (**sis**-toh-you-ree-**THROG**-rah-fee)
- ☐ **Wilms tumor** (**VILMZ**)

LEARNING OBJECTIVES

On completion of this chapter, you should be able to:

1. Describe the major functions and structures of the urinary system.
2. Describe the process of urine formation.
3. Describe the characteristics of urine.
4. Identify the medical specialists who treat disorders of the urinary system.
5. Identify medical word parts of the urinary system.
6. Define the primary terms related to the pathology and the diagnostic and treatment procedures of the urinary system.
7. Spell the primary terms of the urinary system.
8. Pronounce the primary terms of the urinary system.
9. Identify common abbreviations related to the urinary system.

FUNCTIONS OF THE URINARY SYSTEM

The urinary system performs many functions that are important in maintaining homeostasis. ***Homeostasis*** is the process through which the body maintains a constant internal environment (**home/o** means constant, and **-stasis** means control). These functions include:

- Maintaining the proper balance of water, electrolytes, and acids in the body by filtering the blood as it flows through the kidneys.
- Constantly filtering the blood to remove urea, creatinine, uric acid, and other waste materials from the bloodstream. **Urea** (you-**REE**-ah) is the major waste product of protein metabolism. ***Creatinine*** is a waste product of muscle metabolism.
- Converting these waste products and excess fluids into urine in the kidneys and excreting them from the body via the urinary bladder.
- **Urine** is a clear, amber, slightly acidic liquid with an acrid odor that is formed in the kidneys and excreted from the urinary bladder.

STRUCTURES OF THE URINARY SYSTEM

The urinary system, also referred to as the ***urinary tract***, consists of two kidneys, two ureters, one bladder, and one urethra (Figures 10.1 and 10.4). The adrenal glands, which are part of the endocrine system, are located on the top of the kidneys.

The urinary tract is located in close proximity to the reproductive organs, so these two body systems are sometimes referred to together as the ***genitourinary tract***.

The Kidneys

The **kidneys** constantly filter the blood to remove waste products and excess water. These are excreted as urine, which is 95% water and 5% urea and other body wastes.

Roughly 150–200 quarts of blood are processed every day, producing 1–2 quarts of urine. The kidneys also help the body maintain the proper level of fluid, produce hormones that control blood pressure and make red blood cells, and activate vitamin D to maintain healthy bones.

- The term **renal** (**REE**-nal) means pertaining to the kidneys (**ren** means kidney or kidneys, and **-al** means pertaining to).
- The two bean-shaped kidneys are located in the retroperitoneal space, with one on each side of the vertebral column below the diaphragm and the lower edge of the rib cage. ***Retroperitoneal*** means behind the peritoneum, which is the membrane that lines the abdominal cavity.
- The **renal cortex** (**REE**-nal **KOR**-tecks) is the outer region of the kidney. This layer of tissue contains

more than one million microscopic units called nephrons. The term *cortex* means the outer portion of an organ.

- The **medulla** (meh-**DULL**-ah) is the inner region of the kidney, and it contains most of the urine-collecting tubules. A *tubule* is a small tube.

Nephrons

The **nephrons** (**NEF**-ronz) are the microscopic functional units of each kidney. It is here that urine is produced through the processes of filtration, reabsorption, and secretion (Figure 10.2). *Reabsorption* is the return to the blood of some of the substances that were removed during filtration.

- Each nephron contains a **glomerulus** (gloh-**MER**-you-lus), which is a cluster of capillaries (plural, *glomeruli*), surrounded by a cup-shaped membrane called the Bowman's capsule, and a **renal tubule**.
- Blood enters the kidney through the **renal artery** and flows into the nephrons.
- After passing through the filtration system of the glomerulus, the filtered blood containing protein and blood cells leaves the kidney and returns to the bloodstream through the **renal vein**.
- The remaining filtrate flows into the renal tubules, where elements, including some water, sugar, and electrolytes, are returned to the bloodstream via a nearby capillary.
- Remaining waste products are continuously converted into urine, which is transported to the renal pelvis and collected in preparation for entry into the ureters.

If waste products are not efficiently removed from the bloodstream, the body cannot maintain homeostasis, with a stable balance of electrolytes and other substances.

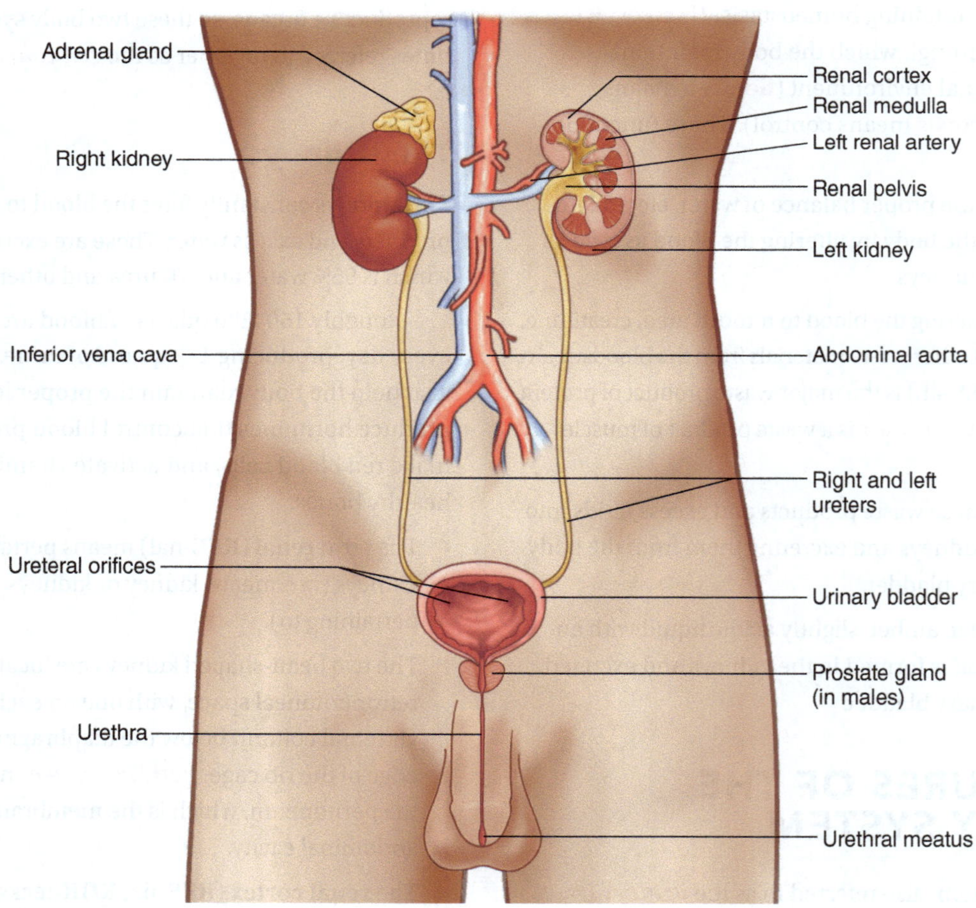

FIGURE 10.1 The primary structures of the urinary system, as shown here in a male, are the kidneys, ureters, urinary bladder, and urethra. The adrenal gland, positioned on top of each kidney, is a structure of the endocrine system. The prostate gland, which is part of the male reproductive system, surrounds the urethra.

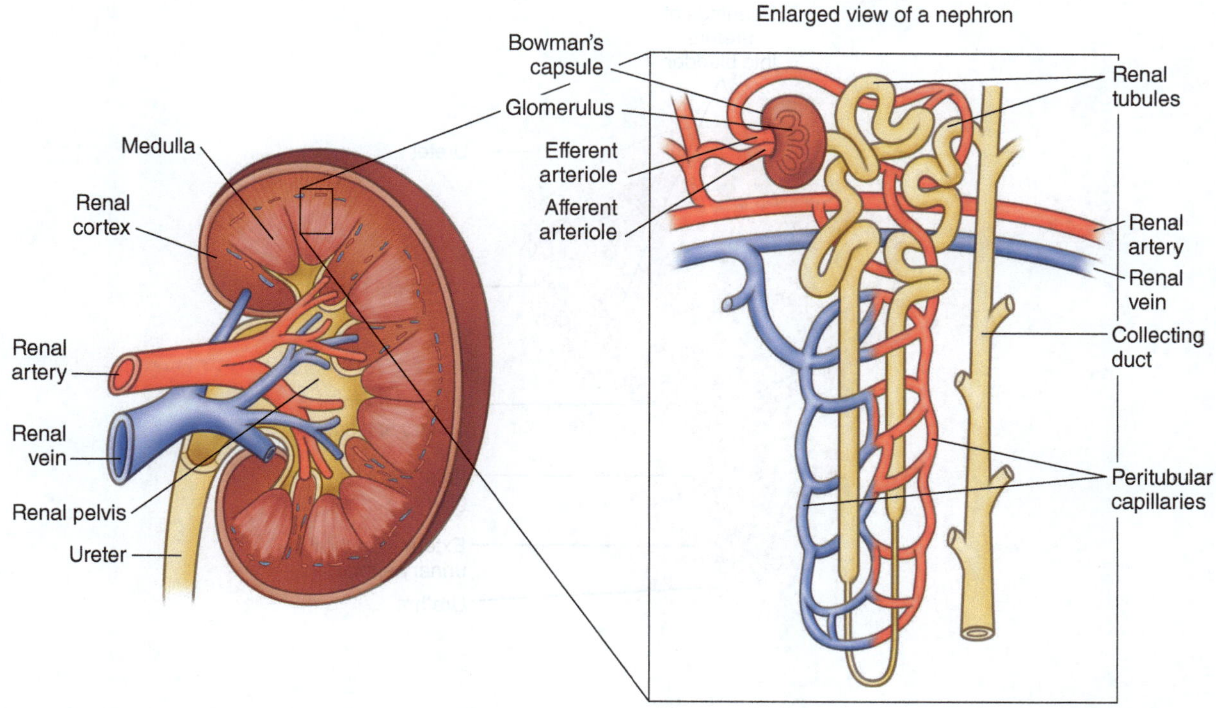

FIGURE 10.2 A kidney, with a nephron in close-up, showing the nephron's associated structures.

The Renal Pelvis

The **renal pelvis** is the funnel-shaped area inside each kidney that is surrounded by the renal cortex and medulla. This is where the newly formed urine from the nephrons collects before it flows into the ureters.

The Ureters

- The **ureters** (you-**REE**-ters) are two narrow tubes, each about 10 to 12 inches long, which transport urine from the kidney to the bladder. ***Peristalsis***, which is a series of wave-like contractions, moves urine down each ureter to the bladder. Peristalsis is also part of the digestive process, as described in Chapter 9.
- Urine drains from the ureters into the bladder through the **ureteral orifices** in the wall of the urinary bladder (Figure 10.1). ***Orifice*** means opening.

The Urinary Bladder

The **urinary bladder** is an oval, hollow, muscular organ that is a reservoir for urine before it is excreted from the body (Figure 10.3).

- The bladder is located in the anterior portion of the pelvic cavity behind the pubic symphysis. The average adult bladder stores more than one pint of urine.
- Like the stomach, the bladder is lined with ***rugae***. These folds allow it to expand when full and contract when empty.

The Urethra

The **urethra** (you-**REE**-thrah) is the tube extending from the bladder to the exterior of the body. *Caution:* The spellings of *ureter* and *urethra* are very similar! You may find it helpful to remember that the ureter comes first, both anatomically and alphabetically.

- There are two ***urinary sphincters***, one located at either end of the urethra. These muscular rings control the flow of urine from the bladder into the urethra and out of the urethra through the urethral meatus. A ***sphincter*** is a ring-like muscle that closes a passageway (Figure 10.3).
- The **urethral meatus** (you-**REE**-thrahl mee-**AY**-tus), also known as the ***urinary meatus***, is the external opening of the urethra. The term ***meatus*** means the external opening of a canal (Figure 10.4).
- The **female urethra** is approximately 1.5 inches long, and the urethral meatus is located between the clitoris and the opening of the vagina (see Chapter 16). In the female, the urethra transports only urine (Figure 10.4).

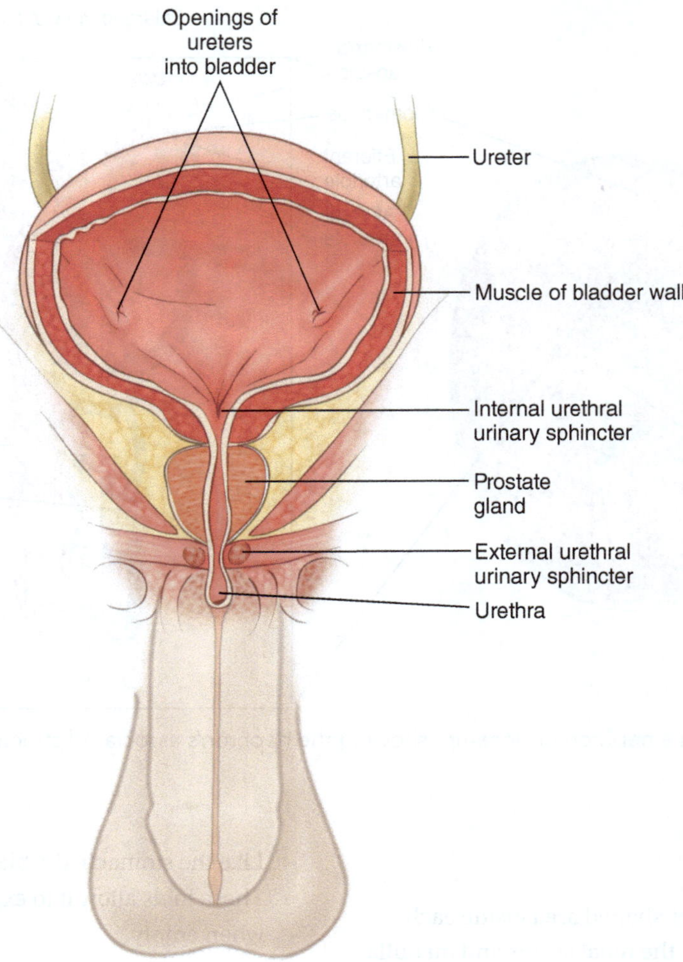

FIGURE 10.3 The structures of the male urinary bladder.

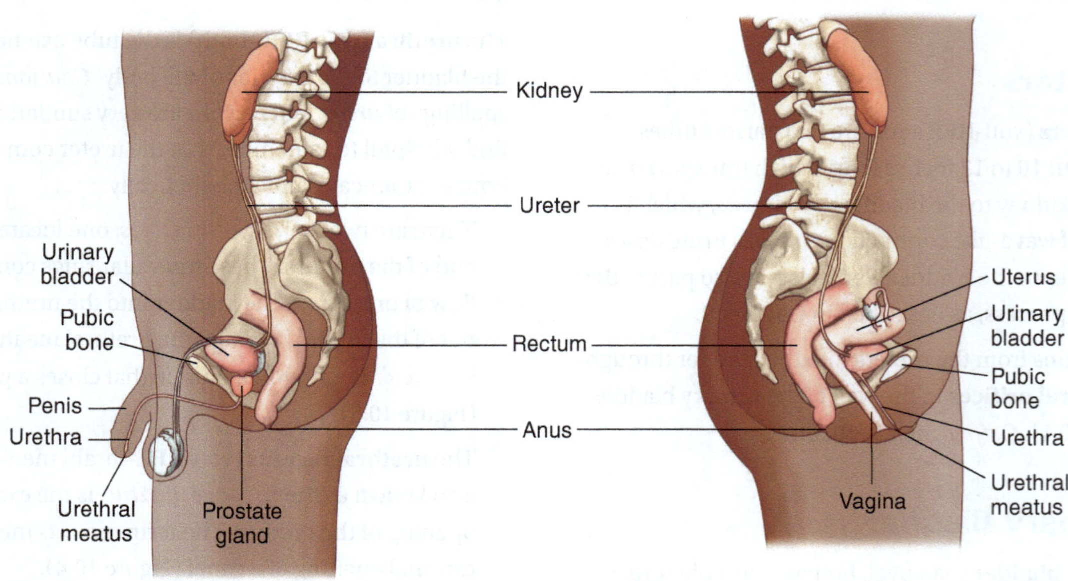

FIGURE 10.4 Cross-sections of the male and female urinary systems.

- The **male urethra** is approximately 8 inches long, and the urethral meatus is located at the tip of the penis (Figures 10.1 and 10.4). This urethra transports both urine and semen.

- The **prostate gland** (**PROS**-tayt), which is part of the male reproductive system, surrounds the urethra (Figures 10.3 and 10.4). Most disorders of the prostate affect the male's ability to urinate. For more information about the role of the prostate gland in reproduction, see Chapter 15.

THE EXCRETION OF URINE

Urination, also known as ***voiding*** or ***micturition***, is the normal process of excreting urine.

- As the bladder fills up with urine, pressure is placed on the base of the urethra, resulting in the urge to **urinate** or ***micturate***.
- Urination requires the coordinated contraction of the bladder muscles and relaxation of the sphincters. This action forces the urine through the urethra and out through the urethral meatus.

MEDICAL SPECIALTIES RELATED TO THE URINARY SYSTEM

- A **nephrologist** (neh-**FROL**-oh-jist) is a physician who specializes in diagnosing and treating diseases and disorders of the kidneys (**nephr** means kidney, and **-ologist** means specialist).
- A **urologist** (you-**ROL**-oh-jist) is a physician who specializes in diagnosing and treating diseases and disorders of the urinary system of females and the genitourinary system of males (**ur** means urine, and **-ologist** means specialist).

PATHOLOGY OF THE URINARY SYSTEM

Nephropathy

The term **nephropathy** (neh-**FROP**-ah-thee) means any disease of the kidney (**nephr/o** means kidney, and **-pathy** means disease). This definition includes both degenerative and inflammatory conditions. ***Diabetic nephropathy*** is kidney disease resulting from poorly controlled diabetes mellitus.

Renal Failure

Renal failure, also known as ***kidney failure***, is the inability of one or both of the kidneys to perform their functions. The body cannot replace damaged nephrons, and when too many nephrons have been destroyed, the result is kidney failure.

- **Azotemia** (ay-zoh-**TEE**-mee-ah) is an elevation of blood urea nitrogen (BUN) caused by a lack of blood flow to each kidney. Uremia can occur when this excess becomes toxic.
- **Uremia** (you-**REE**-mee-ah), also known as ***uremic poisoning***, is a toxic condition resulting from renal failure in which kidney function is compromised and urea and other waste products normally secreted in the urine are retained in the blood (**ur** means urine, and **-emia** means blood condition).
- **Acute renal failure** (ARF) has sudden onset and is characterized by uremia. It can be fatal if not reversed promptly. This condition can be caused by the kidneys not receiving enough blood to filter due to dehydration or a sudden drop in blood volume or blood pressure from injury, burns, or a severe infection.
- **Chronic kidney disease** (CKD) is the progressive loss of renal function over months or years. This common condition, which can be life-threatening, may result from diabetes mellitus, hypertension, or a family history of kidney disease.
- The buildup of waste in the blood from chronic kidney disease can be a contributing factor in heart attacks and strokes.
- **End-stage renal disease** (ESRD), also known as ***kidney failure***, is the final stage of chronic kidney disease, and this condition is fatal unless the functions of the failed kidneys are replaced by dialysis, or with a successful kidney transplant.

Nephrotic Syndrome

Nephrotic syndrome (neh-**FROT**-ick), also known as ***nephrosis***, is a group of conditions in which excessive amounts of protein are lost through the urine. This condition, which is usually caused by damage to the glomeruli, results in abnormally low levels of protein in the blood (**nephr/o** means kidney, and **-tic** means pertaining to).

- **Edema** (eh-**DEE**-mah) is excessive fluid accumulation in body tissues that can be symptomatic of nephrotic syndrome and other kidney diseases. This swelling can be in the area around the eyes, or in the legs and feet.
- **Hyperproteinuria** (**high**-per-**proh**-tee-in-**YOU**-ree-ah) is the presence of abnormally high concentrations of protein in the urine (**hyper-** means excessive, **protein** means protein, and **-uria** means urine).
- **Hypoproteinemia** (**high**-poh-**proh**-tee-in-**EE**-mee-ah) is the presence of abnormally low concentrations

of protein in the blood (**hypo-** means deficient or decreased, **protein** means protein, and **-emia** means blood condition). This condition is often associated with hyperproteinuria.

- Causes of nephrotic syndrome include diabetes mellitus, infection, and kidney disorders. ***Minimal change disease***, so called because the nephrons look normal under a regular microscope, is the most common cause of nephrotic syndrome in children.

Additional Kidney Conditions

- An **ectopic kidney** is a congenital condition in which one kidney is located in an abnormal position or has fused with the other kidney. *Ectopic* means located in an abnormal place or position (**ec-** means out, **top** means place, and **-ic** means pertaining to). This condition can be associated with an increased risk of urinary tract infections and nephroliths.
- **Hydronephrosis** (**high**-droh-neh-**FROH**-sis) is the dilation (swelling) of one or both kidneys (**hydr/o** means water, **nephr** means kidney, and **-osis** means abnormal condition or disease). This condition can be caused by problems associated with the backing up of urine due to an obstruction such as a nephrolith (kidney stone) or a stricture (narrowing) in the ureter (Figure 10.5).
- **Nephritis** (neh-**FRY**-tis) is an inflammation of the kidney or kidneys (**nephr** means kidney, and **-itis** means inflammation). The most common causes of nephritis are toxins, infection, or an autoimmune disease.
- **Glomerulonephritis** (gloh-**mer**-you-loh-neh-**FRY**-tis) is a type of nephritis caused by inflammation of the glomeruli that causes red blood cells and proteins to leak into the urine (**glomerul/o** means glomeruli, **nephr** means kidney, and **-itis** means inflammation).
- **Pyonephrosis** (**pye**-oh-nef-**ROH**-sis), also known as ***nephropyosis***, is suppuration of the kidney (**py/o** means pus, **nephr** means kidney, and **-osis** means abnormal condition or disease), and is often associated with hydronephrosis. ***Suppuration*** means the formation of pus.
- **Polycystic kidney disease** (**pol**-ee-**SIS**-tick) (PKD) is a genetic disorder characterized by the growth of numerous fluid-filled cysts in the kidneys (**poly-** means many, **cyst** means cyst, and **-ic** means pertaining to). These cysts, which slowly replace much of the mass of the kidney, reduce the kidney function, which eventually leads to kidney failure (Figure 10.6).

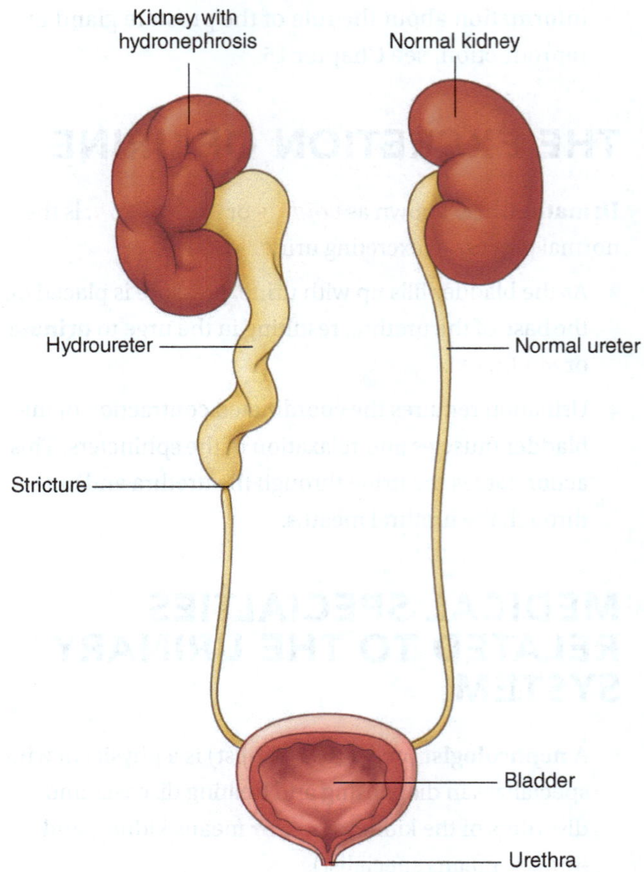

FIGURE 10.5 A stricture of the ureter can cause both hydronephrosis and hydroureter.

- **Renal colic** (**REE**-nal **KOLL**-ick) is an acute pain in the kidney area that is caused by blockage during the passage of a nephrolith (kidney stone). ***Colic*** means spasms of pain in the abdomen. Renal colic pain sometimes comes in waves due to the peristaltic movement of the ureters.
- **Renal cell carcinoma** is the most common form of kidney cancer in adults. It can cause flank pain and blood in the urine, but is most commonly asymptomatic until the tumor has grown enough to impair kidney function.
- A **Wilms tumor** (**VILMZ**), also known as a ***nephroblastoma***, is a rare type of malignant tumor of the kidney that occurs in young children. There is a high cure rate for this condition when treated promptly.

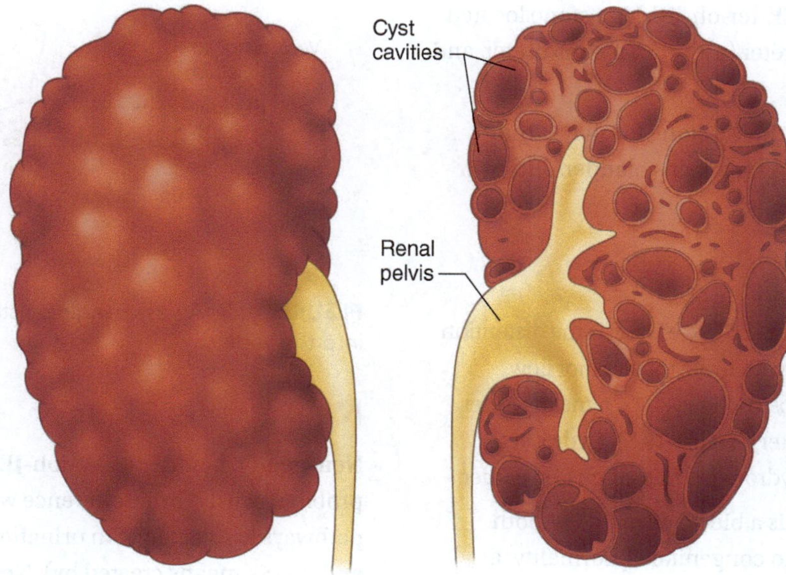

FIGURE 10.6 Polycystic kidney disease: On the left is the exterior of a kidney with polycystic disease. On the right is a cross-section view of a kidney with polycystic disease.

Stones

A **stone**, also known as a ***calculus***, is an abnormal mineral deposit that has formed within the body and is named for the organ or tissue where it is located (plural, *calculi*). These stones vary in size from small sand-like granules that pass through the body unnoticed to stones the size of marbles that can become lodged, causing acute pain and urinary tract obstruction.

- In the urinary system, stones form when waste products in the urine separate and crystallize (Figure 10.7). Normally, urine contains chemicals to prevent this from happening; however, dehydration and other factors may disrupt this balance.
- The term **nephrolithiasis** (**nef**-roh-lih-**THIGH**-ah-sis) describes the presence of stones in the kidney (**nephr/o** means kidney, and **-lithiasis** means the presence of stones). As these stones travel with the flow of urine, they are named for the location where they become lodged.
- A **urinary tract obstruction** is a blockage that prevents the flow of urine in one part of the urinary tract. Obstructions are named for their locations, and are commonly caused by stones, congenital abnormalities, or an enlarged prostate.
- A **nephrolith** (**NEF**-roh-lith), also known as a ***kidney stone*** or ***renal calculus***, is found in the kidney (**nephr/o** means kidney, and **-lith** means stone).

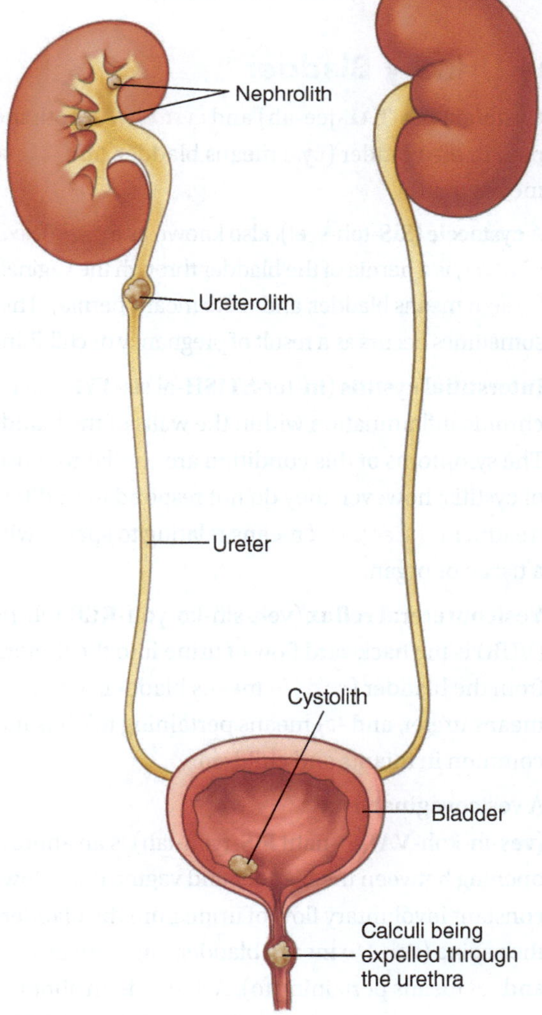

FIGURE 10.7 Potential locations of renal stones (calculi) as they move through the urinary system.

- A **ureterolith** (you-**REE**-ter-oh-**lith**) is a stone located anywhere along the ureter (**ureter/o** means ureter, and **-lith** means stone).
- A **cystolith** (**SIS**-toh-lith) is a stone located within the urinary bladder (**cyst/o** means bladder, and **-lith** means stone).

The Ureters

- **Hydroureter** (**high**-droh-**YOUR**-eh-ter) is the distention (swelling) of the ureter with urine that cannot flow because of a ureteral obstruction (**hydr/o** means water, and **-ureter** means ureter) (Figure 10.5). Hydroureter always accompanies hydronephrosis, discussed earlier.
- **Ureteral obstruction** is a blockage of one or both ureters. It can be due to congenital abnormality, a ureterolith, or other disorders.
- **Ureterorrhagia** (you-**ree**-ter-oh-**RAY**-jee-ah) is the discharge of blood from the ureter (**ureter/o** means ureter, and **-rrhagia** means bleeding).

The Urinary Bladder

- **Cystalgia** (sis-**TAL**-jee-ah) and ***cystodynia*** both mean pain in the bladder (**cyst** means bladder, and **-algia** means pain).
- A **cystocele** (**SIS**-toh-seel), also known as a ***prolapsed bladder***, is a hernia of the bladder through the vaginal wall (**cyst/o** means bladder, and **-cele** means hernia). This sometimes occurs as a result of pregnancy or childbirth.
- **Interstitial cystitis** (**in**-ter-**STISH**-al sis-**TYE**-tis) is a chronic inflammation within the walls of the bladder. The symptoms of this condition are similar to those of cystitis; however, they do not respond to traditional treatment. ***Interstitial*** means relating to spaces within a tissue or organ.
- **Vesicoureteral reflux** (**veh**-sih-ko-you-**REE**-teh-ral) (VUR) is the backward flow of urine into the ureters from the bladder (**vesic/o** means bladder, **ureter** means ureter, and **-al** means pertaining to). It is most common in infants and children.
- A **vesicovaginal fistula** (**ves**-ih-koh-**VAJ**-ih-nahl **FIS**-tyou-lah) is an abnormal opening between the bladder and vagina that allows constant involuntary flow of urine from the bladder into the vagina (**vesic/o** means bladder, **vagin** means vagina, and **-al** means pertaining to). A ***fistula*** is an abnormal passage between two internal organs (Figure 10.8). A vesicovaginal fistula may be caused by prolonged labor during childbirth or surgery such as a hysterectomy.

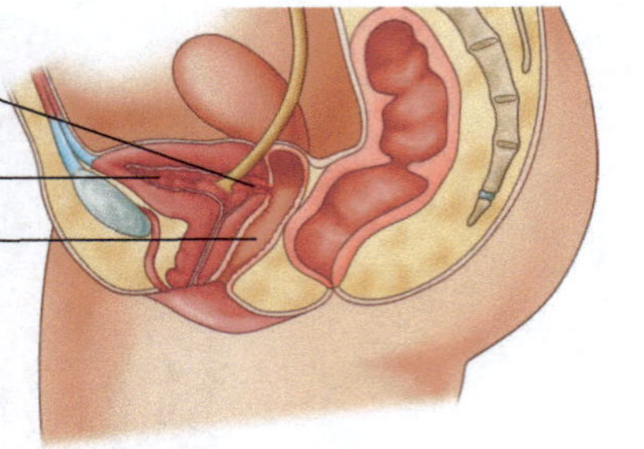

FIGURE 10.8 A vesicovaginal fistula allows urine to flow into the vagina.

Neurogenic Bladder

Neurogenic bladder (new-roh-**JEN**-ick) is a urinary problem caused by interference with the normal nerve pathways associated with urination (**neur/o** means nerve, and **-genic** means created by). Normal urinary function depends on nerves to sense when the bladder is full and to control the muscles that either retain the urine or allow the bladder to empty.

- Depending on the type of neurological disorder causing the problem, the bladder may empty spontaneously, resulting in incontinence, which is discussed in a later section.
- In contrast, the problem can prevent the bladder from emptying at all or from emptying completely. This can result in urinary retention with overflow leakage.
- Some of the causes of this condition are a tumor of the nervous system, trauma, neuropathy, or an inflammatory condition such as multiple sclerosis. ***Neuropathy*** is any disease or damage to a nerve.

The Prostate Gland

- **Benign prostatic hyperplasia** (bee-**NINE** pros-**TAT**-ick **high**-per-**PLAY**-zee-ah) (BPH), also known as ***benign prostatic hypertrophy*** or an ***enlarged prostate***, is an enlargement of the prostate gland that most often occurs in men older than age 50 (Figure 10.9). This condition can make urination difficult and causes other urinary tract problems for men. ***Hyperplasia*** is an increase in cell numbers typically associated with tumor growth; however, in this case, it is not caused by cancer or infection.
- **Prostatism** (**PROS**-tah-tizm) is a disorder resulting from the compression or obstruction of the urethra due to benign prostatic hyperplasia (**prostat** means prostate gland, and **-ism** means condition of). This can produce difficulties with urination, including urinary retention.
- **Prostate cancer** is one of the most common cancers among men. The disease can grow slowly with no

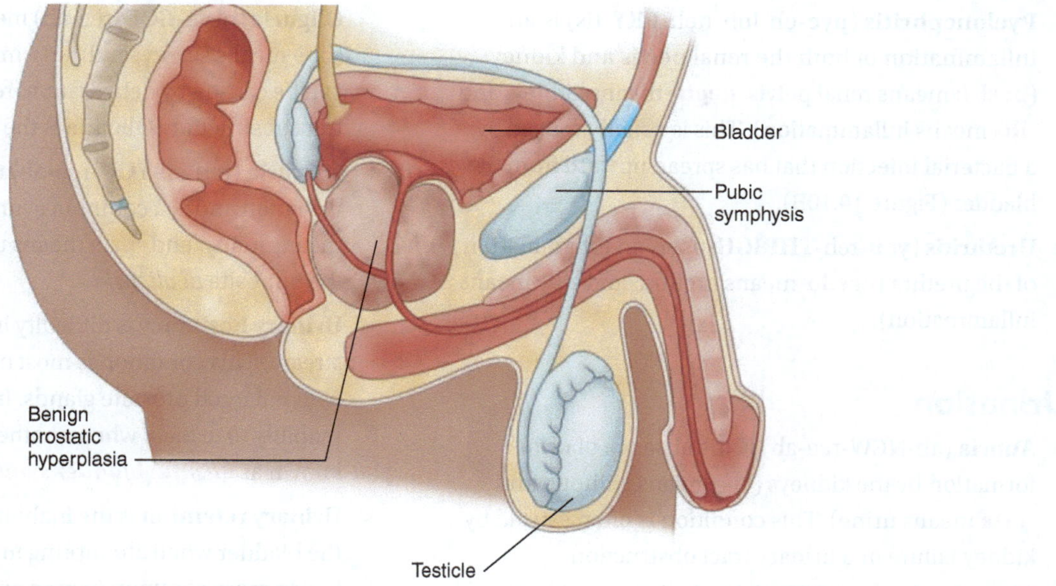

FIGURE 10.9 In benign prostatic hyperplasia, the enlarged prostate presses against the bladder and slows the flow of urine through the urethra.

symptoms, or it can grow aggressively and spread throughout the body.

- **Prostatitis** (**pros**-tah-**TYE**-tis) is a group of disorders characterized by the inflammation of the prostate gland (**prostat** means prostate gland, and **-itis** means inflammation).
- The most common type is ***chronic nonbacterial prostatitis***, with no single known cause.
- ***Bacterial prostatitis*** usually results from bacteria transported in the urine.

The Urethra

- **Urethrorrhagia** (you-**ree**-throh-**RAY**-jee-ah) is bleeding from the urethra (**urethr/o** means urethra, and **-rrhagia** means bleeding).
- **Urethrorrhea** (you-**ree**-throh-**REE**-ah) is an abnormal discharge from the urethra (**urethr/o** means urethra, and **-rrhea** means flow or discharge). This condition is associated with some sexually transmitted diseases (see Chapter 15).
- **Urethrostenosis** (you-**ree**-throh-steh-**NOH**-sis), or ***urethral stricture***, is narrowing of the urethra (**urethr/o** means urethra, and **-stenosis** means tightening or narrowing). This condition occurs almost exclusively in men and is caused by scarring from infection or injury.

Abnormal Urethral Openings

- **Epispadias** (**ep**-ih-**SPAY**-dee-as) is a congenital abnormality of the urethral opening. In the male with epispadias, the urethral opening is located on the upper surface of the penis. In the female with epispadias, the urethral opening is in the region of the clitoris.
- **Hypospadias** (**high**-poh-**SPAY**-dee-as) is a congenital abnormality of the urethral opening. In the male with hypospadias, the urethral opening is on the ventral surface (underside) of the penis. In the female with hypospadias, the urethra opens into the vagina.

Urinary Tract Infections

A **urinary tract infection** (UTI) usually begins in the bladder; however, such an infection can affect all parts of the urinary system. These common infections are caused by bacteria, most often *E. coli*, entering the urinary system through the urethra. They occur more frequently in women because the urethra is short and located near the opening to the rectum. In the elderly, a UTI often causes weakness and confusion rather than urinary symptoms, and can cause urosepsis.

- **Urosepsis** (**you**-roh-**SEP**-sis) is a life-threatening systemic bacterial infection that can occur when a urinary tract infection spreads to the kidneys.
- A **recurrent urinary tract infection** is cystitis that occurs two or more times in six months, or three or more times a year. This chronic bladder infection may require long-term daily antibiotic treatment.
- **Cystitis** (sis-**TYE**-tis) is an inflammation of the bladder (**cyst** means bladder, and **-itis** means inflammation) (Figure 10.10A). See also *interstitial cystitis* in the earlier section "The Urinary Bladder."

- **Pyelonephritis** (**pye**-eh-loh-neh-**FRY**-tis) is an inflammation of both the renal pelvis and kidney (**pyel/o** means renal pelvis, **nephr** means kidney, and **-itis** means inflammation). This is usually caused by a bacterial infection that has spread upward from the bladder (Figure 10.10B).
- **Urethritis** (**you**-reh-**THRIGH**-tis) is an inflammation of the urethra (**urethr** means urethra, and **-itis** means inflammation).

Urination

- **Anuria** (ah-**NEW**-ree-ah) is the absence of urine formation by the kidneys (**an-** means without, and **-uria** means urine). This condition is often caused by kidney failure or a urinary tract obstruction.
- **Diuresis** (**dye**-you-**REE**-sis) is the increased output of urine (**di-** means through, and **-uresis** means urination).
- **Dysuria** (dis-**YOU**-ree-ah) is difficult or painful urination (**dys-** means painful, and **-uria** means urination). This condition is frequently associated with urinary tract infections.
- **Enuresis** (**en**-you-**REE**-sis) is the involuntary discharge of urine (**en-** means into, and **-uresis** means urination).
- **Nocturnal enuresis** (nock-**TER**-nal **en**-you-**REE**-sis) is urinary incontinence during sleep. It is also known as ***bed-wetting***. ***Nocturnal*** means pertaining to night.
- **Nocturia** (nock-**TOO**-ree-ah) is frequent and excessive urination during the night (**noct** means night, and **-uria** means urination).
- **Oliguria** (**ol**-ih-**GOO**-ree-ah) means scanty urination (**olig** means scanty, and **-uria** means urination). This can be caused by dehydration, renal failure, or a urinary tract obstruction. Oliguria is the opposite of *polyuria*.
- **Polyuria** (**pol**-ee-**YOU**-ree-ah) means excessive urination and is a common symptom of diabetes (**poly-** means many, and **-uria** means urination). Polyuria is the opposite of *oliguria*.
- **Urinary hesitancy** is difficulty in starting a urinary stream. This condition is most common in older men with enlarged prostate glands. In younger people, the inability to urinate when another person is present is known as ***bashful bladder syndrome***.
- **Urinary retention** is the inability to completely empty the bladder when attempting to urinate. This condition is also more common in men and is frequently associated with an enlarged prostate gland.

Incontinence

Incontinence (in-**KON**-tih-nents) is the inability to control the excretion of urine, feces, or both.

- **Urinary incontinence** is the inability to control the voiding of urine.
- **Overflow incontinence** is continuous leaking from the bladder either because it is full or because it does not empty completely. It is usually caused by a blocked urethra and is prevalent in older men with enlarged prostates.
- **Stress incontinence** is the inability to control the voiding of urine under physical stress such as running, sneezing, laughing, or coughing. This common condition occurs more often in women than in men.

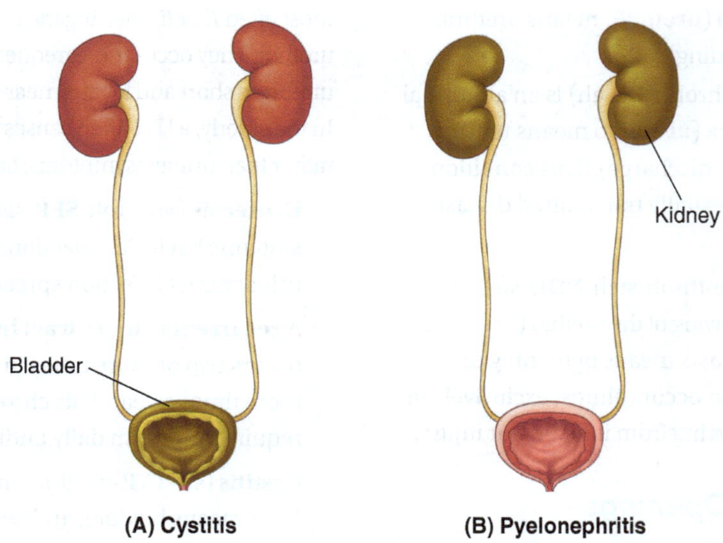

FIGURE 10.10 Infections of the urinary tract, indicated in olive: (A) cystitis and (B) pyelonephritis.

- **Overactive bladder** (OAB), also known as ***urge incontinence***, occurs when the muscles of the bladder contract involuntarily even though the bladder is not actually full enough to indicate the need to urinate. The urinary sphincters' relaxation in response to this urgent need to urinate may result in increased urinary frequency or incontinence.

DIAGNOSTIC PROCEDURES OF THE URINARY SYSTEM

- **Urinalysis** (**you**-rih-**NAL**-ih-sis) (UA) is the examination of urine for the presence of abnormal elements (**urin** means urine, and **-alysis** means a study of the parts). These tests are used to diagnose diseases, kidney damage, and pregnancy, as well as to detect the presence of substances such as illicit drugs and prescription medications. Urinalysis is discussed further in Chapter 21.
- **Glomerular filtration rate** (GFR) is a blood test to check how well the kidneys are functioning at filtering blood. This test can help diagnose chronic kidney disease and kidney failure. The ***blood urea nitrogen (BUN) test***, also an indicator of kidney function, is discussed in Chapter 21.
- A **bladder ultrasound** is the use of a handheld ultrasound transducer to look for stones or for elevation of the bladder by an enlarged prostate and to measure the residual amount of urine remaining in the bladder after urination. A normal bladder holds between 300 and 400 mL of urine. When more than this amount is still present after urination, the bladder is described as being ***distended***, or enlarged.
- *Urinary catheterization* is the insertion of a tube into the bladder to procure a sterile specimen for diagnostic purposes. It is also used to drain urine from the bladder when the patient is unable to urinate for other reasons, or to place medication into the bladder. (See the section "Treatment Procedures of the Urinary System.")
- **Cystoscopy** (sis-**TOS**-koh-pee) is the visual examination of the urinary bladder with the use of a specialized type of endoscope known as a cystoscope (**cyst/o** means bladder, and **-scopy** means visual

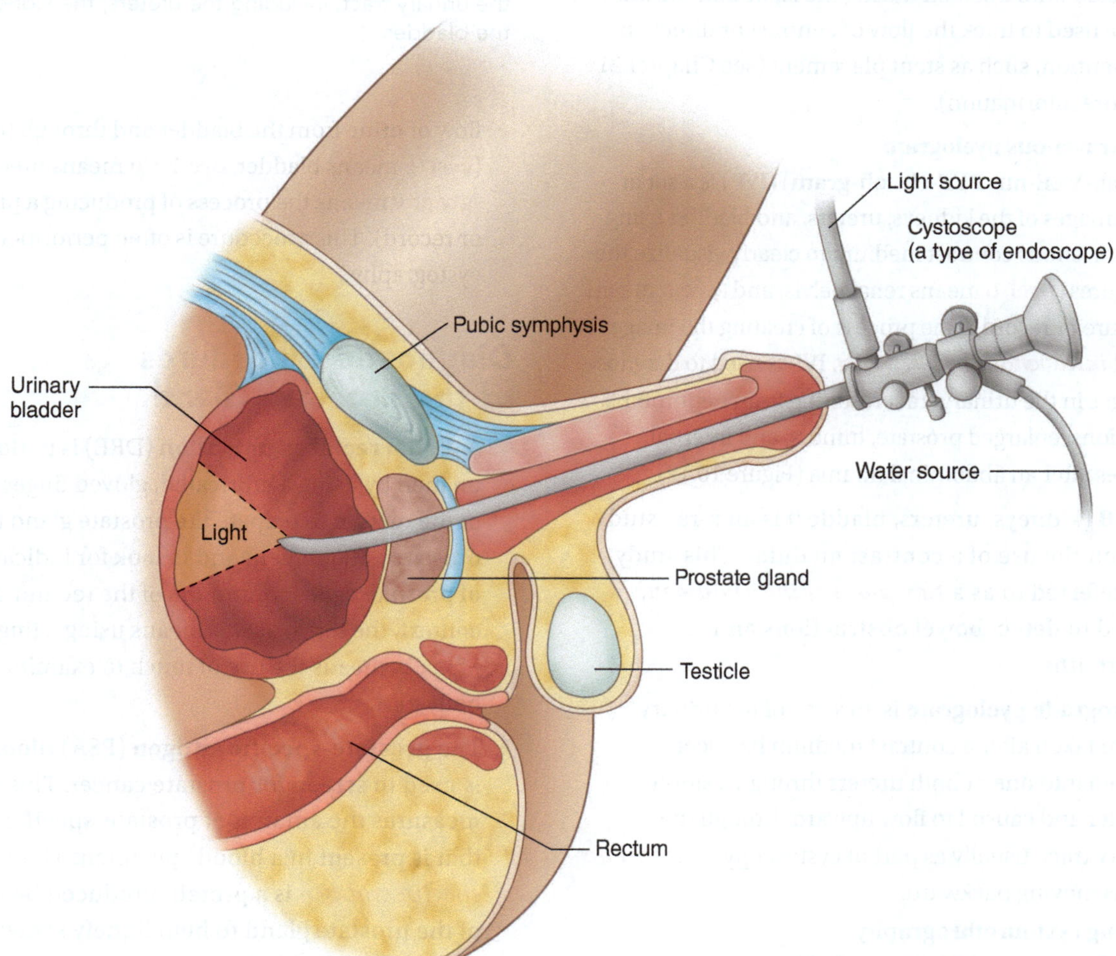

FIGURE 10.11 Use of a cystoscope to examine the interior of the bladder in a male.

examination) (Figure 10.11). An *endoscope* is an instrument used for visual examination of internal structures. A specialized cystoscope is also used for treatment procedures such as the removal of tumors or the reduction of an enlarged prostate gland.

Radiographic Examinations of the Urinary System

- **Computed tomography**, also known as a *CT scan*, is commonly used to evaluate the urinary system because it can be rapidly performed and provides additional radiographic imaging of the abdomen, which may reveal other potential sources for the patient's symptoms.
- **Cystography** (sis-**TOG**-rah-fee) is an x-ray or fluoroscopy examination of the bladder after a contrast medium is instilled via a urethral catheter (**cyst/o** means bladder, and **-graphy** means the process of creating a picture or record). The resulting film is a *cystogram*. *Fluoroscopy* uses continuous x-rays projected onto a screen during the examination, and can be used to track the flow of contrast or direct an intervention, such as stent placement (see Chapter 21 for more information).
- An **intravenous pyelogram** (**in**-trah-**VEE**-nus **PYE**-eh-loh-**gram**) (IVP) is a set of x-ray images of the kidneys, ureters, and bladder using an intravenous contrast medium to clearly visualize the structures (**pyel/o** means renal pelvis, and **-gram** means a picture or record). The process of creating the images is called *intravenous pyelography*. IVP is used to diagnose changes in the urinary tract resulting from nephroliths, infections, enlarged prostate, tumors, and internal injuries after an abdominal trauma (Figure 10.12).
- A **KUB** (kidneys, ureters, bladder) is an x-ray study without the use of a contrast medium. This study, also referred to as a *flat-plate of the abdomen*, is used to detect bowel obstructions and nephroliths.
- A **retrograde pyelogram** is an x-ray of the urinary system taken after a contrast medium has been instilled into one or both ureters through a sterile catheter and caused to flow upward through the urinary tract, usually as part of cystoscopy. *Retrograde* means moving backward.
- **Voiding cystourethrography** (**sis**-toh-you-ree-**THROG**-rah-fee) is a diagnostic procedure in which fluoroscopy is used to examine the flow of urine from the bladder and through the urethra (**cyst/o** means bladder, **urethr/o** means urethra, and **-graphy** means the process of producing a picture or record). This procedure is often performed after cystography.

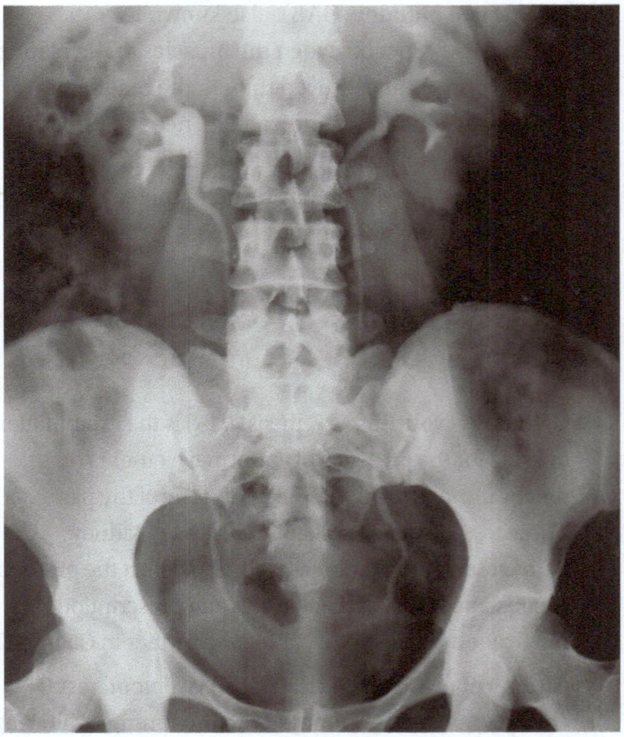
Biophoto Associates/Science Source

FIGURE 10.12 This normal intravenous pyelogram shows the urinary tract, including the ureters, the kidneys, and the bladder.

Diagnostic Procedures of the Prostate Gland

- A **digital rectal examination** (DRE) is performed on men by using a lubricated, gloved finger placed in the rectum to palpate the prostate gland to detect prostate enlargement and to look for indications of prostate cancer or tumors of the rectum. In this context, the term *digital* means using a finger. *Palpate* means the use of touch to examine a body part.
- The **prostate-specific antigen** (PSA) **blood test** is used to screen for prostate cancer. This test measures the amount of prostate-specific antigen that is present in a blood specimen. The *prostate-specific antigen* is a protein produced by the cells of the prostate gland to help liquefy semen. The higher a man's PSA level, the more likely cancer is present.

TREATMENT PROCEDURES OF THE URINARY SYSTEM

Medications

- **Diuretics** (**dye**-you-**RET**-icks) are medications administered to increase urine secretion, primarily to rid the body of excess water and salt. Some foods and drinks, such as coffee, tea, and alcoholic beverages, also have a diuretic effect.
- Other drugs used to treat urinary tract problems include *antibiotics* for urinary tract infections and *antispasmodics* to block the signals that cause urinary incontinence.

Nutritional Interventions

Important dietary considerations for people with kidney disease include monitoring the amounts of sodium, potassium, protein, and phosphorus in their diet.

Dialysis

Dialysis (dye-**AL**-ih-sis) is a procedure to remove waste products, such as urea, creatinine, and excess water, from the blood of a patient whose kidneys no longer function (**dia-** means complete or through, and **-lysis** means separation). The two types of dialysis in common use are *hemodialysis* and *peritoneal dialysis*. Patients can sometimes choose the type of long-term dialysis they prefer.

Hemodialysis

Hemodialysis (**hee**-moh-dye-**AL**-ih-sis) is the process by which waste products are filtered directly from the patient's blood (**hem/o** means blood, **dia** means complete or through, and **-lysis** means separation). Treatment is performed on an external hemodialysis machine, sometimes referred to as an *artificial kidney* (Figure 10.13). Hemodialysis is the most common type of dialysis.

- A shunt implanted in the patient's arm is connected to the hemodialysis unit, and arterial blood flows through the filters of the unit. A *shunt* is an artificial passage that allows the blood to flow between the body and the hemodialysis unit.
- The filters contain *dialysate*, a sterilized solution made up of water and electrolytes. This solution cleanses the blood by removing waste products and excess fluids.

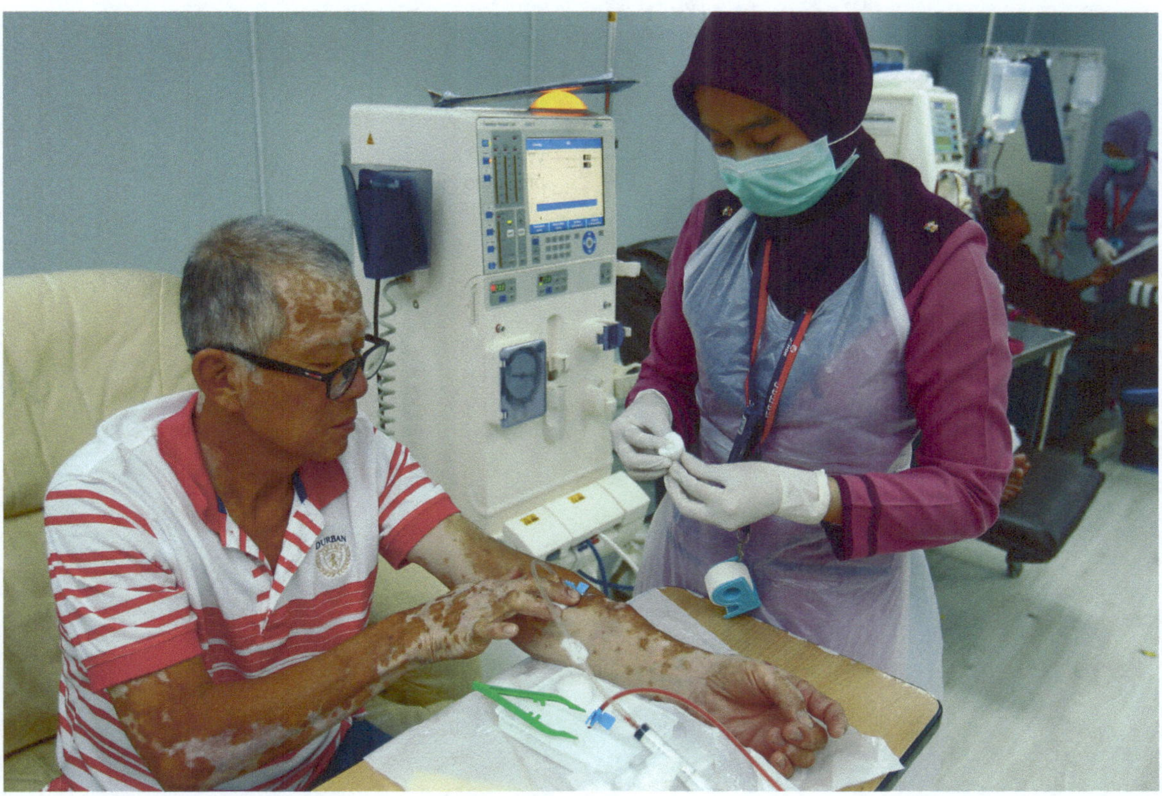

Djohan Shahrin/Shutterstock.com

FIGURE 10.13 In a hemodialysis unit, waste is filtered from the patient's blood. The filtered blood is then returned to the patient's body.

- *Electrolytes* are the minerals that conduct electricity and are found in the body fluid, tissue, and blood.
- The cleansed blood is returned to the body through a vein.
- These treatments each take around four hours and must be repeated about three times a week. They can be done at a hospital, a dialysis clinic, or at home with the necessary equipment.

Peritoneal Dialysis

In **peritoneal dialysis** (**pehr**-ih-toh-**NEE**-al dye-**AL**-ih-sis), the lining of the peritoneal cavity acts as a filter to remove waste from the blood. The sterile dialysate flows into the peritoneal cavity around the intestine through a catheter implanted in the abdominal wall. This fluid is left in for a period of time to absorb waste products and then drained out through the tube.

The process is normally repeated several times during the day and can be done using an automated system. This type of dialysis has some advantages; for example, it can be done at home by the patient. However, it is considered less effective than hemodialysis (Figure 10.14).

- *Continuous ambulatory peritoneal dialysis* (CAPD) provides ongoing dialysis as the patient goes about his or her daily activities. In this procedure, the dialysate solution is instilled from a plastic container worn under

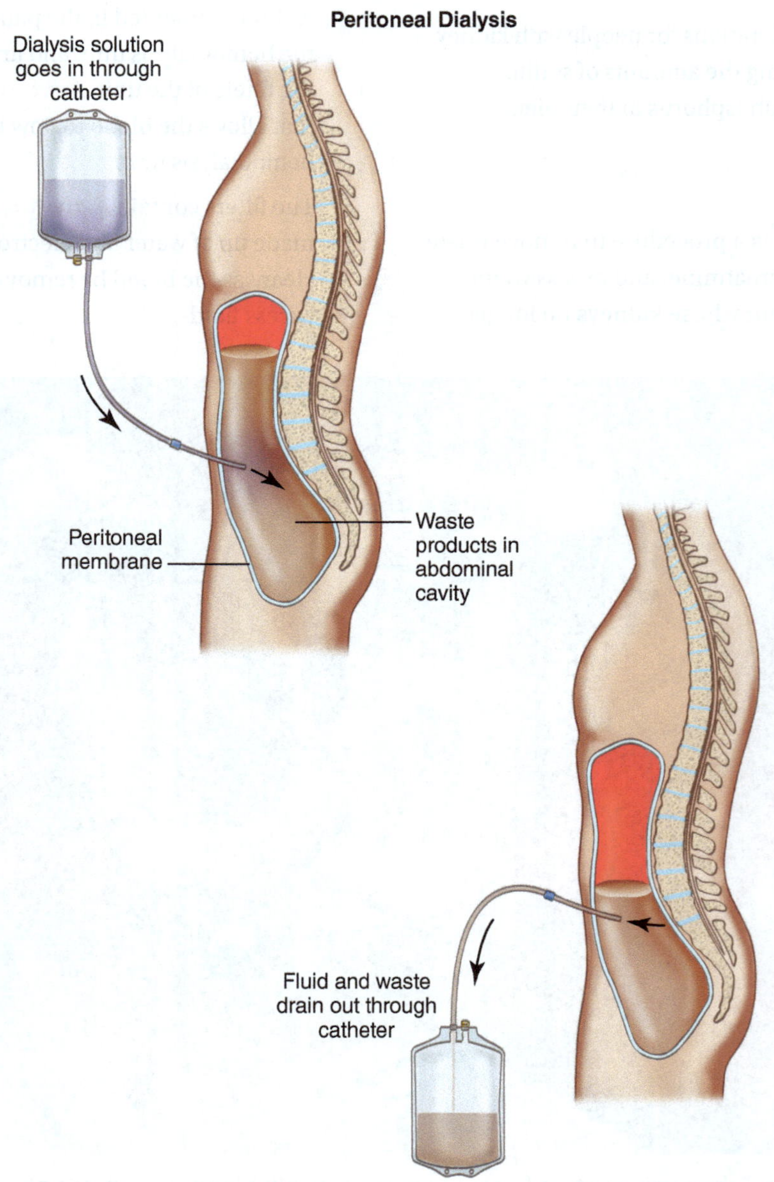

FIGURE 10.14 Peritoneal dialysis removes waste through a fluid exchange in the peritoneal cavity.

the patient's clothing. About every four hours, the used solution is drained back into this bag and the bag is discarded. A new bag is then attached, the solution is instilled, and the process continues.

- *Continuous cycling peritoneal dialysis* (CCPD) or *automated peritoneal dialysis* (APD) uses a machine to cycle the dialysate solution during the night while the patient sleeps.

The Kidneys

- **Nephrolysis** (neh-**FROL**-ih-sis) is the surgical freeing of a kidney from adhesions (**nephr/o** means kidney, and **-lysis** means setting free). An *adhesion* is a band of fibers that holds structures together abnormally.
  Note: The suffix **-lysis** means setting free; however, it also means destruction. Therefore, the term *nephrolysis* can also describe a pathologic condition in which there is destruction of renal cells.
- A **nephrostomy** (neh-**FROS**-toh-mee) is the placement of a catheter to maintain an opening from the pelvis of one or both kidneys to the exterior of the body (**nephr** means kidney, and **-ostomy** means creating an opening). In a kidney affected by hydronephrosis, this allows urine from the kidney to be drained directly through the lower back. Nephrostomy tubes are also used to gain access to the kidneys for diagnostic procedures.
- A **pyelotomy** (**pye-eh-LOT**-oh-mee) is a surgical incision into the renal pelvis (**pyel** means the renal pelvis, and **-otomy** means surgical incision). This procedure is performed to remove obstructions such as a stone lodged in the junction between the renal pelvis and the ureter.
- **Renal transplantation**, commonly known as a *kidney transplant*, is the grafting of a donor kidney, from either a living or nonliving donor, into the body to replace the recipient's failed kidneys. Kidney donors do not need to be genetically related to the recipient, although a tissue match increases the success rate. A single transplanted kidney is capable of adequately performing all kidney functions and frees the patient from the need for dialysis (Figure 10.15).

Treatment of Nephroliths

Most small nephroliths (kidney stones) pass out of the urinary tract naturally over a period of two days to three weeks. This process can be quite painful and is sometimes accompanied by vomiting due to the pain. Larger stones may require surgical intervention.

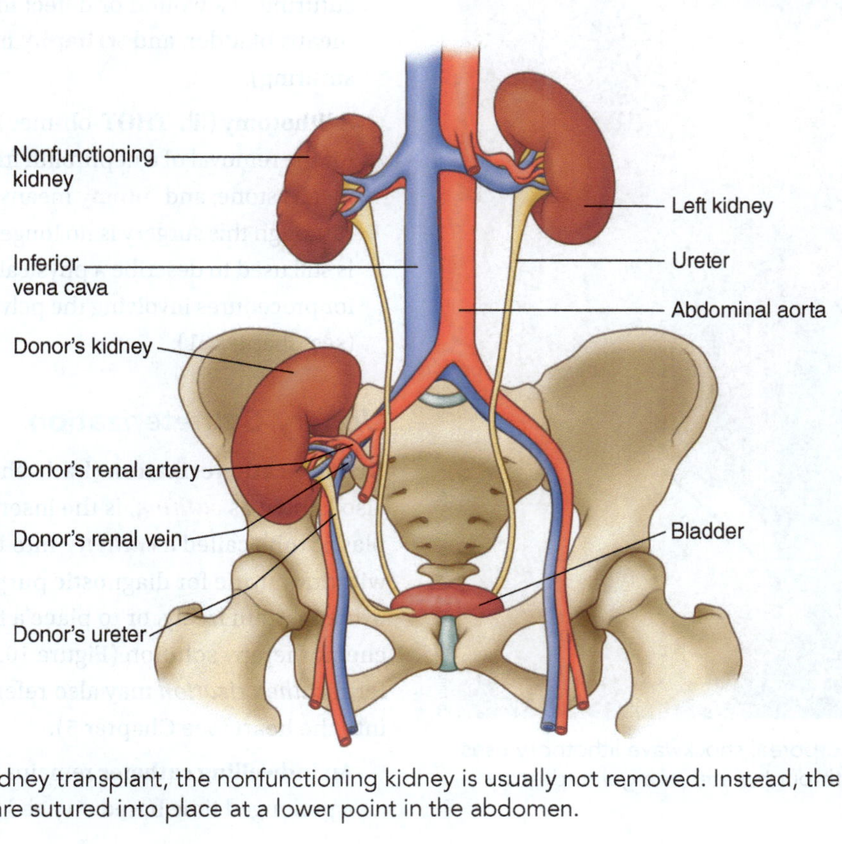

FIGURE 10.15 In a kidney transplant, the nonfunctioning kidney is usually not removed. Instead, the donor kidney and its associated structures are sutured into place at a lower point in the abdomen.

- **Extracorporeal shockwave lithotripsy** (**ecks**-trah-kor-**POUR**-ee-al **shock**-wayv **LITH**-oh-**trip**-see) (ESWL) is the most common kidney stone treatment (**lith/o** means stone, and **-tripsy** means to crush). High-energy ultrasonic waves traveling through water or gel are used to break the stone into fragments, which are then excreted in the urine. ***Extracorporeal*** means situated or occurring outside the body (Figure 10.16).
- Lithotripsy is also used to break up calculi in the ureter, bladder, or urethra.
- A **percutaneous nephrolithotomy** (**per**-kyou-**TAY**-nee-us **nef**-roh-lih-**THOT**-oh-mee) (PCNL) is the surgical removal of a nephrolith through a small incision in the back (**nephr/o** means kidney, **lith** means stone, and **-otomy** means surgical incision). A small tube is temporarily inserted through the incision into the kidney. First urine is removed; then the stone is crushed and the pieces are removed. This procedure is used if ESWL has not been successful, if an infection is present, or if the stone is particularly large. ***Percutaneous*** means performed through the skin.

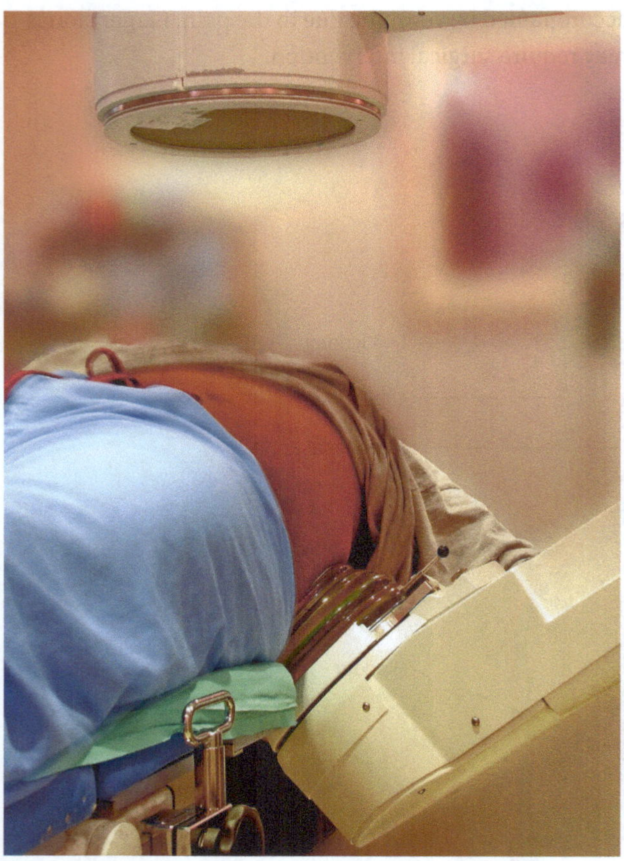
Carolina K. Smith MD/Shutterstock.com

FIGURE 10.16 Extracorporeal shockwave lithotripsy uses shock waves traveling through water or a gel to destroy kidney stones.

The Ureters

- A **ureterectomy** (**you**-reh-ter-**ECK**-toh-mee) is the surgical removal of a ureter (**ureter** means ureter, and **-ectomy** means surgical removal).
- **Ureteroscopy** (you-ree-teh-**ROS**-koh-pee) is a treatment for a nephrolith lodged in the ureter (**ureter/o** means ureter, and **-scopy** means visual examination). A specialized instrument called a ***ureteroscope*** is inserted through the urethra and bladder into the ureter. If possible, the nephrolith is removed intact through the scope. If the stone is too large, a laser is used to break it up and the pieces are then removed.

The Urinary Bladder

- A **cystectomy** (sis-**TECK**-toh-mee) is the surgical removal of all or part of the urinary bladder. This procedure is usually performed to treat bladder cancer (**cyst** means bladder, and **-ectomy** means surgical removal).
- An **ileal conduit** (**ill**-ee-al **KON**-doo-it), or ***urinary ileostomy***, is the use of a small piece of intestine to convey urine to the ureters and to a stoma in the abdomen (**ile** means ileum or small intestine, and **-al** means pertaining to).
- **Cystorrhaphy** (sis-**TOR**-ah-fee) is the surgical suturing of a wound or defect in the bladder (**cyst/o** means bladder, and **-rrhaphy** means surgical suturing).
- A **lithotomy** (lih-**THOT**-oh-mee) is a surgical incision for the removal of a nephrolith from the bladder (**lith** means stone, and **-otomy** means surgical incision). Although this surgery is no longer common, its name is still used to describe a physical examination position for procedures involving the pelvis and lower abdomen (see Chapter 21).

Urinary Catheterization

Urinary catheterization (**kath**-eh-ter-eye-**ZAY**-shun), also known as ***cathing***, is the insertion of a flexible plastic tube called a ***catheter*** into the bladder to withdraw urine for diagnostic purposes, to allow urine to drain freely, or to place a fluid such as a chemotherapy solution (Figure 10.17). Note that the term *catheterization* may also refer to inserting a tube into the heart (see Chapter 5).

- An **indwelling catheter** remains inside the body for a prolonged time based on need (Figure 10.17A).

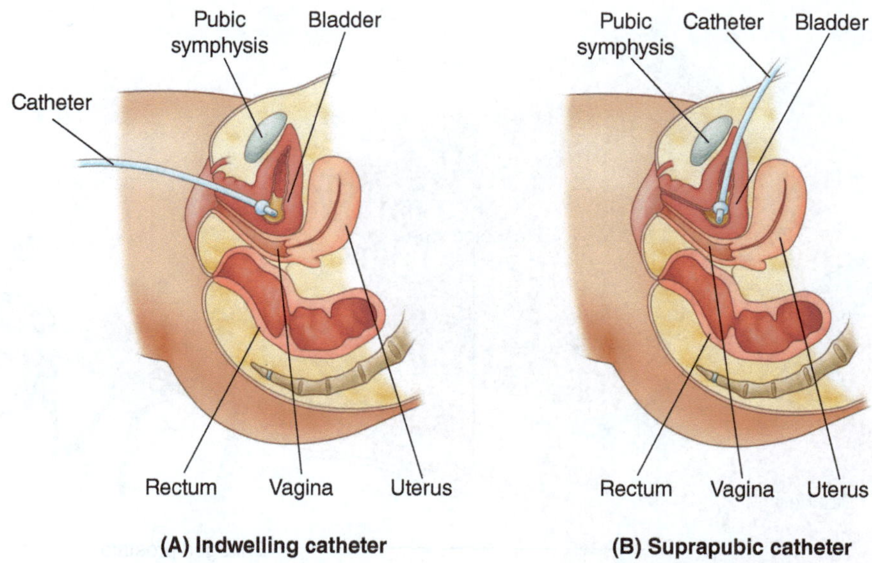

FIGURE 10.17 Types of urinary catheterization.

Indwelling means residing within. This can be either a urethral or a suprapubic catheter.

- **Urethral catheterization** is performed by inserting a catheter though the urethra and into the bladder.
- **Suprapubic catheterization** (**soo**-prah-**PYOU**-bick **kath**-eh-ter-eye-**ZAY**-shun) is the placement of a catheter into the bladder through a small incision made through the abdominal wall just above the pubic bone (Figure 10.17B).
- A **Foley catheter** is the most common type of indwelling catheter. This device is made of a flexible tube with a balloon filled with sterile water at the end to hold it in place in the bladder. It is commonly used on postsurgical patients and is named for its inventor, surgeon Frederic Foley.
- An **intermittent catheter**, also known as a *short-term catheter*, is inserted as needed several times a day to drain urine from the bladder.

The Urethra

- A **meatotomy** (**mee**-ah-**TOT**-oh-mee) is a surgical incision made in the urethral meatus to enlarge the opening (**meat** means meatus, and **-otomy** means surgical incision).
- **Urethroplasty** (you-**REE**-throh-**plas**-tee) is the surgical repair of damage or a defect in the walls of the urethra (**urethr/o** means urethra, and **-plasty** means surgical repair).
- A **urethrotomy** (**you**-reh-**THROT**-oh-mee) is a surgical incision into the urethra for relief of a stricture (**urethr** means urethra, and **-otomy** means surgical incision). A *stricture* is an abnormal narrowing of a bodily passage.

Prostate Treatment

- **Ablation** (ab-**LAY**-shun) is the term used to describe some types of treatment of prostate cancer. This treatment involves the removal of a body part or the destruction of its function through the use of surgery, hormones, drugs, heat, chemicals, electrocautery, or other methods. *Electrocautery* is the use of high-frequency electrical current to destroy tissue.
- A **prostatectomy** (**pros**-tah-**TECK**-toh-mee) is the surgical removal of part or all of the prostate gland (**prostat** means prostate, and **-ectomy** means surgical removal). This procedure is performed to treat prostate cancer or to reduce an enlarged prostate gland; however, this treatment can lead to erectile difficulties. A *radical prostatectomy* is the surgical removal of the entire prostate gland in cases where it is extremely enlarged or when cancer is suspected.
- A **transurethral prostatectomy** (TURP) is the removal of excess tissue from an enlarged prostate gland with the use of a resectoscope. A *resectoscope* is

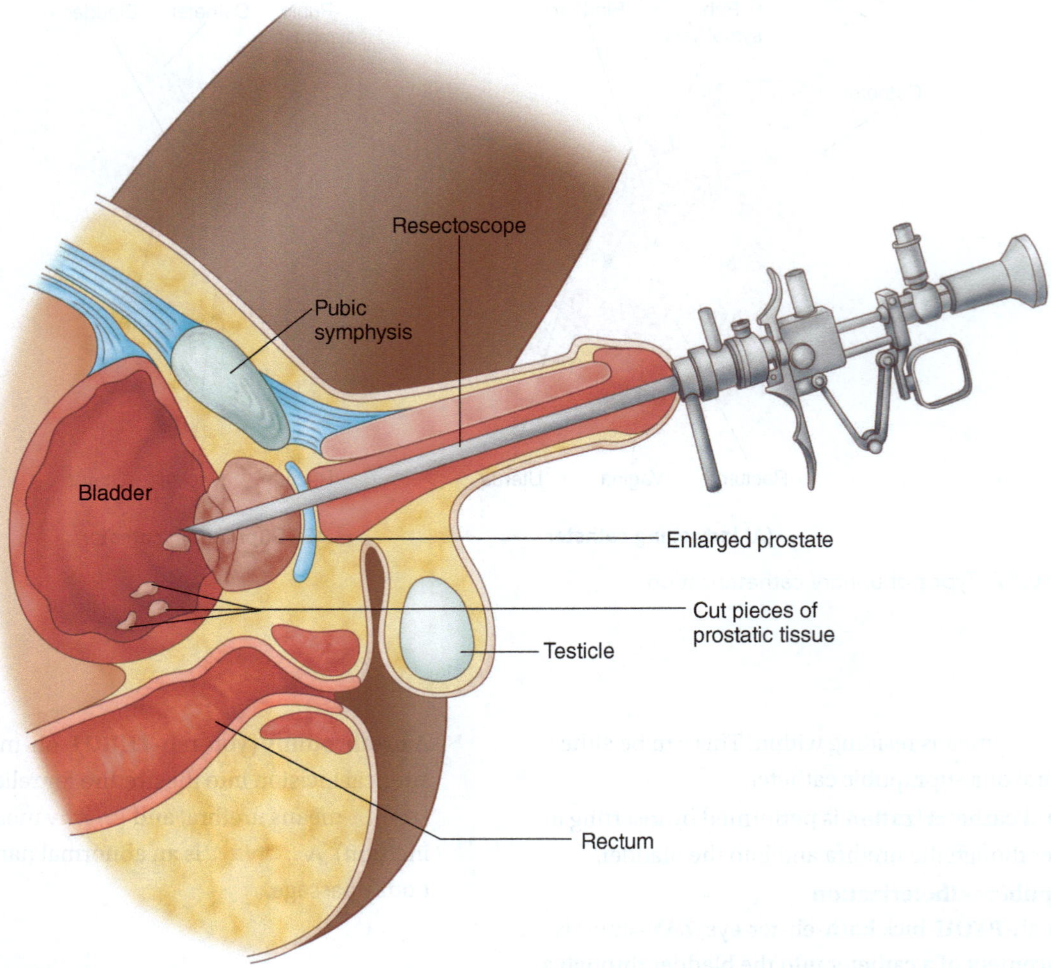

FIGURE 10.18 A transurethral prostatectomy (TURP) being performed with the use of a resectoscope.

a specialized endoscopic instrument that resembles a cystoscope (Figure 10.18). **Retrograde ejaculation** is when an orgasm results in semen flowing backward into the bladder instead of out through the penis. This is the most common long-term complication of a TURP.

- *Radiation therapy* and *hormone therapy* are additional treatments used to control prostate cancer. *Watchful waiting* is often the prescribed course of action in older patients because this disease normally progresses slowly.

Urinary Incontinence Treatment

- **Kegel exercises**, named for Dr. Arnold Kegel, are a series of pelvic muscle exercises used to strengthen the muscles of the pelvic floor. They are used to control urinary stress incontinence in both sexes, in men to treat prostate pain and swelling, and in women to condition the muscles so that they will recover quickly after childbirth.
- **Bladder retraining** is behavioral therapy in which the patient learns to urinate on a schedule, with increasingly longer time intervals as the bladder increases its capacity. The goal is to reestablish voluntary bladder control and to break the cycle of frequency and urgency that results from urge incontinence.

ABBREVIATIONS RELATED TO THE URINARY SYSTEM

Table 10.1 presents an overview of the abbreviations related to the terms introduced in this chapter. *Note:* To avoid errors or confusion, always be cautious when using abbreviations.

TABLE 10.1

Abbreviations Related to the Urinary System

acute renal failure = ARF	**ARF** = acute renal failure
benign prostatic hyperplasia = BPH	**BPH** = benign prostatic hyperplasia
catheterization = cath	**cath** = catheterization
chronic kidney disease = CKD	**CKD** = chronic kidney disease
cystoscopy = cysto	**cysto** = cystoscopy
digital rectal examination = DRE	**DRE** = digital rectal examination
end-stage renal disease = ESRD	**ESRD** = end-stage renal disease
extracorporeal shockwave lithotripsy = ESWL	**ESWL** = extracorporeal shockwave lithotripsy
polycystic kidney disease = PKD	**PKD** = polycystic kidney disease
transurethral resection of the prostate = TURP	**TURP** = transurethral resection of the prostate
urinary tract infection = UTI	**UTI** = urinary tract infection

LEARNING EXERCISES

Matching Word Parts 1

Write the correct answer in the middle column.

	Definition	Correct Answer	Possible Answers
10.1.	bladder	________	-cele
10.2.	glomerulus	________	cyst/o
10.3.	hernia, tumor	________	glomerul/o
10.4.	kidney	________	lith/o
10.5.	stone, calculus	________	nephr/o

Matching Word Parts 2

Write the correct answer in the middle column.

	Definition	Correct Answer	Possible Answers
10.6.	urine, urinary tract	________	-tripsy
10.7.	renal pelvis	________	pyel/o
10.8.	setting free, separation	________	ur/o
10.9.	surgical repair	________	-plasty
10.10.	to crush	________	-lysis

Matching Word Parts 3

Write the correct answer in the middle column.

	Definition	Correct Answer	Possible Answers
10.11.	complete, through	________	-uria
10.12.	water	________	urethr/o

10.13. ureter ______________________ ureter/o

10.14. urethra ______________________ hydr/o

10.15. urination, urine ______________________ dia-

Definitions

Select the correct answer, and write it on the line provided.

10.16. Excessive fluid accumulation in body tissues is called ______________________.

uremia edema nephritis hyperproteinuria

10.17. A stone in the urinary bladder is known as a ______________________.

cholelith cystolith nephrolith ureterolith

10.18. The increased output of urine is known as ______________________.

anuria diuresis dysuria oliguria

10.19. Before entering the ureters, urine collects in the ______________________.

glomeruli renal cortex renal pelvis urinary bladder

10.20. A disorder of the ______________________ gland affects a male's ability to urinate.

prostate kidney ureter urethra

10.21. Urine is produced in microscopic functional units of each kidney called ______________________.

uremia ureters urethra nephrons

10.22. In the male, the ______________________ carries both urine and semen.

prostate gland renal pelvis ureter urethra

10.23. A specialist who treats the genitourinary system of males is a ______________________.

gynecologist nephrologist neurologist urologist

10.24. In ______________________, the urethral opening is on the upper surface of the penis.

epispadias hyperspadias hypospadias urethritis

10.25. The term ______________________ describes treatment in which a body part is removed or its function is destroyed. This type of procedure is frequently used to treat prostate cancer.

ablation adhesion lithotomy meatotomy

Matching Structures

Write the correct answer in the middle column.

	Definition	Correct Answer	Possible Answers
10.26.	the opening through which urine leaves the body	____________	urethral meatus
10.27.	the portion of a nephron that is active in filtering urine	____________	urethra
10.28.	the outer region of the kidney	____________	ureters
10.29.	the tube from the bladder to the outside of the body	____________	renal cortex
10.30.	the tubes that carry urine from the kidney to the bladder	____________	glomerulus

Which Word?

Select the correct answer, and write it on the line provided.

10.31. A surgical incision into the renal pelvis is a ____________________.

pyelotomy pyeloplasty

10.32. The discharge of blood from the ureter is ____________________.

ureterorrhagia urethrorrhagia

10.33. The term meaning excessive urination is ____________________.

incontinence polyuria

10.34. The term meaning inflammation of the bladder is ____________________.

cystitis urethritis

10.35. The major waste product of protein metabolism is ____________________.

urea urine

Spelling Counts

Find the misspelled word in each sentence. Then write that word, spelled correctly, on the line provided.

10.36. A Willms tumor is a malignant tumor of the kidney that occurs in children. ____________________

10.37. Being unable to control excretory functions is known as incontinance. ____________________

10.38. The process of withdrawing urine from the bladder is known as urinary cathaterization.

____

10.39. Keagel exercises are a series of pelvic muscle exercises used to strengthen the muscles of the pelvic floor to control urinary stress incontinence. ________________

10.40. A vesicovaginel fistula is an abnormal opening between the bladder and vagina. ________________

Abbreviation Identification

In the space provided, write the words that each abbreviation stands for.

10.41. **BPH** ________________

10.42. **ESRD** ________________

10.43. **ESWL** ________________

10.44. **GFR** ________________

10.45. **OAB** ________________

Term Selection

Select the correct answer, and write it on the line provided.

10.46. The absence of urine formation by the kidneys is known as ________________.

anuria nocturia oliguria polyuria

10.47. The surgical suturing of the bladder is known as ________________.

cystorrhaphy cystorrhagia urethroplasty nephrorrhaphy

10.48. The term meaning the freeing of a kidney from adhesions is ________________.

nephrolithiasis nephrolysis anuria pyelonephritis

10.49. The term meaning scanty urination is ________________.

diuresis dysuria enuresis oliguria

10.50. The process of artificially filtering waste products from the patient's blood is known as ________________.

diuresis hemodialysis homeostasis hydroureter

Sentence Completion

Write the correct term or terms on the lines provided.

10.51. An inflammation of the kidney, most commonly caused by toxins, infection, or an autoimmune disease, is called ______________________.

10.52. A stone located anywhere along the ureter is known as a ______________________.

10.53. The placement of a catheter into the bladder through a small incision made through the abdominal wall just above the pubic bone is known as ______________________.

10.54. A life-threatening systemic bacterial infection that can occur when a urinary tract infection spreads to the kidneys is known as ______________________.

10.55. A ______________________ (TURP) is the removal of excess tissue from the prostate with the use of a resectoscope.

Word Surgery

Divide each term into its component word parts. Write these word parts, in sequence, on the lines provided. When necessary, use a slash (/) to indicate a combining vowel. (You may not need all of the lines provided.)

10.56. **Hyperproteinuria** is abnormally high concentrations of protein in the urine.

__________ __________ __________ __________

10.57. **Hydronephrosis** is the dilation of one or both kidneys.

__________ __________ __________ __________

10.58. Voiding **cystourethrography** is a diagnostic procedure in which a fluoroscope is used to examine the flow of urine from the bladder and through the urethra.

__________ __________ __________ __________

10.59. A percutaneous **nephrolithotomy** is the surgical removal of a kidney stone through a small incision in the back.

__________ __________ __________ __________

10.60. **Pyelonephritis** is an inflammation of both the renal pelvis and kidney.

__________ __________ __________ __________

True/False

If the statement is true, write **True** on the line. If the statement is false, write **False** on the line.

10.61. ________ Stress incontinence is the inability to control the voiding of urine under physical stress such as running, sneezing, laughing, or coughing.

10.62. ________ Prostatism is a malignancy of the prostate gland.

10.63. ________ Urethrorrhea is bleeding from the urethra.

10.64. ________ Renal colic is an acute pain in the kidney area that is caused by blockage during the passage of a kidney stone.

10.65. ________ Acute renal failure has sudden onset and is characterized by uremia.

Clinical Conditions

Write the correct answer on the line provided.

10.66. Mr. Baldridge suffers from excessive urination during the night. The medical term for this is ____________________.

10.67. Rosita LaPinta inherited ____________________ kidney disease. These cysts slowly reduce kidney function, and this eventually leads to kidney failure.

10.68. Doris Volk has a chronic bladder condition involving inflammation within the wall of the bladder. This is known as ____________________.

10.69. John Danielson has an enlarged prostate gland. This caused narrowing of the urethra, which is known as ____________________.

10.70. Norman Smith was born with the opening of the urethra on the upper surface of the penis. This is known as ____________________.

10.71. Henry Wong's kidneys failed. He is being treated with ____________________, which involves the removal of waste from his blood through a fluid exchange in the abdominal cavity.

10.72. Roberta Gridley is scheduled for surgical repair of the walls of her urethra. This procedure is a/an ____________________.

10.73. When Lenny Nowicki's ______________________ blood test showed a very high PSA level, his physician was concerned about the possibility of prostate cancer.

10.74. Dr. Morita's patient was diagnosed as having ______________________. This is a type of kidney disease caused by inflammation of the glomeruli that causes red blood cells and proteins to leak into the urine.

10.75. Mrs. Franklin has a congenital condition in which one kidney is located in an abnormal position. The medical term for this condition is a/an ______________________.

Which Is the Correct Medical Term?

Select the correct answer, and write it on the line provided.

10.76. Acute renal failure has sudden onset and is characterized by ______________________. This condition can be caused by many factors, including a sudden drop in blood volume or blood pressure due to injury or surgery.

anuria dysuria enuresis uremia

10.77. The term ______________________ means urinary incontinence during sleep. It is also known as bed-wetting.

nocturnal enuresis overactive bladder stress incontinence urinary incontinence

10.78. The term meaning the distention of the ureter is ______________________.

ureteritis hydroureter ureterolith urethrostenosis

10.79. The presence of abnormally *low* concentrations of protein in the blood is known as ______________________.

hyperplasia hyperproteinuria hypocalcemia hypoproteinemia

10.80. A specialist in diagnosing and treating diseases and disorders of the kidneys is a/an ______________________.

gynecologist nephrologist proctologist urologist

Challenge Word Building

These terms are **not** primary terms in the chapter; however, they are made up of the following familiar word parts. If you need help in creating the term, refer to your medical dictionary.

cyst/o	**-cele**
nephr/o	**-itis**
pyel/o	**-lysis**
ureter/o	**-malacia**
urethr/o	**-ostomy**
	-otomy
	-plasty
	-ptosis
	-sclerosis

10.81. The creation of an artificial opening between the urinary bladder and the exterior of the body is a/an ________________.

10.82. A surgical incision into the kidney is a/an ________________.

10.83. Abnormal hardening of the kidney is known as ________________.

10.84. Prolapse of the bladder into the urethra is known as ________________.

10.85. A prolapse of the female urethra is a/an ________________.

10.86. The procedure to separate adhesions around a ureter is a/an ________________.

10.87. Abnormal softening of the kidney is known as ________________.

10.88. The surgical repair of the ureter is known as ________________.

10.89. The surgical creation of an outside excretory opening from the urethra is a/an ________________.

10.90. The surgical repair of the bladder is a/an ________________.

Labeling Exercises

Identify the numbered items on the accompanying figure.

10.91. ______________________ gland

10.92. exterior view of the right ______________________

10.93. inferior ______________________

10.94. ______________________

10.95. renal ______________________

10.96. renal ______________________

10.97. abdominal ______________________

10.98. right and left ______________________

10.99. urinary ______________________

10.100. urethral ______________________

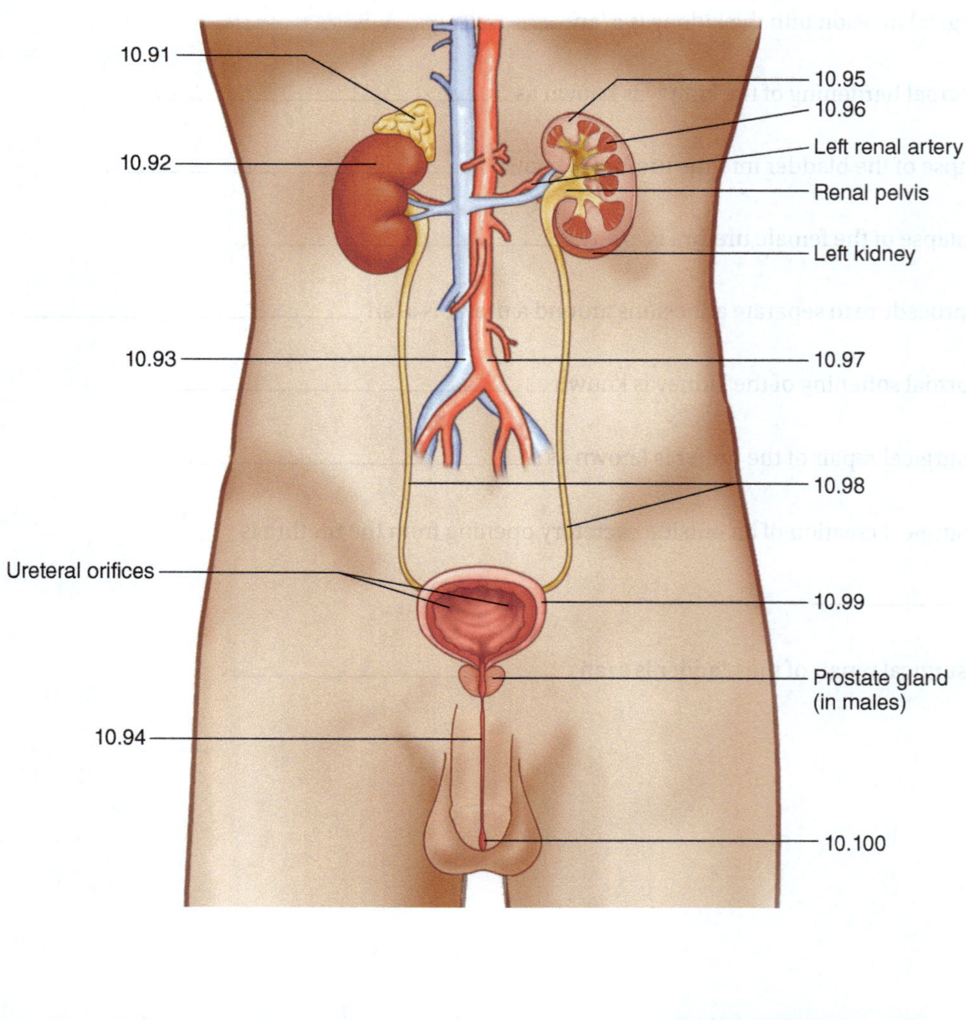

The Human Touch

CRITICAL THINKING EXERCISE

The following story and questions are designed to stimulate critical thinking through class discussion or as a brief essay response. There are no right or wrong answers to these questions.

"Mom, they want me to play for the National Women's Hockey League!" Josie yelled as she ran into the living room. She had just finished practice, and the scouts had told her afterward how impressed they were with her moves. Finally, her lifelong dream of winning an Olympic gold medal for Canada might actually come true! She'd had to make some sacrifices, like living at home after high school, but it looked like that would all pay off. As soon as she saw the looks on the faces of her parents, her smile disappeared.

"Honey, we just got back from the doctor. It turns out that your brother's recurrent bouts of pyelonephritis have led to irreversible kidney damage. The nephrologist is recommending that Xavier have a kidney transplant," her mom explained with a pained look. "We know that he has a better chance if he has a related donor, but he could always go on hemodialysis and wait for a cadaver donor..."

Josie saw her dreams of a hockey career fade away. After Xavier's third bout with nephrotic syndrome, the whole family had been tested for compatibility in case he needed a transplant. Josie was the only one with a positive cross-match. The doctors had explained to her then what it would mean if she decided to donate one of her kidneys, but Josie had brushed it off, assuming that her brother would get better. Now the voices of the doctors came back to her. "No contact sports after a nephrectomy," she heard them say. "There's too big a risk of rupturing the remaining kidney."

Josie was faced with the toughest decision of all: She loved Xavier, but hockey was her life.

Suggested Discussion Topics

1. Discuss the long-term repercussions of being a living organ donor.
2. Imagine that you are Josie's mom or dad and one of your children has the opportunity to save the life of another one of your children. Would you encourage him or her to donate an organ?
3. If Josie decides to donate her kidney and then later chooses to continue playing hockey, what advice should her parents give her?
4. What options might be open to Josie's brother other than having his sister donate a kidney?

CHAPTER 11

THE NERVOUS SYSTEM

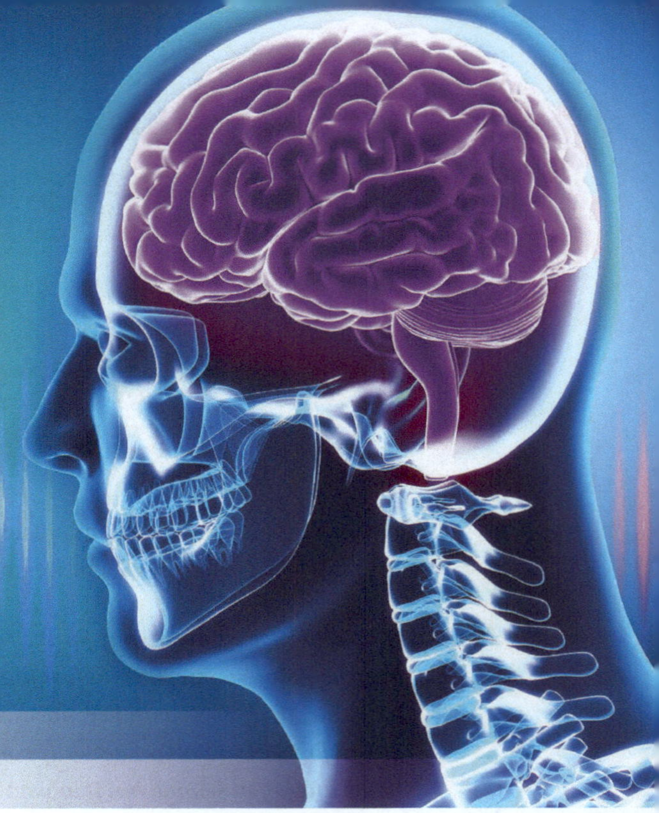

Overview of

STRUCTURES, COMBINING FORMS, AND FUNCTIONS OF THE NERVOUS SYSTEM

Major Structures	Related Combining Forms	Primary Functions
Brain	cerebr/o, encephal/o	Coordinates all body activities by receiving and transmitting messages throughout the body.
Spinal Cord	myel/o	Transmits nerve impulses between the brain, arms and legs, and lower part of the body.
Nerves	neur/i, neur/o	Receive and transmit messages to and from all parts of the body.
Sensory Organs and Receptors		Receive external stimulation and transmit these stimuli to the sensory neurons.
• Eyes (sight)		See Chapter 12.
• Ears (hearing)		See Chapter 12.
• Nose (smell)		See Chapter 8.
• Skin (touch)		See Chapter 13.
• Tongue (taste)		See Chapter 9.

Vocabulary Related to **THE NERVOUS SYSTEM**

This list contains essential word parts and medical terms for this chapter. These and the other important **primary terms** are shown in **boldface** throughout the chapter. *Secondary terms*, which appear in *orange* italics, clarify the meaning of primary terms.

Word Parts

- ☐ **caus/o** burning, burn
- ☐ **cephal/o** head
- ☐ **cerebr/o** cerebrum, brain
- ☐ **concuss/o** shaken together, violently agitated
- ☐ **contus/o** bruise
- ☐ **crani/o** cranium, skull
- ☐ **encephal/o** brain
- ☐ **-esthesia** sensation, feeling
- ☐ **esthet/o** feeling, nervous sensation, sense of perception
- ☐ **mening/o** membranes, meninges
- ☐ **myel/o** spinal cord, bone marrow
- ☐ **neur/i, neur/o** nerve, nerve tissue
- ☐ **-phasia** speak, speech
- ☐ **radicul/o** root, nerve root
- ☐ **-tropic** having an affinity for

Medical Terms

- ☐ **Alzheimer's disease** (**ALTZ**-high-merz)
- ☐ **amnesia** (am-**NEE**-zee-ah)
- ☐ **amyotrophic lateral sclerosis** (ah-**my**-oh-**TROH**-fick **LAT**-er-al skleh-**ROH**-sis)
- ☐ **anesthesiologist** (**an**-es-**thee**-zee-**OL**-oh-jist)
- ☐ **anesthetic** (**an**-es-**THET**-ick)
- ☐ **anesthetist** (ah-**NES**-theh-tist)
- ☐ **Bell's palsy** (**PAWL**-zee)
- ☐ **carotid ultrasonography** (kah-**ROT**-id **ul**-trah-son-**OG**-rah-fee)
- ☐ **causalgia** (kaw-**ZAL**-jee-ah)
- ☐ **central nervous system**
- ☐ **cerebral contusion** (**SER**-eh-bral kon-**TOO**-zhun)
- ☐ **cerebral palsy** (**seh-REE**-bral **PAWL**-zee)
- ☐ **cerebrovascular accident** (**ser**-eh-broh-**VAS**-kyou-lar)
- ☐ **cerebrum** (seh-**REE**-brum)
- ☐ **cervical radiculopathy** (rah-**dick**-you-**LOP**-ah-thee)
- ☐ **cognition** (kog-**NISH**-un)
- ☐ **coma** (**KOH**-mah)
- ☐ **concussion** (kon-**KUSH**-un)
- ☐ **cranial hematoma** (**hee**-mah-**TOH**-mah)
- ☐ **delirium** (deh-**LEER**-ee-um)
- ☐ **dementia** (dih-**MEN**-shah)
- ☐ **dura mater** (**DOO**-rah **MAH**-ter)
- ☐ **dyslexia** (dis-**LECK**-see-ah)
- ☐ **electroencephalography** (ee-**leck**-troh-en-**sef**-ah-**LOG**-rah-fee)
- ☐ **encephalitis** (en-**sef**-ah-**LYE**-tis)
- ☐ **epidural anesthesia** (**ep**-ih-**DOO**-ral **an**-es-**THEE**-zee-ah)
- ☐ **epilepsy** (**EP**-ih-**lep**-see)
- ☐ **ganglion** (**GANG**-glee-on)
- ☐ **hallucination** (hah-**loo**-sih-**NAY**-shun)
- ☐ **hemorrhagic stroke** (**hem**-oh-**RAJ**-ick)
- ☐ **hydrocephalus** (**high**-droh-**SEF**-ah-lus)
- ☐ **hyperesthesia** (**high**-per-es-**THEE**-zee-ah)
- ☐ **ischemic stroke** (iss-**KEE**-mick)
- ☐ **lethargy** (**LETH**-ar-jee)
- ☐ **meningitis** (**men**-in-**JIGH**-tis)
- ☐ **meningocele** (meh-**NING**-goh-**seel**)
- ☐ **migraine headache** (**MY**-grayn)
- ☐ **multiple sclerosis** (skleh-**ROH**-sis)
- ☐ **myelin sheath** (**MY**-eh-lin)
- ☐ **myelitis** (**my**-eh-**LYE**-tis)
- ☐ **myelography** (**my**-eh-**LOG**-rah-fee)
- ☐ **neurologist** (new-**ROL**-oh-jist)
- ☐ **neurons** (**NEW**-ronz)
- ☐ **neurotransmitters** (**new**-roh-trans-**MIT**-erz)
- ☐ **paresthesia** (**pair**-es-**THEE**-zee-ah)
- ☐ **Parkinson's disease**
- ☐ **peripheral nervous system**
- ☐ **peripheral neuropathy** (new-**ROP**-ah-thee)
- ☐ **Reye's syndrome** (**RIZE SIN**-drohm)
- ☐ **sciatica** (sigh-**AT**-ih-kah)
- ☐ **seizure** (**SEE**-zhur)
- ☐ **shaken baby syndrome**
- ☐ **spinal cord**
- ☐ **syncope** (**SIN**-koh-pee)
- ☐ **tetanus** (**TET**-ah-nus)
- ☐ **Tourette syndrome** (tuh-**RET SIN**-drohm)
- ☐ **transient ischemic attack**
- ☐ **tremor**
- ☐ **trigeminal neuralgia** (try-**JEM**-ih-nal new-**RAL**-jee-ah)
- ☐ **unconscious**

LEARNING OBJECTIVES

On completion of this chapter, you should be able to:

1. Describe the functions of the nervous system.
2. Describe the structures of the central nervous system.
3. Describe the structures of the peripheral nervous system.
4. Identify the medical specialists who treat disorders of the nervous system.
5. Identify medical word parts of the nervous system.
6. Define the primary terms related to the pathology and the diagnostic and treatment procedures of the nervous system.
7. Spell the primary terms of the nervous system.
8. Pronounce the primary terms of the nervous system.
9. Identify common abbreviations related to the nervous system.

FUNCTIONS OF THE NERVOUS SYSTEM

The nervous system, with the brain as its center, coordinates and controls all bodily activities. When the brain ceases functioning, the body is no longer able to live on its own.

STRUCTURES OF THE NERVOUS SYSTEM

The major structures of the nervous system are the nerves, brain, spinal cord, and sensory organs. The sensory organs, which are the eyes, ears, nose, skin, and tongue, are discussed in other chapters.

Divisions of the Nervous System

For descriptive purposes, the nervous system is divided into two primary parts: the central nervous system and the peripheral nervous systems (Figure 11.1).

- The **central nervous system** (CNS) includes the brain and spinal cord. The functions of the central nervous system are to receive and process information and to regulate all bodily activity.
- The **peripheral nervous system** (PNS) includes the 12 pairs of cranial nerves extending from the brain and the 31 pairs of peripheral spinal nerves extending outward from the spinal cord. The function of the peripheral nervous system is to transmit nerve signals to and from the central nervous system.

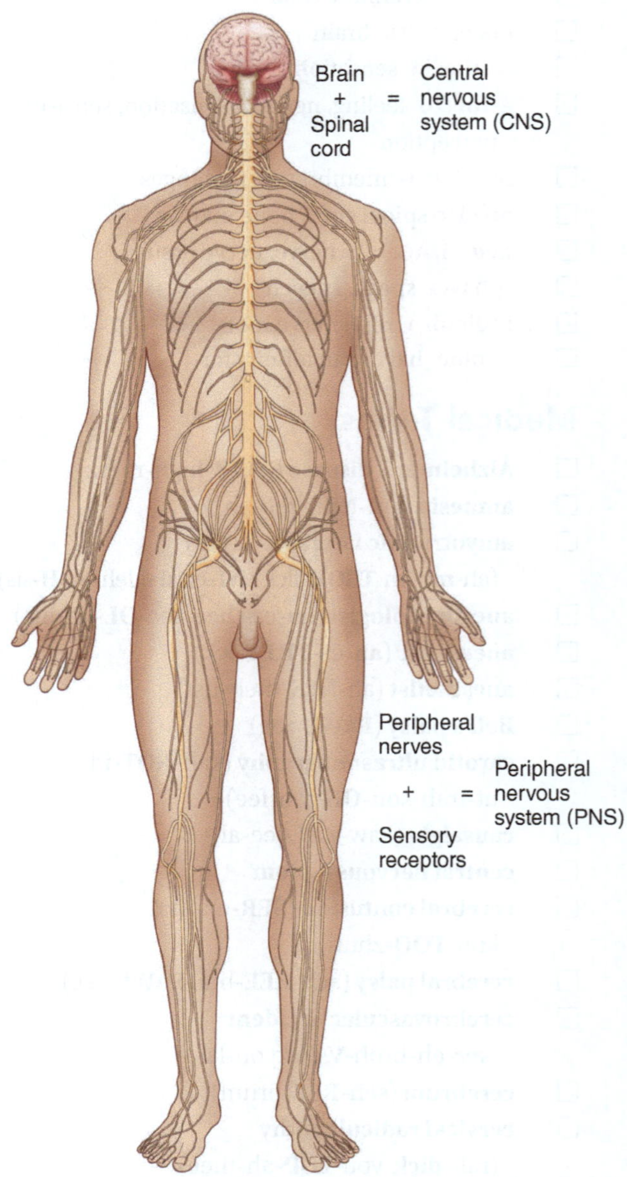

FIGURE 11.1 The structural organization of the central and peripheral nervous systems.

The Nerves

A **nerve** is one or more bundles of *neurons* that connect the brain and spinal cord with other parts of the body. A

tract is a bundle or group of nerve fibers located within the brain or spinal cord.

- *Ascending nerve tracts* carry nerve impulses *toward* the brain.
- *Descending nerve tracts* carry nerve impulses *away from* the brain.
- A **ganglion** (**GANG**-glee-on) is a nerve center made up of a cluster of nerve cell bodies outside the central nervous system (plural, *ganglia* or *ganglions*). *Note:* The term *ganglion* also describes a benign, tumor-like cyst.
- The term **innervation** (**in**-err-**VAY**-shun) means the supply of nerves to a specific body part.
- A **plexus** (**PLECK**-sus) is a network of intersecting spinal nerves (plural, *plexuses*) (Figure 11.8A). This term also describes a network of intersecting blood or lymphatic vessels.
- **Receptors** are sites in the sensory organs (eyes, ears, skin, nose, and taste buds) that receive external stimulation. The receptors send the stimulus through the sensory neurons to the brain for interpretation.
- A **stimulus** is anything that excites (activates) a nerve and causes an impulse (plural, *stimuli*). An *impulse* is a wave of excitation transmitted through nerve fibers and neurons.

The Reflexes

A **reflex** (**REE**-flecks) is an automatic, involuntary response to some change, either inside or outside the body. Examples of reflex actions include:

- Changes in the heart rate, respiratory rate, and blood pressure
- Coughing and sneezing
- Responses to painful stimuli
- Deep tendon reflexes (discussed in Chapter 4)

The Neurons

Neurons (**NEW**-ronz) are the basic cells of the nervous system that allow different parts of the body to communicate with each other.

- The body has billions of neurons carrying nerve impulses throughout the body via an electrochemical process. In the brain, this process creates patterns of neuron electrical activity known as *brain waves*. Different types of brain waves are produced during periods of intense activity, rest, and sleep.
- The three types of neurons are described according to their function. The system of naming the neurons is summarized in Table 11.1. The memory aid **A-C-E** will help you remember their names, and **S-A-M** will help you remember their functions.

Neuron Parts

Each neuron consists of a cell body, several dendrites, a single axon, and terminal end fibers (Figure 11.2).

- The **dendrites** (**DEN**-drytes) are the root-like processes that receive impulses and conduct them to the cell body. A *process* is a structure that extends out from the cell body.
- The **axon** (**ACK**-son) is a process that conducts impulses away from the nerve cell. An axon can be more than 3 feet long. Many, but not all, axons are protected by a myelin sheath, which is a white fatty tissue covering.

TABLE 11.1

Types of Neurons and Their Functions

Types of Neurons	Neuron Functions
A-C-E	**S-A-M**
Afferent neurons (**AF**-er-ent) *Afferent* means toward.	Also known as *sensory neurons*, these neurons emerge from sensory organs and the skin to carry the impulses from the sensory organs *toward* the brain and spinal cord.
Connecting neurons	Also known as *associative neurons*, these neurons link afferent and efferent neurons.
Efferent neurons (**EF**-er-ent) *Efferent* means away from.	Also known as *motor neurons*, these neurons carry impulses *away from* the brain and spinal cord and toward the muscles and glands.

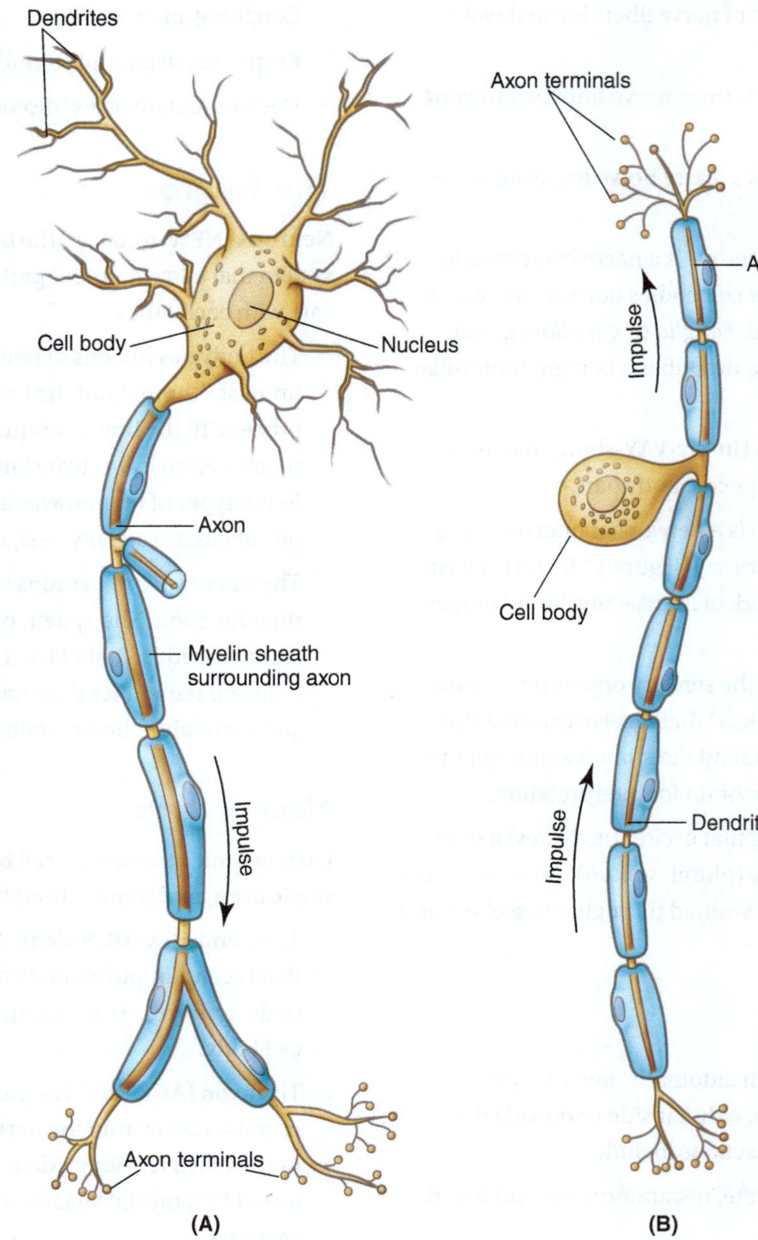

FIGURE 11.2 The structure of two types of neurons. (A) Efferent (motor) neurons. (B) Afferent (sensory) neurons.

- **Terminal end fibers** are the branching fibers at the end of the axon that lead the nerve impulse from the axon to the synapse.
- A **synapse** (**SIN**-apps) is the space between two neurons or between a neuron and a receptor organ. A single neuron can have a few or several hundred synapses.

Neurotransmitters

Neurotransmitters (**new**-roh-trans-**MIT**-erz) are chemical substances that make it possible for messages to cross from the synapse of a neuron to the target receptor. There are between 200 and 300 known neurotransmitters, and each has a specialized function. Here are some examples of neurotransmitters and their roles:

- ***Acetylcholine*** is released at some synapses in the spinal cord and at neuromuscular junctions; it influences muscle action.
- ***Dopamine*** is released within the brain and plays a role in motivation, pleasure, and muscle movement. An excess of dopamine is associated with schizophrenia, mood and thought disorders, and abnormal movement disorders such as Parkinson's disease.

- ***Glutamate*** plays an important role in learning; too little of this chemical can cause psychosis.
- ***Endorphins*** are naturally occurring substances that are produced by the brain to help relieve pain.
- ***Norepinephrine*** affects alertness and arousal, increasing blood pressure and heart rate, and releasing stores of glucose in response to stress. It is also a hormone released by the adrenal gland as part of the body's fight-or-flight response (see Chapter 14).
- ***Serotonin***, which is released in the brain, has roles in sleep, hunger, and pleasure recognition. It is also sometimes linked to mood disorders.

Glial Cells

Glial cells (**GLEE**-ul) provide support and protection for neurons, and their four main functions are (1) to surround neurons and hold them in place, (2) to supply nutrients and oxygen to neurons, (3) to insulate one neuron from another, and (4) to destroy and remove dead neurons.

The Myelin Sheath

A **myelin sheath** (**MY**-eh-lin) is the protective covering made up of glial cells. This white sheath forms the white matter of the brain and covers some parts of the spinal cord and the axon of most peripheral nerves (Figure 11.2).

- The portions of the nerve fibers that are myelinated are known as ***white matter***. The term ***myelinated*** means having a myelin sheath. It is the color of this covering that makes these fibers white.
- The portions of the nerve fibers that are unmyelinated are known as ***gray matter***. The term ***unmyelinated*** means lacking a myelin sheath. The lack of the myelin sheath reveals the brownish-gray color of the cortex of the cerebrum and cerebellum, and the core of the spinal cord.

THE CENTRAL NERVOUS SYSTEM

The **central nervous system** is made up of the brain and spinal cord. These structures are protected externally by the bones of the cranium and the vertebrae of the spinal column, which are discussed in Chapter 3. Within these bony structures, the brain and spinal cord are further protected by the meninges and the cerebrospinal fluid (Figure 11.3).

The Meninges

The **meninges** (meh-**NIN**-jeez) are the system of membranes that enclose the brain and spinal cord (singular, *meninx*). The meninges consist of three layers of connective tissue. These are the dura mater, the arachnoid membrane, and the pia mater (Figure 11.3).

The Dura Mater

The **dura mater** (**DOO**-rah **MAH**-ter) is the thick, tough, outermost membrane of the meninges. ***Dura*** means hard, and ***mater*** means mother.

- The inner surface of the cranium (skull) is lined with the dura mater.
- The inner surface of the vertebral column is known as the ***epidural space***. This space, which is located between the walls of the vertebral column and the dura mater of the meninges, contains fat and supportive connective tissues to cushion the dura mater.
- In both the skull and vertebral column, the ***subdural space*** is located between the dura mater and the arachnoid membrane.

The Arachnoid Membrane

The **arachnoid membrane** (ah-**RACK**-noid), which resembles a spider web, is the second layer of the meninges and is located between the dura mater and the pia mater. ***Arachnoid*** means having to do with spiders.

- The arachnoid membrane is loosely attached to the other meninges to allow space for fluid to flow between the layers.
- The ***subarachnoid space***, which is located below the arachnoid membrane and above the pia mater, contains cerebrospinal fluid.

The Pia Mater

The **pia mater** (**PEE**-ah **MAH**-ter), which is the third layer of the meninges, is located nearest to the brain and spinal cord. It consists of delicate connective tissue that contains a rich supply of blood vessels. ***Pia*** means tender or delicate, and ***mater*** means mother.

Cerebrospinal Fluid

Cerebrospinal fluid (**ser**-eh-broh-**SPY**-nal) (CSF), also known as ***spinal fluid***, is produced by special capillaries within the four ventricles located in the middle region of

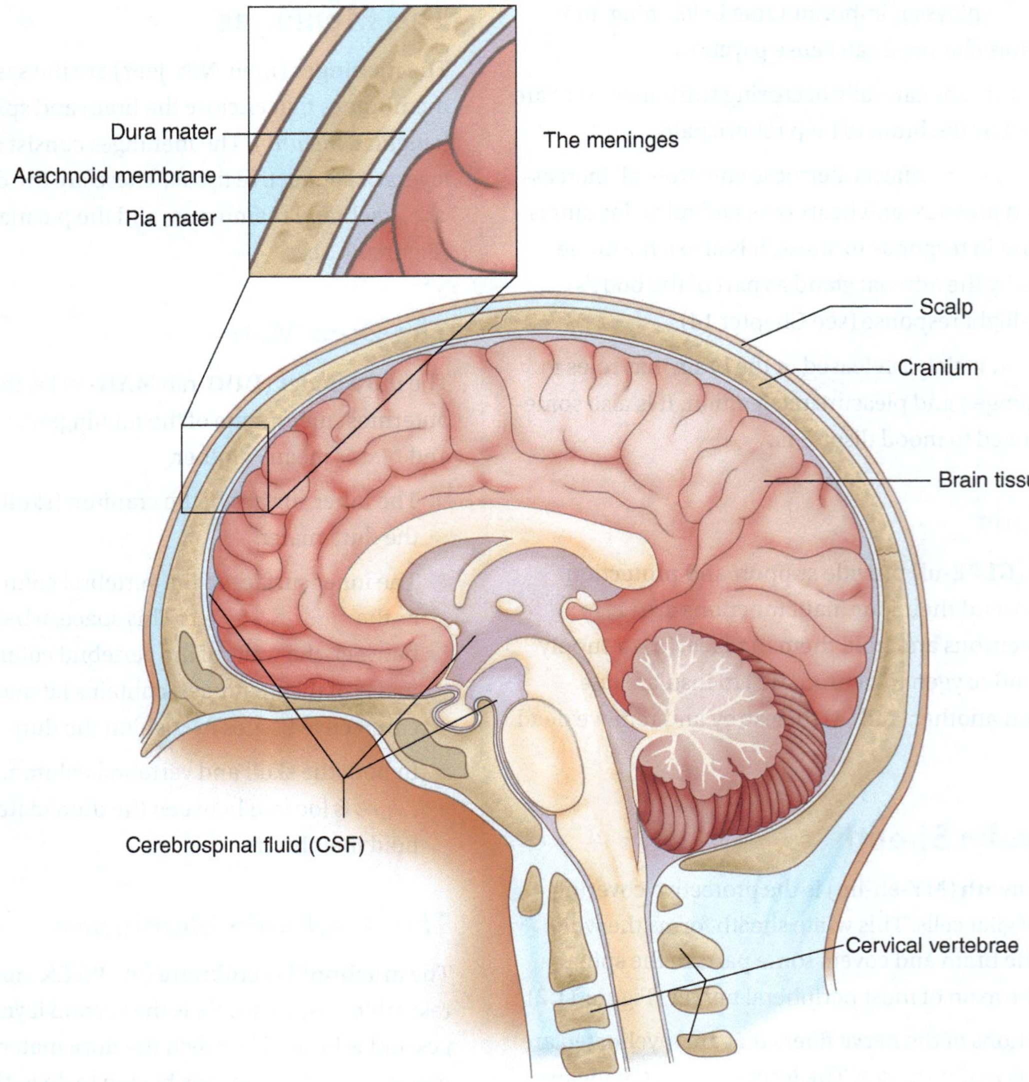

FIGURE 11.3 A cross-section of the brain showing the meninges and the protective coverings. The cerebrospinal fluid is shown in purple.

the cerebrum (Figures 11.3 and 11.4). Cerebrospinal fluid is a clear, colorless, watery fluid that flows throughout the brain and around the spinal cord. The functions of this fluid are to:

- Cool and cushion these organs from shock or injury
- Nourish the brain and spinal cord by transporting nutrients and chemical messengers to these tissues

The Parts of the Brain

The brain parts are shown in Figures 11.4 through 11.6. The body functions that are controlled by these brain parts are summarized in Table 11.2. Notice that the functions most essential to the support of life are located within the most protected portions of the brain.

The Cerebrum

The **cerebrum** (seh-**REE**-brum) is the largest and uppermost portion of the brain. It is responsible for all thought, judgment, memory, and emotion, as well as for controlling and integrating motor and sensory functions. Note that *cerebrum* and *cerebellum* are similar words but refer to very different parts of the brain. *Memory aid:* the cere*bel*lum is *bel*ow the cerebrum.

- The term **cerebral** (seh-**REE**-bral) means pertaining to the cerebrum or to the brain (**cerebr** means brain, and **-al** means pertaining to).
- The **cerebral cortex**, which is made up of gray matter, is the outer layer of the cerebrum and is made up of elevated folds and deep fissures (Figure 11.6).

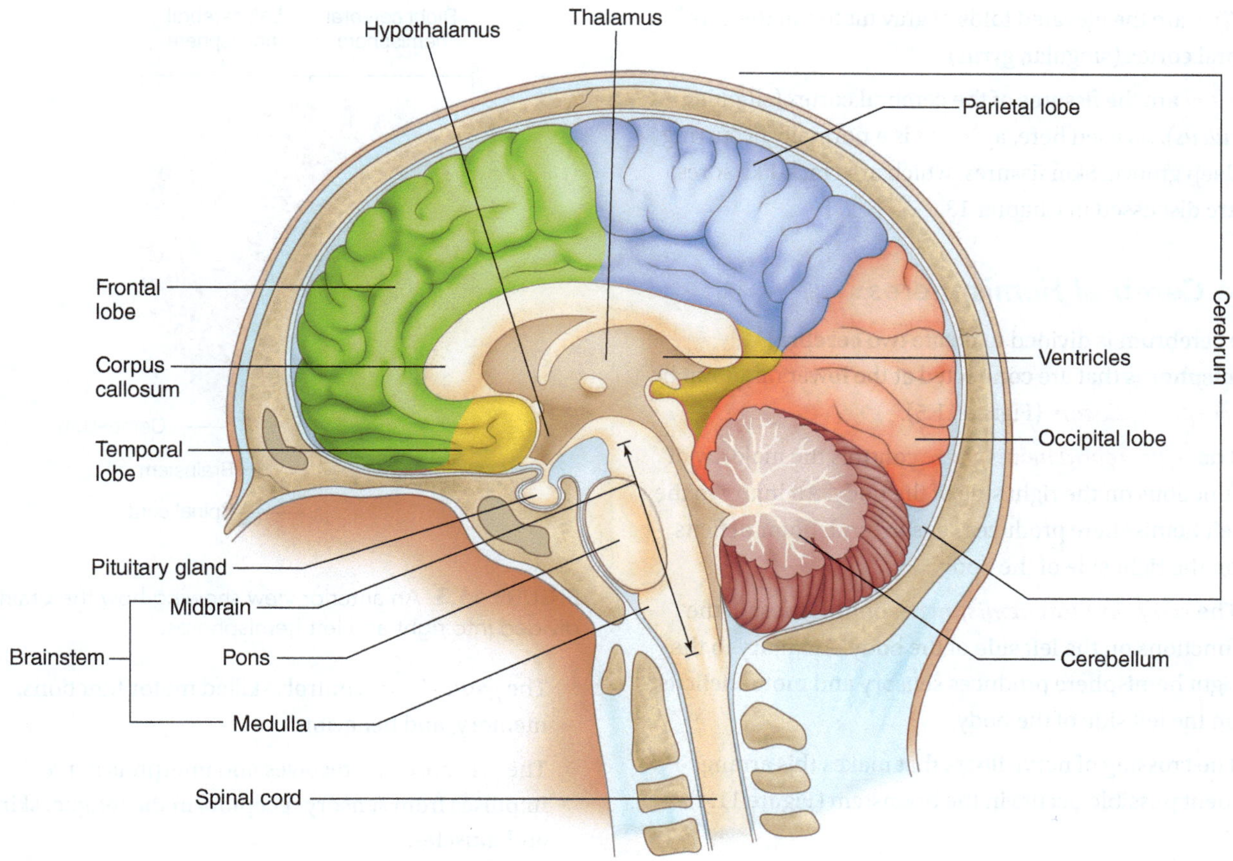

FIGURE 11.4 A cross-section showing the major parts of the brain.

TABLE 11.2

Brain Parts and Their Functions

Brain Part	Functions
The **cerebrum**, which is the largest and uppermost part of the brain, consists of four lobes.	Controls the highest level of thought, including judgment, memory, association, and critical thinking. It also processes sensations and controls all voluntary muscle activity.
The **thalamus** is located below the cerebrum.	Relays sensory stimuli from the spinal cord and midbrain to the cerebral cortex. The thalamus suppresses some stimuli and magnifies others.
The **hypothalamus** is located below the thalamus.	Controls vital bodily functions (Table 11.3).
The **cerebellum** is located in the lower back of the cranium below the cerebrum.	Coordinates muscular activity and balance for smooth and steady movements.
The **brainstem** is located in the base of the brain and forms the connection between the brain and spinal cord. It consists of the: • Midbrain • Pons • Medulla oblongata	Controls the functions necessary for survival (breathing, digestion, heart rate, and blood pressure) and for arousal (being awake and alert).

- *Gyri* are the elevated folds of gray matter in the cerebral cortex (singular, *gyrus*).
- *Sulci* are the fissures of the cerebral cortex (singular, *sulcus*). As used here, a *fissure* is a normally occurring deep groove. Skin fissures, which are crack-like sores, are discussed in Chapter 13.

The Cerebral Hemispheres

The cerebrum is divided to create two **cerebral hemispheres** that are connected at the lower midpoint by the *corpus callosum* (Figure 11.5).

- The *left cerebral hemisphere* controls the majority of functions on the right side of the body. An injury to the left hemisphere produces sensory and motor deficits on the right side of the body.
- The *right cerebral hemisphere* controls most of the functions on the left side of the body. An injury to the right hemisphere produces sensory and motor deficits on the left side of the body.
- The crossing of nerve fibers that makes this arrangement possible occurs in the brainstem (Figure 11.4).

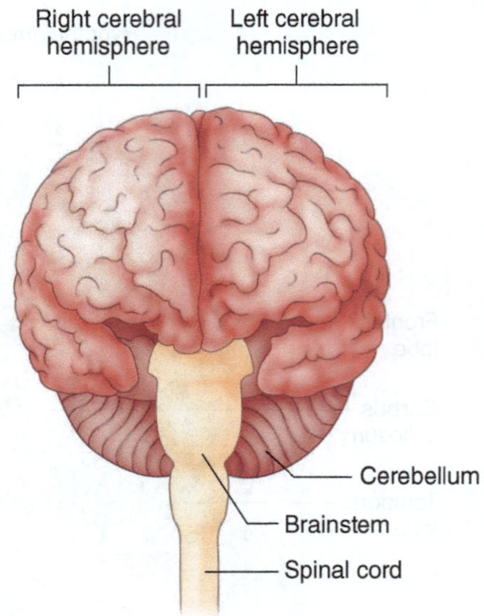

FIGURE 11.5 An anterior view showing how the brain is divided into right and left hemispheres.

The Cerebral Lobes

Each cerebral hemisphere is subdivided to create pairs of **cerebral lobes**. Each lobe is named for the bone of the cranium that covers it (Figure 11.6).

- The *frontal lobe* controls skilled motor functions, memory, and behavior.
- The *parietal lobe* receives and interprets nerve impulses from sensory receptors in the tongue, skin, and muscles.
- The *occipital lobe* controls eyesight.
- The *temporal lobe* controls the senses of hearing and smell, and the ability to create, store, and access new information.

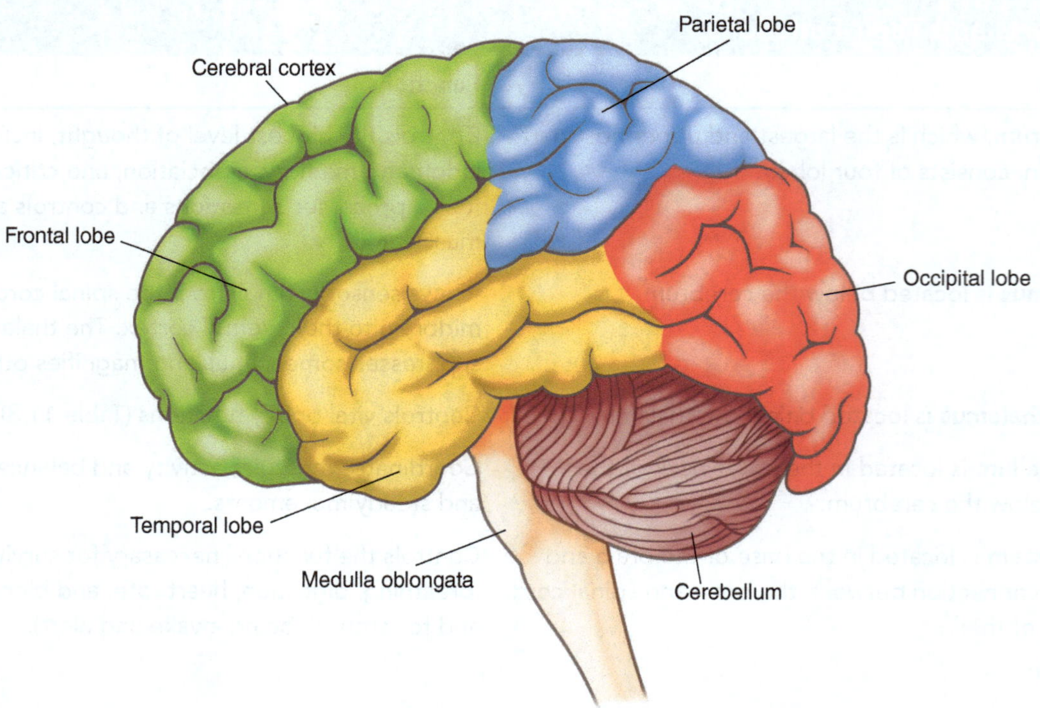

FIGURE 11.6 A left lateral view of the exterior of the brain showing the four lobes of the cerebrum plus the medulla oblongata and the cerebellum. The cerebral cortex is the outer layer of the cerebrum.

The Thalamus

The **thalamus** (**THAL**-ah-mus), which is located below the cerebrum, produces sensations by relaying impulses to and from the cerebrum and the sense organs of the body.

The Hypothalamus

The **hypothalamus** (**high**-poh-**THAL**-ah-mus) is located below the thalamus (Figure 11.4). The seven major regulatory functions of the hypothalamus are summarized in Table 11.3.

The Cerebellum

The **cerebellum** (**ser**-eh-**BELL**-um) is the second-largest part of the brain. It is located at the back of the head below the posterior portion of the cerebrum (Figures 11.4 through 11.6).

- The cerebellum receives incoming messages regarding movement within joints, muscle tone, and positions of the body. From here, messages are relayed to the different parts of the brain that control the motions of skeletal muscles.
- The general functions of the cerebellum are to produce smooth and coordinated movements, to maintain equilibrium, and to sustain normal postures.

The Brainstem

The **brainstem** is the stalk-like portion of the brain that connects the cerebral hemispheres with the spinal cord. It is made up of three parts: the midbrain, pons, and medulla oblongata (Figure 11.4).

- The **midbrain** and **pons** (**PONZ**) provide conduction pathways to and from the higher and lower centers in the brain. They also control reflexes for movements of the eyes and head in response to visual and auditory stimuli. *Pons* is the Latin word for bridge.
- The **medulla oblongata** (meh-**DULL**-ah **ob**-long-**GAH**-tah), which is located at the lowest part of the brainstem, is connected to the spinal cord. It controls basic survival functions, including the muscles that make possible respiration, heart rate, and blood pressure, as well as reflexes for coughing, sneezing, swallowing, and vomiting.

The Spinal Cord

The **spinal cord** is a long, fragile, tube-like structure that begins at the end of the brainstem and continues down almost to the bottom of the spinal column (Figure 11.1).

- The spinal cord contains all the nerves that affect the limbs and lower part of the body, and serves as the pathway for impulses traveling to and from the brain.
- The spinal cord is surrounded and protected by cerebrospinal fluid and the meninges.

THE PERIPHERAL NERVOUS SYSTEM

The **peripheral nervous system** consists of the 12 pairs of cranial nerves that extend from the brain, plus 31 pairs of spinal nerves that extend from the spinal cord. ***Peripheral*** means pertaining to body parts that are away from the center of the body.

TABLE 11.3

Regulatory Functions of the Hypothalamus

1. Regulates and integrates the autonomic nervous system, including controlling heart rate, blood pressure, respiratory rate, and digestive tract activity
2. Regulates emotional responses, including fear and pleasure
3. Regulates body temperature
4. Regulates food intake by controlling hunger sensations
5. Regulates water balance by controlling thirst sensations
6. Regulates sleep–wakefulness cycles
7. Regulates the pituitary gland and endocrine system activity (see Chapter 14)

Three types of specialized peripheral nerves transmit signals to and from the central nervous system. These are autonomic, sensory, and somatic nerve fibers.

- ***Autonomic nerve fibers*** carry instructions to the organs and glands from the autonomic nervous system.
- ***Sensory nerve fibers*** receive external stimuli, such as how something feels, and transmit this information to the brain, where it is interpreted.
- ***Somatic nerve fibers***, which are also known as ***motor nerve fibers***, convey information that controls the body's voluntary muscular movements.

The Cranial Nerves

The 12 pairs of **cranial nerves** originate from the under-surface of the brain. The two nerves of a pair are identical in function and structure, and each nerve of a pair serves half of the body. These cranial nerves are identified by Roman numerals and are named for the area or function they serve (Figure 11.7).

The Peripheral Spinal Nerves

The 31 pairs of **peripheral spinal nerves** are grouped together and named based on the region of the body they innervate.

- Within each region, the nerves are referred to by number. The cervical nerves are C1–C8, the thoracic nerves are T1–T12, the lumbar nerves are L1–L5, and the sacral nerves are S1–S5 (Figure 11.8B).
- Spinal nerves sometimes join with others to form a plexus to innervate a certain area. The lumbar plexus, as shown in Figure 11.8A, is made up of the first four lumbar nerves (L1–L4) and serves the lower back.

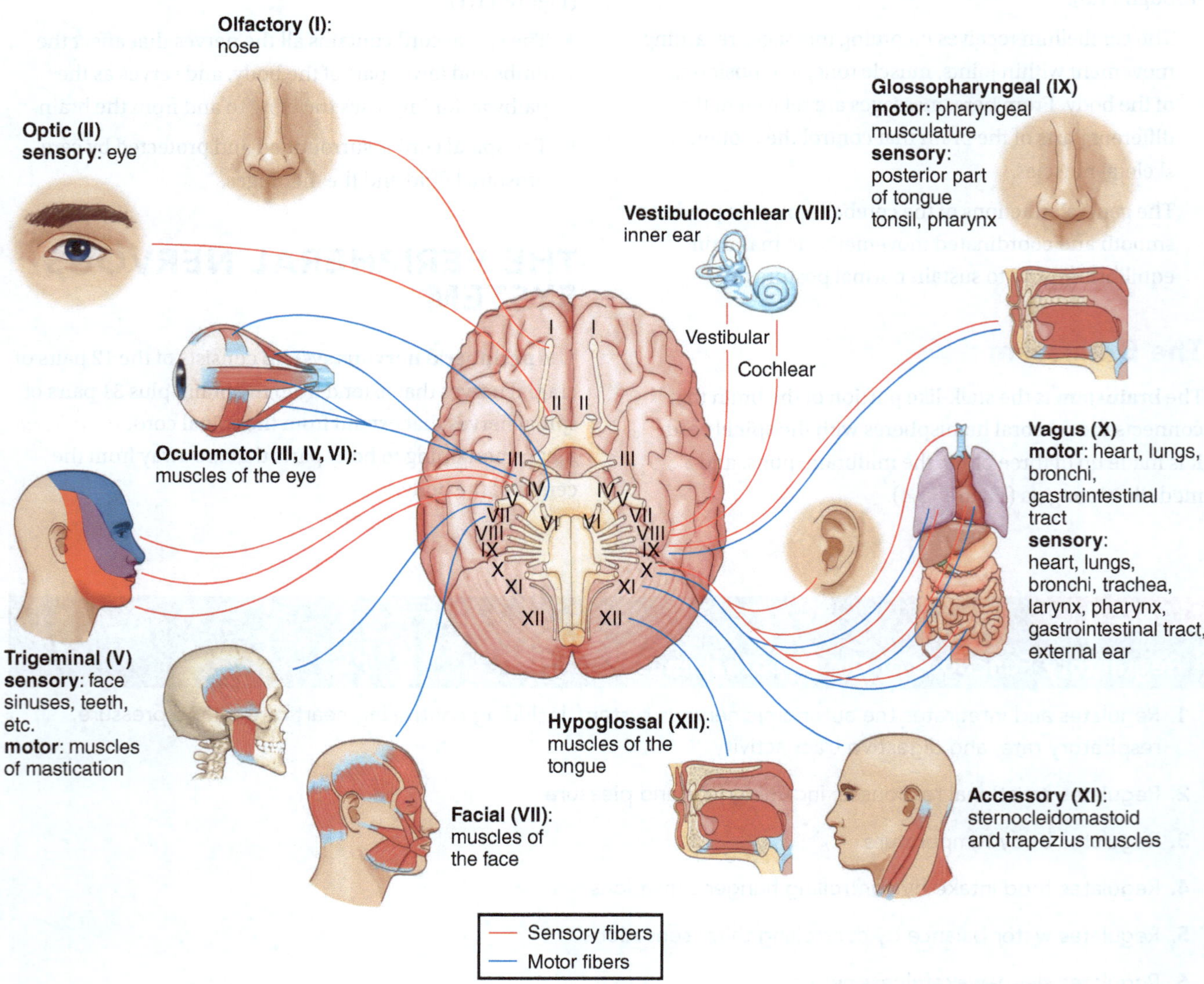

FIGURE 11.7 Cranial nerves are identified with Roman numerals and are named for the area or function they serve.

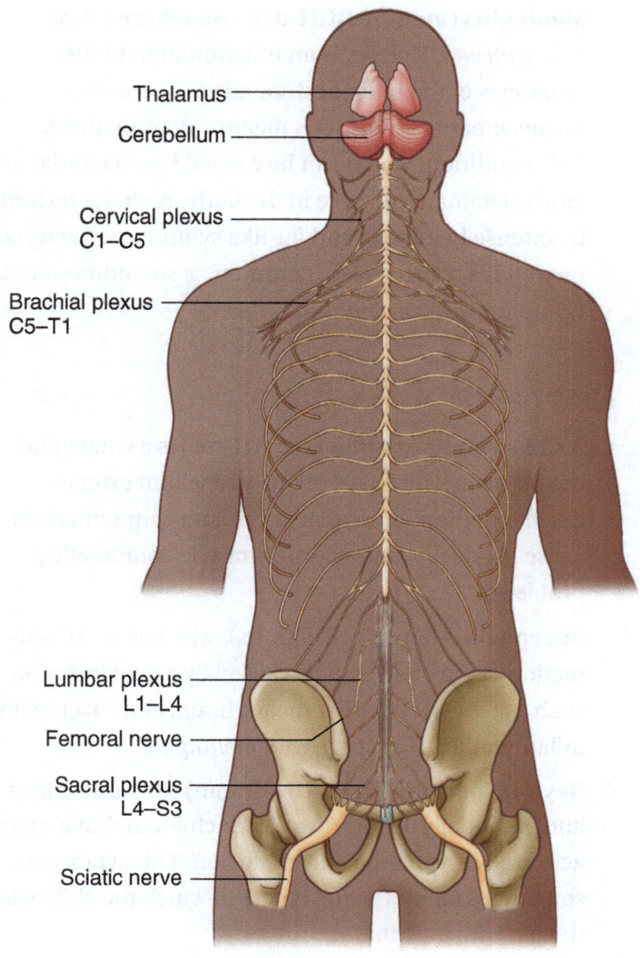

FIGURE 11.8A Most spinal cord plexuses are named for the corresponding vertebrae.

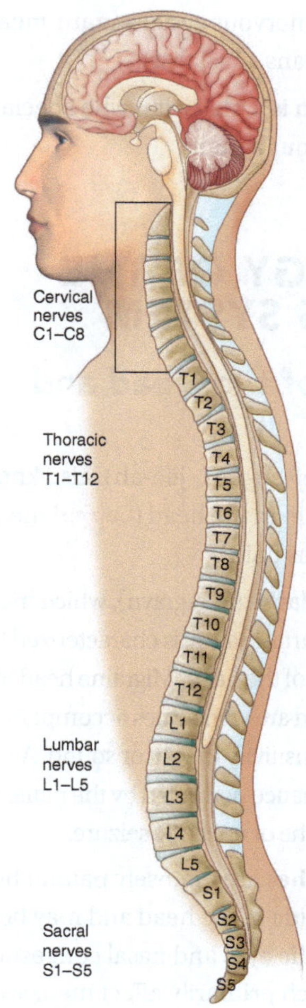

FIGURE 11.8B Within each spinal region, the nerves are referred to by number..

The Autonomic Nervous System

The **autonomic nervous system** is organized into two divisions, one comprising *sympathetic nerves* and the other *parasympathetic nerves*. The autonomic nervous system controls the involuntary actions of the body such as the functioning of internal organs. To maintain homeostasis within the body, each division balances the activity of the other division. ***Homeostasis*** is the process of maintaining the constant internal environment of the body.

- The **sympathetic nerves** prepare the body for emergencies and stress by increasing the respiratory rate, heart rate, and blood flow to muscles. These nerves become aroused as part of the ***fight-or-flight response***, which is the body's natural reaction to real or imaginary danger.
- The **parasympathetic nerves** return the body to normal after a response to stress. They also maintain normal body functions during ordinary circumstances that are not emotionally or physically stressful.

MEDICAL SPECIALTIES RELATED TO THE NERVOUS SYSTEM

- An **anesthesiologist** (**an**-es-**thee**-zee-**OL**-oh-jist) is a physician who specializes in administering anesthetic agents before and during surgery (**an-** means without, **esthesi** means feeling, and **-ologist** means specialist).
- An **anesthetist** (ah-**NES**-theh-tist) is a medical professional who specializes in administering anesthesia but is not a physician, for example, a nurse anesthetist (**an-** means without, **esthet** means feeling, and **-ist** means specialist).
- A **neurologist** (new-**ROL**-oh-jist) is a physician who specializes in diagnosing and treating diseases and

disorders of the nervous system (**neur** means nerve, and **-ologist** means specialist).

- A **neurosurgeon** is a physician who specializes in surgery of the nervous system.

PATHOLOGY OF THE NERVOUS SYSTEM

Conditions of the Head and Meninges

- **Cephalalgia** (**sef**-ah-**LAL**-jee-ah), also known as a ***headache***, is pain in the head (**cephal** means head, and **-algia** means pain).
- A **migraine headache** (**MY**-grayn), which may be preceded by a warning aura, is characterized by throbbing pain on one side of the head. Migraine headaches primarily affect women and are sometimes accompanied by nausea, vomiting, and sensitivity to light or sound. A ***warning aura*** is a visual disturbance perceived by the patient preceding a migraine headache or epileptic seizure.
- **Cluster headaches** are intensely painful headaches that affect one side of the head and may be associated with tearing of the eyes and nasal congestion. These headaches, which primarily affect men, are named for their repeated occurrence in groups or clusters.
- An **encephalocele** (en-**SEF**-ah-loh-**seel**), also known as a ***craniocele***, is a congenital herniation of brain tissue through a gap in the skull (**encephal/o** means brain, and **-cele** means hernia). ***Congenital*** means present at birth, and ***herniation*** means protrusion of a structure from its normal position. Compare this with a *meningocele*.
- A **meningocele** (meh-**NING**-goh-**seel**) is the congenital herniation of the meninges through a defect in the skull or spinal column (**mening/o** means meninges, and **-cele** means hernia). Compare this with an *encephalocele*.
- **Hydrocephalus** (**high**-droh-**SEF**-ah-lus) is a condition in which excess cerebrospinal fluid accumulates in the ventricles of the brain (**hydr/o** means water, **cephal** means head, and **-us** is a singular noun ending). This condition can occur at birth (this is called congenital) or develop later in life from obstructions related to meningitis, brain tumors, or other causes.
- A **meningioma** (meh-**nin**-jee-**OH**-mah) is a common, slow-growing, and usually benign tumor of the meninges (**mening/i** means meninges, and **-oma** means tumor).
- **Meningitis** (**men**-in-**JIGH**-tis), also referred to as ***infectious meningitis***, is an inflammation of the meninges of the brain and spinal cord (**mening** means meninges, and **-itis** means inflammation). This condition, which can be caused by a bacterial or viral infection elsewhere in the body, is characterized by intense headache and flu-like symptoms. Bacterial meningitis, which is less common, is sometimes fatal. Compare with *encephalitis*.

Disorders of the Brain

- A **Chiari malformation** (kee-**AH**-ree) is a congenital condition in which part of the cerebellum extends down into the spinal canal. It can be asymptomatic or cause headache, neck pain, or muscle coordination problems.
- **Encephalitis** (en-**sef**-ah-**LYE**-tis), which is an inflammation of the brain, can be caused by a viral infection such as rabies (**encephal** means brain, and **-itis** means inflammation). Compare with *meningitis*.
- **Reye's syndrome** (**RIZE SIN**-drohm) (RS) is a serious and potentially deadly disorder in children that is characterized by vomiting and confusion. This syndrome sometimes follows a viral illness in which the child was treated with aspirin.
- **Tetanus** (**TET**-ah-nus), also known as ***lockjaw***, is an acute and potentially fatal infection of the central nervous system caused by a toxin produced by the tetanus bacteria. Tetanus can be prevented through immunization. In unimmunized people, this condition is typically acquired through a deep puncture wound.
- **Tourette syndrome** (tuh-**RET SIN**-drohm) (TS) is a complex neurological disorder characterized by involuntary tics, grunts, and compulsive utterances that sometimes include obscenities.
- The term **cognition** (kog-**NISH**-un) describes the mental activities associated with thinking, learning, and memory. ***Mild cognitive impairment*** is decline from normal function characterized by short-term memory loss, which may be an early predictor of dementia.
- **Dementia** (dih-**MEN**-shah) is a slowly progressive decline in mental abilities, including memory, thinking, and judgment, that is often accompanied by personality changes. ***Senile dementia*** is dementia of the aged. ***Sundowning*** refers to a group of symptoms leading to a state of confusion that can happen toward the end of the day in patients with dementia.

- **Vascular dementia** is a form of dementia caused by a stroke or other restriction of the flow of blood to the brain. Although Alzheimer's disease is the primary cause of dementia, vascular dementia accounts for about 10–20% of all cases.

Congenital Nervous System Disorders

Congenital disorders are those that are present at birth. In the nervous system these are birth defects of the structures of the brain or spinal cord that occur while the fetus is growing. These include Chiari malformation, hydrocephalus, encephalocele, meningocele, and cerebral palsy (all discussed elsewhere in this chapter) as well as *neural tube defects*: congenital disorders of the brain and spine such as spina bifida and anencephaly (see Chapter 18). To help prevent neural tube defects, pregnant women should take *folic acid* supplements during pregnancy.

Neurodegenerative Diseases

The term **neurodegenerative disease** (**new**-roh-deh-**JEN**-er-ah-tiv), also called *degenerative nerve disease*, is an umbrella term for disorders in which there is a progressive loss of the structure or functions of the neurons.

- **Alzheimer's disease** (**ALTZ**-high-merz) (AD) is a group of disorders involving the parts of the brain that control thought, memory, and language (Figure 11.9). It is the leading form of dementia and is marked by progressive deterioration that affects both the memory and reasoning capabilities of an individual.
- *Huntington's disease* is a genetic disorder that is classified as a neurodegenerative disease (see Chapter 2).
- **Parkinson's disease** (PD) is a chronic, degenerative central nervous disorder characterized by fine muscle tremors, rigidity, and a slow or shuffling gait. *Gait* describes the manner of walking. This slow or shuffling gait is caused by gradual progressive loss of control over movements due to inadequate levels of the neurotransmitter dopamine in the brain.
- A **tremor** is a repetitive, involuntary muscle movement usually involving the hands, arms, head, or face. There are multiple types of tremors, which cause different types of movements and can be differentiated by their causes and presentation. For example, a *Parkinsonian tremor* is characterized by a "pill-rolling" movement of the hands while at rest, while an *essential tremor* causes shakiness of the arms, hands, or head, which worsens during voluntary movements.
- *Lewy body dementia*, which is the second most common type of dementia, occurs when abnormal proteins interfere with cell function in the brain. It is named for neurologist Frederic Lewy.
- **Amyotrophic lateral sclerosis** (ah-**my**-oh-**TROH**-fick **LAT**-er-al skleh-**ROH**-sis) (ALS), also known as *Lou Gehrig's disease*, is a rapidly progressive neurological disease that attacks the nerve cells responsible for controlling voluntary muscles. Patients affected with this condition become progressively weaker until they are completely paralyzed and die.

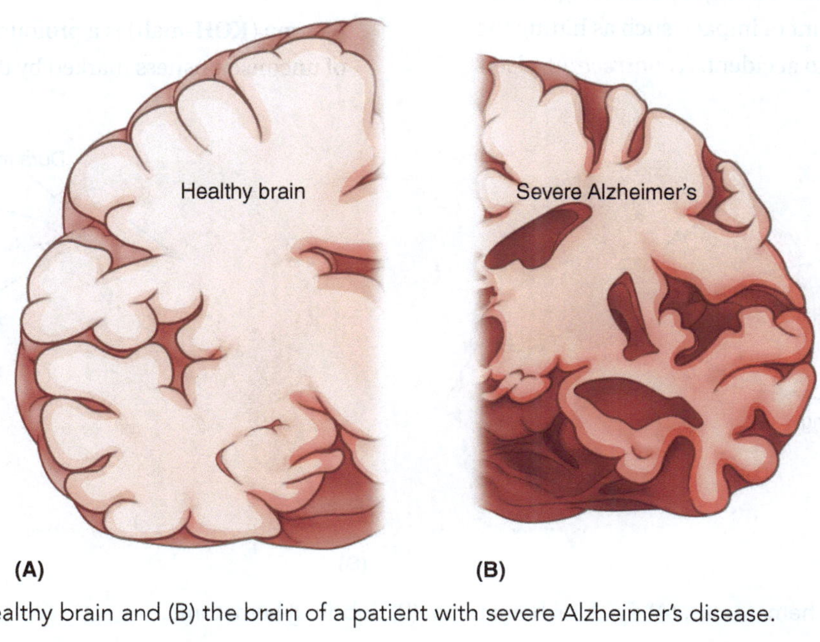

FIGURE 11.9 (A) A healthy brain and (B) the brain of a patient with severe Alzheimer's disease.

Brain Injuries

- **Amnesia** (am-**NEE**-zee-ah) is a memory disturbance characterized by a total or partial inability to recall past experiences. This condition can be caused by a brain injury, an illness, or a psychological disturbance.
- A **concussion** (kon-**KUSH**-un) is a violent shaking up or jarring of the brain (**concuss** means shaken together, and **-ion** means condition or state of). A concussion may result in a temporary loss of awareness and function. Compare with a *cerebral contusion.*
- A **cerebral contusion** (**SER**-eh-bral kon-**TOO**-zhun) is the bruising of brain tissue as the result of a head injury that causes the brain to bounce against the rigid bone of the skull (**contus** means bruise, and **-ion** means condition). Compare with *concussion.*
- A **cranial hematoma** (hee-mah-**TOH**-mah) is a collection of blood trapped in the tissues of the brain (**hemat** means blood, and **-oma** means tumor). Named for their location, the types of cranial hematomas include an ***epidural hematoma*** located above the dura mater, and a ***subdural hematoma***, which is located below the dura mater (Figure 11.10). Cranial hematomas may be caused by a major or minor head injury.

Traumatic Brain Injury

A **traumatic brain injury** (TBI) is a blow to the head or a penetrating head injury that damages the brain. Not all blows to the head result in damage to the brain. When an injury does occur, it can range from mild, with only a brief change in mental status, to severe, with longer-lasting effects.

- The term ***coup*** describes an injury occurring within the skull near the point of impact, such as hitting the windshield in an auto accident. A ***contrecoup***, also described as a ***counterblow***, is an injury that occurs beneath the skull opposite to the area of impact (Figure 11.11).
- **Shaken baby syndrome** describes the results of a child being violently shaken by someone. This action can cause brain injury, blindness, fractures, seizures, paralysis, and death.

Levels of Consciousness

Levels of consciousness (LOC) describe the measurement of response to arousal and stimulus. ***Altered levels of consciousness*** (ALOC) refer to a decrease in consciousness due to injury, disease, or substances such as medication, drugs, or alcohol. Exercise caution when using LOC, as the abbreviation can also mean *loss of consciousness.*

- Being **conscious** is the state of being awake, alert, aware, and responding appropriately.
- Being **unconscious** is a state of being unaware and unable to respond to any stimuli, including pain.
- **Lethargy** (**LETH**-ar-jee) is a lowered level of consciousness marked by listlessness, drowsiness, and apathy. As used here, ***apathy*** means indifference and a reduced level of activity. The term ***lethargic*** refers to a person who is at this level of consciousness.
- A **stupor** (**STOO**-per) is an unresponsive state from which a person can be aroused only briefly despite vigorous, repeated attempts.
- **Syncope** (**SIN**-koh-pee), also known as ***fainting***, is the brief loss of consciousness caused by a decreased flow of blood to the brain.
- A **coma** (**KOH**-mah) is a profound (deep) state of unconsciousness marked by the absence of

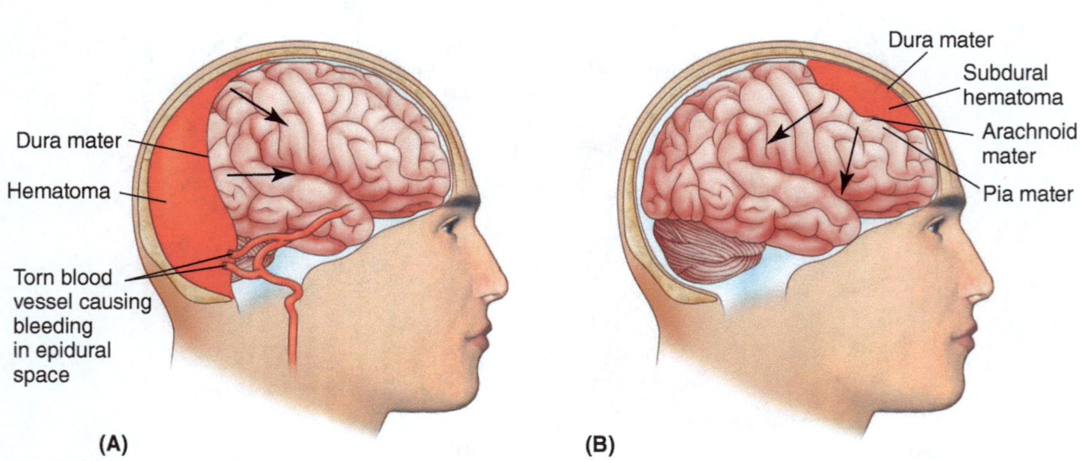

FIGURE 11.10 Cranial hematomas. (A) Epidural hematoma. (B) Subdural hematoma.

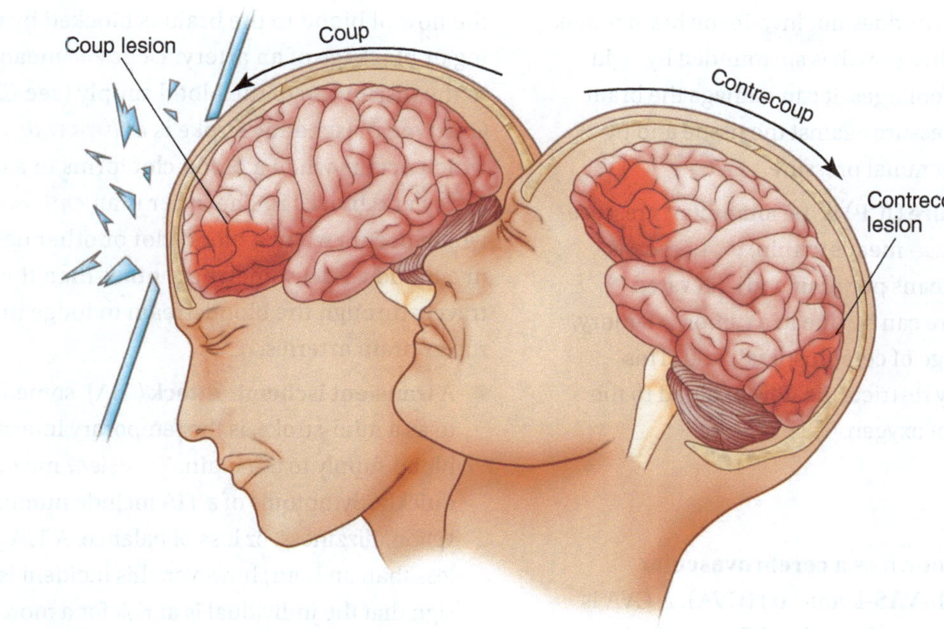

FIGURE 11.11 Coup and contrecoup traumatic brain injuries.

spontaneous eye movements, no response to painful stimuli, and the lack of speech. The term ***comatose*** refers to a person who is in a coma.

- A **persistent vegetative state** is a type of coma in which the patient exhibits alternating sleep and wake cycles; however, due to severe damage to certain areas of the brain, the person is unconscious even when appearing to be awake.
- A person is considered brain dead when the brain has ceased functioning. Vital functions such as breathing can sometimes be maintained artificially to allow for organ donation.

Delirium

Delirium (deh-**LEER**-ee-um) is an acute condition of confusion, disorientation, disordered thinking and memory, agitation, and hallucinations. This is classified as a ***neurocognitive disorder*** in *The Diagnostic and Statistical Manual of Mental Disorders* (DSM-5). For more information about the DSM-5, see Chapter 17.

This condition is usually caused by a treatable physical condition, such as a high fever. An individual suffering from this condition is described as being ***delirious***.

Brain Tumors

A **brain tumor** is an abnormal growth located inside the skull (Figure 11.12).

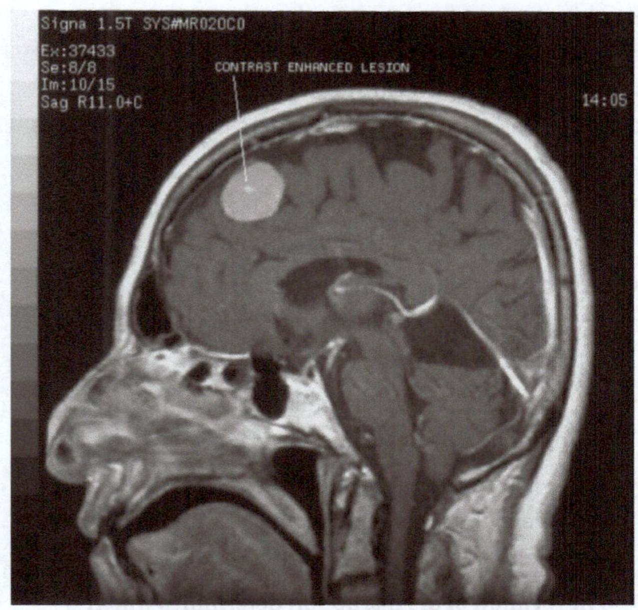

FIGURE 11.12 A brain tumor visualized by magnetic resonance imaging (MRI).

- **Glioblastoma** (**glee**-oh-blas-**TOH**-mah), also known as ***glioblastoma multiforme***, is a type of fast-growing, malignant brain tumor that forms from glial cells.
- An invasive ***malignant brain tumor*** destroys brain tissue. When this cancer originates in the brain, it is considered to be the primary site. If this cancer metastasizes (spreads) to the brain from another body system, it is considered to be a secondary site (see Chapter 20).

- A ***benign brain tumor*** does not invade the brain tissue; however, because this growth is surrounded by rigid bone, as the tumor enlarges, it can damage the brain tissue by placing pressure against the tissue and by increasing the intracranial pressure.
- **Intracranial pressure** (ICP) is the amount of pressure inside the skull (**intra-** means within, **crani** means cranium, and **-al** means pertaining to). Elevated intracranial pressure can be due to a tumor, an injury, or improper drainage of cerebrospinal fluid. This pressure potentially restricts the flow of blood to the brain, depriving it of oxygen.

Strokes

A ***stroke*** is properly known as a **cerebrovascular accident** (**ser**-eh-broh-**VAS**-kyou-lar) (CVA). A CVA is brain damage that occurs when blood flow to the brain is disrupted because a blood vessel either is blocked or has ruptured. Strokes are currently the third-leading cause of death and the primary cause of long-term disability. The ***Cincinnati Prehospital Stroke Scale*** is a three-question scale used to recognize CVA using the mnemonic ***FAST***. This test can be used by members of the public as well as first responders to see if a stroke is occurring:

- ***Facial droop***: one side of the face droops or does not move equally when the person smiles.
- ***Arm drift***: weakness on one side of the body, demonstrated by one arm drifting down when both arms are extended.
- ***Speech abnormality***: slurred speech, using the wrong words, or unable to speak.
- ***Time***: if any of the signs are present, immediate conveyance to the emergency room is essential for critical treatments such as thrombolytics (see Chapter 5).
- The location of the disruption determines which symptoms will be present.
- Damage to the right side of the brain produces symptoms on the left side of the body (Figures 11.13A and 11.13B).
- Damage to the left side of the brain produces symptoms on the right side of the body (Figures 11.13A and 11.13B).

Ischemic Stroke

An **ischemic stroke** (iss-**KEE**-mick), which is the most common type of stroke in older people, occurs when the flow of blood to the brain is blocked by the narrowing or blockage of an artery. ***Ischemic*** means pertaining to the disruption of the blood supply (see Chapter 5). One type of ischemic stroke is a ***thrombotic stroke***, which occurs when a blood clot forms in a carotid artery and blocks it. The other is an ***embolic stroke***, which occurs when a blood clot or other debris forms in a blood vessel somewhere other than the brain and travels through the bloodstream to lodge in the narrower brain arteries.

- A **transient ischemic attack** (TIA), sometimes referred to as a mini-stroke, is the temporary interruption in the blood supply to the brain. ***Transient*** means passing quickly. Symptoms of a TIA include numbness, blurred vision, dizziness, or loss of balance. A TIA passes in less than an hour; however, this incident is a warning sign that the individual is at risk for a more serious and debilitating stroke.
- **Aphasia** (ah-**FAY**-zee-ah), which is often caused by brain damage associated with a stroke, is the loss of the ability to speak, write, and/or comprehend the written or spoken word (**a-** means without, and **-phasia** means speech).

Hemorrhagic Stroke

A hemorrhagic stroke (**hem**-oh-**RAJ**-ick), also known as a ***bleed***, occurs when a blood vessel in the brain leaks. A bleed also occurs when an aneurysm within the brain ruptures. An ***aneurysm*** is a localized, weak, balloon-like enlargement of an artery wall. This type of stroke is less common than ischemic strokes and is often fatal. A hemorrhagic stroke affects the area of the brain damaged by the leaking blood (Figures 11.14 and 11.15). An ***intracerebral hemorrhage***, the most common type of hemorrhagic stroke, occurs within the brain, while a ***subarachnoid hemorrhage*** (SAH) occurs between the brain and the arachnoid membrane.

Arteriovenous malformation (ar-**tee**-ree-oh-**VEE**-nus) (AVM) is one of the causes of hemorrhagic strokes. This abnormal connection between the arteries and veins in the brain is usually congenital and can rupture suddenly at any age (**arteri/o** means artery, **ven** means vein, and **-ous** means pertaining to).

The Spinal Cord

- **Myelitis** (**my**-eh-**LYE**-tis) is an inflammation of the spinal cord (**myel** means spinal cord or bone marrow, and **-itis** means inflammation). The term *myelitis* also means inflammation of bone marrow.

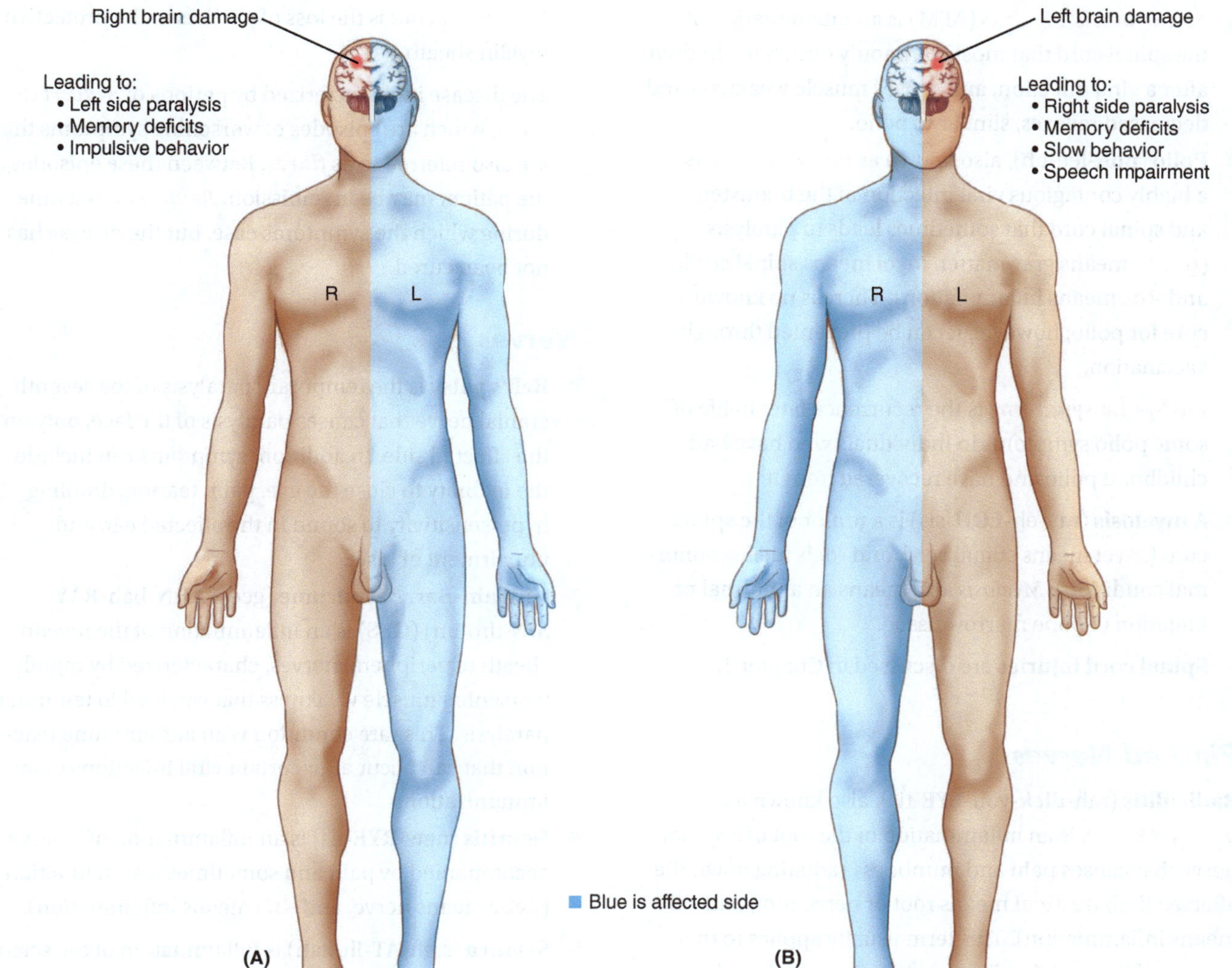

FIGURE 11.13 The location of the damage caused by a cerebrovascular accident depends upon which side of the brain is affected.

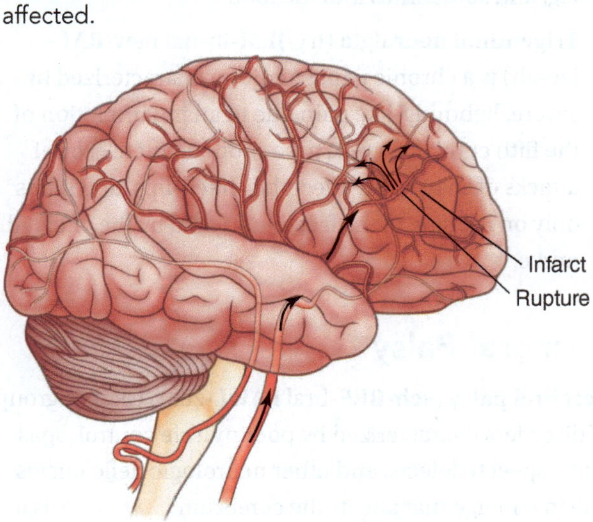

FIGURE 11.14 In a hemorrhagic stroke, the rupture of a blood vessel causes decreased blood flow to an area of the brain tissue. An *infarct* is a localized area of dead tissue caused by a lack of blood (see Chapter 5).

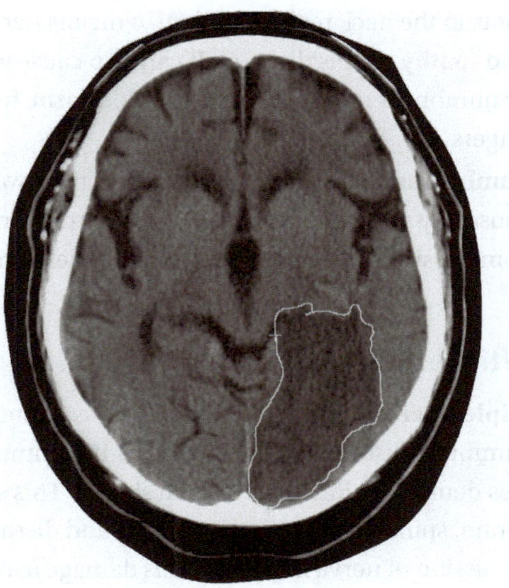

FIGURE 11.15 Magnetic resonance image of a brain with the area of a bleed visible in the lower right.

- *Acute flaccid myelitis* (AFM) is an inflammation of the spinal cord that most commonly occurs in children after a viral infection, and causes muscle weakness and decreased reflexes, similar to polio.
- **Polio** (**poh**-lee-oh), also known as *poliomyelitis*, is a highly contagious viral infection of the brainstem and spinal cord that sometimes leads to paralysis (**poli/o** means gray matter, **myel** means spinal cord, and **-itis** means inflammation). There is no known cure for polio; however, it can be prevented through vaccination.
- *Post-polio syndrome* is the recurrence later in life of some polio symptoms in individuals who have had childhood polio and have recovered from it.
- A **myelosis** (**my**-eh-**LOH**-sis) is a tumor of the spinal cord (**myel** means spinal cord, and **-osis** means abnormal condition). *Myelosis* also means an abnormal proliferation of bone marrow tissue.
- **Spinal cord injuries** are discussed in Chapter 4.

Pinched Nerves

Radiculitis (rah-**dick**-you-**LYE**-tis), also known as a *pinched nerve*, is an inflammation of the root of a spinal nerve that causes pain and numbness radiating down the affected limb (**radicul** means root or nerve root, and **-itis** means inflammation). This term usually applies to that portion of the root that lies between the spinal cord and the intervertebral canal of the spinal column. Figure 3.18 in Chapter 3 shows one cause of this condition.

- **Cervical radiculopathy** (rah-**dick**-you-**LOP**-ah-thee) is nerve pain caused by pressure on the spinal nerve roots in the neck region (**radicul/o** means nerve root, and **-pathy** means disease). It can also cause weakness or numbness radiating to the shoulder, arm, hand, or fingers.
- **Lumbar radiculopathy** is nerve pain in the lower back caused by muscle spasms or nerve root irritation from the compression of vertebral disks such as a herniated disk.

Multiple Sclerosis

Multiple sclerosis (skleh-**ROH**-sis) (MS) is a progressive autoimmune disorder characterized by inflammation that causes demyelination of the myelin sheath. This scars the brain, spinal cord, and optic nerves and disrupts the transmission of nerve impulses. This damage leaves the patient with varying degrees of pain plus physical and cognitive problems.

- *Demyelination* is the loss of patches of the protective myelin sheath.
- The disease is characterized by periods of *exacerbations*, which are episodes of worsening symptoms that are also referred to as *flares*. Between these episodes, the patient may be in remission. *Remission* is a time during which the symptoms ease, but the disease has not been cured.

Nerves

- **Bell's palsy** is the temporary paralysis of the seventh cranial nerve that causes paralysis of the face, only on the affected side. In addition, symptoms can include the inability to close the eye, pain, tearing, drooling, hypersensitivity to sound in the affected ear, and impairment of taste.
- **Guillain-Barré syndrome** (gee-**YAHN**-bah-**RAY SIN**-drohm) (GBS) is an inflammation of the myelin sheath of peripheral nerves, characterized by rapidly worsening muscle weakness that can lead to temporary paralysis. This rare condition is an autoimmune reaction that can occur after certain viral infections or an immunization.
- **Neuritis** (new-**RYE**-tis) is an inflammation of a nerve accompanied by pain and sometimes loss of function (**neur** means nerve, and **-itis** means inflammation).
- **Sciatica** (sigh-**AT**-ih-kah) is inflammation of the sciatic nerve (Figure 11.8A) caused by pressure on the nerve roots that results in pain, burning, and tingling along the course of the affected nerve through the thigh, the leg, and sometimes into the foot.
- **Trigeminal neuralgia** (try-**JEM**-ih-nal new-**RAL**-jee-ah) is a chronic pain condition characterized by severe, lightning-like pain due to an inflammation of the fifth cranial nerve. These sudden, intense, brief attacks of sharp pain affect the cheek, lips, and gums only on the side of the face innervated by the affected nerve.

Cerebral Palsy

Cerebral palsy (**seh-REE**-bral **PAWL**-zee) (CP) is a group of disorders characterized by poor muscle control, spasticity, speech defects, and other neurologic deficiencies due to damage that affects the cerebrum. *Spasticity* is a condition in which certain muscles are continuously contracted. *Palsy* means weakness of a body part that is often accompanied by loss of feeling and uncontrolled body movements, such as shaking.

- Cerebral palsy occurs most frequently in premature or low birth-weight infants.
- Cerebral palsy is usually caused by a brain injury that occurs during pregnancy, at birth, or soon after birth.

Epilepsy and Seizures

Epilepsy (**EP**-ih-**lep**-see) is a chronic neurological condition characterized by recurrent episodes of seizures of varying severity. Also known as a ***seizure disorder***, epilepsy can usually be controlled with medication.

A **seizure** (**SEE**-zhur) (Sz) is a sudden surge of electrical activity in the brain that affects how a person feels or acts for a short time. Some seizures can hardly be noticed, whereas others cause a brief loss of consciousness. Seizures are symptoms of different disorders that can affect the brain and also can be caused by extreme high fever, brain injury, or brain lesions.

- A **tonic–clonic seizure**, also called a ***grand mal seizure***, involves the entire body. In the tonic phase of the seizure, the body becomes rigid, and in the clonic phase, there is uncontrolled jerking.
- An **absence seizure**, also called a ***petit mal seizure***, is a brief disturbance in brain function in which there is a loss of awareness often described as a staring episode.
- A **focal seizure**, also called a ***partial seizure***, is a seizure involving part of the brain, which may involve absence seizure–like symptoms and repetitive muscle movements.
- A **febrile seizure** is a tonic–clonic seizure that occurs in infants and young children in response to a fever. It is not indicative of a seizure disorder, and most children outgrow febrile seizures by age 5.
- ***Sudden unexpected death in epilepsy*** (SUDEP) refers to the death of someone with epilepsy, usually during or immediately following a seizure. The cause of SUDEP is unknown, but may be related to respiratory failure or cardiac arrhythmias caused by a prolonged seizure.

Abnormal Sensations

- **Causalgia** (kaw-**ZAL**-jee-ah) is persistent, severe burning pain that usually follows an injury to a sensory nerve (**caus** means burning, and **-algia** means pain).
- **Complex regional pain syndrome** (CRPS) is chronic nerve pain affecting one limb usually following an injury. Characteristics of CRPS include causalgia, changes in skin color and temperature, and swelling of the affected limb.
- **Hyperesthesia** (**high**-per-es-**THEE**-zee-ah) is a condition of abnormal and excessive sensitivity to touch, pain, or other sensory stimuli (**hyper-** means excessive, and **-esthesia** means sensation or feeling).
- **Paresthesia** (**pair**-es-**THEE**-zee-ah) refers to a burning or prickling sensation with no apparent physical cause that is usually felt in the hands, arms, legs, or feet but can also occur in other parts of the body (**par-** means abnormal, and **-esthesia** means sensation or feeling). These sensations may be the first symptoms of peripheral neuropathy or may be a drug side effect.
- **Peripheral neuropathy** (new-**ROP**-ah-thee) is a disorder of the peripheral nerves that carry information to and from the brain and spinal cord (**neur/o** means nerve, and **-pathy** means disease). This produces pain, the loss of sensation, and the inability to control muscles, particularly in the hands or feet. ***Diabetic neuropathy*** is peripheral neuropathy caused by poorly controlled diabetes.
  - ***Neuropathy*** is any disease or damage to a nerve.
  - ***Mononeuropathy*** is damage to a singular peripheral nerve, as in carpal tunnel syndrome (see Chapter 4).
  - ***Polyneuropathy*** is when multiple peripheral nerves are damaged. Diabetes is a common cause of polyneuropathy, along with trauma, vitamin deficiencies, and alcoholism.
- **Restless legs syndrome** (RLS) is a neurological disorder of unknown cause characterized by uncomfortable feelings in the legs, producing a strong urge to move them. The sensation is usually most noticeable at night or when trying to rest.

DIAGNOSTIC PROCEDURES OF THE NERVOUS SYSTEM

- **Magnetic resonance imaging** (MRI), **magnetic resonance angiography** (MRA), and **computed tomography** (CT) are important neuroimaging tools because they facilitate the examination of the soft tissue structures of the brain and spinal cord (Figures 11.12 and 11.15). These diagnostic techniques are discussed further in Chapter 21.
- A **functional MRI** (fMRI) detects changes in blood flow in the brain when the patient is asked to perform a specific task. This gives a clearer picture of the brain tissue relevant to accomplishing this task.
- **Carotid ultrasonography** (kah-**ROT**-id **ul**-trah-son-**OG**-rah-fee) is an ultrasound study of the carotid

artery (**ultra-** means beyond, **son/o** means sound, and **-graphy** means the process of producing a picture or record). This diagnostic test is performed to detect plaque buildup in the artery to predict or diagnose an ischemic stroke.

- **Electroencephalography** (ee-**leck**-troh-en-**sef**-ah-**LOG**-rah-fee) (EEG) is the process of recording the electrical activity of the brain through the use of electrodes attached to the scalp (**electr/o** means electric, **encephal/o** means brain, and **-graphy** means the process of producing a picture or record). The resulting record is an *electroencephalogram*. This electrical activity may also be displayed on a monitor as brain waves.
- **Myelography** (**my**-eh-**LOG**-rah-fee) is a fluoroscopic and CT study of the spinal cord after the injection of a contrast medium through a lumbar puncture (**myel/o** means spinal cord, and **-graphy** means the process of producing a picture or record). The resulting record is a *myelogram*. Since this is an invasive procedure, it is done only if the spine is not adequately visualized in an MRI.
- **Electromyography** (EMG) uses electrodes taped to or inserted into the skin to measure the transfer of electrical signals in peripheral nerves to the muscles. This is often paired with *nerve conduction studies*, which measure the speed of an electrical signal through a nerve.
- A **lumbar puncture** (LP), also known as a *spinal tap*, is the process of obtaining a sample of cerebrospinal fluid by inserting a needle into the subarachnoid space of the lumbar region to withdraw fluid. Changes in the composition of the cerebrospinal fluid can be an indication of injury, infection, or disease.

TREATMENT PROCEDURES OF THE NERVOUS SYSTEM

Sedative and Hypnotic Medications

- A **hypnotic** depresses the central nervous system and usually produces sleep.
- An **anticonvulsant** (**an**-tih-kon-**VUL**-sant) is administered to prevent seizures such as those associated with epilepsy.
- **Barbiturates** (bar-**BIT**-you-raytz) are a class of drugs whose major action is a calming or depressed effect on the central nervous system.
  - *Phenobarbital* is a barbiturate used as a sedative and as an anticonvulsant.
- A **sedative** depresses the central nervous system to produce calm and diminished responsiveness without producing sleep. *Sedation* is the effect produced by a sedative.

Anesthesia

Anesthesia (**an**-es-**THEE**-zee-ah) is the absence of normal sensation, especially sensitivity to pain, that is induced by the administration of an anesthetic agent (**an-** means without, and **-esthesia** means feeling).

- An **anesthetic** (**an**-es-**THET**-ick) is the medication used to induce anesthesia. The anesthetic may be topical, local, regional, or general (**an-** means without, **esthet** means feeling, and **-ic** means pertaining to).
- **Epidural anesthesia** (**ep**-ih-**DOO**-ral **an**-es-**THEE**-zee-ah) is regional anesthesia produced by injecting medication into the epidural space of the lumbar or sacral region of the spine. When administered during childbirth, it numbs the nerves from the uterus and birth passage without stopping labor (Figure 11.16).
- *General anesthesia* involves the total loss of body sensation and consciousness induced by anesthetic agents administered primarily by inhalation or intravenous injection.
- *Conscious sedation* is a type of short-acting, shallow general anesthesia where the patient is still able to breathe on their own and respond to verbal commands, but is sleepy and unlikely to remember the sedation. It is achieved by use of both sedative and anesthetic medications usually administered through an IV, and is often used for brief procedures such as re-aligning a broken bone.
- *Local anesthesia* causes the loss of sensation in a limited area by injecting an anesthetic solution near that area. It is used to numb small areas, such as a finger.
- *Regional anesthesia*, the temporary interruption of nerve conduction, is produced by injecting an anesthetic solution near the nerves to be blocked. It is used to numb a larger area than local anesthesia, such as an entire limb.
- **Spinal anesthesia**, also called a *spinal block*, is regional anesthesia produced by injecting medication into the subarachnoid space. As with epidural anesthesia, the patient remains conscious. Spinal anesthesia provides numbness from the toes to the waist or lower chest.
- *Topical anesthesia* numbs only the tissue surface and is applied as a liquid, an ointment, or a spray.

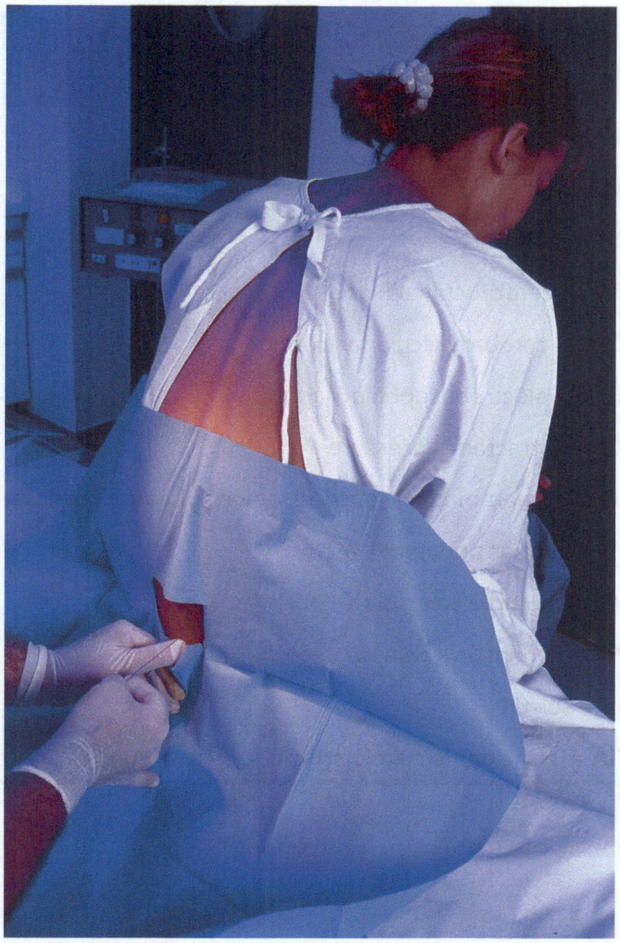

FIGURE 11.16 Epidural anesthesia administered during childbirth numbs the nerves from the uterus and birth passage without stopping labor.

The Brain

- **Deep brain stimulation** (DBS) is a neurosurgical procedure used in the treatment of dystonia, tremors, and Parkinson's disease. A device to stimulate the brain with mild electrical signals is implanted in the brain and is connected to a stimulator implanted near the collar bone. ***Dystonia*** is the impairment of voluntary muscle movement (see Chapter 4).
- **Stereotactic radiosurgery** (SRS) uses a three-dimensional coordinate system to accurately find small tumors within the body, such as in the brain or breast, and deliver radiation directly to them while minimizing damage to the surrounding tissue. One example of this is gamma knife surgery.
- **Gamma knife surgery** is a type of radiation treatment for brain tumors performed without a knife or an incision. The surgeon uses gamma radiation to destroy diseased tissue while preserving the healthy tissue around the tumor. ***Gamma radiation***, which is characterized by high energy and a short wavelength, is also used in nuclear medicine (see Chapter 21).
- **Electroconvulsive therapy** (ee-**leck**-troh-kon-**VUL**-siv) (ECT), also known as ***electroshock therapy***, is a procedure in which small amounts of electric current are passed through the brain, deliberately triggering a brief seizure in order to reverse symptoms of certain mental illnesses or to improve motor function in Parkinson's disease.
- A **lobectomy** (loh-**BECK**-toh-mee) is surgical removal of a portion of the brain to treat brain cancer or seizure disorders that cannot be controlled with medication.
- A **thalamotomy** (**thal**-ah-**MOT**-oh-mee) is a surgical incision into the thalamus (**thalam** means thalamus, and **-otomy** means surgical incision). This procedure, which destroys brain cells, is primarily performed to quiet the tremors of Parkinson's disease.
- **Transcranial magnetic stimulation** (TMS) uses brief, powerful electromagnetic pulses to alter electrical pathways in the brain. This noninvasive procedure is used to treat severe depression, and is being studied for use with Parkinson's disease and other neurologic conditions.

Nerves

- **Radiofrequency ablation** (RFA), also known as ***rhizotomy***, is a minimally invasive procedure that relieves chronic nerve pain by burning part of the nerves, preventing the transmission of pain signals. RFA is often used for chronic pain and arthritis pain.
- **Neurotomy** (new-**ROT**-oh-mee) is the surgical division or dissection (cutting) of a nerve (**neur** means nerve, and **-otomy** means a surgical incision). This procedure is used to relieve pain or suppress tremors.

ABBREVIATIONS RELATED TO THE NERVOUS SYSTEM

Table 11.4 presents an overview of the abbreviations related to the terms introduced in this chapter. *Note:* To avoid errors or confusion, always be cautious when using abbreviations.

TABLE 11.4

Abbreviations Related to the Nervous System

Alzheimer's disease = AD	**AD** = Alzheimer's disease
amyotrophic lateral sclerosis = ALS	**ALS** = amyotrophic lateral sclerosis
cerebral palsy = CP	**CP** = cerebral palsy
cerebrospinal fluid = CSF	**CSF** = cerebrospinal fluid
cerebrovascular accident = CVA	**CVA** = cerebrovascular accident
electroencephalography = EEG	**EEG** = electroencephalography
intracranial pressure = ICP	**ICP** = intracranial pressure
levels of consciousness *or* **loss of consciousness** = LOC	**LOC** = levels of consciousness *or* loss of consciousness
lumbar puncture = LP	**LP** = lumbar puncture
multiple sclerosis = MS	**MS** = multiple sclerosis
Parkinson's disease = PD	**PD** = Parkinson's disease
seizure = Sz	**Sz** = seizure
transient ischemic attack = TIA	**TIA** = transient ischemic attack

CHAPTER 11

LEARNING EXERCISES

Matching Word Parts 1

Write the correct answer in the middle column.

	Definition	Correct Answer	Possible Answers
11.1.	feeling	________________________	**cephal/o**
11.2.	brain	________________________	**encephal/o**
11.3.	bruise	________________________	**contus/o**
11.4.	head	________________________	**concuss/o**
11.5.	shaken together	________________________	**esthet/o**

Matching Word Parts 2

Write the correct answer in the middle column.

	Definition	Correct Answer	Possible Answers
11.6.	membrane covering the brain	________________________	**-esthesia**
11.7.	process of producing a picture	________________________	**-graphy**
11.8.	sensation, feeling	________________________	**radicul/o**
11.9.	spinal cord, bone marrow	________________________	**mening/o**
11.10.	nerve root	________________________	**myel/o**

Matching Word Parts 3

Write the correct answer in the middle column.

	Definition	Correct Answer	Possible Answers
11.11.	cranium, skull	________________	-tropic
11.12.	burning sensation	________________	crani/o
11.13.	brain	________________	neur/o
11.14.	nerve, nerves	________________	cerebr/o
11.15.	having an affinity for	________________	caus/o

Definitions

Select the correct answer, and write it on the line provided.

11.16. The space between two neurons or between a neuron and a receptor organ is known as a ________________.

dendrite ganglion plexus synapse

11.17. The white protective covering over some parts of the spinal cord and the axon of most peripheral nerves is the ________________.

myelin sheath neuroglia neurotransmitter pia mater

11.18. The ________________ are the root-like structures of a nerve that receive impulses and conduct them to the cell body.

axons dendrites ganglions neurotransmitters

11.19. The ________________ is the layer of the meninges that is located nearest to the brain and spinal cord.

arachnoid membrane dura mater meninx pia mater

11.20. Seven vital body functions are regulated by the ________________.

cerebral cortex cerebellum hypothalamus thalamus

11.21. The ________________ nerves are the division of the autonomic nervous system that prepare the body for emergencies and stress.

afferent parasympathetic peripheral sympathetic

11.22. A ______________________ is a network of intersecting nerves.

ganglion   plexus   synapse   tract

11.23. Cranial nerves are part of the ______________________ nervous system.

autonomic   central   cranial   peripheral

11.24. The ______________________ relays sensory stimuli from the spinal cord and midbrain to the cerebral cortex.

cerebellum   hypothalamus   medulla oblongata   thalamus

11.25. The ______________________ neurons carry impulses away from the brain and spinal cord.

afferent   associative   efferent   sensory

Matching Structures

Write the correct answer in the middle column.

	Definition	Correct Answer	Possible Answers
11.26.	connects the brain and spinal cord	______________________	medulla oblongata
11.27.	controls vital body functions	______________________	hypothalamus
11.28.	coordinates muscular activity	______________________	cerebrum
11.29.	controls basic survival functions	______________________	cerebellum
11.30.	uppermost layer of the brain	______________________	brainstem

Which Word?

Select the correct answer, and write it on the line provided.

11.31. A physician who specializes in administering anesthetic agents is an ______________________.

anesthetist   anesthesiologist

11.32. A ______________________ is a profound state of unconsciousness marked by the absence of spontaneous eye movements, no response to painful stimuli, and the lack of speech.

coma   stupor

11.33. An ______________________ drug is also known as a tranquilizer.

antipsychotic anxiolytic

11.34. A ______________________ is a type of congenital disorder that can be prevented in part by the use of folic acid by a woman during pregnancy.

neural tube defect hydrocephalus

11.35 Brain damage that occurs when blood flow to the brain is disrupted is a ______________________ accident, also called a stroke; this is currently the leading cause of disability.

cerebrovascular transient ischemic

Spelling Counts

Find the misspelled word in each sentence. Then write that word, spelled correctly, on the line provided.

11.36. A migrane headache is characterized by throbbing pain on one side of the head. ________________

11.37. Alzhiemer's disease is a group of disorders involving the parts of the brain that control thought, memory, and language. ________________

11.38. An anasthetic is the medication used to induce anesthesia. ________________

11.39. Epalepsy is a chronic neurological condition characterized by recurrent episodes of seizures of varying severity. ________________

11.40. Siatica is a nerve inflammation that results in pain, burning, and tingling through the thigh, leg, and foot. ________________

Abbreviation Identification

In the space provided, write the words that each abbreviation stands for.

11.41. **CP** ______________________

11.42. **CSF** ______________________

11.43 **MS** ______________________

11.44 **CVA** ______________________

11.45. **TIA** ______________________

Term Selection

Select the correct answer, and write it on the line provided.

11.46. The acute condition that is characterized by confusion, disorientation, disordered thinking and memory, agitation, and hallucinations is known as ______________________.

delirium | dementia | lethargy | stupor

11.47. The term meaning inflammation of the spinal cord is ______________________. This term also means inflammation of bone marrow.

encephalitis | myelitis | myelosis | radiculitis

11.48 Abnormal sensitivity to touch or pain is known as ______________________.

paresthesia | hyperesthesia | restless leg syndrome | causalgia

11.49. The condition known as ______________________ is characterized by severe, lightning-like pain due to an inflammation of the fifth cranial nerve.

Bell's palsy | Guillain-Barré syndrome | Lou Gehrig's disease | trigeminal neuralgia

11.50 The process of collecting a sample of cerebrospinal fluid is called a ______________________.

spinal anesthesia | neurotomy | lumbar puncture | myelography

Sentence Completion

Write the correct term or terms on the lines provided.

11.51. A/An ______________________ is the bruising of brain tissue as the result of a head injury.

11.52 A common slow growing tumor of the meninges is known as a/an ______________________.

11.53 Spina bifida is a type of ______________________, which is a congenital disorder that affects the brain and spine.

11.54 The amount of pressure inside the skull is called ______________________ pressure.

11.55 A/An ______________________ is a surgical procedure to remove a portion of the brain.

Word Surgery

Divide each term into its component word parts. Write these word parts, in sequence, on the lines provided. When necessary, use a slash (/) to indicate a combining vowel. (You may not need all of the lines provided.)

11.56. An **anesthetic** is the medication used to induce anesthesia.

__________ __________ __________ __________

11.57 An **arteriovenous malformation** is an abnormal connection between the arteries and veins in the brain that can cause hemorrhagic stroke.

__________ __________ __________ __________

11.58. **Electroencephalography** is the process of recording the electrical activity of the brain through the use of electrodes attached to the scalp.

__________ __________ __________ __________

11.59. **Paresthesia** refers to a burning or prickling sensation that is usually felt in the hands, arms, legs, or feet.

__________ __________ __________ __________

11.60. **Hydrocephalus** is a condition in which excess cerebrospinal fluid accumulates in the ventricles of the brain.

__________ __________ __________ __________

True/False

If the statement is true, write **True** on the line. If the statement is false, write **False** on the line.

11.61. __________ A hemorrhagic stroke occurs when a blood vessel in the brain leaks.

11.62. __________ An absence seizure is a brief disturbance in brain function in which there is a loss of awareness.

11.63. __________ A sedative is administered to prevent the seizures associated with epilepsy.

11.64. __________ A patient in a persistent vegetative state sleeps through the night and is awake and conscious during the day.

11.65 __________ Temporary paralysis of the seventh cranial nerve that causes paralysis on one side of the face is called Bell's palsy.

Clinical Conditions

Write the correct answer on the line provided.

11.66. The viral infection of the spinal cord called ______________________ can be prevented by vaccination.

11.67. In an auto accident, Anthony DeNicola hit his head on the windshield. The paramedics were concerned that this jarring of the brain had caused a/an ______________________.

11.68. Georgia Houghton suffered a/an ______________________ attack (TIA), and her doctors were concerned that this was a warning of an increased stroke risk.

11.69. To control her patient's tremors caused by Parkinson's disease, Dr. Wang performed a/an ______________________. This is a surgical incision into the thalamus.

11.70. Mary Beth Cawthorn was diagnosed as having ______________________. This progressive autoimmune disease is characterized by inflammation that causes demyelination of the myelin sheath.

11.71. An unresponsive state from which a person can be aroused only briefly is called a/an ______________________.

11.72. After her stroke, Rosita Valladares was unable to understand written or spoken words. This condition is known as ______________________.

11.73. Jill Beck said she fainted. The medical term for this brief loss of consciousness caused by the decreased blood flow to the brain is ______________________.

11.74. The Baily baby was born with congenital ______________________. This condition is an abnormally increased amount of cerebrospinal fluid in the ventricles of the brain.

11.75. The MRI indicated that Mrs. Hoshi had a collection of blood trapped in the tissues of her brain. This condition, which was caused by a head injury, is called a cranial ______________________.

Which Is the Correct Medical Term?

Select the correct answer, and write it on the line provided.

11.76. Persistent, severe burning pain that usually follows an injury to a sensory nerve is known as ______________________.

causalgia hyperesthesia hypoesthesia paresthesia

11.77. The classification of drug that depresses the central nervous system and usually produces sleep is known as a/an ______________.

anesthetic barbiturate hypnotic sedative

11.78 Ester's children were afraid that she had developed ______________ after her stroke since she was exhibiting problems with memory and judgement lately.

vascular dementia Alzheimer's disease senile dementia delirium

11.79. During childbirth, ______________ anesthesia is administered to numb the nerves from the uterus and birth passage without stopping labor.

epidural local regional topical

11.80. The condition known as ______________ is a rapidly progressive neurological disease that attacks the nerve cells responsible for controlling voluntary muscles.

amyotrophic lateral sclerosis cerebral palsy epilepsy multiple sclerosis

Challenge Word Building

These terms are *not* primary terms in the chapter; however, they are made up of the following familiar word parts. If you need help in creating the term, refer to your medical dictionary.

poly-	**encephal/o**	**-algia**
	mening/o	**-itis**
	myel/o	**-malacia**
	neur/o	**-oma**
		-pathy

11.81. Based on word parts, the term meaning inflammation of the nerves and spinal cord is ______________.

11.82. Abnormal softening of the meninges is known as ______________.

11.83. A benign neoplasm made up of nerve tissue is a/an ______________.

11.84. Based on word parts, the term meaning any degenerative disease of the brain is ______________.

11.85. Pain affecting many nerves is known as ______________________.

11.86. Abnormal softening of nerve tissue is known as ______________________.

11.87. Inflammation of the meninges and the brain is known as ______________________.

11.88. Based on word parts, the term meaning any pathological condition of the spinal cord is ______________________.

11.89. Abnormal softening of the brain is known as ______________________.

11.90. Inflammation of the meninges, brain, and spinal cord is known as ______________________.

Labeling Exercises

Identify the numbered items on the accompanying figures.

11.91. ______________________ cortex

11.92. ______________________ lobe

11.93. ______________________ lobe

11.94. ______________________ lobe

11.95. ______________________ lobe

11.96. ______________________

11.97. ______________________

11.98. ______________________

11.99. ______________________ cord

11.100. ______________________

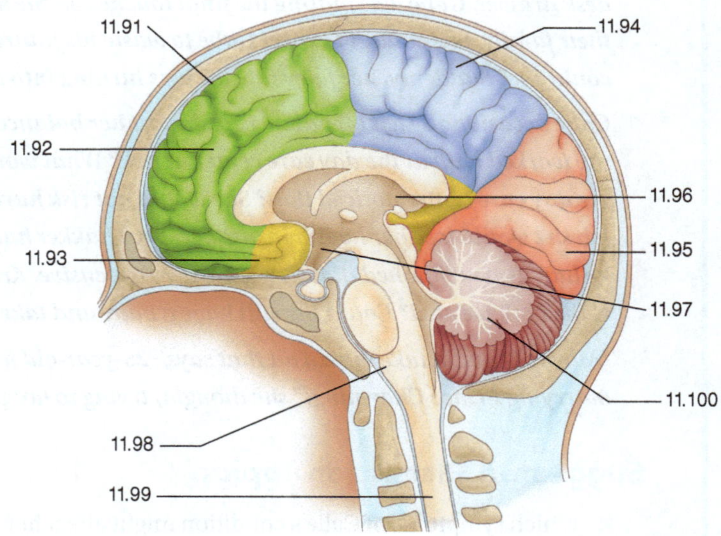

The Human Touch

CRITICAL THINKING EXERCISE

The following story and questions are designed to stimulate critical thinking through class discussion or as a brief essay response. There are no right or wrong answers to these questions.

Calle Washington read the information Dr. Thakker gave her with numb disbelief. "Multiple sclerosis (MS) is a neurological disorder characterized by demyelination of nerve fibers in the brain and spinal column. This disease may be progressively debilitating with symptoms that could include numbness, paralysis, ataxia, pain, and blindness. Some patients do experience life-threatening complications. This disease attacks young adults. It affects more women than men."

"Well, I sure fit the profile," thought Calle bitterly. She took a deep breath, trying to quiet the fluttering in her stomach. How could this happen now? Everything was so perfect. Her wedding gown was getting its last alterations, and the tickets for their honeymoon to Jamaica were in the desk drawer. Gabe was putting the final touches on the house where they planned on raising their family. She couldn't expect Gabe to waste his future caring for someone in a wheelchair, could she? Suddenly, her fairy tale life was turning into a nightmare.

Calle occasionally felt off balance. If she lost her balance suddenly, would this put the children she worked with at the day care center at risk? What would happen once her fellow teachers at the day care center noticed that? She would not risk hurting one of the children, but if she lost her job she would lose her health insurance. Dr. Thakker had said there were new drugs for MS, but he had also mentioned that they were very expensive. And what about the children that she and Gabe both wanted? Could she still have a baby and take care of it?

"Maybe I should take out an ad that says, '25-year-old female seeks cure for deadly disease before marrying Prince Charming,'" she thought, trying to laugh through her tears...!

Suggested Discussion Topics

1. Which symptoms of Calle's condition might affect her job? She has been working with the youngest children. Should she consider resigning, or could she ask for a different assignment?
2. Calle and Gabe decide to go ahead with the wedding. If they have children, is there a risk that Calle will transmit this condition? If Calle cannot have children, what other options would enable them to have the family they both want?
3. After their marriage, Calle will be covered by her husband's health insurance, but she has questions about what the insurance will actually cover. Where could Calle get information as to whether or not the insurance company will cover her expensive medications for this disease?
4. Calle is an excellent teacher and the children love her. In the past, her coworkers have commented, "I wish I could learn to be as good at this as you are." Even with multiple sclerosis, could Calle have a future in training other teachers? What other positive steps might she contemplate taking?

CHAPTER 12

SPECIAL SENSES: THE EYES AND EARS

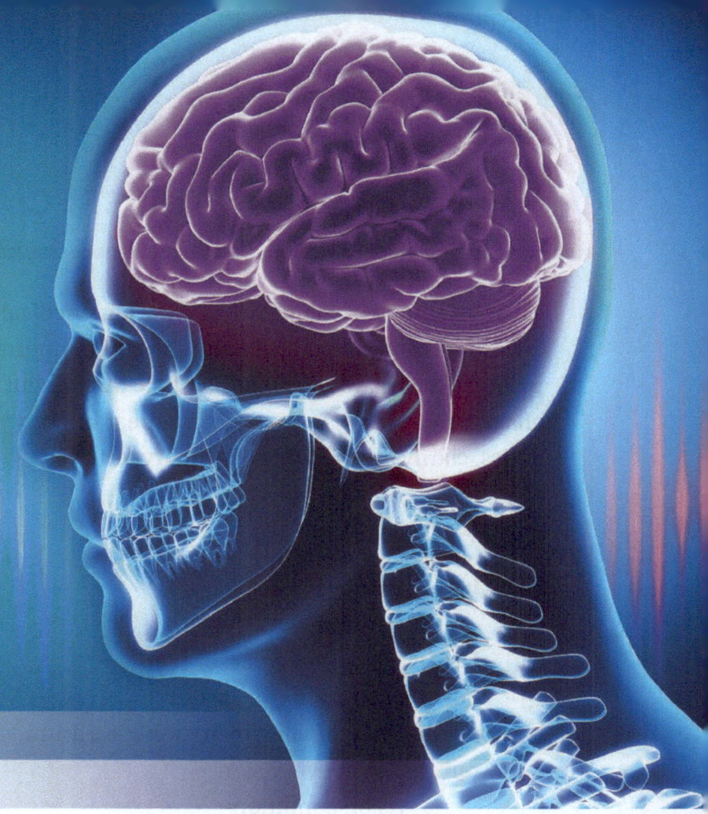

Overview of

STRUCTURES, COMBINING FORMS, AND FUNCTIONS OF THE EYES AND EARS

Major Structures	Related Combining Forms	Primary Functions
Eyes	opt/i, opt/o, optic/o, ophthalm/o	Receptor organs for the sense of sight.
Iris	ir/i, ir/o, irid/o, irit/o	Controls the amount of light entering the eye.
Lens	phac/o, phak/o	Focuses rays of light on the retina.
Retina	retin/o	Converts light images into electrical impulses and transmits them to the brain.
Lacrimal Apparatus	dacryocyst/o, lacrim/o	Accessory structures of the eyes that produce, store, and remove tears.
Ears	acous/o, acoust/o, audi/o, audit/o, ot/o	Receptor organs for the sense of hearing; also help maintain balance.
Outer Ear	pinn/i	Transmits sound waves to the middle ear.
Middle Ear	myring/o, tympan/o	Transmits sound waves to the inner ear.
Inner Ear	labyrinth/o	Receives sound vibrations and transmits them to the brain.

Vocabulary Related to **THE SPECIAL SENSES**

This list contains essential word parts and medical terms for this chapter. These and the other important **primary terms** are shown in **boldface** throughout the chapter. *Secondary terms*, which appear in *orange* italics, clarify the meaning of primary terms.

Word Parts

- ☐ **blephar/o** eyelid
- ☐ **-cusis** hearing
- ☐ **irid/o** iris, colored part of eye
- ☐ **kerat/o** horny, hard, cornea
- ☐ **myring/o** tympanic membrane, eardrum
- ☐ **ophthalm/o** eye, vision
- ☐ **-opia** vision condition
- ☐ **opt/o** eye, vision
- ☐ **ot/o** ear, hearing
- ☐ **phak/o** lens of eye
- ☐ **presby/o** old age
- ☐ **retin/o** retina, net
- ☐ **scler/o** sclera, white of eye, hard
- ☐ **trop/o** turn, change
- ☐ **tympan/o** tympanic membrane, eardrum

Medical Terms

- ☐ **adnexa** (ad-**NECK**-sah)
- ☐ **amblyopia** (**am**-blee-**OH**-pee-ah)
- ☐ **ametropia** (**am**-eh-**TROH**-pee-ah)
- ☐ **anisocoria** (**an**-ih-so-**KOH**-ree-ah)
- ☐ **astigmatism** (ah-**STIG**-mah-tizm)
- ☐ **audiometry** (**aw**-dee-**OM**-eh-tree)
- ☐ **cataract** (**KAT**-ah-rakt)
- ☐ **chalazion** (kah-**LAY**-zee-on)
- ☐ **cochlear implant** (**KOCK**-lee-ar)
- ☐ **conjunctivitis** (kon-**junk**-tih-**VYE**-tis)
- ☐ **dacryoadenitis** (**dack**-ree-oh-ad-eh-**NIGH**-tis)
- ☐ **diplopia** (dih-**PLOH**-pee-ah)
- ☐ **ectropion** (eck-**TROH**-pee-on)
- ☐ **emmetropia** (em-eh-**TROH**-pee-ah)
- ☐ **entropion** (en-**TROH**-pee-on)
- ☐ **esotropia** (**es**-oh-**TROH**-pee-ah)
- ☐ **exotropia** (**eck**-soh-**TROH**-pee-ah)
- ☐ **fluorescein angiography** (**flew**-oh-**RES**-ee-in an-jee-**OG**-rah-fee)
- ☐ **glaucoma** (glaw-**KOH**-mah)
- ☐ **hemianopia** (**hem**-ee-ah-**NOH**-pee-ah)
- ☐ **hordeolum** (hor-**DEE**-oh-lum)
- ☐ **hyperopia** (**high**-per-**OH**-pee-ah)
- ☐ **infectious myringitis** (**mir**-in-**JIGH**-tis)
- ☐ **iritis** (eye-**RYE**-tis)
- ☐ **keratitis** (**ker**-ah-**TYE**-tis)
- ☐ **labyrinthectomy** (**lab**-ih-rin-**THECK**-toh-mee)
- ☐ **laser iridotomy** (**ir**-ih-**DOT**-oh-mee)
- ☐ **laser trabeculoplasty** (trah-**BECK**-you-loh-**plas**-tee)
- ☐ **mastoidectomy** (**mas**-toy-**DECK**-toh-mee)
- ☐ **mydriasis** (mih-**DRY**-ah-sis)
- ☐ **myopia** (my-**OH**-pee-ah)
- ☐ **myringotomy** (**mir**-in-**GOT**-oh-mee)
- ☐ **nyctalopia** (**nick**-tah-**LOH**-pee-ah)
- ☐ **nystagmus** (nis-**TAG**-mus)
- ☐ **ophthalmoscopy** (**ahf**-thal-**MOS**-koh-pee)
- ☐ **optometrist** (op-**TOM**-eh-trist)
- ☐ **otitis media** (oh-**TYE**-tis **MEE**-dee-ah)
- ☐ **otomycosis** (**oh**-toh-my-**KOH**-sis)
- ☐ **otopyorrhea** (**oh**-toh-**pye**-oh-**REE**-ah)
- ☐ **otorrhea** (**oh**-toh-**REE**-ah)
- ☐ **otosclerosis** (**oh**-toh-skleh-**ROH**-sis)
- ☐ **papilledema** (**pap**-ill-eh-**DEE**-mah)
- ☐ **periorbital edema** (**pehr**-ee-**OR**-bih-tal eh-**DEE**-mah)
- ☐ **photophobia** (**foh**-toh-**FOH**-bee-ah)
- ☐ **pneumatic retinopexy** (**RET**-ih-noh-**peck**-see)
- ☐ **presbycusis** (**pres**-beh-**KOO**-sis)
- ☐ **presbyopia** (**pres**-bee-**OH**-pee-ah)
- ☐ **ptosis** (**TOH**-sis)
- ☐ **radial keratotomy** (**ker**-ah-**TOT**-oh-mee)
- ☐ **scleritis** (skleh-**RYE**-tis)
- ☐ **sensorineural hearing loss** (sen-suh-ree-**NOOR**-al)
- ☐ **stapedectomy** (**stay**-peh-**DECK**-toh-mee)
- ☐ **strabismus** (strah-**BIZ**-mus)
- ☐ **tarsorrhaphy** (tahr-**SOR**-ah-fee)
- ☐ **tinnitus** (tih-**NIGH**-tus)
- ☐ **tonometry** (toh-**NOM**-eh-tree)
- ☐ **tympanometry** (**tim**-pah-**NOM**-eh-tree)
- ☐ **vertigo** (**VER**-tih-go)
- ☐ **vitrectomy** (vih-**TRECK**-toh-mee)
- ☐ **xerophthalmia** (**zeer**-ahf-**THAL**-mee-ah)

LEARNING OBJECTIVES

On completion of this chapter, you should be able to:

1. Describe the functions and structures of the eyes and their accessory organs.
2. Explain the process of vision.
3. Identify the medical specialists who treat disorders of the eyes.
4. Identify the medical word parts related to the eyes and vision.
5. Define the primary terms related to the pathology and the diagnostic and treatment procedures of the eyes and vision.
6. Describe the functions and structures of the ears.
7. Explain the process of hearing.
8. Identify the medical specialists who treat disorders of the ears.
9. Identify the medical word parts related to the ears and hearing.
10. Define the primary terms related to the pathology and the diagnostic and treatment procedures of the ears and hearing.
11. Spell the primary terms related to the special senses.
12. Pronounce the primary terms related to the special senses.
13. Identify common abbreviations related to the special senses.

FUNCTIONS OF THE EYES

The eyes are the receptor organs of sight, and their functions are to receive images and transmit them to the brain.

The abbreviations relating to the eyes, with the Latin words from which they originate, are shown in Table 12.1. *Oculus* means eye, and the plural is *oculi*. *Note:* **The Joint Commission**, the largest American standards-setting and accrediting body in health care, recommends writing out these terms instead of using abbreviations.

STRUCTURES OF THE EYES

The structures of the eye include the eyeball and the adnexa that are attached to or surround the eyeball (Figure 12.1).

The Adnexa of the Eyes

The **adnexa of the eyes**, also known as *adnexa oculi*, are the structures outside the eyeball. These include the orbit, eye muscles, eyelids, eyelashes, conjunctiva, and lacrimal apparatus. **Adnexa** (ad-**NECK**-sah) means the accessory or adjoining anatomical parts of an organ. The term *adnexa* is plural.

The Orbit

The **orbit**, also known as the *eye socket*, is the bony cavity of the skull that contains and protects the eyeball and its associated muscles, blood vessels, and nerves.

Muscles of the Eye

Six major **eye muscles**, which are arranged in three pairs, are attached to each eye (Figure 12.2). These are the:

- Superior and inferior oblique muscles
- Superior and inferior rectus muscles
- Lateral and medial rectus muscles

These muscles make a wide range of very precise eye movements possible. *Oblique* describes an angle that is slanted but is not perpendicular or parallel. *Rectus* means straight.

Binocular vision (**bin-** means two, **ocul** means eye, and **-ar** means pertaining to) occurs when the muscles of both eyes work together in coordination to make normal depth perception possible. *Depth perception* is the ability to see things in three dimensions.

TABLE 12.1

Abbreviations Relating to the Eyes

The Adnexa of the Eyes	
OD	Right eye (*oculus dexter*)
OS	Left eye (*oculus sinister*)
OU	Each eye (*oculus uterque*) or both eyes (*oculi uterque*)

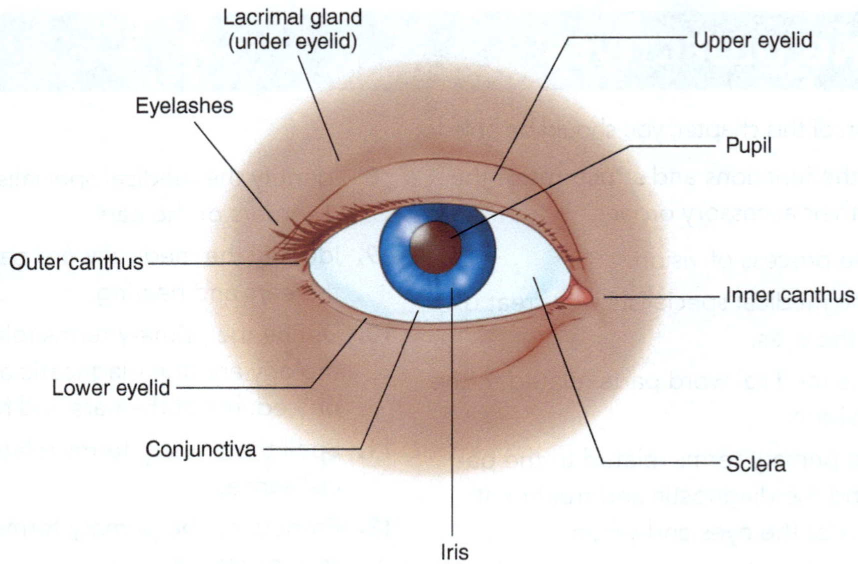

FIGURE 12.1 Major structures of the adnexa and eyeball.

The Eyelids, Eyebrows, and Eyelashes

The **upper** and **lower eyelids**, together with the **eyebrows** and **eyelashes**, help protect the eyeball from foreign matter, excessive light, and injuries due to other causes (Figure 12.1).

- The **canthus** (**KAN**-thus) is the angle where the upper and lower eyelids meet (**canth** means corner of the eye, and **-us** is a singular noun ending). The plural of canthus is *canthi*.
- The edges of the eyelids contain oil-producing sebaceous glands. These glands are discussed in Chapter 12.
- The **cilia** (**SIL**-ee-ah), which are small hairs, make up the eyebrows and eyelashes. Cilia are also present in the nose to prevent foreign matter from being inhaled.
- The **tarsus** (**TAHR**-suhs), also known as the ***tarsal plate***, is the framework within the upper and lower eyelids that provides the necessary stiffness and shape (**tars** means edge of the eyelid, and **-us** is a singular noun ending). The plural of tarsus is *tarsi. Note: Tarsus* also refers to the cluster of seven tarsal bones of the foot's instep.

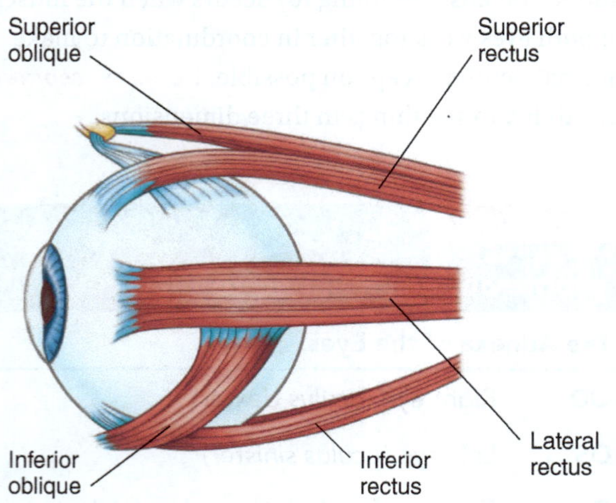

FIGURE 12.2 Six muscles, arranged as three pairs, make major eye movement possible. The medial rectus muscle is not visible here.

The Conjunctiva

The **conjunctiva** (**kon**-junk-**TYE**-vah) is the transparent mucous membrane that lines the underside of each eyelid and continues to form a protective covering over the exposed surface of the eyeball. The plural of *conjunctiva* is *conjunctivae* (Figure 12.1).

The Lacrimal Apparatus

The **lacrimal apparatus** (**LACK**-rih-mal), also known as the ***tear apparatus***, consists of the structures that produce, store, and remove tears. ***Lacrimation*** is the secretion of tears.

- The **lacrimal glands**, which secrete lacrimal fluid (tears), are located on the underside of the upper eyelid just above the outer corner of each eye (Figure 12.1).
- The function of **lacrimal fluid**, commonly known as ***tears***, is to maintain moisture on the anterior surface of the eyeball. Blinking distributes the lacrimal fluid across the eye.
- The **lacrimal canal** consists of a duct at the inner corner of each eye. These ducts collect tears and empty them into the lacrimal sacs. Crying is the overflowing of tears from the lacrimal canals.
- The **lacrimal sac**, also known the ***tear sac***, is an enlargement of the upper portion of the lacrimal duct.

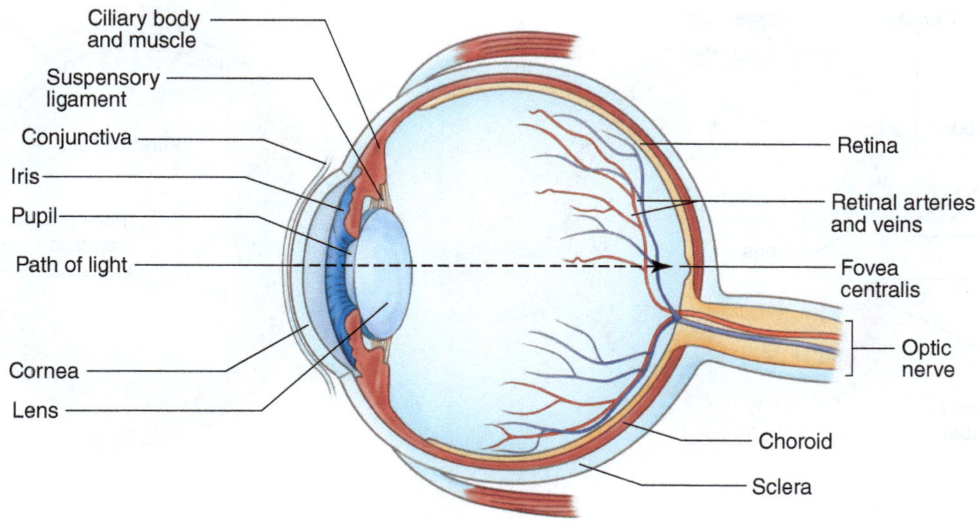

FIGURE 12.3 The structures of the eyeball shown in cross-section.

- The **lacrimal duct**, also known as the ***nasolacrimal duct***, is the passageway that drains excess tears into the nose.

The Eyeball

The **eyeball**, also known as the ***globe***, is a one-inch sphere with only about one-sixth of its surface visible (Figure 12.3).

- The term **optic** (**OP**-tik) means pertaining to the eye or sight (**opt** means vision, and **-ic** means pertaining to).
- **Ocular** (**OCK**-you-lar) means pertaining to the eye (**ocul** means eye, and **-ar** means pertaining to).
- **Extraocular** (eck-strah-**OCK**-you-lar) means outside the eyeball (**extra-** means on the outside, **ocul** means eye, and **-ar** means pertaining to).
- **Intraocular** (**in**-trah-**OCK**-you-lar) means within the eyeball (**intra-** means within, **ocul** means eye, and **-ar** means pertaining to).

Walls of the Eyeball

The walls of the eyeball are made up of three layers: the sclera, choroid, and retina (Figure 12.4).

- The **sclera** (**SKLEHR**-ah), also known as the ***white of the eye***, maintains the shape of the eye and protects the delicate inner layers of tissue. This tough, fibrous tissue forms the outer layer of the eye, except for the part covered by the cornea. *Note:* The combining form **scler/o** means the white of the eye, and it also means hard.
- The **choroid** (**KOH**-roid), also known as the ***choroid coat***, is the opaque middle layer of the eyeball that contains many blood vessels and provides the blood supply for the entire eye. ***Opaque*** means that light cannot pass through this substance.

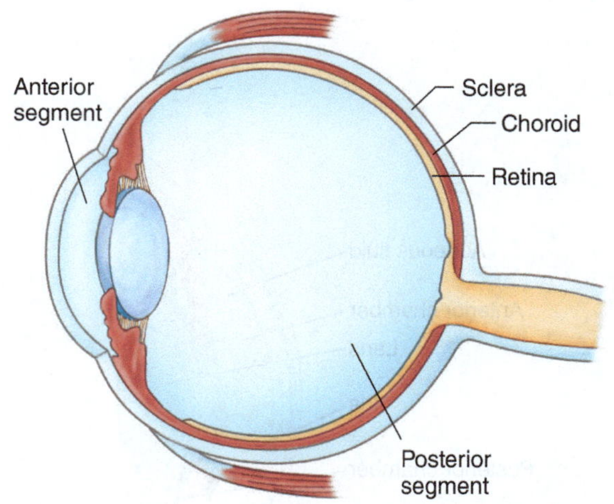

FIGURE 12.4 The walls of the eyeball are made up of the sclera, choroid, and retina.

- The **retina** (**RET**-ih-nah) is the sensitive innermost layer that lines the posterior segment of the eye. The retina receives nerve impulses and transmits them to the brain via the ***optic nerve***. This is also known as the ***second cranial nerve*** and is discussed in Chapter 11.

Segments of the Eyeball

The interior of the eyeball is divided into the anterior and posterior segments (Figures 12.4 and 12.5A and B).

Anterior Segment of the Eye

The anterior segment makes up the front one-third of the eyeball. This segment is divided into anterior and posterior chambers (Figures 12.5A and 12.6).

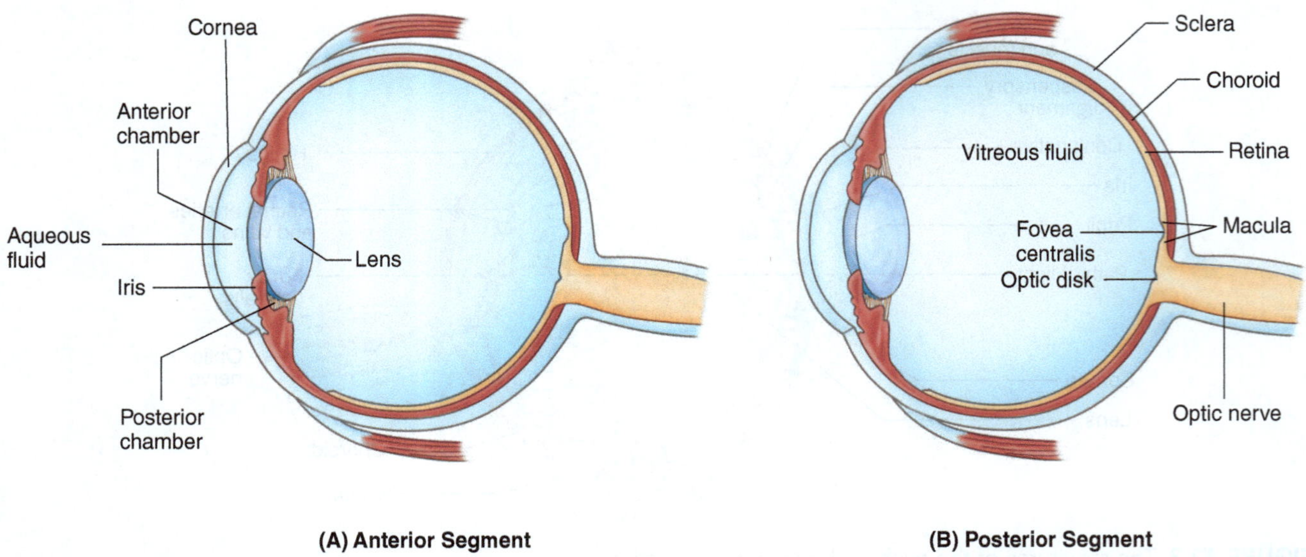

FIGURE 12.5 The segments of the eyeball. (A) The anterior segment is divided into anterior and posterior chambers. (B) The posterior segment.

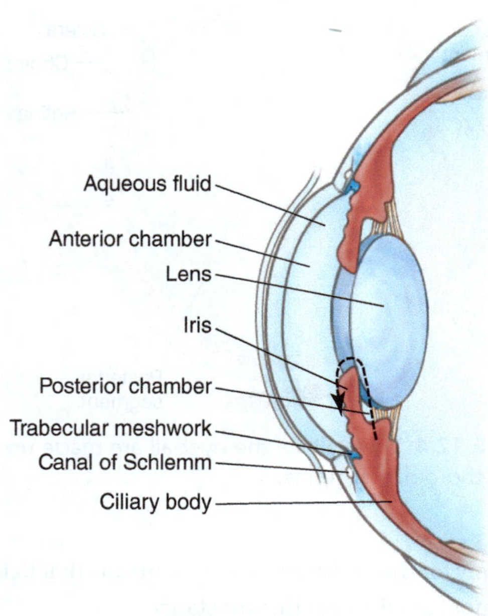

FIGURE 12.6 Close-up of the anterior segment of the eye with an arrow indicating the flow of aqueous humor.

- The anterior chamber is located behind the cornea and in front of the iris. The posterior chamber is located behind the iris and in front of the ligaments holding the lens in place. *Note:* Don't confuse the posterior *chamber* with the posterior *segment*.
- **Aqueous humor** (**AH**-kwee-uhs), which is also known as ***aqueous fluid***, fills both of these chambers. The term *aqueous* means watery or containing water. As used here, the term ***humor*** describes any clear body liquid or semifluid substance.
- The aqueous humor helps the eye maintain its shape and nourishes the intraocular structures. This fluid is constantly filtered and drained through the ***trabecular meshwork*** and the ***canal of Schlemm*** (Figure 12.6).
- **Intraocular pressure** (IOP) is a measurement of the fluid pressure inside the eye. This pressure is regulated by the rate at which aqueous humor enters and leaves the eye.

Posterior Segment of the Eye

The **posterior segment**, which makes up the remaining two-thirds of the eyeball, is lined with the retina and filled with **vitreous humor** (**VIT**-ree-us). Also known as ***vitreous gel***, this is a soft, clear, jelly-like mass that contains millions of fine fibers. These fibers, which are attached to the surface of the retina, help the eye maintain its shape (Figures 12.3, 12.4, and 12.5B).

Structures of the Retina

- The **rods** and **cones** of the retina receive images that have passed through the lens of the eye. These images are converted into nerve impulses and transmitted to the brain via the optic nerve. *Rods* are the black and white receptors, and *cones* are the color receptors.
- The **macula** (**MACK**-you-lah), also known as the ***macula lutea***, is the clearly defined light-sensitive area in the center of the retina that is responsible for sharp central vision. Note that the term *macula* means a small spot. A macula, also known as a macule, can also

refer to a small, discolored spot on the skin, such as a freckle (see Chapter 13).

- The **fovea centralis** (**FOH**-vee-ah sen-**TRAH**-lis) is a pit in the middle of the macula. Color vision is best in this area because it contains a high concentration of cones and no rods.
- The **optic disk**, also known as the *blind spot*, is a small region in the eye where the nerve endings of the retina enter the optic nerve. This is called the blind spot, because it does not contain any rods or cones to convert images into nerve impulses.
- The **optic nerve** transmits these nerve impulses from the retina to the brain.

The Uvea

The **uvea** (**YOU**-vee-ah) is the pigmented layer of the eye. It has a rich blood supply and consists of the choroid, ciliary body, and iris (Figure 12.3).

The Ciliary Body

The **ciliary body** (**SIL**-ee-ehr-ee), which is located within the choroid, is a set of muscles and suspensory ligaments that adjust the thickness of the lens to refine the focus of light rays on the retina (Figure 12.6).

- The ciliary body produces the aqueous humor that fills the anterior segment of the eye.
- To focus on nearby objects, these muscles adjust the lens to make it *thicker*.
- To focus on distant objects, these muscles stretch the lens so it is *thinner*.

The Iris

The **iris** is the colorful circular structure that surrounds the pupil (Figure 12.3). The muscles within the iris control the amount of light that is allowed to enter the eye through the pupil.

- To *decrease* the amount of light entering the eye, the muscles of the iris contract, making the opening of the pupil smaller.
- To *increase* the amount of light entering the eye, the muscles of the iris relax, or *dilate*, making the opening of the pupil larger. See *dilation* in the section "Diagnostic Procedures for Vision and the Eyes." Note that the term *dilate* refers to expanding any opening of the body, for example, the dilating of the cervix during childbirth (see Chapter 16).

The Cornea, Pupil, and Lens

- The **cornea** (**KOR**-nee-ah) is the transparent outer surface of the eye covering the iris and pupil. It is the primary structure focusing light rays entering the eye (Figure 12.3).
- The **pupil** is the black circular opening in the center of the iris that permits light to enter the eye.
- The **lens** is the clear, flexible, curved structure that focuses images on the retina. The lens is contained within a clear capsule located behind the iris and pupil.

Normal Action of the Eyes

The process of normal vision occurs when light rays pass through the cornea to the pupil, hitting the lens. From here the rays pass through the vitreous humor before reaching the retina. The retina inverts the image and the optic nerve sends the information to the brain.

- **Accommodation** (ah-**kom**-oh-**DAY**-shun) is the process whereby the eyes make adjustments for seeing objects at various distances. These adjustments include contraction (narrowing) and dilation (widening) of the pupil, movement of the eyes, and changes in the shape of the lens.
- **Convergence** (kon-**VER**-jens) is the simultaneous inward movement of the eyes toward each other. This occurs in an effort to maintain single binocular vision as an object comes nearer.
- **Emmetropia** (em-eh-**TROH**-pee-ah) is the normal relationship between the refractive power of the eye and the shape of the eye that enables light rays to focus correctly on the retina (**emmetr** means in proper measure, and **-opia** means vision condition).
- **Refraction**, also known as *refractive power*, is the ability of the lens to bend light rays so they focus on the retina. Normal refraction is shown in Figure 12.10A.
- **Visual acuity** (ah-**KYOU**-ih-tee) (VA) is the ability to distinguish object details and shape at a distance. *Acuity* means sharpness (Figure 12.8A).

MEDICAL SPECIALTIES RELATED TO THE EYES AND VISION

- An **ophthalmologist** (ahf-thal-**MOL**-oh-jist) is a physician who specializes in diagnosing and treating the full spectrum of diseases and disorders of the eyes, from vision correction to eye surgery (**ophthalm** means eye, and **-ologist** means specialist).

- An **optometrist** (op-**TOM**-eh-trist) holds a doctor of optometry degree and provides primary eye care, including diagnosing eye diseases and conditions, and measuring the accuracy of vision to determine whether corrective lenses are needed (**opt/o** means vision, and **-metrist** means one who measures). A ***certified paraoptometric*** sometimes plays a support role to an optometrist.
- An **optician** (op-**TISH**-uhn) is a health care practitioner who designs, fits, and dispenses lenses for vision correction.

PATHOLOGY OF THE EYES AND VISION

The Eyelids

- **Ptosis** (**TOH**-sis) is the drooping of the upper eyelid that is usually due to muscle weakness or paralysis (**ptosis** means drooping or sagging). The term ***blepharoptosis*** has the same meaning.
- A **chalazion** (kah-**LAY**-zee-on) is a nodule or cyst, usually on the upper eyelid, caused by obstruction of a sebaceous gland. The plural of chalazion is *chalazia*. Compare with a *hordeolum*.
- A **hordeolum** (hor-**DEE**-oh-lum), also known as a ***stye***, is a pus-filled and often painful lesion on the eyelid resulting from an acute infection in a sebaceous gland. Compare with a *chalazion*.
- **Blepharitis** is swelling of the eyelid, often at the location of the eyelash hair follicles (**blephar** means eyelid, and **-itis** means inflamation).
- **Ectropion** (eck-**TROH**-pee-on) is the eversion of the edge of an eyelid (**ec-** means out, **trop** means turn, and **-ion** means condition). ***Eversion*** means turning outward. This usually affects the lower lid, thereby exposing the inner surface of the eyelid to irritation and preventing tears from draining properly (Figure 12.7A). Ectropion is the opposite of *entropion*.
- **Entropion** (en-**TROH**-pee-on) is the inversion of the edge of an eyelid (**en-** means in, **trop** means turn, and **-ion** means condition). ***Inversion*** means turning inward. This usually affects the lower eyelid and causes the eyelashes to rub against the cornea (Figure 12.7B). Entropion is the opposite of *ectropion*.
- **Periorbital edema** (**pehr**-ee-**OR**-bih-tal eh-**DEE**-mah) is swelling of the tissues surrounding the eye or eyes (**peri-** means surrounding, **orbit** means eyeball, and **-al** means pertaining to). This can give the face a bloated appearance and cause the eyes to be partially covered by the swollen eyelids. This swelling is associated with conditions such as allergic reaction (see Chapter 7), nephrotic syndrome (see Chapter 10), or cellulitis (see Chapter 13).

Additional Adnexa Pathology

- **Conjunctivitis** (kon-**junk**-tih-**VYE**-tis), also known as ***pinkeye***, is an inflammation of the conjunctiva that is usually caused by a viral infection, allergy, or irritants (**conjunctiv** means conjunctiva, and **-itis** means inflammation).
- **Dacryoadenitis** (**dack**-ree-oh-ad-eh-**NIGH**-tis) is an inflammation of the lacrimal gland caused by a bacterial, viral, or fungal infection (**dacry/o** means tear, **aden** means gland, and **-itis** means inflammation). Signs and symptoms of this condition include sudden severe pain, redness, and pressure above the eye.
- **Dacryocystitis** (**dack**-ree-oh-sis-**TYE**-tis) is an inflammation of the lacrimal sac usually caused by blockage of the lacrimal duct, often accompanied by a

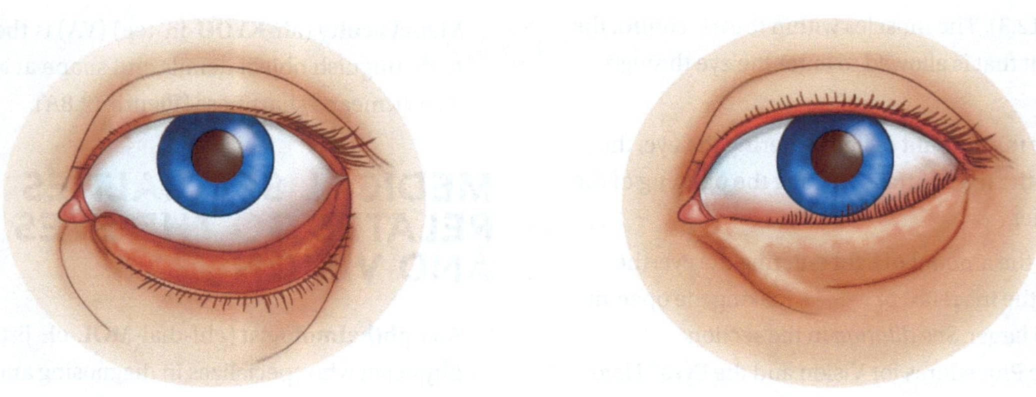
(A) (B)

FIGURE 12.7 Disorders of the eyelid. (A) Ectropion. (B) Entropion.

bacterial infection (**dacry/o** means tear, **cyst** means sac of fluid, and **-itis** means inflammation).

- **Subconjunctival hemorrhage** (**sub**-kon-junk-**TIH**-val **HEM**-or-idj) is bleeding between the conjunctiva and the sclera. This condition, which is usually caused by an injury, creates a red area over the white of the eye.
- **Xerophthalmia** (**zeer**-ahf-**THAL**-mee-ah), also known as *dry eye*, is drying of eye surfaces, including the conjunctiva, because the tear glands do not produce enough tears (**xer** means dry, **ophthalm** means eye, and **-ia** means abnormal condition). This condition is often associated with aging. It can also be due to systemic diseases such as rheumatoid arthritis or caused by a lack of vitamin A.

Uvea, Cornea, and Sclera

- **Uveitis** (you-vee-**EYE**-tis) is an inflammation of the uvea causing swelling and irritation (**uve** means uvea, and **-itis** means inflammation). Complications from uveitis can potentially lead to permanent vision loss.
- **Iritis** (eye-**RYE**-tis) is the most common form of uveitis. This inflammation of the uvea affects primarily structures in the front of the eye (**ir** means iris, and **-itis** means inflammation). This condition has a sudden onset and may last six to eight weeks.
- A **corneal abrasion** (ah-**BRAY**-zhun) is an injury, such as a scratch or irritation, to the outer layers of the cornea (**corne** means cornea, and **-al** means pertaining to). Compare with *corneal ulcer*.
- A **corneal ulcer** is an open sore on the cornea caused by an infection or injury. Although these ulcers heal with treatment, they can leave a cloudy scar that impairs vision. Compare with *corneal abrasion*.
- **Keratitis** (**ker**-ah-**TYE**-tis) is an inflammation of the cornea (**kerat** means cornea, and **-itis** means inflammation). This condition can be due to many causes, including bacterial, viral, or fungal infections. *Note:* **kerat/o** also means hard.
- **Keratoconus** (ker-**uh**-toh-**KOH**-nus) occurs when the cornea becomes irregular and cone-shaped, causing blurring and distortion of vision.
- **Scleritis** (skleh-**RYE**-tis) is an inflammation of the sclera (**scler** means white of the eye, and **-itis** means inflammation). This condition is usually associated with infections, chemical injuries, or autoimmune diseases.

The Eye

- **Anisocoria** (**an**-ih-so-**KOH**-ree-ah) is a condition in which the pupils are unequal in size (**anis/o** means unequal, **cor** means pupil, and **-ia** means abnormal condition). This condition can be congenital or caused by a head injury, an aneurysm, or pathology of the central nervous system.
- A **cataract** (**KAT**-ah-rakt) is the loss of transparency of the lens that causes a progressive loss of visual clarity. The formation of most cataracts is associated with aging; however, this condition can be congenital or due to an injury or disease (Figure 12.8B).
- **Diabetic retinopathy** is damage to the retina as a complication of uncontrolled diabetes. This is discussed in the section "Diabetic Complications" in Chapter 14. As diabetic retinopathy progresses, *diabetic macular edema* can occur.
- **Endophthalmitis** (**end**-op-thahl-**MYE**-tis) is inflammation of the intraocular fluids (**end-** means inside, **ophthalm** means eye, and **-itis** means inflammation). It can be caused by infection or as a complication of eye surgery.
- **Floaters**, also known as *vitreous floaters*, are particles of cellular debris that float in the vitreous humor and cast shadows on the retina. Floaters often occur normally but may be an indication of retinal detachment, especially when accompanied by photopsia.
- **Photopsia** (foh-**TOP**-see-ah) is the presence of what appear to be flashes of light, or *flashers* (**phot** means light, and **-opsia** means view of). These are often caused by damage to the eye or migraine headaches.
- **Miosis** (mye-**OH**-sis) is the contraction of the pupil, normally in response to exposure to light but also possibly due to the use of prescription or illegal drugs (**mio-** means smaller, and **-sis** means abnormal condition).
- **Mydriasis** (mih-**DRY**-ah-sis), the dilation of the pupil, is the opposite of *miosis* (**mydrias** means the dilation of the pupil, and **-is** means abnormal condition). The causes of mydriasis include diseases, trauma (injury), and drugs.
- **Nystagmus** (nis-**TAG**-mus) is an involuntary, constant, rhythmic movement of the eyeball that can be congenital or caused by a neurological injury or drug use.
- **Papilledema** (**pap**-ill-eh-**DEE**-mah), also known as a *choked disk*, is swelling and inflammation of the optic nerve at the point of entrance into the eye through the optic disk (**papill** means nipple-like, and **-edema**

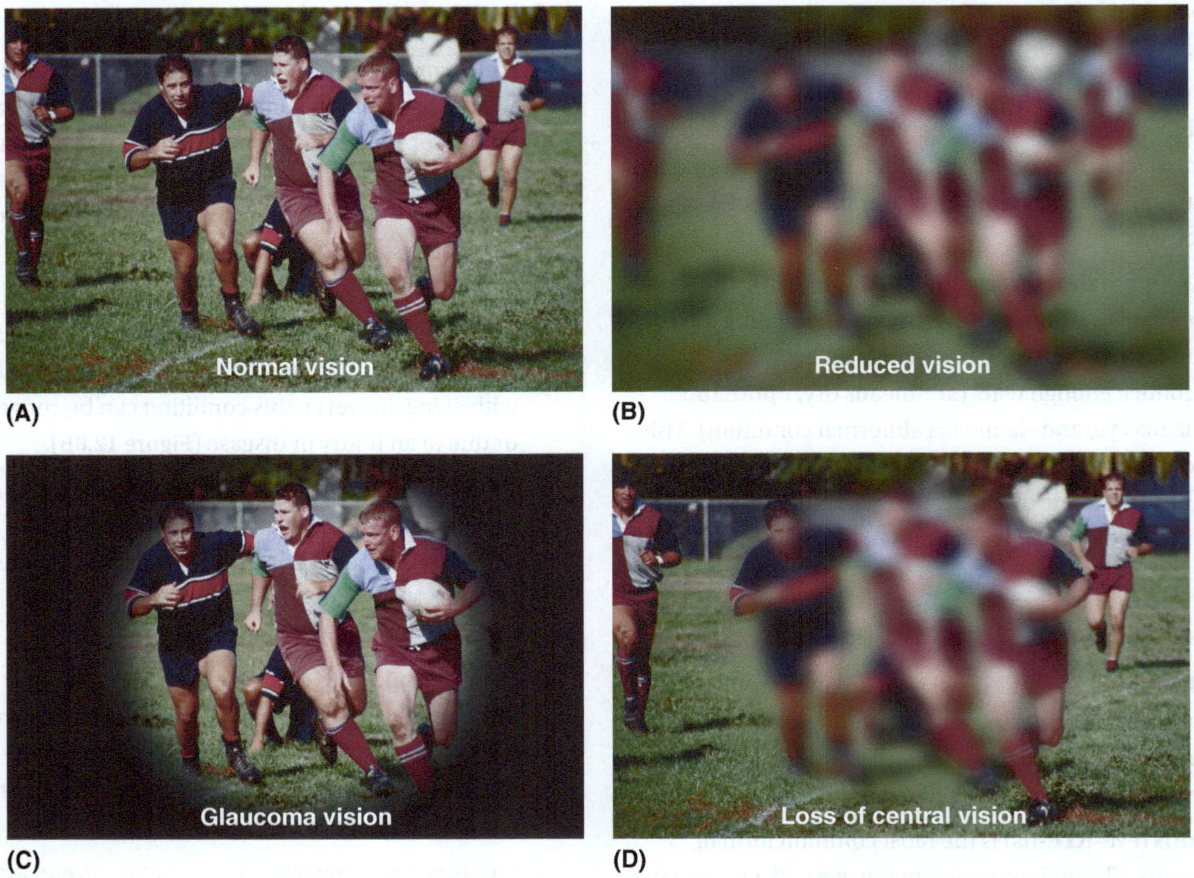

FIGURE 12.8 Normal vision and pathologic vision changes. (A) Normal vision. (B) Vision reduced by cataracts. (C) The loss of peripheral vision due to untreated glaucoma. (D) The loss of central vision due to macular degeneration.

means swelling). This swelling is caused by increased intracranial pressure and can be due to a tumor pressing on the optic nerve.

- **Retinal detachment**, also known as a *detached retina*, and **retinal tears** are the separation of some or all of the light-sensitive retina from the choroid. If not treated, the entire retina can detach, causing blindness. Risk factors for these conditions include head trauma, severe myopia, diabetic retinopathy, and complications from eye surgery (Figure 12.9).
- **Retinitis pigmentosa** (**ret**-ih-**NIGH**-tis pig-men-**TOH**-sah) is a progressive degeneration of the retina that affects night and peripheral vision. It can be detected by the presence of dark pigmented spots in the retina.
- **Retinoblastoma** (**ret**-ih-noh-blas-**TOH**-ma) is an eye cancer caused by the abnormal growth of retinal cells. While rare, it is the most common type of intraocular cancer in children.
- *Temporal arteritis* is a form of vasculitis that can cause a sudden vision loss, usually in one eye (see Chapter 5).

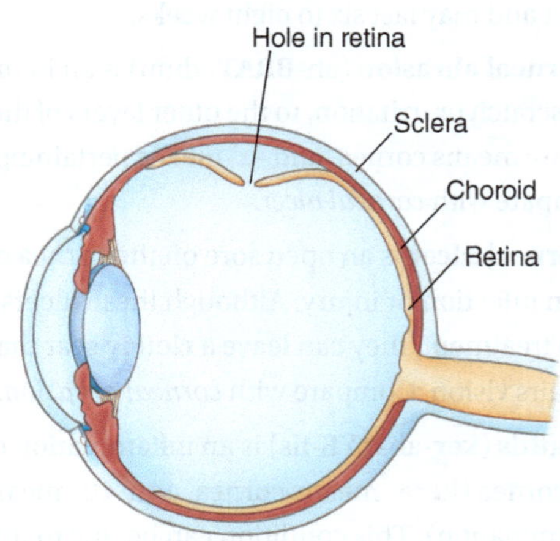

FIGURE 12.9 A retinal detachment.

Glaucoma

Glaucoma (glaw-**KOH**-mah) is a group of diseases characterized by increased intraocular pressure that causes damage to the retinal nerve fibers and the optic nerve (Figure 12.8C). This increase in pressure is caused by a blockage in the flow of fluid out of the eye. If untreated, this pressure can cause the loss of peripheral vision and eventually blindness.

- **Open-angle glaucoma**, also known as *chronic glaucoma*, is by far the most common form of this condition. The trabecular meshwork gradually becomes blocked, causing a buildup of pressure. Symptoms of this condition are not noticed by the patient until the optic nerve has been damaged; however, it can be detected earlier through regular eye examinations, including tonometry and visual field testing. See the section "Diagnostic Procedures for Vision and the Eyes."
- In **closed-angle glaucoma**, also known as *acute glaucoma*, the opening between the cornea and iris narrows so that fluid cannot reach the trabecular meshwork. This narrowing can cause a sudden increase in the intraocular pressure that produces severe pain, nausea, redness of the eye, and blurred vision. Without immediate treatment, blindness can occur in as little as two days.

Macular Degeneration

Macular degeneration (**MACK**-you-lar) (MD) is a gradually progressive condition in which the macula at the center of the retina is damaged, resulting in the loss of central vision but not in total blindness (**macul** means spot, and **-ar** mean pertaining to) (Figure 12.8D).

- *Age-related macular degeneration* (AMD) occurs most frequently in older people and is the leading cause of severe vision loss in those over age 60. While the symptoms often start in one eye, there is a high risk that AMD will also develop in the other eye.
- *Dry macular degeneration*, which accounts for 90% of all AMD cases, is caused by the slow deterioration of the cells of the macula over time.
- *Wet macular degeneration* is an advanced form of dry AMD. New blood vessels growing beneath the retina leak blood and fluid, damaging the macular cells. These small hemorrhages usually result in rapid and severe vision loss.

Functional Defects

- **Diplopia** (dih-**PLOH**-pee-ah), also known as *double vision*, is the perception of two images of a single object (**dipl** means double, and **-opia** means vision condition). It is sometimes a symptom of a serious underlying disorder such as multiple sclerosis or a brain tumor.
- **Hemianopia** (**hem**-ee-ah-**NOH**-pee-ah) is blindness in one-half of the visual field (**hemi-** means half, **an** means without, and **-opia** means vision condition).
- **Color blindness** is a general term referring to the inability to perceive certain colors in a normal manner due to the absence or abnormal function of cones. There are multiple types of color blindness, the most common of which is red-green color blindness.
- **Nyctalopia** (**nick**-tah-**LOH**-pee-ah), also known as *night blindness*, is a condition in which an individual with normal daytime vision has difficulty seeing at night (**nyctal** means night, and **-opia** means vision condition).
- **Photophobia** (**foh**-toh-**FOH**-bee-ah) means excessive sensitivity to light and can be the result of migraines, excessive wearing of contact lenses, drug use, or inflammation (**phot/o** means light, and **-phobia** means abnormal fear).
- **Presbyopia** (**pres**-bee-**OH**-pee-ah) is the condition of common changes in the eyes that occur with aging (**presby** means old age, and **-opia** means vision condition). With age, near vision declines noticeably as the lens becomes less flexible and the muscles of the ciliary body become weaker. The result is that the eyes are no longer able to focus the image properly on the retina.

Strabismus

Strabismus (strah-**BIZ**-mus) is a disorder in which the eyes point in different directions or are not aligned correctly, because the eye muscles are unable to focus together.

- **Esotropia** (**es**-oh-**TROH**-pee-ah) (ET), also known as *cross-eyes*, is strabismus characterized by an inward deviation of one or both eyes (**eso-** means inward, **trop** means turn, and **-ia** means abnormal condition). Esotropia is the opposite of *exotropia*.
- **Exotropia** (**eck**-soh-**TROH**-pee-ah), also known as *walleye*, is strabismus characterized by the outward deviation of one eye relative to the other (**exo-** means outward, **trop** means turn, and **-ia** means abnormal condition). Exotropia is the opposite of *esotropia*.

Refractive Disorders

A **refractive disorder** is a focusing problem that occurs when the lens and cornea do not bend light so that it focuses properly on the retina (Figure 12.10).

- **Ametropia** (**am**-eh-**TROH**-pee-ah) is any error of refraction in which images do not focus properly on the retina (**ametr** means out of proportion, and **-opia** means vision condition). Astigmatism, hyperopia, and myopia are all forms of ametropia.

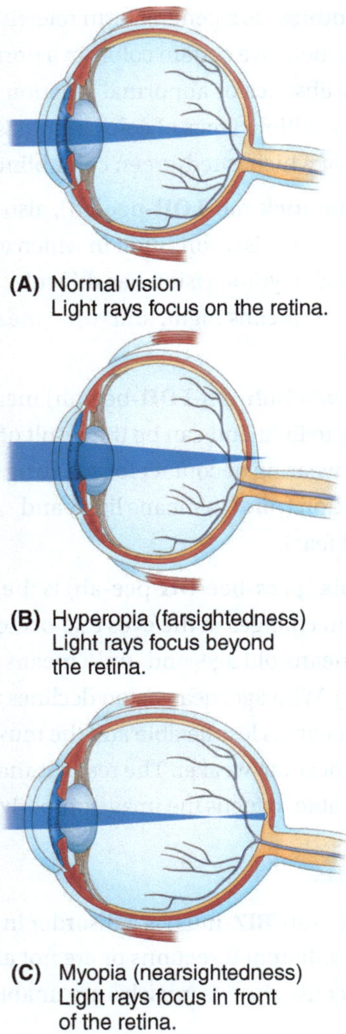

FIGURE 12.10 Refraction. (A) Normal vision. (B) Hyperopia. (C) Myopia.

- **Astigmatism** (ah-**STIG**-mah-tizm) is a condition in which the eye does not focus properly because of uneven curvatures of the cornea.
- **Hyperopia** (**high**-per-**OH**-pee-ah), also known as ***farsightedness***, is a defect in which light rays focus beyond the retina (**hyper-** means excessive, and **-opia** means vision condition). This condition can occur in childhood but usually causes difficulty after age 40 (Figure 12.10B). Hyperopia is the opposite of *myopia*.
- **Myopia** (my-**OH**-pee-ah), also known as ***nearsightedness***, is a defect in which light rays focus in front of the retina (**my** is from the Greek word for shortsighted, and **-opia** means vision condition). This condition occurs most commonly around puberty (Figure 12.10C). Myopia is the opposite of *hyperopia*.

Blindness

Blindness is the inability to see. Although some sight remains, ***legal blindness*** is the point at which, under law, an individual is considered to be blind. A commonly used standard is that a person is legally blind when his or her best-corrected vision is reduced to 20/200 or less.

- **Amblyopia** (**am**-blee-**OH**-pee-ah) is a dimness of vision or the partial loss of sight, especially in one eye, without detectable disease of the eye (**ambly** means dim or dull, and **-opia** means vision condition).
- **Scotoma** (skoh-**TOH**-mah), also known as ***blind spot***, is an abnormal area of diminished vision surrounded by an area of normal vision.

DIAGNOSTIC PROCEDURES FOR VISION AND THE EYES

Diagnostic Procedures for Vision

- A **Snellen chart** (SC) is used to measure visual acuity. The results for each eye are recorded as a fraction with 20/20 being considered normal.
  - The *first number* indicates the standard distance from the chart, which is 20 feet.
  - The *second number* indicates the deviation from the norm based on the ability to read progressively smaller lines of letters on the chart.
- A **refraction test** is done to determine an eye's refractive error so that the best corrective lenses can be prescribed. This term also refers to the ability of the lens to bend light rays so they focus on the retina.
- A **diopter** (dye-**AHP**-tur) is the unit of measurement of a lens's refractive power.
- The **cover test** is an examination of how the two eyes work together and is used to assess binocular vision. One eye at a time is covered while the patient focuses on an object across the room.
- **Visual field testing**, also known as ***perimetry***, is performed to determine losses in peripheral vision. *Peripheral* means occurring away from the center. Blank sections in the visual field can be symptomatic of glaucoma or an optic nerve disorder. This test is done by having the patient look straight ahead and indicate whether or not they can see an object or flash of light when it is presented in their periphery.

Diagnostic Procedures for the Eyes

- **Ophthalmoscopy** (**ahf**-thal-**MOS**-koh-pee), also known as ***funduscopy***, is the use of an ophthalmoscope to visually examine the fundus (back part) of the eye. This examination includes the retina, optic disk, choroid, and blood vessels.
- **Dilation** (dye-**LAY**-shun) of the eyes is required in preparation for the ophthalmoscopic examination of the interior of the eye. Artificial enlargement of the pupils is achieved through the use of mydriatic drops.
- **Mydriatic drops** (**mid**-ree-**AT**-ick) are placed into the eyes to produce temporary paralysis, forcing the pupils to remain dilated even in the presence of bright light.
- **Slit-lamp ophthalmoscopy** (**ahf**-thal-**MOS**-koh-pee) is a diagnostic procedure in which a narrow beam of light is focused onto parts of the eye to permit the ophthalmologist to examine the structures at the front of the eye, including the cornea, iris, and lens (Figure 12.11). Often fluorescein staining is used to help detect foreign bodies or an infected or injured area of the eye.
- **Fluorescein staining** (**flew**-oh-**RES**-ee-in) is the application of fluorescent dye to the surface of the eye via eye drops or a strip applicator. This dye causes a corneal abrasion to temporarily appear bright green.
- **Fluorescein angiography** (**flew**-oh-**RES**-ee-in **an**-jee-**OG**-rah-fee) (FA) is a photographic study of the blood vessels in the back of the eye following the intravenous injection of a fluorescein dye as a contrast medium. The resulting ***angiograms*** are used to determine whether there is proper circulation in the retinal vessels.
- **PERRLA** is an acronym meaning **P**upils are **E**qual, **R**ound, **R**eactive to **L**ight and **A**ccommodation. This is a diagnostic observation, and any abnormality here could indicate a head injury or damage to the brain. *Accommodation* refers to the eyes' ability to focus on objects that are both close up and far away.
- **Tonometry** (toh-**NOM**-eh-tree) is the measurement of intraocular pressure (**ton/o** means tension, and **-metry** means to measure). Abnormally high pressure can be an indication of glaucoma.

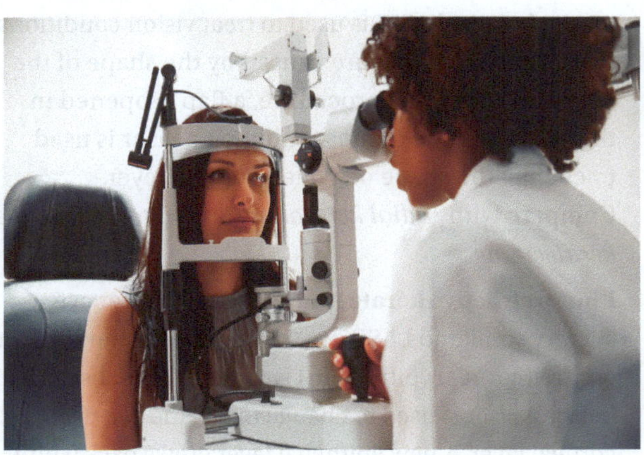

iStock.com/AMR Image

FIGURE 12.11 A routine eye exam using a slit lamp.

TREATMENT PROCEDURES OF THE EYES AND VISION

The Orbit and Eyelids

- An **orbitotomy** (**or**-bih-**TOT**-oh-mee) is a surgical incision into the orbit (**orbit** means bony socket, and **-otomy** means surgical incision). This procedure is performed for biopsy, abscess drainage, or removal of a tumor or foreign object.
- **Tarsorrhaphy** (tahr-**SOR**-ah-fee) is the partial or complete suturing together of the upper and lower eyelids to protect the eye when the lids are paralyzed and unable to close normally, or to help corneal lesions heal (**tars/o** means eyelid, and **-rrhaphy** means surgical suturing).
- Cosmetic procedures relating to the eyelids are discussed in Chapter 13.

The Conjunctiva and Eyeball

- **Anti-VEGF injections** (**V**ascular **E**ndothelial **G**rowth **F**actor) are intravitreal injections used to treat wet macular degeneration by slowing the growth of abnormal blood vessels in the eye (**intra-** means within, **vitre** means vitreous humor, and **-al** means pertaining to).
- A **corneal transplant**, also known as ***keratoplasty***, is the surgical replacement of a scarred or diseased cornea with clear corneal tissue from a donor. It is currently the most common and successful transplant procedure in the United States.
- **Enucleation** (ee-**new**-klee-**AY**-shun) is the removal of the eyeball, leaving the eye muscles intact (**e-** means out of, **nucle** means nucleus, and **-ation** means action).
- An **ocular prosthesis** (pros-**THEE**-sis), also known as an ***artificial eye***, may be fitted to wear over a malformed eye or to replace an eyeball that is either congenitally missing or has been surgically removed. A ***prosthesis*** is an artificial substitute for a diseased or missing body part.

- A **radial keratotomy** (**ker**-ah-**TOT**-oh-mee) (RK) is a surgical procedure to treat myopia (**kerat** means cornea, and **-otomy** means surgical incision). During the surgery, incisions are made in the cornea to cause it to flatten. These incisions allow the sides of the cornea to bulge outward and thereby flatten the central portion of the cornea. This brings the focal point of the eye closer to the retina and improves distance vision. Compare with *LASIK* and *photorefractive keratectomy*, in the section "Laser Treatments of the Eyes."
- A **scleral buckle** (**SKLER**-al) is a silicone band or sponge used to repair a detached retina. The detached layers are brought closer together by attaching this band onto the sclera, or outer wall, of the eyeball, creating an indentation or buckle effect inside the eye.
- **Vitrectomy** (vih-**TRECK**-toh-mee) is the removal of the vitreous humor and its replacement with a saline solution (**vitr** means vitreous humor, and **-ectomy** means removal). This procedure is sometimes performed to provide access to treat a retinal detachment or when diabetic retinopathy causes blood to leak and cloud the vitreous humor.

Cataract Surgery

- **Cataract surgery** is the general term used to describe the surgical removal of a cataract-clouded lens and its replacement with an artificial intraocular lens.
- **Phacoemulsification** (**fack**-koh-ee-**mul**-sih-fih-**KAY**-shun) is the use of ultrasonic vibration to shatter and remove the lens clouded by a cataract. This is performed through a very small opening, and the same opening is used to slide the intraocular lens into place.
- An **intraocular lens** (IOL) is a surgically implanted replacement for a natural lens that has been removed (**intra-** means within, **ocul** means eye, and **-ar** means pertaining to). There are two types of IOLs, ***monofocal*** and ***multifocal***, which was designed to eliminate the need for additional corrective lenses.

Corrective Lenses

Refractive errors in the eye can often be corrected with lenses that alter the angle of light rays before they reach the cornea. Glasses with ***concave lenses*** (curved inward) are used for myopia, or nearsightedness, and glasses with ***convex lenses*** (curved outward) for hyperopia (farsightedness).

- Corrective lenses can combine two or three different refractive powers, one above the other, to allow for better distance vision when looking up and near vision when looking down. ***Bifocals*** are lenses with two powers. ***Trifocals*** are lenses with three powers.
- Strabismus is sometimes treated with corrective lenses or an eye patch covering the stronger eye and thus strengthening the muscles in the weaker eye.
- ***Contact lenses*** are refractive lenses that float directly on the tear film in front of the eye. Rigid gas-permeable lenses cover the central part of the cornea, and disposable soft lenses cover the entire cornea. Contact lenses can be single focus, have multiple refractive powers, or be weighted at the bottom to correct astigmatism.

Laser Treatments of the Eyes

In the treatment of eye disorders, lasers have many uses. More details on how lasers work can be found in Chapter 13.

- A **laser iridotomy** (**ir**-ih-**DOT**-oh-mee) uses a focused beam of light to create a hole in the iris of the eye (**irid** means iris, and **-otomy** means surgical incision). This procedure is performed to treat closed-angle glaucoma by creating an opening that allows the aqueous humor to flow between the anterior and posterior chambers of the anterior segment of the eye.
- A **laser trabeculoplasty** (trah-**BECK**-you-loh-**plas**-tee) is used to treat open-angle glaucoma by creating openings in the trabecular meshwork to allow the fluid to drain properly.
- **LASIK** is the acronym for **L**aser-**A**ssisted in **SI**tu **K**eratomileusis (**kerat/o** means cornea, and **-mileusis** means carving). ***In situ*** means in its original place. LASIK is used to treat vision conditions, such as myopia, that are caused by the shape of the cornea. During this procedure, a flap is opened in the surface of the cornea, and then a laser is used to change the shape of a deep corneal layer. Compare with *radial keratotomy* and *photorefractive keratectomy*.
- **Photorefractive keratectomy** (PRK) is a laser eye surgery similar to LASIK, in which the outer layer of the cornea (corneal epithelium) is removed and discarded before a laser is used to change the shape of a deep corneal layer. A new epithelial layer grows back within a few days of surgery.

- **Laser photocoagulation** (**foh**-toh-koh-**ag**-you-**LAY**-shun) is the use of a laser to treat diabetic retinopathy and age-related macular degeneration by sealing leaking or damaged blood vessels. This technique is also used to repair small retinal tears by intentionally forming scar tissue to seal the holes.
- **Pneumatic retinopexy** (**RET**-ih-noh-**peck**-see) is a surgery in which a gas bubble is injected into the vitreous cavity to put pressure on the detached area in a retinal detachment while it heals (**retin/o** means retina, and **-pexy** means surgical fixation). The bubble gradually dissipates.
- Lasers are used to remove clouded tissue that may have formed in the posterior portion of the lens capsule after cataract extraction.

FUNCTIONS OF THE EARS

The ears are the receptor organs of hearing, and their functions are to receive sound impulses and transmit them to the brain. The inner ear also helps maintain balance.

The abbreviations relating to the ears, with the Latin words from which they originated, are shown in Table 12.2. (*Note:* The Joint Commission recommends writing out these terms instead of using abbreviations.)

TABLE 12.2
Abbreviations Relating to the Ears

AD	Right ear (*auris dexter*)
AS	Left ear (*auris sinister*)
AU	Each ear (*auris uterque*) or both ears (*auris unitas*)

- The term **auditory** (**AW**-dih-**tor**-ee) means pertaining to the sense of hearing (**audit** means hearing or sense of hearing, and **-ory** means pertaining to).
- **Acoustic** (ah-**KOOS**-tick) means pertaining to sound or hearing (**acous** means hearing or sound, and **-tic** means pertaining to).

STRUCTURES OF THE EARS

The ear is divided into three separate regions: the outer ear, the middle ear, and the inner ear (Figure 12.12).

The Outer Ear

- The **pinna** (**PIN**-nah), also known as the ***auricle*** or ***outer ear***, is the external portion of the ear. The pinna captures sound waves and transmits them into the external auditory canal.

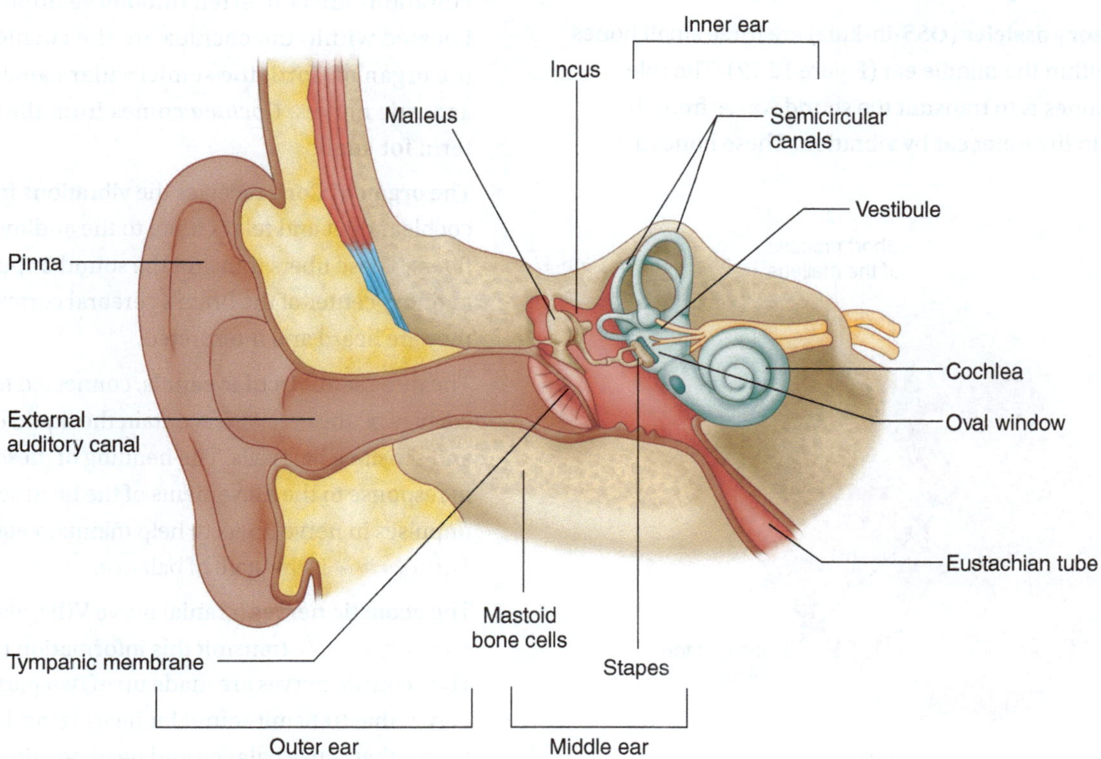

FIGURE 12.12 Structures of the ear shown in cross-section.

- The **external auditory canal** transmits these sound waves to the tympanic membrane (eardrum) of the middle ear.
- **Cerumen** (seh-**ROO**-men), also known as ***earwax***, is secreted by ceruminous glands that line the auditory canal. This sticky yellow-brown substance has protective functions because it traps small insects, dust, debris, and some bacteria to prevent them from entering the middle ear.

The Middle Ear

The **middle ear**, which is located between the outer ear and the inner ear, transmits sound across the space between these two parts (Figure 12.12).

- The **tympanic membrane** (tim-**PAN**-ick), also known as the ***eardrum***, is located between the outer and middle ear (Figure 12.13). The word parts **myring/o** and **tympan/o** both mean tympanic membrane. When sound waves reach the eardrum, this membrane transmits the sound by vibrating.
- The **mastoid process** is the temporal bone containing hollow air space that surrounds the middle ear. As used here, a *process* is a projection on a structure such as a bone.

The Auditory Ossicles

The **auditory ossicles** (**OSS**-ih-kulz) are three small bones located within the middle ear (Figure 12.12). The role of these bones is to transmit the sound waves from the eardrum to the inner ear by vibration. These bones are named for the Latin terms that describe their shapes. They are as follows:

- **Malleus** (**MAL**-ee-us), also known as the ***hammer***
- **Incus** (**ING**-kus), also known as the ***anvil***
- **Stapes** (**STAY**-peez), also known as the ***stirrup***

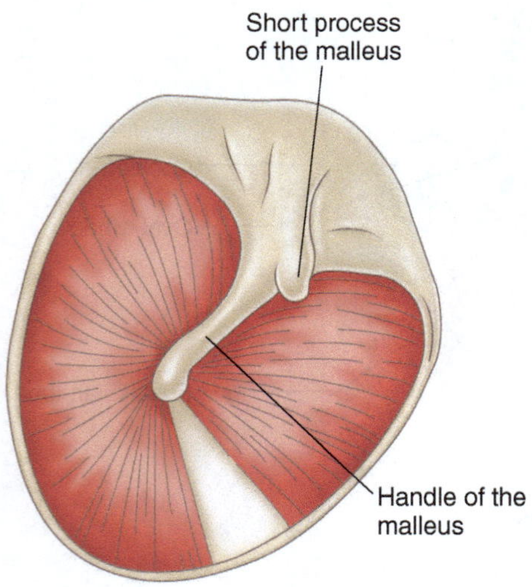

FIGURE 12.13 Schematic of the normal tympanic membrane as viewed from the external auditory canal.

The Eustachian Tubes

The **eustachian tubes** (you-**STAY**-shun), also known as the ***auditory tubes***, are narrow tubes that lead from the middle ear to the nasal cavity and the throat. The purpose of these tubes is to equalize the air pressure within the middle ear with that of the outside atmosphere.

The Inner Ear

The **inner ear** contains the sensory receptors for hearing and balance (Figure 12.12). The structures of the inner ear are a maze-like system known as the **labyrinth** (**LAB**-ih-rinth).

- The **oval window**, which is located under the base of the stapes, is the membrane that separates the middle ear from the inner ear. Vibrations enter the inner ear through this structure.
- The **cochlea** (**KOCK**-lee-ah) is the snail-shaped structure of the inner ear and is where sound vibrations are converted into nerve impulses. Located within the cochlea are the cochlear duct, the organ of Corti, the semicircular canals, and the acoustic nerves. *Cochlea* comes from the Greek term for snail.
- The **organ of Corti** receives the vibrations from the cochlear duct and relays them to the auditory nerve fibers. These fibers transmit the sound impulses to the auditory center of the brain's cerebral cortex, where they are heard and interpreted.
- The three **semicircular canals**, connected to the cochlea by the ***vestibule***, contain the liquid ***endolymph*** and sensitive hair cells. The bending of these hair cells in response to the movements of the head sets up impulses in nerve fibers to help maintain equilibrium. ***Equilibrium*** is the state of balance.
- The **acoustic nerves** (cranial nerve VIII), also called ***auditory nerves***, transmit this information to the brain. The acoustic nerves are made up of two parts: ***cochlear nerves*** that transmit sound for hearing, and ***vestibular nerves*** that sense balance and head position. These nerves are discussed in Chapter 11.

Normal Action of the Ears

- **Air conduction** (AC) is the process by which sound waves enter the ear through the pinna and then travel down the external auditory canal until they strike the tympanic membrane, which is located between the outer ear and middle ear.
- **Bone conduction** (BC) occurs as the eardrum vibrates and causes the auditory ossicles of the middle ear to vibrate. The vibration of these bones transmits the sound waves through the middle ear to the oval window of the inner ear.
- **Sensorineural conduction** (**sen**-suh-ree-**NOOR**-al) occurs when these sound vibrations reach the inner ear. The structures of the inner ear receive the sound waves and relay them to the auditory nerve for transmission to the brain.

MEDICAL SPECIALTIES RELATED TO THE EARS AND HEARING

- An **audiologist** (**aw**-dee-**OL**-oh-jist) specializes in the measurement of hearing function and in the rehabilitation of persons with hearing impairments (**audi** means hearing, and **-ologist** means specialist). An otolaryngologist (ear, nose, and throat physician) is discussed in Chapter 8.
- A **speech-language pathologist** (SLP) can be involved in numerous medical areas including audiology. These practitioners help patients who have problems related to swallowing, speech, and communication disorders.

PATHOLOGY OF THE EARS AND HEARING

The Outer Ear

- **Impacted cerumen** is an accumulation of earwax that forms a solid mass by adhering to the walls of the external auditory canal. ***Impacted*** means lodged or wedged firmly in place. Impacted cerumen can cause otalgia, tinnitus, and temporary hearing loss.
- **Otalgia** (oh-**TAL**-gee-ah), also known as an ***earache***, is pain in the ear (**ot** means ear, and **-algia** means pain).
- **Otitis** (oh-**TYE**-tis) means any inflammation of the ear (**ot** means ear, and **-itis** means inflammation). The second part of the term gives the location of the inflammation. For example, ***otitis externa*** is an inflammation of the external auditory canal, also known as ***swimmer's ear***.
- **Otomycosis** (**oh**-toh-my-**KOH**-sis) is a fungal infection of the external auditory canal (**ot/o** means ear, **myc** means fungus, and **-osis** means abnormal condition).
- **Otopyorrhea** (**oh**-toh-**pye**-oh-**REE**-ah) is the flow of pus from the ear (**ot/o** means ear, **py/o** means pus, and **-rrhea** means flow or discharge).
- **Otorrhea** (**oh**-toh-**REE**-ah) is any discharge from the ear (**ot/o** means ear, and **-rrhea** means discharge). In rare cases this could include leakage of cerebrospinal fluid.
- **Otorrhagia** (**oh**-toh-**RAY**-jee-ah) is bleeding from the ear (**ot/o** means ear, and **-rrhagia** means bleeding).

The Middle Ear

- **Barotrauma** (**bar**-oh-**TRAW**-mah) is a pressure-related ear condition (**bar/o** means pressure, and **-trauma** means injury). These conditions can be caused by pressure changes when flying, driving in the mountains, scuba diving, or when the eustachian tube is blocked.
- A **cholesteatoma** (koh-**les**-tee-ah-**TOH**-mah), also known as a ***pearly tumor***, is a destructive epidermal cyst in the middle ear and/or the mastoid process made up of epithelial cells and cholesterol (**cholesteat** refers to cholesterol, and **-oma** means tumor). It can be congenital or a serious complication of chronic otitis media (discussed in this section).
- **Mastoiditis** (**mas**-toy-**DYE**-tis) is an inflammation of any part of the mastoid bone (**mastoid** means mastoid process, and **-itis** means inflammation). This condition may develop when acute otitis media that cannot be controlled with antibiotics spreads to the mastoid process.
- **Infectious myringitis** (**mir**-in-**JIGH**-tis) is a contagious inflammation that causes painful blisters on the eardrum (**myring** means eardrum, and **-itis** means inflammation). This condition is associated with a middle ear infection. It is not to be confused with *infectious meningitis*, which is an inflammation of the brain and spinal cord (see Chapter 11).
- **Otitis media** (oh-**TYE**-tis **MEE**-dee-ah) is an inflammation of the middle ear.

- *Acute otitis media* is usually associated with an upper respiratory infection and is most commonly seen in young children. This condition can lead to a ruptured eardrum due to the buildup of pus or fluid in the middle ear.
- *Serous otitis media* is a fluid buildup in the middle ear without symptoms of an infection. This condition can follow acute otitis media or can be caused by dysfunction of the eustachian tube. It is more common in infants and small children.

- **Otosclerosis** (**oh**-toh-skleh-**ROH**-sis) is the ankylosis of the bones of the middle ear, resulting in a conductive hearing loss (**ot/o** means ear, and **-sclerosis** means abnormal hardening). *Ankylosis* means fused together. If severe, this condition is treated with a stapedectomy.

The Inner Ear

- **Labyrinthitis** (**lab**-ih-rin-**THIGH**-tis) is an inflammation of the labyrinth that can result in vertigo and deafness (**labyrinth** means labyrinth, and **-itis** means inflammation).
- **Vertigo** (**VER**-tih-goh) is a sense of whirling, dizziness, and loss of balance that is often combined with nausea and vomiting. Although it is a symptom of many disorders, recurrent vertigo is sometimes associated with inner ear problems such as Ménière's disease. It can be treated with vestibular rehabilitation therapy; see "Treatment Procedures of the Ear and Hearing" for more information.
- **Benign paroxysmal positional vertigo** (BPPV) is a common cause of vertigo that occurs when there is a shift in the location of small crystals in the semicircular canals. BPPV, labyrinthitis, and Ménière's disease are examples of *vestibular disorders*, which are disorders of the body's balance-controlling vestibular system in the inner ear.
- **Ménière's disease** (men-**YEHRS**) is a relatively rare chronic disorder in which the amount of fluid in the inner ear increases intermittently, producing attacks of vertigo, a fluctuating hearing loss (usually in one ear), and tinnitus.
- **Tinnitus** (tih-**NITE**-us), also commonly pronounced (**TIN**-ih-tus), is a condition of a ringing, buzzing, or roaring sound in one or both ears. It is often associated with hearing loss and is more likely to occur when there has been prolonged exposure to loud noises.

Hearing Loss

- An **acoustic neuroma** (new-**ROH**-mah) is a benign brain tumor that develops adjacent to the cranial nerve running from the brain to the inner ear (**acous** means hearing, and **-tic** means pertaining to; **neur** means nerve, and **-oma** means tumor). This is one of the most common types of brain tumors and can cause hearing loss, vertigo, and tinnitus.
- **Deafness** is the complete or partial loss of the ability to hear. It can range from the inability to hear sounds of a certain pitch or intensity, to a complete loss of hearing.
  - **Presbycusis** (pres-beh-**KOO**-sis) is a gradual loss of sensorineural hearing that occurs as the body ages (**presby** means old age, and **-cusis** means hearing).
  - **Conductive hearing loss** occurs when sound waves are prevented from passing from the air to the fluid-filled inner ear. Causes of this hearing loss include a buildup of earwax, infection, fluid in the middle ear, a punctured eardrum, otosclerosis, and scarring. This type of hearing loss can often be treated.
  - **Sensorineural hearing loss** (sen-suh-ree-**NOOR**-al), also known as *nerve deafness*, develops when the auditory nerve or hair cells in the inner ear are damaged. This is usually due to age, noise exposure, or an acoustic neuroma. The source of this hearing loss can be located in the inner ear, in the nerve from the inner ear to the brain, or in the brain.

Noise-Induced Hearing Loss

Noise-induced hearing loss (NIHL) is a type of nerve deafness caused by repeated exposure to extremely loud noises such as a gunshot or to moderately loud noises that continue for long periods of time.

- These noises can permanently damage the hair cells in the cochlea, and at least partial hearing loss occurs. Unfortunately, this gradual hearing loss usually isn't noticed until some hearing has been permanently destroyed.
- Any sound above 85 decibels (dB) can cause some hearing loss if the exposure is prolonged (Figure 12.14). Most portable music players and smartphones can produce sounds up to 105 dB, which is louder than a lawn mower or a chain saw and is equivalent to an ambulance siren.
- A **decibel** (**DES**-ih-bell) (dB) is commonly used as the measurement of the loudness of sound.

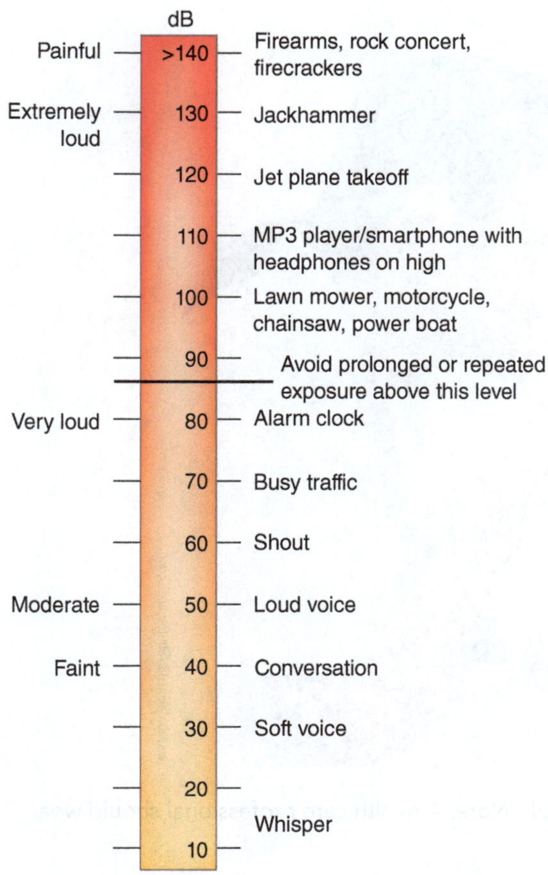

FIGURE 12.14 A decibel scale of frequently heard sounds.

DIAGNOSTIC PROCEDURES OF THE EARS AND HEARING

- An **audiological evaluation**, also known as ***speech audiometry***, is the measurement of the ability to hear and understand speech sounds based on their pitch and loudness. This testing is best achieved in a sound-treated room with earphones. The resulting graph is an ***audiogram*** that represents the ability to hear a variety of sounds at various loudness levels.
- **Audiometry** (aw-dee-**OM**-eh-tree) is the use of an audiometer to measure hearing acuity (**audi/o** means hearing, and **-metry** means to measure). An ***audiometer*** is an electronic device that produces acoustic stimuli of a set frequency and intensity.
- Sound is measured in two different ways, in hertz and decibels. A **hertz** (Hz) is a measure of sound frequency that determines how high or low a pitch is. *Note:* The singular and plural of *hertz* are the same.
- An **otoscope**, which is an instrument used to examine the external ear canal, is discussed further in Chapter 21 (Figure 12.15). A ***pneumatic otoscope*** has the attachment of a bulb filled with air; during an exam with an otoscope the bulb is pressed to visualize whether or not the tympanic membrane is immobile, indicating possible otitis media.
- **Monaural testing** (mon-**AW**-rahl) involves one ear (**mon-** means one, **aur** means hearing, and **-al** means pertaining to). Compare with *binaural testing.*
- **Binaural testing** (bye-**NAW**-rul *or* bin-**AW**-rahl) involves both ears (**bin-** means two, **aur** means hearing, and **-al** means pertaining to). Compare with *monaural testing.*
- **Tympanometry** (**tim**-pah-**NOM**-eh-tree) is the use of air pressure in the ear canal to test for disorders of the middle ear (**tympan/o** means eardrum, and **-metry** means to measure). The resulting record is a ***tympanogram***. This is used to test for middle-ear fluid buildup or eustachian tube obstruction, or to evaluate a conductive hearing loss.
- **Acoustic reflectometry** (AR) measures how much sound is reflected back from the eardrum, a way to test how much fluid is in the middle ear to diagnose otitis media.
- **Weber and Rinne tests** use a tuning fork to distinguish between conductive and sensorineural hearing losses. The patient's perception of the tuning fork's vibrations helps evaluate his or her hearing ability by air conduction compared to that of bone conduction.

TREATMENT PROCEDURES OF THE EARS AND HEARING

The Outer Ear

- **Otoplasty** (**OH**-toh-**plas**-tee) is the surgical repair, restoration, or alteration of the pinna of the ear (**ot/o** means ear, and **-plasty** means surgical repair). This is sometimes done as a cosmetic surgery called ***ear pinning*** to bring protruding ears closer to the head.

The Middle Ear

- **Ear tubes**, formally known as ***tympanostomy tubes***, are tiny ventilating tubes placed through the eardrum of a child prone to repeated ear infections to provide ongoing drainage for fluids and to relieve pressure. Fluid buildup can lead to hearing problems and speech delays (Figure 12.16).

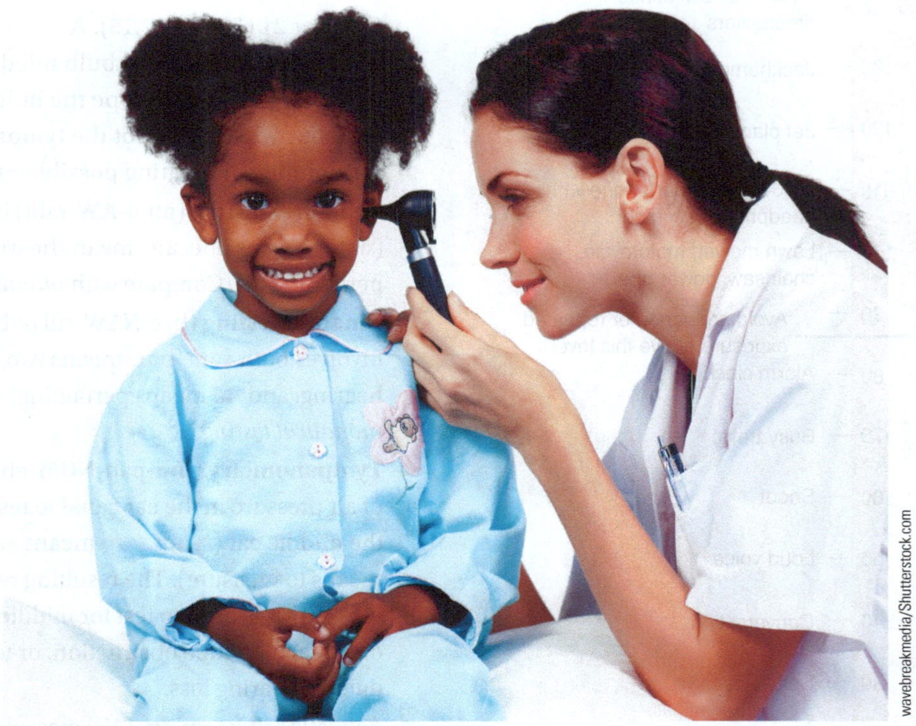

FIGURE 12.15 An otoscope is used to examine the external ear canal. (*Note:* A health care professional should wear gloves during all medical procedures.)

- A **mastoidectomy** (**mas**-toy-**DECK**-toh-mee) is the surgical removal of part of the mastoid process (**mastoid** means mastoid process, and **-ectomy** means surgical removal). This procedure is used to treat mastoiditis that cannot be controlled with antibiotics or in preparation for the placement of a cochlear implant.
- A **myringotomy** (**mir**-in-**GOT**-oh-mee) is a small surgical incision in the eardrum to relieve pressure from excess pus or fluid or to create an opening for the placement of ear tubes (**myring** means eardrum, and **-otomy** means surgical incision).
- A **stapedectomy** (**stay**-peh-**DECK**-toh-mee) is the surgical removal of the stapes bone and the insertion of a small prosthetic device to conduct sound vibrations to the inner ear (**staped** means stapes, and **-ectomy** means surgical removal).

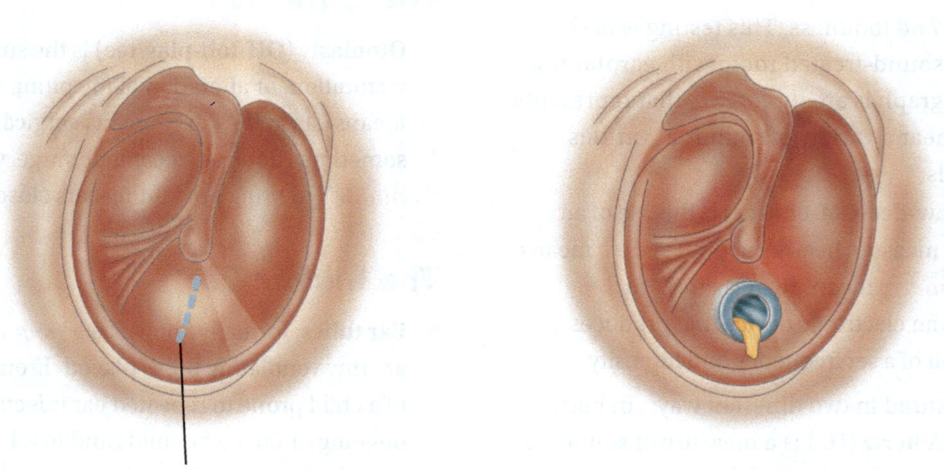

FIGURE 12.16 Tympanic membrane incision and the placement of a pediatric ear tube.

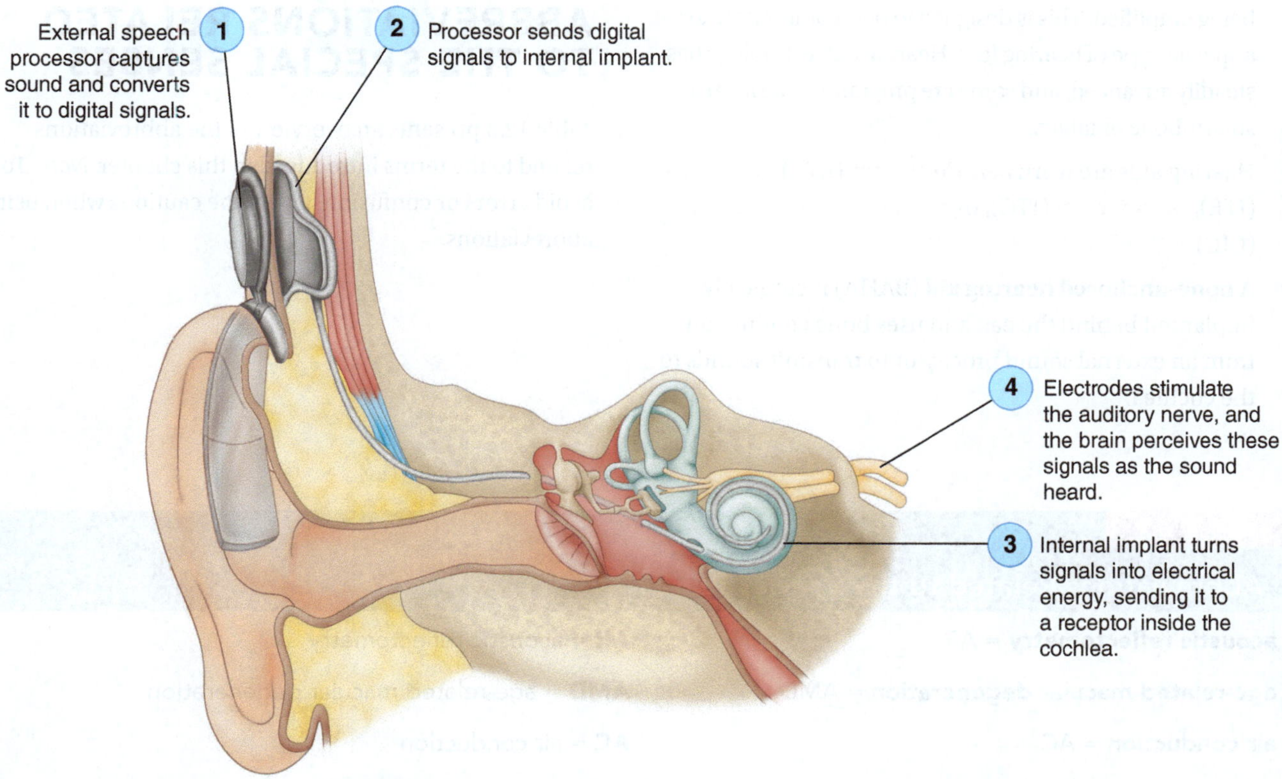

FIGURE 12.17 A cochlear implant transmits signals to electrodes that are implanted in the cochlea. This provides limited hearing for an individual who has been deaf since birth or an adult who has a profound hearing loss.

- **Tympanoplasty** (**tim**-pah-noh-**PLAS**-tee) is the surgical correction of a hole in the eardrum, either to cure chronic inflammation or to restore function (**tympan/o** means eardrum, and **-plasty** means a surgical repair).

The Inner Ear

- A **labyrinthectomy** (**lab**-ih-rin-**THECK**-toh-mee) is the surgical removal of all or a portion of the labyrinth (**labyrinth** means labyrinth, and **-ectomy** means surgical removal). This procedure is performed to relieve uncontrolled vertigo; however, it causes complete hearing loss in the affected ear.
- **Vestibular rehabilitation therapy** (ves-**TIB**-you-lar) (VRT) is a form of physical therapy designed to treat a wide variety of balance disorders, including dizziness, the majority of which are caused by problems in the inner ear and vestibular nerve (**vestibul** means an entrance, and **-ar** means pertaining to).

Treatments for Hearing Loss

- An **assistive listening device** (ALD) transmits, processes, or amplifies sound and can be used with or without a hearing aid. An ALD can be helpful in eliminating distracting background noise. The Americans with Disabilities Act (ADA) requires that many public places provide assistive listening devices.
- A **cochlear implant** (**KOCK**-lee-ar) is an electronic device that bypasses the damaged portions of the ear and directly stimulates the auditory nerve (Figure 12.17). The external speech processor captures sounds and converts them into digital signals. Electrodes that are implanted into the cochlea receive the signals and stimulate the auditory nerve. The brain receives these signals and perceives them as sound; however, it may take several months to adjust to the difference in speech when it is received in this manner.

Hearing Aids

Hearing aids are electronic devices that are worn to correct a hearing loss.

- An ***analog hearing aid*** is an external electronic device that uses a microphone to detect and amplify sounds.
- A ***digital hearing aid*** uses a computer chip to convert the incoming sound into a code that can be filtered before

being amplified. This is designed to best compensate for a specific type of hearing loss. Hearing aid technology has steadily advanced, and some are programmable from a smartphone or tablet.

- Hearing aids are worn ***behind the ear*** (BTE), ***in the ear*** (ITE), ***in the canal*** (ITC), or ***completely in the canal*** (CIC).
- A **bone-anchored hearing aid** (BAHA) is surgically implanted behind the ear, and uses bone conduction from an external sound processor to transmit sounds to the cochlea.

ABBREVIATIONS RELATED TO THE SPECIAL SENSES

Table 12.3 presents an overview of the abbreviations related to the terms introduced in this chapter. *Note:* To avoid errors or confusion, always be cautious when using abbreviations.

TABLE 12.3

Abbreviations Related to the Special Senses

acoustic reflectometry = AR	**AR** = acoustic reflectometry
age-related macular degeneration = AMD	**AMD** = age-related macular degeneration
air conduction = AC	**AC** = air conduction
assistive listening device = ALD	**ALD** = assistive listening device
benign paroxysmal positional vertigo = BPPV	**BPPV** = benign paroxysmal positional vertigo
bone conduction = BC	**BC** = bone conduction
decibel = dB	**dB** = decibel
fluorescein angiography = FA	**FA** = fluorescein angiography
intraocular lens = IOL	**IOL** = intraocular lens
macular degeneration = MD	**MD** = macular degeneration
noise-induced hearing loss = NIHL	**NIHL** = noise-induced hearing loss
photorefractive keratectomy = PRK	**PRK** = photorefractive keratectomy
radial keratotomy = RK	**RK** = radial keratotomy
visual acuity = VA	**VA** = visual acuity

CHAPTER 12

LEARNING EXERCISES

Matching Word Parts 1

Write the correct answer in the middle column.

	Definition	Correct Answer	Possible Answers
12.1.	cornea, hard	________________	opt/o
12.2.	eyelid	________________	-metry
12.3.	eye, vision	________________	kerat/o
12.4.	hearing	________________	-cusis
12.5.	to measure	________________	blephar/o

Matching Word Parts 2

Write the correct answer in the middle column.

	Definition	Correct Answer	Possible Answers
12.6.	eardrum	________________	presby/o
12.7.	eye, vision	________________	-opia
12.8.	iris of the eye	________________	ophthalm/o
12.9.	old age	________________	myring/o
12.10.	vision condition	________________	irid/o

Matching Word Parts 3

Write the correct answer in the middle column.

	Definition	Correct Answer	Possible Answers
12.11.	ear	________________	tympan/o
12.12.	eardrum	________________	trop/o

12.13. hard, white of eye ______________________ scler/o

12.14. retina ______________________ retin/o

12.15. turn ______________________ ot/o

Definitions

Select the correct answer, and write it on the line provided.

12.16. The ______________________ is the structure that maintains the shape of the eye and protects the delicate inner layers of tissue.

choroid conjunctiva cornea sclera

12.17. The ______________________ is the snail-shaped structure of the inner ear.

cochlea incus tarsus stapes

12.18. The ______________________ is also known as the blind spot of the eye.

fovea centralis macula optic disk optic nerve

12.19. The ______________________ lie(s) between the outer ear and the middle ear.

mastoid cells oval window posterior segment tympanic membrane

12.20. The ______________________ separates the middle ear from the inner ear.

eustachian tube inner canthus oval window tympanic membrane

12.21. The auditory ossicle, which is also known as the anvil, is the ______________________.

incus labyrinth malleus stapes

12.22. The term meaning common changes in the eyes that occur with aging is ______________________.

ametropia amblyopia presbyopia presbycusis

12.23. In ______________________, a laser is used to repair a detached retina.

keratoplasty photocoagulation retinopexy trabeculoplasty

12.24. The turning inward of the edge of the eyelid is known as ______________________.

ectropion emmetropia entropion esotropia

12.25. An inflammation of the middle ear is also called ______________________.

mastoiditis otitis media infectious myringitis otalgia

Matching Conditions

Write the correct answer in the middle column.

	Definition	Correct Answer	Possible Answers
12.26.	cross-eyes	________________	exotropia
12.27.	double vision	________________	myopia
12.28.	farsightedness	________________	hyperopia
12.29.	nearsightedness	________________	esotropia
12.30.	walleye	________________	diplopia

Which Word?

Select the correct answer, and write it on the line provided.

12.31. A ________________ is the unit of measurement of a lens's refractive power.

decibel diopter

12.32. In the process of normal hearing, ________________ conduction occurs when sound vibrations reach the inner ear.

sensorineural air

12.33. A ________________ is the surgical incision of the eardrum to create an opening for the placement of ear tubes.

myringotomy tympanoplasty

12.34. A visual field test to determine losses in peripheral vision is used to diagnose ________________.

cataracts glaucoma

12.35. An inflammation of the uvea, causing swelling and irritation, is called ________________.

corneal abrasion uveitis

Spelling Counts

Find the misspelled word in each sentence. Then write that word, spelled correctly, on the line provided.

12.36. The eustashian tubes lead from the middle ear to the nasal cavity and the throat. ______________________

12.37. Cerunem, also known as earwax, is secreted by glands that line the external auditory canal. ______________________

12.38. Astegmatism is a condition in which the eye does not focus properly because of uneven curvatures of the cornea. ______________________

12.39. Laberinthitis is an inflammation of the labyrinth that can result in vertigo and deafness. ______________________

12.40. A Snellan chart is used to measure visual acuity. ______________________

Abbreviation Identification

In the space provided, write the words that each abbreviation stands for.

12.41. **BPPV** ______________________

12.42. **IOL** ______________________

12.43. **OD** ______________________

12.44. **IOP** ______________________

12.45. **MD** ______________________

Term Selection

Select the correct answer, and write it on the line provided.

12.46. A radial keratotomy is performed to treat ______________________.

cataracts hyperopia myopia strabismus

12.47. The condition in which the pupils are unequal in size is known as ______________________.

anisocoria choked disk macular degeneration astigmatism

12.48. A ______________ is performed in preparation for the placement of a cochlear implant.

keratoplasty labyrinthectomy mastoidectomy myringoplasty

12.49. Normal vision begins when light rays first reach the ______________.

retina cornea pupil iris

12.50. A fungal infection of the external auditory canal is ______________.

otalgia otitis otomycosis otopyorrhea

Sentence Completion

Write the correct term or terms on the lines provided.

12.51. The ability of the lens to bend light rays so they focus on the retina is known as ______________.

12.52. A sense of whirling, dizziness, and the loss of balance is called ______________.

12.53. A/An ______________ is a specialist in measuring the accuracy of vision.

12.54. An inflammation of the cornea that can be due to many causes, including bacterial, viral, or fungal infections, is known as ______________.

12.55. The medical term meaning color blindness is ______________.

Word Surgery

Divide each term into its component word parts. Write these word parts, in sequence, on the lines provided. When necessary, use a slash (/) to indicate a combining vowel. (You may not need all of the lines provided.)

12.56. **Anisocoria** is a condition in which the pupils are unequal in size.

________ ________ ________ ________

12.57. **Emmetropia** is the normal relationship between the refractive power of the eye and the shape of the eye that enables light rays to focus correctly on the retina.

________ ________ ________ ________

12.58. **Otopyorrhea** is the flow of pus from the ear.

________ ________ ________ ________

12.59. **Presbycusis** is a gradual loss of sensorineural hearing that occurs as the body ages.

__________ __________ __________ __________

12.60. **Xerophthalmia** is drying of eye surfaces, including the conjunctiva, that is often associated with aging.

__________ __________ __________ __________

True/False

If the statement is true, write **True** on the line. If the statement is false, write **False** on the line.

12.61. _______ Rods in the retina are the receptors for color.

12.62. _______ Aqueous humor is drained through the canal of Schlemm.

12.63. _______ Visual field testing is performed to determine the presence of cataracts.

12.64. _______ Dacryoadenitis is an inflammation of the lacrimal gland caused by a bacterial, viral, or fungal infection.

12.65. _______ A speech-language pathologist specializes in the measurement of hearing function.

Clinical Conditions

Write the correct answer on the line provided.

12.66. Following a boxing match, Jack Lawson required __________________ to repair the injured pinna of his ear.

12.67. During his scuba diving expedition, Jose Ortega suffered from pressure-related ear discomfort. The medical term for this condition is __________________.

12.68. Margo Spencer was diagnosed with closed-angle glaucoma affecting her left eye. She is scheduled to have a/an __________________ performed to treat this condition.

12.69. Edward Cooke was diagnosed as having __________________. This condition is characterized by blindness in one-half of the visual field.

12.70. While gathering branches after the storm, Vern Passman scratched the cornea of his eye. To diagnose the damage, his ophthalmologist performed __________________ staining, which caused the corneal abrasions to appear bright green.

12.71. Ted Milligan was treated for an allergic reaction to being stung by a wasp. His reaction was swelling of the tissues around his eyes, and this is known as ____________ edema.

12.72. Adrienne Jacobus is unable to drive at night because she suffers from night blindness. The medical term for this condition is ____________.

12.73. James Escobar complained of a ringing sound in his ears. His physician refers to this condition as ____________.

12.74. The obstruction of a sebaceous gland caused the ____________ to form on Ingrid Clareus's upper eyelid.

12.75. Susie Harris was diagnosed as having ____________. Her mother referred to this condition as pinkeye.

Which Is the Correct Medical Term?

Select the correct answer, and write it on the line provided.

12.76. Commonly known as choked disk, ____________ is swelling and inflammation of the optic nerve at the point of entrance into the eye through the optic disk.

dilation papilledema tinnitus xerophthalmia

12.77. The presence of what appear to be flashes of light is known as ____________.

blind spot retinal detachment floaters photopsia

12.78. The term ____________ describes any error of refraction in which images do not focus properly on the retina.

ametropia diplopia esotropia hemianopia

12.79. An ____________ is a physician who specializes in diagnosing and treating disorders of the eye.

optometrist ophthalmologist optician audiologist

12.80. The term ____________ describes an accumulation of earwax that forms a solid mass by adhering to the walls of the external auditory canal.

canthus impacted cerumen otitis externa mastoiditis

Challenge Word Building

These terms are *not* primary terms in the chapter; however, they are made up of the following familiar word parts. If you need help in creating the term, refer to your medical dictionary.

blephar/o	**-algia**
irid/o	**-ectomy**
labyrinth/o	**-edema**
lacrim/o	**-itis**
ophthalm/o	**-ology**
retin/o	**-otomy**
	-pathy

12.81. Pain felt in the iris is known as ______________________.

12.82. Removal of all or part of the eyelid is known as ______________________.

12.83. Inflammation of the lacrimal duct is ______________________.

12.84. Based on word parts, the term ______________________ means any disease of the eyelid.

12.85. The medical specialty concerned with the eye, its diseases, and refractive errors is known as ______________________.

12.86. Swelling of the eyelid is known as ______________________.

12.87. A surgical incision into the lacrimal duct is a/an ______________________.

12.88. A surgical incision into the labyrinth of the inner ear is a/an ______________________.

12.89. The term meaning any disease of the iris is ______________________.

12.90. The surgical removal of the retina is known as a/an ______________________.

Labeling Exercises

Identify the numbered items on the accompanying figures.

12.91. ____________________

12.92. anterior ____________________

12.93. crystalline ____________________

12.94. ____________________

12.95. ____________________ centralis

12.96. ____________________ or auricle

12.97. external ____________________ canal

12.98. ____________________ membrane

12.99. ____________________ tube

12.100. ____________________

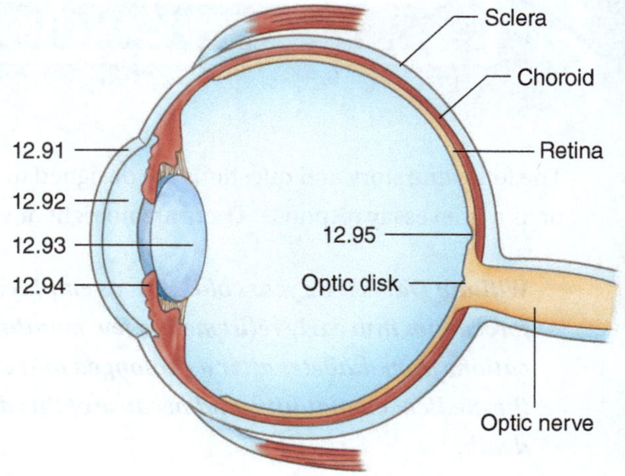

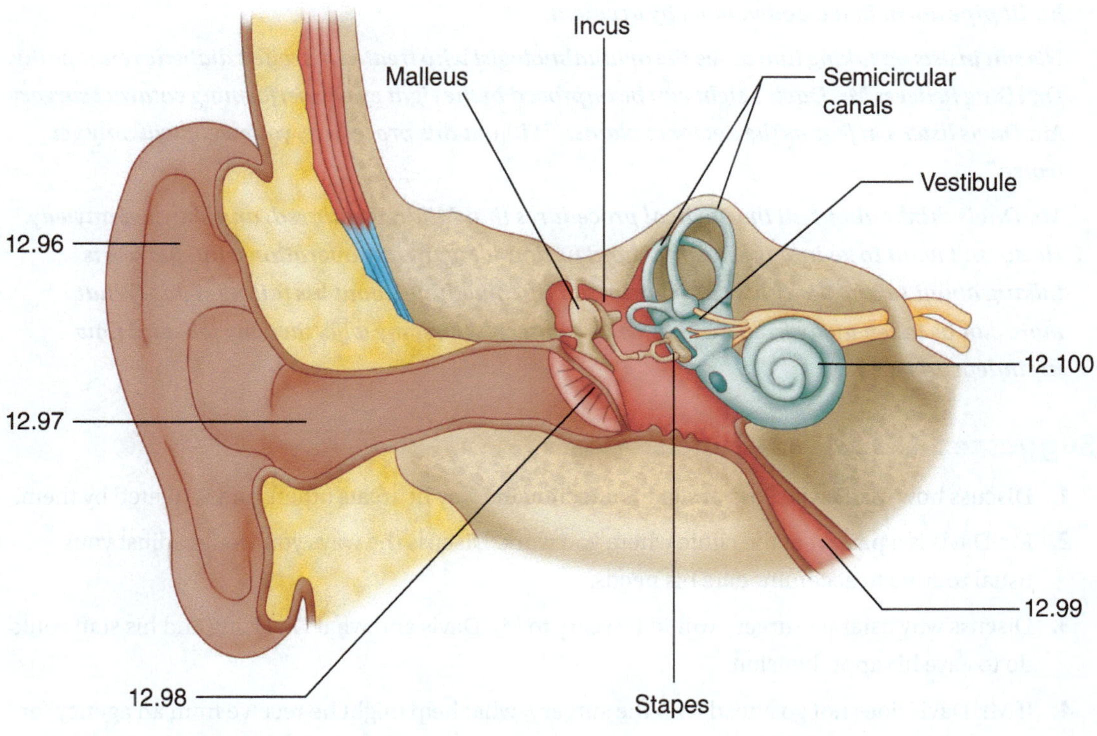

The Human Touch

CRITICAL THINKING EXERCISE

The following story and questions are designed to stimulate critical thinking through class discussion or as a brief essay response. There are no right or wrong answers to these questions.

William Davis is 62 years old. He was employed as a postal worker until his declining eyesight forced him into early retirement a few months ago. His wife, Mildred, died last year of complications from diabetes after a prolonged and expensive hospitalization. Mr. Davis does not trust the medical community, and because of this distrust, he has not been to a doctor since his wife's death.

Mr. Davis is not considered legally blind, but his presbyopia and an advancing cataract in his right eye are starting to interfere with his ability to take care of himself. He still drives to the market once a week, but other drivers get angry and honk at him. He pays for his groceries with a credit card because he is afraid the cashier will cheat him if he accidentally gives her the wrong bills. He complains that the cleaning lady hides things from him and deliberately leaves the furniture out of place. When she leaves, he can't find his slippers or an ashtray. Yesterday, he put his lit pipe down in a wooden bowl by accident.

His son insists on taking him to see the ophthalmologist who treated his wife's diabetic retinopathy. Dr. Hsing believes Mr. Davis's sight can be improved in the right eye by performing cataract surgery. Mr. Davis listens in fear as the doctor explains. "Without this procedure, your sight will only get worse."

Mr. Davis thinks about all the medical procedures that Mildred endured, and she died anyway. He doesn't want to go into the hospital, and he doesn't want any operations. But his son is talking about taking away his car if he doesn't do something about his failing sight. "What more can be taken away from me?" he thinks bitterly. "First my wife, then my job, and now my independence."

Suggested Discussion Topics

1. Discuss how Mr. Davis's loss of sight is affecting the way he treats others and is treated by them.
2. Mr. Davis is a patient at the clinic where you work. Discuss the ways you would adjust your usual routine to accommodate his needs.
3. Discuss why cataract surgery would be scary to Mr. Davis and what Dr. Hsing and his staff could do to ease his apprehension.
4. If Mr. Davis does not go ahead with the surgery, what help might he receive from an agency for the visually impaired? What other services might be available to help him deal with his grief and depression?

CHAPTER 13

SKIN: THE INTEGUMENTARY SYSTEM

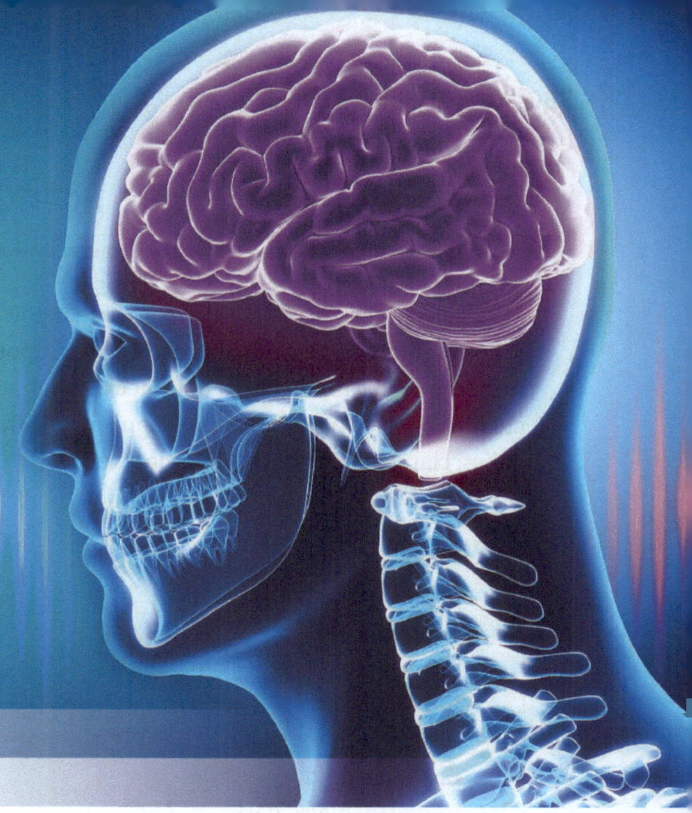

Overview of STRUCTURES, COMBINING FORMS, AND FUNCTIONS OF THE INTEGUMENTARY SYSTEM

Major Structures	Related Combining Forms	Primary Functions
Skin	cutane/o, dermat/o, derm/o	Intact skin is the first line of defense for the immune system. Skin waterproofs the body and is the major receptor for the sense of touch.
Sebaceous Glands	seb/o	Secrete sebum (oil) to lubricate the skin and discourage the growth of bacteria on the skin.
Sweat Glands	hidr/o	Secrete sweat to regulate body temperature and water content and excrete some metabolic waste.
Hair	pil/i, pil/o	Aids in controlling the loss of body heat.
Nails	onych/o, ungu/o	Protect the dorsal surface of the last bone of each finger and toe.

Vocabulary Related to **THE INTEGUMENTARY SYSTEM**

This list contains essential word parts and medical terms for this chapter. These and the other important **primary terms** are shown in **boldface** throughout the chapter. *Secondary terms*, which appear in *orange* italics, clarify the meaning of primary terms.

Word Parts

- ☐ **cry/o** cold
- ☐ **cutane/o** skin
- ☐ **derm/o**, **dermat/o** skin
- ☐ **hidr/o** sweat
- ☐ **hirsut/o** hairy, rough
- ☐ **lip/o** fat, lipid
- ☐ **melan/o** black, dark
- ☐ **myc/o** fungus
- ☐ **onych/o** fingernail or toenail
- ☐ **pil/i**, **pil/o** hair
- ☐ **py/o** pus
- ☐ **rhytid/o** wrinkle
- ☐ **seb/o** sebum
- ☐ **urtic/o** rash, hives
- ☐ **xer/o** dry

Medical Terms

- ☐ **actinic keratosis** (ack-**TIN**-ick **kerr**-ah-**TOH**-sis)
- ☐ **albinism** (**AL**-bih-**niz**-um)
- ☐ **alopecia** (**al**-oh-**PEE**-shee-ah)
- ☐ **blepharoplasty** (**BLEF**-ah-roh-**plas**-tee)
- ☐ **bulla** (**BULL**-ah)
- ☐ **capillary hemangioma** (**KAP**-uh-**ler**-ee hee-**man**-jee-**OH**-mah)
- ☐ **carbuncle** (**KAR**-bung-kul)
- ☐ **cellulitis** (**sell**-you-**LYE**-tis)
- ☐ **cicatrix** (sick-**AY**-tricks)
- ☐ **comedo** (**KOM**-eh-doh)
- ☐ **debridement** (dah-**BREED**-ment)
- ☐ **dermatitis** (**der**-mah-**TYE**-tis)
- ☐ **diaphoresis** (**dye**-ah-foh-**REE**-sis)
- ☐ **dysplastic nevi** (dis-**PLAS**-tick **NEE**-vye)
- ☐ **ecchymosis** (**eck**-ih-**MOH**-sis)
- ☐ **eczema** (**ECK**-zeh-mah)
- ☐ **erythema** (**er**-ih-**THEE**-mah)
- ☐ **erythroderma** (eh-**rith**-roh-**DER**-mah)
- ☐ **exanthem** (eck-**ZAN**-thum)
- ☐ **exfoliative dermatitis** (ecks-**FOH**-lee-**ay**-tiv **der**-mah-**TYE**-tis)
- ☐ **folliculitis** (foh-**lick**-you-**LYE**-tis)
- ☐ **furuncles** (**FYOU**-rung-kulz)
- ☐ **hematoma** (**hee**-mah-**TOH**-mah)
- ☐ **hirsutism** (**HER**-**soot**-izm)
- ☐ **ichthyosis** (**ick**-thee-**OH**-sis)
- ☐ **impetigo** (**im**-peh-**TYE**-goh)
- ☐ **keloid** (**KEE**-loid)
- ☐ **keratosis** (**kerr**-ah-**TOH**-sis)
- ☐ **koilonychia** (**koy**-loh-**NICK**-ee-ah)
- ☐ **lipedema** (lip-eh-**DEE**-mah)
- ☐ **lipoma** (lih-**POH**-mah)
- ☐ **macule** (**MACK**-youl)
- ☐ **malignant melanoma** (mel-ah-**NOH**-mah)
- ☐ **melasma** (muh-**LAZ**-mah)
- ☐ **necrotizing fasciitis** (**NECK**-roh-**tie**-zing **fas**-ee-**EYE**-tis)
- ☐ **onychocryptosis** (**on**-ih-koh-krip-**TOH**-sis)
- ☐ **onychomycosis** (**on**-ih-koh-my-**KOH**-sis)
- ☐ **papilloma** (**pap**-ih-**LOH**-mah)
- ☐ **papule** (**PAP**-youl)
- ☐ **paronychia** (**par**-oh-**NICK**-ee-ah)
- ☐ **pediculosis** (pee-**dick**-you-**LOH**-sis)
- ☐ **petechiae** (peh-**TEE**-kee-eye)
- ☐ **pressure ulcer**
- ☐ **pruritus** (proo-**RYE**-tus)
- ☐ **psoriasis** (soh-**RYE**-uh-sis)
- ☐ **purpura** (**PUR**-pew-rah)
- ☐ **purulent** (**PYOU**-roo-lent)
- ☐ **rhytidectomy** (**rit**-ih-**DECK**-toh-mee)
- ☐ **rosacea** (roh-**ZAY**-shee-ah)
- ☐ **scabies** (**SKAY**-beez)
- ☐ **scleroderma** (**sklehr**-oh-**DER**-mah)
- ☐ **seborrheic dermatitis** (**seb**-oh-**REE**-ick **der**-mah-**TYE**-tis)
- ☐ **squamous cell carcinoma** (**SKWAY**-mus)
- ☐ **systemic lupus erythematosus** (sis-**TEH**-mik **LOO**-pus er-ih-**thee**-mah-**TOH**-sus)
- ☐ **tinea** (**TIN**-ee-ah)
- ☐ **urticaria** (**ur**-tih-**KARE**-ee-ah)
- ☐ **verrucae** (veh-**ROO**-kee)
- ☐ **vitiligo** (**vit**-ih-**LYE**-goh)
- ☐ **wheal** (**WHEEL**)
- ☐ **xeroderma** (zee-roh-**DER**-mah)

LEARNING OBJECTIVES

On completion of this chapter, you should be able to:

1. Describe the functions and structures of the integumentary system.
2. Identify the medical specialists who treat disorders of the integumentary system.
3. Identify the medical word parts of the integumentary system.
4. Differentiate lesion types.
5. Define the primary terms related to the pathology and the diagnostic and treatment procedures of the integumentary system.
6. Spell the primary terms of the integumentary system.
7. Pronounce the primary terms of the integumentary system.
8. Identify common abbreviations related to the integumentary system.

FUNCTIONS OF THE INTEGUMENTARY SYSTEM

The **integumentary system** (in-**teg**-you-**MEN**-tah-ree), which is made up of the skin and its related structures, performs important functions in maintaining the health of the body. The term ***integument*** comes from the Latin word meaning to cover or enclose.

Functions of the Skin

The **skin** forms the protective outer layer covering the external surfaces of the entire body.

- The skin waterproofs the body and prevents fluid loss.
- Intact (unbroken) skin plays an important role in the immune system by blocking the entrance of pathogens into the body (see Chapter 7).
- Skin is the major receptor for the sense of touch.
- Skin helps the body synthesize vitamin D, an essential nutrient, from the sun's ultraviolet light, while screening out some harmful ultraviolet radiation.
- The average adult has 22 square feet of skin, making it the largest bodily organ.

Functions of Related Structures

The related structures of the integumentary system are the sebaceous glands, sweat glands, hair, and nails (Figure 13.1).

- The **sebaceous glands** (seh-**BAY**-shus) secrete sebum (oil) that lubricates the skin and discourages the growth of bacteria on the skin.
- The **sweat glands** help regulate body temperature and water content by secreting sweat. A small amount of metabolic waste is also excreted through the sweat glands.
- **Hair** helps control the loss of body heat.
- **Nails** protect the dorsal surface of the last bone of each toe and finger.

THE STRUCTURES OF THE SKIN AND ITS RELATED STRUCTURES

The Skin

The skin is a complex system of specialized tissues made up of three basic layers: the *epidermis*, *dermis*, and *subcutaneous* layers (Figure 13.1). The term **cutaneous** (kyou-**TAY**-nee-us) means pertaining to the skin (**cutane** means skin, and **-ous** means pertaining to).

The Epidermis

The **epidermis** (**ep**-ih-**DER**-mis), which is the outermost layer of the skin, is made up of several specialized epithelial tissues (**epi-** means above or upon, **derm** means skin, and **-is** is a noun ending).

The epidermis does not contain any blood vessels or connective tissue. It is therefore dependent on lower layers for nourishment.

- **Epithelial tissues** (**ep**-ih-**THEE**-lee-al) form a protective covering for all of the internal and external surfaces of the body.

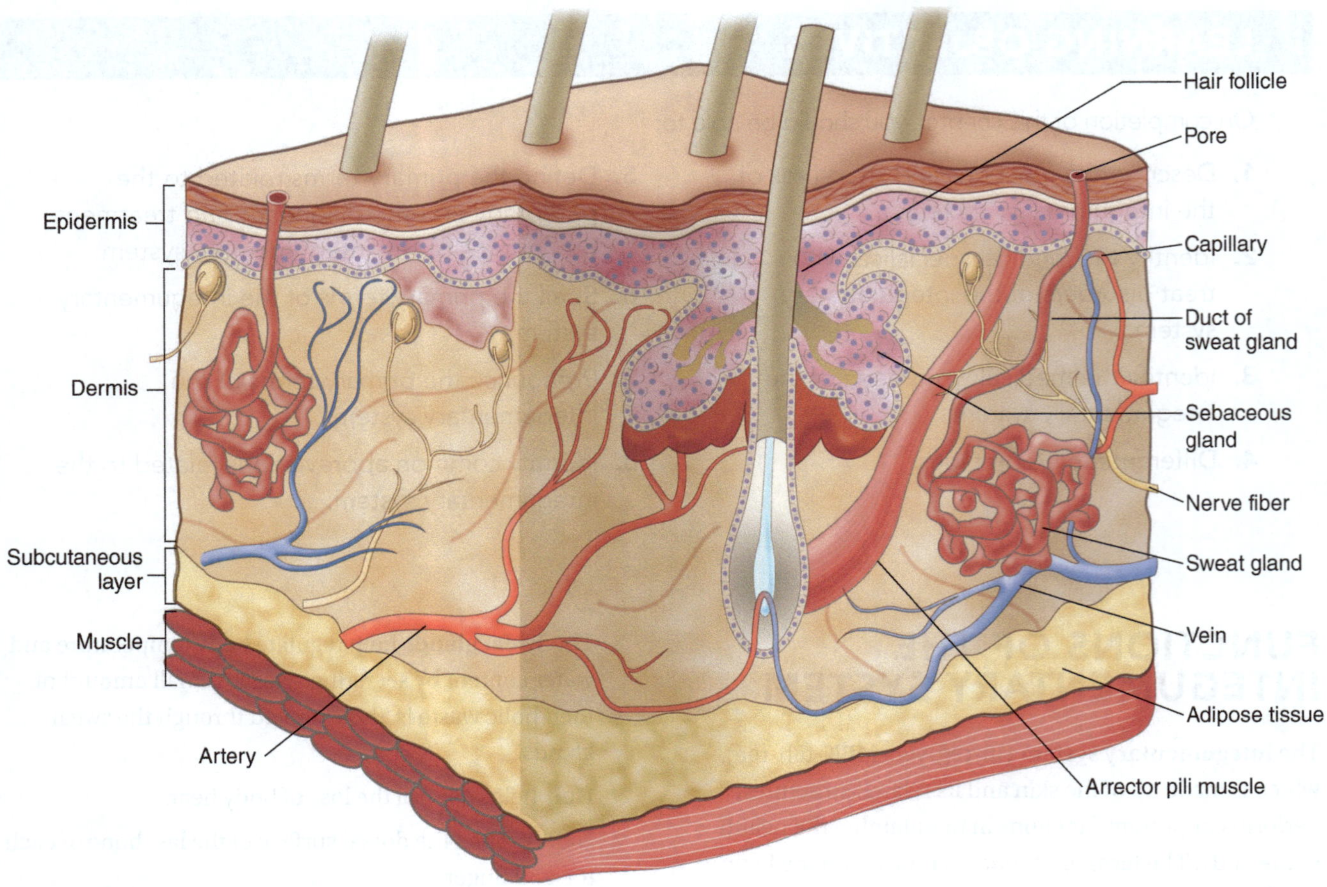

FIGURE 13.1 Structures of the skin. The sweat and sebaceous glands are associated structures of the skin.

- **Squamous epithelial tissue** (**SKWAY**-mus) forms the upper layer of the epidermis. ***Squamous*** means scale-like. This layer consists of flat, scaly cells that are continuously shed.
- The **basal layer** (**BAY**-suhl) is the lowest layer of the epidermis. It is here that new cells are produced and then pushed upward. When these cells reach the surface, they die and become filled with keratin.
- **Keratin** (**KER**-ah-tin) is a fibrous, water-repellent protein. Soft keratin is a primary component of the epidermis. Hard keratin is found in the hair and nails.
- **Melanocytes** (meh-**LA**-noh-sites) are special cells that are found in the basal cell layer. These cells produce and contain a dark brown to black pigment known as melanin.
- **Melanin** (**MEL**-ah-nin) is the pigment that determines the color of the skin, which depends upon the type and amount of this pigment that is present (Figure 13.2). Melanin also produces spots of color such as freckles and age spots, which are discussed in the section "Pathology of the Integumentary System."
- Melanin has the important function of protecting the skin against some of the harmful ultraviolet rays of the sun. ***Ultraviolet*** (UV) refers to light that is beyond the visible spectrum at the violet end. Some UV rays help the skin produce vitamin D; however, other rays damage the skin.

The Dermis

The **dermis** (**DER**-mis), also known as the ***corium***, is the thick layer of living tissue directly below the epidermis. It contains connective tissue, blood and lymph vessels, and nerve fibers. Also found in the dermis are the *hair follicles*, *sebaceous glands*, and *sweat glands*, which are the related structures of the integumentary system (as well as the *nails*).

Sensory nerve endings in the dermis are the sensory receptors for stimuli such as touch, temperature, pain, and pressure.

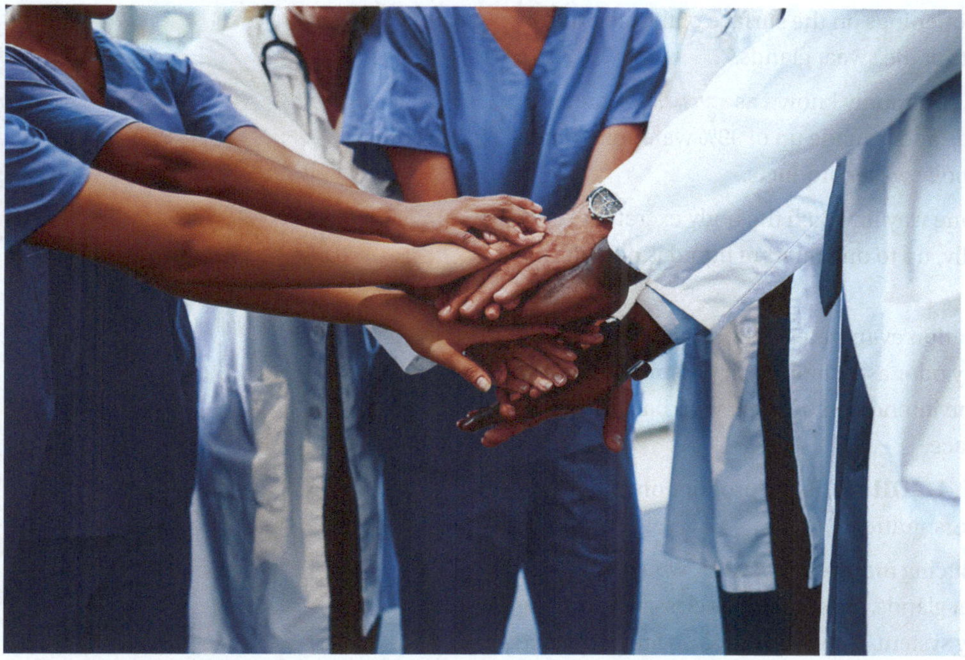

FIGURE 13.2 The amount of melanin present determines the color of the skin.

Tissues Within the Dermis

- **Collagen** (**KOL**-ah-jen), which means glue, is a tough yet flexible fibrous protein material found in the skin and also in the bones, cartilage, tendons, and ligaments.
- **Mast cells**, which are found in the connective tissue of the dermis, respond to injury, infection, or allergy by producing and releasing substances, including heparin and histamine.
- **Heparin** (**HEP**-ah-rin), which is released in response to an injury, is an anticoagulant. An ***anticoagulant*** prevents blood clotting.
- **Histamine** (**HISS**-tah-meen), which is released in response to allergens, causes the symptoms of an allergic response, including itching and increased mucus secretion.

The Subcutaneous Layer

The **subcutaneous layer** (sub-kyou-**TAY**-nee-us) is located just below the layers of the skin and connects the skin to the surface muscles.

- This layer is made up of loose connective tissue and **adipose tissue** (**AD**-ih-pohs). ***Adipose*** means fat.
- ***Cellulite*** is a term used to describe deposits of dimpled fat around the buttocks and thighs. This is not a scientific term, and medical authorities agree that cellulite is simply ordinary fatty tissue. *Note:* Do not confuse cellulite with *cellulitis*, which is discussed later in this chapter.
- **Lipocytes** (**LIP**-oh-sights), also known as ***fat cells***, are predominant in the subcutaneous layer, where they manufacture and store large quantities of fat (**lip/o** means fat, and **-cytes** means cells).

The Sebaceous Glands

Sebaceous glands (seh-**BAY**-shus) are located in the dermis layer of the skin and are closely associated with hair follicles (Figure 13.1).

- These glands secrete **sebum** (**SEE**-bum), which is an oily substance that is released through ducts opening into the hair follicles. From here, the sebum moves onto the surface and lubricates the skin.
- Because sebum is slightly acidic, it discourages the growth of bacteria on the skin.

The Sweat Glands

Sweat glands, also known as ***sudoriferous glands***, are tiny, coiled glands found on almost all body surfaces. There are two types, ***apocrine*** glands, which are found at hair follicles, and ***eccrine*** glands, which open onto the skin and are most numerous in the palms of the hands, the soles of the feet, and the forehead.

- **Pores** are the openings on the surface of the skin that act as the ducts of the sweat glands.
- **Perspiration**, commonly known as ***sweat***, is secreted by sweat glands and is made up of 99% water plus some salt and metabolic waste products.
- Perspiring is one way in which the body excretes excess water. Normally, up to one quart of liquid is perspired daily.
- As the perspiration evaporates into the air, it also cools the body. Body odor associated with perspiration comes from the interaction of sweat with bacteria on the skin's surface.
- **Hidrosis** (high-**DROH**-sis) is the production and excretion of perspiration.
- The milk-producing **mammary glands**, which are modified sweat glands, are sometimes classified with the integumentary system. However, they also are part of the reproductive system and are discussed in Chapter 16.

The Hair

Hair fibers are rod-like structures composed of tightly fused, dead protein cells filled with hard keratin. The darkness and color of the hair is determined by the amount and type of melanin produced by the melanocytes that surround the core of the hair shaft.

- **Hair follicles** (**FOL**-lick-kulz) are the sacs that hold the root of the hair fibers. The shape of the follicle determines whether the hair is straight or curly.
- Although hair is dead tissue, it appears to grow because the cells at the base of the follicle divide rapidly and push the old cells upward. As these cells are pushed upward, they harden and undergo pigmentation.
- The **arrector pili** (ah-**RECK**-tor **PYE**-lye) are tiny muscle fibers attached to the hair follicles that cause the hair to stand erect. In response to cold or fright, these muscles contract, causing raised areas of skin known as goose bumps. This action reduces heat loss through the skin.

The Nails

An **unguis** (**UNG**-gwis), which is commonly known as a fingernail or toenail, is the keratin plate that protects the dorsal surface of the last bone of each finger and toe (plural, *ungues*). Each nail consists of the following parts (Figure 13.3):

- The ***nail plate***, which is translucent, is closely molded to the surface of the underlying tissues. It is made up of hard, keratinized plates of epidermal cells.

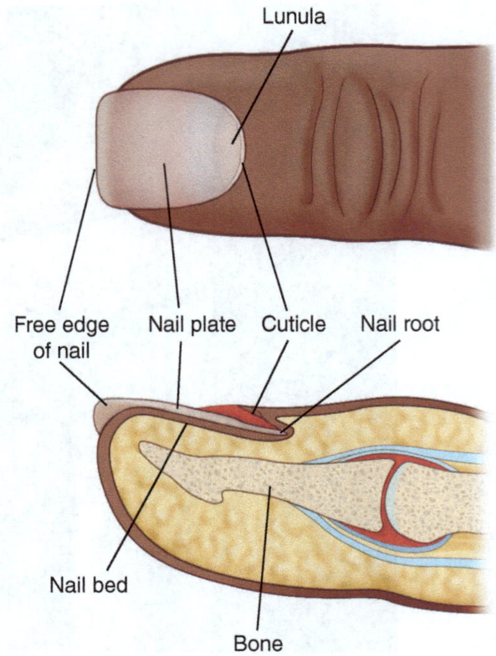

FIGURE 13.3 Structures of the fingernails and toenails.

- The ***nail bed*** is the skin underneath the nail plate, which joins the nail body to the underlying connective tissue and nourishes the nail. The blood vessels here give the nail its characteristic pink color.
- The ***free edge***, which is the portion of the nail not attached to the nail bed, extends beyond the tip of the finger or toe.
- The **lunula** (**LOO**-new-lah) is a pale half-moon-shaped region at every nail root, which is generally most easily seen in the thumbnail (plural, *lunulae*). This is the active area of the nail, where new keratin cells form (**lun** means moon, and **-ula** means little).
- The **cuticle** is a narrow band of epidermis attached to the surface of the nail just in front of the root, protecting the new keratin cells as they form.
- The **nail root** fastens the nail to the finger or toe by fitting into a groove in the skin.

MEDICAL SPECIALTIES RELATED TO THE INTEGUMENTARY SYSTEM

- A **dermatologist** (der-mah-**TOL**-oh-jist) is a physician who specializes in diagnosing and treating disorders of the skin (**dermat** means skin, and **-ologist** means specialist).

- A **plastic surgeon** is a physician who specializes in the surgical restoration and reconstruction of body structures. The term ***plastic*** is related to the suffix **-plasty**, meaning surgical repair.
- ***Cosmetic surgeons*** are plastic surgeons who perform operations such as breast augmentation, liposuction, and facelifts that are usually done for aesthetic rather than medical reasons.

PATHOLOGY OF THE INTEGUMENTARY SYSTEM

The Sebaceous Glands

- **Acne vulgaris** (**ACK**-nee vul-**GAY**-ris), commonly known as ***acne***, is a chronic inflammatory disease characterized by pustular eruptions of the skin caused by an overproduction of sebum around the hair shaft. Although often triggered by hormones in puberty and adolescence, it also occurs in adults. ***Vulgaris*** is a Latin term meaning common.
- A **comedo** (**KOM**-eh-doh) is a noninfected lesion formed by the buildup of sebum and keratin in a hair follicle often associated with acne vulgaris (plural, *comedones*). A comedo with an obstructed opening is called a ***whitehead*** (a closed comedo). A sebum plug that is exposed to air often oxidizes and becomes a ***blackhead*** (an open comedo).
- An **epidermoid cyst** (**ep**-ih-**DER**-moyd **SIST**), often referred to as a ***sebaceous cyst***, is a closed sac that is found just under the skin. These cysts contain yellow, fatty material and are usually found on the face, neck, or trunk.
- **Seborrheic dermatitis** (**seb**-oh-**REE**-ick **der**-mah-**TYE**-tis) is an inflammation sometimes resulting from overactivity of the sebaceous glands that causes scaling and itching of the upper layers of the skin or scalp (**seb/o** means sebum, and **-rrheic** means pertaining to flow or discharge). Extensive ***dandruff*** is a form of seborrheic dermatitis, as is the scalp rash in infants known as ***cradle cap***. In contrast, mild dandruff is usually caused by a yeast-like fungus on the scalp.
- A **seborrheic keratosis** (**seb**-oh-**REE**-ick **kerr**-ah-**TOH**-sis) is a benign skin growth that has a waxy or "pasted-on" look. These growths, which can vary in color from light tan to black, occur most commonly in adults over the age of 50.

The Sweat Glands

- **Anhidrosis** (**an**-high-**DROH**-sis), also known as ***hypohidrosis***, is the abnormal condition of lacking sweat in response to heat (**an-** means without, **hidr** means sweat, and **-osis** means abnormal condition). People with anhidrosis are at risk for heat stroke.
- **Diaphoresis** (**dye**-ah-foh-**REE**-sis) is profuse sweating (**dia-** means through or complete, **phor** means movement, and **-esis** means abnormal condition). This is a normal condition when brought on by heat or exertion but can also be the body's response to emotional or physical distress.
- **Heat rash**, also known as ***prickly heat***, is an intensely itchy rash caused by blockage of the sweat glands by bacteria and dead cells.
- **Heat stroke**, also known as ***sunstroke***, is a medical emergency caused by prolonged exposure to high temperatures. It is characterized by a core temperature of at least 104°F, altered mental state, and racing heart rate, and can cause organ swelling and death.
- **Hyperhidrosis** (**high**-per-high-**DROH**-sis) is a condition of excessive sweating in one area or over the whole body (**hyper-** means excessive, **hidr** means sweat, and **-osis** means abnormal condition).
- **Sleep hyperhidrosis**, commonly known as ***night sweats***, is the occurrence of hyperhidrosis during sleep. There are many potential causes of this condition including menopause, certain medications, and some infectious diseases.

The Hair

- **Folliculitis** (foh-**lick**-you-**LYE**-tis) is an inflammation of the hair follicles (**follicul** means the hair follicle, and **-itis** means inflammation). This condition is especially common on arms, legs, and in the beard area of men. One of the causes of folliculitis is a bacterium found in poorly chlorinated hot tubs or whirlpools. This leads to a condition called ***hot tub folliculitis***.
- **Trichomycosis axillaris** (**try**-koh-my-**KOH**-sis **ak**-sih-**LAR**-is) is a superficial bacterial infection of the hair shafts in areas with extensive sweat glands, such as the armpits (**trich/o** means hair, **myc** means fungus, and **-osis** means abnormal condition). *Axillaris* is Latin for axillary (**axill** means armpit, and **-ary** means pertaining to).

Excessive Hairiness

- **Hirsutism** (**HER-soot**-izm) is the presence of excessive body and facial hair in women, usually occurring in a male pattern (**hirsut** means hairy, and **-ism** means condition). This condition can be hereditary or caused by a hormonal imbalance.

Abnormal Hair Loss

- **Alopecia** (**al**-oh-**PEE**-shee-ah), also known as ***baldness***, is the partial or complete loss of hair, most commonly on the scalp (**alopec** means baldness, and **-ia** means abnormal condition).
- **Alopecia areata** (ah-ree-**AY**-tuh) is an autoimmune disorder that attacks the hair follicles, causing well-defined bald areas on the scalp or elsewhere on the body (Figure 13.4). This condition often begins in childhood. ***Areata*** means occurring in patches.
- **Alopecia totalis** (toh-**TAL**-is) (AT) is an uncommon condition characterized by the loss of all the hair on the scalp.
- **Alopecia universalis** (**yoo**-nih-vers-**AHL**-is) (AU) is the total loss of hair on all parts of the body. ***Universalis*** means universal.

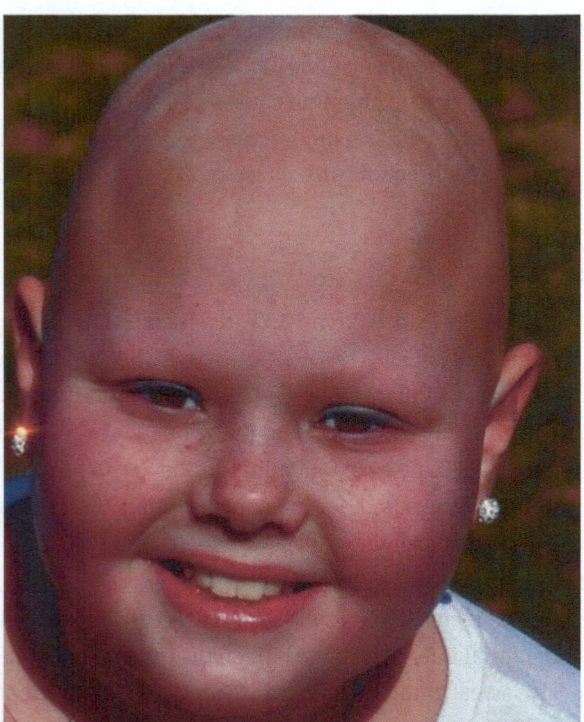

Used with permission from the Children's Alopecia Project

FIGURE 13.4 Alopecia areata is an autoimmune disorder that often begins in childhood.

- **Androgenic alopecia** (an-**DROH**-jen-ik **al**-oh-**PEE**-shee-ah) is the most common type of hair loss. Androgenic means referring to ***androgens***, the hormones involved in the development and maintenance of masculine characteristics (see Chapter 15).
  - In men it is called ***male pattern baldness***, with the hairline receding from the front to the back until only a horseshoe-shaped area of hair remains in the back and at the temples.
  - When it occurs in women it is called ***female pattern baldness***, and is characterized by the hair thinning in the front and on the sides of the scalp and sometimes on the crown. This condition rarely leads to total hair loss.

The Nails

- **Clubbing** is the abnormal curving of the nails that is often accompanied by enlargement of the fingertips. This condition can be hereditary but is usually caused by changes associated with oxygen deficiencies related to coronary or pulmonary diseases such as lung cancer.
- **Koilonychia** (**koy**-loh-**NICK**-ee-ah), also known as ***spoon nail***, is a malformation of the nails in which the outer surface is concave or scooped out like the bowl of a spoon (**koil** means hollow or concave, **onych** means fingernail or toenail, and **-ia** means abnormal condition). This condition is often an indication of iron-deficiency anemia (see Chapter 5).
- **Onychia** (oh-**NICK**-ee-ah), also known as ***onychitis***, is an inflammation of the bed of the nail that often results in the loss of the nail (**onych** means fingernail or toenail, and **-ia** means abnormal condition).
- **Onychocryptosis** (**on**-ih-koh-krip-**TOH**-sis) is commonly known as an ***ingrown toenail*** (**onych/o** means fingernail or toenail, **crypt** means hidden, and **-osis** means abnormal condition). The edges of a toenail, usually on the big toe, curve inward and cut into the skin. The affected area is prone to inflammation or infection.
- **Onychomycosis** (**on**-ih-koh-my-**KOH**-sis) is a fungal infection of the nail (**onych/o** means fingernail or toenail, **myc** means fungus, and **-osis** means abnormal condition). Depending on the type of fungus involved, this condition can cause the nails to turn white, yellow, green, or black and to become thick or brittle.

- **Onycholysis** (**on**-ih-koh-**LYE**-sis) is the separation of the nail plate from the nail bed (**onych/o** means fingernail or toenail, and **-lysis** means separation). It is usually painless, and can be caused by a localized allergic reaction, fungal infection, or psoriasis.
- **Paronychia** (**par**-oh-**NICK**-ee-ah) is an acute or chronic infection of the skin fold around a nail (**par-** means near, **onych** means fingernail or toenail, and **-ia** means abnormal condition).

Skin Pigmentation

- **Acanthosis nigricans** (ak-an-**THO**-sis **NIG**-rih-kans) is a condition where one or more areas of the skin develop dark, velvety areas of discoloration, usually in skin folds. This can be a sign of a disease such as cancer or type 2 diabetes or a reaction to a medication.
- **Age spots**, also known as ***solar lentigines*** (singular, *lentigo*) or ***liver spots***, are discolorations caused by sun exposure. Although harmless, these spots sometimes resemble skin cancer growths.
- **Albinism** (**AL**-bih-**niz**-um) is a genetic condition characterized by a deficiency or the absence of pigment in the skin, hair, and irises of the eyes (**albin** means white, and **-ism** means condition). This condition is the result of a missing enzyme that is necessary for the production of melanin. A person with this condition is known as an ***albino***.
- **Melasma** (muh-**LAZ**-mah), also known as ***chloasma*** or the ***mask of pregnancy***, is a pigmentation disorder characterized by brownish spots on the face. This can occur during pregnancy, especially among women with dark hair and fair skin, and usually disappears after delivery.
- **Vitiligo** (**vit**-ih-**LYE**-goh) is a skin condition resulting from the destruction of the melanocytes due to unknown causes. Vitiligo causes irregular patches of white skin, a process known as ***depigmentation***. Hair growing in an affected area may also turn white.

Bleeding into the Skin

- A **contusion** (kon-**TOO**-zhun) is an injury to underlying tissues without breaking the skin and is characterized by discoloration and pain (**contus** means bruise, and **-ion** means condition). This discoloration is caused by an accumulation of blood within the skin.
- An **ecchymosis** (**eck**-ih-**MOH**-sis), commonly known as a ***bruise***, is a large, irregular area of purplish discoloration due to bleeding under the skin (**ecchym** means pouring out of juice, and **-osis** means abnormal condition) (Figure 13.5). The plural form is *ecchymoses*.
- **Purpura** (**PUR**-pew-rah) is the appearance of multiple purple discolorations on the skin caused by bleeding underneath the skin (**purpur** means purple, and **-a** is a noun ending). These areas of discoloration are smaller than an ecchymosis and larger than petechiae.
- **Petechiae** (peh-**TEE**-kee-eye) are very small, pinpoint hemorrhages that are less than 2 mm in diameter (singular, *petechia*). These hemorrhages sometimes result from high fevers.
- A **hematoma** (hee-mah-**TOH**-mah), which is usually caused by an injury, is a swelling of clotted blood trapped in the tissues (**hemat** means blood, and **-oma** means tumor). The body eventually reabsorbs this blood. A hematoma is often named for the area where it occurs. For example, a ***subungual hematoma*** is blood trapped under a finger or toenail.

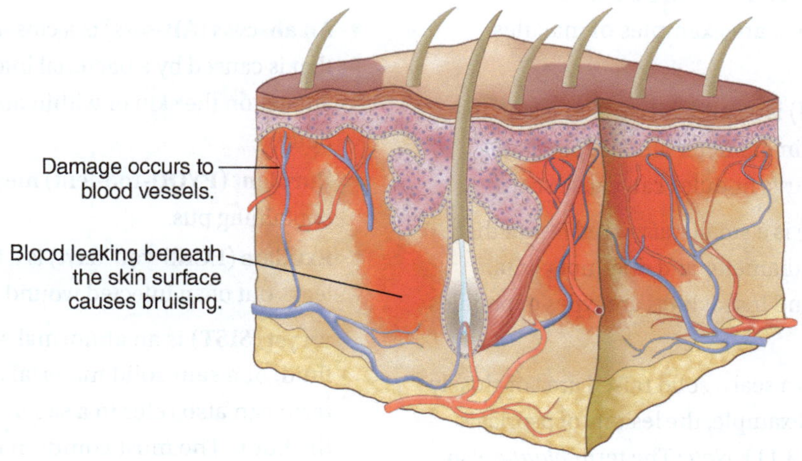

FIGURE 13.5 A cross-section of the skin showing the bleeding under the skin causing ecchymosis.

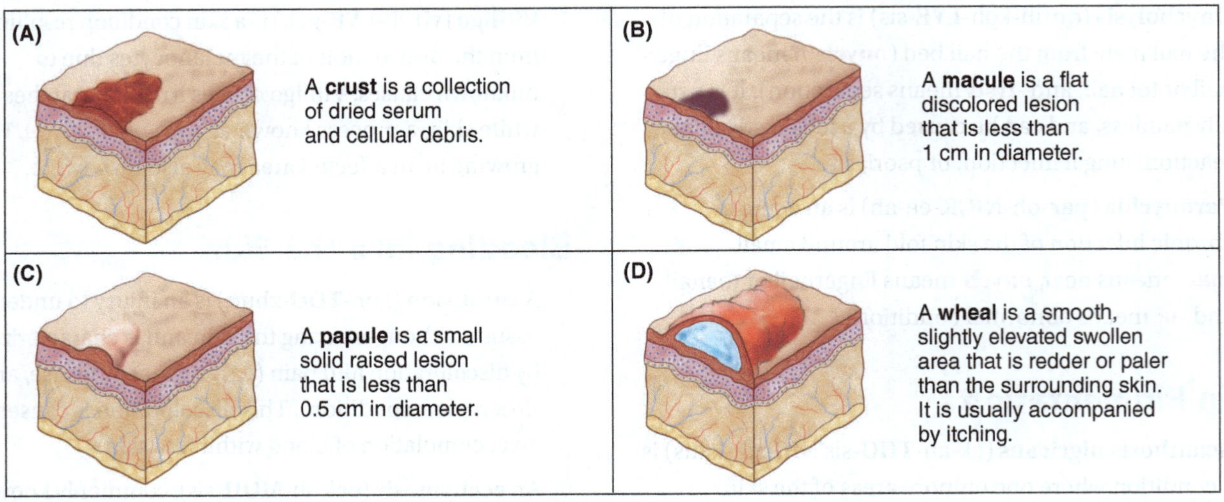

FIGURE 13.6 Surface lesions of the skin. (A) Crust. (B) Macule. (C) Papule. (D) Wheal.

Surface Lesions

A **lesion** (LEE-zhun) is a pathologic change of the tissues due to disease or injury. Skin lesions are described by their appearance, location, color, and size as measured in centimeters (cm).

- A **crust**, also known as ***scab***, is a collection of hard, dried serum and blood that forms as a barrier over a partial-thickness wound (Figure 13.6A).
- **Eschar** (**ES**-kar) is dead crust-like tissue found in a full-thickness wound. It is usually brown or black, and is often a natural stage of wound healing.
- **Erosion** (eh-**ROH**-zhun) is the wearing away of a surface, such as the epidermis of the skin or the outer layer of a mucous membrane. This term can also describe the progressive loss of dental enamel.
- A **macule** (**MACK**-youl), also known as a ***macula***, is a discolored flat spot that is less than 1 cm in diameter. Freckles, or flat moles, are examples of macules (Figure 13.6B).
- A **nodule** (**NOD**-youl) is a solid, raised skin lesion that is *larger than* 0.5 cm in diameter and deeper than a papule. In acne vulgaris, nodules can cause scarring.
- A **papule** (**PAP**-youl) is a small, raised red lesion that is *less than* 0.5 cm in diameter and does not contain pus. Small pimples and insect bites are types of papules (Figure 13.6C).
- A **plaque** (**PLACK**) is a scaly, solid raised area of closely spaced papules. For example, the lesions of psoriasis are plaques (Figure 13.11). *Note:* The term *plaque* also means a fatty buildup in the arteries (see Chapter 5) and a soft substance that forms on the teeth (see Chapter 9).
- **Scales** are flakes or dry patches made up of excess dead epidermal cells. Some shedding of these scales is normal; however, excessive shedding is associated with skin disorders such as psoriasis.
- **Verrucae** (veh-**ROO**-kee), also known as ***warts***, are small, hard skin lesions caused by the *human papillomavirus* (singular, *verruca*). ***Plantar warts*** are verrucae that develop on the sole of the foot. See Chapter 15 for more information on the *human papillomavirus*.
- A **wheal** (**WHEEL**), also known as a ***welt***, is a small bump that itches. Wheals can appear as *urticaria*, or hives, as a symptom of an allergic reaction (Figure 13.6D).

Fluid-Filled Lesions

- An **abscess** (**AB**-sess) is a closed pocket containing pus that is caused by a bacterial infection. An abscess can appear on the skin or within other structures of the body.
- **Purulent** (**PYOU**-roo-lent) means producing or containing pus.
- **Exudate** (**ECKS**-you-dayt) is a fluid, such as pus, that leaks out of an infected wound.
- A **cyst** (**SIST**) is an abnormal sac containing gas, fluid, or a semisolid material (Figure 13.7A). The term can also refer to a sac or vesicle elsewhere in the body. The most common type of skin cyst is a sebaceous cyst.

- A **pustule** (**PUS**-tyoul), also known as a ***pimple***, is a small, circumscribed lesion containing pus (Figure 13.7B). ***Circumscribed*** means contained within a limited area. Pustules can be caused by acne vulgaris, impetigo, or other skin infections.
- A **vesicle** (**VES**-ih-kul) is a small blister, *less than* 0.5 cm in diameter, containing watery fluid (Figure 13.7C). For example, the rash of poison ivy consists of vesicles (Figure 13.10).
- A **bulla** (**BULL**-ah) is a large blister that is usually *more than* 0.5 cm in diameter (plural, *bullae*) (Figure 13.7D).

Lesions Through the Skin

- An **abrasion** (ah-**BRAY**-zhun) is an injury in which superficial layers of skin are scraped or rubbed away.
- A **fissure** (**FISH**-ur) is a groove or crack-like break in the skin. Fissures are, for example, the breaks in the skin between the toes caused by tinea pedis, or athlete's foot (Figure 13.8A). The term *fissure* also describes folds in the contours of the brain.
- A **laceration** (**lass**-er-**AY**-shun) is a torn or jagged wound or an accidental cut wound.
- A **pressure ulcer**, also known as a ***decubitus ulcer*** or ***bedsore***, is an open ulcerated wound that is caused by prolonged pressure on an area of skin over a bony prominence, such as heels, elbows, hips, and spine. Without proper care, these sores quickly become seriously infected and can result in tissue death. A pressure ulcer often starts as a ***deep tissue injury***, or damage to the tissues under intact skin, which looks like an area of redness or bruising that does not change color when touched.
- A **needlestick injury** is an accidental puncture wound caused by a used hypodermic needle, potentially transmitting an infection. A ***puncture wound*** is an injury caused by a pointed object piercing the skin.
- An **ulcer** (**UL**-ser) is an open lesion of the skin or mucous membrane resulting in tissue loss around the edges (Figure 13.8B). *Note:* Ulcers also occur inside the body. Those associated with the digestive system are discussed in Chapter 9.

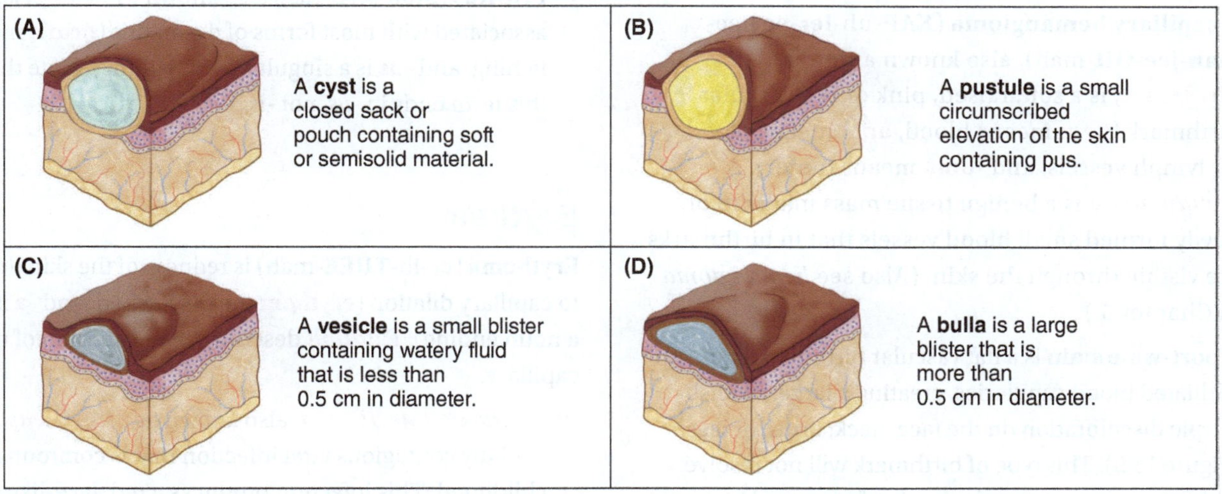

FIGURE 13.7 Fluid-filled lesions in the skin. (A) Cyst. (B) Pustule. (C) Vesicle. (D) Bulla.

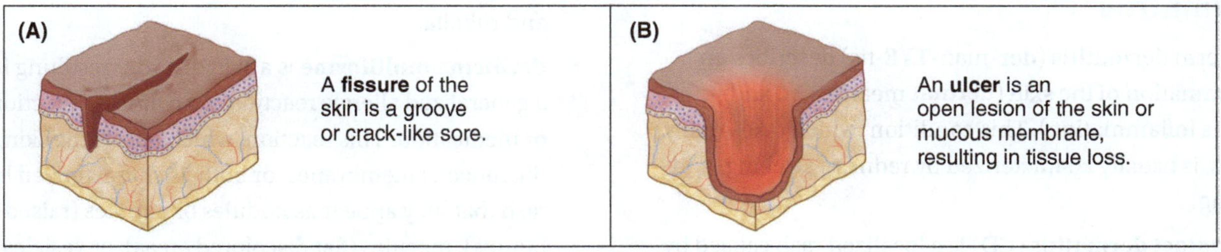

FIGURE 13.8 Lesions extending through the skin. (A) Fissure. (B) Ulcer.

Birthmarks

A birthmark is a mole or blemish on the skin present at birth or shortly thereafter. Some birthmarks fade as a child gets older.

- **Pigmented birthmarks** include **nevi**, also known as ***moles***, as well as café-au-lait spots and other irregularities in skin color.
- A ***slate grey nevus*** is a benign blue-grey birthmark commonly found on the back, buttocks, or shoulders of Asian, African American, Polynesian, and Native American babies. It is caused by melanocytes that did not migrate to the surface of the skin before birth, and can resemble a bruise. It usually fades by puberty, and is also known as a ***Mongolian spot***.
- **Vascular birthmarks** are caused by blood vessels close to the skin's surface. These are the most common type of birthmarks and include macular stains, hemangiomas, and port-wine stains.
- **Macular stains** are flat, red irregularly shaped birthmarks that are also called ***salmon patches*** for their shape, or ***angel kisses*** depending on their location.
- A **capillary hemangioma** (**KAP**-uh-**ler**-ee hee-**man**-jee-**OH**-mah), also known as a ***strawberry birthmark***, is a soft, raised, pink or red vascular birthmark (**hem** means blood, **angi** means blood or lymph vessels, and **-oma** means tumor). A ***hemangioma*** is a benign tissue mass made up of newly formed small blood vessels that in birthmarks are visible through the skin. (Also see *hemangioma* in Chapter 5.)
- A **port-wine stain** is a flat vascular birthmark made up of dilated blood capillaries, creating a large, reddish-purple discoloration on the face, neck, arms, or legs (Figure 13.9). This type of birthmark will not resolve without treatment. See the section "Laser and Light Source Treatments of Skin Conditions."

Dermatitis

The term **dermatitis** (**der**-mah-**TYE**-tis) describes an inflammation of the skin (**dermat** means skin, and **-itis** means inflammation). This condition, which takes many forms, is usually characterized by redness, swelling, and itching.

- **Contact dermatitis** (CD) is a localized rash caused by repeated contact with an irritant, such as harsh cleaning chemicals, or an allergen, such as latex gloves or poison ivy (Figure 13.10). Contact dermatitis can cause localized redness, blisters, swelling, and itching.
- **Intertrigo** (**in**-ter-**TRYE**-goh) is dermatitis caused by the friction of skin rubbing together in skin folds, such as those in the armpits, groin, and under the breasts. The damage makes the skin more susceptible to fungal or bacterial infections.
- **Eczema** (**ECK**-zeh-mah), also known as ***atopic dermatitis***, is a form of persistent or recurring dermatitis usually characterized by redness, itching, and dryness, with possible blistering, cracking, oozing, or bleeding. This chronic condition, most often seen in infants and children, appears to be the result of a malfunction of the body's immune system.
- **Exfoliative dermatitis** (ecks-**FOH**-lee-**ay**-tiv **der**-mah-**TYE**-tis) is a condition in which there is widespread scaling of the skin. It is often accompanied by pruritus, erythroderma (redness), and hair loss. It may occur in severe cases of many common skin conditions, including eczema, psoriasis, and allergic reactions.
- **Pruritus** (proo-**RYE**-tus), also known as ***itching***, is associated with most forms of dermatitis (**prurit** means itching, and **-us** is a singular noun ending). Note that this term ends in *-us*, not *-is*.

Erythema

Erythema (**er**-ih-**THEE**-mah) is redness of the skin due to capillary dilation (**erythem** means flushed, and **-a** is a noun ending). ***Dilation*** describes the expansion of the capillary.

- ***Erythema infectiosum***, also known as ***fifth disease***, is a mildly contagious viral infection that is common in childhood. This infection produces a red, lace-like rash on the child's face that looks as if the child has been slapped. It is called fifth disease for its place on a list of six common childhood diseases that can cause an exanthem (widespread rash). Others include measles and rubella.
- **Erythema multiforme** is a skin disorder resulting from a generalized allergic reaction to an illness, infection, or medication. This reaction, which affects the skin, the mucous membranes, or both, is characterized by a rash that may appear as nodules or papules (raised red bumps), macules (flat discolored areas), or vesicles or bullae (blisters).

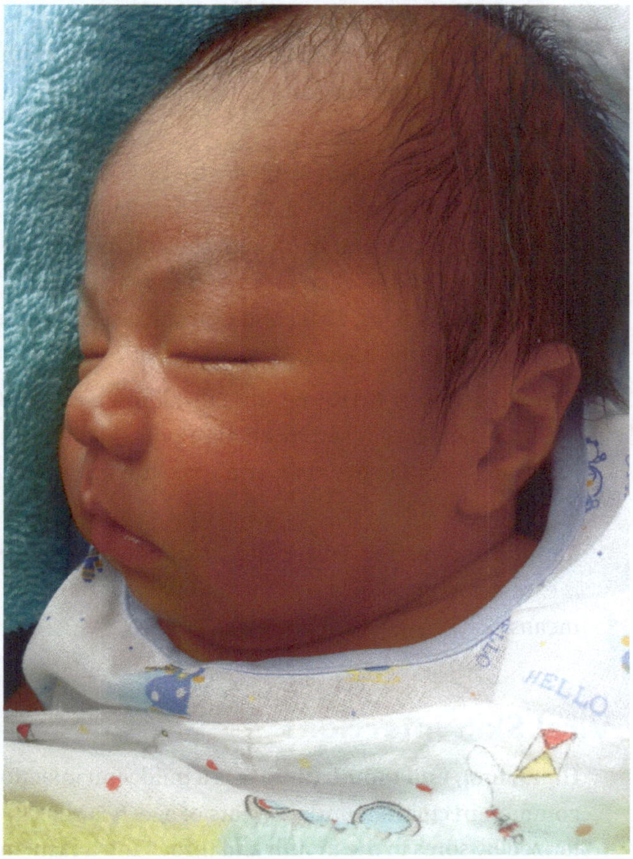

jaojormami/Shutterstock.com

FIGURE 13.9 A port-wine stain is a flat vascular birthmark made up of dilated blood capillaries.

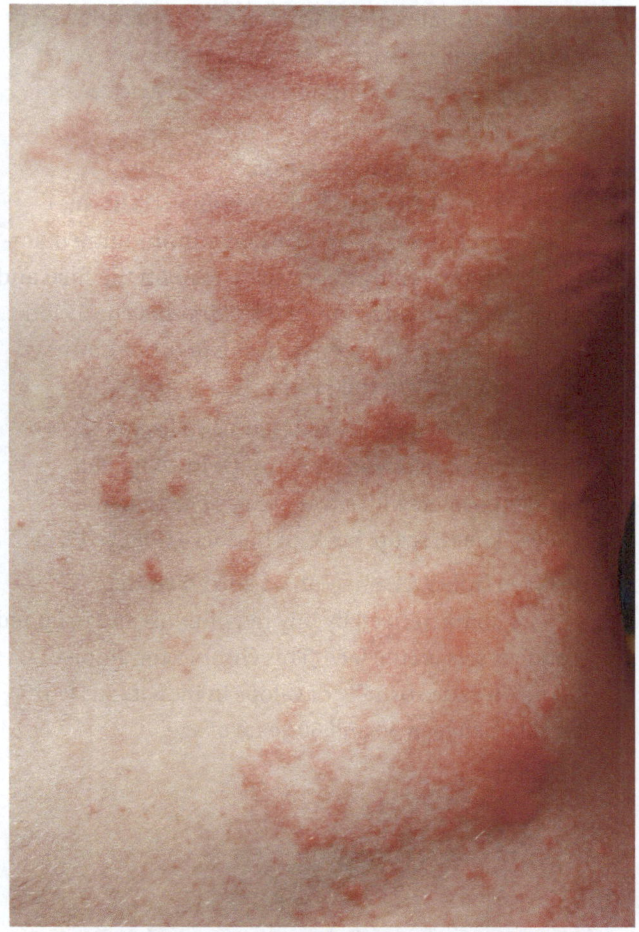

Joy Brown/Shutterstock.com

FIGURE 13.10 Contact dermatitis on a young man's torso caused by poison ivy.

- ***Erythema pernio***, also known as ***chilblains***, is a purple-red inflammation that occurs when the small blood vessels below the skin are damaged, usually due to exposure to cold and damp weather. When warmth restores full circulation, the affected areas begin to itch; however, they usually heal without treatment.
- ***Sunburn*** is a form of erythema in which skin cells are damaged by exposure to the ultraviolet rays in sunlight. This damage increases the chances of later developing skin cancer.
- **Erythroderma** (eh-**rith**-roh-**DER**-mah) is abnormal redness of the entire skin surface (**erythr/o** means red, and **-derma** means skin).
- **Exanthem** (eck-**ZAN**-thum) refers to a widespread rash, usually in children. A ***rash*** is a breaking out, or eruption, that changes the color or texture of the skin.

General Skin Conditions

- **Dermatosis** (**der**-mah-**TOH**-sis) is a general term used to denote skin lesions or eruptions of any type that are *not* associated with inflammation (**dermat** means skin, and **-osis** means abnormal condition).
- **Ichthyosis** (**ick**-thee-**OH**-sis) is a group of disorders characterized by dry, thickened, and scaly skin (**ichthy** means dry or scaly, and **-osis** means abnormal condition). These conditions are caused either by the slowing of the skin's natural shedding process or by a rapid increase in the production of the skin's cells.
- **Lipedema** (lip-eh-**DEE**-mah), also known as ***painful fat syndrome***, is a chronic abnormal condition that is characterized by the accumulation of fat and fluid in the tissues just under the skin of the hips and legs (**lip** means fat, and **-edema** means swelling). This

condition usually affects women and even with weight loss this localized excess fat does not go away. *Note:* Don't confuse this condition with *lymphedema*, discussed in Chapter 7.

- **Systemic lupus erythematosus** (sis-**TEH**-mik **LOO**-pus er-ih-**thee**-mah-**TOH**-sus) (SLE), also known as ***lupus***, is an autoimmune disorder characterized by a red, scaly rash on the face and upper trunk. In addition to the skin, this condition also attacks the connective tissue in other body systems, especially in the joints.
- **Psoriasis** (soh-**RYE**-uh-sis) (Ps) is a common skin disorder characterized by flare-ups in which red papules covered with silvery scales occur on the elbows, knees, scalp, back, or buttocks (Figure 13.11).
- **Rosacea** (roh-**ZAY**-shee-ah), also known as ***adult acne***, is characterized by tiny red pimples and enlarged blood vessels on the face. This chronic condition of unknown cause usually develops in individuals with fair skin between 30 and 60 years of age.

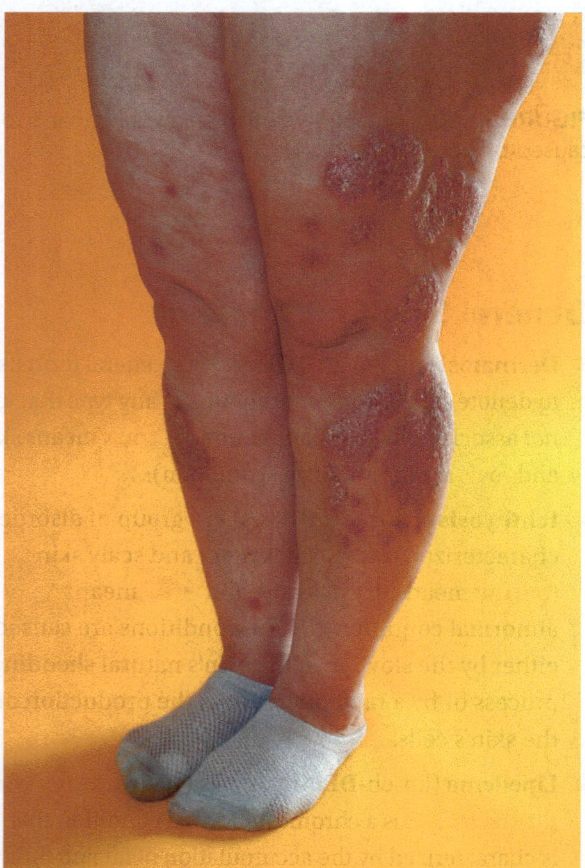

Egor_Kulinich/Shutterstock.com

FIGURE 13.11 Psoriasis is characterized by red papules covered with silvery scales.

- **Rhinophyma** (**rye**-noh-**FIGH**-muh), also known as ***bulbous nose***, usually occurs in older men (**rhin/o** means nose, and **-phyma** means growth). This condition is characterized by hyperplasia (overgrowth) of the tissues of the nose and is associated with advanced rosacea.
- **Scleroderma** (**sklehr**-oh-**DER**-mah) (SCD) is an autoimmune disorder in which the connective tissues become thickened and hardened, causing the skin to become hard and swollen (**scler/o** means hard, and **-derma** means skin). This condition can also affect the joints and internal organs.
- **Urticaria** (**ur**-tih-**KARE**-ee-ah), also known as ***hives***, are itchy wheals caused by an allergic reaction (**urtic** means rash, and **-aria** means connected with).
- **Xeroderma** (zee-roh-**DER**-mah), also known as ***xerosis***, is excessively dry skin (**xer/o** means dry, and **-derma** means skin).

Viral Skin Infections

- **Hand, foot, and mouth disease** is a mild viral infection common in children under 5 years of age. It is characterized by sores in the mouth and throat and a rash on the hands and feet.
- **Molluscum contagiosum** (moh-**LUS**-kum kon-**tay**-gee-**OH**-sum) is a viral infection that causes small, raised lesions, called ***mollusca***. Mollusca are white, pink, or flesh colored with a dimpled center, and may occur anywhere on the body.

Bacterial Skin Infections

- **Cellulitis** (**sell**-you-**LYE**-tis) is an acute, rapidly spreading bacterial infection within the connective tissues that is characterized by malaise, swelling, warmth, and red streaks. *Note:* Do not confuse cellulitis with *cellulite*, which is discussed earlier in this chapter.
- **Furuncles** (**FYOU**-rung-kulz), also known as ***boils***, are large, tender, swollen areas caused by a staphylococcal infection around hair follicles or sebaceous glands.
- A **carbuncle** (**KAR**-bung-kul) is a cluster of connected furuncles.
- **Gangrene** (**GANG**-green), which is death of tissue, is most commonly caused by a loss of circulation to the affected tissues. The tissue death is followed by

bacterial invasion that causes putrefaction, and if this infection enters the bloodstream, it can be fatal. *Putrefaction* is decay that produces foul-smelling odors.

- **Impetigo** (**im**-peh-**TYE**-goh) is a highly contagious bacterial skin infection that commonly occurs in children. This condition is characterized by isolated pustules that become crusted and rupture.
- **Necrotizing fasciitis** (**NECK**-roh-**tie**-zing **fas**-ee-**EYE**-tis) (NF) is a rare, severe infection caused by group A strep bacteria, which are also known as *flesh-eating bacteria*. These bacteria normally live harmlessly on the skin; however, if they enter the body through a skin wound, this serious, sometimes fatal, infection can result.
- **Pyoderma** (**pye**-oh-**DER**-mah) is any acute, inflammatory, pus-forming bacterial skin infection such as impetigo (**py/o** means pus, and **-derma** means skin).

Fungal Skin Infections

- **Mycosis** (my-**KOH**-sis) describes any abnormal condition or disease caused by a fungus (**myc** means fungus, and **-osis** means abnormal condition or disease).

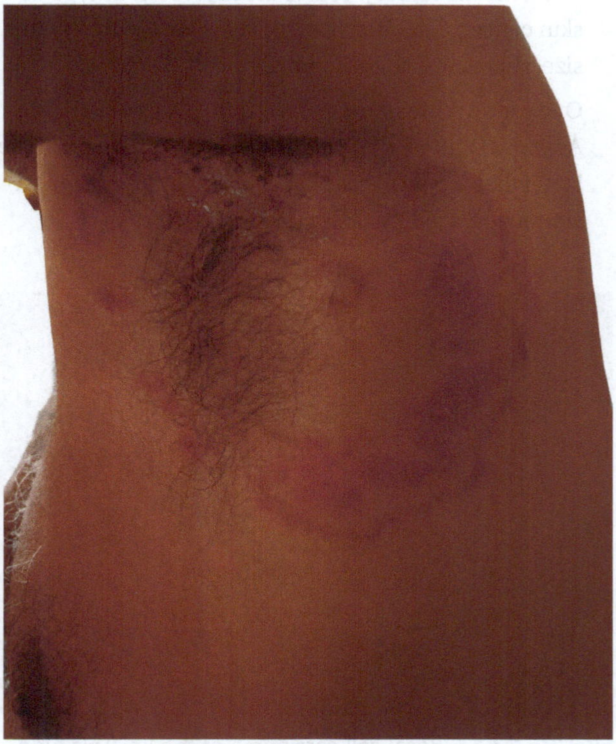
RandomizeTH/Shutterstock.com

FIGURE 13.12 Tinea is a fungal infection also known as ringworm.

- **Tinea** (**TIN**-ee-ah) is a fungal infection that can grow on the skin, hair, or nails. This condition is also known as *ringworm*, not because a worm is involved, but because as the fungus grows on the skin, it spreads out in a worm-like circle (Figure 13.12). Tinea does not create this pattern when it grows on the nails.
- *Tinea capitis* is found on the scalps of children. *Capitis* means head.
- *Tinea corporis* is a fungal infection of the skin on the body. *Corporis* means body.
- *Tinea cruris*, also known as *jock itch*, is found in the genital area.
- *Tinea pedis*, also known as *athlete's foot*, is most commonly found between the toes. *Pedis* means feet.
- *Tinea versicolor*, also known as *pityriasis versicolor*, is a fungal infection that causes painless, discolored areas on the skin. *Versicolor* means a variety of color.

Parasitic Skin Infestations

An **infestation** is the dwelling of microscopic parasites on external surface tissue. Some parasites live temporarily on the skin. Others lay eggs and reproduce there.

- **Pediculosis** (pee-**dick**-you-**LOH**-sis) is an infestation with *lice* (**pedicul** means lice, and **-osis** means abnormal condition). In order to get rid of the infestation, the lice eggs, which are known as *nits*, must be destroyed. There are three types of lice, each attracted to a specific part of the body:
  - *Pediculosis capitis* is an infestation with head lice.
  - *Pediculosis corporis* is an infestation with body lice.
  - *Pediculosis pubis* is an infestation with lice in the pubic hair and pubic region.
- **Scabies** (**SKAY**-beez) is a skin infection caused by an infestation of *itch mites*. These tiny mites cause small, itchy bumps and blisters by burrowing into the top layer of human skin to lay their eggs. Medications applied to the skin kill the mites; however, itching may persist for several weeks.

Skin Growths

- A **callus** (**KAL**-us) is a thickening of part of the skin on the hands or feet caused by repeated rubbing. Compare with *callus* in Chapter 3. A *clavus*, or *corn*, is a callus in the keratin layer of the skin covering the joints of the toes, usually caused by ill-fitting shoes.

- A **cicatrix** (sick-**AY**-tricks) is a normal scar resulting from the healing of a wound (plural, *cicatrices*).
- **Granulation tissue** is the tissue that normally forms during the healing of a wound. This tissue eventually forms the scar.
- A **keloid** (**KEE**-loid) is an abnormally raised or thickened scar that expands beyond the boundaries of the original incision (**kel** means growth or tumor, and **-oid** means resembling). A tendency to form keloids is often inherited and is more common among people with dark-pigmented skin.
- A **keratosis** (**kerr**-ah-**TOH**-sis) is any skin growth, such as a wart or a callus, in which there is overgrowth and thickening of the skin (**kerat** means hard or horny, and **-osis** means abnormal condition) (plural, *keratoses*). Patches of keratosis in the mouth are known as *leukoplakia*.
  Note: **kerat/o** also refers to the cornea of the eye (see Chapter 11).
- A **lipoma** (lih-**POH**-mah) is a benign, slow-growing fatty tumor located between the skin and the muscle layer (**lip** means fatty, and **-oma** means tumor). This fatty tumor is usually harmless, and treatment is rarely necessary unless the tumor is in a bothersome location, is painful, or is growing rapidly.
- **Nevus** (**NEE**-vus), also known as a *mole*, is a small, dark skin growth that develops from melanocytes in the skin (plural, *nevi*). Normally, these growths are benign.
- In contrast, **dysplastic nevi** (dis-**PLAS**-tick **NEE**-vye) are atypical moles that can develop into skin cancer.
- A **papilloma** (**pap**-ih-**LOH**-mah) is a benign, superficial, wart-like growth on the epithelial tissue or elsewhere in the body, such as in the bladder (**papill** means resembling a nipple, and **-oma** means tumor).
- **Polyp** (**POL**-up) is a general term used most commonly to describe a mushroom-like growth from the surface of a mucous membrane, such as a polyp in the nose. These growths have many causes and are not necessarily malignant.
- **Skin tags**, also known as *achrocordon*, are small, flesh-colored or light-brown polyps that hang from the body by fine stalks. Skin tags are benign and usually develop in skin folds of the neck, groin, or armpits.

Skin Cancer

Skin cancer is a malignant growth on the skin which can have many causes, including repeated severe sunburns or long-term exposure to the sun. Skin cancer is becoming very common, affecting about one in five Americans in his or her lifetime. There are three main types of skin cancer: basal cell carcinoma, squamous cell carcinoma, and melanoma.

- An **actinic keratosis** (ack-**TIN**-ick **kerr**-ah-**TOH**-sis) (AK), also called a *solar keratosis*, is a precancerous skin growth that occurs on sun-damaged skin. It often looks like a red, tan, or pink scaly patch and feels like sandpaper. *Precancerous* describes a growth that is not yet malignant; however, if not treated, it is likely to become malignant.
- A **basal cell carcinoma** (**BAYS**-al) (BCC) is a malignant tumor of the basal cell layer of the epidermis. This is the most common and least harmful type of skin cancer because it is slow growing and rarely spreads to other parts of the body. The lesions, which occur mainly on the face or neck and tend to bleed easily, are usually pink and smooth and are raised with a depression in the center (Figure 13.13).
- **Squamous cell carcinoma** (**SKWAY**-mus) (SCC) originates as a malignant tumor of the scaly squamous cells of the epithelium; however, it can quickly spread to other body systems. These cancers begin as skin lesions that appear to be sores that will not heal or that have a crusted look (Figure 13.14).
- **Malignant melanoma** (mel-ah-**NOH**-mah) (MM), also known as *melanoma*, is a type of skin cancer that occurs in the melanocytes (**melan** means black, and **-oma** means tumor). This is the most serious type of skin cancer, and often the first signs are changes in the size, shape, or color of a mole.

  One way to remember this is by thinking of A-B-C-D-E: *Asymmetry*, *Border irregularity*, *Color variation*, *Diameter* larger than a pencil eraser, and *Evolving* by changing in size, shape, shade, or color (Figure 13.15).

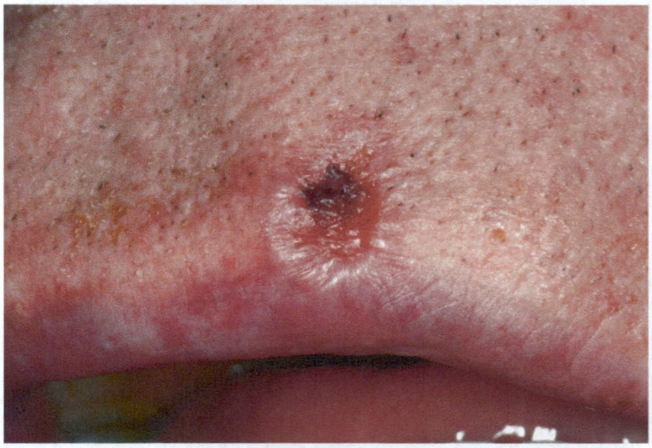
Dr. P. Marazzi/Science Source

FIGURE 13.13 Basal cell carcinoma of the lip. This type of malignant tumor occurs in the basal cell layer of the epidermis.

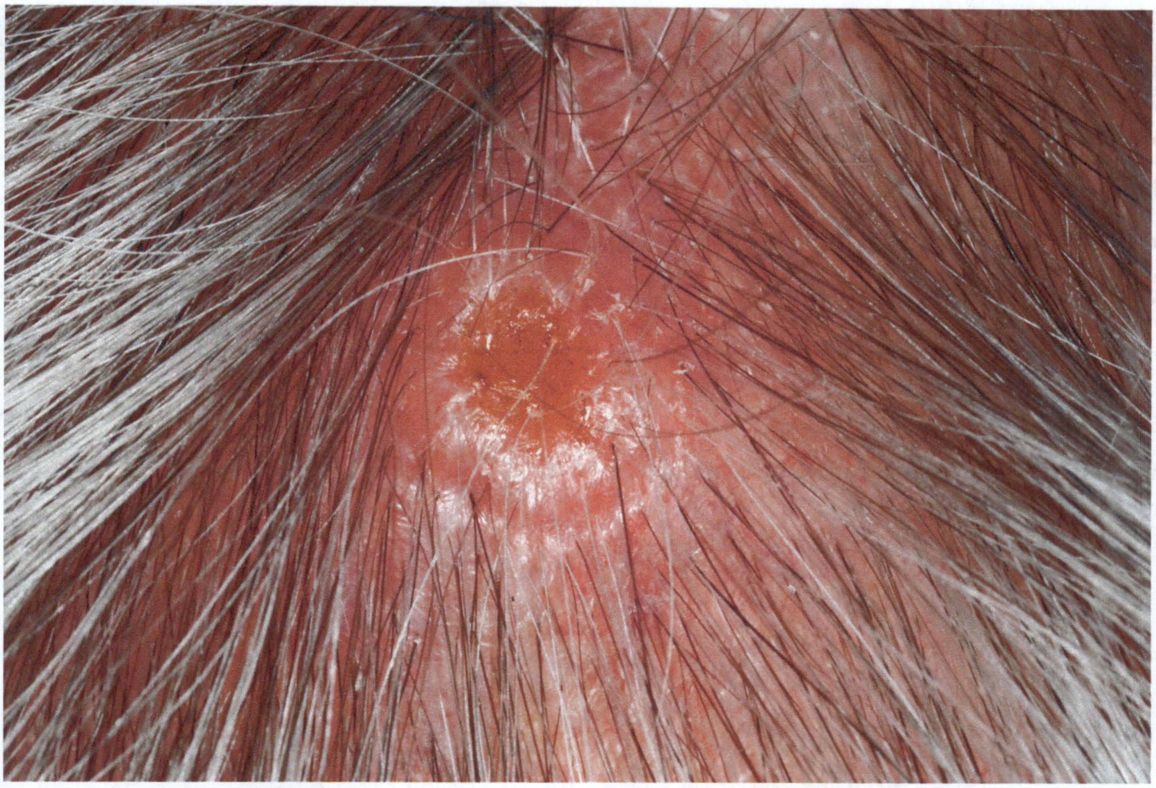

Dr. P. Marazzi/Science Source

FIGURE 13.14 Squamous cell carcinoma of the scalp.

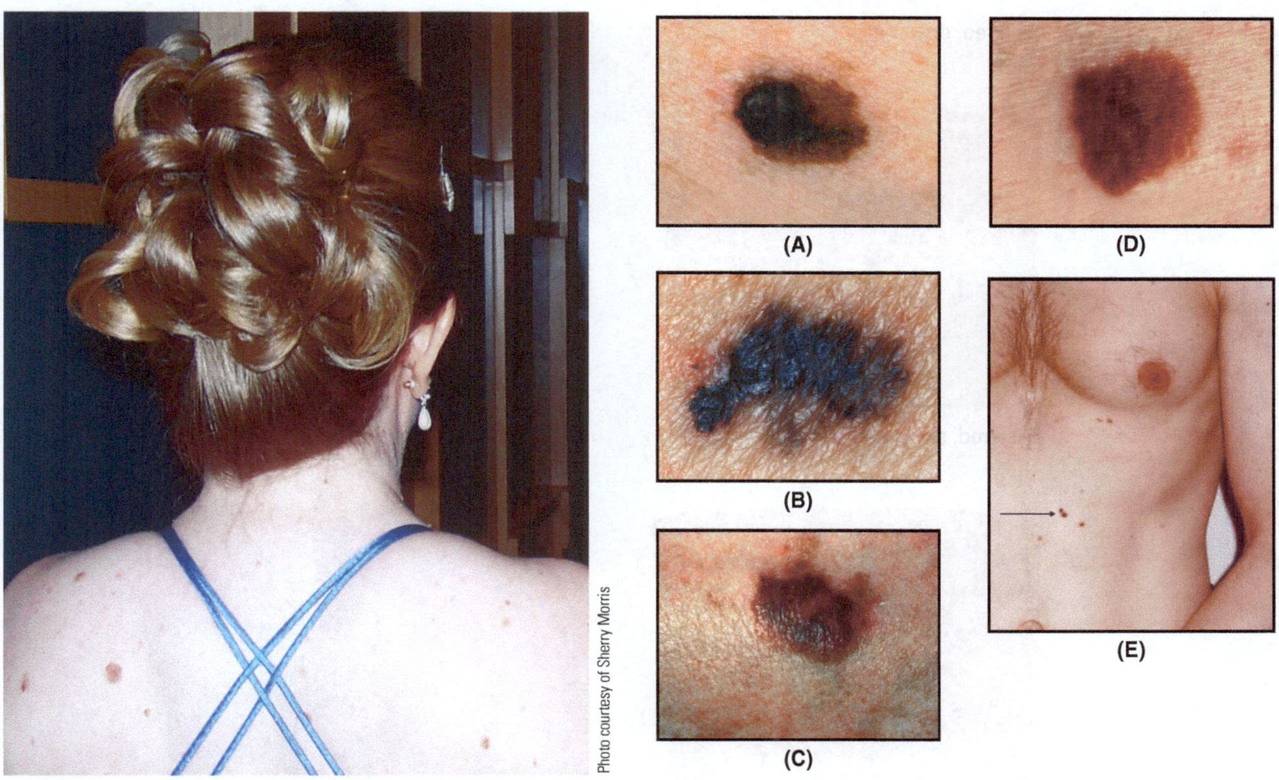

Photo courtesy of Sherry Morris

The Skin Cancer Foundation www.skincancer.org

FIGURE 13.15 Left: Melanoma visible on the left shoulder blade. Right: The A-B-C-D-E signs of melanoma are (A) asymmetry, (B) border irregularity, (C) color variation, (D) diameter larger than a pencil eraser, and (E) evolving, or changing in size, shape, or shade of color.

TABLE 13.1 Classification of Burn Severity		
Type of Burn	**Also Known As**	**Layers of Skin Involved**
First-degree burn	*Superficial burn*	No blisters; superficial damage to the epidermis
Second-degree burn	*Partial thickness burn*	Blisters, damage to the epidermis and dermis
Third-degree burn	*Full thickness burn*	Damage to the epidermis, dermis, and subcutaneous layers, and possibly also the muscle and bone below

Burns

A **burn** is an injury to body tissues caused by heat, flame, electricity, sun, chemicals, or radiation. The severity of a burn is described according to the percentage of the total body skin surface affected (more than 15% is considered serious). It is also described according to the depth or layers of skin involved (Table 13.1 and Figure 13.16).

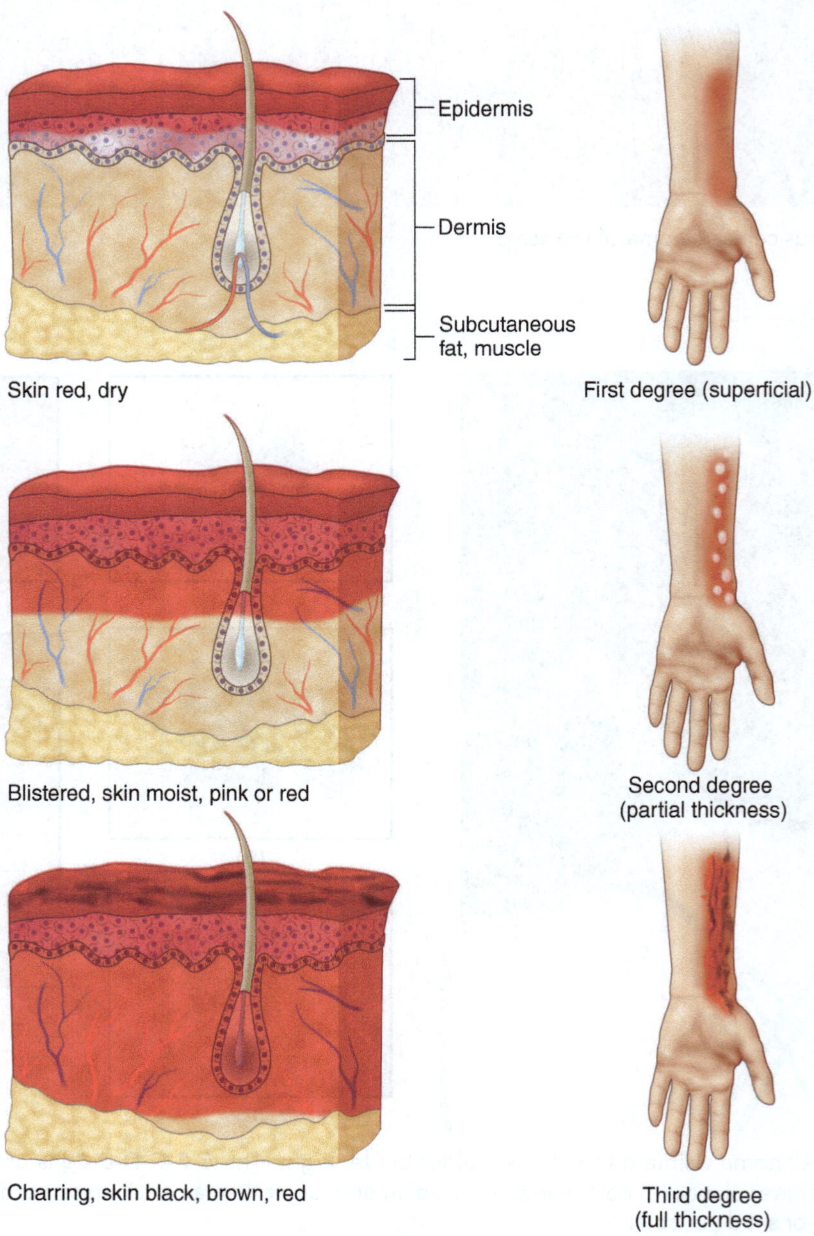

FIGURE 13.16 The degree of a burn is determined by the layers of skin involved.

DIAGNOSTIC PROCEDURES OF THE INTEGUMENTARY SYSTEM

A **biopsy** (**BYE**-op-see) is the removal of a small piece of living tissue for examination to confirm or establish a diagnosis (**bi** means pertaining to life, and **-opsy** means view of).

- In an ***incisional biopsy***, a piece, but not all, of the tumor or lesion is removed.
- In an ***excisional biopsy***, the entire tumor or lesion and a margin of surrounding tissue are removed. ***Excision*** means the complete removal of a lesion or organ.
- In a ***needle biopsy***, a hollow needle is used to remove a core of tissue for examination.
- **Exfoliative cytology** (ecks-**FOH**-lee-**ay**-tiv sigh-**TOL**-oh-jee), also referred to as ***skin scraping***, is a technique in which cells are scraped from the tissue and examined under a microscope. ***Exfoliation*** is the removal of dead epidermal cells, often through sanding or chemabrasion (which is discussed in the next section), and is sometimes done for cosmetic purposes.

TREATMENT PROCEDURES OF THE INTEGUMENTARY SYSTEM

Preventive Measures

Sunscreen that blocks out the harmful ultraviolet B (UVB) rays is sometimes measured in terms of the strength of the ***sun protection factor*** (SPF). Some sunscreens also give protection against ultraviolet A (UVA) rays.

Burn Treatment

The type of treatment for a burn depends on its degree and the percentage of the body surface involved. A hospital ***burn center*** provides care for serious burns, including pain relief, debridement and skin grafts, IV fluids and nutritional supplements, antibiotics, cosmetic reconstruction, and rehabilitation.

- **Skin grafts**, also known as ***dermatoplasty***, are the replacement of damaged skin with healthy tissue taken from a donor site on the patient's body (**dermat/o** means skin, and **-plasty** means surgical repair).

Tissue Removal

- **Cauterization** (**kaw**-ter-eye-**ZAY**-shun) is the destruction of tissue by burning.
- **Chemabrasion** (**kem**-ah-**BRAY**-zhun), also known as a ***chemical peel***, is the use of chemicals to remove the outer layers of skin to treat acne scarring, fine wrinkling, and keratoses.
- **Cryosurgery** (**krye**-oh-**SIR**-jur-ee), also called freezing, is the destruction or elimination of abnormal tissue cells, such as warts or tumors, through the application of extreme cold by using liquid nitrogen (**cry/o** means cold, and **-surgery** means operative procedure).
- **Curettage** (**kyou**-reh-**TAHZH**) is the removal of material from the surface by scraping. One use of this technique is to remove basal cell tumors.
- **Debridement** (dah-**BREED**-ment) is the removal of dirt, foreign objects, damaged tissue, and cellular debris from a wound to prevent infection and to promote healing.
- In an **irrigation and debridement** (I&D) procedure, pressurized fluid is used to clean out wound debris.
- **Dermabrasion** (**der**-mah-**BRAY**-zhun) is a form of abrasion involving the use of a revolving wire brush or sandpaper. It is used to remove acne and chickenpox scars as well as for facial skin rejuvenation. ***Microdermabrasion*** removes only a fine layer of skin, so the results are temporary.
- **Electrodesiccation** (ee-**leck**-troh-des-ih-**KAY**-shun) is a surgical technique performed in conjunction with curettage in which layers of tissue are destroyed using an electric spark and then scraped away. It is primarily used to eliminate small superficial growths and to seal off blood vessels, and is also known as ***electrodesiccation and curettage*** (EDC).
- An **incision** is a cut made with a surgical instrument. ***Incision and drainage*** (I&D) is an incision (cutting open) of a lesion, such as an abscess, and the draining of the contents. *Note:* The abbreviation I&D is used for both irrigation and debridement, and incision and drainage.
- **Mohs surgery** is a technique used to treat various types of skin cancer. Individual layers of cancerous tissue are removed and examined under a microscope one at a time until a margin that is clear of all cancerous tissue has been achieved.

Laser and Light Source Treatments of Skin Conditions

The term **laser** is an acronym in which the letters stand for **L**ight **A**mplification by **S**timulated **E**mission of **R**adiation. Lasers are used to treat skin conditions and other disorders of the body.

A laser tube can be filled with a solid, liquid, or gas substance that is stimulated to emit light at a specific wavelength. Some wavelengths are capable of destroying all skin tissue; others target tissue of a particular color.

- Port-wine stain is treated using short pulses of laser light to remove the birthmark. Treatment can require many sessions because only a small section is treated at a time.
- Rhinophyma is treated by using a laser to reshape the nose by vaporizing the excess tissue.
- Tattoos are removed by using lasers that target particular colors.
- Some skin cancers, precancer of the lip, and warts that recur around nails and on the soles of feet are treated using lasers.
- **Phototherapy** is the use of natural or artificial light to treat skin conditions such as vitiligo and eczema. One type of phototherapy is *photodynamic therapy*.
- **Photodynamic therapy** (**foh**-toh-dye-**NAH**-mik) (PDT), also known as *blue-light therapy*, is a technique used to treat damaged and precancerous skin, as well as various types of cancer.
    - A *photosensitizing drug* is administered topically or by injection. An incubation period is followed by exposure to a specific wavelength of light, administered either externally or endoscopically.
    - When the photosensitizers are activated, they produce a form of oxygen that kills nearby cells. PDT is used to treat tumors on or near the surface of the skin, or in the lining of internal organs such as the lungs and esophagus.

Medications for Treatment of the Skin

Fluorouracil is a topical chemotherapy cream used to treat basal cell carcinoma and actinic keratoses by targeting fast-growing cells. It is applied regularly for 2 to 12 weeks, and causes localized irritation, redness, and swelling.

Retinoids (**RET**-ih-noydz) are a class of chemical compounds derived from vitamin A that are used in skin care and treatment because of their effect on epithelial cell growth. The use of retinoids can, however, make the skin burn more easily.

- *Isotretinoin*, known by its trade name of Accutane, is a powerful retinoid taken in pill form for the treatment of severe acne.
- *Tretinoin* is the active ingredient in Retin-A and Renova, which are used to treat sun-damaged skin, acne, and wrinkles.

Topical steroids such as hydrocortisone and other more potent variations are used in the treatment of various skin disorders and diseases. These drugs, which are derivatives of the natural corticosteroid hormones produced by the adrenal glands, must be used cautiously to avoid potential side effects, which can include irreversible thinning of the skin.

Many over-the-counter face washes recommended for treating acne contain salicylic acid or benzoyl peroxide. These are considered *noncomedogenic*, meaning that they do not clog pores.

Cosmetic Procedures

- **Blepharoplasty** (**BLEF**-ah-roh-**plas**-tee), also known as a *lid lift*, is the surgical reduction of the upper and lower eyelids by removing sagging skin (**blephar/o** means eyelid, and **-plasty** means surgical repair) (Figure 13.17). A small amount of fat from the patient's thighs or buttocks is sometimes injected in the hollow below the eye to improve appearance. This procedure is also sometimes performed to improve eyesight limited by drooping eyelids.
- **Botox** is a formulation of *botulinum toxin*. This is the same neurotoxin responsible for the form of food poisoning known as botulism. When small, sterile doses are injected into muscles on the forehead, it can temporarily block the nerve signals to the injected muscle for up to three to four months, reducing moderate to severe *frown lines* between the eyebrows. Botox is also used therapeutically to treat migraines, overactive bladder, strabismus, and muscle spasms.
- **Collagen replacement therapy** is a form of soft-tissue augmentation used to soften facial lines or scars or to make lips appear fuller. Tiny quantities of collagen are injected under a line or scar to boost the skin's natural supply of collagen. The effect usually lasts for 3 to 12 months.
- **Electrolysis** (ee-leck-**TROL**-ih-sis) is the use of electric current to destroy hair follicles in order to produce

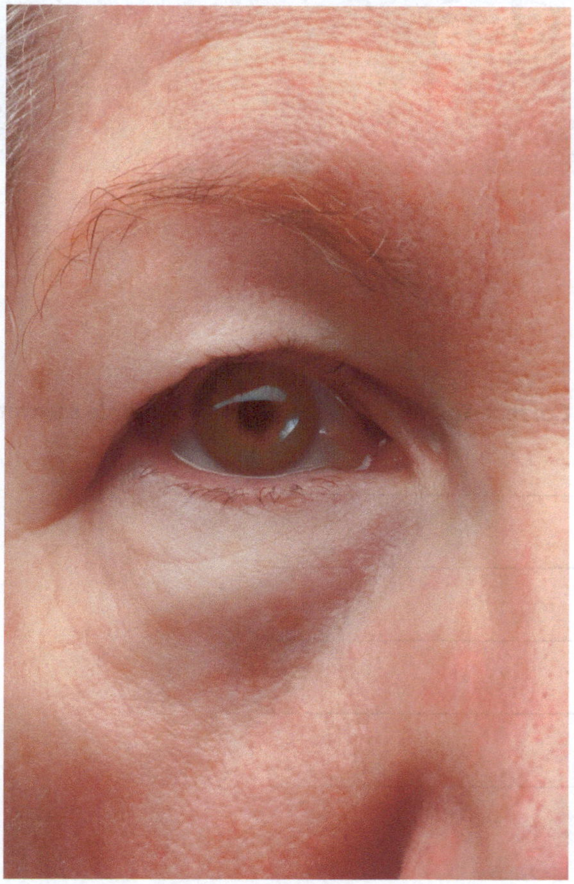

iStock.com/ElFlacodelNorte

FIGURE 13.17 Blepharoplasty is the surgical reduction of the eyelids by removing sagging skin that can interfere with the field of vision.

the relatively permanent removal of unwanted hair (**electr/o** means electric, and **-lysis** means destruction). ***Laser hair removal*** is the use of lasers to damage hair follicles in order to produce the relatively permanent removal of unwanted hair, such as for patients with hirsutism.

- **Lipectomy** (lih-**PECK**-toh-mee) is the surgical removal of fat from beneath the skin to improve physical appearance (**lip** means fat, and **-ectomy** means surgical removal).
- **Liposuction** (**LIP**-oh-**suck**-shun), also known as ***suction-assisted lipectomy***, is the surgical removal of fat beneath the skin with the aid of suction.
- **Rhytidectomy** (**rit**-ih-**DECK**-toh-mee), also known as a ***facelift***, is the surgical removal of excess skin and fat from the face to eliminate wrinkles (**rhytid** means wrinkle, and **-ectomy** means surgical removal).
- **Sclerotherapy** (**sklehr**-oh-**THER**-ah-pee) is the treatment of spider veins by injecting a saline sclerosing solution into the vein. This solution irritates the tissue, causing the veins to collapse and disappear. ***Spider veins*** are small, nonessential veins that can be seen through the skin, often on the legs.

ABBREVIATIONS RELATED TO THE INTEGUMENTARY SYSTEM

Table 13.2 presents an overview of the abbreviations related to the terms introduced in this chapter. *Note:* To avoid errors or confusion, always be cautious when using abbreviations.

TABLE 13.2

Abbreviations Related to the Integumentary System

alopecia totalis = AT	**AT** = alopecia totalis
basal cell carcinoma = BCC	**BCC** = basal cell carcinoma
contact dermatitis = CD	**CD** = contact dermatitis
incision and drainage; irrigation and debridement = I&D	**I&D** = incision and drainage; irrigation and debridement
malignant melanoma = MM	**MM** = malignant melanoma
necrotizing fasciitis = NF	**NF** = necrotizing fasciitis
photodynamic therapy = PDT	**PDT** = photodynamic therapy
psoriasis = Ps	**Ps** = psoriasis
scleroderma = SCD	**SCD** = scleroderma
squamous cell carcinoma = SCC	**SCC** = squamous cell carcinoma
systemic lupus erythematosus = SLE	**SLE** = systemic lupus erythematosus

LEARNING EXERCISES

Matching Word Parts 1

Write the correct answer in the middle column.

	Definition	Correct Answer	Possible Answers
13.1.	skin	____________	urtic/o
13.2.	rash	____________	rhytid/o
13.3.	red	____________	hidr/o
13.4.	sweat	____________	erythr/o
13.5.	wrinkle	____________	cutane/o

Matching Word Parts 2

Write the correct answer in the middle column.

	Definition	Correct Answer	Possible Answers
13.6.	black, dark	____________	pedicul/o
13.7.	fat, lipid	____________	melan/o
13.8.	horny, hard	____________	lip/o
13.9.	lice	____________	kerat/o
13.10.	skin	____________	dermat/o

Matching Word Parts 3

Write the correct answer in the middle column.

	Definition	Correct Answer	Possible Answers
13.11.	dry	____________	xer/o
13.12.	fungus	____________	seb/o

13.13. hairy, rough ________________ **onych/o**

13.14. nail ________________ **myc/o**

13.15. sebum ________________ **hirsut/o**

Definitions

Select the correct answer, and write it on the line provided.

13.16. An acute, rapidly spreading bacterial infection within the connective tissues is known as ________________.

abscess cellulitis fissure ulcer

13.17. Atypical moles that can develop into skin cancer are known as ________________.

dysplastic nevi lipomas malignant keratosis papillomas

13.18. The autoimmune disorder in which there are well-defined bald areas is known as ________________.

alopecia areata alopecia capitis alopecia universalis psoriasis

13.19. A/An ________________ is a swelling of clotted blood trapped in the tissues.

abscess contusion hematoma petechiae

13.20. The term ________________ means profuse sweating.

anhidrosis diaphoresis hidrosis ecchymosis

13.21. A normal scar resulting from the healing of a wound is called a ________________.

cicatrix keloid keratosis papilloma

13.22. A large blister that is usually more than 0.5 cm in diameter is known as a/an ________________.

abscess bulla pustule vesicle

13.23. The removal of dirt, foreign objects, damaged tissue, and cellular debris from a wound is called ________________.

cauterization curettage debridement dermabrasion

13.24. A ________________ burn has blisters plus damage only to the epidermis and dermis.

first-degree fourth-degree second-degree third-degree

13.25. Commonly known as warts, ____________ are small, hard skin lesions caused by the human papillomavirus.

nevi petechiae scabies verrucae

Matching Structures

Write the correct answer in the middle column.

	Definition	Correct Answer	Possible Answers
13.26.	fibrous protein found in hair, nails, and skin	____________	unguis
13.27.	fingernail or toenail	____________	sebaceous glands
13.28.	glands secreting sebum	____________	mammary glands
13.29.	milk-producing glands	____________	keratin
13.30.	the layer of tissue below the epidermis	____________	dermis

Which Word?

Select the correct answer, and write it on the line provided.

13.31. The medical term for the condition commonly known as an ingrown toenail is ____________.

onychomycosis onychocryptosis

13.32. The bacterial skin infection characterized by isolated pustules that become crusted and rupture is known as ____________. This highly contagious condition commonly occurs in children.

impetigo xeroderma

13.33. A torn or jagged wound or an accidental cut wound is known as a ____________.

laceration lesion

13.34. The lesions of ____________ carcinoma tend to bleed easily.

basal cell squamous cell

13.35. Group A strep, also known as flesh-eating bacteria, causes ____________.

systematic lupus erythematosus necrotizing fasciitis

Spelling Counts

Find the misspelled word in each sentence. Then write that word, spelled correctly, on the line provided.

13.36. Soriasus is a disease of the skin characterized by itching and by red papules covered with silvery scales. ______________

13.37. Exema is an inflammatory skin disease with possible blistering, cracking, oozing, or bleeding. ______________

13.38. An absess is a localized collection of pus. ______________

13.39. Onichia is an inflammation of the nail bed that usually results in the loss of the nail. ______________

13.40. Schleroderma is an autoimmune disorder in which the connective tissues become thickened and hardened, causing the skin to become hard and swollen. ______________

Abbreviation Identification

In the space provided, write the words that each abbreviation stands for.

13.41. **BCC** ______________

13.42. **I&D** ______________

13.43. **SLE** ______________

13.44. **MM** ______________

13.45. **SCC** ______________

Term Selection

Select the correct answer, and write it on the line provided.

13.46. ______________ is dermatitis caused by the friction of skin rubbing together in skin folds.

Eczema Intertrigo Keratosis Erythema

13.47. An infestation of lice is known as ______________.

pediculosis itch mites cicatrix scabies

13.48. The term ________________ is used to describe any redness of the skin due to dilated capillaries.

dermatitis ecchymosis erythema urticaria

13.49. Flakes or dry patches made up of excess dead epidermal cells are known as ________________.

bullae macules plaques scales

13.50. A cluster of connected boils is known as a/an ________________.

acne vulgaris carbuncle comedo furuncle

Sentence Completion

Write the correct term or terms on the lines provided.

13.51. The term meaning producing or containing pus is ________________.

13.52. The term meaning a fungal infection of the nail is ________________.

13.53. A physician who specializes in diagnosing and treating disorders of the skin is known as a/an ________________.

13.54. A genetic condition characterized by a deficiency or absence of pigment in the skin, hair, and irises is known as ________________.

13.55. The role of ________________ tissues is to form a protective covering for the surfaces of the body.

Word Surgery

Divide each term into its component word parts. Write these word parts, in sequence, on the lines provided. When necessary use a slash (/) to indicate a combining vowel. (You may not need all of the lines provided.)

13.56. A **rhytidectomy** is the surgical removal of excess skin for the elimination of wrinkles.

________ ________ ________ ________

13.57. **Onychomycosis** is a fungal infection of the nail.

________ ________ ________ ________

13.58. **Folliculitis** is an inflammation of the hair follicles that is especially common on the limbs and in the beard area of men.

________ ________ ________ ________

13.59. **Pruritus**, which is commonly known as itching, is associated with most forms of dermatitis.

________ ________ ________ ________

13.60. **Ichthyosis** is a group of hereditary disorders that are characterized by dry, thickened, and scaly skin.

________ ________ ________ ________

True/False

If the statement is true, write **True** on the line. If the statement is false, write **False** on the line.

13.61. ________ An actinic keratosis is a precancerous skin growth that occurs on sun-damaged skin.

13.62. ________ A skin tag is a malignant skin enlargement commonly found on older adults.

13.63. ________ The arrector pili cause the raised areas of skin known as goose bumps.

13.64. ________ A keratosis is an abnormally raised scar.

13.65. ________ Lipedema, which is also known as painful fat syndrome, affects mostly women.

Clinical Conditions

Write the correct answer on the line provided.

13.66. Carmella Espinoza underwent ________________ for the treatment of spider veins.

13.67. Jordan Caswell is an albino. This disorder, which is known as ________________, is due to a missing enzyme necessary for the production of melanin.

13.68. Soon after Ying Li hit his thumb with a hammer, a collection of blood formed beneath the nail. This condition is a subungual ________________.

13.69. Trisha Bell fell off her bicycle and scraped off the superficial layers of skin on her knees. This type of injury is known as a/an ________________.

13.70. Molly Malone had a severe fever, and then she developed very small, pinpoint hemorrhages under her skin. The doctor described these as being ________________.

13.71. Many of the children in the Happy Hours Day Care Center required treatment for ________________, a skin infection caused by an infestation of itch mites.

13.72. Dr. Liu treated Jeanette Isenberg's skin cancer with ______________________________ surgery. With this technique, individual layers of cancerous tissue are removed and examined under a microscope until all cancerous tissue has been removed.

13.73. Mrs. Garrison had cosmetic surgery that is commonly known as a lid lift. The medical term for this surgical treatment is a/an ______________________________.

13.74. Manuel Fernandez developed a/an ______________________________. This condition is a closed pocket containing pus that is caused by a bacterial infection.

13.75. Agnes Farrington calls them night sweats; however, the medical term for this condition is ______________________________.

Which Is the Correct Medical Term?

Select the correct answer, and write it on the line provided.

13.76. The term that refers to an acute infection of the fold of skin around a nail is ______________________________.

onychia onychocryptosis paronychia vitiligo

13.77. When the sebum plug of a ______________________________ is exposed to air, it oxidizes and becomes a blackhead.

chloasma comedo macule pustule

13.78. The condition known as ______________________________ is a skin disorder characterized by flare-ups of red papules covered with silvery scales.

melasma eczema psoriasis rosacea

13.79. The medical term referring to a malformation of the nail is ______________________________. This condition is also called spoon nail.

clubbing koilonychia onychomycosis paronychia

13.80. Commonly known as a mole, a ______________________________ is a small, dark, skin growth that develops from melanocytes in the skin.

keloid nevus papilloma verrucae

Challenge Word Building

These terms are *not* primary terms in the chapter; however, they are made up of the following familiar word parts. If you need help in creating the term, refer to your medical dictionary.

an-	**dermat/o**	**-derma**
hypo-	**hidr/o**	**-ectomy**
	melan/o	**-ia**
	myc/o	**-itis**
	onych/o	**-malacia**
	py/o	**-oma**
		-osis
		-pathy
		-plasty

13.81. Abnormal softening of the nails is known as ______________________.

13.82. An abnormal condition resulting in the diminished flow of perspiration is known as ______________________.

13.83. The plastic surgery procedure to change the shape or size of the nose is a/an ______________________.

13.84. A tumor arising from the nail bed is known as ______________________.

13.85. The term meaning any disease marked by abnormal pigmentation of the skin is ______________________.

13.86. The surgical removal of a fingernail or toenail is a/an ______________________.

13.87. The term meaning pertaining to the absence of fingernails or toenails is ______________________.

13.88. The term meaning any disease of the skin is ______________________.

13.89. A fungal irritation of the skin is ______________________.

13.90. An excess of melanin present in an area of inflammation of the skin is known as ______________________.

Labeling Exercises

Identify the numbered items on the accompanying figures.

13.91. ______________________________

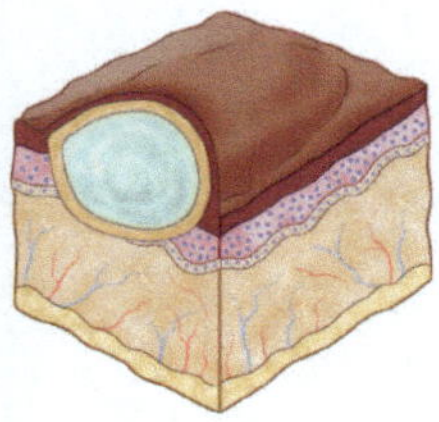

A **13.91** is a closed sack or pouch containing soft or semisolid material.

13.94. ______________________________

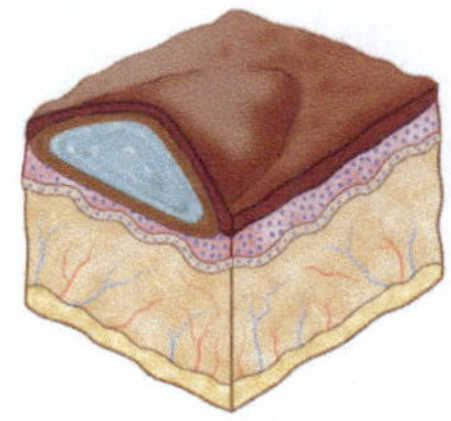

A **13.94** is a large blister that is more than 0.5 cm in diameter.

13.92. ______________________________

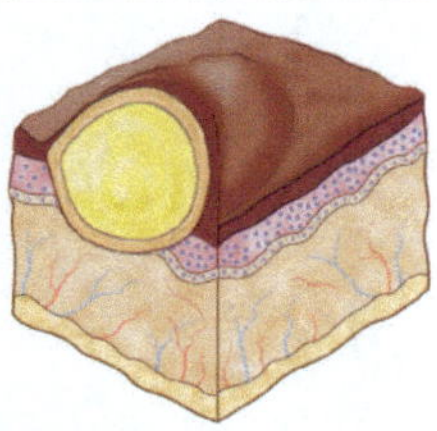

A **13.92** is a small circumscribed elevation of the skin containing pus.

13.95. ______________________________

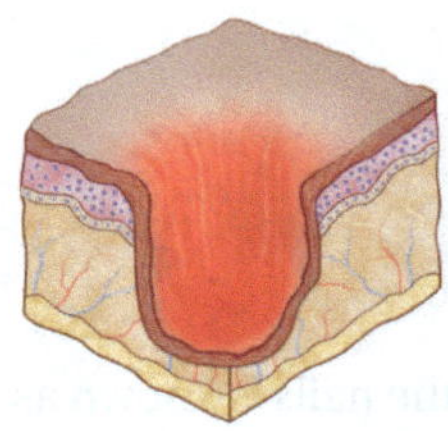

A **13.95** is an open lesion of the skin or mucous membrane, resulting in tissue loss.

13.93. ______________________________

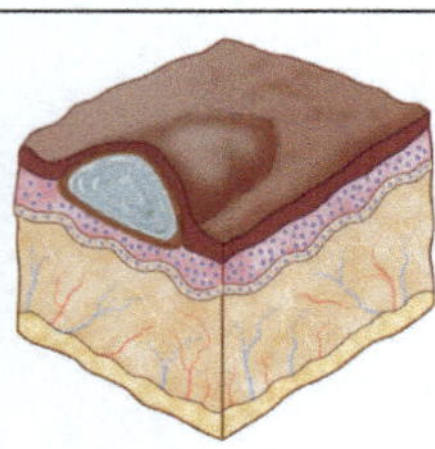

A **13.93** is a small blister containing watery fluid that is less than 0.5 cm in diameter.

13.96. ________________

13.97. ________________

13.98. ________________ layer

13.99. ________________ gland

13.100. ________________ gland

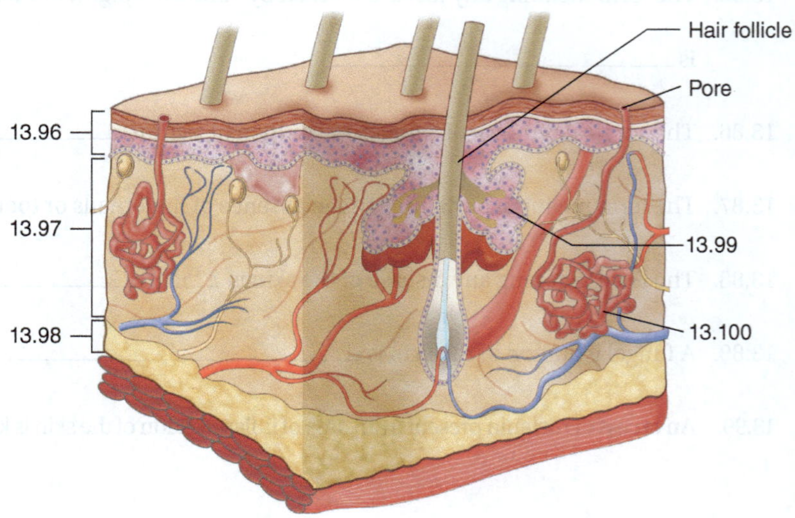

The Human Touch

CRITICAL THINKING EXERCISE

The following story and questions are designed to stimulate critical thinking through class discussion or as a brief essay response. There are no right or wrong answers to these questions.

"OK, guys, we're late again." Shaylene Boulay calls out to her two oldest sons, Nathan Jr., 10, and Carl, 12. Grabbing the lunches Nate Sr. packed, she walks out the back door. "Come on, Michael, school time!" Shaylene peers under the porch for her 5-year-old. Their house is only a mile from the waterfront, and he loves to race cars between their dog Bubba's big paws in the cool sand underneath the porch. "Look at you!" As Shaylene dusts him off and heads to the truck, she notices that the rash of blisters on his leg is still bright red. "Must be ant bites," she thinks.

"Have a good day!" Shaylene hands Nathan and Carl their lunches as they hop out of the truck at the middle school. Next stop, Oak Creek Elementary. As Michael starts to get out, clutching his brown lunch bag tightly, his kindergarten teacher comes rushing over. "Michael, what are you doing here today? Didn't you give your mother the note from the nurse?"

"What note? Michael, honey, did you forget to give Mama something from school?" Michael smiles sheepishly and reaches into his shorts pocket for a wadded up piece of paper. The note says: "We believe Michael has impetigo. Since this condition is very contagious, please consult your doctor as soon as possible. We will need a note from the doctor before we can allow Michael to reenter class."

"Oh, no," Shaylene thinks. "I'm due for my shift at the diner in 15 minutes. Nobody's home to watch Michael, and we don't have the money to see Dr. Gaines again. And what if this rash on my arm is that thing Michael has?" She sits clutching the wheel of the old pickup, asking herself over and over, "What am I gonna do?"

Suggested Discussion Topics

1. Discuss why the school wants Michael to have completed treatment before he returns to class.
2. You work in Dr. Gaines's office and you know that the Boulays' appointment today is about a potential contagious rash. What precautions should you take when the family arrives?
3. Discuss how you might explain to Shaylene what impetigo is, how it spreads, and what she can do to prevent her other children from getting it.
4. Shaylene is in a very difficult, and all too common, situation. Discuss possible answers to her question, "What am I gonna do?"

CHAPTER 14

THE ENDOCRINE SYSTEM

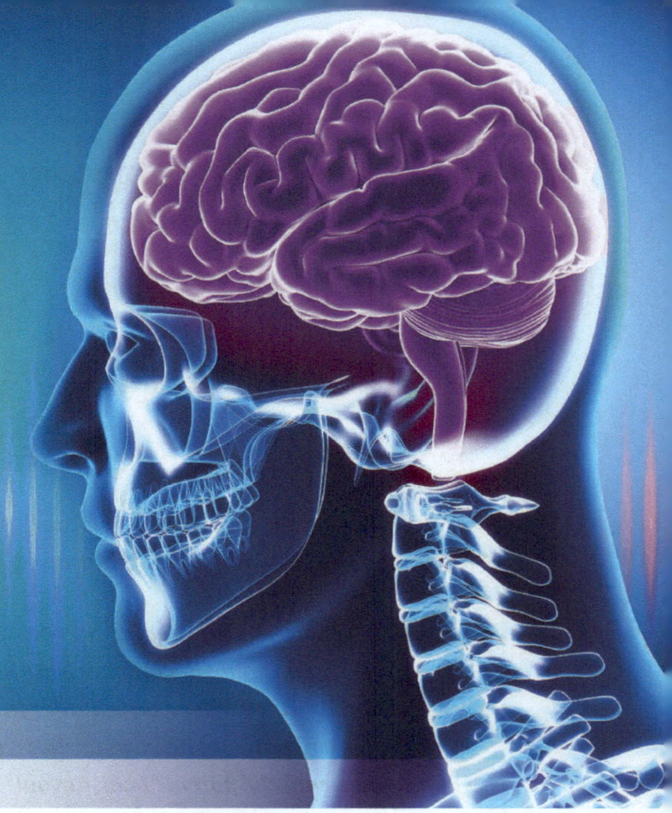

Overview of

STRUCTURES, COMBINING FORMS, AND FUNCTIONS OF THE ENDOCRINE SYSTEM

Major Structures	Related Combining Forms	Primary Functions
Adrenal Glands	adren/o	Regulate electrolyte levels, influence metabolism, and respond to stress.
Gonads	gonad/o	Gamete (sex cell)-producing glands.
Male: Testicles	testic/o	Sperm-producing glands.
Female: Ovaries	ovari/o	Ova (egg)-producing glands.
Pancreas	pancreat/o	Controls blood sugar levels and glucose metabolism.
Parathyroid Glands	parathyroid/o	Regulate calcium levels throughout the body.
Pineal Gland	pineal/o	Influences the sleep–wakefulness cycle.
Pituitary Gland	pituit/o, pituitar/o	Secretes hormones that control the activity of the other endocrine glands.
Thymus	thym/o	Plays a major role in the immune reaction.
Thyroid Gland	thyr/o, thyroid/o	Stimulates metabolism, growth, and the activity of the nervous system.

Vocabulary Related to **THE ENDOCRINE SYSTEM**

This list contains essential word parts and medical terms for this chapter. These and the other important **primary terms** are shown in **boldface** throughout the chapter. ***Secondary terms***, which appear in ***orange*** italics, clarify the meaning of primary terms.

Word Parts

- ☐ **acr/o** extremities (hands and feet), top, extreme point
- ☐ **adren/o** adrenal glands
- ☐ **crin/o** secrete
- ☐ **-dipsia** thirst
- ☐ **glyc/o** glucose, sugar
- ☐ **gonad/o** gonad, sex glands
- ☐ **-ism** condition, state of
- ☐ **pancreat/o** pancreas
- ☐ **parathyroid/o** parathyroid glands
- ☐ **pineal/o** pineal gland
- ☐ **pituitar/o** pituitary gland
- ☐ **poly-** many
- ☐ **somat/o** body
- ☐ **thym/o** thymus gland
- ☐ **thyr/o, thyroid/o** thyroid gland

Medical Terms

- ☐ **acromegaly** (**ack**-roh-**MEG**-ah-lee)
- ☐ **Addison's disease** (**AD**-ih-sonz)
- ☐ **adrenalitis** (ah-**dree**-nal-**EYE**-tis)
- ☐ **aldosteronism** (al-**DOSS**-teh-roh-**niz**-em)
- ☐ **antidiuretic hormone** (**an**-tih-dye-you-**RET**-ick)
- ☐ **calcitonin** (**kal**-sih-**TOH**-nin)
- ☐ **corticosteroids** (**kor**-tih-koh-**STEHR**-oidz)
- ☐ **cortisol** (**KOR**-tih-sol)
- ☐ **cretinism** (**CREE**-tin-izm)
- ☐ **Cushing's syndrome** (**KUSH**-ingz)
- ☐ **diabetes insipidus** (**dye**-ah-**BEE**-teez in-**SIP**-ih-dus)
- ☐ **diabetes mellitus** (**dye**-ah-**BEE**-teez **MEL**-ih-tus)
- ☐ **diabetic ketoacidosis** (**kee**-toh-**ah**-seh-**DOH**-sis)
- ☐ **diabetic retinopathy** (**ret**-ih-**NOP**-ah-thee)
- ☐ **electrolytes** (ee-**LECK**-troh-lytes)
- ☐ **epinephrine** (**ep**-ih-**NEF**-rin)
- ☐ **estrogen** (**ES**-troh-jen)
- ☐ **exophthalmos** (**eck**-sof-**THAL**-mos)
- ☐ **follicle-stimulating hormone** (**FOL**-lick-kul)
- ☐ **fructosamine test** (fruck-**TOHS**-ah-meen)
- ☐ **gestational diabetes mellitus** (jes-**TAY**-shun-al **dye**-ah-**BEE**-teez **MEL**-ih-tus)
- ☐ **gigantism** (jigh-**GAN**-tiz-em)
- ☐ **glucagon** (**GLOO**-kah-gon)
- ☐ **glucose** (**GLOO**-kohs)
- ☐ **Graves' disease** (**GRAYVZ**)
- ☐ **growth hormone**
- ☐ **gynecomastia** (**guy**-neh-koh-**MAS**-tee-ah)
- ☐ **Hashimoto's disease** (hah-shee-**MOH**-tohz)
- ☐ **hypercalcemia** (**high**-per-kal-**SEE**-mee-ah)
- ☐ **hyperglycemia** (**high**-per-glye-**SEE**-mee-ah)
- ☐ **hyperinsulinism** (**high**-per-**IN**-suh-lin-izm)
- ☐ **hyperpituitarism** (**high**-per-pih-**TOO**-ih-tah-rizm)
- ☐ **hyperthyroidism** (**high**-per-**THIGH**-roid-izm)
- ☐ **hypoglycemia** (**high**-poh-gly-**SEE**-mee-ah)
- ☐ **hypothyroidism** (**high**-poh-**THIGH**-roid-izm)
- ☐ **insulin** (**IN**-suh-lin)
- ☐ **insulinoma** (**in**-suh-lin-**OH**-mah)
- ☐ **ketosis** (kee-**TOH**-sis)
- ☐ **laparoscopic adrenalectomy** (**lap**-ah-roh-**SKOP**-ick ah-**dree**-nal-**ECK**-toh-mee)
- ☐ **leptin** (**LEP**-tin)
- ☐ **luteinizing hormone** (**LOO**-tee-in-eye-zing)
- ☐ **myxedema** (**mick**-seh-**DEE**-mah)
- ☐ **norepinephrine** (**nor**-ep-ih-**NEF**-rin)
- ☐ **oxytocin** (**ock**-see-**TOH**-sin)
- ☐ **pancreatitis** (**pan**-kree-ah-**TYE**-tis)
- ☐ **parathyroidectomy** (**par**-ah-**thigh**-roi-**DECK**-toh-mee)
- ☐ **pituitary adenoma** (pih-**TOO**-ih-**tair**-ee **ad**-eh-**NOH**-mah)
- ☐ **polydipsia** (**pol**-ee-**DIP**-see-ah)
- ☐ **polyphagia** (**pol**-ee-**FAY**-jee-ah)
- ☐ **polyuria** (**pol**-ee-**YOU**-ree-ah)
- ☐ **prediabetes** (**pree**-**dye**-ah-**BEE**-teez)
- ☐ **progesterone** (proh-**JES**-ter-ohn)
- ☐ **prolactinoma** (proh-**lack**-tih-**NOH**-mah)
- ☐ **puberty** (**PYU**-ber-tee)
- ☐ **radioactive iodine treatment**
- ☐ **steroids** (**STEHR**-oidz)
- ☐ **testosterone** (tes-**TOS**-teh-rohn)
- ☐ **thymectomy** (thigh-**MECK**-toh-mee)
- ☐ **thymosin** (**THIGH**-moh-sin)
- ☐ **thyroxine** (thigh-**ROCK**-sin)

LEARNING OBJECTIVES

On completion of this chapter, you should be able to:

1. Describe the role of the endocrine glands in maintaining homeostasis.
2. Identify each gland of the endocrine system.
3. Describe the functions of the primary hormones secreted by each of the endocrine glands.
4. Identify the medical specialists who treat disorders of the endocrine system.
5. Identify the medical word parts of the endocrine system.
6. Describe the various types of diabetes.
7. Define the primary terms related to the pathology and the diagnostic and treatment procedures of the endocrine system.
8. Spell the primary terms of the endocrine system.
9. Pronounce the primary terms of the endocrine system.
10. Define common abbreviations related to the endocrine system.

FUNCTIONS OF THE ENDOCRINE SYSTEM

The primary function of the endocrine system is to produce hormones that work together to maintain homeostasis. **Homeostasis** is the process through which the body maintains a constant internal environment (**home/o** means constant, and **-stasis** means control) (see Chapter 2).

- **Hormones** are chemical messengers that are secreted by endocrine glands directly into the bloodstream (see Chapter 2). This enables them to reach targeted cells and organs throughout the body.
- Each hormone has specialized functions in regulating the activities of specific cells, organs, or both. The hormones of the endocrine system affect almost every organ and cell in the body.
- Blood or urine tests are used to measure hormone levels. These tests are discussed in Chapter 21.

STRUCTURES OF THE ENDOCRINE SYSTEM

Endocrine glands (EN-doh-krin), which produce hormones, do not have ducts (**endo-** means within, and **-crine** means to secrete).

There are 13 major glands that make up the endocrine system (Figure 14.1):

- One **pituitary gland** (divided into two lobes)
- One **pineal gland**
- One **thyroid gland**
- Four **parathyroid glands**
- One **thymus**
- One **pancreas**
- Two **adrenal glands**
- Two **gonads** (either a pair of ovaries in females or a pair of testicles in males)

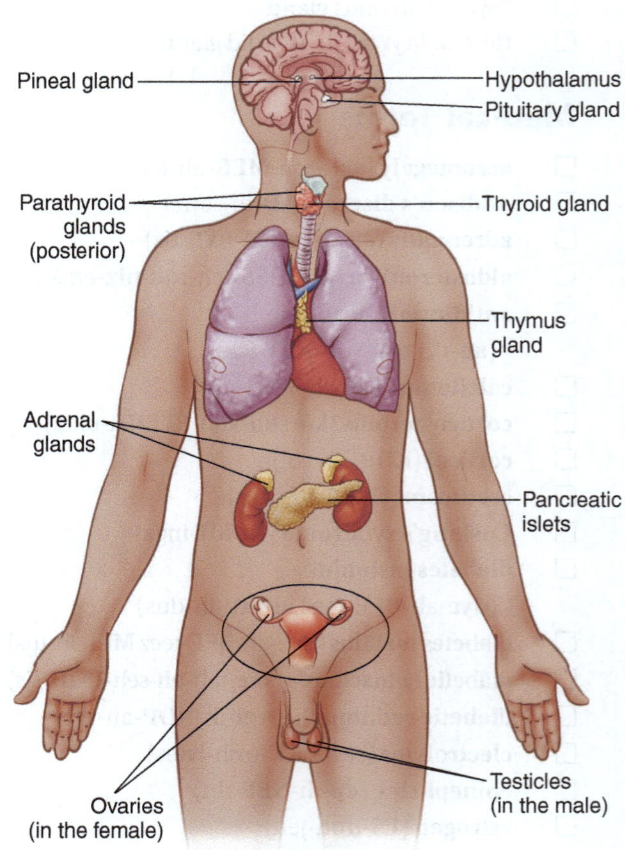

FIGURE 14.1 Structures of the endocrine system.

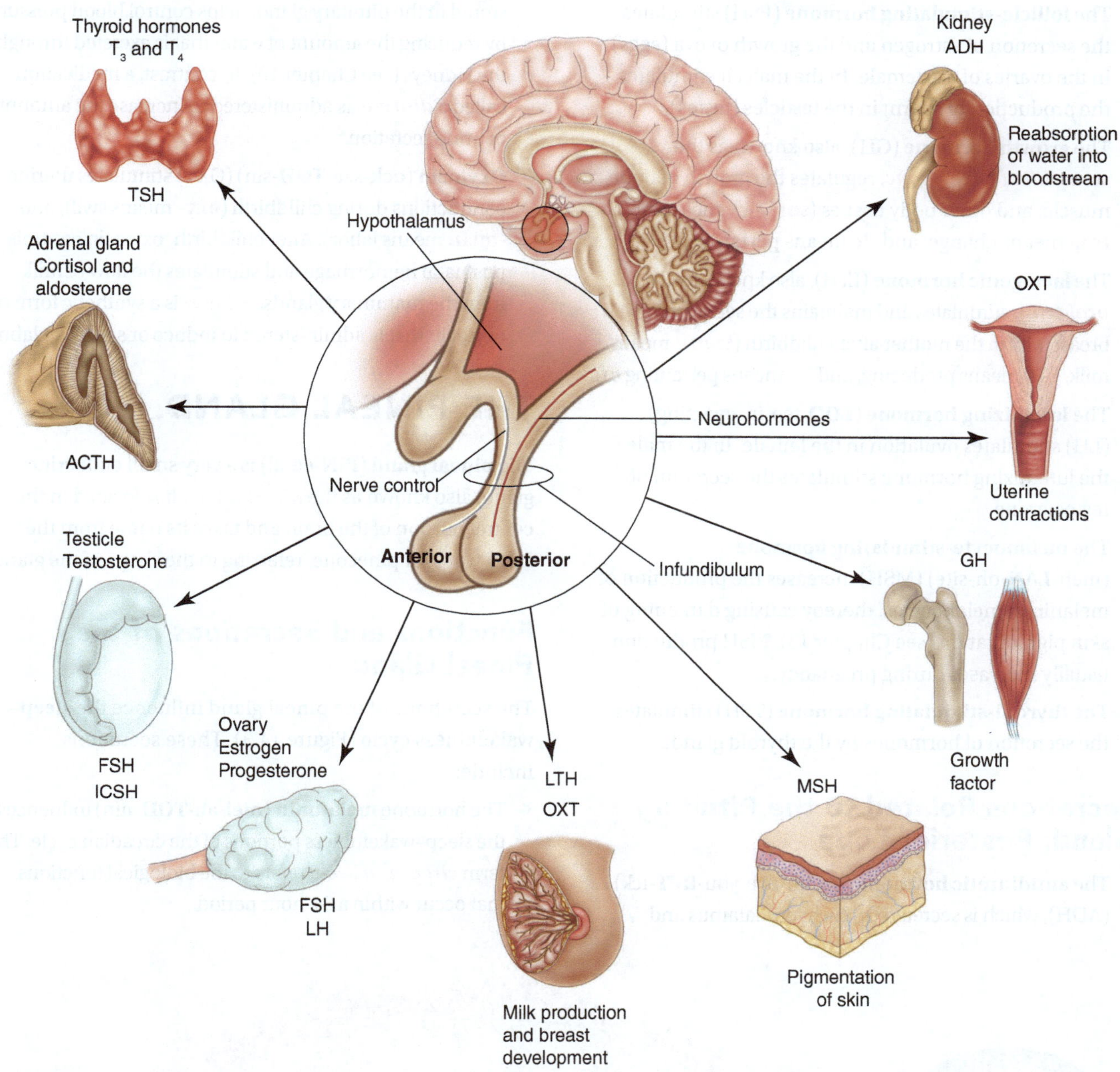

FIGURE 14.2 The pituitary gland secretes hormones that control the activity of other endocrine glands. Hormones are often referred to by their abbreviations, all of which are explained in the following sections.

THE PITUITARY GLAND

The **pituitary gland** (pih-**TOO**-ih-**tair**-ee), or ***hypophysis***, is a pea-sized gland that is divided into two parts, the anterior and the posterior lobes. These lobes hang from a stalk-like structure located below the hypothalamus in the brain (Figure 14.2). The hypothalamus is part of the nervous system that produces hormones that control many body functions (see Chapter 11).

Functions of the Pituitary Gland

The primary function of the pituitary gland is to secrete hormones that control the activity of other endocrine glands.

The pituitary gland acts in response to stimuli from neurohormones secreted by the hypothalamus. This creates a system of checks and balances to maintain an appropriate blood level of each hormone.

Secretions of the Pituitary Gland: Anterior Lobe

- The **adrenocorticotropic hormone** (ah-**DREE**-noh-**kor**-tih-koh-**TROP**-ik) (ACTH) stimulates the growth and secretions of the adrenal cortex (**adren/o** means adrenal, **cortic/o** means cortex, **trop** means change, and **-ic** means pertaining to).

- The **follicle-stimulating hormone** (FSH) stimulates the secretion of estrogen and the growth of ova (eggs) in the ovaries of the female. In the male, it stimulates the production of sperm in the testicles (testes).
- The **growth hormone** (GH), also known as the ***somatotropic hormone***, regulates the growth of bone, muscle, and other body tissues (**somat/o** means body, **trop** means change, and **-ic** means pertaining to).
- The **lactogenic hormone** (LTH), also known as ***prolactin***, stimulates and maintains the secretion of breast milk in the mother after childbirth (**lact/o** means milk, **gen** means producing, and **-ic** means pertaining to).
- The **luteinizing hormone** (**LOO**-tee-in-**eye**-zing) (LH) stimulates ovulation in the female. In the male, the luteinizing hormone stimulates the secretion of testosterone.
- The **melanocyte-stimulating hormone** (meh-**LAN**-oh-site) (MSH) increases the production of melanin in melanocytes, thereby causing darkening of skin pigmentation (see Chapter 13). MSH production usually increases during pregnancy.
- The **thyroid-stimulating hormone** (TSH) stimulates the secretion of hormones by the thyroid gland.

Secretions Related to the Pituitary Gland: Posterior Lobe

- The **antidiuretic hormone** (**an**-tih-dye-you-**RET**-ick) (ADH), which is secreted by the hypothalamus and stored in the pituitary gland, helps control blood pressure by reducing the amount of water that is excreted through the kidneys (see Chapter 10). In contrast, a medication called a ***diuretic*** is administered to increase the amount of urine secretion.
- **Oxytocin** (**ock**-see-**TOH**-sin) (OXT) stimulates uterine contractions during childbirth (**oxy-** means swift, and **-tocin** means labor). After childbirth, oxytocin controls postnatal hemorrhage and stimulates the flow of milk from the mammary glands. ***Pitocin*** is a synthetic form of oxytocin that is administered to induce or speed up labor.

THE PINEAL GLAND

The **pineal gland** (**PIN**-ee-al) is a very small endocrine gland, also known as the ***pineal body***. It is located in the central portion of the brain and takes its name from the Latin word for pinecone, referring to the shape of the gland.

Functions and Secretions of the Pineal Gland

The secretions of the pineal gland influence the sleep–wakefulness cycle (Figure 14.3). These secretions include:

- The hormone **melatonin** (**mel**-ah-**TOH**-nin) influences the sleep-wakefulness portions of the circadian cycle. The term ***circadian cycle*** refers to the biological functions that occur within a 24-hour period.

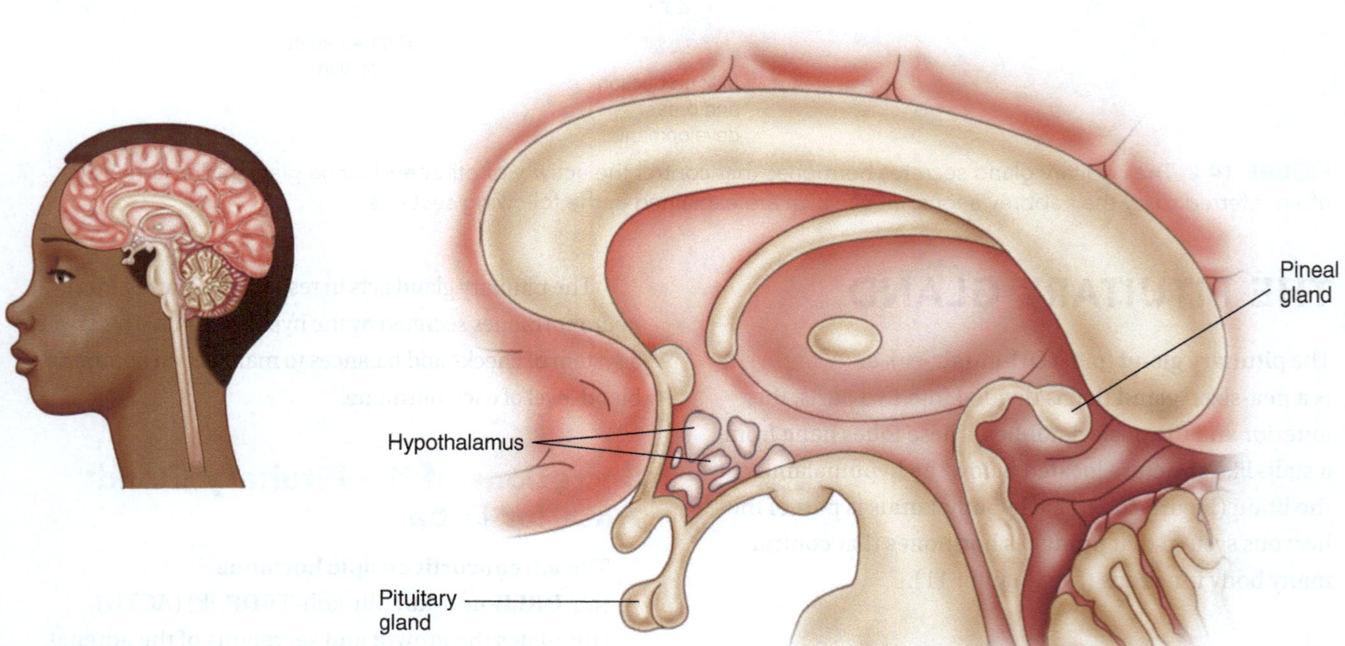

FIGURE 14.3 The pineal gland is located within the brain.

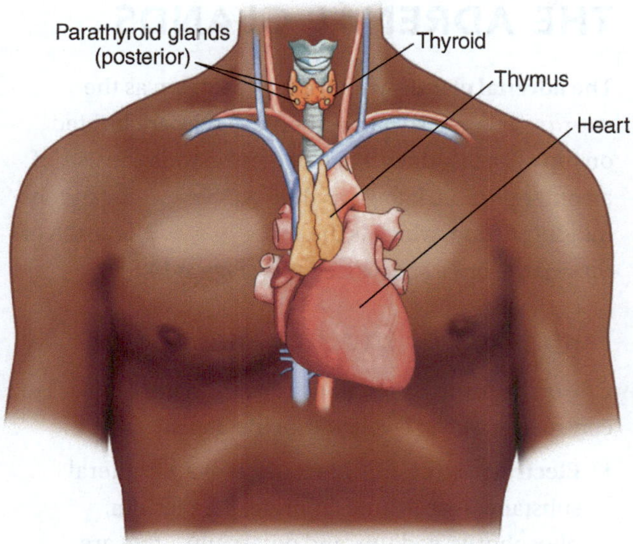

FIGURE 14.4 The thyroid, parathyroid, and thymus glands.

THE THYROID GLAND

The butterfly-shaped **thyroid gland** lies on either side of the larynx, just below the thyroid cartilage (Figure 14.4).

Functions and Secretions of the Thyroid Gland

One of the primary functions of the thyroid gland is to regulate the body's metabolism. The term ***metabolism*** describes all of the processes involved in the body's use of nutrients, including the rate at which they are used. Thyroid secretions also influence growth and the functioning of the nervous system.

- The two primary thyroid hormones regulate the rate of metabolism and affect the growth and rate of function of many other body systems. They are:
  - **Thyroxine** (thigh-**ROCK**-seen) (T_4)
  - **Triiodothyronine** (try-**eye**-oh-doh-**THIGH**-roh-neen) (T_3)
- The rate of secretion of these two hormones is controlled by the *thyroid-stimulating hormone* produced by the anterior lobe of the pituitary gland.
- **Calcitonin** (**kal**-sih-**TOH**-nin), which is produced by the thyroid gland, is a hormone that works with the parathyroid hormone to decrease calcium levels in the blood and tissues by moving calcium into storage in the bones and teeth.

THE PARATHYROID GLANDS

The four **parathyroid glands**, each of which is about the size of a grain of rice, are embedded in the posterior surface of the thyroid gland (Figure 14.4).

Functions and Secretions of the Parathyroid Glands

The primary function of the parathyroid glands is to regulate calcium levels throughout the body. These calcium levels are important to the smooth functioning of the muscular and nervous systems. The secretions of the parathyroid glands include:

- The **parathyroid hormone** (PTH), which works with the hormone *calcitonin* that is secreted by the thyroid gland. Together, they regulate the calcium levels in the blood and tissues.
- Higher-than-normal levels of parathyroid hormone can increase calcium levels in the blood by mobilizing the release of calcium stored in bones and teeth.

THE THYMUS

- The **thymus** (**THIGH**-mus) is located near the midline in the anterior portion of the thoracic cavity. It is posterior to (behind) the sternum and slightly superior to (above) the heart (Figure 14.4).

Functions and Secretions of the Thymus

The thymus functions as part of the endocrine system by secreting a hormone that functions as part of the immune system, helping develop the body's immune system before birth and in childhood. Its function is greatly reduced after puberty, and it slowly turns into fatty tissue. The secretions of the thymus include:

- **Thymosin** (**THIGH**-moh-sin), which plays an important part in the immune system by stimulating the maturation of lymphocytes into T cells (see Chapter 7).

THE PANCREAS

The **pancreas** (**PAN**-kree-as) is a feather-shaped organ located posterior to the stomach that functions as part of both the digestive and the endocrine systems (Figure 14.1).

The **pancreatic islets** (**pan**-kree-**AT**-ick **EYE**-lets) are those parts of the pancreas that have endocrine functions. An ***islet*** is a small isolated mass, or island, of one type of tissue within a larger mass of a different type.

Functions and Secretions of the Pancreatic Islets

The endocrine functions of these islets are to control the blood glucose levels and glucose metabolism throughout the body. The secretions of the pancreatic islets include:

- **Glucose** (**GLOO**-kohs) is the basic form of energy used by the body. Glucose in the bloodstream is also known as ***blood sugar***.
- **Glucagon** (**GLOO**-kah-gon) (GCG) is the hormone secreted by the ***alpha cells*** of the pancreatic islets in response to low levels of glucose in the bloodstream. Glucagon increases the glucose level by stimulating the liver to convert glycogen into glucose for release into the bloodstream. (*Note: Glucagon* and *glycogen* are similar words, and the prefixes **gluc/o** and **glyc/o** both refer to glucose or sugar. It may help to remember that glucagon is a hormone secreted in the pancreas, and glycogen is excess carbohydrate stored in the liver.)
- **Insulin** (**IN**-suh-lin) is the hormone secreted by the ***beta cells*** of the pancreatic islets in response to high levels of glucose in the bloodstream. Insulin functions in two ways:
    1. When energy is needed, insulin allows glucose to enter the cells to be used as energy.
    2. When additional glucose is *not* needed, insulin stimulates the liver to convert glucose into glycogen for storage.

THE ADRENAL GLANDS

The **adrenal glands**, which are also known as the ***suprarenals***, are so named because they are located on top of each kidney. Each of these glands consists of an outer portion, known as the ***adrenal cortex***, and the middle portion, which is the ***adrenal medulla***. Each of these parts has a specialized role (Figure 14.5).

Functions of the Adrenal Glands

One of the primary functions of the adrenal glands is to control electrolyte levels within the body.

- **Electrolytes** (ee-**LECK**-troh-lytes) are mineral substances—calcium, chloride, magnesium, phosphorus, sodium, and potassium—that are normally found in the blood and other bodily fluids.
- Other important functions of the adrenal glands include helping regulate metabolism and interacting with the sympathetic nervous system in response to stress (see Chapter 11).

Secretions of the Adrenal Cortex

- **Androgens** are sex hormones secreted by the gonads, the adrenal cortex, and fat cells.
- **Corticosteroids** (**kor**-tih-koh-**STEHR**-oidz) are the steroid hormones produced by the adrenal cortex. The same term describes synthetically produced equivalents that are administered as medications.
    - **Aldosterone** (al-**DOSS**-ter-ohn) (ALD) is a corticosteroid that regulates the sodium and water levels in the body by increasing sodium reabsorption and potassium excretion by the kidneys. ***Reabsorption*** means returning a substance to the bloodstream.

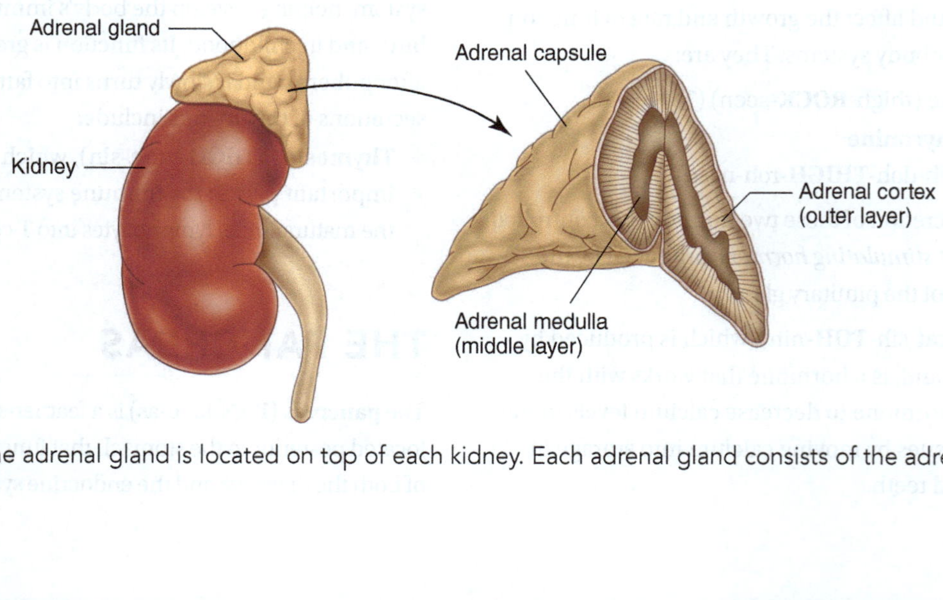

FIGURE 14.5 One adrenal gland is located on top of each kidney. Each adrenal gland consists of the adrenal cortex and adrenal medulla.

- **Cortisol** (**KOR**-tih-sol), also known as *hydrocortisone*, is a corticosteroid that has an anti-inflammatory action. It also helps regulate the metabolism of carbohydrates, fats, and proteins in the body.

Secretions of the Adrenal Medulla

- **Epinephrine** (**ep**-ih-**NEF**-rin) (Epi, EPI), also known as *adrenaline*, stimulates the sympathetic nervous system in response to physical injury or to mental stress such as fear. It makes the heart beat faster and can raise blood pressure. It also helps the liver release glucose and limits the release of insulin.
- **Norepinephrine** (**nor**-ep-ih-**NEF**-rin) is both a hormone and a neurohormone. It is released as a hormone by the adrenal medulla and as a neurohormone by the sympathetic nervous system. It plays an important role in the "fight-or-flight response" by raising blood pressure, strengthening the heartbeat, and stimulating muscle contractions.

THE GONADS

The **gonads** (**GOH**-nadz) are gamete-producing glands. These are ovaries in females and testicles in males.

Functions of the Gonads

The gonads secrete the hormones that are responsible for the development and maintenance of the secondary sex characteristics that develop during puberty. *Secondary sex characteristics* refer to features that distinguish the two sexes but are not directly related to reproduction. The additional functions of the gonads are discussed in Chapter 15.

- **Puberty** (**PYU**-ber-tee) is the process of physical changes by which a child's body becomes an adult body that is capable of reproducing (Figure 14.6). It is marked by maturing of the genital organs, the development of secondary sex characteristics, and the first occurrence of menstruation in the female. In the United States the average age is 12 for girls and 11 for boys.
- *Precocious puberty* is the early onset of the changes of puberty, usually before age 8 in girls and age 9 in boys. *Precocious* means exceptionally early in development or occurrence.

Secretions of the Gonads

- **Estrogen** (**ES**-troh-jen) (E) is a hormone secreted by the ovaries that is important for the development and maintenance of the female secondary sex characteristics and in regulation of the menstrual cycle.
- **Progesterone** (proh-**JES**-ter-ohn) is the hormone released during the second half of the menstrual cycle by the corpus luteum in the ovary. Its function is to complete the preparation of the uterus for possible pregnancy (see Chapter 16).

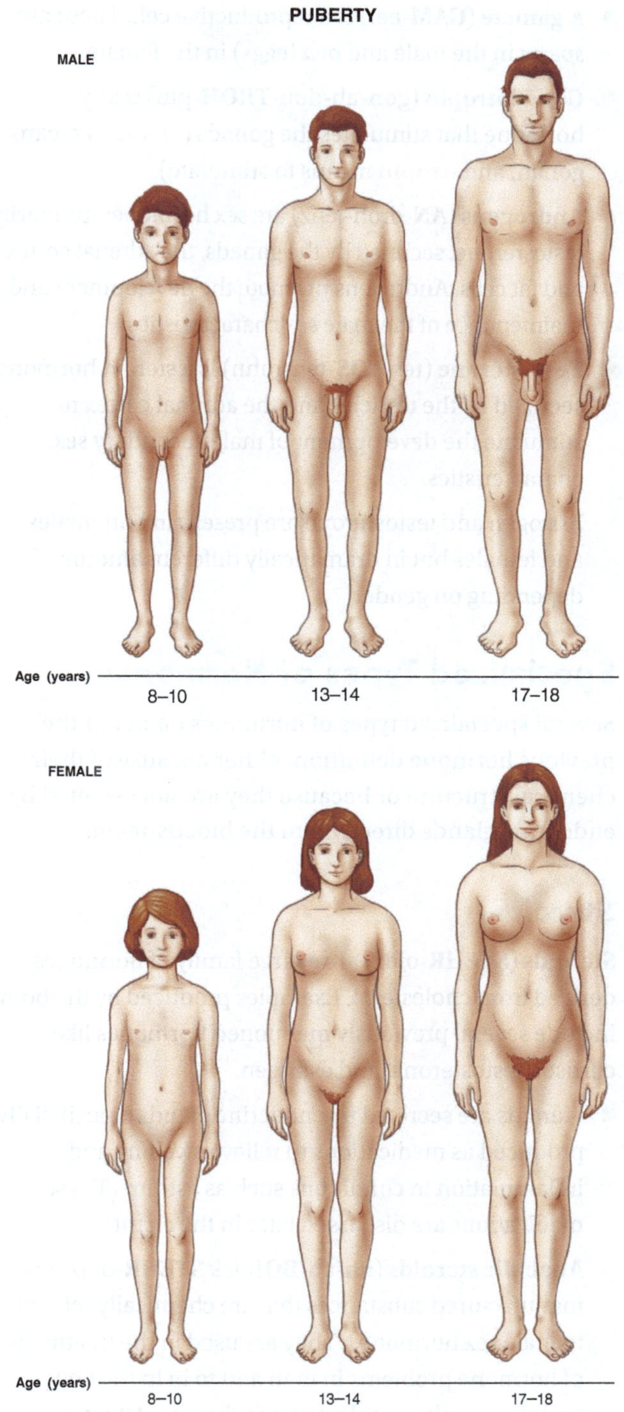

FIGURE 14.6 Puberty is the process through which secondary sex characteristics are gradually developed.

- A **gamete** (**GAM**-eet) is a reproductive cell. These are *sperm* in the male and *ova* (eggs) in the female.
- **Gonadotropin** (**gon**-ah-doh-**TROH**-pin) is any hormone that stimulates the gonads (**gonad/o** means gonad, and **-tropin** means to stimulate).
- **Androgens** (**AN**-droh-jenz) are sex hormones, primarily testosterone, secreted by the gonads, the adrenal cortex, and fat cells. Androgens promote the development and maintenance of the male sex characteristics.
- **Testosterone** (tes-**TOS**-teh-rohn) is a steroid hormone secreted by the testicles and the adrenal cortex to stimulate the development of male secondary sex characteristics.
- Estrogen and testosterone are present in both males and females but in dramatically different amounts depending on gender.

Specialized Types of Hormones

Several specialized types of hormones do not fit the previous hormone definition, either because of their chemical structure or because they are not secreted by endocrine glands directly into the bloodstream.

Steroids

Steroids (**STEHR**-oidz) are a large family of hormones derived from cholesterol. Examples produced by the body include several previously mentioned hormones like cortisol, testosterone, and estrogen.

- Steroids are secreted by endocrine glands or artificially produced as medications to relieve swelling and inflammation in conditions such as asthma. These medications are discussed later in the chapter.
- **Anabolic steroids** (**an**-ah-**BOL**-ick **STEHR**-oidz) are manufactured substances that are chemically related to male sex hormones. They are used in the treatment of hormone problems in men and to help the body replace muscle mass lost due to disease. Athletes may use anabolic steroids illegally to build muscle mass, a dangerous practice that can lead to lasting damage to the body.

Hormones Secreted by Fat Cells

Adipose tissue is not commonly thought of as an endocrine gland; however, research has shown that fat cells do secrete at least one and possibly more hormones that play important roles in the balance and health of the body.

- **Leptin** (**LEP**-tin) is a hormone secreted by fat cells that is involved in the regulation of appetite.
- Leptin leaves the fat cells and travels in the bloodstream to the brain, where it acts on the hypothalamus to suppress appetite and burn fat stored in adipose tissue.
- In contrast, **ghrelin** (**GREL**-in) is a hormone produced in the gastrointestinal tract. Sometimes referred to as the hunger hormone, research is ongoing to flesh out the role that leptin and ghrelin play in rising levels of obesity. Ghrelin is a recent term created from the words **G**rowth **H**ormone **REL**easing with the suffix **-in**.

Neurohormones

Neurohormones (**new**-roh-**HOR**-mohnz) are produced and released by neurons in the brain, rather than by the endocrine glands, and delivered to organs and tissues through the bloodstream. One example is neurohormones secreted by the hypothalamus that control the secretions of the pituitary gland (Figure 14.2).

MEDICAL SPECIALTIES RELATED TO THE ENDOCRINE SYSTEM

- An **endocrinologist** (**en**-doh-krih-**NOL**-oh-jist) is a physician who specializes in diagnosing and treating diseases and malfunctions of the endocrine glands (**endocrin** means to secrete within, and **-ologist** means specialist).
- A **certified diabetes educator** (CDE) is a health care professional qualified to teach people with diabetes how to manage their disease.

PATHOLOGY OF THE ENDOCRINE SYSTEM

The Pituitary Gland

- **Acromegaly** (**ack**-roh-**MEG**-ah-lee) is a rare hormonal disorder characterized by abnormal enlargement of the extremities (hands and feet) caused by the excessive secretion of growth hormone *after* puberty (**acr/o** means extremities, and **-megaly** means enlargement). Contrast with *gigantism*.
- **Gigantism** (jigh-**GAN**-tiz-em) is abnormal growth of the entire body that is caused by excessive secretion of growth hormone *before* puberty. Contrast with *acromegaly*.

- **Hyperpituitarism** (**high**-per-pih-**TOO**-ih-tah-rizm) is the excess secretion of growth hormone that causes both acromegaly and gigantism (**hyper-** means excessive, **pituitar** means pituitary, and **-ism** means condition). This condition is usually caused by a pituitary adenoma.
- **Hypopituitarism** (**high**-poh-pih-**TOO**-ih-tah-rizm) is a condition in which the pituitary gland does not produce enough growth hormone (**hypo-** means deficient, **pituitar** means pituitary, and **-ism** means condition). This is one of the causes of **short stature**, formerly known as *dwarfism* (see Chapter 3).
- A **pituitary adenoma** (pih-**TOO**-ih-**tair**-ee ad-eh-**NOH**-mah) is also known as a ***pituitary tumor***. This is a slow-growing benign tumor of the pituitary gland. ***Functional*** pituitary tumors often produce hormones in large and unregulated amounts. These hormones might include ACTH, growth hormones, prolactin, or TSH.
- **Galactorrhea** is a condition in which an excess of prolactin causes the breasts to produce milk spontaneously, not due to childbirth (see Chapter 16).
- A **prolactinoma** (proh-**lack**-tih-**NOH**-mah) is a benign functional pituitary tumor (**pro-** means on behalf of, **lactin** means milk, and **-oma** means tumor). This type of tumor causes the pituitary gland to produce too much of the lactogenic hormone known as prolactin. It can cause infertility in women, erectile dysfunction in men, and can also impair vision.

Antidiuretic Hormone Conditions

- **Diabetes insipidus** (**dye**-ah-**BEE**-teez in-**SIP**-ih-dus) (DI), which is not related to *diabetes mellitus*, is an uncommon disorder caused by an insufficient production of the antidiuretic hormone ADH or by the inability of the kidneys to respond appropriately to this hormone. This causes an imbalance of fluids in the body, leading to extreme thirst and frequent urination.
- **Syndrome of inappropriate antidiuretic hormone** (SIADH) is caused by the overproduction of the antidiuretic hormone ADH. This is often as a result of cancer or its treatment. High amounts of ADH keep the kidneys from excreting water, resulting in bloating and water retention that can dilute the blood, causing electrolyte imbalances, particularly hyponatremia (low levels of sodium).

The Pineal Gland

- A **pinealoma** (pin-ee-ah-**LOH**-mah) is a tumor of the pineal gland that can disrupt the production of melatonin (**pineal** means pineal gland, and **-oma** means tumor). This tumor can also cause insomnia by disrupting the circadian cycle.

The Thyroid Gland

Thyroid carcinoma is the most common cancer of the endocrine system and is the most rapidly increasing cancer in the United States. Thyroid carcinoma, which has a high survival rate, affects significantly more women than men and is commonly diagnosed between ages 20 and 55.

Insufficient Thyroid Secretion

- **Hypothyroidism** (**high**-poh-**THIGH**-roid-izm), also known as an ***underactive thyroid***, is caused by a deficiency of thyroid secretion (**hypo-** means deficient, **thyroid** means thyroid, and **-ism** means condition). Symptoms include fatigue, depression, sensitivity to cold, and a decreased metabolic rate.
- **Hashimoto's disease** (hah-shee-**MOH**-tohz), also known as ***Hashimoto's thyroiditis***, is an autoimmune disease in which the body's own antibodies attack and destroy the cells of the thyroid gland. This inflammation often leads to hypothyroidism.
- **Cretinism** (**CREE**-tin-izm) is a congenital form of hypothyroidism. If thyroid hormone replacement is not started soon after birth, cretinism causes arrested physical and mental development.
- **Myxedema** (**mick**-seh-**DEE**-mah), which is also known as ***adult hypothyroidism***, is caused by an extreme deficiency of thyroid secretion. Symptoms include swelling, particularly around the eyes and cheeks, fatigue, and a subnormal temperature.

Excessive Thyroid Secretion

- **Hyperthyroidism** (**high**-per-**THIGH**-roid-izm), also known as ***thyrotoxicosis***, is the overproduction of thyroid hormones (**hyper-** means excessive, **thyroid** means thyroid, and **-ism** means condition), which causes an imbalance of metabolism. This causes symptoms including an increased metabolic rate, sweating, nervousness, and weight loss. The most common cause of hyperthyroidism is Graves' disease.
- **Graves' disease** (**GRAYVZ**) (GD) is a disorder of unknown cause in which the immune system attacks the thyroid gland and stimulates it to make excessive amounts of thyroid hormone. This results in hyperthyroidism and can also cause goiter, exophthalmos, or both.

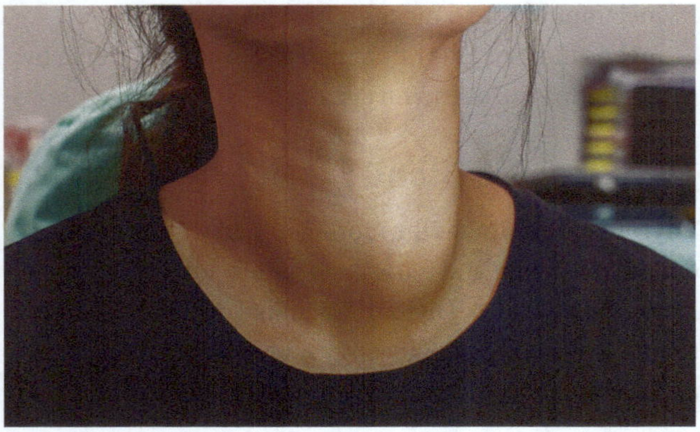

FIGURE 14.7 Graves' disease can cause goiter.

- **Goiter** (**GOI**-ter), also known as *thyromegaly*, is an abnormal, benign enlargement of the thyroid gland (**thyr/o** means thyroid, and **-megaly** means abnormal enlargement) (Figure 14.7). This enlargement produces a swelling in the front of the neck. A goiter usually occurs when the thyroid gland is not able to produce enough thyroid hormone to meet the body's needs, either due to Graves' disease, other medical conditions, or an iodine deficiency.
- **Exophthalmos** (**eck**-sof-**THAL**-mos) is an abnormal protrusion of the eyeball out of the orbit (**ex-** means out, **ophthalm/o** means eye, and **-s** is a noun ending).
- *Thyroid nodules* are lumps in the thyroid that can grow large enough to cause a goiter. Most nodules are benign; however, some are malignant or produce too much thyroxine.
- A **thyroid storm**, also known as a *thyrotoxic crisis*, is a relatively rare, life-threatening condition caused by exaggerated hyperthyroidism. Patients experiencing a thyroid storm may complain of fever, chest pain, palpitations, shortness of breath, tremors, increased sweating, disorientation, and fatigue.

The Parathyroid Glands

- **Hyperparathyroidism** (**high**-per-**par**-ah-**THIGH**-roid-izm), which is the overproduction of the parathyroid hormone, causes the condition known as hypercalcemia (**hyper-** means excessive, **parathyroid** means parathyroid, and **-ism** means condition). Hyperparathyroidism can result from a disorder of the parathyroid gland or from a disorder elsewhere in the body, such as kidney failure. Hyperparathyroidism is the opposite of *hypoparathyroidism*.
- **Hypoparathyroidism** (**high**-poh-**par**-ah-**THIGH**-roid-izm) is caused by an insufficient or absent secretion of the parathyroid hormone (**hypo-** means deficient, **parathyroid** means parathyroid, and **-ism** means condition). This condition causes hypocalcemia, and in severe cases, it leads to tetany. *Tetany* is the condition of periodic, painful muscle spasms and tremors. Hypoparathyroidism is the opposite of *hyperparathyroidism*.
- **Hypercalcemia** (**high**-per-kal-**SEE**-mee-ah) is characterized by abnormally *high* concentrations of calcium circulating in the blood instead of being stored in the bones and teeth (**hyper-** means excessive, **calc** means calcium, and **-emia** means blood condition). This can lead to weakened bones and the formation of kidney stones. Hypercalcemia is the opposite of *hypocalcemia*.
- **Hypocalcemia** (**high**-poh-kal-**SEE**-mee-ah) is characterized by abnormally *low* levels of calcium in the blood (**hypo-** means deficient, **calc** means calcium, and **-emia** means blood condition). Hypocalcemia is the opposite of *hypercalcemia*.

The Thymus

- **Myasthenia gravis**, discussed on Chapter 4, can be characterized by an abnormally large thymus, with or without a **thymoma**, a tumor on the thymus.

The Pancreas

- An **insulinoma** (**in**-suh-lin-**OH**-mah) is a benign tumor of the pancreas that secretes additional insulin, causing hypoglycemia (low blood glucose) (**insulin** means insulin, and **-oma** means tumor).
- **Pancreatitis** (**pan**-kree-ah-**TYE**-tis) is an inflammation of the pancreas (**pancreat** means pancreas, and **-itis** means inflammation). Alcohol abuse is a leading cause of pancreatitis.

Abnormal Blood Glucose Levels

- **Hyperglycemia** (**high**-per-glye-**SEE**-mee-ah) is an abnormally high concentration of glucose in the blood (**hyper-** means excessive, **glyc** means sugar, and **-emia** means blood condition). Hyperglycemia is seen primarily in patients with diabetes mellitus. The symptoms include polydipsia, polyphagia, and polyuria. Hyperglycemia is the opposite of *hypoglycemia*.

- **Polydipsia** (**pol**-ee-**DIP**-see-ah) is excessive thirst (**poly-** means many, and **-dipsia** means thirst).
- **Polyphagia** (**pol**-ee-**FAY**-jee-ah) is excessive hunger (**poly-** means many, and **-phagia** means eating).
- **Polyuria** (**pol**-ee-**YOU**-ree-ah) is excessive urination (**poly-** means many, and **-uria** means urination).

- **Hyperinsulinism** (**high**-per-**IN**-suh-lin-izm) is the condition of excessive secretion of insulin in the bloodstream (**hyper-** means excessive, **insulin** means insulin, and **-ism** means condition). Hyperinsulinism can cause hypoglycemia.
- **Hypoglycemia** (**high**-poh-glye-**SEE**-mee-ah) is an abnormally low concentration of glucose (sugar) in the blood (**hypo-** means deficient, **glyc** means sugar, and **-emia** means blood condition). Symptoms include nervousness and shakiness, confusion, perspiration, or feeling anxious or weak. Hypoglycemia is the opposite of *hyperglycemia*.

Diabetes Mellitus

Diabetes mellitus (**dye**-ah-**BEE**-teez **MEL**-ih-tus) (DM), the most common endocrine system disease, is a group of metabolic disorders characterized by hyperglycemia resulting from defects in the body's production of insulin (type 1) or its ability to use it properly (type 2). *Diabetes mellitus* is not related to *diabetes insipidus*.

- These conditions are classified as type 1, type 2, and latent autoimmune diabetes in adults.
- In the past, when a child developed diabetes, this condition was referred to as ***juvenile diabetes***; however, the condition in children is now described as being either type 1 or type 2.
- The treatment goals for all types of diabetes are to effectively control blood glucose levels and prevent complications.

Type 1 Diabetes

Type 1 diabetes is an autoimmune insulin deficiency disorder caused by the destruction of pancreatic islet beta cells. ***Insulin deficiency*** means that the pancreatic beta cells do not secrete enough insulin. For more information about autoimmune disorders, see Chapter 7.

- Symptoms of type 1 diabetes include polydipsia, polyphagia, polyuria, weight loss, blurred vision, extreme fatigue, and slow healing.
- The onset of type 1 diabetes is often triggered by a viral infection.
- Treatment for type 1 diabetes involves a combination of diet, exercise, and carefully regulated ***insulin replacement therapy*** administered by injection or insulin pump (Figure 14.8). An ***insulin pump*** is a small computerized device attached to the body designed to deliver insulin continuously into the subcutaneous tissue in the abdomen.

Type 2 Diabetes

Type 2 diabetes is an insulin resistance disorder. ***Insulin resistance*** means that insulin is being produced, but the body does not use it effectively. In an attempt to compensate for this lack of response, the body secretes more insulin. With the rise of childhood obesity, type 2 diabetes is increasingly common in children and young adults. Obese adults are also at high risk for this condition.

- **Prediabetes** is a condition in which the blood glucose level is higher than normal, but not high enough to be classified as type 2 diabetes. However, this condition indicates an increased risk of developing type 2 diabetes, heart disease, and stroke.

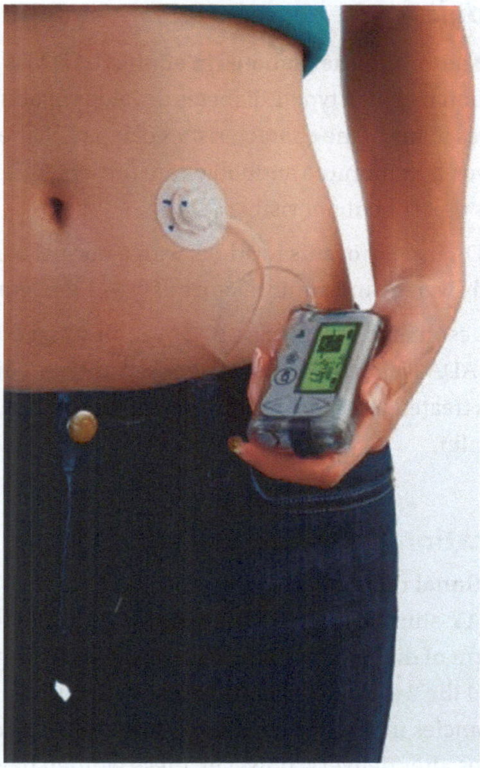

Photo courtesy of Medtronic, Inc.

FIGURE 14.8 An insulin pump can be worn on the patient's pants, administering controlled insulin replacement therapy.

A person with type 2 diabetes might be asymptomatic for years. ***Asymptomatic*** means showing no symptoms. When symptoms do occur, they include those of type 1 diabetes listed above plus recurring infections, irritability, and a tingling sensation in the hands or feet. ***Metabolic syndrome***, which increases a person's risk of heart disease, stroke, and type 2 diabetes, is discussed in Chapter 2.

- Treatment for type 2 diabetes usually includes diet, exercise, and oral medications, which might include the following:
  - A low glycemic index diet, using the ***glycemic index*** to consume foods that will not raise the blood sugar more than necessary.
  - ***Oral hypoglycemics***, which lower blood glucose by causing the pancreas to release more insulin or by increasing the body's sensitivity to insulin.
  - ***Metformin***, which works within the cells to combat insulin resistance and to help insulin let blood glucose into the cells.
  - Depending on the severity of symptoms, insulin replacement therapy may also be prescribed.

Latent Autoimmune Diabetes in Adults

Latent autoimmune diabetes in adults (LADA) is a condition in which type 1 diabetes develops in adults. It shares many of the characteristics of type 2 diabetes; however, autoimmune antibodies are present. ***Latent*** means present but not visible.

- LADA usually occurs in adults with a normal or low body weight and family history of type 1 diabetes.
- It is estimated that at least 10% of adult-onset diabetes is LADA which can be misdiagnosed as type 2 diabetes. It is treated with diet, exercise, oral medications, and insulin.

Gestational Diabetes Mellitus

Gestational diabetes mellitus (jes-**TAY**-shun-al **dye**-ah-**BEE**-teez **MEL**-ih-tus) (GDM) is a form of diabetes mellitus with onset occurring around the 24th week of approximately 2–10% of pregnancies in the United States. This condition usually resolves after delivery; however, these women have an increased risk of developing type 2 diabetes later in life.

Diabetic Emergencies

Diabetic emergencies are due to either too high or too low levels of blood glucose. Treatment depends on accurately diagnosing the cause of the emergency (Figures 14.9A and 14.9B).

- A **diabetic coma** is caused by very high blood glucose (hyperglycemia) or very low blood glucose (hypoglycemia) resulting in a stupor or coma. This causes a person to become unconscious and can be fatal if untreated.
- **Diabetic ketoacidosis** (**kee**-toh-**ah**-seh-**DOH**-sis) (DKA) is a life-threatening diabetes complication caused by a buildup of acids (called ketones) in the blood. Treatment includes the administration of insulin and the replacement of fluids and electrolytes.
- **Severe hypoglycemia**, which is also known as ***insulin shock***, ***diabetic shock***, or ***insulin reaction***, is caused by very low blood glucose levels. ***Oral glucose***, in the format of tablets, gel, or liquid, is a sugary substance that can quickly be absorbed into the bloodstream. This is consumed to rapidly raise the blood sugar level. Alternatively, the hormone glucagon can be administered via injection if the person is unable to take glucose by mouth.

Diabetic Complications

Most diabetic complications result from the damage to capillaries and other blood vessels due to long-term exposure to excessive blood glucose.

- **Diabetic retinopathy** (**ret**-ih-**NOP**-ah-thee) occurs when diabetes damages the tiny blood vessels in the retina. This causes blood to leak into the posterior segment of the eyeball and produces the damage that causes the loss of vision (see Chapter 12).
- ***Heart disease*** occurs because excess blood glucose makes the walls of the blood vessels sticky and rigid. This encourages hypertension and atherosclerosis (see Chapter 5) and increases the risk of stroke (see Chapter 11).
- **Ketosis** (kee-**TOH**-sis) is a normal metabolic process that helps the body utilize stored fat when other sources of energy are lacking. An excessively high level of ketosis may indicate that the body is not producing enough insulin to convert glucose into energy. A ***ketogenic diet*** which is high in fat and low in carbohydrates has been shown to be helpful in managing epileptic seizures.

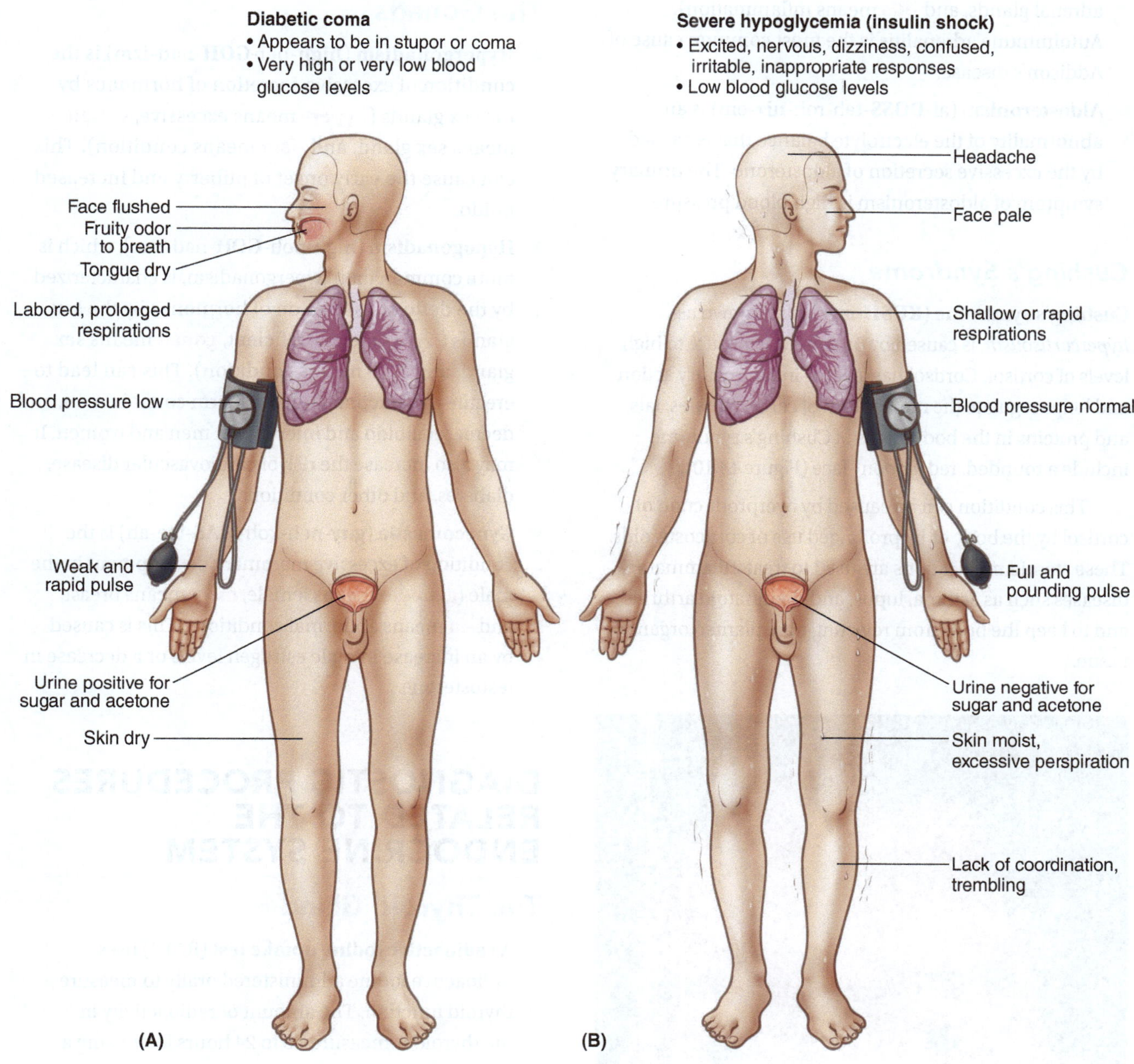

FIGURE 14.9 (A) Diabetic coma. (B) Severe hypoglycemia (insulin shock).

- ***Kidney disease*** can lead to renal failure because damage to the blood vessels reduces blood flow through the kidneys (see Chapter 10).
- ***Peripheral neuropathy*** is damage to the nerves affecting the hands and feet which makes it harder to feel a cut or other injury (see Chapter 11).
- Poorly controlled blood glucose can also slow wound healing and increase the likelihood of wound infections. This can make minor injuries worse and lead to ulcers and gangrene, requiring amputation, particularly in the feet and legs.

The Adrenal Glands

- **Addison's disease** (**AD**-ih-sonz) occurs when the adrenal glands do not produce enough of the hormones cortisol or aldosterone. This potentially life-threatening condition is characterized by chronic, worsening fatigue and muscle weakness; loss of appetite; low blood pressure; and weight loss. Many patients also develop patches of dark skin.
- **Adrenalitis** (ah-**dree**-nal-**EYE**-tis) is inflammation of one or both of the adrenal glands (**adrenal** means

adrenal glands, and **-itis** means inflammation). Autoimmune adrenalitis is the most common cause of Addison's disease.

- **Aldosteronism** (al-**DOSS**-teh-roh-**niz**-em) is an abnormality of the electrolyte balance that is caused by the excessive secretion of aldosterone. The primary symptom of aldosteronism is high blood pressure.

Cushing's Syndrome

Cushing's syndrome (**KUSH**-ingz), also known as *hypercortisolism*, is caused by prolonged exposure to high levels of cortisol. Cortisol has an anti-inflammatory action and helps regulate the metabolism of carbohydrates, fats, and proteins in the body. Signs of Cushing's syndrome include a rounded, red "moon" face (Figure 14.10).

This condition can be caused by overproduction of cortisol by the body or by prolonged use of corticosteroids. These steroid medications are used to treat inflammatory diseases such as asthma, lupus, and rheumatoid arthritis and to keep the body from rejecting transplanted organs or tissue.

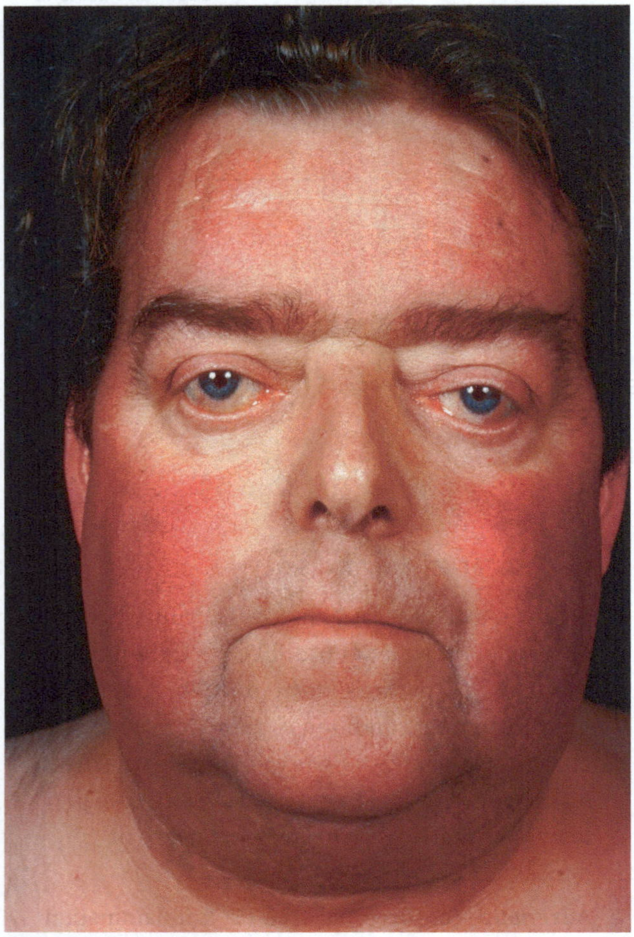

Biophoto Associates/Science Source

FIGURE 14.10 Cushing's syndrome causes a characteristic rounded, red "moon" face.

The Gonads

- **Hypergonadism** (**high**-per-**GOH**-nad-izm) is the condition of excessive secretion of hormones by the sex glands (**hyper-** means excessive, **gonad** means sex gland, and **-ism** means condition). This can cause the early onset of puberty and increased libido.
- **Hypogonadism** (**high**-poh-**GOH**-nad-izm), which is more common than hypergonadism, is characterized by the deficient secretion of hormones by the sex glands (**hypo-** means deficient, **gonad** means sex gland, and **-ism** means condition). This can lead to erectile dysfunction and low sperm count in men, and decreased libido and infertility in men and women. It may also increase the risk of cardiovascular disease, diabetes, and other conditions.
- **Gynecomastia** (**guy**-neh-koh-**MAS**-tee-ah) is the condition of excessive mammary development in the male (**gynec/o** means female, **mast** means breast, and **-ia** means abnormal condition). This is caused by an increase in male estrogen levels or a decrease in testosterone.

DIAGNOSTIC PROCEDURES RELATED TO THE ENDOCRINE SYSTEM

The Thyroid Gland

- A **radioactive iodine uptake test** (RAIU) uses radioactive iodine administered orally to measure thyroid function. The amount of radioactivity in the thyroid is measured 6 to 24 hours later using a handheld instrument called a gamma probe.
- A **thyroid-stimulating hormone assay** is a diagnostic test to measure the circulating blood level of TSH. This test is used to detect abnormal thyroid activity resulting from excessive pituitary stimulation.
- A **thyroid scan**, which measures thyroid function, is a form of nuclear medicine that is discussed in Chapter 21.

Diabetes Mellitus

- A **fasting blood sugar test** (FBS), also known as a *fasting plasma glucose test*, measures the blood glucose levels after the patient has not eaten for 8 to 12 hours. This test is used to screen for diabetes as well as to monitor treatment of this condition.

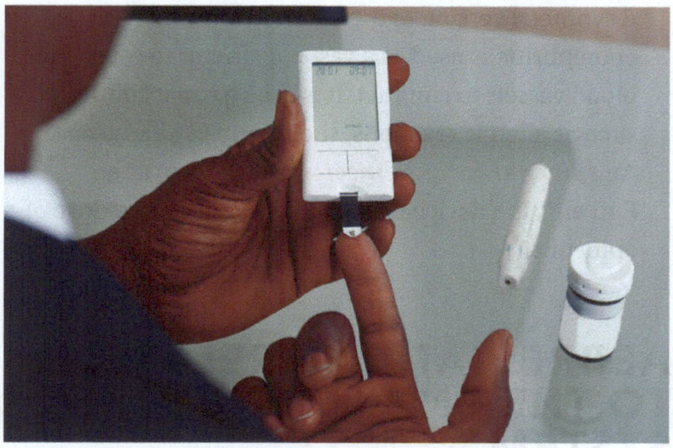

FIGURE 14.11 Home blood glucose monitoring allows the patient to measure their blood glucose level multiple times per day.

- An **oral glucose tolerance test** (OGTT) is most commonly performed to diagnose type 2 or gestational diabetes. After fasting at least eight hours, the patient has a baseline blood draw, then drinks a liquid containing a high concentration of sugar, and the blood glucose level is tested after one hour and again after two hours.
- **Home blood glucose monitoring** measures the current blood glucose level using a drop of blood and is often performed by the patient multiple times per day (Figure 14.11).
- **Continuous glucose monitoring** (CGM) is a method of tracking glucose levels 24 hours a day through a tiny sensor inserted under the skin on the abdomen or arm. The sensor measures the glucose levels in the cellular fluid just under the skin, with data continuously transmitted wirelessly to a smartphone or other device. An alert signals when glucose levels are too high or low.
- **Hemoglobin A1c testing**, also known as ***HbA1c***, pronounced as "H-B A-one-C," is a blood test that measures the average blood glucose level over the previous three to four months. (*Note:* The name of this test is sometimes shortened to *A1c.*)
- **The fructosamine test** (fruck-**TOHS**-ah-meen) measures average glucose levels over the previous three weeks. The fructosamine test is able to detect changes more rapidly than the HbAlc test.

TREATMENT PROCEDURES RELATED TO THE ENDOCRINE SYSTEM

The Pituitary Gland

- The **human growth hormone** (HGH) is a synthetic version of the growth hormone that is administered to stimulate growth when the natural supply of growth hormone is insufficient for normal development. This drug is sometimes abused by athletes in an attempt to increase lean body mass and decrease body fat.
- A **hypophysectomy** (high-**pof**-ih-**SECK**-toh-mee) is the surgical removal of the pituitary gland, performed to treat cancerous or benign tumors (**hypophys** refers to the pituitary gland, and **-ectomy** means removal). This surgery is performed through the nose or an opening in the skull.

The Thyroid Gland

- An **antithyroid drug** is a medication administered to slow the ability of the thyroid gland to produce thyroid hormones.
- **Radioactive iodine treatment** (RAI) is the oral administration of radioactive iodine to destroy thyroid cells. This nuclear medicine procedure, which disables at least part of the thyroid gland, is used to treat thyroid cancer and chronic hyperthyroid disorders such as Graves' disease. For more information on nuclear medicine, see Chapter 21.
- A **lobectomy** (loh-**BECK**-toh-mee) is the surgical removal of one lobe of the thyroid gland. This term is also used to describe the removal of a lobe of the liver, brain, or lung.
- **Thyroid replacement therapy** is the use of ***synthetic thyroid hormones***, which are oral medications administered to replace lost thyroid function.

The Parathyroid Glands

- A **parathyroidectomy** (**par**-ah-**thigh**-roi-**DECK**-toh-mee), which is the surgical removal of one or more of the parathyroid glands, is performed to control hyperparathyroidism or remove parathyroid tumors (**parathyroid** means parathyroid glands, and **-ectomy** means surgical removal).

The Thymus

- A **thymectomy** (thigh-**MECK**-toh-mee) is the surgical removal of the thymus gland (**thym** means thymus, and **-ectomy** means surgical removal).

The Pancreas

- A **pancreatectomy** (**pan**-kree-ah-**TECK**-toh-mee) is the surgical removal of all or part of the pancreas (**pancreat** means pancreas, and **-ectomy** means surgical removal).

A ***total pancreatectomy*** is performed to treat pancreatic cancer. This procedure also involves removing the spleen, gallbladder, common bile duct, and portions of the small intestine and stomach.

The Adrenal Glands

- A **laparoscopic adrenalectomy** (**lap**-ah-roh-**SKOP**-ick ah-**dree**-nal-**ECK**-toh-mee) is a minimally invasive surgical procedure to remove one or both adrenal glands (**adrenal** means adrenal gland, and **-ectomy** means surgical removal).
- **Cortisone** (**KOR**-tih-sohn) is the synthetic equivalent of corticosteroids produced by the adrenal glands. Cortisone, and the synthetic corticosteroid ***prednisone***, are administered to suppress inflammation and as an immunosuppressant (see Chapter 7).
- A synthetic version of the adrenal hormone epinephrine is used as a vasoconstrictor to cause the blood vessels to contract. It is used to treat conditions such as allergic reactions, shock, and cardiac arrest. An ***epinephrine autoinjector***, also known as an EpiPen®, is a device used to inject a measured dose of epinephrine.

ABBREVIATIONS RELATED TO THE ENDOCRINE SYSTEM

Table 14.1 presents an overview of the abbreviations related to the terms introduced in this chapter. *Note:* To avoid errors or confusion, always be cautious when using abbreviations.

TABLE 14.1

Abbreviations Related to the Endocrine System

adrenocorticotropic hormone = ACTH	**ACTH** = adrenocorticotropic hormone
aldosterone = ALD	**ALD** = aldosterone
antidiuretic hormone = ADH	**ADH** = antidiuretic hormone
diabetic ketoacidosis = DKA	**DKA** = diabetic ketoacidosis
diabetes mellitus = DM	**DM** = diabetes mellitus
epinephrine = EPI, Epi	**EPI, Epi** = epinephrine
fasting blood sugar = FBS	**FBS** = fasting blood sugar
follicle-stimulating hormone = FSH	**FSH** = follicle-stimulating hormone
Graves' disease = GD	**GD** = Graves' disease
human growth hormone = HGH	**HGH** = human growth hormone
latent autoimmune diabetes in adults = LADA	**LADA** = latent autoimmune diabetes in adults
oral glucose tolerance test = OGTT	**OGTT** = oral glucose tolerance test
radioactive iodine treatment = RAI	**RAI** = radioactive iodine treatment
thyroid-stimulating hormone = TSH	**TSH** = thyroid-stimulating hormone

CHAPTER 14

LEARNING EXERCISES

Matching Word Parts 1

Write the correct answer in the middle column.

	Definition	Correct Answer	Possible Answers
14.1.	adrenal glands	______________	acr/o
14.2.	extremities	______________	adren/o
14.3.	ovaries or testicles	______________	crin/o
14.4.	thirst	______________	-dipsia
14.5.	to secrete	______________	gonad/o

Matching Word Parts 2

Write the correct answer in the middle column.

	Definition	Correct Answer	Possible Answers
14.6.	condition	______________	pituitar/o
14.7.	pancreas	______________	pineal/o
14.8.	parathyroid glands	______________	parathyroid/o
14.9.	pineal gland	______________	pancreat/o
14.10.	pituitary gland	______________	-ism

Matching Word Parts 3

Write the correct answer in the middle column.

	Definition	Correct Answer	Possible Answers
14.11.	body	______________	thym/o
14.12.	many	______________	thyroid/o

14.13. sugar	______________________	somat/o
14.14. thyroid	______________________	poly-
14.15. thymus	______________________	glyc/o

Definitions

Select the correct answer, and write it on the line provided.

14.16. The ______________________ hormone stimulates ovulation in the female.

estrogen | follicle-stimulating | lactogenic | luteinizing

14.17. The ______________________ gland secretes hormones that control the activity of the other endocrine glands.

adrenal | hypothalamus | pituitary | thymus

14.18. The ______________________ hormone stimulates the growth and secretions of the adrenal cortex.

adrenocorticotropic | growth | melanocyte-stimulating | thyroid-stimulating

14.19. The ______________________ gland functions as part of the endocrine system by secreting a hormone that functions as part of the immune system.

adrenal | parathyroid | pineal | thymus

14.20. The ______________________ hormone works with the parathyroid hormone to decrease calcium levels in the blood and tissues.

aldosterone | calcitonin | glucagon | leptin

14.21. Cortisol is secreted by the ______________________.

adrenal cortex | adrenal medulla | pituitary gland | thyroid gland

14.22. The amount of glucose in the bloodstream is increased by the hormone ______________________.

adrenaline | glucagon | hydrocortisone | insulin

14.23. Norepinephrine is secreted by the ______________________.

adrenal cortex | adrenal medulla | pancreatic islets | pituitary gland

14.24. The hormone ______________________ stimulates uterine contractions during childbirth.

estrogen | oxytocin | progesterone | testosterone

14.25. The development of the male secondary sex characteristics is stimulated by the hormone

____________________.

parathyroid pitocin progesterone testosterone

Matching Structures

Write the correct answer in the middle column.

	Definition	Correct Answer	Possible Answers
14.26.	controls blood glucose levels	____________________	thyroid gland
14.27.	controls the activity of other endocrine glands	____________________	pituitary glands
14.28.	influences the sleep–wakefulness cycle	____________________	pineal gland
14.29.	regulates electrolyte levels	____________________	pancreatic islets
14.30.	stimulates metabolism	____________________	adrenal glands

Which Word?

Select the correct answer, and write it on the line provided.

14.31. The hormonal disorder that results from too much growth hormone in adults is known

as ____________________.

acromegaly gigantism

14.32. The growth hormone is secreted by the ____________________ lobe of the pituitary gland.

anterior posterior

14.33. Type 2 diabetes is an ____________________ disorder.

insulin deficiency insulin resistance

14.34. Insufficient production of ADH causes ____________________.

diabetes insipidus Graves' disease

14.35. ____________________ is caused by prolonged exposure to high levels of cortisol.

Addison's disease Cushing's syndrome

Spelling Counts

Find the misspelled word in each sentence. Then write that word, spelled correctly, on the line provided.

14.36. The lutinizing hormone stimulates ovulation in the female. ______

14.37. Diabetes mellitas is a group of diseases characterized by defects in insulin secretion, insulin action, or both. ______

14.38. Myxedemia is also known as adult hypothyroidism. ______

14.39. The hormone progestarone is released during the second half of the menstrual cycle. ______

14.40. Thymoxin is secreted by the thymus gland. ______

Abbreviation Identification

In the space provided, write the words that each abbreviation stands for.

14.41. **ACTH** ______

14.42. **ADH** ______

14.43. **DM** ______

14.44. **FBS** ______

14.45. **FSH** ______

Term Selection

Select the correct answer, and write it on the line provided.

14.46. A rare, life-threatening condition caused by exaggerated hyperthyroidism is called ______.

thyroid nodules | goiter | thyroid storm | Graves' disease

14.47. The condition known as ______ is characterized by abnormally high concentrations of calcium circulating in the blood instead of being stored in the bones.

hypercalcemia | hyperthyroidism | hypocalcemia | polyphagia

14.48. The four ______________ glands, each of which is about the size of a grain of rice, are embedded in the posterior surface of the thyroid gland.

adrenal | pancreatic | parathyroid | pineal

14.49. A/An ______________ is a benign tumor of the pituitary gland that causes it to produce too much prolactin.

insuloma | thymoma | pituitary adenoma | prolactinoma

14.50. The average blood glucose levels over the past three weeks is measured by the ______________ test.

blood glucose monitoring | fructosamine | glucose tolerance | hemoglobin A1c

Sentence Completion

Write the correct term on the line provided.

14.51. The mineral substances known as ______________ are found in the blood and include sodium and potassium.

14.52. The two primary hormones secreted by the thyroid gland are triiodothyronine (T_3) and ______________ (T_4).

14.53. Damage to the retina of the eye caused by diabetes mellitus is known as diabetic ______________.

14.54. The medical specialist who treats disorders of the endocrine system is known as a/an ______________.

14.55. Abnormal protrusion of the eye out of the orbit is known as ______________.

Word Surgery

Divide each term into its component word parts. Write these word parts, in sequence, on the lines provided. When necessary, use a slash (/) to indicate a combining vowel. (You may not need all of the lines provided.)

14.56. **Hyperpituitarism** is the excess secretion of growth hormone by the pituitary gland, causing acromegaly and gigantism.

______ ______ ______ ______

14.57. **Homeostasis** is the process through which the body maintains a constant internal environment.

__________ __________ __________ __________

14.58. **Hyperinsulinism** is the condition of excessive secretion of insulin in the bloodstream.

__________ __________ __________ __________

14.59. **Gynecomastia** is the condition of excessive mammary development in the male.

__________ __________ __________ __________

14.60. **Hypocalcemia** is characterized by abnormally low levels of calcium in the blood.

__________ __________ __________ __________

True/False

If the statement is true, write **True** on the line. If the statement is false, write **False** on the line.

14.61. ________ The beta cells of the pancreatic islets secrete glucagon in response to low blood glucose levels.

14.62. ________ Hyperglycemia is a life-threatening diabetes complication caused by a buildup of acids.

14.63. ________ The hormone melatonin is secreted by the adrenal cortex.

14.64. ________ An insulinoma is a malignant tumor of the pancreas that causes hypoglycemia by secreting insulin.

14.65. ________ Polyuria is excessive urination.

Clinical Conditions

Write the correct answer on the line provided.

14.66. During his nursing studies, Rodney Milne learned that the ____________________ helps control blood pressure by reducing the amount of water that is excreted through the kidneys.

14.67. Eduardo Chavez complained of being thirsty all the time. His doctor noted this excessive thirst on his chart as ____________________.

14.68. Mrs. Wei's symptoms included chronic, worsening fatigue, muscle weakness, loss of appetite, and weight loss because her adrenal glands do not produce enough cortisol. Her doctor diagnosed this condition as ____________________.

14.69. Linda Thomas was diagnosed as having a/an ______________________. This is a benign tumor of the pancreas that causes hypoglycemia by secreting insulin.

14.70. Patrick Edward has the autoimmune disorder known as ______________________ in which the body's own antibodies attack and destroy the cells of the thyroid gland.

14.71. Because Joe Dean's ultimate goal was to swim in the Olympics, he was tempted to make illegal use of ______________________ steroids to increase his strength and muscle mass.

14.72. Holly Yates was surprised to learn that ______________________, which is a hormone secreted by fat cells, travels to the brain and controls the balance of food intake and energy expenditure.

14.73. As a result of a congenital lack of thyroid secretion, the Vaugh-Eames child suffers from ______________________, which is a condition of arrested physical and mental development.

14.74. Ray Grovenor is excessively tall and large. This condition, which was caused by excessive secretion of growth hormone before puberty, is known as ______________________.

14.75. Rosita DeAngelis required the surgical removal of her pancreas. The medical term for this procedure is a/an ______________________.

Which Is the Correct Medical Term?

Select the correct answer, and write it on the line provided.

14.76. Hormone(s) called ______________________ is/are produced and released by neurons in the brain, rather than by the endocrine glands, and delivered to organs and tissues through the bloodstream.

oxytocin neurohormones neurotransmitters steroids

14.77. A ______________________ is a slow-growing, benign tumor of the pituitary gland.

hyperpituitarism hypophysectomy pituitary adenoma prolactinoma

14.78. ______________________ disease, which is an autoimmune disorder caused by hyperthyroidism, is often characterized by goiter, exophthalmos, or both.

Addison's Cushing's Graves' Hashimoto's

14.79. The diabetic emergency caused by very high blood glucose causing a person to become unconscious is a/an ______________________.

diabetic coma | severe hypoglycemia | insulin shock | insuloma

14.80. The hormone ______________________, which is secreted by the pineal gland, influences the sleep–wakefulness cycle.

glucagon | melatonin | parathyroid | thymosin

Challenge Word Building

These terms are *not* found in this chapter; however, they are made up of the following familiar word parts. If you need help in creating the term, refer to your medical dictionary.

endo-	**adren/o**	**-emia**
	crin/o	**-itis**
	insulin/o	**-megaly**
	pancreat/o	**-ology**
	pineal/o	**-oma**
	thym/o	**-otomy**
	thyroid/o	**-pathy**

14.81. The term meaning any disease of the adrenal glands is ______________________.

14.82. The study of endocrine glands and their secretions is known as ______________________.

14.83. Abnormal enlargement of the adrenal glands is known as ______________________.

14.84. The term meaning any disease of the thymus gland is ______________________.

14.85. Inflammation of the thyroid gland is known as ______________________.

14.86. A surgical incision into the pancreas is a/an ______________________.

14.87. A surgical incision into the thyroid gland is a/an ______________________.

14.88. The term meaning any disease of the pineal gland is ______________________.

14.89. Abnormally high levels of insulin in the blood are known as ______________________.

14.90. Inflammation of the adrenal glands is known as ______________________.

Labeling Exercises

Identify the numbered items on the accompanying figure.

14.91. ______________________ gland

14.92. ______________________ glands

14.93. ______________________ gland

14.94. ______________________ of the female

14.95. ______________________

14.96. ______________________ gland

14.97. ______________________ gland

14.98. ______________________ glands

14.99. ______________________ islets

14.100. ______________________ of the male

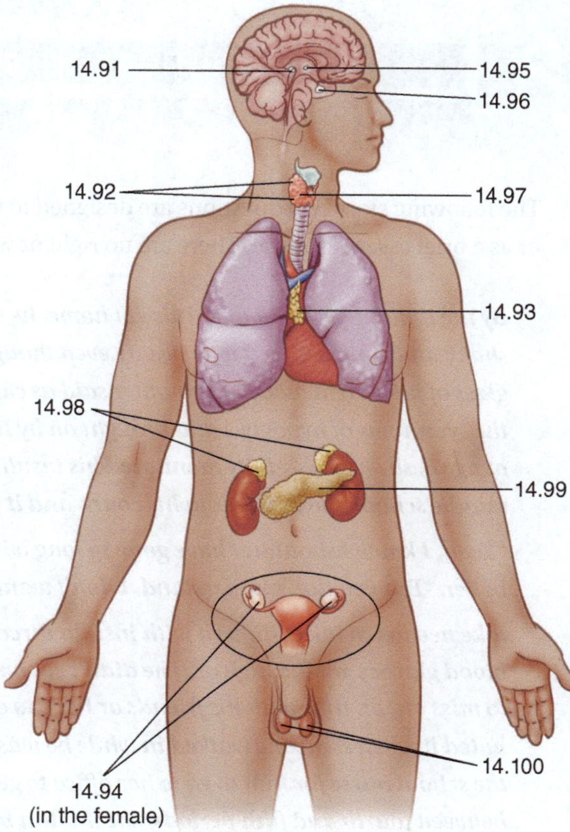

The Human Touch

CRITICAL THINKING EXERCISE

The following story and questions are designed to stimulate critical thinking through class discussion or as a brief essay response. There are no right or wrong answers to these questions.

By the time 14-year-old Jake Tuls got home, he was sick enough for his mom to notice. He seemed shaky and confused and was sweaty even though the fall weather was cool. "Jake, let's get you a glass of juice right away," his mother said as calmly as she could. She was all too familiar with the symptoms of hypoglycemia brought on by Jake's type 1 diabetes. Ever since he was diagnosed at age 6, she had carefully monitored his insulin, eating, and exercise. But now that he was in middle school, the ball was in his court, and it really worried her that he often seemed to mess up.

"Yeah, I know I shouldn't have gone so long without eating," Jake muttered once he was feeling better. "But you don't understand. I don't want to be different from the other kids."

Jake needed to inject himself with insulin three times a day. He knew what happened when his blood glucose got too high or if he didn't eat on schedule and it got too low. But he didn't want to miss out on time with his friends or have to eat what his mom packed him for lunch. And he hated it when someone walked in while he was injecting. His mom had made arrangements with the school nurse for him to go to her office to get some privacy, and whenever he didn't show up between fourth and fifth periods, she made a big deal about having to come into the classroom to get him.

He was tired of having this disease, sick of shots, and angry that he could not sleep late and skip meals like other kids. He made a face at his mother as she sat down to call the school nurse, and turned on the TV.

Suggested Discussion Topics

1. Why is it more difficult for Jake to maintain his injection routine in middle school than it was in elementary school?
2. Knowing that missing an insulin injection could cause a diabetic coma and possibly death, why do you think Jake is not more conscientious in his self-care?
3. Do you think Jake's schoolmates talk about him, or does he just think they do? Discuss both possibilities. What steps can Jake take to help his classmates understand his condition?
4. An insulin pump or continuous glucose monitor might be an option for Jake. What are some of the factors that will help his doctor decide if he's a good candidate?

CHAPTER 15

THE MALE REPRODUCTIVE SYSTEM

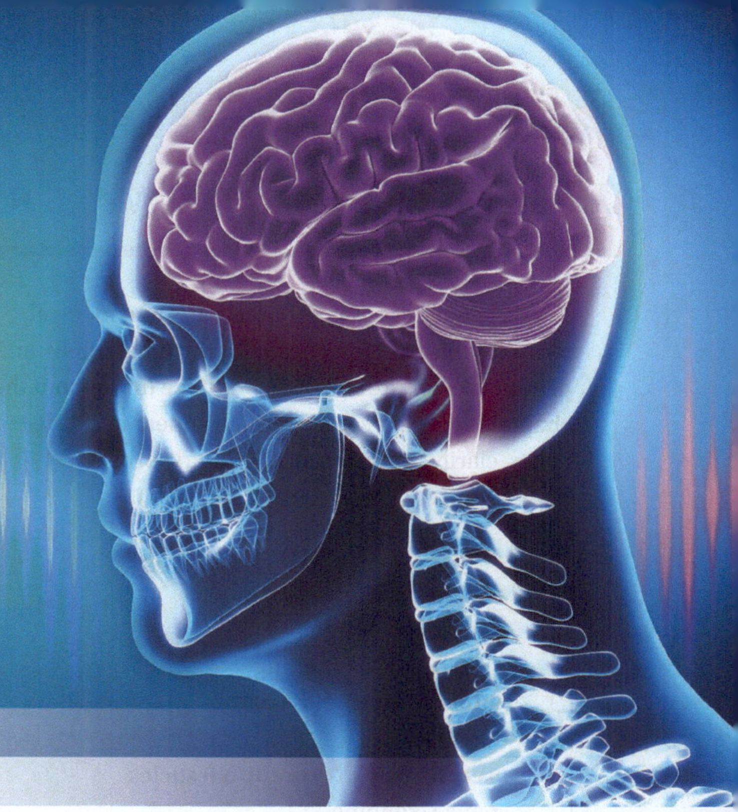

Overview of

STRUCTURES, COMBINING FORMS, AND FUNCTIONS OF THE MALE REPRODUCTIVE SYSTEM

Major Structures	Related Combining Forms	Primary Functions
Penis	**pen/i, phall/i**	Used for sexual intercourse and urination.
Testicles	**orch/o, orchid/o, test/i**	Produce spermatozoa and the hormone testosterone.
Spermatozoa	**sperm/o, spermat/o**	These male gametes are necessary for the fertilization of an ovum.

Vocabulary Related to THE MALE REPRODUCTIVE SYSTEM

This list contains essential word parts and medical terms for this chapter. These and the other important **primary terms** are shown in **boldface** throughout the chapter. *Secondary terms*, which appear in *orange* italics, clarify the meaning of primary terms.

Word Parts

- ☐ **andr/o** male, masculine
- ☐ **balan/o** glans penis
- ☐ **-cele** hernia or swelling
- ☐ **epididym/o** epididymis
- ☐ **olig/o** few
- ☐ **orch/o, orchid/o, orchi/o** testicles
- ☐ **-pause** stopping
- ☐ **pen/i** penis
- ☐ **phall/i** penis
- ☐ **prostat/o** prostate gland
- ☐ **semin/i** semen, sperm
- ☐ **sperm/o, spermat/o** spermatozoa
- ☐ **test/i** testicle, testis
- ☐ **varic/o** varicose veins
- ☐ **venere/o** venereal, sexual intercourse

Medical Terms

- ☐ **androgen replacement therapy** (**AN**-droh-jen)
- ☐ **andrologist** (an-**DROL**-oh-jist)
- ☐ **azoospermia** (ay-**zoh**-oh-**SPER**-mee-ah)
- ☐ **balanitis** (**bal**-ah-**NIGH**-tis)
- ☐ **bilateral orchiectomy** (bye-**LAT**-er-ahl or-key-**EK**-toh-mee)
- ☐ **bulbourethral glands** (**bul**-boh-you-**REE**-thral)
- ☐ **chancre** (**SHANK**-er)
- ☐ **chlamydia** (klah-**MID**-ee-ah)
- ☐ **circumcision** (**ser**-kum-**SIZH**-un)
- ☐ **cryopreservation**
- ☐ **cryptorchidism** (krip-**TOR**-kih-dizm)
- ☐ **ejaculation** (eh-**jack**-you-**LAY**-shun)
- ☐ **ejaculatory duct**
- ☐ **epididymitis** (**ep**-ih-did-ih-**MY**-tis)
- ☐ **erectile dysfunction**
- ☐ **foreskin**
- ☐ **gamete** (**GAH**-meet)
- ☐ **genital herpes** (**HER**-peez)
- ☐ **genitourinary** (**jen**-ih-toh-**YOUR**-in-air-ee)
- ☐ **glans penis** (**GLANZ PEE**-nis)
- ☐ **gonorrhea** (**gon**-oh-**REE**-ah)
- ☐ **hematospermia** (**hee**-mah-toh-**SPER**-mee-ah)
- ☐ **human immunodeficiency virus**
- ☐ **human papillomavirus** (pa-pih-**LOH**-mah)
- ☐ **hydrocele** (**HIGH**-droh-seel)
- ☐ **inguinal hernia** (**ING**-gwih-nal)
- ☐ **male hypogonadism** (**high**-poh-**GOH**-nad-izm)
- ☐ **orchiectomy** (**or**-kee-**ECK**-toh-mee)
- ☐ **oligospermia** (**ol**-ih-goh-**SPER**-mee-ah)
- ☐ **orchiopexy** (**or**-kee-oh-**PECK**-see)
- ☐ **penis** (**PEE**-nis)
- ☐ **perineum** (pehr-ih-**NEE**-um)
- ☐ **Peyronie's disease** (pay-roh-**NEEZ**)
- ☐ **phimosis** (fih-**MOH**-sis)
- ☐ **priapism** (**PRYE**-ah-**piz**-em)
- ☐ **prostate gland** (**PROS**-tayt)
- ☐ **pubic lice**
- ☐ **scrotum** (**SKROH**-tum)
- ☐ **semen** (**SEE**-men)
- ☐ **seminal vesicles** (**SEM**-ih-nal)
- ☐ **seminiferous tubules** (**see**-mih-**NIF**-er-us **TOO**-byouls)
- ☐ **sexually transmitted diseases**
- ☐ **sexually transmitted infections**
- ☐ **sperm count**
- ☐ **spermatogenesis** (**sper**-mah-toh-**JEN**-eh-sis)
- ☐ **spermatozoa** (**sper**-mah-toh-**ZOH**-ah)
- ☐ **syphilis** (**SIF**-ih-lis)
- ☐ **testes** (**TEH**-steez)
- ☐ **testicular torsion**
- ☐ **testis** (**TEH**-stis)
- ☐ **testosterone** (tes-**TOS**-teh-rohn)
- ☐ **trichomoniasis** (**trick**-oh-moh-**NYE**-ah-sis)
- ☐ **urethral meatus** (mee-**ATE**-is)
- ☐ **urologist** (you-**ROL**-oh-jist)
- ☐ **varicocele** (**VAR**-ih-koh-**seel**)
- ☐ **vas deferens** (**VAS DEF**-er-enz)
- ☐ **vasectomy** (vah-**SECK**-toh-mee)
- ☐ **vasovasostomy** (**vay**-soh-vah-**ZOS**-toh-mee)
- ☐ **varicocelectomy** (**var**-ih-koh-sih-**LECK**-toh-mee)
- ☐ **venereologist** (veh-**neer**-ee-**OL**-oh-jist)

LEARNING OBJECTIVES

On completion of this chapter, you should be able to:

1. Describe the major functions and structures of the male reproductive system.
2. Identify the medical specialists who treat disorders of the male reproductive system.
3. Identify the medical word parts of the male reproductive system.
4. Define the primary terms related to the pathology and the diagnostic and treatment procedures of the male reproductive system.
5. Compare and contrast the most common sexually transmitted diseases.
6. Spell the primary terms of the male reproductive system.
7. Pronounce the primary terms of the male reproductive system.
8. Define common abbreviations related to the male reproductive system.
9. Define abbreviations used for sexually transmitted diseases.

FUNCTIONS OF THE MALE REPRODUCTIVE SYSTEM

The primary function of the male reproductive system is to produce sperm and deliver them into the female body so that one sperm can unite with a single ovum (egg) to create a new life. Some structures of the male reproductive system also function as part of the urinary system. These are discussed in Chapter 10.

STRUCTURES OF THE MALE REPRODUCTIVE SYSTEM

- The *external male genitalia* are the penis and the scrotum, which contains two testicles.
- The *internal male genitalia* include the remaining structures of the male reproductive system (Figures 15.1 and 15.2).

The Scrotum and Testicles

The **scrotum** (**SKROH**-tum) is the sac-like structure that surrounds, protects, and supports the testicles. The scrotum is suspended from the pubic arch behind the penis and lies between the thighs. The area between the scrotum and anus is called the **perineum** (pehr-ih-**NEE**-um).

The **testicles**, also known as **testes** (**TEH**-steez), are the two small, egg-shaped glands that produce the sperm. The singular of testes is **testis** (**TEH**-stis). These glands develop within the abdomen of the male fetus and normally descend into the scrotum before or soon after birth.

- Sperm are formed within the **seminiferous tubules** (**see**-mih-**NIF**-er-us **TOO**-byouls) of each testicle (Figure 15.2).
- The **epididymis** (**ep**-ih-**DID**-ih-mis) is a coiled tube at the upper part of each testicle. This tube runs down the length of the testicle, then turns upward toward the body. Here, it narrows to form the tube known as the *vas deferens*.
- The **spermatic cord** extends upward from the epididymis and is attached to each testicle. Each cord contains a vas deferens plus the arteries, veins, nerves, and lymphatic vessels required by each testicle.
- **Testosterone** (tes-**TOS**-teh-rohn) is a steroid hormone secreted by the testicles and the adrenal cortex (see Chapter 14).
- **Androgens** (**AN**-droh-jens) are male sex hormones. Testosterone and androstenedione are the principal androgens. Androgens are present in both men and women; however, they normally occur in much higher levels in men.

Semen Formation

Spermatozoa (**sper**-mah-toh-**ZOH**-ah), also known as **sperm**, are the male gametes necessary to fertilize a female gamete. A **gamete** (**GAH**-meet) is a male or female reproductive cell, that is, a sperm or an ovum. The singular of spermatozoa is *spermatozoon.*

- **Semen** (**SEE**-men) is the whitish fluid containing sperm that is ejaculated through the urethra at the peak of male sexual excitement. The verb

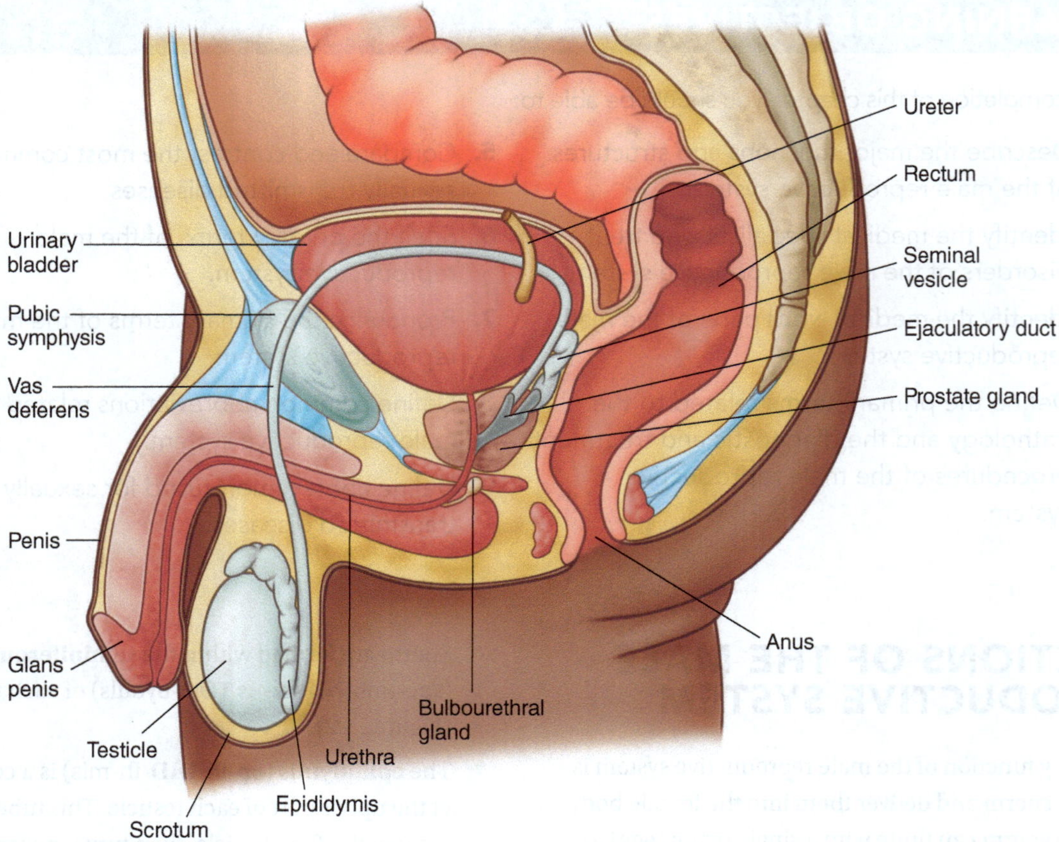

FIGURE 15.1 Organs and ducts of the male reproductive system shown in a lateral cross-section view.

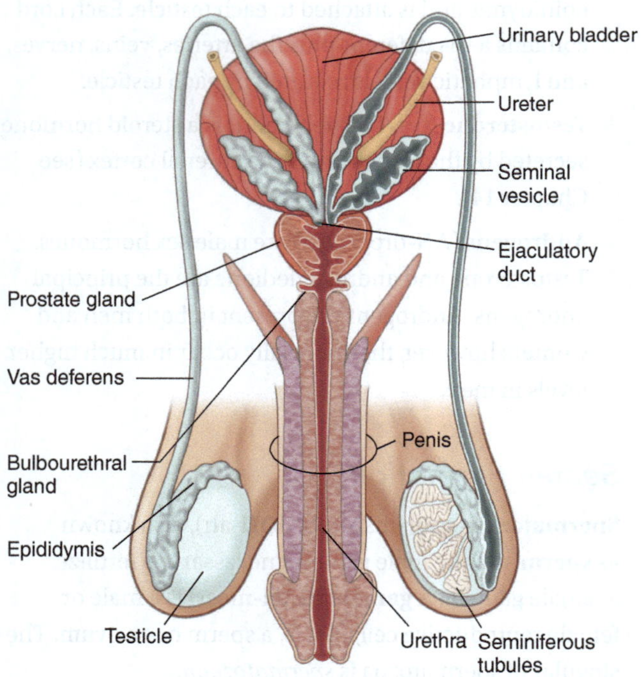

FIGURE 15.2 Structures of the male reproductive system as shown in an anterior cross-section view.

ejaculate (eh-**JACK**-you-**late**) means to expel suddenly, and the noun *ejaculate* (eh-**JACK**-you-**lat**) is another word for semen. Note that the verb and noun are spelled the same way.

- **Spermatogenesis** (**sper**-mah-toh-**JEN**-eh-sis) is the process of sperm formation (**spermat/o** means sperm, and **-genesis** means creation).
- The ideal temperature for sperm formation is 93.2°F. The scrotum aids in maintaining this temperature by adjusting how closely it holds the testicles to the body.
- Sperm are formed in the seminiferous tubules of the testicles.
- From here, the sperm move into the epididymis, where they become motile and are temporarily stored. *Motile* means capable of movement.
- From the epididymis, the sperm travel upward into the body and enter the vas deferens. Here, the seminal vesicles and the prostate gland add their secretions to form semen.

The Penis

The **penis** (**PEE**-nis) is the male sex organ that transports the sperm out of the body. The penis is composed of three columns of erectile tissue (Figures 15.1 and 15.2).

- During sexual stimulation, the erectile tissue fills with blood under high pressure. This causes the swelling, hardness, and stiffness known as an *erection*.
- The adjectives *penile* and *phallic* both mean relating to the penis (both **pen/i** and **phall/i** mean penis).
- The **glans penis** (**GLANZ PEE**-nis), also known as the *head of the penis*, is the sensitive region located at the tip of the penis (Figure 15.1).
- The **urethral meatus** (mee-**ATE**-is) is the external opening for the urethra at the tip of the glans penis.
- The **foreskin**, also known as the *prepuce*, is a retractable double-layered fold of skin and mucous membrane that covers and protects the glans penis.

The Vas Deferens, Seminal Vesicles, and Ejaculatory Duct

The **vas deferens** (**VAS DEF**-er-enz), also known as the *ductus deferens*, are the long, narrow continuations of each epididymis. These structures lead upward and eventually join the urethra (Figures 15.1 and 15.2). *Vas* means vessel, and *deferens* is a Latin term meaning carrying down.

- The **seminal vesicles** (**SEM**-ih-nal) are glands that secrete a thick, yellow substance to nourish the sperm cells. This secretion forms 60% of the fluid found in semen. These glands are located at the base of the urinary bladder and open into the vas deferens as it joins the urethra.
- The **ejaculatory duct**, which begins at the vas deferens, passes through the prostate gland and empties into the urethra. During ejaculation, which is a reflex action caused by these ducts, semen passes into the urethra, which exits the body via the penis. **Ejaculation**(eh-**jack**-you-**LAY**-shun) is the act of discharging semen from the body.

The Prostate Gland

The **prostate gland** (**PROS**-tayt) lies under the bladder and surrounds the end of the urethra in the region where the vas deferens enters the urethra (Figures 15.1 and 15.2).

During ejaculation, the prostate gland secretes a thick, alkaline fluid into the semen that aids the motility of the sperm. *Motility* means ability to move independently. Disorders and treatment of the prostate gland are discussed in Chapter 10.

The Bulbourethral Glands

The two **bulbourethral glands** (**bul**-boh-you-**REE**-thral) are located just below the prostate gland. One of these glands is located on either side of the urethra, and they open into the urethra (Figures 15.1 and 15.2).

During sexual arousal, these glands secrete a fluid known as *pre-ejaculate* or *precum*. This fluid helps flush out any residual urine or foreign matter in the urethra. It also lubricates the urethra for sperm to pass through. This fluid can contain sperm and is able to cause pregnancy even if ejaculation does not occur.

The Urethra

The **urethra** passes through the penis to the outside of the body. In the male, the urethra serves both the reproductive and the urinary systems. Disorders of the urethra are discussed in Chapter 10.

MEDICAL SPECIALTIES RELATED TO THE MALE REPRODUCTIVE SYSTEM

- An **andrologist** (an-**DROL**-oh-jist) is a doctor focusing on the treatment of conditions affecting male fertility and sexuality (**andr** means male, and **-ologist** means specialist).
- A **urologist** (you-**ROL**-oh-jist) is a physician who specializes in diagnosing and treating diseases and disorders of the genitourinary system of males and the urinary system of females (**ur** means urine, and **-ologist** means specialist). The term **genitourinary** (**jen**-ih-toh-**YOUR**-in-air-ee) means relating to both the genital and urinary organs (**genit/o** means reproduction, **urin** means urine, and **-ary** means pertaining to).
- A **venereologist** (veh-**neer**-ee-**OL**-oh-jist) is a doctor who specializes in the treatment of sexually transmitted diseases and infections (**venere** means venereal, and **-ologist** means specialist).

PATHOLOGY OF THE MALE REPRODUCTIVE SYSTEM

The Penis

- **Balanitis** (bal-ah-**NIGH**-tis) is an inflammation of the glans penis that is usually caused by poor hygiene in men who have not had the foreskin removed by circumcision (**balan** means glans penis, and **-itis** means inflammation).

- *Epispadias* and *hypospadias* are congenital abnormalities of the urethral opening on the penis (see Chapter 10).
- **Phimosis** (fih-**MOH**-sis) is a narrowing of the opening of the foreskin so it cannot be retracted (pulled back) to expose the glans penis. This condition can be present at birth or become apparent during childhood.
- **Erectile dysfunction** (ED), also known as *impotence*, is the inability of the male to achieve or maintain a penile erection. A penis that is not erect is referred to as being *flaccid*, or limp.
- **Male hypogonadism** (**high**-poh-**GOH**-nad-izm) is also known as a *testosterone deficiency*. Deficient secretions from the gonads (see Chapter 14) can cause symptoms that may include impaired sexual development or erectile dysfunction, depending on the age of onset (**hypo-** means deficient, **gonad** means gonad, and **-ism** means condition).
- **Peyronie's disease** (pay-roh-**NEEZ**) (PD), also known as *penile curvature*, is a form of sexual dysfunction in which the penis is bent or curved during erection. This condition is usually the result of fibrous scar tissue inside the penis. It is named after the 18th-century French surgeon François Gigot de la Peyronie.
- **Priapism** (**PRYE**-ah-**piz**-em) is a painful and persistent erection that lasts four hours or more, but is either not caused by sexual excitement or does not go away after sexual stimulation has ended. The condition can be caused by medications or by blood-related diseases such as sickle cell anemia or leukemia.
- **Premature ejaculation** is a condition in which the male reaches climax too soon, usually before or shortly after penetration. *Penetration* during vaginal intercourse refers to the penis entering the vagina.

The Testicles and Related Structures

- Andropause (**AN**-droh-pawz), a condition sometimes referred to as *male menopause*, is marked by the decrease of the male hormone testosterone (**andr/o** means masculine, and **-pause** means stopping). This gradual hormonal change usually begins when a man is in his 40s, and can cause low energy, depression, a reduction in muscle mass, and difficulty sleeping or concentrating.
- **Cryptorchidism** (krip-**TOR**-kih-dizm), also known as an *undescended testicle*, is a developmental defect seen in newborns in which one or both of the testicles have failed to descend into their normal position in the scrotum (**crypt** means hidden, **orchid** means testicle, and **-ism** means abnormal condition).
- **Epididymitis** (**ep**-ih-did-ih-**MY**-tis) is a painful inflammation of the epididymis resulting from a bacterial infection (**epididym** means epididymis, and **-itis** means inflammation). The most common cause is sexually transmitted diseases such as gonorrhea or chlamydia; however, urinary tract infections can also cause epididymitis (Figure 15.3A).
- A **hydrocele** (**HIGH**-droh-seel) is a fluid-filled sac in the scrotum along the spermatic cord leading from the testicles (**hydr/o** means relating to water, and **-cele** means a hernia or swelling). It is most common in newborns, especially premature infants, and usually disappears without treatment. *Note:* The term *hydrocele* is also used to describe the accumulation of fluid in any body cavity.
- **Testicular cancer** is cancer that originates in the testicles. It is the most common cancer in American men between the ages of 15 and 35 years. This cancer is highly treatable at all stages.
  - Almost all testicular cancer originates with a **germ cell tumor**, usually in the testicles. *Germ cells* are the sperm- or egg-producing cells. In women, germ cell tumors can occur in the ovaries.
- **Testicular torsion** is the twisting of the spermatic cord leading into the testicle, causing sharp pain in the scrotum. *Torsion* means twisting.
- **Orchitis** (or-**KYE**-tis), also known as *testitis*, is inflammation of one or both testicles (**orch** means testicle, and **-itis** means inflammation) (Figure 15.3B).
- A **varicocele** (**VAR**-ih-koh-**seel**) is a knot of widening varicose veins in one side of the scrotum (**varic/o** means varicose veins, and **-cele** means a hernia or swelling). This is can lead to low sperm production and male infertility. *Varicose veins* are abnormally swollen veins (Figure 15.3C) that can also occur in the legs and feet.

Hernias

An **inguinal hernia** (**ING**-gwih-nal), also called a *groin hernia*, is a protrusion of tissue, often part of the small intestine, through the inguinal canal. The *inguinal canal* is a passage through the abdominal wall on either side of the midline through which the spermatic cord passes. The term *inguinal* means referring to the groin.

- Inguinal hernias, which can occur from muscle strain or the progressive weakening of the abdominal muscles with age, sometimes extend into the scrotum, causing pain and swelling. See Figure 15.4.
- Congenital inguinal hernias in male infants are more common in those born prematurely.

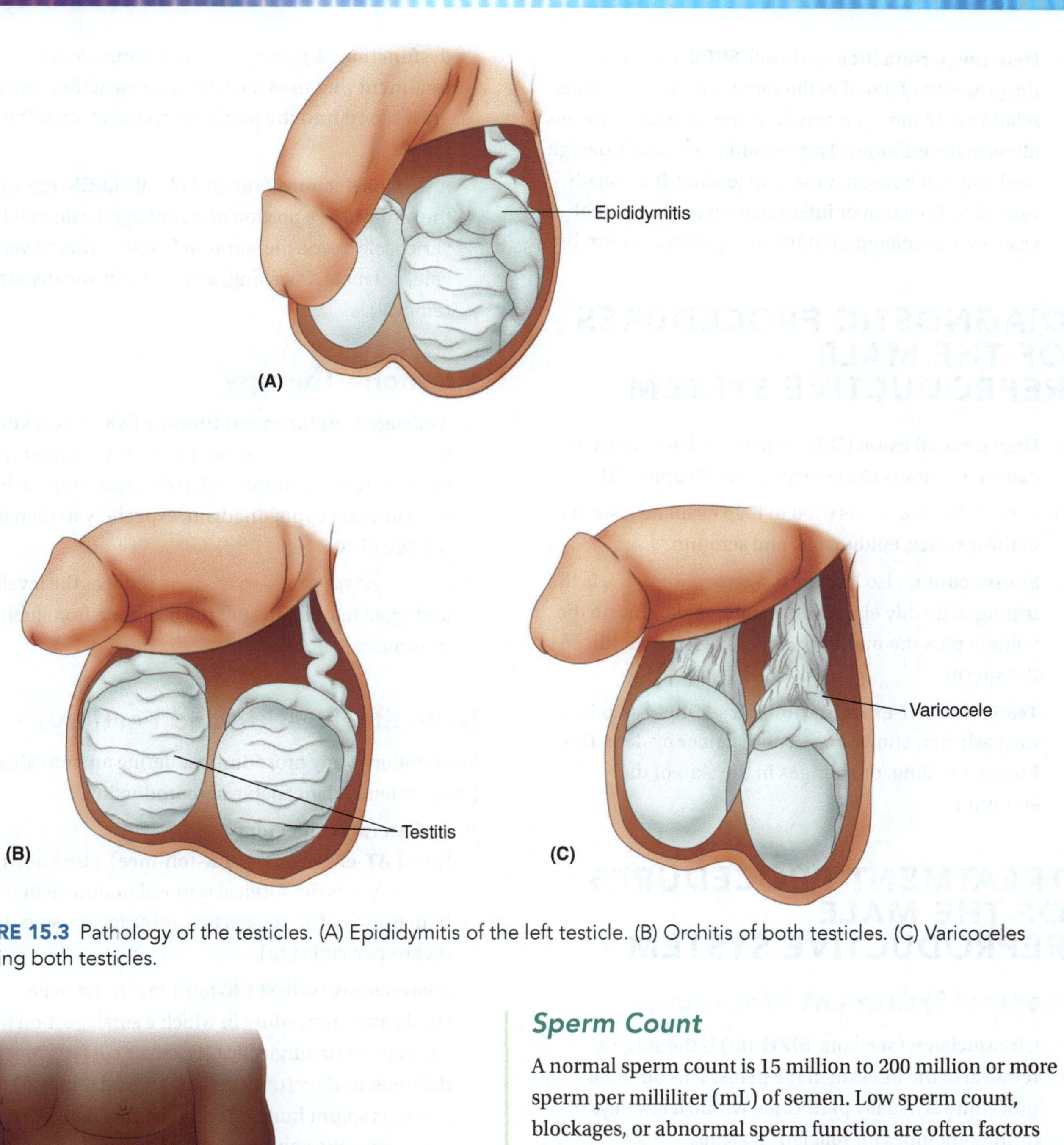

FIGURE 15.3 Pathology of the testicles. (A) Epididymitis of the left testicle. (B) Orchitis of both testicles. (C) Varicoceles affecting both testicles.

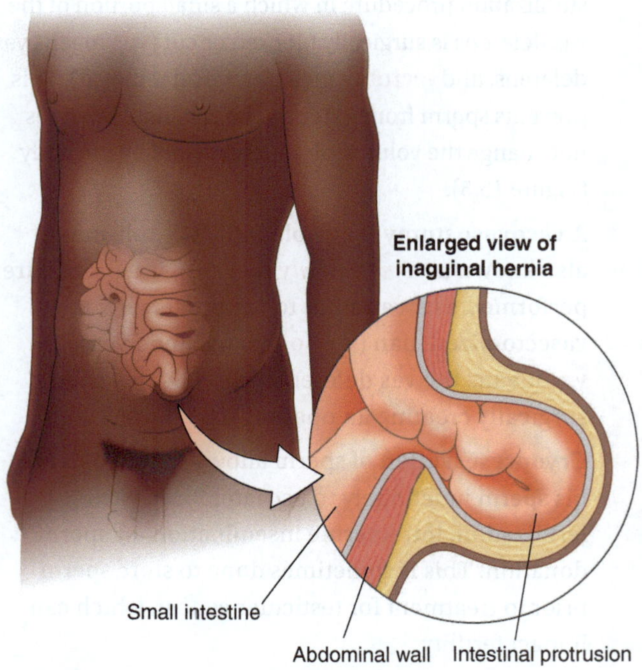

FIGURE 15.4 An inguinal hernia.

Sperm Count

A normal sperm count is 15 million to 200 million or more sperm per milliliter (mL) of semen. Low sperm count, blockages, or abnormal sperm function are often factors in male infertility. ***Male infertility*** is defined as the inability to conceive a child after a year or more of unprotected sexual intercourse.

- **Azoospermia** (ay-**zoh**-oh-**SPER**-mee-ah) is the absence of sperm in the semen (**a-** means without, **zoo** means (animal) life, **sperm** means sperm, and **-ia** means abnormal condition). This may be caused by the testicles not producing sperm normally or by a problem preventing the sperm from reaching the penis.
- **Oligospermia** (**ol**-ih-goh-**SPER**-mee-ah) is a sperm count of below 15 million/mL (**olig/o** means few, **sperm** means sperm, and **-ia** means abnormal condition). This is also known as a ***low sperm count*** and is a common cause of male infertility.

- **Hematospermia** (**hee**-mah-toh-**SPER**-mee-ah) is the presence of blood in the semen (**hemat/o** means relating to blood, **sperm** means sperm, and **-ia** means abnormal condition). This condition is usually benign, and may not have an impact on fertility. It is usually caused by infection or inflammation of the seminal vesicles, vas deferens, epididymis, prostate, or urethra.

DIAGNOSTIC PROCEDURES OF THE MALE REPRODUCTIVE SYSTEM

- **Digital rectal exam** (DRE) is used to detect prostate cancer or tumors of the rectum (see Chapter 10).
- ***Scrotal ultrasound*** is used to help evaluate disorders of the testicles, epididymis, and scrotum.
- **Sperm count**, also known as a ***semen analysis***, is the testing of freshly ejaculated semen to determine the volume plus the number, shape, size, and motility of the sperm.
- **Testicular self-examination** is a self-help step in the early detection of testicular cancer by detecting lumps, swelling, or changes in the skin of the scrotum.

TREATMENT PROCEDURES OF THE MALE REPRODUCTIVE SYSTEM

General Treatment Procedures

- **Circumcision** (**ser**-kum-**SIZH**-un) is the surgical removal of the foreskin of the penis. This optional procedure is usually performed within a few days of birth, sometimes for religious reasons.
- An **orchiectomy** (**or**-kee-**ECK**-toh-mee), also known as an ***orchidectomy***, is the surgical removal of one or both testicles (**orchi** means testicle, and **-ectomy** means surgical removal).
- **Orchiopexy** (**or**-kee-oh-**PECK**-see) is the repair of cryptorchidism, which is an undescended testicle (**orchi/o** means testicle, and **-pexy** means surgical fixation). This is an endoscopic surgery performed on infants before the age of 1 year to move the testicle into its normal position in the scrotum. Orchiopexy is also used to resolve testicular torsion.
- ***Penile implants*** are semirigid or inflatable devices surgically inserted into the penis to treat erectile dysfunction. A ***penis pump*** is a noninvasive treatment that uses a vacuum constriction device to draw blood into the penis, temporarily creating an erection.
- A **varicocelectomy** (**var**-ih-koh-sih-**LECK**-toh-mee) is the removal of a portion of an enlarged vein to relieve a varicocele inside the scrotum (**varic/o** means varicose vein, **cel** means swelling, and **-ectomy** means surgical removal).

Hormone Therapy

- **Androgen replacement therapy** (ART), also known as ***testosterone replacement therapy***, is sometimes used to treat conditions related to testosterone loss such as male hypogonadism, especially in men over the age of 40.
- ***Androgen suppression therapy*** reduces the levels of androgen in order to stop the hormone from fueling prostate cancer cells.

Male Sterilization and Fertility

Sterilization is any procedure rendering an individual (male or female) incapable of reproduction.

- A **bilateral orchiectomy** (bye-**LAT**-er-ahl or-key-**EK**-toh-mee), also known as ***castration***, is the surgical removal or destruction of both testicles (**bi-** means two, **later** means side, and **-al** means pertaining to).
- A **vasectomy** (vah-**SECK**-toh-mee) is the male sterilization procedure in which a small portion of the vas deferens is surgically blocked or cut (**vas** means vas deferens, and **-ectomy** means surgical removal). This prevents sperm from entering the ejaculate but does not change the volume of semen created by the body (Figure 15.5).
- A **vasovasostomy** (**vay**-soh-vah-**ZOS**-toh-mee), also known as a ***vasectomy reversal***, is a procedure performed as an attempt to restore fertility to a vasectomized man (**vas/o** means blood vessel, **vas** means the vas deferens, and **-ostomy** means surgically creating an opening).
- **Cryopreservation** of sperm allows a man to freeze his sperm indefinitely to use later for in vitro fertilization, intrauterine insemination, or sperm donation. This is sometimes done to store sperm prior to treatment for testicular cancer, which can impact fertility.

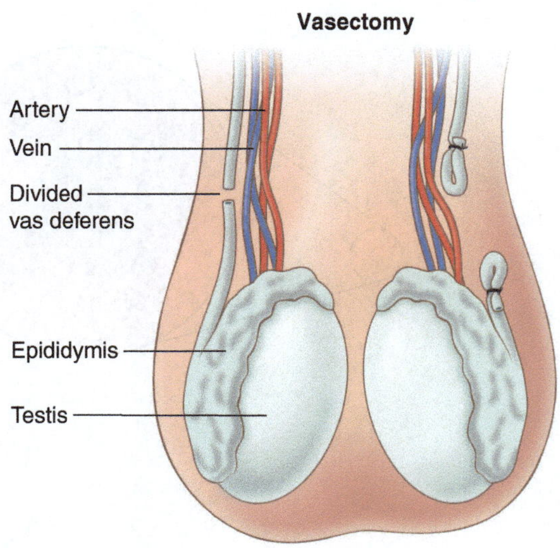

FIGURE 15.5 In a vasectomy, a portion of the vas deferens is removed to prevent sperm from entering the semen.

- ***PDE5 inhibitors*** are drugs such as Viagra used to treat erectile dysfunction by causing vasodilation in the penis.

SEXUALLY TRANSMITTED DISEASES

Sexually transmitted diseases (STDs) are infections caused by either bacteria or viruses that affect both males and females. (See Chapter 16 for more information about STDs in women.) These conditions are commonly spread through sexual intercourse or other genital contact. An older term for an STD is ***venereal disease***, which is a reference to Venus, the Roman goddess of love.

- Although all STDs are caused by infections, not all **sexually transmitted infections** (STIs) develop into a disease. Someone who has an STI can be a carrier for an STD without ever developing any disease. These individuals often have no symptoms, and therefore do not know that they are infected and contagious.
- A pregnant woman who is infected with one of these diseases can transmit it to her baby during birth. For this reason, all newborns receive an antibiotic ointment in each eye within an hour after birth to prevent ***neonatal conjunctivitis***. This condition is caused by the bacteria responsible for chlamydia or gonorrhea.

There are more than 20 types of STDs. The following are several of the more common diseases.

Chlamydia

Chlamydia (klah-**MID**-ee-ah), which is caused by the bacterium *Chlamydia trachomatis*, is the most commonly reported STD in the United States. It is highly contagious and requires early treatment with antibiotics. See Figure 15.6 for symptoms of chlamydia.

- In females, chlamydia can damage the reproductive organs. Even though symptoms are usually mild or absent, serious complications can cause irreversible damage, including infertility.
- In males, chlamydia is one of the causes of ***urethritis***, an inflammation of the urethra (see Chapter 10).

Genital Herpes and HPV

Genital herpes and the human papillomavirus (HPV) have similar symptoms, leaving some people unsure as to which one they have.

- **Genital herpes** (**HER**-peez) is caused by the *herpes simplex virus type 1 (HSV-1)* or *herpes simplex virus type 2 (HSV-2)*. Symptoms include itching or burning before the appearance of ***lesions*** (sores) on the genitals or rectum (Figure 15.7). This condition is highly

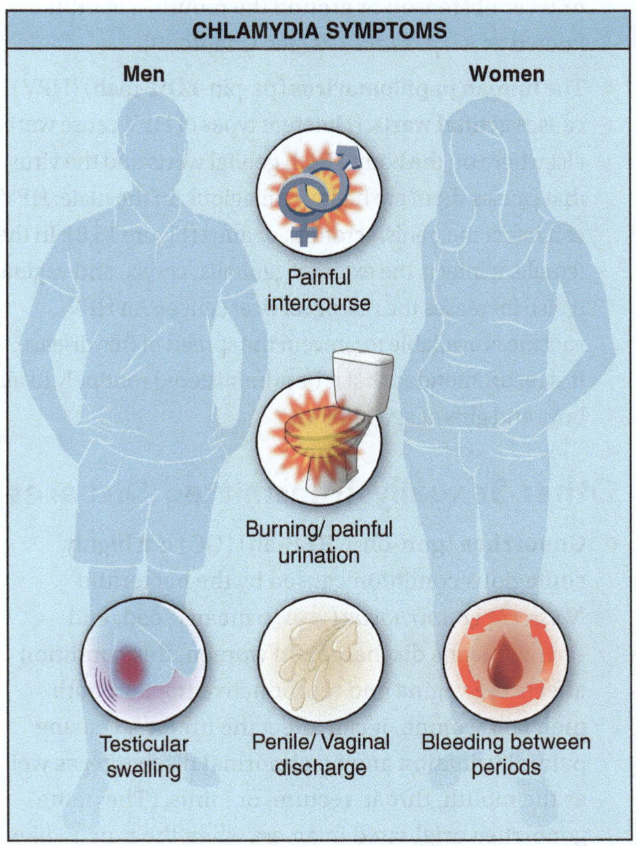

FIGURE 15.6 Chlamydia symptoms in men and women.

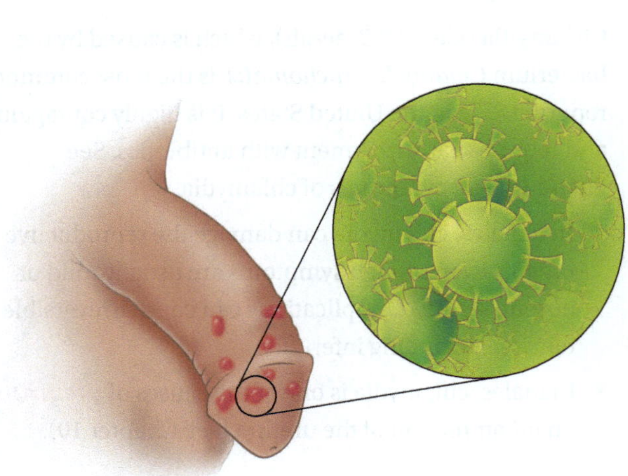

FIGURE 15.7 Genital herpes lesions and a close-up view of the herpes simplex viruses.

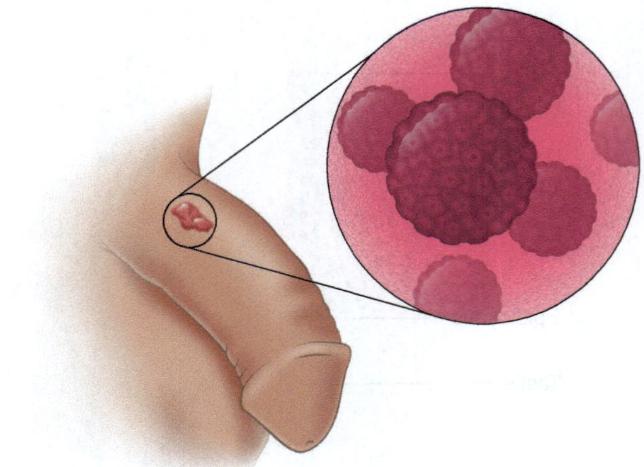

FIGURE 15.8 One common location of a genital wart, with a close-up view of HPV.

contagious, even when visible lesions are not present. Antiviral drugs ease symptoms and can suppress future outbreaks; however, currently there is no cure. The herpes simplex virus type 1 can also cause cold sores or fever blisters on or around the mouth, a condition known as ***herpes labialis*** (see Chapter 9).

- The **human papillomavirus** (pa-pih-**LOH**-mah) (HPV) causes **genital warts**. (Different types of HPV cause warts elsewhere on the body.) Both genital warts and the virus that causes them are highly contagious. In the male, HPV can infect the penis, scrotum, or anus (Figure 15.8). In the female, it infects the external genitalia, cervix, and vagina. It also increases the risk of cervical cancer. An HPV vaccine is available to prevent the spread of this disease. It is recommended that it be administered routinely to all boys and girls at age 11 or 12.

Other Sexually Transmitted Diseases

- **Gonorrhea** (**gon**-oh-w**REE**-ah) (GC) is a highly contagious condition caused by the bacterium *Neisseria gonorrhoeae* (**gon/o** means seed, and **-rrhea** means discharge). In women, this condition affects the vagina and reproductive tract. In both men and women, it can affect the urethra, causing painful urination and an abnormal discharge, as well as the mouth, throat, rectum, or joints. (The name gonorrhea originated in an era when the mucus-like discharge was mistaken for semen.)
- The **human immunodeficiency virus** (HIV) is transmitted through exposure to infected body fluids, particularly through sexual intercourse with an infected partner. HIV and AIDS (acquired immunodeficiency syndrome) are discussed in Chapter 7.
- **Pubic lice**, also known as ***crabs***, are small parasites that can be transmitted during sexual contact or via bed linens. They are usually found in the skin and hair around the genitals; however, pubic lice can turn up in eyelashes, eyebrows, chest hair, armpits, or facial hair. An infection of pubic lice, called ***pthiriasis***, is a common STD that can usually be cured using over-the-counter treatments.
- **Syphilis** (**SIF**-ih-lis), which is caused by the bacterium *Treponema pallidum*, has many symptoms that are difficult to distinguish from other STDs. Syphilis is highly contagious and is passed from person to person through direct contact with a **chancre** (**SHANK**-er), which is a sore caused by syphilis. This condition can be detected through the VDRL (**V**enereal **D**isease **R**esearch **L**aboratory) blood test before the lesions appear. The RPR test (**R**apid **P**lasma **R**eagin) is another blood test for syphilis. When treated early, syphilis is highly curable.
- **Trichomoniasis** (**trick**-oh-moh-**NYE**-ah-sis), also known as ***trich***, is an infection caused by the parasite *Trichomonas vaginalis*. One of the most common symptoms in infected women is a thin, foul-smelling

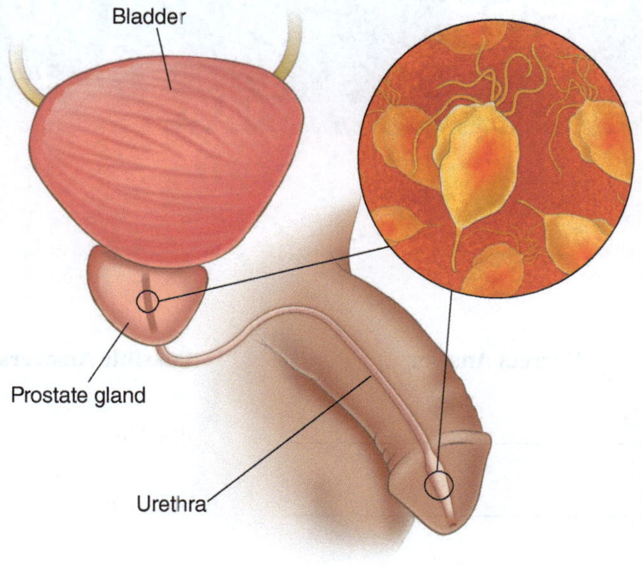

FIGURE 15.9 The parasite trichomonas vaginalis can cause urethritis.

vaginal discharge. Infected men often do not have symptoms; however, when symptoms are present, they include painful urination or a clear discharge from the penis (Figure 15.9).

- **Bacterial vaginosis** (**vaj**-ih-**NOH**-sis) (BV) is not an STD; however, the risk seems to increase with multiple sexual partners. See Chapter 16 for more information about bacterial vaginosis and the pathology of the vagina.

ABBREVIATIONS RELATED TO THE MALE REPRODUCTIVE SYSTEM AND SEXUALLY TRANSMITTED DISEASES

Table 15.1 presents an overview of the abbreviations related to the terms introduced in this chapter. *Note:* To avoid errors or confusion, always be cautious when using abbreviations.

TABLE 15.1

Abbreviations Related to the Male Reproductive System and Sexually Transmitted Diseases

androgen replacement therapy = ART	**ART** = androgen replacement therapy
digital rectal exam = DRE	**DRE** = digital rectal exam
erectile dysfunction = ED	**ED** = erectile dysfunction
gonorrhea = GC	**GC** = gonorrhea
herpes simplex virus = HSV	**HSV** = herpes simplex virus
human papillomaviruses = HPV	**HPV** = human papillomaviruses
sexually transmitted diseases = STDs	**STDs** = sexually transmitted diseases
sexually transmitted infections = STIs	**STIs** = sexually transmitted infections
trichomoniasis = trich	**trich** = trichomoniasis

LEARNING EXERCISES

Matching Word Parts 1

Write the correct answer in the middle column.

	Definition	Correct Answer	Possible Answers
15.1.	epididymis	____________	andr/o
15.2.	hernia	____________	balan/o
15.3.	glans penis	____________	-cele
15.4.	few	____________	epididym/o
15.5.	male	____________	olig/o

Matching Word Parts 2

Write the correct answer in the middle column.

	Definition	Correct Answer	Possible Answers
15.6.	penis	____________	orch/o
15.7.	semen	____________	-pause
15.8.	stopping	____________	pen/i
15.9.	testicles	____________	prostat/o
15.10.	prostate gland	____________	semin/i

Matching Word Parts 3

Write the correct answer in the middle column.

	Definition	Correct Answer	Possible Answers
15.11.	testicles	____________________	**phall/i**
15.12.	penis	____________________	**spermat/o**
15.13.	varicose veins	____________________	**test/i**
15.14.	venereal	____________________	**varic/o**
15.15.	spermatozoa	____________________	**venere/o**

Definitions

Select the correct answer, and write it on the line provided.

15.16. Sperm are formed within the ____________________.

spermatic cord | seminiferous tubules | vas deferens | perineum

15.17. The external opening for the urethra is the ____________________.

glans penis | foreskin | ejaculatory duct | urethral meatus

15.18. The condition in which the opening of the foreskin cannot be retracted to expose the glans penis is called ____________________.

balanitis | Peyronie's disease | priapism | phimosis

15.19. Genital warts are caused by the ____________________.

human immunodeficiency virus | herpes simplex virus | human papillomavirus | trichomonas vaginalis

15.20. The presence of blood in the semen is referred to as ____________________.

hematospermia | azoospermia | oligospermia | phimosis

15.21. Twisting of the spermatic cord leading into a testicle is called ____________________.

a hydrocele | cryptorchidism | testicular torsion | andropause

15.22. The medical terms for a painful and persistent erection lasting 4 hours or more is ____________________.

Peyronie's disease | priapism | male hypogonadism | balanitis

15.23. The surgical removal of one or both testicles is called a/an ______________________.

orchiectomy   orchiopexy   varicocelectomy   vasectomy

15.24. In the male, the region between the scrotum and the anus is known as the ______________________.

epididymis   vas deferens   perineum   prostate

15.25. The developmental condition in which one testicle has not descended is called ______________________.

cryptorchidism   testicular torsion   orchitis   inguinal hernia

Matching Structures

Write the correct answer in the middle column.

	Definition	Correct Answer	Possible Answers
15.26.	the external opening for the urethra	______________________	spermatic cord
15.27.	surrounds the testicles	______________________	scrotum
15.28.	contains a vas deferens	______________________	seminal vesicles
15.29.	protects the tip of the penis	______________________	foreskin
15.30.	secrete a substance to nourish the sperm cells	______________________	urethral meatus

Which Word?

Select the correct answer, and write it on the line provided.

15.30. A male *or* female reproductive cell is a ______________________.

spermatozoa   gamete

15.31. A deficiency in testosterone is known as ______________________.

priapism   male hypogonadism

15.32. The singular form of *testicles* is ______________________.

testes   testis

15.34. The viral STD transmitted through exposure to infected body fluids is ______________________.

human papillomavirus   human immunodeficiency virus

15.35. A physician who specializes in the diseases and disorders of the genitourinary system is called a /an

______________________.

urologist andrologist

Spelling Counts

Find the misspelled word in each sentence. Then write that word, spelled correctly, on the line provided.

15.36. The prostrate gland secretes a thick fluid that aids the motility of the sperm. ______________________

15.37. Payronie's disease is a form of sexual dysfunction in which the penis is bent or curved during erection.

____

15.38. Chryopreservation of sperm allows a man to freeze his sperm indefinitely. ______________________

15.39. Chlamidia is the most commonly reported STD in the United States. ______________________

15.40. The surgical removal of the foreskin of the penis is known as curcimcizun. ______________________

Abbreviation Identification

In the space provided, write the words that each abbreviation stands for.

15.41. **DRE** ______________________

15.42. **HSV** ______________________

15.43. **HPV** ______________________

15.44. **STDs** ______________________

15.45. **STIs** ______________________

Term Selection

Select the correct answer, and write it on the line provided.

15.46. A treatment sometimes used for conditions related to testosterone loss is ______________________.

cryopreservation androgen replacement therapy orchiectomy varicocelectomy

15.47. A ______________________ is a knot of widening varicose veins in one side of the scrotum.

hydrocele phimosis priapism varicocele

15.48. The inflammation of one or both testicles is called ______________.

balanitis epididymitis phimosis orchitis

15.49. The removal of a portion of an enlarged vein to relieve a varicocele inside the scrotum is called

______________.

varicocelectomy orchiopexy vasovasostomy bilateral orchiectomy

15.50. The ______________ secrete a fluid known as pre-ejaculate.

testicles seminal vesicles vas deferens bulbourethral glands

Sentence Completion

Write the correct term or terms on the lines provided.

15.51. A doctor focusing on the treatment of conditions affecting male fertility and sexuality is a/an

______________.

15.52. A protrusion of tissue, often part of the small intestine, through the inguinal canal is called a/an

______________.

15.53. Small parasites that can be transmitted during sexual contact and are usually found in the skin and hair around the genitals are ______________.

15.54. A sore caused by syphilis is called a ______________.

15.55. Someone who has a/an ______________ can be a carrier for an STD without ever developing any disease.

Word Surgery

Divide each term into its component word parts. Write these word parts, in sequence, on the lines provided. When necessary use a slash (/) to indicate a combining vowel. (You may not need all of the lines provided.)

15.56. A **vasovasostomy** is a procedure performed as an attempt to restore fertility to a vasectomized man.

__________ __________ __________ __________

15.57. **Male hypogonadism** is a condition caused by deficient secretions from the gonads.

__________ __________ __________ __________

15.58. **Spermatogenesis** is the process of sperm formation.

_____________ _____________ _____________ _____________

15.59. A **urologist** is a physician who specializes in diagnosing and treating diseases and disorders of the genito-urinary system of males.

_____________ _____________ _____________ _____________

15.60. **Azoospermia** is the absence of sperm in the semen.

_____________ _____________ _____________ _____________

True/False

If the statement is true, write **True** on the line. If the statement is false, write **False** on the line.

15.61. ________ Gonorrhea is a highly contagious condition caused by pthiriasis.

15.62. ________ Testicular self-examination is a self-help step in the detection of STDs.

15.63. ________ Genitourinary means relating to both the genital and urinary organs.

15.64. ________ Syphilis is caused by the bacterium *Treponema pallidum.*

15.65. ________ Premature ejaculation is a condition in which the male reaches climax too soon.

Clinical Conditions

Write the correct answer on the line provided.

15.66. Baby Ortega's left testicle had not descended into his scrotum by the time he was 7 months old, so a/an ______________________________ was performed.

15.67. Gabe Wagner took comfort in the fact that ______________________________, a condition in which the male reaches climax too soon, is a common sexual complaint in men his age.

15.68. The urologist performed a ______________________________ in order to check for signs of prostate cancer or tumors of the rectum.

15.69. Christopher Osman's primary physician prescribed ______________________________ to help counteract the effects of testosterone loss.

15.70. Enrico Flores had a portion of each vas deferens removed. The medical term for this sterilization procedure is _______________________________.

15.71. An analysis of Zack Schmidt's freshly ejaculated semen called a/an _______________________________ was done to explore possible causes of the fertility issues he and his partner were experiencing.

15.72. Mr. Wolford, who is age 70, has been reading a lot about the decrease of testosterone in older men. His physician told him that the medical term for this condition is _______________________________.

15.73. The cause of Kyle Ahamad's urethritis was a common bacterial STD called _______________________________.

15.74. Dr. Wang ran tests to determine the cause of Joe Majhi's recent inability to achieve or maintain an erection, a condition known as _______________________________.

15.75. The Takahashis' newborn son had one testicle that had not descended into the scrotum, a condition known as _______________________________.

Which Is the Correct Medical Term?

Select the correct answer, and write it on the line provided.

15.76. The surgical removal of one or both testicles is called a/an _______________________________.

varicocelectomy orchiopexy orchiectomy vasovasostomy

15.77. The STD caused by the bacterium *Treponema pallidum* is called _______________________________.

gonorrhea syphilis trichomoniasis genital herpes

15.78. The term that describes an inflammation of the glans penis is _______________________________.

phimosis balanitis epididymitis orchitis

15.79. The term _______________________________ refers to a step in the early detection of testicular cancer.

orchiopexy sperm count digital rectal exam testicular self-examination

15.80. Someone who has a/an _______________________________ can be a carrier for an STD without ever developing any disease.

chancre genital wart sexually transmitted infection priapism

Challenge Word Building

These terms are *not* primary terms in the chapter; however, they are made up of the following familiar word parts. If you need help in creating the term, refer to your medical dictionary.

an-	**andr/o**	**-cele**
hyper-	**epididym/o**	**-cide**
	gonad/o	**-ectomy**
	orch/o, orchid/o, orchi/o	**-genous**
	pen/i, phall/i	**-ic**
	semin/o	**-ism**
	sperm/o, spermat/o	**-itis**
	test/i, test/o	**-ology**
	varic/o	**-oma**
	venere/o	**-otomy**

15.81. The term meaning the branch of medicine concerned with venereal diseases is

____________________.

15.82. The term for an incision into a testis is ____________________.

15.83. The term for the condition in which the gonads overproduce hormones is ____________________.

15.84. The adjective meaning relating to the penis is ____________________.

15.85. The term meaning a contraceptive substance that immobilizes or kills sperm is

____________________.

15.86. The term meaning surgery to remove varicose veins in the scrotum is ____________________.

15.87. The term meaning a tumor that originates in the sperm-producing cells is ____________________.

15.88. The term meaning surgery to remove the epididymis is ____________________.

15.89. The term meaning the absence of testes is ____________________.

15.90. Another word for orchialgia, or pain in the testes, is ____________________.

Labeling Exercises

Identify the numbered items on the accompanying figure.

15.91. ______________________ bladder

15.91. ______________________ deferens

15.93. ______________________ penis

15.94. ______________________

15.95. ______________________

15.96. ______________________

15.97. ______________________

15.98. ______________________ gland

15.99. ______________________ duct

15.100. ______________________ vesicle

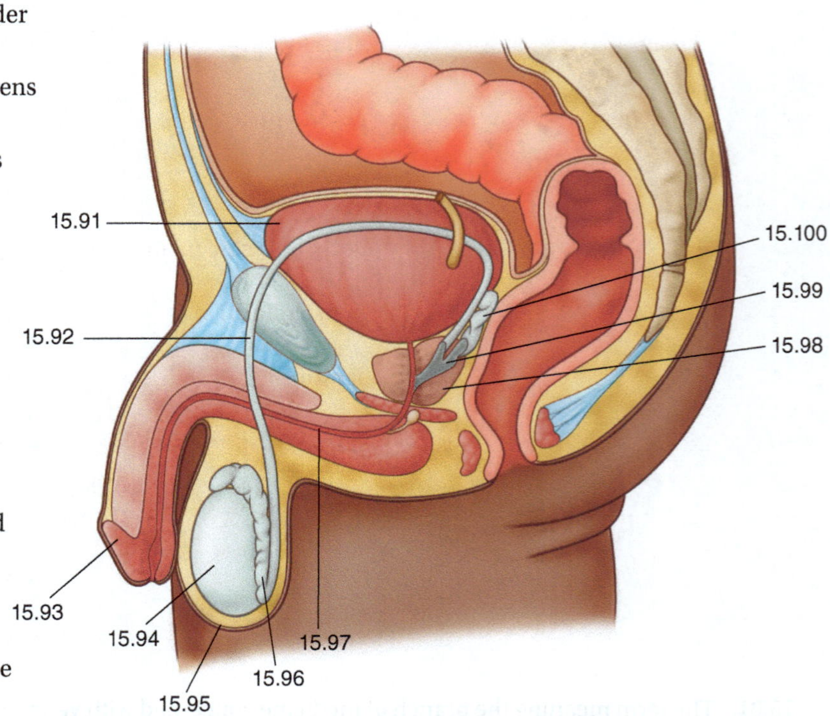

The Human Touch

CRITICAL THINKING EXERCISE

The following story and questions are designed to stimulate critical thinking through class discussion or as a brief essay response. There are no right or wrong answers to these questions.

Clayton and Lucy agreed early in their marriage that they didn't want to have children, so Clayton agreed to have a vasectomy. Tragically, Lucy died at the age of 32 from inflammatory breast cancer. A few years after her death, Clayton met Juanita through an online dating service. During their second dinner together, Juanita mentioned that she had been married once before.

"I really wanted to have children," she said after taking a slow slip of wine. "But Jon wasn't that interested. I think that was one reason that our marriage didn't last."

The prospect of motherhood was clearly very important to Juanita. Clayton had started to warm to the idea of becoming a father as he saw how much his friends enjoyed having children. So he was willing to consider undergoing vasovasostomy surgery if he and Juanita ended up getting married—even though he knew the procedure was not always successful. But there was another problem that weighed on his mind.

When he was in college, a casual sexual encounter had resulted in Clayton contracting chlamydia. He knew that this STD could have caused genetic damage to his sperm, so it was possible that he might be infertile even if he had the surgery.

The more he got to know Juanita, the more he knew that he wanted this relationship to last. But he just wasn't sure how to talk to her about his worries regarding their ability to have children together.

Suggested Discussion Topics

1. Chlamydia is one of the most common STDs in the U.S. What could Clayton have done to prevent contracting it?
2. What are some of the issues regarding family planning that a couple might discuss before becoming sexually active?
3. If Clayton is infertile, are there other options open to them to become parents?
4. Since having children is important to Juanita, how soon do you think Clayton should tell her about the vasectomy?

CHAPTER 16

THE FEMALE REPRODUCTIVE SYSTEM AND OBSTETRICS

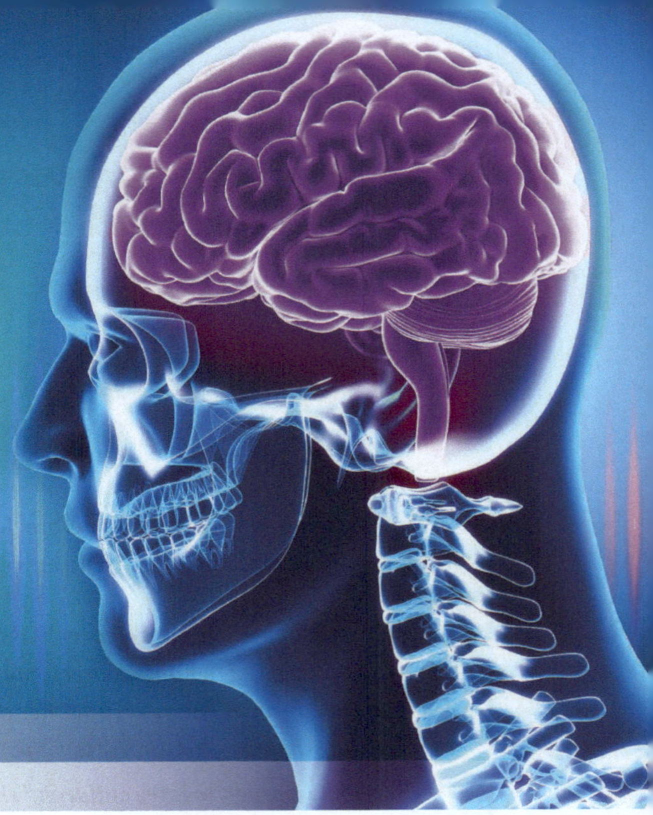

Overview of

STRUCTURES, COMBINING FORMS, AND FUNCTIONS OF THE FEMALE REPRODUCTIVE SYSTEM

Major Structures	Related Combining Forms	Primary Functions
Ovaries	oophor/o, ovari/o	Produce ova (eggs) and female hormones.
Fallopian Tubes	salping/o	Catch the mature ovum (egg) and transport it to the uterus. Also the site of fertilization.
Uterus	hyster/o, metr/o, metri/o, uter/o	Protects and supports the developing child.
Vagina	vagin/o, colp/o	Used for sexual intercourse, acts as channel for menstrual flow, and functions as the birth canal.
Placenta	placent/o	Exchanges nutrients and waste between the mother and fetus during pregnancy.

Vocabulary Related to **THE REPRODUCTIVE SYSTEMS AND OBSTETRICS**

This list contains essential word parts and medical terms for this chapter. These and the other important **primary terms** are shown in **boldface** throughout the chapter. ***Secondary terms***, which appear in ***orange*** italics, clarify the meaning of primary terms.

Word Parts

- ☐ **cervic/o** cervix
- ☐ **colp/o** vagina
- ☐ **gynec/o** woman, female
- ☐ **hyster/o** uterus
- ☐ **mast/o** breast
- ☐ **men/o** menstruation
- ☐ **metr/o** uterus
- ☐ **nat/o** birth
- ☐ **oophor/o** ovary
- ☐ **ov/o** egg, ovum
- ☐ **ovari/o** ovary
- ☐ **placent/o** placenta
- ☐ **salping/o** fallopian tube
- ☐ **vagin/o** vagina
- ☐ **vulv/o** vulva

Medical Terms

- ☐ **abruptio placentae** (ah-**BRUP**-shee-oh plah-**SEN**-tee)
- ☐ **amenorrhea** (ah-**men**-oh-**REE**-ah)
- ☐ **bacterial vaginosis** (**vaj**-ih-**NOH**-sis)
- ☐ **cauterization** (**kaw**-ter-eye-**ZAY**-shun)
- ☐ **cephalic presentation** (seh-**FAL**-ick)
- ☐ **cervical dysplasia** (**SER**-vih-kal dis-**PLAY**-see-ah)
- ☐ **cervicitis** (**ser**-vih-**SIGH**-tis)
- ☐ **chorionic villus sampling** (**kor**-ee-**ON**-ick **VIL**-us)
- ☐ **coitus** (**KOH**-ih-tus)
- ☐ **colostrum** (kuh-**LOS**-trum)
- ☐ **colporrhaphy** (kol-**POR**-ah-fee)
- ☐ **colposcopy** (kol-**POS**-koh-pee)
- ☐ **conization** (**kon**-ih-**ZAY**-shun)
- ☐ **corpus luteum** (**KOR**-pus **LOO**-tee-um)
- ☐ **dysmenorrhea** (**dis**-men-oh-**REE**-ah)
- ☐ **eclampsia** (eh-**KLAMP**-see-ah)
- ☐ **ectopic pregnancy** (eck-**TOP**-ick)
- ☐ **endometriosis** (**en**-doh-**mee**-tree-**OH**-sis)
- ☐ **epidural block** (**ep**-ih-**DOO**-ral)
- ☐ **episiotomy** (eh-**piz**-ee-**OT**-oh-mee)
- ☐ **fibroadenoma** (**figh**-broh-**ad**-eh-**NOH**-mah)
- ☐ **galactorrhea** (gah-**lack**-toh-**REE**-ah)
- ☐ **gynecologist** (**guy**-neh-**KOL**-oh-jist)
- ☐ **hypomenorrhea** (**high**-poh-men-oh-**REE**-ah)
- ☐ **hysterectomy** (**hiss**-teh-**RECK**-toh-mee)
- ☐ **hysterosalpingography** (**hiss**-ter-oh-**sal**-pin-**GOG**-rah-fee)
- ☐ **hysteroscopy** (**hiss**-ter-**OSS**-koh-pee)
- ☐ **in vitro fertilization** (**VEE**-troh)
- ☐ **lactation** (lack-**TAY**-shun)
- ☐ **leukorrhea** (**loo**-koh-**REE**-ah)
- ☐ **lochia** (**LOH**-kee-ah)
- ☐ **luteal phase** (**LOO**-tee-al)
- ☐ **mastalgia** (mass-**TAL**-jee-ah)
- ☐ **mastopexy** (**MAS**-toh-**peck**-see)
- ☐ **meconium** (meh-**KOH**-nee-um)
- ☐ **menarche** (**MEN**-ar-kee)
- ☐ **metrorrhagia** (**mee**-troh-**RAY**-jee-ah)
- ☐ **myometrium** (my-oh-**MEE**-tree-um)
- ☐ **neonate** (**NEE**-oh-nayt)
- ☐ **nullipara** (nuh-**LIP**-ah-rah)
- ☐ **obstetrician** (ob-steh-**TRISH**-un)
- ☐ **oligomenorrhea** (**ol**-ih-goh-**men**-oh-**REE**-ah)
- ☐ **oophorectomy** (**oh**-ahf-oh-**RECK**-toh-mee)
- ☐ **ovulation** (**ov**-you-**LAY**-shun)
- ☐ **pelvic inflammatory disease**
- ☐ **perimenopause** (pehr-ih-**MEN**-oh-pawz)
- ☐ **perinatologist** (**pehr**-ee-nay-**TOL**-oh-jist)
- ☐ **placenta previa** (plah-**SEN**-tah **PREE**-vee-ah)
- ☐ **polycystic ovary syndrome** (**pol**-ee-**SIS**-tick)
- ☐ **postpartum** (pohst-**PAR**-tum)
- ☐ **preeclampsia** (**pree**-ee-**KLAMP**-see-ah)
- ☐ **premenstrual syndrome**
- ☐ **primigravida** (**prye**-mih-**GRAV**-ih-dah)
- ☐ **primipara** (prye-**MIP**-ah-rah)
- ☐ **salpingo-oophorectomy** (sal-**ping**-goh- oh-**ahf**-oh-**RECK**-toh-mee)
- ☐ **speculum** (**SPECK**-you-lum)
- ☐ **transvaginal ultrasound** (**trans**-**VAJ**-ih-nal)
- ☐ **uterine prolapse** (**YOU**-ter-ihn proh-**LAPS**)
- ☐ **vaginismus** (**VAJ**-ih-**nihz**-mis)
- ☐ **vulvodynia** (vul-voh-**DIN**-ee-ah)

LEARNING OBJECTIVES

On completion of this chapter, you should be able to:

1. Describe the functions and structures of the female reproductive system.
2. Identify the phases of the average menstrual cycle.
3. Discuss the stages of pregnancy and childbirth.
4. Identify the medical word parts related to obstetrics.
5. Define the primary terms related to obstetrics: pregnancy and childbirth.
6. Identify the medical specialties related to the female reproductive system and obstetrics.
7. Identify the medical word parts of the female reproductive system.
8. Define the primary terms related to the pathology and the diagnostic and treatment procedures of the female reproductive system.
9. Define the primary terms related to the pathology and complications that impact pregnancy, childbirth, and the postpartum period.
10. Define the primary terms related to the diagnostic and treatment procedures for pregnancy and childbirth.
11. Spell the primary terms related to the female reproductive system and obstetrics.
12. Pronounce the primary terms related to the female reproductive system and obstetrics.
13. Define common abbreviations related to the female reproductive system and obstetrics.

TERMS RELATED TO THE REPRODUCTIVE SYSTEM

The **genitalia (jen**-ih-**TAY**-lee-ah) are the organs of reproduction and their associated structures.

- *External genitalia* are reproductive organs located outside of the body cavity.
- *Internal genitalia* are reproductive organs protected within the body.

The **perineum** (pehr-ih-**NEE**-um) is the external surface region in both males and females between the pubic symphysis and the coccyx. The tissue of the *female perineum* extends from the pubic symphysis to the area around the anus (Figure 16.1).

FUNCTIONS OF THE FEMALE REPRODUCTIVE SYSTEM

The primary function of the female reproductive system is the creation and support of new life.

- The ovaries produce mature eggs to be fertilized by the sperm.
- The uterus provides the environment and support for the developing child.
- After birth, the breasts produce milk to feed the child.

STRUCTURES OF THE FEMALE REPRODUCTIVE SYSTEM

The structures of the female reproductive system include the external female genitalia and the internal female reproductive organs (Figure 16.2).

The *external female genitalia* are located posterior to the **mons pubis** (**MONZ PYOU**-bis), which is a rounded, fleshy prominence located over the pubic symphysis. The *pubic symphysis* is the area where the pubic bones meet (Figure 16.2). These structures are known collectively as the **vulva** (**VUL**-vah) or the *pudendum*. The vulva consists of the labia, clitoris, Bartholin's glands, and vaginal orifice.

- The **labia majora** and **labia minora** (**LAY**-bee-ah mah-**JOR**-ah and **LAY**-bee-ah mih-**NOR**-ah) are the vaginal lips that protect the other external genitalia and the urethral meatus (singular, *labium*). The *urethral meatus*, which is the external opening of the urethra, is discussed in Chapter 10.
- The **clitoris** (**KLIT**-oh-ris) is an organ of sensitive erectile tissue located anterior to the urethral meatus and the vaginal orifice.
- **Bartholin's glands** produce a mucus secretion to lubricate the vagina. These two small, round glands are located on either side of the vaginal orifice.

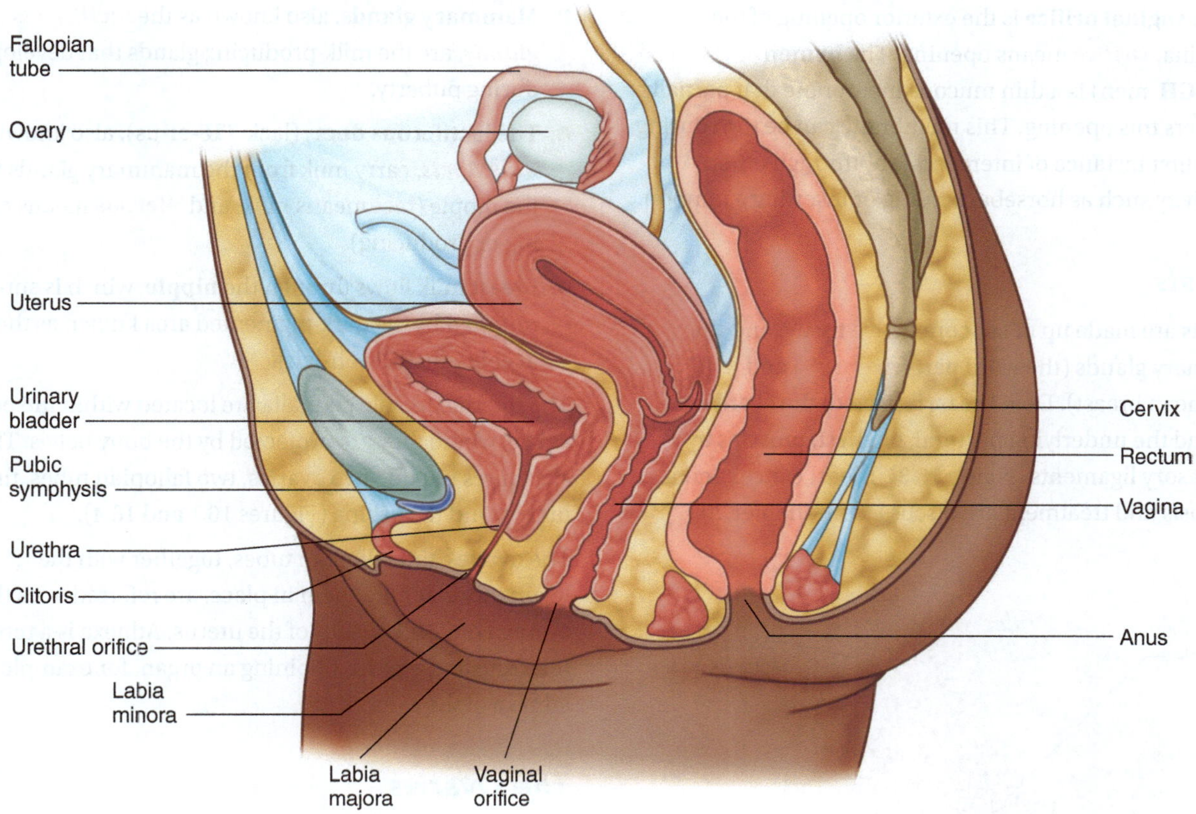

FIGURE 16.1 The structures of the female genitalia.

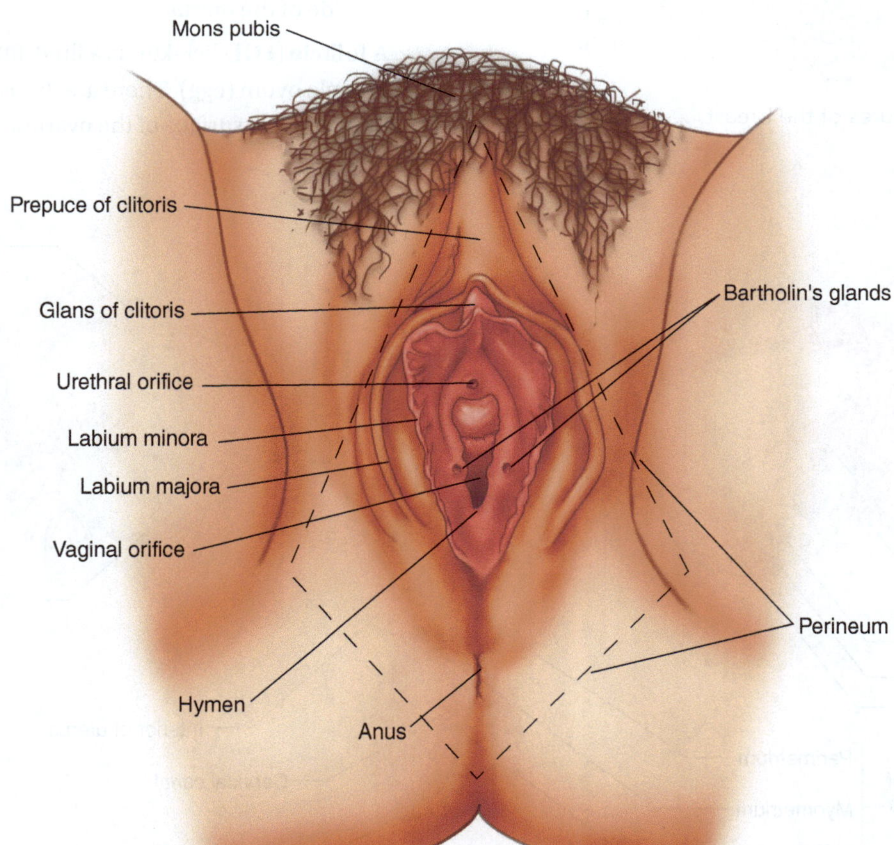

FIGURE 16.2 The external female genitalia.

- The **vaginal orifice** is the exterior opening of the vagina. ***Orifice*** means opening. The **hymen** (**HIGH**-men) is a thin mucous membrane that partially covers this opening. This membrane can be torn during the first instance of intercourse, or through other activity such as horseback riding or inserting a tampon.

Breasts

Breasts are made up of fat, connective tissue, and the mammary glands (the word parts **mamm/o** and **mast/o** both mean breast). Each breast is fixed to the overlying skin and the underlying pectoral, or chest, muscles by suspensory ligaments (Figure 16.3). Breast cancer and its diagnosis and treatment are discussed in Chapter 20.

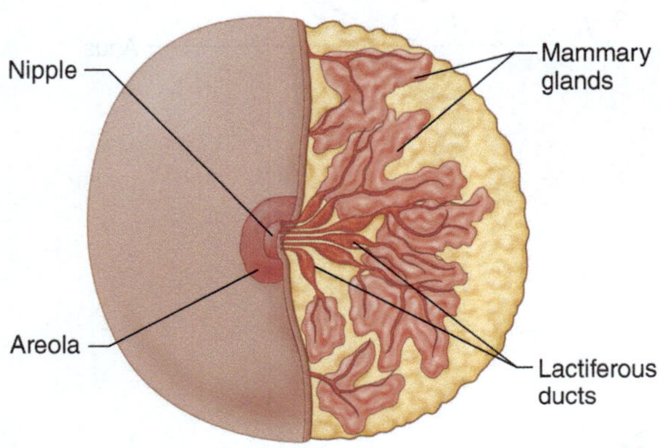

FIGURE 16.3 Structures of the breast.

- **Mammary glands**, also known as the ***lactiferous glands***, are the milk-producing glands that develop during puberty.
- The **lactiferous ducts** (lack-**TIF**-er-us), also known as ***milk ducts***, carry milk from the mammary glands to the nipple (**lact** means milk, and **-iferous** means carrying or producing).
- Breast milk flows through the **nipple**, which is surrounded by the dark-pigmented area known as the **areola** (ah-**REE**-oh-lah).

The internal female genitalia are located within the pelvic cavity, where they are protected by the bony pelvis. These structures include two ovaries, two fallopian tubes, the uterus, and the vagina (Figures 16.1 and 16.4).

The ovaries and fallopian tubes, together with the ligaments that hold them in place, are referred to as the **adnexa** (ad-**NECK**-sah) of the uterus. Adnexa is a term referring to the parts adjoining an organ, for example, the adnexa of the eyes.

The Ovaries

The **ovaries** (**OH**-vah-rees) are a pair of small, almond-shaped glands located in the lower abdomen, one on either side of the uterus.

- A **follicle** (**FOL**-lick-kul) is a fluid-filled sac containing a single ovum (egg). There are thousands of these sacs on the inside surface of the ovaries.

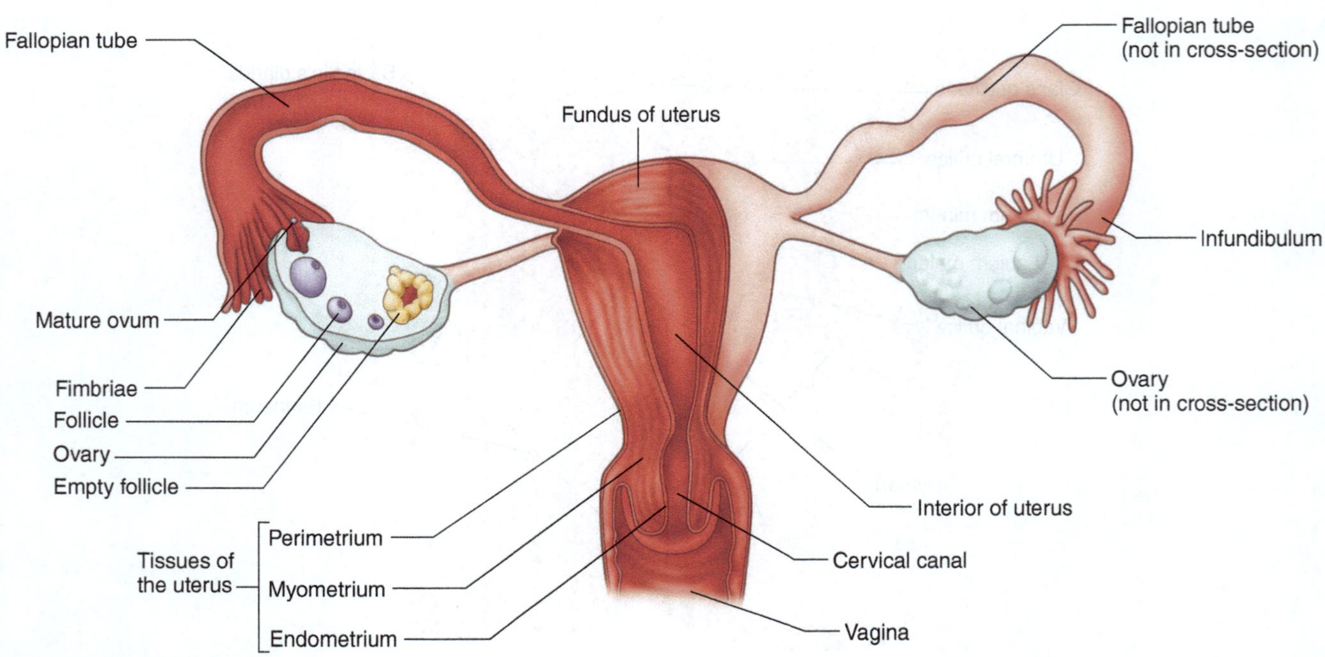

FIGURE 16.4 An anterior schematic view of the female reproductive organs.

- The **ova** (**OH**-vah), also known as *eggs*, are the female gametes (singular, ovum). These immature ova are present at birth. Normally, after puberty, one ovum matures and is released each month. A *gamete* is a sperm or an egg cell.
- The ovaries also produce the sex hormones estrogen and progesterone, which are discussed in Chapter 14.

The Fallopian Tubes

There are two **fallopian tubes** (fah-**LOH**-pee-an), which are also known as *uterine tubes*. These tubes extend from the upper end of the uterus to a point near but not attached to an ovary.

- The **infundibulum** (**in**-fun-**DIB**-you-lum) is the funnel-shaped opening into the fallopian tube near the ovary.
- The **fimbriae** (**FIM**-bree-ee) are the fringed, finger-like extensions of this opening. Their role is to catch the mature ovum when it leaves the ovary (singular, *fimbria*).
- During menstruation, one of these tubes carries a mature ovum from the ovary to the uterus (Figure 16.4). These tubes also carry sperm upward from the uterus toward the descending mature ovum so that fertilization can occur.

The Uterus

The **uterus** (**YOU**-ter-us), formerly known as the *womb*, is a pear-shaped organ with muscular walls and a mucous membrane lining filled with a rich supply of blood vessels (Figure 16.4).

- The uterus is located between the urinary bladder and the rectum, and midway between the sacrum and the pubic bone.
- In its normal position, which is known as **anteflexion** (**an**-tee-**FLECK**-shun), the body of the uterus is bent forward (**ante-** means forward, **flex** means bend, and **-ion** means condition) (Figure 16.1).

The Parts of the Uterus

The body of the uterus consists of three major anatomic areas:

- The **fundus** (**FUN**-dus) is the bulging, rounded part above the entrance of the fallopian tubes. Because the fundus rises during pregnancy, measuring the fundal height in relation to the pubic bone helps determine the baby's growth.
- The **corpus** (**KOR**-pus), also known as the *body of the uterus*, is the middle portion.
- The **cervix** (**SER**-vicks), also known as the *cervix uteri*, is the lower, narrow portion that extends into the vagina. Within the cervix is the *cervical canal*, which ends at the *cervical os* at the vagina.

The Tissues of the Uterus

The uterus is composed of three major layers of tissue:

- The **perimetrium** (pehr-ih-**MEE**-tree-um) is the tough, membranous outer layer (**peri-** means surrounding, **metri** means uterus, and **-um** is a singular noun ending). *Membranous* means pertaining to a thin layer of tissue.
- The **myometrium** (my-oh-**MEE**-tree-um) is the muscular middle layer (**my/o** means muscle, **metri** means uterus, and **-um** is a singular noun ending).
- The **endometrium** (en-doh-**MEE**-tree-um) is the inner layer, and it consists of specialized epithelial mucosa that is rich in blood vessels (**endo-** means within, **metri** means uterus, and **-um** is a singular noun ending). *Mucosa* means referring to mucous membrane.

Vagina

The **vagina** (vah-**JIGH**-nah) is the muscular tube lined with mucosa that extends from the cervix to the outside of the body. The word parts **colp/o** and **vagin/o** both mean vagina (Figures 16.2 and 16.4).

Menstruation

- **Menstruation** (**men**-stroo-**AY**-shun), also known as *menses*, is the normal periodic discharge of the endometrial lining and unfertilized egg from uterus. The average *menstrual cycle* consists of 28 days. These days are grouped into four phases, which are summarized in Table 16.1:
  1. **Menstrual phase**
  2. **Follicular phase**, also called the *postmenstrual phase*
  3. **Ovulation phase**
  4. **Luteal phase** (**LOO**-tee-al), also called the *premenstrual phase*
- **Menarche** (**MEN**-ar-kee) is the beginning of menstruation (**men** means menstruation, and **-arche** means beginning). This begins after the maturation that occurs during puberty. In the United States the average age of menarche is 12½.

TABLE 16.1

Phases of the Menstrual Cycle

Approximately Days 1–5	***Menstrual phase***. These are the days when the endometrial lining of the uterus is sloughed off and discharged through the vagina as the menstrual flow.
Approximately Days 6–12	***Follicular phase***. From the first day of menstruation until ovulation, the pituitary gland releases follicle-stimulating hormone (FSH), causing an ovum to mature. Estrogen stimulates the endometrium of the uterus to regenerate in preparation for a zygote (fertilized egg).
Approximately Days 13–14	***Ovulation phase***. On approximately the 13th or 14th day of the cycle, ovulation occurs. Ovulation is the release of a mature ovum. The mature egg leaves the ovary and travels slowly down the fallopian tube toward the uterus. During this time, the female is fertile and can become pregnant.
Approximately Days 15–28	***Luteal phase***. If fertilization does not occur, hormone levels change to cause the breakdown of the uterine endometrium and the beginning of a new menstrual cycle.

- The term **climacteric** (kly-MAK-ter-ik) describes the time during which ovarian activity declines. Perimenopause, menopause, and postmenopause are all part of this period of life. Climacteric, which also refers to the decline in male reproductive ability, comes from a Greek word meaning a critical point in life.
- **Menopause** (MEN-oh-pawz) is the normal termination of menstruation in a woman during middle age (**men/o** means menstruation, and **-pause** means stopping). Menopause is defined as the absence of menstruation for one year. The average age of menopause in the U.S. is now 51, although its onset can vary by 10 or more years.
- **Premature menopause** describes menopause starting before the age of 40. This can occur abruptly as the result of a surgery such as a hysterectomy removing both ovaries. Other factors that can lead to premature menopause include certain health conditions such as HIV, damage to the ovaries from medications, chemotherapy or radiation, and smoking.
- **Perimenopause** (pehr-ih-MEN-oh-pawz) is the term used to designate the transition phase between regular menstrual periods and no periods at all (**peri-** means surrounding, **men/o** means menstruation, and **-pause** means stopping). During this phase, which can last as long as a decade, changes in hormone production can cause symptoms including irregular menstrual cycles, hot flashes, mood swings, and disturbed sleep.
- **Postmenopausal** describes a woman who has not had a menstrual cycle for one year or more.

OBSTETRICS: PREGNANCY AND CHILDBIRTH

The study of pregnancy, childbirth, and the period immediately after birth is referred to as **obstetrics**.

Origin of Oocytes

Women are born with all of the all of the **oocytes** (**OH**-oh-sites), or immature egg cells, they will ever have—approximately 1 to 2 million. Due to a natural process called ***ovarian follicle atresia***, only about 300,000 of the egg cells are still present at puberty.

Oogenesis

Oogenesis (oh-oh-**JEN**-eh-sis) is a process called differentiation during which an oocyte becomes an **ovum** (**OH**-vum), or mature egg cell, ready to be released for potential fertilization (**o/o** means egg, and **-genesis** means creation). During ***differentiation***, young, immature cells reach their mature form and specialized function.

Ovulation

Ovulation (ov-you-**LAY**-shun) is the release of a mature egg from a follicle on the surface of one of the ovaries that happens on approximately the 13th or 14th day of a woman's menstrual cycle.

- After the ovum is released, it is caught up by the fimbriae of the fallopian tube. Wave-like peristaltic actions move the ovum down the fallopian tube toward the uterus.

- It usually takes an ovum about five days to pass through the fallopian tube. If sperm are present at that time, one may fertilize the ovum within the fallopian tube.
- After the ovum has been released, the ruptured follicle enlarges, takes on a yellow fatty substance, and becomes the corpus luteum.
- The **corpus luteum** (**KOR**-pus **LOO**-tee-um) secretes the hormone progesterone during the luteal phase of the menstrual cycle. This maintains the growth of the uterine lining in preparation for the fertilized egg.
- If the ovum is not fertilized, the corpus luteum degenerates during the luteal phase, and the endometrium lining of the uterus sloughs off as the menstrual flow occurs. If the ovum is fertilized, the corpus luteum continues to secrete the hormones required to maintain the pregnancy.

Fertilization

- During penetrative **coitus** (**KOH**-ih-tus), also known as ***sexual intercourse*** or ***copulation***, the male ejaculates approximately 100 million sperm per milliliter of fluid into the female's vagina. The sperm travel upward through the vagina, into the uterus, and on into the fallopian tubes. The adjective ***coital*** means relating to sexual intercourse.
- **Conception** occurs when one sperm penetrates and fertilizes the descending ovum. This union, which is the beginning of a new life, forms a single cell known as a **zygote** (**ZYE**-goht).
- After fertilization occurs in the fallopian tube, the zygote travels to the uterus, where it is implanted. ***Implantation*** is the embedding of the zygote into the lining of the uterus.
- From implantation through the eighth week of pregnancy, the developing baby is known as an **embryo** (**EM**-bree-oh).
- From the ninth week of pregnancy to the time of birth, the baby in utero is known as a **fetus** (**fet** means unborn child, and **-us** is a singular noun ending). The plural of fetus is *fetuses*. ***In utero*** means within the uterus (Figure 16.5).

Multiple Births

If more than one egg is passing down the fallopian tube when sperm are present, the fertilization of more than one egg is possible.

- **Fraternal twins** result from the fertilization of separate ova by separate sperm. The medical term for this is ***polyzygotic***, meaning more than one zygote is involved. These fertilized ova develop into two separate embryos (Figure 16.6). Fraternal twins tend to run in families through a genetic link on the mother's side.
- **Identical twins** are formed by the fertilization of a single egg cell by a single sperm that divides to form two embryos. The medical term for this is ***monozygotic***, because only one zygote is involved. Each of these twins receives exactly the same genetic information from the parents.
- The term **multiples** describes more than one baby born at the same time.
- ***Higher-order multiples*** refers to three or more infants born at the same time. Triplets, quadruplets, and larger numbers of multiples can be fraternal, identical or a combination of the two.

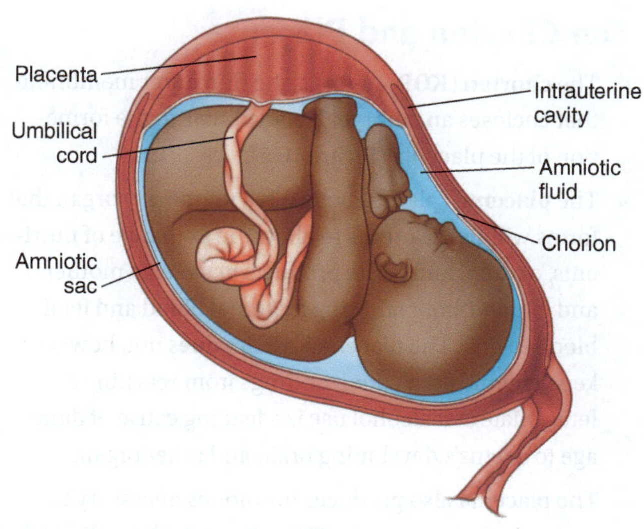

FIGURE 16.5 A fetus in utero.

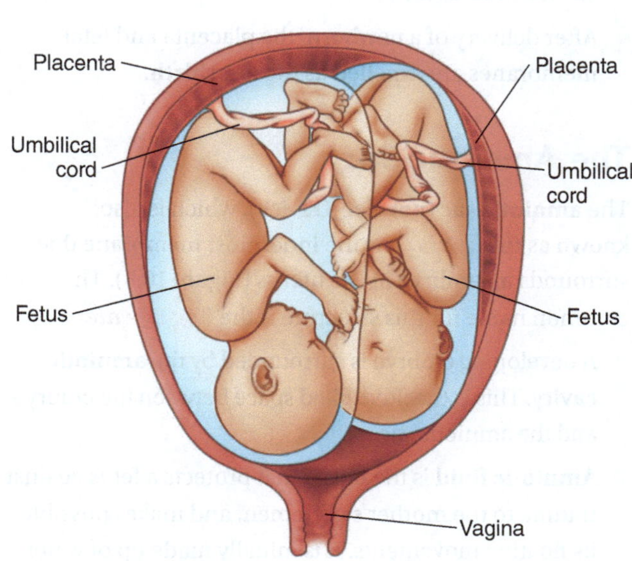

FIGURE 16.6 Fraternal twins in utero.

The Chorion and Placenta

- The **chorion** (**KOR**-ee-on) is the thin outer membrane that encloses an embryo. It contributes to the formation of the placenta (Figure 16.5).
- The **placenta** (plah-**SEN**-tah) is a temporary organ that forms within the uterus to allow the exchange of nutrients, oxygen, and waste products between a mother and fetus without allowing maternal blood and fetal blood to mix. The placental barrier does not, however, keep chemicals, alcohol, or drugs from reaching a fetus. Maternal alcohol use is a leading cause of damage to a fetus's developing brain and other organs.
- The placenta also produces hormones necessary to maintain the pregnancy. These hormones are discussed in Chapter 14.
- After delivery of a newborn, the placenta and fetal membranes are expelled as the **afterbirth**.

The Amniotic Sac

The **amniotic sac** (am-nee-**OT**-ick), which is also known as the *amnion*, is the innermost membrane that surrounds an embryo in the uterus (Figure 16.5). The common name for this structure is the *bag of waters*.

- A developing embryo is surrounded by the **amniotic cavity**. This is the fluid-filled space between the embryo and the amniotic sac.
- **Amniotic fluid** is the liquid that protects a fetus against trauma to the mother's abdomen, and makes possible its floating movements. It is initially made up of water from the mother; however, as the fetus swallows and "inhales" the fluid, it is gradually replaced by fetal urine and lung secretions.

The Umbilical Cord

The **umbilical cord** (um-**BILL**-ih-kal) is the tube that carries blood, oxygen, and nutrients from the placenta to a developing baby. It also transports waste from the fetus to be disposed of through the mother's excretory system. This cord is cut soon after the birth of the infant and before the delivery of the placenta.

- After birth, the **navel**, also known as the *belly button*, is formed where the umbilical cord was attached to the fetus.

Gestation

Gestation (jes-**TAY**-shun), which lasts approximately 280 days (40 weeks), is the period of development of the fetus in the mother's uterus. Upon completion of this developmental time, the fetus is described as being *at term* and should be ready for birth (Figure 16.7).

- The term **pregnancy**, which is often used interchangeably with *gestation*, means the condition of having a developing fetus in the uterus.
- The length of pregnancy is described according to the number of weeks of gestation (usually 40 weeks total). For descriptive purposes, pregnancy can also be divided into three **trimesters** of about 13 weeks each. These trimesters make up the stages of pregnancy.
  - **First trimester** (first day of last menstrual period to week 13): The mother's body goes through hormonal changes as it adapts to being pregnant. The embryo becomes a fetus as it develops a body structure and organ systems.
  - **Second trimester** (weeks 14 to 27): The growing fetus puts pressure on the mother's back, abdomen, and internal organs. The first movements of the fetus can be felt.
  - **Third trimester** (weeks 28 to 40): The increased size of the fetus pushes against the mother's diaphragm and bladder. The fetus—which can now kick, stretch, and hiccup—drops lower in the abdomen as the time of birth approaches. Contractions indicating real or false labor (Braxton Hicks contractions) may occur.
- The **due date**, or *estimated date of delivery* (EDD), is calculated by taking the first day of the *last menstrual period* (LMP), adding one year, subtracting three months, and adding seven days.
- **Quickening** is the first movement of the fetus in the uterus that can be felt by the mother. This usually occurs between the 16th and 20th weeks of pregnancy.
- The fetus is described as being **viable** when it is capable of surviving outside the uterus. Viability depends on the developmental age, birth weight, and developmental stage of the lungs of the fetus. In general, a fetus must have reached 24 weeks of gestation to be considered viable.
- The term **antepartum** (**an**-tee-**PAHR**-tum) refers to the final stage of pregnancy just before the onset of labor.

The Mother

- **Advanced maternal age** (AMA) refers to women who are 35 or older at the time of pregnancy. AMA can contribute to a higher risk of complications.

- **Gravida** (**GRAH**-vid-ah) is a term referring to the number of pregnancies a woman has experienced.
- A **primigravida** (**prye**-mih-**GRAV**-ih-dah) is a woman during her first pregnancy (**primi-** means first, and **-gravida** means pregnant). Compare with *primipara*.
- **Para** refers to a pregnancy that has gone to 20 weeks gestation or beyond.
- A **nullipara** (nuh-**LIP**-ah-rah) is a woman who has never borne a viable child (**nulli-** means none, and **-para** means to give birth).
- A **primipara** (prye-**MIP**-ah-rah) is a woman who has borne one viable child (**primi-** means first, and **-para** means to give birth). Compare with *primigravida*.
- A **multipara** (mul-**TIP**-ah-rah) is a woman who has given birth to a viable child two or more times (**multi-** means many, and **-para** means to give birth).

Childbirth

The term **parturition** (**par**-cher-**ISH**-un) means the act of giving birth. During the last months prior to parturition, a woman may experience *false labor*, with painless, irregular contractions of the uterus, but no dilation of the cervix.

- These **Braxton Hicks contractions** occur with increasing frequency as the pregnancy progresses. The contractions are named after British doctor John Braxton Hicks, who first described them in 1872.

Labor and delivery, also known as *childbirth*, occurs in three stages, shown in Figure 16.7. The stages of labor and delivery are as follows:

1. Dilation
2. Delivery of the baby
3. Expulsion of the afterbirth

The First Stage of Labor

The first (and longest) stage of labor begins when regular contractions begin to dilate the cervix. *Active labor* describes the period of more rapid labor progression between 6 and 10 centimeters (cm) dilation. **Contractions** during childbirth are the regular tightening and relaxing of the uterine muscle that help push the baby down the birth canal.

- The changes that occur during this stage include the gradual **dilation** (dye-**LAY**-shun) and effacement of the cervix and the rupture of the amniotic sac. **Effacement** (eh-**FAYS**-ment) is the process by which the cervix prepares for delivery as it gradually softens, shortens, and becomes thinner (Figure 16.7B).
- The **rupture of the amniotic sac**, also referred to as the *water breaking*, often occurs on its own. If not, the membrane may be ruptured artificially. When the amniotic sac ruptures prior to the onset of labor, medical evaluation is recommended.

The Second Stage of Labor

The second stage begins when the cervix has fully dilated (10 cm) and ends with the delivery of the infant. As the uterine contractions become stronger and more frequent, the mother pushes to help expel the child through the *birth canal* (vagina). Normally, the baby's head presents first.

Cephalic presentation (seh-**FAL**-ick), or *crowning*, describes when the baby is coming head first. The head can be seen at the vaginal opening (Figure 16.7C).

The Third Stage of Labor

The third stage is the expulsion, or delivery, of the placenta as the *afterbirth* (Figure 16.7D). *Umbilical cord blood* can be collected at this time so that its stem cells can be saved and used in future medical treatments.

- *Recovery*, which is the period during which the mother and baby are reunited, is sometimes referred to as the fourth stage of labor. The baby may be ready to nurse during this time, an action which triggers uterine contractions. These contractions, which may continue for two or three days, help the uterus return to its pre-pregnancy size.

Postpartum

The term **postpartum** (pohst-**PAR**-tum) means after childbirth (*post* means after, and *partum* means childbirth).

The Mother

- **Puerperium** (**pyoor**-**PEER**-ee-um) is the time from the delivery of the placenta through approximately the first six weeks after the delivery. By the end of this period, most of the changes in the mother's body due to pregnancy have resolved, and her reproductive organs have reverted to their nonpregnant state.
- **Lochia** (**LOH**-kee-ah) is the postpartum vaginal discharge that typically continues for up to four to six weeks after childbirth (**loch** means childbirth, and **-ia** means pertaining to). It consists primarily of blood and mucus.
- **Uterine involution** is the return of the uterus to its normal size and former condition after delivery. *Involution* means the return of an enlarged organ to its normal size.

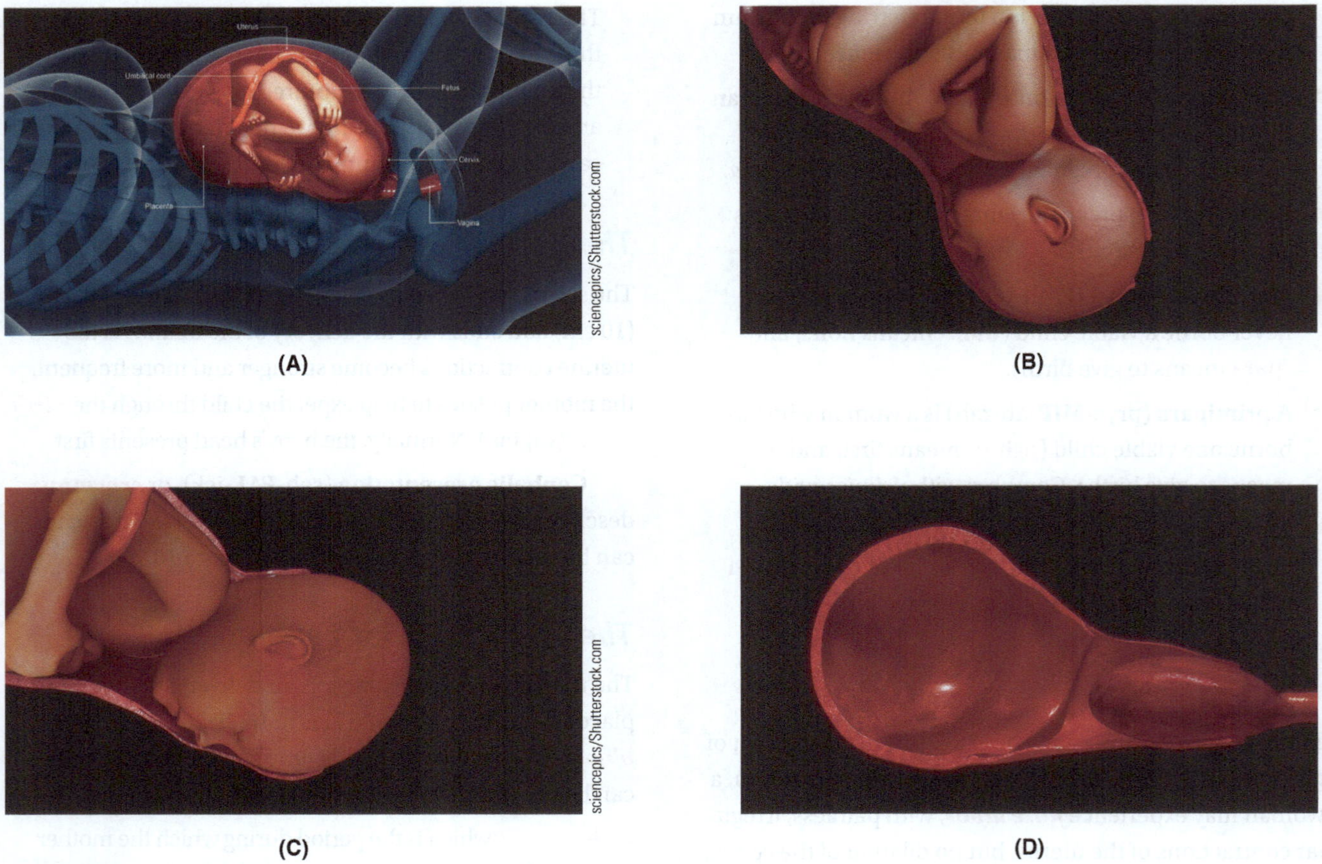

FIGURE 16.7 The three stages of labor. (A) Position of the fetus before labor. (B) First stage of labor, cervical dilation. (C) Second stage of labor, fetal delivery. (D) Third stage of labor, delivery of the afterbirth (placenta and fetal membrane).

The Baby

The newborn infant is known as a **neonate** (**NEE**-oh-nayt) during the first four weeks after birth. See Chapter 18 for further information.

- **Vernix** (**VER**-nicks) is a greasy substance that protects a fetus in utero and can still be present at birth. It is made up of sebum and discarded epidermal cells from the skin of the fetus (see Chapter 13).
- **Meconium** (meh-**KOH**-nee-um) is the greenish material that collects in the intestines of a fetus and forms the first feces of a newborn. ***Meconium aspiration syndrome*** is a condition that can occur when a newborn passes meconium during labor or delivery, and then inhales it via the amniotic fluid, causing difficulty breathing.

Lactation

Lactation (lack-**TAY**-shun) is the process of forming and secreting milk from the breasts as nourishment for the infant. The breast milk develops a few days after giving birth to replace the colostrum. **Colostrum** (kuh-**LOS**-trum) is a specialized form of breast milk that delivers essential nutrients and antibodies in a form that the newborn can digest. Colostrum is produced by the mammary glands in late pregnancy and during the first few days after giving birth.

- When the baby sucks at the breast, the hormones prolactin and oxytocin are released into the mother's bloodstream, causing the ***let-down reflex*** to make the breast milk flow.

MEDICAL SPECIALTIES RELATED TO THE FEMALE REPRODUCTIVE SYSTEM AND OBSTETRICS

- A **gynecologist** (**guy**-neh-**KOL**-oh-jist) (GYN) is a physician who specializes in diagnosing and treating diseases and disorders of the female reproductive system (**gynec** means female, and **-ologist** means specialist). This specialty is referred to as ***gynecology***.
- An **obstetrician** (**ob**-steh-**TRISH**-un) (OB) is a physician who specializes in providing medical care to women during pregnancy, during childbirth, and

immediately thereafter. The combined obstetrics and gynecology specialties are often referred to as *OB/GYN*.

- A **certified midwife** (CM) assists in labor and delivery. A *certified nurse midwife* (CNM) is an RN with specialized training in obstetrics and gynecology who provides primary care in normal pregnancies and deliveries. A *doula* is an experienced birth coach, usually without formal obstetric training, hired to provide added support and guidance during labor, delivery, and the postpartum period.
- A **neonatologist** (**nee**-oh-nay-**TOL**-oh-jist) is a physician who specializes in diagnosing and treating disorders of the newborn (**neo-** means new, **nat** means birth, and **-ologist** means specialist). The **neonatal intensive care unit** (NICU) is a nursery offering specialized care for premature or critically ill infants. Those who have progressed out of the NICU may go into a *special care nursery*, which is also where infants with less acute medical needs are treated.
- A **perinatologist** (**pehr**-ee-nay-**TOL**-oh-jist), also known as a *maternal-fetal medicine specialist*, works with women whose pregnancy is considered high risk (**peri-** means around, **nat** means birth, and **-ologist** means specialist).
- An **infertility specialist**, also known as a *reproductive endocrinologist*, helps couples by diagnosing and treating problems associated with conception and maintaining pregnancy.

PATHOLOGY OF THE FEMALE REPRODUCTIVE SYSTEM

The Ovaries, Fallopian Tubes, and Ovulation

- **Anovulation** (**an**-ov-you-**LAY**-shun) is the absence of ovulation when it would be normally expected (**an-** means without, and **ovulation** means the release of a mature egg). This condition can be caused by high levels of stress, inadequate nutrition, obesity, or hormonal imbalances. Menstruation continues even if an ovum is not released.
- *Blocked fallopian tubes*, which is a potential cause of infertility, can result from scarring, or conditions such as fibroids, endometriosis, or pelvic inflammatory disease.
- A **dermoid cyst** (**DER**-moyd), also called a *teratoma*, is a benign tumor containing various tissues such as teeth, bone, skin, glands, or hair. It is present at birth, and may be found on the face, inside the skull, on the lower back, in or on the ovaries (**derm** means skin, and **-oid** means resembling). Some dermoid cysts require surgical removal.
- **Ovarian cysts** are fluid-filled sacs in or on the surface of an ovary. These are generally harmless unless they rupture.
- **Ovarian cancer** originates within the cells of the ovaries. These cancer cells can break away from the ovary and spread (metastasize) to other tissues and organs within the abdomen or travel through the bloodstream to other parts of the body. It is difficult to detect ovarian cancer in its earliest stages, when treatment is most effective.
- **Pelvic inflammatory disease** (PID) is any inflammation of the female reproductive organs that is not associated with surgery or pregnancy. This condition occurs most frequently as a complication of a sexually transmitted disease and can lead to infertility, ectopic pregnancy, and other serious disorders.
- **Polycystic ovary syndrome** (**pol**-ee-**SIS**-tick) (PCOS) is a condition characterized by an imbalance of reproductive hormones resulting in irregular menstrual cycles, hirsutism (excessive body and facial hair), and acne. High levels of insulin and the male hormone androgen, normally found in small amounts in women, are often present in those with PCOS.
- **Primary ovarian insufficiency** (POI), also known as *premature ovarian failure*, is when the ovaries stop functioning normally before the age of 40. This can be caused by chemotherapy or radiation treatments, as well as chromosomal defects. This condition, which causes premature menopause, often leads to infertility.
- **Pyosalpinx** (**pye**-oh-**SAL**-pinks) is an accumulation of pus in a fallopian tube, sometimes as a result of pelvic inflammatory disease (**py/o** means pus, and **-salpinx** means fallopian tube).
- **Salpingitis** (**sal**-pin-**JIGH**-tis) is an inflammation of a fallopian tube caused by a bacterial infection, usually as a result of an STD (**salping** means fallopian tube, and **-itis** means inflammation).
- *Sexually transmitted diseases* (STDs) and *sexually transmitted infections* (STIs) are discussed with the Male Reproductive System in Chapter 15; however, most STDs can be transmitted by both men or women.

The Uterus

- **Endometriosis** (**en**-doh-**mee**-tree-**OH**-sis) is a condition in which patches of endometrial tissue escape the uterus and become attached to other structures in the pelvic cavity (**endo-** means within, **metri** means uterus, and **-osis** means abnormal condition). The cause of this painful condition is not known.

- **Endometrial cancer** (en-doh-**MEE**-tree-al) involves a cancerous growth that begins in the lining of the uterus and can spread to the ovaries and fallopian tubes. Symptoms include vaginal bleeding after menopause, bleeding between menstrual periods, and pelvic pain.
- **Uterine fibroids**, also known as ***myomas***, are benign tumors composed of muscle and fibrous tissue that occur in the wall of the uterus (Figure 16.8). These common growths are not associated with an increased risk of uterine cancer. ***Fibroid*** means characterized by fibrous tissue.
- A **uterine prolapse** (**YOU**-ter-ihn proh-**LAPS**), also known as a ***pelvic floor hernia***, is a condition in which the weakening of pelvic muscles and supportive tissues allows the uterus to slide from its normal position in the pelvic cavity and sag into the vagina. ***Prolapse*** (also pronounced **PROH**-laps) means the falling or dropping down of an organ or internal part.

The Cervix

- **Cervical cancer** is a slow-growing squamous cell cancer (see Chapter 13). It is caused by human papillomavirus (HPV) infection, which is spread through sexual contact. Carcinoma of the cervix is usually diagnosed between ages 35 and 50, and is more common among women with multiple sexual partners and those who smoke. An HPV vaccine is now available to help prevent certain types of infection, and it works most effectively when administered to girls and boys at ages 11 or 12. See Chapter 18 for more information.

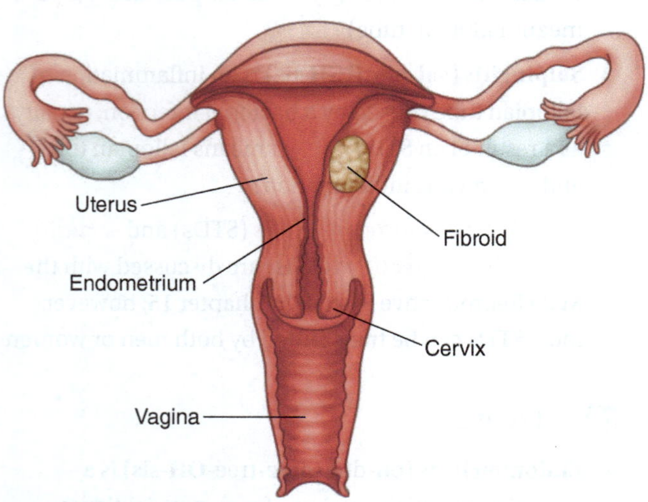

FIGURE 16.8 A uterine fibroid.

- **Cervical dysplasia** (**SER**-vih-kal dis-**PLAY**-see-ah) is the presence of precancerous changes in the cells that make up the inner lining of the cervix. Without early detection and treatment, these cells can become malignant.
- **Cervicitis** (**ser**-vih-**SIGH**-tis) is an inflammation of the cervix that is usually caused by infection, irritation, or allergies (**cervic** means cervix, and **-itis** means inflammation). It can also be the result of a sexually transmitted infection such as chlamydia or gonorrhea (see Chapter 15).

The Vagina

- **Bacterial vaginosis** (**vaj**-ih-**NOH**-sis) (BV) is a condition in which there is an abnormal overgrowth of certain bacteria in the vagina (**vagin** means vagina, and **-osis** means abnormal condition or disease). This condition is not an STD; however, the risk seems to increase with multiple sexual partners. It can cause complications during pregnancy and an increased risk of infection if there is exposure to HIV. Symptoms sometimes include discharge, odor, pain, itching, or burning.
- A **cystocele** (**SIS**-toh-seel) is a hernia of the bladder through the vaginal wall (**cyst/o** means bladder, and **-cele** means hernia). This sometimes occurs as a result of pregnancy or childbirth.
- **Dyspareunia** (**dis**-pah-**ROO**-nee-ah) is pain during sexual intercourse (**dys** means painful, and **-pareunia** means coitus).
- **Leukorrhea** (**loo**-koh-**REE**-ah) is a profuse whitish mucus discharge from the uterus and vagina (**leuk/o** means white, and **-rrhea** means flow or discharge). Women normally may have some vaginal discharge; however, leukorrhea describes a change and increase in this discharge that may be due to an infection or hormonal imbalance.
- **Toxic shock syndrome** is a rare but potentially fatal bacterial infection caused by an overgrowth of the bacteria *Staphylococcus aureus*. Although it can affect either men or women, it is sometimes linked to the use of super-absorbent tampons, diaphragms, or cervical caps.
- **Vaginal atrophy**, also known as ***genitourinary syndrome of menopause***, is a thinning, drying, and inflammation of the vaginal walls caused by hormonal changes. It affects about half of all postmenopausal women and can be treated with vaginal moisturizers, lubricants, or estrogen therapy.

- **Vaginal candidiasis** (**kan**-dih-**DYE**-ah-sis), also known as a ***yeast infection***, is a common vaginal infection caused by the yeast-like fungus *Candida albicans* (see Chapter 7). The growth of this fungus is usually controlled by bacteria normally present in the vagina. Symptoms of vaginal candidiasis include burning, itching, and a "cottage cheese-like" vaginal discharge.
- **Vaginismus** (**VAJ**-ih-**nihz**-mis) is an involuntary spasm of the pelvic floor muscles, which close off the vagina (**vagin** means vagina, and **-ismus** means spasm or contraction). This spasm can cause dyspareunia and difficulty tolerating the insertion of a tampon or a speculum for a gynecological exam.
- **Vaginitis** (**vaj**-ih-**NIGH**-tis) is an inflammation of the lining of the vagina (**vagin** means vagina, and **-itis** means inflammation). The most common causes of a vaginal inflammation are bacterial vaginosis, trichomoniasis, and vaginal candidiasis.

The External Genitalia

- **Vulvodynia** (vul-voh-**DIN**-ee-ah) is a painful syndrome of unknown cause that lasts at least three months (**vulv/o** means vulva, and **-dynia** means pain). It is characterized by chronic burning, dyspareunia, itching, or stinging irritation of the vulva.
- **Vulvitis** (vul-**VYE**-tis) is an inflammation of the vulva (**vulv** means vulva, and **-itis** means inflammation). Possible causes include fungal or bacterial infections, chafing, skin conditions, or allergies to products such as soaps and bubble bath.

Breast Diseases

- **Breast cancer**, along with its diagnosis and treatment, is discussed in Chapter 20.
- A **fibroadenoma** (**figh**-broh-**ad**-eh-**NOH**-mah) is a round, firm, rubbery mass that arises from excess growth of glandular and connective tissue in the breast (**fibr/o** means fibrous tissue, **aden** means gland, and **-oma** means tumor) (Figure 16.9). These masses, which occur most often between ages 15 and 35, are benign and usually painless. Fibroadenomas often enlarge during pregnancy and shrink after menopause due to changes in hormone levels.
- **Fibrocystic breasts** (**figh**-broh-**SIS**-tick) is a term used to describe the presence of fibrous tissue and benign cysts in the breasts. This common condition usually occurs in premenopausal women. A ***cyst*** is a closed sac containing fluid or semisolid material.

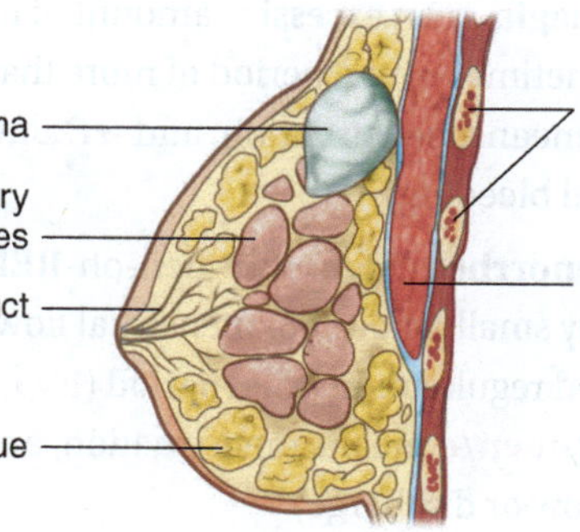

FIGURE 16.9 A fibroadenoma of the breast.

- **Galactorrhea** (gah-**lack**-toh-**REE**-ah) is the production of breast milk in a woman who is not breastfeeding (**galact/o** means milk, and **-rrhea** means flow or discharge). This condition is caused by a malfunction of the pituitary gland. In men, galactorrhea is a nipple discharge associated with a testosterone deficiency.
- **Mastalgia** (mass-**TAL**-jee-ah) is pain or tenderness in the breast (**mast** means breast, and **-algia** means pain).
- **Mastitis** (mas-**TYE**-tis) is a breast infection that is caused by bacteria that enter the mammary glands, most frequently during breastfeeding (**mast** means breast, and **-itis** means inflammation).

Menstrual Disorders

- **Amenorrhea** (ah-**men**-oh-**REE**-ah) is an abnormal absence of menstrual periods for 90 days or more (**a-** means without, **men/o** means menstruation, and **-rrhea** means flow or discharge). This condition, which is normal only before puberty, during pregnancy, while breastfeeding, and after menopause, can be caused by stress, hormonal problems, inadequate nutrition, or excessive exercise.
- **Dysmenorrhea** (**dis**-men-oh-**REE**-ah), or ***menstrual cramps***, is pain caused by uterine contractions during a menstrual period (**dys-** means bad, **men/o** means menstruation, and **-rrhea** means flow or discharge). This pain, which occurs in the lower abdomen, can be sharp, intermittent, dull, or aching.
- **Abnormal uterine bleeding**, also known as ***dysfunctional uterine bleeding***, is a condition characterized by abnormal bleeding during or outside of the menstrual period. This can be caused by fibroids, hormone problems, or other conditions.

- **Menorrhagia**, is an excessive amount of menstrual flow, sometimes over a period of more than seven days (**men/o** means menstruation, and **-rrhagia** means abnormal bleeding).
- **Hypomenorrhea** (**high**-poh-men-oh-**REE**-ah) is an unusually small amount of menstrual flow during a shortened regular menstrual period (**hypo-** means deficient, **men/o** means menstruation, and **-rrhea** means flow or discharge).
- **Metrorrhagia** (**mee**-troh-**RAY**-jee-ah), also known as ***intermenstrual bleeding***, is irregular uterine bleeding outside of regular menstrual periods (**metr/o** means uterus, and **-rrhagia** means abnormal bleeding).
- **Oligomenorrhea** (**ol**-ih-goh-**men**-oh-**REE**-ah), also called ***infrequent menstruation***, is the term used to describe irregular or very light menstruation in a woman with previously normal periods (**olig/o** means scanty, **men/o** means menstruation, and **-rrhea** means flow or discharge). Oligomenorrhea is the opposite of *polymenorrhea*.
- **Polymenorrhea** (**pol**-ee-**men**-oh-**REE**-ah) is the occurrence of menstrual cycles more frequently than is normal (**poly-** means many, **men/o** means menstruation, and **-rrhea** means flow or discharge). Polymenorrhea is the opposite of *oligomenorrhea*.
- **Premature menopause** is a condition in which the ovaries cease functioning before age 40 due to disease, a hormonal disorder, or surgical removal. This causes infertility and often brings on menopausal symptoms.
- **Premenstrual syndrome** (PMS) is a group of symptoms experienced by some women within the two-week period before menstruation. These symptoms can include bloating, swelling, headaches, mood swings, and breast discomfort.
- **Premenstrual dysphoric disorder** (PMDD) is a condition associated with severe emotional and physical problems that are closely linked to the menstrual cycle. Symptoms occur regularly in the second half of the cycle and end when menstruation begins or shortly thereafter.

PATHOLOGY OF PREGNANCY AND CHILDBIRTH

Termination of Pregnancy

- An **abortion** (ah-**BOR**-shun) is the interruption or termination of pregnancy before the fetus is viable.
- A ***spontaneous abortion***, also known as a ***miscarriage***, usually occurs early in the pregnancy and may be due to an abnormality or genetic disorder.
- An ***induced abortion*** is one caused by human intervention. When done for medical purposes, it is known as a ***therapeutic abortion***. Abortion is achieved through either the use of an ***abortifacient*** medication within the first weeks after conception or a surgical procedure called suction aspiration.
- An **ectopic pregnancy** (eck-**TOP**-ick), also known as an ***extrauterine pregnancy***, is a dangerous condition in which a fertilized egg is implanted and begins to develop outside of the uterus. ***Ectopic*** means out of place, and Figure 16.10 illustrates some of these potential locations.

Challenges of Conceiving

Infertility is the inability of a couple to achieve pregnancy after one year of regular, unprotected intercourse, or the inability of a woman to carry a pregnancy to a live birth. ***Secondary infertility*** means the inability to become pregnant or to carry a baby to term after previously having given birth.

Complications of Pregnancy

A ***complication*** is an unanticipated problem that develops as a result of a primary condition, in this case being pregnant.

- **Cervical insufficiency**, also known as an ***incompetent cervix***, refers to weakened tissue in the cervix. In pregnancy, this condition may cause the cervix to open too soon, leading to late miscarriage or a premature birth.

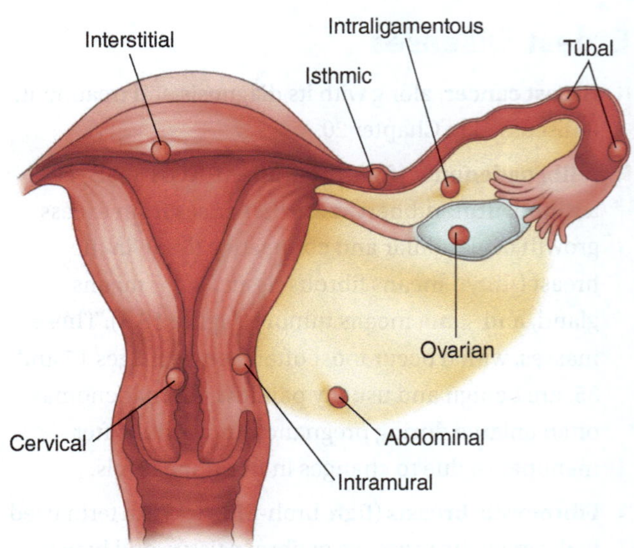

FIGURE 16.10 Potential sites of an ectopic pregnancy.

- **Gestational diabetes mellitus**, a form of diabetes that occurs during pregnancy, is discussed in Chapter 14. *Gestational* is an adjective referring to the time between conception and birth.
- **Placental disorders** can impact the safety of the fetus during pregnancy and delivery.
  - **Abruptio placentae** (ah-**BRUP**-shee-oh plah-**SEN**-tee), or *placental abruption*, is a disorder in which the placenta separates from the uterine wall before the birth of the fetus. *Abruption* means breaking off. This condition can cause fetal death or long-term health complications.
  - **Placenta previa** (plah-**SEN**-tah **PREE**-vee-ah) is the abnormal implantation of the placenta in the lower portion of the uterus, partially or completely covering the cervix. *Previa* means appearing before or in front of. Symptoms include painless sudden-onset bleeding during the third trimester, and possibly also severe bleeding during delivery.
  - **Placenta accreta** (ah-**KREE**-tah) occurs when the placenta attaches itself too deeply into the uterine wall, making it difficult for the placenta to separate during childbirth. This increases the risk of hemorrhage. *Accreta* is a Latin word meaning encased in.
- **Eclampsia** (eh-**KLAMP**-see-ah), a serious condition characterized by seizures and coma that can develop from uncontrolled preeclampsia.
  - **Gestational hypertension**, also known as *pregnancy-induced hypertension*, is high blood pressure that sometimes develops after 20 weeks of pregnancy, and usually goes away within 12 weeks after giving birth. Hypertension is discussed in Chapter 5. Gestational hypertension can lead to preeclampsia.
  - **Preeclampsia** (**pree**-ee-**KLAMP**-see-ah) is a complication of pregnancy characterized by hypertension (high blood pressure) and proteinuria (an abnormally high level of protein in the urine). This condition is a common cause of preterm birth and other maternal and other complications for the mother and fetus.
  - **HELLP syndrome** is a life-threatening pregnancy complication characterized by **H**emolysis (breakdown of red blood cells), **E**levated **L**iver enzymes, and **L**ow **P**latelet count. It occurs in 10–20% of women with severe preeclampsia and can cause damage to the liver and blood cells.
- **Hyperemesis gravidarum** (**high**-per-**EM**-ih-sis **grav**-ih-**DAHR**-um) means excessive vomiting during pregnancy (**hyper** means excessive, and **-emesis** means vomiting). *Gravidarum* is a Latin word meaning associated with pregnancy. Many women experience bouts of nausea and vomiting, often referred to as *morning sickness*, in the first trimester. But with hyperemesis gravidarum, medical treatment is required to prevent severe ongoing vomiting from causing dehydration and weight loss.
- **Implantation bleeding** is light vaginal bleeding that sometimes occurs 10 to 14 days after conception. This is normal; however, heavy or persistent bleeding is a cause of concern.
- **Melasma** (meh-**LAZ**-ma), also known as the *mask of pregnancy*, is a darkening of patches of the skin on the forehead, cheeks, and neck that sometimes occurs when estrogen and progesterone levels stimulate excess melanin production. This **hyperpigmentation** can also result in a darkening of freckles, moles, and the areolas of the breasts, as well as a dark line down the center of the abdomen known as the *linea nigra* (**hyper-** means excessive, **pigment** means color, and **-ation** means state).
- A **molar pregnancy**, also known as a as *hydatidiform mole*, is a rare and serious condition caused by the abnormal division of the fertilized egg. Most molar pregnancies end spontaneously with a miscarriage. Women younger than 20 and older than 35 are more likely to experience a molar pregnancy.
- **Oligohydramnios** (**al**-ih-go-hy-**DRAM**-nee-os) is a condition in which there is less amniotic fluid than normal. This usually occurs when the amniotic sac ruptures; however, it can also be caused by a problem with fetal urine production. The opposite is a less common condition called *polyhydramnios*, in which there is more amniotic fluid than normal.

The Rh Factor

The **Rh factor** defines the presence or absence of the Rh antigen on red blood cells (see Chapter 6). The Rh factor can cause difficulties when an Rh negative (Rh–) mother is pregnant with an Rh positive (Rh+) baby. If a small amount of the baby's blood enters the mother's bloodstream, she can develop antibodies in an allergic response.

- A man who is Rh+ can father a baby that is either Rh+ or Rh–, potentially causing a reaction if the mother is Rh–. (If both parents are Rh–, there is no danger of incompatibility.)

- The antibodies that develop in the mother's body during pregnancy can cause anemia and other problems for the baby and can also be a risk factor in subsequent pregnancies if the mother is not treated.
- Blood tests of both parents can identify this potential problem. If it exists, the mother is vaccinated with a blood product called ***Rho(D) immune globulin***.
- The abbreviation Rh comes from the fact that blood samples from rhesus monkeys were used in the experiments that lead to the discovery of the Rh factor in 1940.

CHILDBIRTH AND POSTPARTUM

- **Breech presentation** occurs when the buttocks or feet of the fetus, instead of the head, are positioned to enter the birth canal first. ***Abnormal presentations***, which may also include the shoulder presenting first, can lead to birth injuries. A cesarean delivery is often performed to prevent this.
- **Labor induction** is the stimulation of uterine contractions before labor begins on its own. Labor may be induced due to health concerns for the mother or baby, or in order to try to achieve a vaginal birth. Medication may be used to thin or soften the cervix, and the amniotic sac may be ruptured, prior to the intravenous administration of a synthetic version of the hormone oxytocin such as Pitocin®. The rupturing of the amniotic sac is called an ***amniotomy***.
- **Preterm labor**, also known as ***early labor***, is when regular contractions begin as the result of the opening of the cervix after the 20th week and before the 37th week of a pregnancy. This can result in the baby being born prematurely.
- The **premature rupture of membranes** (PROM) is when the amniotic sac ruptures before the 37th week of pregnancy. Labor is often induced in order to avoid the risk of infection.
- A **premature infant**, also known as a ***preemie***, is a fetus born before the 37th week of gestation. This is referred to as a ***preterm birth***.
- A baby born after 42 weeks is considered ***postmature***. This is a rare occurrence.
- A **stillbirth** is the birth of a fetus that died before or during delivery.
- **Peripartum onset depression**, often referred to as ***postpartum depression***, is a mood disorder characterized by feelings of sadness and the loss of pleasure in normal activities that can occur shortly after giving birth. One cause of this depression is the rapid change in the hormone levels that occurs after giving birth. Treatment may be required if the depression is severe, or lasts beyond the two weeks of normal ***baby blues*** that often follows delivery.

DIAGNOSTIC PROCEDURES OF THE FEMALE REPRODUCTIVE SYSTEM

- **Colposcopy** (kol-**POS**-koh-pee) is the direct visual examination of the tissues of the cervix, vagina, and vulva (**colp/o** means vagina, and **-scopy** means direct visual examination). This examination is performed using a binocular magnifier known as a ***colposcope***.
- In an **endometrial biopsy**, a small amount of the tissue from the lining of the uterus is removed for microscopic examination. This test is most often used to determine the cause of abnormal uterine bleeding.
- **Transvaginal ultrasound** (**trans**-**VAJ**-ih-nal) (TVS), also known as an ***endovaginal ultrasound***, is performed to determine the cause of pelvic pain, infertility, or abnormal vaginal bleeding (**trans-** means through, **vagin** means vagina, and **-al** means pertaining to). This test is performed by placing an ultrasound transducer in the vagina so that the sound waves can create images of the uterus and ovaries.
- **Hysterosalpingography** (**hiss**-ter-oh-**sal**-pin-**GOG**-rah-fee) (HSG) is an x-ray examination of the uterus and fallopian tubes (**hyster/o** means uterus, **salping/o** means fallopian tube, and **-graphy** means the process of producing a picture or record). This test requires the instillation of radiopaque contrast material into the uterine cavity and fallopian tubes to make them visible. ***Instillation*** means the slow introduction of a liquid into a body part by pouring or injection.
- **Hysteroscopy** (**hiss**-ter-**OSS**-koh-pee) (HYS) is the direct visual examination of the inside of the uterus and cervix (**hyster/o** means uterus, and **-scopy** means direct visual examination). This examination, used to diagnose and treat abnormal bleeding, is performed by using the lighted magnification of a ***hysteroscope***.
- A **Pap smear**, or ***Pap test***, is an exfoliative biopsy of the cervix developed by Dr. George Papanicolaou. It is performed to detect conditions that can be early indicators of cervical cancer (Figure 16.11). As used here, ***exfoliative*** means that cells are scraped from the tissue and examined under a microscope. A **speculum**

(**SPECK**-you-lum) is an instrument used to enlarge the opening of the vagina during the examination of the cervix and vagina.

- *Ultrasound* and *laparoscopy*, which are also used to diagnose disorders of the reproductive system, are discussed further in Chapter 21.

Diagnostic Procedures Related to Pregnancy and Childbirth

- A **pregnancy test** is performed to detect an unusually high level of the *human chorionic gonadotropin* (HCG) hormone in either a blood or urine specimen, which is usually an indication of pregnancy. A home pregnancy test uses a urine specimen, whereas a pregnancy test based on a blood specimen at a doctor's office usually provides more reliable results.
- There are three categories for signs of pregnancy: *presumptive*, *probable*, and *positive*.
  - Presumptive signs include amenorrhea, fatigue, frequent urination, nausea, and/or sore or enlarged breasts.
  - Probable signs include a positive pregnancy test; however, there is the possibility of a false negative. The softening of the cervix known as *Goodell's sign* is considered a probable indicator of pregnancy.
  - Positive signs include detecting a fetal heartbeat and movement, and ultrasound imaging of the fetus.
- **Fetal ultrasound** testing is discussed in Chapter 21.
- **First trimester screening**, also known as *combined screening*, is performed between 11 and 13 weeks of pregnancy and involves an ultrasound and a blood test. The combined results of these two measurements, plus the mother's age, detect if the fetus is at increased risk for a chromosome abnormality such as Down syndrome, which is discussed in Chapter 2. Diagnostic tests, such as amniocentesis or chorionic villus sampling, are recommended for those at increased risk for this condition.
- **Chorionic villus sampling** (**kor**-ee-**ON**-ick **VIL**-us) (CVS) is the examination of cells retrieved from the *chorionic villi*, which are minute, vascular projections on the chorion. This test is performed between the 11th and 14th weeks of pregnancy to search for genetic abnormalities in the developing fetus.
- **Amniocentesis** (**am**-nee-oh-sen-**TEE**-sis) (AMN) is a surgical puncture with a needle to obtain a specimen of amniotic fluid (**amni/o** means the amniotic sac, and **-centesis** means a surgical puncture to remove fluid). This specimen, which is usually obtained after the 15th week of pregnancy, is used to evaluate fetal health and to diagnose certain congenital disorders.

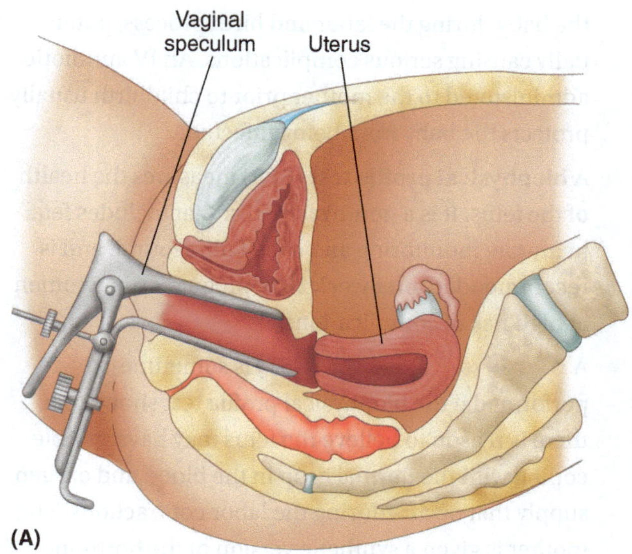

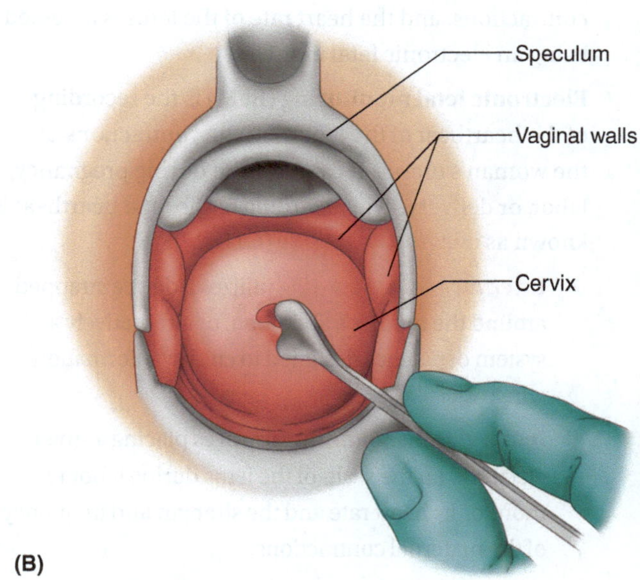

FIGURE 16.11 For a Pap smear, a speculum is used to enlarge the vaginal opening (A), and a few cervical cells are removed for sudy under a microscope (B).

- A **glucose tolerance test** is an oral test used to diagnose gestational diabetes during pregnancy, and sometimes to screen for type 2 diabetes. Two hours after drinking a syrupy glucose solution, a blood glucose test is done to see if the body has processed the glucose normally. Glucose screening is normally performed between 24 and 28 weeks of pregnancy.
- A **group B strep test** (GBS test), performed during the third trimester, is a vaginal and rectal swab test. If *group B streptococcus* is present, it can be passed to

the baby during the labor and birth process, potentially causing serious complications. An IV antibiotic administered to the mother prior to childbirth usually protects the baby from being infected.

- A **biophysical profile test** (BPP) measures the health of the fetus. It is a noninvasive test that includes fetal heart rate monitoring and a fetal ultrasound, and is recommended after week 28 of pregnancy for women at high risk of complications.
- A ***contraction stress test*** (CST) is sometimes performed if the biophysical profile test shows that there is reason to believe the fetus may have trouble coping with the normal drop in the blood and oxygen supply that occurs during the labor contractions. The mother is given a synthetic version of the hormone oxytocin intravenously to temporarily induce contractions, and the heart rate of the fetus is assessed using an electronic fetal monitor.
- **Electronic fetal monitoring** (EFM) is the recording of the heartbeat of the fetus and the contractions of the woman's uterus. It can be done during pregnancy, labor, or delivery. The recording of the fetal heartbeat is known as ***cardiotocography*** (CTG).
    - ***External fetal monitoring*** utilizes a device strapped around the mother's abdomen, or alternatively a system of patches designed to convey information wirelessly.
    - ***Internal fetal monitoring*** involves placing a small electrode on the scalp of the fetus during labor to monitor its heart rate and the strength and frequency of the maternal contractions.
- ***Fetal scalp pH testing*** is a procedure during active labor in which a small blood sample is taken from the scalp of the fetus to analyze for oxygen content. If a problem is detected, a forceps delivery or cesarean birth may be necessary.

TREATMENT PROCEDURES OF THE FEMALE REPRODUCTIVE SYSTEM

Birth Control

- A **contraceptive** is a measure taken to lessen the likelihood of pregnancy. *Note:* Some forms of contraception are used by men, some by women, and some by both. See Chapter 15 for more information about male birth control and sterilization.
- ***Family planning*** refers to controlling whether to have a child and deciding on the ideal intervals between births. Both contraception and means of becoming pregnant are aspects of family planning.
- **Birth control pills** are the hormones estrogen and progestin administered as an oral contraceptive. This type of contraceptive is also available as an injection, a skin patch, an arm implant, and a vaginally inserted ring.
- A ***contraceptive implant*** is a thin rod containing the hormone progestin that is placed under the skin of the upper arm. It can be left in place for up to three years, during which time it releases a slow, steady dose of the hormone.
- ***Morning-after pills*** are emergency contraception taken to prevent pregnancy when a woman has had unprotected intercourse, or if her method of birth control failed. They are most effective when taken within 72 hours, and work primarily by delaying or preventing ovulation.
- ***Abstinence*** means avoiding pregnancy by not having sexual relations.
- ***Barrier methods of contraception*** block the sperm from entering the uterus after sexual intercourse. Diaphragms, cervical caps, and condoms are barrier methods.
    - A **diaphragm** is a barrier contraceptive inserted into the vagina to cover the cervix, preventing the sperm from reaching and fertilizing the egg. A ***spermicide*** is a gel, lube, or foam that can be added to kill sperm or stop sperm from moving.
    - A ***cervical cap*** is a smaller covering for the cervix that can remain in place longer than a diaphragm.
    - A **condom** will prevent pregnancy when used correctly. It is the only contraceptive method mentioned here that will also prevent the transmission of sexually transmitted diseases (STDs).
- An **intrauterine device** (IUD) is a molded plastic contraceptive inserted through the cervix into the uterus to prevent pregnancy (**intra-** means within, and **uterine** means uterus). ***Intrauterine*** means situated within the uterus. There are two types of IUDs: one is copper-coated (copper is toxic to sperm), and the other releases the hormone progestin, which thickens cervical mucus to prevent sperm from reaching the egg. An IUD is a form of ***long-acting, reversible contraception*** (LARC).
- **Tubal ligation**, sometimes referred to has having the ***tubes tied***, is a surgical sterilization procedure in which the fallopian tubes are sealed or cut to prevent sperm from reaching a mature ovum. **Sterilization** is any procedure rendering an individual (male or female) incapable of reproduction.

Hormone Treatments

- **Hormone replacement therapy** (HRT) is the use of the hormones estrogen and progesterone to replace those the body no longer produces during and after perimenopause. The goal of this treatment is to relieve severe menopausal symptoms such as hot flashes and vaginal dryness. ***Estradiol*** and ***progestin*** are commonly used synthetic forms of estrogen and progesterone, respectively.
- Menorrhagia is sometimes treated with oral progestin and NSAIDs.
- Amenorrhea can often be treated with hormone replacement therapy when caused by a lack of estrogen, and with birth control pills when caused by polycystic ovary syndrome.

The Ovaries and Fallopian Tubes

- An **oophorectomy** (**oh**-ahf-oh-**RECK**-toh-mee), also known as an ***ovariectomy***, is the surgical removal of one or both ovaries (**oophor** mean ovary, and **-ectomy** means surgical removal). If both ovaries are removed in a premenopausal woman, the patient will experience ***surgical menopause*** because the hormone estrogen is no longer being produced. Surgical menopause refers to menopausal symptoms being induced by the abrupt cessation of ovarian hormones.
- A **salpingectomy** (**sal**-pin-**JECK**-toh-mee) is the surgical removal of one or both fallopian tubes (**salping** means fallopian tube, and **-ectomy** means surgical removal).
- A **salpingo-oophorectomy** (sal-**ping**-goh-oh-**ahf**-oh-**RECK**-toh-mee) (SO) is the surgical removal of a fallopian tube and ovary (**salping/o** means fallopian tube, **oophor** means ovary, and **-ectomy** means surgical removal). A ***bilateral salpingooophorectomy*** is the removal of both of the fallopian tubes and ovaries. This procedure is sometimes used to treat ovarian cancer, or to reduce the risk of ovarian cancer occurring.

The Uterus, Cervix, and Vagina

- A **sacrocolpopexy** (sa-kroh-**KOL**-poh-**peck**-see) is the surgical fixation of a prolapsed vagina to a surrounding structure such as the sacrum (**sacr/o** means sacrum, **colp/o** means vagina, and **-pexy** means surgical fixation).
- **Cauterization** (**kaw**-ter-eye-**ZAY**-shun) is the destruction of pre-cancerous cervical cells through the use of heat, electricity, or chemicals. Cauterization means to destroy tissue by burning.
- **Conization** (**kon**-ih-**ZAY**-shun), also known as a ***cone biopsy***, is the surgical removal of a cone-shaped specimen of tissue from the cervix. This is performed as a diagnostic procedure or to remove abnormal tissue.
- **Colporrhaphy** (kol-**POR**-ah-fee) is the surgical suturing of a tear in the vaginal wall (**colp/o** means vagina, and **-rrhaphy** means surgical suturing).
- **Dilation and curettage** (dye-**LAY**-shun and **kyou**-reh-**TAHZH**), commonly known as a ***D & C***, is a surgical procedure in which the cervix is dilated and the endometrium of the uterus is scraped away. This can be performed as a diagnostic procedure to research the cause of abnormal uterine bleeding, or a treatment to remove tissue after a miscarriage, abortion, or childbirth. ***Dilation*** means the expansion of an opening. ***Curettage*** is the removal of material from the surface by scraping with an instrument known as a curette.
- A **myomectomy** (**my**-oh-**MECK**-toh-mee) is the surgical removal of uterine fibroids (**myom** means a tumor of muscle tissue, and **-ectomy** means surgical removal).
- A **pessary** (**PESS**-ah-ree) is a soft, flexible device inserted into the vagina to support its internal structure. This is a non-surgical means of treating urinary incontinence or a pelvic organ prolapse. The term *pessary* can also refer to a vaginal suppository such as a cervical cap used for contraception.

Hysterectomies

A **hysterectomy** (**hiss**-teh-**RECK**-toh-mee) is the surgical removal of the uterus, often due to problems caused by uterine fibroids, gynecological cancer, endometriosis, or uterine prolapse (**hyster** means uterus, and **-ectomy** means surgical removal). The procedure is further described by the structures that are removed (Figure 16.12).

- In a **total hysterectomy**, also known as a ***complete hysterectomy***, the uterus and cervix are removed. This procedure can be performed through the vagina or laparoscopically through the abdomen (Figure 16.12A).
- A **radical hysterectomy** is the removal of the uterus, ligaments, cervix, and a portion of the vagina. It is most commonly performed to treat cervical cancer (Figure 16.12B).

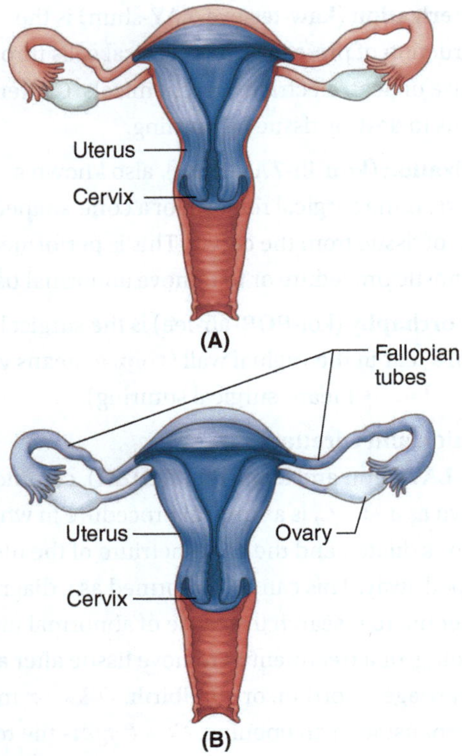

FIGURE 16.12 Types of hysterectomies, with the areas removed shown in blue. (A) In a total hysterectomy, the uterus and cervix are removed. (B) In a radical hysterectomy with a bilateral salpingo-oophorectomy, the ovaries, fallopian tubes, uterus, and cervix are removed.

- In a **partial hysterectomy**, the uterus is removed and the cervix is left in place.
- A ***bilateral salpingo-oophorectomy*** (BSO) is the surgical removal of both of the ovaries and fallopian tubes, which is usually performed during a hysterectomy. If done before natural menopause, the patient will immediately experience surgical menopause (see above).

Mammoplasty

Mammoplasty (**MAM**-oh-**plas**-tee), also spelled *mammaplasty*, is a general term for a cosmetic operation on the breasts (**mamm/o** means breast, and **-plasty** means surgical repair).

- **Breast augmentation** is mammoplasty performed to increase breast size, often for cosmetic reasons. *Augmentation* means the process of adding to make larger.
- **Breast reduction** is mammoplasty performed to decrease and reshape excessively large, heavy breasts. This surgery can be done for cosmetic reasons, or to relieve back, neck and shoulder pain.
- **Mastopexy** (**MAS**-toh-**peck**-see), also called a breast lift, is elective surgery to affix sagging breasts in a more elevated position (**mast/o** means breast, and **-pexy** means surgical fixation).
- **Breast reconstruction surgery** is the creation of the shape of a missing breast for women who have undergone a mastectomy (see Chapter 20). Instead of wearing an external prosthesis to simulate the shape of the breast inside a bra, breast cancer patients often elect to have this surgery.
  - ***Immediate breast reconstruction*** begins during the same surgery as the mastectomy when an "expander" is placed to replace the tissue that was removed.
  - ***Delayed breast reconstruction*** may be necessary if the surgery is to be followed by radiation treatment. Several different techniques are used to restore the size and shape of the missing breast.

Treatment Procedures Related to Pregnancy and Childbirth

- **Cervical cerclage** (sir-**KLAZH**) is a procedure in which sutures or a type of synthetic tape are used to reinforce the cervix in order to prevent premature birth.
- A **cesarean section** (seh-**ZEHR**-ee-un), also known as a *C-section*, is the delivery of the baby through an incision in the maternal abdominal and uterine walls. This is usually performed when a vaginal birth would be unsafe for either the mother or child.
- *VBAC* is the acronym used to describe **V**aginal **B**irth **A**fter a **C**esarean. Many women whose baby was delivered via cesarean section are able to give birth vaginally in subsequent pregnancies.
- An **episiotomy** (eh-**piz**-ee-**OT**-oh-mee) is a surgical incision made into the perineum to enlarge the vaginal orifice to prevent tearing of the tissues as the infant moves out of the birth canal (**episi** means vulva, and **-otomy** means a surgical incision).
- An **incubator** (**IN**-kyou-**bate**-or) is an apparatus for maintaining an environment of controlled temperature, humidity, and oxygen concentration for a premature or ill newborn.

Pain Relief During Childbirth

For labor and delivery, a combination of analgesics and anesthetics may be used for pain relief. The goal is to provide relief without the loss of consciousness or a total loss of feeling, and with a minimal impact on the fetus during the birthing process.

- An **epidural block** (**ep**-ih-**DOO**-ral) (EDB) is regional anesthesia that blocks the nerve impulses from the lower segments of the spine to the lower half of the body, lessening the pain of contractions. A needle is inserted into the epidural space, and a catheter put in place so that additional doses of the anesthesia can be given as needed. This is the most common form of pain relief during childbirth.
- A **spinal block** is a single injection given into the fluid surrounding the spinal cord. Pain relief from this injection lasts an hour or two. A spinal block is often used during a cesarean section.
- **Nitrous oxide** is an inhalation analgesic that can be used during labor. It is administered using a handheld face mask.
- **Natural childbirth** uses relaxation, alternative birthing positions, and/or breathing techniques to make the mother comfortable during an unmedicated birth. ***Lamaze*** is a well-known method of exercises; massage; and controlled, rhythmic breathing popularized by French obstetrician Dr. Fernand Lamaze beginning in the 1950s.

Assisted Reproduction

The science of helping an infertile couple or individual achieve a viable pregnancy is called **assisted reproduction**.

The term **assisted reproductive technology** (ART) describes techniques in which ova and embryos are treated outside the woman's body. Medication is often used to stimulate egg production before the retrieval process.

- **Artificial insemination**, most commonly ***intrauterine insemination*** (IUI), is a technique in which sperm from a woman's partner or from a donor are introduced into the vagina or uterus during the ovulatory phase of her menstrual cycle.
- **In vitro fertilization** (**VEE**-troh) (IVF) is a procedure in which mature ova are removed from the mother to be fertilized. The resulting healthy embryos are transferred into the uterus with the hope that they will implant and continue to develop as a normal pregnancy. ***In vitro*** means in an artificial environment such as a test tube.
- ***Intracytoplasmic sperm injection*** (ICSI) is a form of IVF in which a single sperm is injected into a mature ovum. This technique is sometimes used when low sperm count is a factor in infertility.
- A ***surrogate*** is a woman who agrees to become pregnant and give birth on behalf of a person or couple. Artificial insemination or surgical implantation of an in vitro fertilized egg may be used.

ABBREVIATIONS RELATED TO THE REPRODUCTIVE SYSTEM AND OBSTETRICS

Table 16.2 presents an overview of the abbreviations related to the terms introduced in this chapter. *Note:* To avoid errors or confusion, always be cautious when using abbreviations.

TABLE 16.2

Abbreviations Related to the Female Reproductive System and Obstetrics

amniocentesis = AMN	**AMN** = amniocentesis
bacterial vaginosis = BV	**BV** = bacterial vaginosis
cesarean section = C-section	**C-section** = cesarean section
hormone replacement therapy = HRT	**HRT** = hormone replacement therapy
hysterosalpingography = HSG	**HSG** = hysterosalpingography
hysteroscopy = HYS	**HYS** = hysteroscopy
in vitro fertilization = IVF	**IVF** = in vitro fertilization
intrauterine device = IUD	**IUD** = intrauterine device
neonatal intensive care unit = NICU	**NICU** = neonatal intensive care unit
pelvic inflammatory disease = PID	**PID** = pelvic inflammatory disease
premenstrual syndrome = PMS	**PMS** = premenstrual syndrome
polycystic ovary syndrome = PCOS	**PCOS** = polycystic ovary syndrome

CHAPTER 16

LEARNING EXERCISES

Matching Word Parts 1

Write the correct answer in the middle column.

	Definition	Correct Answer	Possible Answers
16.1.	cervix	________________	men/o
16.2.	female	________________	gynec/o
16.3.	menstruation	________________	-gravida
16.4.	pregnant	________________	colp/o
16.5.	vagina	________________	cervic/o

Matching Word Parts 2

Write the correct answer in the middle column.

	Definition	Correct Answer	Possible Answers
16.6.	egg	________________	vagin/o
16.7.	ovary	________________	test/i
16.8.	testicle	________________	ov/o
16.9.	uterus	________________	ovari/o
16.10.	vagina	________________	hyster/o

Matching Word Parts 3

Write the correct answer in the middle column.

	Definition	Correct Answer	Possible Answers
16.11.	breast	________	salping/o
16.12.	none	________	-pexy
16.13.	surgical fixation	________	-para
16.14.	to give birth	________	nulli-
16.15.	fallopian tube	________	mast/o

Definitions

Select the correct answer, and write it on the line provided.

16.16. The term that describes the inner layer of the uterus is ________.

corpus endometrium myometrium perimetrium

16.17. The term describing the single cell formed immediately after conception is ________.

embryo fetus gamete zygote

16.18. The mucus that lubricates the vagina is produced by the ________.

Bartholin's glands bulbourethral glands Cowper's glands hymen

16.19. The finger-like structures of the fallopian tube that catch the ovum are the ________.

fimbriae fundus infundibulum oviducts

16.20. The term ________ is used to designate the transition phase between regular menstrual periods and no periods at all.

menarche menopause perimenopause puberty

16.21. The medical term for the condition also known as a yeast infection is ________.

oligomenorrhea leukorrhea vaginitis vaginal candidiasis

16.22. During the ________ phase of the menstrual cycle, hormone levels change to cause the breakdown of the uterine endometrium.

menstrual follicular luteal ovulation

16.23. During puberty, the term ________________ describes the beginning of the menstrual function.

menarche menopause menses menstruation

16.24. In the female, the region between the vaginal orifice and the anus is known as the

________________________.

clitoris mons pubis perineum vulva

16.25. The release of a mature egg by the ovary is known as ________________________.

coitus fertilization menstruation ovulation

Matching Structures

Write the correct answer in the middle column.

	Definition	Correct Answer	Possible Answers
16.26.	carry milk from the mammary glands	________________	vulva
16.27.	partially covers the vaginal orifice	________________	hymen
16.28.	external female genitalia	________________	lactiferous ducts
16.29.	the opening into the fallopian tube	________________	infundibulum
16.30.	sensitive tissue near the vaginal opening	________________	clitoris

Which Word?

Select the correct answer, and write it on the line provided.

16.31. The term used to describe a woman during her first pregnancy is ____________________.

primigravida primipara

16.32. The fluid produced by the mammary glands during the first few days after giving birth is

____________________.

colostrum meconium

16.33. The term ____________________ describes an inflammation of the cervix that is usually caused by an infection.

cervicitis cervical dysplasia

16.34. From implantation through the eighth week of pregnancy, the developing child is known as a/an

______________________.

embryo fetus

16.35. Uterine ______________________ is the return of the uterus to its normal size and former condition after delivery.

prolapse involution

Spelling Counts

Find the misspelled word in each sentence. Then write that word, spelled correctly, on the line provided.

16.36. Malazma is a darkening of patches of the skin on the face during pregnancy.

____

16.37. A biphysical profile test measures the health of the fetus.

____

16.38. The third stage of labor and delivery is the expulsion of the plasenta as the afterbirth.

____

16.39. Maconium is the greenish material that forms the first feces of a newborn.

____

16.40. Gestational diabetes millitus is a form of diabetes that occurs during pregnancy.

____

Abbreviation Identification

In the space provided, write the words that each abbreviation stands for.

16.41. **AMA** ______________________

16.42. **PID** ______________________

16.43. **PMDD** ______________________

16.44. **IUD** ______________________

16.45. **HSG** ______________________

Term Selection

Select the correct answer, and write it on the line provided.

16.46. An accumulation of pus in the fallopian tube is known as ____________________.

endometriosis | pelvic inflammatory disease | pyosalpinx | salpingitis

16.47. The abnormal implantation of the placenta in the lower portion of the uterus is called ____________________.

placenta previa | eclampsia | placenta accreta | abruptio placentae

16.48. The direct visual examination of the tissues of the cervix and vagina using a binocular magnifier is known as ____________________.

colposcopy | transvaginal ultrasound | hysterosalpingography | hysteroscopy

16.49. The term used to describe infrequent or very light menstruation in a woman with previously normal periods is ____________________.

amenorrhea | hypomenorrhea | oligomenorrhea | dysmenorrhea

16.50. The examination of cells retrieved from the edge of the thin outer membrane that encloses an embryo between the 11th and 14th weeks of pregnancy is known as ____________________.

amniocentesis | chorionic villus sampling | electronic fetal monitoring | hysterosalpingography

Sentence Completion

Write the correct term or terms on the lines provided.

16.51. The dark-pigmented area surrounding the nipple is known as the ____________________.

16.52. Postmenopausal thinning, drying, and inflammation of the vaginal walls is called ____________________.

16.53. The serious complication of pregnancy that is characterized by convulsions and sometimes coma is known as ____________________. The treatment for this condition is delivery of the fetus.

16.54. Surgical suturing of a tear in the vagina is known as ____________________.

16.55. The ____________________ is the tube that carries blood, oxygen, and nutrients from the placenta to the developing child.

Word Surgery

Divide each term into its component word parts. Write these word parts, in sequence, on the lines provided. When necessary use a slash (/) to indicate a combining vowel. (You may not need all of the lines provided.)

16.56. **Vulvodynia** is a painful syndrome in the external female genitalia of unknown cause that lasts at least three months.

______ ______ ______ ______

16.57. **Metrorrhagia** is irregular uterine bleeding outside of the menstrual periods.

______ ______ ______ ______

16.58. **Hysterosalpingography** is an x-ray examination of the uterus and fallopian tubes.

______ ______ ______ ______

16.59. **Galactorrhea** is the production of breast milk in a woman who is not breastfeeding.

______ ______ ______ ______

16.60. **Fibroadenoma** is a mass that arises from excess growth of tissue in the breast.

______ ______ ______ ______

True/False

If the statement is true, write **True** on the line. If the statement is false, write **False** on the line.

16.61. ______ A neonatologist assists in labor and delivery.

16.62. ______ Braxton Hicks contractions are the first true labor pains.

16.63. ______ HELLP syndrome is a life-threatening pregnancy complication.

16.64. ______ Breast augmentation is mammoplasty that is performed to reduce breast size.

16.65. ______ An ectopic pregnancy is a potentially dangerous condition in which a fertilized egg is implanted and begins to develop outside of the uterus.

Clinical Conditions

Write the correct answer on the line provided.

16.66. Dr. Potter suspected cervical cancer, so she requested that Armine Bakir undergo the surgical removal of a specimen of tissue from the cervix called ______.

16.67. When she went into labor with her first child, Mrs. Hoshi's baby was in a breech presentation. Because of risks associated with this, her obstetrician delivered the baby surgically by performing a/an ____________________.

16.68. Dawn Grossman was diagnosed as having uterine fibroids that required surgical removal. Her gynecologist scheduled Dawn for a/an ____________________.

16.69. Rita Chen, who is 25 years old and knows that she is not pregnant, is concerned because she has not had a menstrual period for three months. Her doctor described this condition as ____________________.

16.70. To test for genetic abnormalities in her developing fetus, the obstetrician scheduled Lexie Campos to come in at week 12 of her pregnancy for ____________________.

16.71. Joni Nguyen is scheduled to undergo a type of surgery called ____________________ to remove one fallopian tube and ovary.

16.72. In order to reinforce Athena Wood's cervix so that her baby wasn't born prematurely, her doctor recommended ____________________.

16.73. Just before the delivery of her baby, Barbara Klein's obstetrician performed a/an ____________________ to prevent tearing of the tissues.

16.74. Jane Marsal showed signs of hypertension and proteinuria while pregnant with twins. The medical term for this condition is ____________________.

16.75. Immediately after birth, the Reicher baby was described as being a newborn or a/an ____________________.

Which Is the Correct Medical Term?

Select the correct answer, and write it on the line provided.

16.76. The postpartum vaginal discharge during the first several weeks after childbirth is known as ____________________.

colostrum involution lochia meconium

16.77. Abdominal pain caused by uterine cramps during a menstrual period is known as ____________________.

dysmenorrhea amenorrhea metrorrhagia polymenorrhea

16.78. The condition in which there is less amniotic fluid than normal is called ______________________.

oligohydramnios balanitis molar pregnancy preeclampsia

16.79. An inflammation of the lining of the vagina is known as ______________________. The most common causes of this condition are bacterial vaginosis, trichomoniasis, and vaginal candidiasis.

cervical dysplasia cervicitis chancre vaginitis

16.80. The term that describes a profuse whitish mucus discharge from the uterus and vagina is ______________________. This type of discharge can be due to an infection or hormonal imbalance.

vaginal candidiasis leukorrhea lochia vaginitis

Challenge Word Building

These terms are *not* primary terms in the chapter; however, they are made up of the following familiar word parts. If you need help in creating the term, refer to your medical dictionary.

endo-	**hyster/o**	**-cele**
	lact/o	**-dynia**
	metr/o	**-gravida**
	null/i	**-itis**
	oophor/o	**-ose**
	ov/o	**-pexy**
	vagin/o	**-rrhaphy**
	vulv/o	**-rrhexis**

16.81. The term meaning a hernia protruding into the vagina is ________________.

16.82. A woman who has never been pregnant. ________________

16.83. The term meaning an inflammation of the endometrium is ________________.

16.84. The adjective meaning pertaining to milk is ________________.

16.85. The term meaning inflammation of an ovary is ________________.

16.86. The term meaning surgical suturing of the uterus is ________________.

16.87. The term meaning a hernia of the uterus, particularly during pregnancy, is a/an ________________.

16.88. The term meaning the surgical fixation of a displaced ovary is ________________.

16.89. The term meaning the rupture of the uterus, particularly during pregnancy, is ________________.

16.90. The term meaning inflammation of the vulva and the vagina is ________________.

Labeling Exercises

Identify the numbered items in these accompanying figures.

16.91. ________________ tube

16.92. ________________

16.93. ________________

16.94. ________________ bladder

16.95. ________________

16.96. ________________

16.97. ________________ orifice

16.98. ________________

16.99. ________________

16.100. ________________

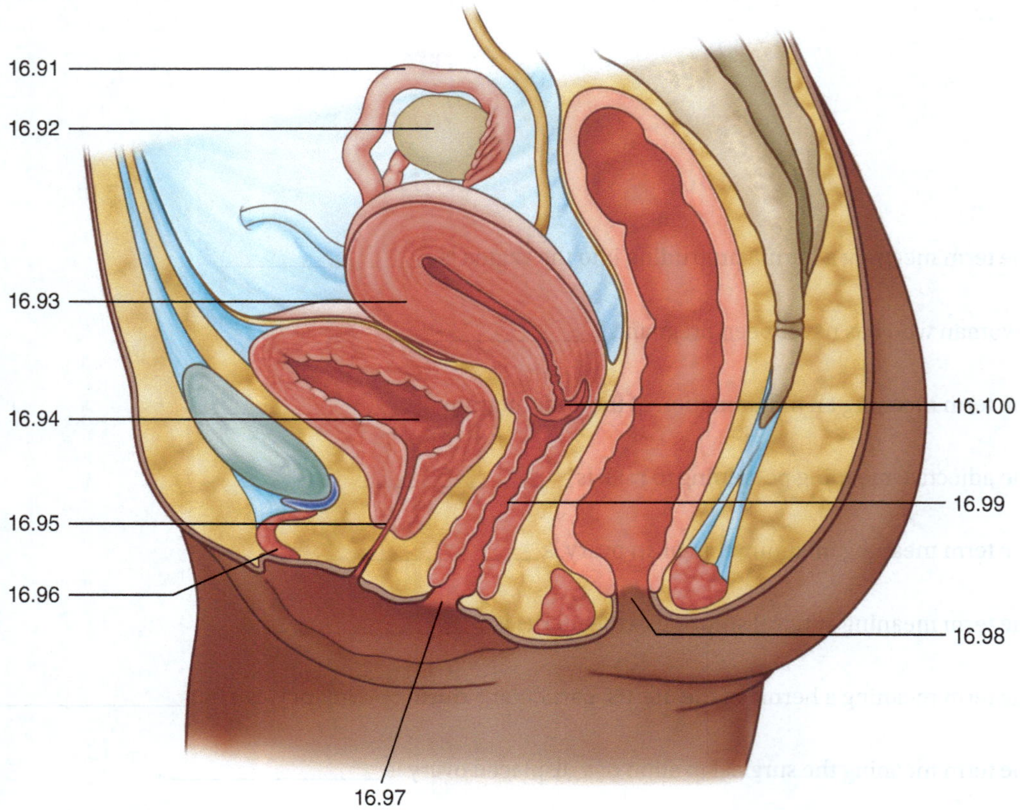

The Human Touch

CRITICAL THINKING EXERCISE

The following story and questions are designed to stimulate critical thinking through class discussion or as a brief essay response. There are no right or wrong answers to these questions.

Eloise was in her late 30s when she finally decided to become a mother on her own. She was tired of dating, wondering each time whether she'd find a partner to raise a child with and then being disappointed when she didn't. At age 37, she realized that she was already considered a primigravida who would require some additional monitoring due to her advanced maternal age. She felt confident that while she could live without romance, she didn't want to go through life without being a mother.

Joining a local Single Mothers by Choice (SMC) group on Facebook made her feel like part of the SMC community before she even started the "trying to conceive" stage. She knew that there were many challenges ahead, including the fact that her health insurance wouldn't cover IVF if she needed it.

Happily, her very first round of artificial insemination was successful. Eloise was delighted to learn that her parents couldn't wait to become grandparents, and were willing to support her despite the fact that she'd become pregnant in a less traditional way. She knew that she'd need them as a major part of her emotional and childcare support system.

During the first few weeks of her pregnancy, Eloise experienced light vaginal bleeding and some pelvic pain. She also had an upset stomach occasionally; however, she assumed that this was morning sickness. But when Eloise woke up early one morning to find that she was bleeding heavily, she made an urgent appointment with her obstetrician.

Dr. Sims performed a transvaginal ultrasound, which confirmed that Eloise was experiencing an ectopic pregnancy. Dr. Sims explained to Eloise that her fertilized egg was implanted and growing in a fallopian tube rather than inside the main cavity of the uterus. "I'm so sorry," she said gently, "but the egg cannot survive outside the uterus. If we don't terminate your pregnancy, the growing tissue could cause dangerous bleeding, risking your health and your chance of having children in the future. I know how hard and emotional this situation must be." She added, "is there someone you can call to be with you?"

Suggested Discussion Topics

1. Why is it important that Eloise have a good support system?
2. What sorts of challenges do people face in raising a child alone?
3. If Eloise's fallopian tube has ruptured or become severely damaged, it might be removed during the surgery. How will that impact her plans to have a baby?
4. Would it help to join a support group of other women who have experienced pregnancy loss?

CHAPTER 17

MENTAL HEALTH

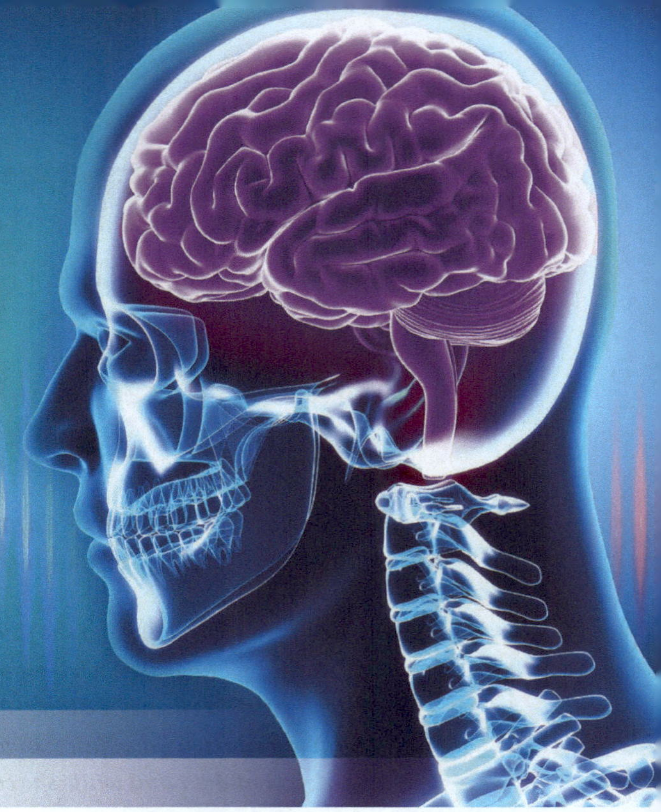

Overview of THE BASICS OF MENTAL HEALTH

Mental illness is extremely common and affects people of all ages, races, genders, and body types. Mental health can affect a person's emotions, behaviors, and well-being and can be influenced by genetics, congenital abnormalities, brain chemistry, medical problems, prescription or illicit drug use, stress, trauma, or other life experiences. Mental health disorders are classified by *The Diagnostic and Statistical Manual of Mental Disorders* (DSM-5) in order to improve diagnoses, treatment, and research.

Vocabulary Related to MENTAL HEALTH

This list contains essential word parts and medical terms for this chapter. These and the other important **primary terms** are shown in **boldface** throughout the chapter. *Secondary terms*, which appear in *orange* italics, clarify the meaning of primary terms.

Word Parts

- ☐ **anxi/o** anxiety
- ☐ **anti-** against
- ☐ **claustr/o** barrier, enclosed space
- ☐ **-mania** madness or obsessive preoccupation
- ☐ **narc/o** sleep, stupor
- ☐ **para-** around, abnormal
- ☐ **-phobia** abnormal fear
- ☐ **phren/o** mind, diaphragm
- ☐ **post-** after
- ☐ **psych/o** mind
- ☐ **schiz/o** split
- ☐ **somn/o** sleep
- ☐ **-tic** pertaining to
- ☐ **traumat/o** injury
- ☐ **-tropic** having an affinity for

Medical Terms

- ☐ **acrophobia** (**ack**-roh-**FOH**-bee-ah)
- ☐ **affect**
- ☐ **agoraphobia** (**ag**-oh-rah-**FOH**-bee-ah)
- ☐ **alcoholism** (**AL**-kuh-hall-izm)
- ☐ **anorexia nervosa** (**an**-oh-**RECK**-see-ah ner-**VOH**-sah)
- ☐ **antidepressant**
- ☐ **anxiety disorders**
- ☐ **anxiolytic drug** (**ang**-zee-oh-**LIT**-ick)
- ☐ **autism spectrum disorder** (**AW**-tizm)
- ☐ **attention deficit/hyperactivity disorder**
- ☐ **bipolar disorder**
- ☐ **binge eating disorder**
- ☐ **biofeedback**
- ☐ **body dysmorphic disorder**
- ☐ **borderline personality disorder**
- ☐ **bulimia nervosa** (buh-**LEE**-mee-ah ner-**VOH**-sah)
- ☐ **claustrophobia** (**klaws**-troh-**FOH**-bee-ah)
- ☐ **cognitive behavioral therapy**
- ☐ **delirium tremens** (deh-**LEER**-ee-um **TREE**-mens)
- ☐ **delusion** (dih-**LOO**-zhun)
- ☐ **depression**
- ☐ **dissociative disorders**
- ☐ **dyslexia** (dis-**LECK**-see-ah)
- ☐ **electroconvulsive therapy** (ee-**leck**-troh-kon-**VUL**-siv)
- ☐ **emotion**
- ☐ **exposure therapy**
- ☐ **factitious disorder** (fack-**TISH**-us)
- ☐ **gender dysphoria** (**JEN**-der dis-**FOR**-ee-ah)
- ☐ **hallucination** (hah-**loo**-sih-**NAY**-shun)
- ☐ **hoarding disorder**
- ☐ **hypnotherapy**
- ☐ **intellectual disability**
- ☐ **limbic system**
- ☐ **mania**
- ☐ **mental illness**
- ☐ **mood**
- ☐ **narcolepsy** (**NAR**-koh-**lep**-see)
- ☐ **neurodevelopmental disorders**
- ☐ **obsessive-compulsive disorder**
- ☐ **oppositional defiant disorder**
- ☐ **panic attack**
- ☐ **paranoia** (**pair**-ah-**NOY**-ah)
- ☐ **paraphilic disorders** (**pair**-ah-**FILL**-ic)
- ☐ **parasomnia** (**pair**-ah-**SOM**-nee-ah)
- ☐ **personality disorder**
- ☐ **phobia** (**FOH**-bee-ah)
- ☐ **posttraumatic stress disorder**
- ☐ **psychiatrist** (sigh-**KYE**-ah-trist)
- ☐ **psychology** (sigh-**KOL**-oh-gee)
- ☐ **psychopharmacology** (**sigh**-koh-farm-uh-**KOL**-oh-gee)
- ☐ **psychosis** (sigh-**KOH**-sis)
- ☐ **psychotic disorder** (sigh-**KOT**-ick)
- ☐ **psychotherapy**
- ☐ **psychotropic drug** (**sigh**-koh-**TROP**-ick)
- ☐ **schizophrenia** (**skit**-soh-**FREE**-nee-ah)
- ☐ **self-harm**
- ☐ **sexual dysfunctions**
- ☐ **stimulant**
- ☐ **suicide** (**SOO**-uh-side)
- ☐ **trauma**

LEARNING OBJECTIVES

On completion of this chapter, you should be able to:

1. Describe factors that contribute to mental health disorders.
2. Identify the structures in the brain related to mental health.
3. Identify medical terms that are applied to the assessment of mental health disorders.
4. Identify the medical specialists within the mental health field.
5. Identify medical word parts related to mental health.
6. List the major signs and symptoms of specific mental health disorders.
7. Define the primary terms related to the pathology and the diagnostic and treatment procedures of mental health disorders.
8. Spell the primary terms of mental health disorders.
9. Pronounce the primary terms of mental health disorders.
10. Identify common abbreviations related to mental health.

FACTORS IMPACTING MENTAL HEALTH

Mental health can affect a person's emotions, behaviors, and well-being. It can be influenced by a combination of factors including but not limited to genetics, congenital abnormalities, brain chemistry, medical problems, prescription or illicit drug use, stress, and trauma or other life experiences. **Mental illness** is extremely common, affecting as many as one in five adults in the United States. Mental illness affects people of all ages, races, genders, and body types. Anxiety and depression are the most common types of mental illness in the U.S.

- The *genes* that a person inherits from their parents may make them more prone to developing mental illness. Certain mental illnesses, such as depression and bipolar disorder, run in families.
- Certain medical problems, such as thyroid imbalance, can cause symptoms of mental illness.
- The use of drugs and alcohol can alter brain chemistry in such a way as to cause mental illness, and substance addiction (itself a mental illness) often occurs in conjunction with other mental illnesses such as anxiety and depression.
- A person's life experience, such as physical or emotional abuse, neglect, loss, or other trauma, can be a source of mental illness. **Trauma** is physical or emotional shock or injury.

As mentioned in Chapter 11, the brain contains hundreds of **neurotransmitters** (**new**-roh-trans-**MIT**-erz), which are chemical substances that make it possible for messages to cross from the synapse of a neuron to the target receptor. An imbalance or disruption of some of these chemicals can lead to mental illness.

- *Dopamine* is released within the brain. An excess of dopamine is associated with schizophrenia, mood and thought disorders, and abnormal movement disorders such as Parkinson's disease.
- *Endorphins* are naturally occurring substances that are produced by the brain to help relieve pain.
- *Norepinephrine* affects alertness and arousal, increasing blood pressure and heart rate, and releasing stores of glucose in response to stress. It is also a hormone released by the adrenal glands as part of the body's fight-or-flight response (see Chapter 14).
- *Serotonin*, which is released in the brain, has roles in sleep, hunger, and pleasure recognition. It is also sometimes linked to mood disorders.
- *Glutamate* plays an important role in learning; too little of this chemical can cause psychosis.
- *Gamma-aminobutyric acid* (GABA) inhibits some nerve cell impulses in the brain to provide an increased sense of calm. People with depression may have decreased GABA levels.

STRUCTURES OF THE BRAIN RELATED TO MENTAL HEALTH

While some mental illnesses can have physical manifestations, such as the wasting associated with anorexia nervosa or the heart palpitations associated with a panic attack, the main structures of mental health reside within the brain. The **limbic system** is a group of structures in the brain generally associated with thought, mood, and emotion (Figure 17.1). These structures help to regulate the body's response to emotions.

- The ***hypothalamus*** helps regulate sexual and behavioral function.
- The ***amygdala*** plays an important part in experiencing positive and negative emotions including anxiety, fear processing, evaluating events for importance, and memory.
- The ***hippocampus*** is responsible for long-term memory and learning.
- The ***thalamus*** produces sensations by relaying impulses to and from the cerebrum and the sense organs of the body.

PSYCHOLOGY

Psychology (sigh-**KOL**-oh-gee) is the scientific study of the mind (**psych** means mind, and **-ology** means the science or study of). **Psychiatry** (sigh-**KYE**-ah-tree) is the study and treatment of mental illness (**psych** means mind, and **-iatry** means field of medicine). The following terms are associated with the study of the mind and mental health:

- **Psyche** (**SIGH**-kee) means the mind, spirit, or soul. Psyche was the Greek goddess of the soul.
- According to the theories of famous neurologist Sigmund Freud, the ***id***, ***ego***, and ***superego*** are the three elements that make up a person's personality. **Personality** is a person's unique characteristics that affect how they think and behave.
- **Emotion** is a current state of feeling which may include a release of chemicals in the brain. Emotions include anger, fear, and love. **Mood** is a current state of emotion.
- **Affect**, used in psychology as a noun, is the outward appearance of a person's mood or emotional state. Affect is sometimes referred to as ***flat*** (showing little or no emotion) or ***appropriate*** for a given situation.
- **Defense mechanisms** are unconscious defenses used to avoid negative emotion.
    - ***Denial*** is the refusal to accept an experience or something else as fact.
    - ***Displacement*** is the direction of emotion onto an alternative subject.

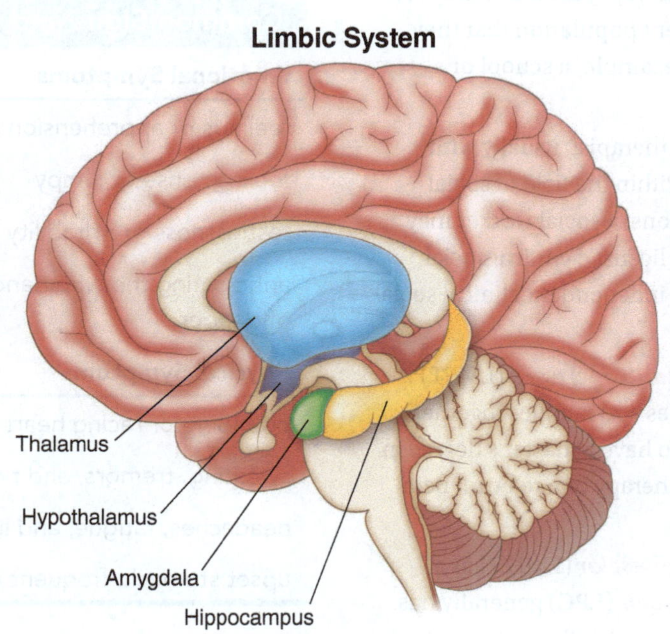

FIGURE 17.1 Structures of the limbic system.

- *Projection* is attributing one's own unacceptable thoughts to someone else.
- *Regression* is the return to a previous state of development or psychological well-being.
- *Repression* is the pushing away of negative experiences or thoughts into the unconscious. These repressed thoughts or experiences can still influence behavior.
- *Sublimation* is the socially acceptable satisfaction of an unacceptable impulse or desire.

MEDICAL SPECIALTIES RELATED TO MENTAL HEALTH

- A **psychiatrist** (sigh-**KYE**-ah-trist) is a physician who specializes in diagnosing and treating chemical dependencies, emotional problems, and mental illness (**psych** means mind, and **-iatrist** means specialist). A psychiatrist can prescribe medications. Within the profession of psychiatry, there are subspecialists such as a ***child and adolescent psychiatrist*** who specializes in diagnosing and treating children and teens, and a ***forensic psychiatrist*** who specializes in the overlap of psychiatry and the legal system.
- A **psychologist** (sigh-**KOL**-oh-jist) has a doctoral degree (PhD or PsyD) but is not a medical doctor (**psych** means mind, and **-ologist** means specialist). This specialist evaluates and treats emotional problems and mental illness. A psychologist may also have a subspecialty or patient population that they focus on working with, for example, a school or a clinical psychologist.
- A ***social worker*** is a trained therapist, usually with a master's degree (MSW). Within the field of social work there are state regulations; a social worker may be required to be an LCSW (licensed clinical social worker) or LICSW (licensed independent clinical social worker).
- A ***licensed marriage and family therapist*** (LMFT) specializes in treating couples and families together. Most states require LMFTs to have a master's degree in either marriage and family therapy or a relevant field such as psychology.
- A ***licensed mental health counselor*** (LMHC) or a ***licensed professional counselor*** (LPC) generally has a master's degree and is licensed at the state level to provide counseling and therapy.

PATHOLOGY OF MENTAL HEALTH

Mental health disorders are classified in ***The Diagnostic and Statistical Manual of Mental Disorders*** (DSM-5), currently in its fifth edition. Hundreds of international mental health experts collaborate on each edition of this handbook that defines and classifies mental disorders in order to improve diagnoses, treatment, and research.

Anxiety Disorders

- **Anxiety disorders** are mental conditions characterized by excessive, irrational dread of everyday situations or fear that is out of proportion to the real danger in a situation. There are many emotional and physical symptoms of anxiety (see Table 17.1). Without treatment, an anxiety disorder can become chronic.
- **Generalized anxiety disorder** (GAD) is characterized by chronic, excessive worrying. Physical symptoms associated with this condition can include muscle tension, sleep disturbance, irritability, trouble concentrating, and restlessness.
- A **panic attack** is an unexpected, sudden experience of fear in the absence of danger, accompanied by physical symptoms such as heart palpitations, shortness of breath, chest tightness, dizziness, sweating or chills, nausea,

TABLE 17.1
Common Signs and Symptoms of Anxiety

Emotional Symptoms
feelings of apprehension or dread
feeling tense or jumpy
restlessness or irritability
anticipating the worst and being watchful for signs of danger
Physical Symptoms
pounding or racing heart and shortness of breath
sweating, tremors, and twitches
headaches, fatigue, and insomnia
upset stomach, frequent urination, or diarrhea

Source: National Alliance on Mental Illness (NAMI). 2020. www.nami.org.

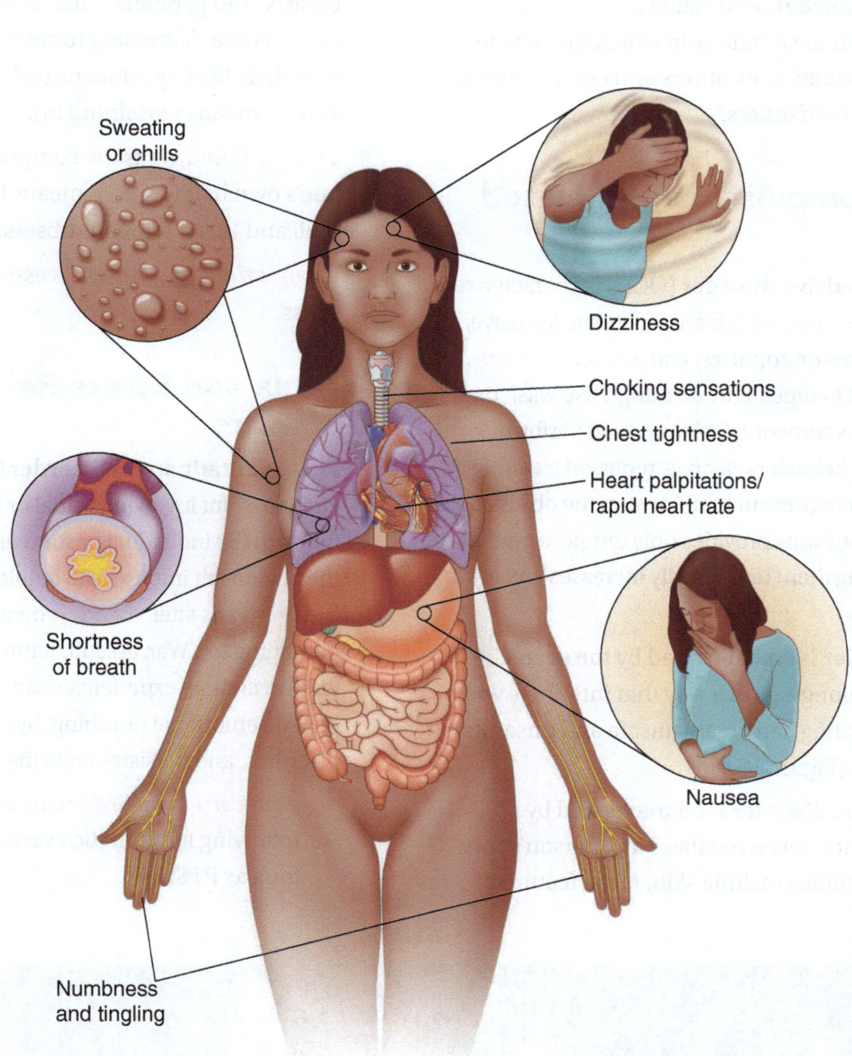

FIGURE 17.2 A panic attack can affect several of the body's systems.

numbness and tingling, choking sensations, or a combination of these (Figure 17.2). A panic attack is the unnecessary activation of the body's fight-or-flight response.

- **Panic disorder** is characterized by a fear of panic attacks. Panic disorder can cause people to develop agoraphobia or other phobias.
- **Selective mutism** (**MEW**-tizm) is an anxiety disorder where a child who is capable of speech is unable to speak or communicate in certain settings.

Phobias

A **phobia** (**FOH**-bee-ah) is a persistent, irrational fear of a specific thing or situation, strong enough to cause significant distress, interfere with functioning, and lead to the avoidance of the thing or situation that causes this reaction. There are countless types of phobias, named by adding **-phobia** to the name of the feared thing or situation.

- **Acrophobia** (**ack**-roh-**FOH**-bee-ah) is an excessive fear of heights (**acr/o** means top, and **-phobia** means abnormal fear).
- **Agoraphobia** (**ag**-oh-rah-**FOH**-bee-ah) is an excessive fear of environments where the person fears a panic attack might occur. In order to avoid these situations, someone suffering from agoraphobia might not even be able to leave home (**agor/a** means marketplace, and **-phobia** means abnormal fear).
- **Claustrophobia** (**klaws**-troh-**FOH**-bee-ah) is an abnormal fear of being in small or enclosed spaces (**claustr/o** means enclosed space, and **-phobia** means abnormal fear).

- **Social anxiety disorder**, also called ***social phobia***, is an excessive fear of situations in which the person fears negative evaluation by others and embarrassing themselves in front of others.

Obsessive-Compulsive and Related Disorders

- **Obsessive-compulsive disorder** (OCD) is characterized by recurrent ***obsessions***, which are repetitive, intrusive, distressing thoughts or impulses, and/or ***compulsions***, feeling compelled to repeatedly do things, like wash or count. OCD makes someone feel they must perform these compulsive behaviors, such as repeated cleaning or checking, in order to prevent harm or stop the obsession. Performing compulsions provides only temporary relief, but *not* performing them temporarily increases anxiety or agitation.
- **Hoarding disorder** is characterized by the overaccumulation of belongings in a way that interferes with daily living. Hoarding can create unsafe and unsanitary living conditions (Figure 17.3).
- **Body dysmorphic disorder** is characterized by a preoccupation with perceived flaws in a person's own appearance. Examples include skin, facial features, breasts, and genitalia. This severe negative body image can become distressing to such a point that it interferes with daily life (**dys-** means bad, **morph** means shape, and **-ic** means pertaining to).
- ***Trichotillomania*** is the compulsive pulling out of one's own hair (**trich/o** means hair, **till/o** means to pull, and **-mania** means obsessive preoccupation).
- ***Excoriation disorder*** is excessive skin picking due to stress.

Trauma and Stress-Related Disorders

- **Posttraumatic stress disorder** (PTSD) may develop after an event involving actual or threatened death or injury to the individual or someone else, during which the person felt intense fear, helplessness, or horror (**post-** means after, **traumat** means injury, and **-ic** means pertaining to). War, assault, natural disasters, and other life-threatening experiences can cause PTSD. Symptoms include emotional numbing, hyperarousal, anxiety, sleep disorders, and persistent reliving of the event.
  - ***Acute stress disorder*** can occur immediately following a traumatic event and does not last as long as PTSD.

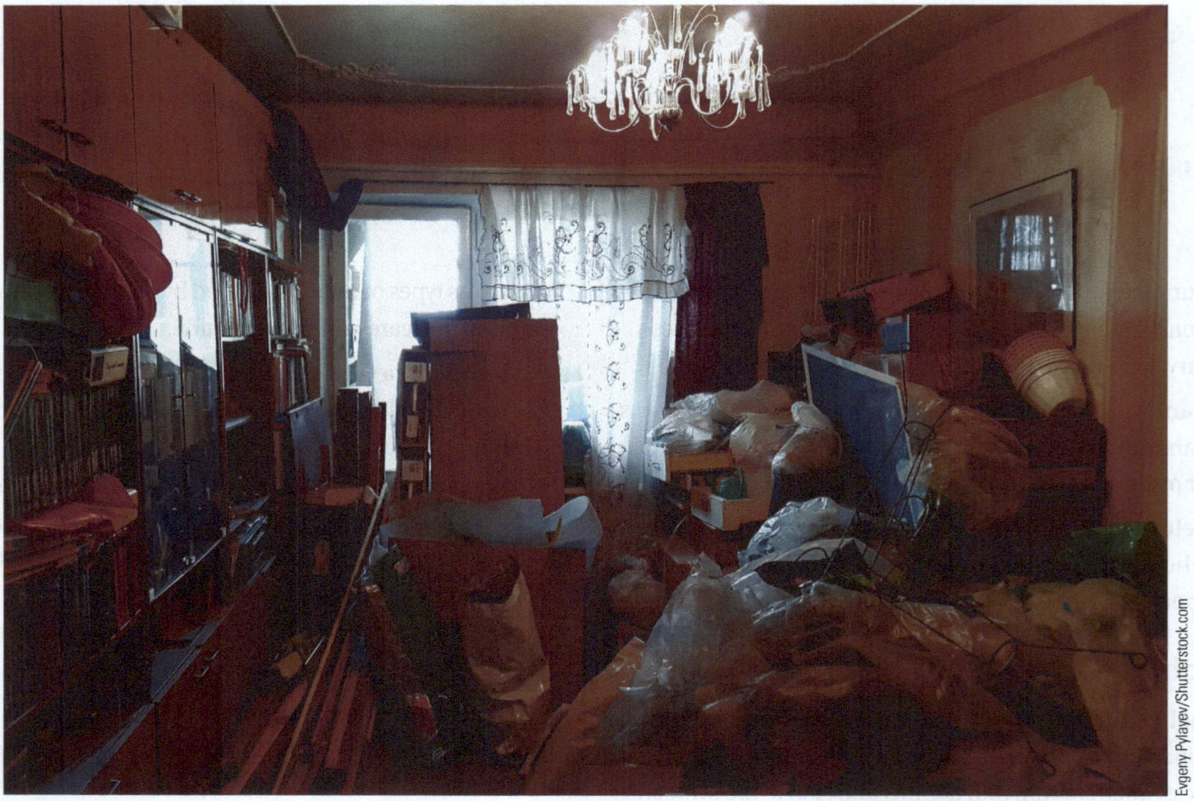

FIGURE 17.3 An example of hoarding disorder creating an unsafe or unsanitary living environment.

- *Adjustment disorder* is caused by feelings of sadness or hopelessness after a stressful life event such as a loved one's death, loss of a job, or divorce.

Neurodevelopmental Disorders

Neurodevelopmental disorders are disorders with childhood onset which are characterized by a disturbance in the central nervous system. More than one neurodevelopmental disorder can co-occur. *Childhood onset* means that the first appearance of the signs or symptoms of an illness is usually before the age of 13.

- An **attention deficit/hyperactivity disorder** (ADHD) is characterized by a short attention span and impulsive behavior that is inappropriate for the child's developmental age. *Hyperactivity* is restlessness or a continuing excess of movement. The term *attention deficit disorder* (ADD) is sometimes used if hyperactivity is not present. Some symptoms of these conditions persist into adulthood.
- **Dyslexia** (dis-**LECK**-see-ah), also known as a *developmental reading disorder*, is a learning disability characterized by substandard reading achievement due to the inability of the brain to process symbols correctly.
- **Learning disabilities** (LD) are disorders found in children of normal intelligence who have difficulties in learning specific skills such as processing language or grasping mathematical concepts.
- **Intellectual disability**, also called *intellectual developmental disorder*, is a diagnosis of significant below-average intellectual and adaptive functioning present from birth or early infancy. An *IQ test* (intelligence quota) is used for testing relative intelligence.
- **Autism spectrum disorder** (**AW**-tizm) (ASD) describes a condition with different levels of symptom severity in which a young child has difficulty developing normal social relationships and communication skills; may compulsively follow repetitive routines; and has narrowly focused, intense interests that are sometimes unusual. Children with **autism** have significant developmental delays, including speech and language. Most children with autism have very minimal verbal skills and lack normal social relationships (Figure 17.4). *Asperger's syndrome* is no longer a diagnosis on its own but is sometimes used to characterize a high-functioning group of individuals with ASD who have normal or above-average intelligence but are impaired in social interactions and nonverbal communication.

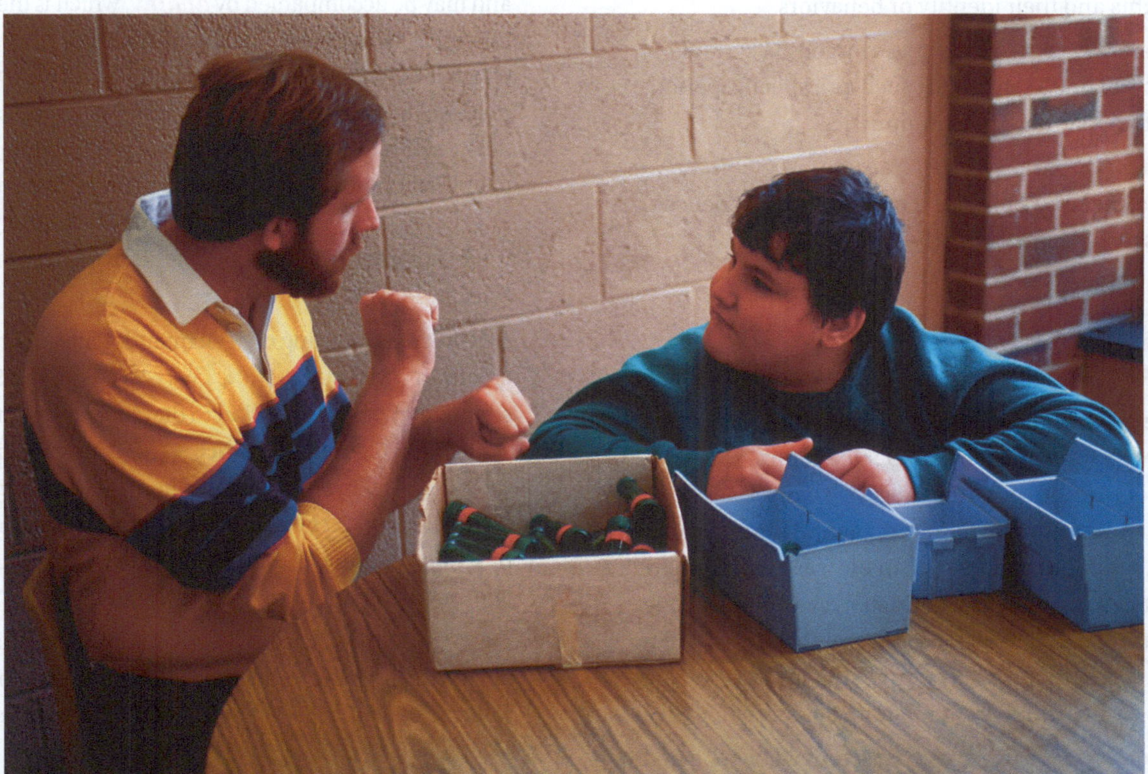

FIGURE 17.4 A therapist works with a boy with autism to develop communication skills.

- **Tourette syndrome** is characterized by uncontrollable physical and/or verbal "tics" such as shrugging shoulders, blinking eyes, or yelling offensive words. It is more common in males, with onset normally occurring in childhood.
- **Communication disorders**, which are common in childhood, are characterized by difficulty either comprehending or communicating with others. ***Childhood-onset fluency disorder***, formerly known as ***stuttering***, is one such disorder. ***Social (pragmatic) communication disorder*** (SCD) is another, and is characterized by difficulties following conversational rules, not adjusting language level to the listener, and only taking words literally.

Dissociative Disorders

Dissociative disorders occur when normal thought is separated from consciousness.

- **Dissociative identity disorder** (DID), formerly referred to as ***multiple personality disorder***, is a mental illness characterized by the presence of two or more distinct personalities, each with its own characteristics, which appear to exist within the same individual. Early childhood trauma and abuse are leading causes of DID. ***Dissociation*** is a disconnect between a person's thoughts and their identity or behaviors.
- ***Dissociative amnesia*** involves forgetting certain aspects of one's self or past such as a specific period of time that may have been traumatic.
- ***Depersonalization/derealization disorder*** is characterized by a persistent out-of-body experience of observing oneself from the outside.

Disruptive and Impulse Control Disorders

Impulse control disorders are a group of psychiatric disorders characterized by a repeated failure to resist an impulse despite potential negative consequences. Psychological trauma, addiction, mental illness, and low levels of serotonin can lead to an increase in impulsive behaviors. An ***impulse*** is a sudden overwhelming urge. The suffix **-mania** means obsessive preoccupation. An impulse is different than a compulsion in that the consequences of the action are often not considered.

- ***Kleptomania*** is a disorder characterized by repeatedly stealing objects neither for personal use nor for their monetary value.
- ***Pyromania*** is a disorder characterized by repeated, deliberate fire setting in order to release pent-up emotion.
- **Oppositional defiant disorder** (ODD) is characterized by a child or adolescent's persistent angry, uncooperative, and disruptive behavior directed toward authority figures, which disrupts daily activities. ***Conduct disorder*** is a more severe version that can include physical altercations, destruction, and violation of rules. This is a childhood diagnosis that can become *antisocial personality disorder* if untreated (see the "Personality Disorders" section).

Bipolar and Depressive Disorders

- **Bipolar disorder** is a condition characterized by cycles of severe mood changes shifting between highs called **mania** (manic behavior, sometimes including a feeling of ***euphoria***, meaning intense happiness and excitement) and either ***hypomania*** (milder manic symptoms) or ***major depressive episode*** (severe depression) that affect a person's attitude, energy, and ability to function.
    - **Manic behavior** includes an abnormally elevated, expansive, or irritable mood, including increased energy and activity, severe insomnia, poor judgment, and inappropriate social behavior.
- **Depression** is a common mood disorder characterized by sadness, changes in sleep, energy, and concentration and may be accompanied by ***apathy***, which is the lack of interest in formerly pleasurable activities, or ***anhedonia***, which is the inability to enjoy oneself. ***Severe depression*** may lead to feelings of worthlessness and thoughts of death, self-harm, or suicide. It is estimated that one in six people will experience depression in their lifetime. ***Major depressive disorder*** is feeling depressed most days of the week. Common signs and symptoms of depression are listed in Table 17.2.
- **Self-harm** is harming oneself intentionally and ranges greatly in severity. ***Non-suicidal self-injury*** (NSSI) is self-injury with no intention to die, such as by cutting or scratching (Figure 17.5). **Suicide** (**SOO**-uh-side) is the intentional taking of one's own life. ***Suicidal ideation*** (SI) is the thought of taking one's own life and can be described as passive (with no plan) or active (with a laid-out plan for how to execute the suicide).
- ***Peripartum onset depression***, or depression that occurs during or immediately after childbirth (often referred to as ***postpartum depression***), is discussed in Chapter 16.
- **Persistent depressive disorder** (PDD), previously known as ***dysthymia***, is a low-grade, chronic

TABLE 17.2

Common Signs and Symptoms of Depression
Changes in sleep
Changes in appetite
Lack of concentration
Loss of energy
Lack of interest in activities
Hopelessness or guilty thoughts
Changes in movement (less activity or agitation)
Physical aches and pains
Suicidal thoughts

Source: National Alliance on Mental Illness (NAMI). 2020. www.nami.org.

depression with symptoms that are milder than those of severe depression but are present on a majority of days for two or more years.

- ***Disruptive mood dysregulation disorder*** (DMDD) is a newer diagnosis for children and adolescents who have frequent, severe temper outbursts and are chronically irritable.
- **Seasonal affective disorder** (SAD), or ***seasonal depression***, is a bout of depression associated with the decrease in hours of daylight during winter months. One method of treatment is ***light therapy***, using a special electric light to simulate sunlight.

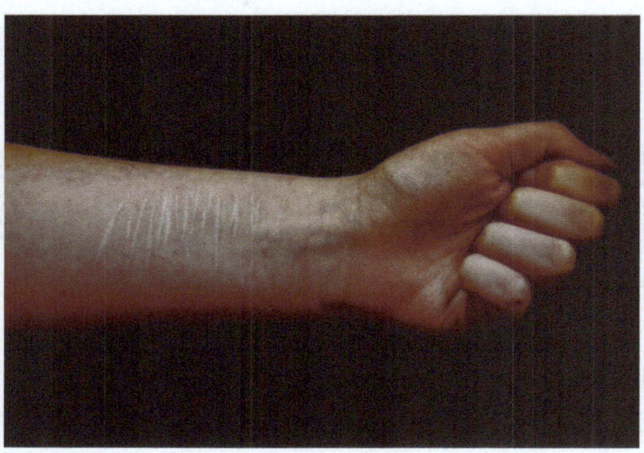

Neal Bryant/Shutterstock.com

FIGURE 17.5 Self-harm can take many forms; here, a history of self-harm can be seen in the scars on the patient's arm from cutting.

Feeding and Eating Disorders

- **Avoidant restrictive food intake disorder** (ARFID) is a feeding and eating disorder most often found in children and adolescents characterized by extreme pickiness and can interfere with adequate nutrition, appropriate growth, and social functioning. These food aversions can be caused by a negative previous experience (such as choking or food poisoning) or sensory issues.
- **Anorexia nervosa** (**an**-oh-**RECK**-see-ah ner-**VOH**-sah) is characterized by a false perception of body appearance. This leads to an intense fear of gaining weight and inability to maintain a healthy body weight (Figure 17.6). Extreme caloric restriction and/or excessive exercising can cause the patient to become emaciated and malnourished. ***Emaciated*** means abnormally thin.
- **Bulimia nervosa** (buh-**LEE**-mee-ah ner-**VOH**-sah) is an eating disorder characterized by frequent episodes

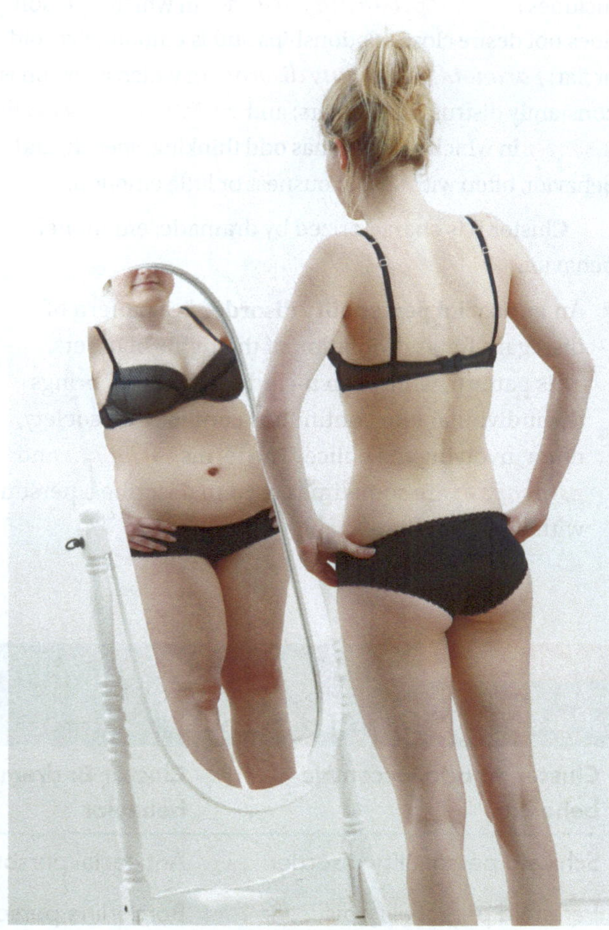

FIGURE 17.6 Anorexia nervosa is characterized by a false perception of body appearance, intense fear of weight gain, and voluntary starvation.

of binge eating followed by compensatory behaviors to purge the food such as self-induced vomiting; excessive exercising; or the misuse of laxatives, diuretics, or other medications. ***Purge*** means to get rid of something that is unwanted.

- **Binge eating disorder** (BED) is characterized by frequent episodes of eating large quantities of food, accompanied by a sense of loss of control and feelings of guilt or shame afterward.

Personality Disorders

A **personality disorder** (PD) is a chronic pattern of inner experience and behavior that causes serious problems with relationships and work. This pattern is pervasive and inflexible, has its onset in adolescence or early adulthood, is stable over time, and leads to distress or impairment. These disorders are classified by three distinct clusters featuring similar behaviors: cluster A, cluster B, and cluster C (see Table 17.3).

Cluster A features odd, eccentric behavior. This cluster includes ***schizoid personality disorder*** in which a person does not desire close relationships and is emotionally cold or flat; ***paranoid personality disorder*** in which a person is constantly distrustful of others; and ***schizotypal personality disorder*** in which a person has odd thinking, speech, and behavior, often with suspiciousness or little emotion.

Cluster B is characterized by dramatic, emotional behavior.

- An **antisocial personality disorder** is a pattern of disregard for and violation of the rights of others. This pattern, which can include aggression, brings the individual into continuous conflict with society, often involving the police. The terms ***sociopath*** and ***psychopath*** are sometimes used to describe a person with this disorder.
- A **borderline personality disorder** is characterized by impulsive actions, often with the potential for self-harm, as well as mood instability and chaotic relationships.
- A **narcissistic personality disorder** is a pattern of extreme preoccupation with the self and complete lack of empathy for others. ***Empathy*** is the ability to recognize and understand another person's mental and emotional state.

Cluster C is characterized by anxious, fearful behavior. This includes ***avoidant personality disorder*** in which a person is shy and overly sensitive, ***dependent personality disorder*** in which a person depends too much on other people for emotional and physical needs, and ***obsessive-compulsive personality disorder*** in which a person has rigid rules they follow and feels that others should follow them as well. This is different from obsessive-compulsive disorder, in which a person is distressed by the rigid rules that they follow.

Psychotic Disorders

A **psychotic disorder** (sigh-**KOT**-ick) is characterized by the loss of contact with reality and deterioration of normal social functioning.

- **Psychosis** (sigh-**KOH**-sis) is a disrupted thought pattern that makes it difficult for a person to distinguish what is real and what is not. This is a symptom of serious mental illness and can include delusions and hallucinations.
- **Catatonic behavior** (**kat**-ah-**TON**-ick) is marked by a lack of responsiveness, stupor, and a tendency to remain in a fixed posture.
- A **delusion** (dih-**LOO**-zhun) is a false personal belief that is maintained despite obvious proof or evidence to the contrary. The belief is not one ordinarily accepted by other members of the individual's culture or religious faith. **Paranoia** (**pair**-ah-**NOY**-ah) is intense anxiety caused by persistent suspicion and mistrust of someone or something.

TABLE 17.3

Personality Disorder Clusters

Cluster A: odd, eccentric behavior	Cluster B: dramatic, emotional behavior	Cluster C: anxious, fearful behavior
Schizoid personality disorder	Antisocial personality disorder	Avoidant personality disorder
Paranoid personality disorder	Borderline personality disorder	Dependent personality disorder
Schizotypal personality disorder	Narcissistic personality disorder	Obsessive-compulsive personality disorder

- A **hallucination** (hah-**loo**-sih-**NAY**-shun) is a sensory perception (i.e., sight, touch, sound, smell, or taste) experienced in the absence of any actual external stimulus.
- **Schizophrenia** (**skit**-soh-**FREE**-nee-ah) is a psychotic disorder usually characterized by withdrawal from reality, illogical patterns of thinking, delusions, and hallucinations and accompanied in varying degrees by other emotional, behavioral, or intellectual disturbances (**schiz/o** means split, **phren** means mind, and **-ia** means condition).
- **Schizoaffective disorder** (**skit**-soh-ah-**FECK**-tiv) is a combination of schizophrenia symptoms with bipolar or depressive disorder symptoms.

Somatic Symptom and Related Disorders

A **somatic symptom disorder** (soh-**MAT**-ick) (SSD) is characterized by distress and excessive focus on physical complaints or symptoms that are out of proportion to any physical findings or disease.

Illness anxiety disorder is characterized by recurring anxiety and excessive worry that a physical illness may be present. The worry is only temporarily relieved by normal results from a medical examination.

A **factitious disorder** (fack-**TISH**-us) is a condition in which an individual acts as if they have a physical or mental illness when they are not really sick. The term ***factitious*** means artificial, self-induced, or not naturally occurring. Visible symptoms are self-inflicted and seem motivated by a desire for attention and sympathy rather than for external benefits like malingering. This can also be referred to as ***Munchausen syndrome***.

- A ***factitious disorder imposed on another***, formerly referred to as ***Munchausen syndrome by proxy***, is a form of child abuse. Although seeming very concerned about the child's well-being, the parent with the mental illness will falsify an illness in a child by making up or inducing symptoms and then seeking medical treatment, even surgery, for the child.
- **Functional neurologic disorders** are characterized by neurologic symptoms without a physical cause. One example is pseudoseizures, where a person exhibits seizure symptoms, but has normal brain waves on EEG. It is important to note that the patient is unaware that these symptoms are psychologically caused. One type of functional neurologic disorder is conversion disorder.
- ***Conversion disorder*** is characterized by serious temporary or ongoing changes in function, such as paralysis or blindness, that are triggered by psychological factors rather than by any physical cause.
- **Malingering** (mah-**LING**-ger-ing), which is not a mental illness, is characterized by the intentional creation of false or grossly exaggerated physical or psychological symptoms. In contrast to a factitious disorder, this condition is motivated by incentives such as avoiding work.

Substance-Related and Addictive Disorders

Substance abuse is the addictive use of tobacco, alcohol, medications, or illicit drugs. This abuse leads to significant impairment in functioning, danger to one's self or others, and recurrent legal and/or interpersonal problems. ***Addiction*** means having a strong dependence on a substance. ***Substance*** can refer to prescription and over-the-counter drugs, street drugs, alcohol, stimulants, and tobacco. These disorders are classified by the type of substance involved, such as alcohol, caffeine, hallucinogen, opioid, or stimulant.

The use and abuse of substances can also be significant causes of other mental illness. For example, chronic ***marijuana*** use is associated with schizophrenia and social anxiety. Substance use is also higher in those who have mental illness, potentially as a self-coping method.

- **Alcoholism** (**AL**-kuh-hall-izm) is chronic alcohol dependence with specific signs and symptoms upon withdrawal. ***Withdrawal*** is a psychological or physical syndrome (or both) caused by the abrupt ***cessation***, or stopping, of the use of alcohol or drugs in an addicted individual.
- **Delirium tremens** (deh-**LEER**-ee-um **TREE**-mens) (DTs) is a disorder involving sudden and severe mental changes or seizures caused by abruptly stopping the use of alcohol.
- ***Methadone*** is a synthetic opiate used to treat addiction to heroin or prescription narcotics.
- **Drug abuse** is the excessive use of illegal or recreational drugs, or the misuse of prescription drugs.
- A ***recreational drug*** is one normally used for personal pleasure or satisfaction rather than medical purposes. Some recreational drugs are ***illicit***, or illegal, whereas others, such as nicotine, alcohol, and marijuana (in some states), are subject to government regulation.

- A **drug overdose** is the potentially fatal, accidental, or intentional use of an illegal drug or prescription medicine in an amount higher than what is safe or normal.
- *Narcan®* is a brand-name medication that is used as an emergency treatment for opioid overdose. Narcan blocks the effects of opioids, which can reverse or reduce the respiratory depression associated with opioid overdose. The generic name for Narcan is *naloxone*.
- *Gambling disorder* is an addiction to gambling which causes distress and personal problems. It is characterized by an inability to stop gambling despite negative consequences and the need to lie about it to family and friends.

Gender Identity

Gender dysphoria (JEN-der dis-FOR-ee-ah) (GD) is a condition where a person's sex at birth does not match the gender with which they currently identify, causing significant amounts of distress. *Dysphoria* means dissatisfaction. These feelings can begin in early childhood. The inclusion of gender dysphoria in the DSM-5 is somewhat controversial and was updated from previous editions of the DSM to clarify that gender non-conformity is not a disorder; rather, some people might experience distress due to their experience with gender.

The term **transgender** (trans-JEN-der) refers to a person whose **gender identity** does not match their sex assigned at birth; *cisgender* refers to a person whose gender identity does match their sex assigned at birth. A transgender person may choose to *transition* their body to align with their identified gender by taking hormones and/or having surgery. Some people believe that gender identity and gender expression exist on a spectrum and refer to themselves as *non-binary* rather than exclusively male or female (Figure 17.7).

Sexual Dysfunctions and Paraphilic Disorders

Sexual dysfunctions are conditions which prevent a person from experiencing satisfaction from sexual activity. *Delayed ejaculation*, *erectile disorder*, and *female orgasmic disorder* are sexual dysfunctions that may be characterized by low sexual desire or difficulty achieving orgasm.

Paraphilic disorders (pair-ah-FILL-ic) are characterized by altered sexual fantasies, urges, or behaviors (**para-** means abnormal, **phil** means attraction to, and **-ic** means pertaining to). They are classified as disorders because of either personal distress or psychological or physical distress that they can cause to others. Sexual desires outside the ordinary that do not cause distress or harm to oneself or others are not considered disorders.

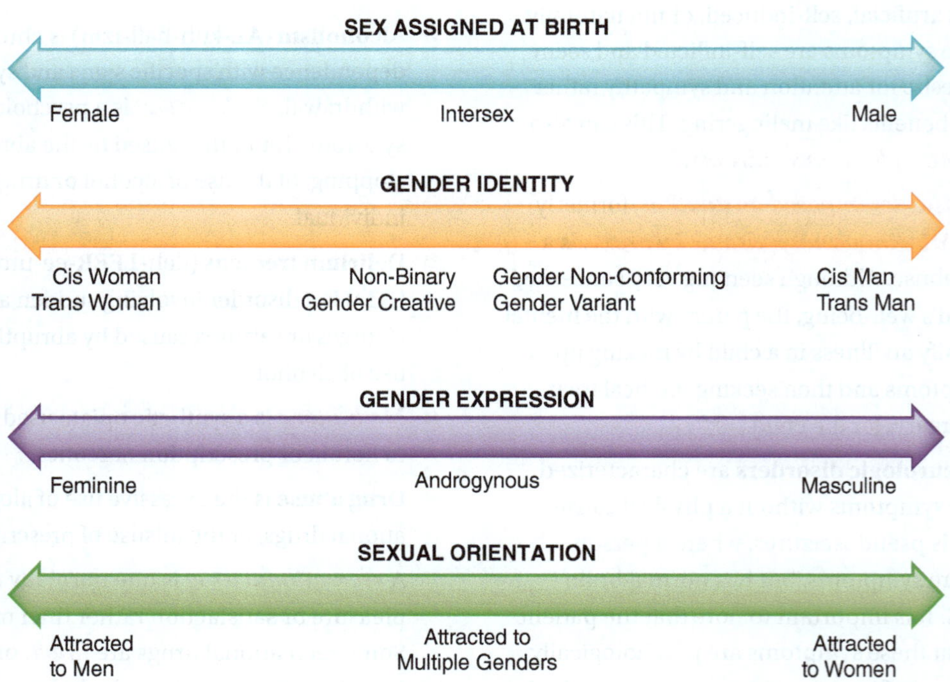

FIGURE 17.7 Gender identity and gender expression, shown on a spectrum.

- Someone with ***voyeuristic disorder*** is consistently sexually aroused by watching others and this either causes significant distress to the person or causes harm to the other person or people who have not provided consent. ***Consent*** is approval or permission for action.
- ***Exhibitionistic disorder*** is characterized by distress caused to oneself or others by the arousal gained from exposing one's genitals to others.
- ***Pedophilic disorder*** is characterized by recurrent sexual fantasies, urges, or behaviors with children under the age of 13. Mental health providers are ***mandated reporters***. This means that if they suspect someone of having abused a child, they are required by law to report it to authorities.
- ***Sexual masochism disorder*** and ***sexual sadism disorder*** are characterized by sexual arousal from receiving or inflicting pain (respectively). They are considered disorders if they cause significant distress to oneself or harm to others.

Sleep Disorders

- **Insomnia** is the prolonged or abnormal inability to sleep. This condition is usually a symptom of another problem such as depression, pain, or consuming an excessive amount of caffeine (**in-** means without, **somn** means sleep, and **-ia** means abnormal condition).
- **Narcolepsy** (**NAR**-koh-**lep**-see) is a potentially dangerous sleep disorder consisting of sudden and uncontrollable brief episodes of falling asleep during the day (**narc/o** means stupor or sleep, and **-lepsy** means seizure).
- **Sleep deprivation** is a sufficient lack of restorative sleep over a cumulative period so as to cause physical or psychological symptoms and affect routine performance or tasks.
- **Parasomnia** (**pair**-ah-**SOM**-nee-ah) is a general term for several categories of sleep disorders that occur while falling asleep, during sleep, or while waking from sleep (**para-** means around, **somn** means sleep, and **-ia** means abnormal condition). *Somnambulism* is one type of parasomnia.
- **Somnambulism** (som-**NAM**-byou-lizm), also known as ***sleepwalking***, is the condition of walking or performing some other activity without awakening (**somn** means sleep, **ambul** means to walk, and **-ism** means condition of).

DIAGNOSTIC PROCEDURES OF MENTAL HEALTH

The Diagnostic and Statistical Manual of Mental Disorders (DSM-5) is the gold standard for assessing and diagnosing mental health disorders. A qualified mental health professional can determine if a patient meets criteria for a disorder or subthreshold disorder. ***Subthreshold*** means some, but not all, of the diagnostic criteria are met.

Screening Tools

Additionally, there are validated assessment questionnaires, sometimes called **screening tools**, available to use when diagnosing certain disorders. ***Validated*** means that the questionnaire has been proven to measure what it is attempting to measure. These assessments might be done by a trained therapist or given in a medical or school setting to determine whether there is the need to refer someone to a mental health professional. They assess for a variety of factors, such as personality traits, intelligence, and risk of harm to oneself or others. There are hundreds of screening tools available for a variety of disorders, some of which are listed here.

- ***PHQ-9*** stands for Patient Health Questionnaire and is a measure of the nine diagnostic criteria for depression.
- ***Minnesota Multiphasic Personality Inventory*** (MMPI) is an extensive personality test used to assess for several mental health disorders.
- ***GAD-7*** stands for Generalized Anxiety Disorder and contains seven questions used to assess for several anxiety disorders as well as posttraumatic stress disorder.
- ***Wechsler Adult Intelligence Scale*** (WAIS) and the ***Stanford-Binet Intelligence Scale*** are both intelligence (IQ) tests used to test cognitive ability.
- ***Vanderbilt ADHD Diagnostic Rating Scale*** assesses for attention deficit/hyperactivity disorder. This rating scale is used in addition to interviews with those close to the person being assessed, such as family members and teachers.
- The **Rorschach test** was developed as a way to assess a person's personality and emotional functioning by analyzing their interpretation of inkblot images (Figure 17.8).

Larch _tree/Shutterstock.com

FIGURE 17.8 A Rorschach inkblot test illustration.

TREATMENT PROCEDURES OF MENTAL HEALTH

Levels of Psychiatric Care

- An **outpatient** level of care is performed in an office setting or via telehealth using a video platform.
- In an ***intensive outpatient program*** (IOP), therapy occurs several times per week, potentially in a group setting. Patients live at home and can often continue working or attending school while actively participating in the program for several hours per week.
- In a ***partial hospitalization program*** (PHP), or ***day treatment***, patients spend several days per week at the program in a combination of group and individual activities, as well as using alternative types of therapy such as art or dance therapy. They return to their own home in the evenings and may have one or two days per week that they do not attend the program, such as weekends.
- ***Residential*** level of care provides 24/7 monitoring and treatment but without full-time medical care. Patients live and sleep at the facility.
- **Inpatient** level of care may be voluntary or involuntary depending on the condition of the patient. If a person is at risk of harming themselves or others, they may be involuntarily committed to a hospital for evaluation, sometimes called ***sectioning***. Each state has its own laws pertaining to involuntary commitment. These units are often referred to as ***locked units*** because patients cannot come and go independently. Inpatient care can also be necessary for medical reasons, if a person is not medically stable.

Drug Therapies

Drug therapy for mental disorders is called **psychopharmacology** (**sigh**-koh-farm-uh-**KOL**-oh-gee). A **psychotropic drug** (**sigh**-koh-**TROP**-ick) acts primarily on the central nervous system, where it produces temporary changes affecting the mind, emotions, and behavior (**psych/o** means mind, and **-tropic** means affinity for). These medications are also used to control pain and to treat narcolepsy and attention disorders.

- An **antidepressant** is administered to prevent or relieve depression. Some of these medications are also used to treat obsessive-compulsive and generalized anxiety disorders and to help relieve chronic pain. Often these medications are named for the brain chemical they are targeting.
  - An **SSRI** (**S**elective **S**erotonin **R**euptake **I**nhibitor) is the most popular type of antidepressant and is commonly used as a first-line treatment against depression.
  - **MAOIs** (**M**ono**a**mine **O**xidase **I**nhibitors) are mainly used to treat treatment-resistant depression.
  - **SNRIs** (**S**erotonin and **N**orepinephrine **R**euptake **I**nhibitors) are used to treat depression and anxiety.
- An **antipsychotic drug** (**an**-tih-sigh-**KOT**-ick), or ***neuroleptic***, is administered to treat symptoms of severe disorders of thinking and mood that are associated with neurological and psychiatric illnesses such as schizophrenia, mania, and delusional disorders (**anti-** means against, **psych/o** means mind, and **-tic** means pertaining to).
- An **anxiolytic drug** (**ang**-zee-oh-**LIT**-ick), also known as an ***antianxiety drug*** or ***tranquilizer***, is administered to temporarily relieve anxiety and to reduce tension (**anxi/o** means anxiety, and **-lytic** means to destroy). An anxiolytic can be used as a sedative before anesthesia. ***Benzodiazepines*** are one category of anxiolytics.
- A **mood stabilizer**, such as lithium, is used to treat mood instability and bipolar disorders.
- A **stimulant** works by increasing activity in certain areas of the brain to increase concentration and wakefulness. Drug therapies using stimulants have been effective in treating ADHD and narcolepsy. The overuse of stimulants, including caffeine, can cause insomnia and heart palpitations.

Side effects of psychotropic drugs are variable but the most common include nausea, vomiting, diarrhea, weight gain, fatigue, and sexual dysfunction. Some psychotropic drugs have been shown to cause suicidal thoughts. There is some trial and error involved in finding the correct dosage for each patient in order to improve symptoms while minimizing physical or psychological side effects.

Psychological Therapies

Mental disorders are often treated with individual or group therapy by a qualified psychotherapist or other mental health professional. These therapies may be performed while someone is inpatient (hospitalized), or in an outpatient setting.

- **Psychotherapy**, sometimes called ***talk therapy*** or ***supportive psychotherapy***, is used to treat many mental illnesses by providing insights into a person's thoughts, emotions, and behaviors.
- **Psychoanalysis** (**sigh**-koh-ah-**NAL**-ih-sis) is based on the idea that mental disorders have underlying causes stemming from childhood and can only be overcome by gaining insight into one's feelings and patterns of behavior.
- **EMDR** (**E**ye **M**ovement **D**esensitization and **R**eprocessing) is an evidence-based therapy for PTSD that involves revisiting traumatic memories while simultaneously focusing on specific bilateral physical stimuli.
- **Behavioral therapy** focuses on changing behavior by identifying problem behaviors, replacing them with appropriate behaviors, and using rewards or other consequences to make the changes.
- **Cognitive behavioral therapy** (CBT) focuses on changing thoughts and behaviors that are affecting a person's emotions and functioning (Figure 17.9). Unhelpful thoughts and actions are identified, challenged with logic and evidence, and tested in action. The emphasis is on what is currently happening in the person's life.
  - A modified version of CBT, called ***dialectical behavior therapy*** (DBT), is used to treat people with suicidal thoughts, self-harm, or borderline personality disorder.
  - Another therapy based on CBT is ***acceptance and commitment therapy*** (ACT), which can be used to treat people with anxiety, depression, OCD, and psychosis.
- **Hypnotherapy** is the use of hypnosis to produce an altered state of focused attention in which the patient may be more willing to believe and act on suggestions. It is used for many purposes, among them pain relief, anxiety reduction, and behavioral modification.
- **Biofeedback** involves monitoring a person's physical reaction to relaxation techniques such as deep breathing. By showing an ability to reduce heart rate, for example, the subject learns that they have the ability to control symptoms of anxiety or panic. This is also used for some physical disorders (Figure 17.10).
- **Exposure therapy** can be used for treating anxiety disorders including phobias. It involves repeated exposure to a fear in a safe and controlled setting.

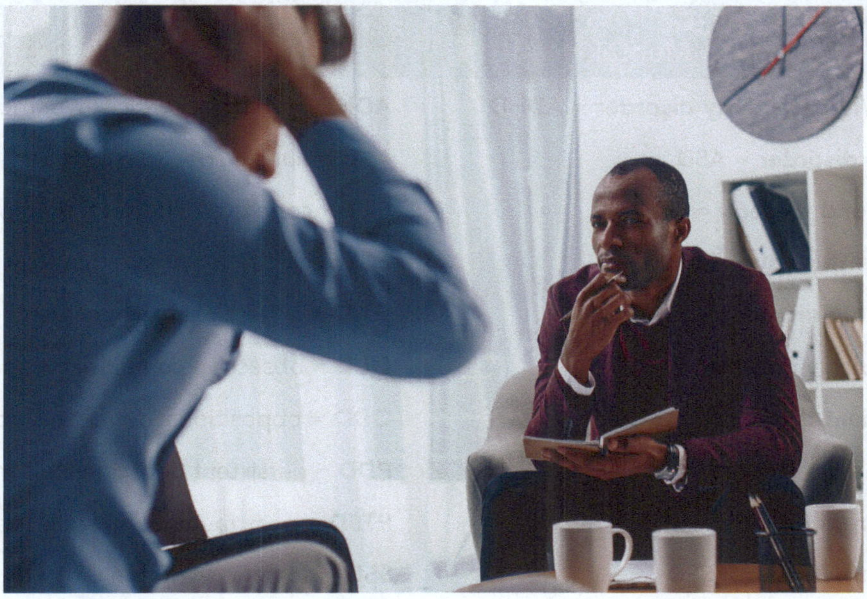

FIGURE 17.9 Cognitive behavioral therapy focuses on changing thoughts that are affecting a person's emotions and actions.

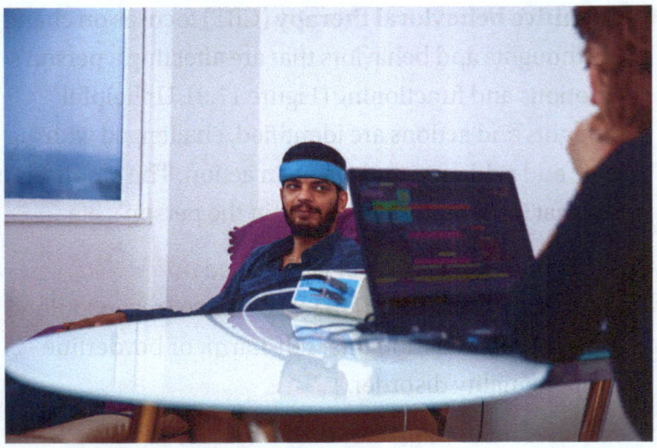

Malt Digital Agency/Shutterstock.com

FIGURE 17.10 A patient receiving biofeedback from a trained therapist in order to control anxiety symptoms.

Systematic desensitization is therapy which works to replace a thought or emotion associated with something feared with an alternative positive thought or emotion.

- **Marriage and family therapy** is a type of therapy involving two or more members of a family interested in learning to work through issues, cope with trauma, or improve communication and relationships with one another.
- In **group therapy**, people with similar issues meet together with one or more counselors for support and to learn coping skills.
- **Play therapy** is targeted therapy for children where coping and communication skills are gained through the use of play with a trained therapist.
- Artistic therapy such as *art therapy, dance therapy*, and *music therapy* can help people cope with and process their emotions by utilizing artistic expression.

Other Treatments

Electroconvulsive therapy (ee-**leck**-troh-kon-**VUL**-siv) (ECT), also known as *electroshock therapy*, is a procedure in which small amounts of electric current are passed through the brain, deliberately triggering a brief seizure in order to reverse symptoms of certain mental illnesses. It is a safe, effective treatment for life-threatening depression.

Transcranial magnetic stimulation (TMS) uses brief, powerful, repetitive electromagnetic pulses to alter electrical pathways in the brain. This noninvasive procedure is used to treat severe depression.

ABBREVIATIONS RELATED TO MENTAL HEALTH

Table 17.4 presents an overview of the abbreviations related to the terms introduced in this chapter. *Note:* To avoid errors or confusion, always be cautious when using abbreviations.

TABLE 17.4

Abbreviations Related to Mental Health

attention deficit/hyperactivity disorder = ADHD	**ADHD** = attention deficit/hyperactivity disorder
autism spectrum disorder = ASD	**ASD** = autism spectrum disorder
cognitive behavioral therapy = CBT	**CBT** = cognitive behavioral therapy
electroconvulsive therapy = ECT	**ECT** = electroconvulsive therapy
generalized anxiety disorder = GAD	**GAD** = generalized anxiety disorder
obsessive-compulsive disorder = OCD	**OCD** = obsessive-compulsive disorder
oppositional defiant disorder = ODD	**ODD** = oppositional defiant disorder
persistent depressive disorder = PDD	**PDD** = persistent depressive disorder
posttraumatic stress disorder = PTSD	**PTSD** = posttraumatic stress disorder
somatic symptom disorder = SSD	**SSD** = somatic symptom disorder
suicidal ideation = SI	**SI** = suicidal ideation

LEARNING EXERCISES

Matching Word Parts 1

Write the correct answer in the middle column.

	Definition	Correct Answer	Possible Answers
17.1.	against	___________	-tic
17.2.	around, abnormal	___________	post-
17.3.	after	___________	para-
17.4.	pertaining to	___________	schiz/o
17.5.	split	___________	anti-

Matching Word Parts 2

Write the correct answer in the middle column.

	Definition	Correct Answer	Possible Answers
17.6.	anxiety	___________	-phobia
17.7.	abnormal fear	___________	-mania
17.8.	madness or obsessive preoccupation	___________	traumat/o
17.9.	injury	___________	phren/o
17.10.	mind, diaphragm	___________	anxi/o

Matching Word Parts 3

Write the correct answer in the middle column.

	Definition	Correct Answer	Possible Answers
17.11.	barrier, enclosed space	___________	somn/o
17.12.	sleep, stupor	___________	narc/o

17.13. mind	______________	**-tropic**
17.14. sleep	______________	**claustr/o**
17.15. having an affinity for	______________	**psych/o**

Definitions

Select the correct answer, and write it on the line provided.

17.16. Serotonin is a ______________ which has a role in pleasure recognition.

norepinephrine | neurotransmitter | mental illness | defense mechanism

17.17. Irrational dread of everyday situations is a characteristic of ______________ disorders.

panic | dissociative | paraphilic | anxiety

17.18. Children with ______________ have significant developmental delays, minimal verbal skills, and few normal social relationships.

Tourette syndrome | autism | intellectual disability | dyslexia

17.19. A/An ______________ disability can be assessed using an IQ test.

learning | intellectual | adjustment | hyperactivity

17.20. An excessive fear of heights is known as ______________.

acrophobia | agoraphobia | claustrophobia | social phobia

17.21. The outward appearance of a person's mood is referred to as ______________ in psychology.

personality | affect | emotion | psyche

17.22. A preoccupation with perceived flaws in appearance which can interfere with daily life is known as ______________.

dissociative disorder | bulimia nervosa | oppositional defiant disorder | body dysmorphic disorder

17.23. Kleptomania and pyromania are examples of ______________ disorders.

bipolar | impulse control | persistent depressive | seasonal affective

17.24. ADHD is an example of a ______________ disorder, which has childhood onset.

personality | neurodevelopmental | communication | dissociative

17.25. Denial, displacement, and projection are all examples of ______________.

mental illness | emotion | defense mechanisms | endorphins

Matching Disorders

Write the correct answer in the middle column.

	Disorder	Correct Answer	Possible Answers
17.26.	psychosis	______________	feeding and eating disorder
17.27.	factitious disorder	______________	bipolar and depressive disorder
17.28.	seasonal affective disorder	______________	psychotic disorder
17.29.	oppositional defiant disorder	______________	disruptive and impulse control disorder
17.30.	anorexia nervosa	______________	somatic symptom and related disorder

Which Word?

Select the correct answer, and write it on the line provided.

17.31. A number of factors can affect a person's mental health including ______________, genes, and a chemical imbalance.

trauma psyche

17.32. A person's unique characteristics that effect how they behave is known as their ______________.

affect personality

17.33. Someone who is ______________ may choose to transition their body to align with their identified gender by taking hormones and/or having surgery.

transgender non-binary

17.34. A ______________ is a sensory perception that has no basis in external stimulation.

delusion hallucination

17.35. A fear of having a panic attack such that a person might not leave the house is ______________.

acrophobia agoraphobia

Spelling Counts

Find the misspelled word in each sentence. Then write that word, spelled correctly, on the line provided.

17.36. A parafilick disorder is characterized by distress over sexual fantasies, urges, or behaviors.

____

17.37. A general term for several categories of sleep disorders is pearasomnea. ________________________

17.38. An anzeolitic drug is administered to relieve anxiety. ________________________

17.39. Pyschalogy is the scientific study of the mind. ________________________

17.40. Fear of enclosed spaces is known as clastrafobia. ________________________

Abbreviation Identification 1

In the space provided, write the words that each abbreviation stands for.

17.41. **GAD** ________________________

17.42. **SI** ________________________

17.43. **OCD** ________________________

17.44. **PTSD** ________________________

17.45. **CBT** ________________________

Term Selection

Select the correct answer, and write it on the line provided.

17.46. Common emotional signs and symptoms of ____________ include feelings of apprehension, restlessness, and anticipating the worst.

depression panic disorder anxiety phobia

17.47. Intentionally taking one's own life is known as ____________.

self-harm suicide depression mania

17.48. The medical term meaning an abnormal fear of being in small or enclosed spaces is ____________.

acrophobia claustrophobia kleptomania pyromania

17.49. Intense anxiety caused by persistent mistrust is a characteristic of ____________.

hallucination delusion psychosis paranoia

17.50. The medical term for the condition also known as a developmental reading disorder is ____________.

autism dissociative disorder dyslexia intellectual disability

Sentence Completion 1

Write the correct term or terms on the lines provided.

17.51. One example of a ____________ neurologic disorder is pseudoseizures.

17.52. The group of mental conditions characterized by excessive, irrational dread of everyday situations or fear that is out of proportion to the real danger in a situation is known as ____________.

17.53. A low-grade, chronic depression with symptoms that are milder than those of severe depression but are present on a majority of days for two or more years is known as ____________.

17.54. The intense fear of gaining weight associated with voluntary starvation is known as ____________.

17.55. A/An ____________ drug is administered to treat symptoms of severe disorders of thinking and mood that are associated with neurological and psychiatric illnesses such as schizophrenia, mania, and delusional disorders.

Word Surgery

Divide each term into its component word parts. Write these word parts, in sequence, on the lines provided. When necessary, use a slash (/) to indicate a combining vowel. (You may not need all of the lines provided.)

17.56. **Schizophrenia** is a psychotic disorder characterized by withdrawal from reality, illogical patterns of thinking, delusions, and hallucinations.

____________ ____________ ____________ ____________

17.57. **Somnambulism** is commonly known as sleepwalking.

____________ ____________ ____________ ____________

17.58. **Acrophobia** is an excessive fear of heights

_____________ _____________ _____________ _____________

17.59. A **psychologist** evaluates and treats emotional problems and mental illness.

_____________ _____________ _____________ _____________

17.60. **Insomnia** is the inability to sleep which can be a symptom of another problem such as depression or pain.

_____________ _____________ _____________ _____________

True/False 1

If the statement is true, write **True** on the line. If the statement is false, write **False** on the line.

17.61. ________ A borderline personality disorder is a pattern of extreme preoccupation with the self and complete lack of empathy for others.

17.62. ________ Schizoaffective disorder is a combination of schizophrenia symptoms with bipolar or depressive disorder symptoms.

17.63. ________ Delirium tremens is chronic alcohol dependence.

17.64. ________ A psychologist is a physician who prescribes medication for mental health disorders.

17.65. ________ A psychotropic drug acts primarily on the central nervous system, where it produces temporary changes affecting the mind, emotions, and behavior.

Clinical Conditions

Write the correct answer on the line provided.

17.66. Harvey Ikeman has mood shifts from highs to severe lows that affect his attitude, energy, and ability to function. Harvey's doctor describes this condition as a/an ____________________ disorder.

17.67. The case file for Benji Jones described several episodes of instigating violence with schoolmates as well as smashing a window in the cafeteria. He is being assessed by the school psychologist for ____________________ personality disorder.

17.68. Gundhram Ahmad was excited about his new relationship but worried that Joaquin wouldn't understand his ____________________ stress disorder, which he was diagnosed with after he was assaulted in college.

17.69. Celia Burgess was having trouble sleeping due to worrying, increased muscle soreness, and a pestering feeling of restlessness. Her doctor suggested that she see a therapist for ____________________ anxiety disorder.

17.70. Rene Ruiz tried hiding her ____________________ from her roommate by only smoking when he wasn't home, but when she began stealing from him to pay for cigarettes, she knew she had to disclose her addiction to him.

17.71. After several months of being unable to sleep well, Wayne Ladner visited his doctor about this problem. His doctor recorded this condition as being ____________________.

17.72. When she noticed her son's hands were raw, Jacquelyn McBride knew he was washing them excessively, a sign that his ____________________ was flaring.

17.73. Hayami Kenshin knew he had a family history of mental illness so wasn't surprised when his therapist diagnosed him with ____________________ when he described his apathy, anhedonia, and persistent sadness.

17.74. After she experienced heart palpitations, sweating, and a tingling in her fingers during her first ____________________ attack, Beria Kerimoglu became fearful it would happen again.

17.75. Sophia Perez's parents are concerned because large quantities of food have gone missing from the kitchen and they have found empty boxes of laxatives in her trash can. They suspect she might have ____________________.

Which Is The Correct Medical Term?

Select the correct answer, and write it on the line provided.

17.76. Lithium is an example of a/an ________________ used to treat bipolar disorders.

stimulant	anxiolytic drug	mood stabilizer	antipsychotic drug

17.77. The type of therapy that focuses on changing thoughts and behaviors affecting a person's emotions and functioning is called ________________.

EMDR	biofeedback	hypnotherapy	cognitive behavioral therapy

17.78. A/An __________ disorder is characterized by a person acting as though they are sick despite no medical evidence to support an illness, often for attention or sympathy.

anxiety | conversion | factitious | panic

17.79. The most common type of antidepressant prescribed, a/an __________, is named for the brain chemicals it targets.

MAOI | SSRI | SNRI | EMDR

17.80. The term __________ can describe delayed ejaculation, erectile disorder, and female orgasmic disorder.

sexual dysfunctions | paraphilic disorders | exhibitionistic disorder | sexual masochism disorder

Abbreviation Identification 2

In the space provided, write the words that each abbreviation stands for.

17.81. **ODD** __________

17.82. **SSD** __________

17.83. **ECT** __________

17.84. **ADHD** __________

17.85. **ASD** __________

True/False 2

If the statement is true, write **True** on the line. If the statement is false, write **False** on the line.

17.86. __________ Social anxiety disorder is characterized by the overaccumulation of belongings.

17.87. __________ Also known as developmental reading disorder, dyslexia is characterized by substandard reading achievement.

17.88. __________ The high feeling that someone with bipolar disorder might experience during shifting mood changes is called apathy.

17.89. ________ In an inpatient level of psychiatric care, a patient can continue with their normal job or school and can live at home.

17.90. ________ Biofeedback uses hypnosis to produce an altered state of focused attention.

Sentence Completion 2

Write the correct term or terms on the lines provided.

17.91. The group of structures in the brain generally associated with thought, mood, and emotion is called the ________________ system.

17.92. Referred to as the DSM-5, *The* ________________ *of Mental Disorders* is used by qualified clinicians to diagnose mental illness.

17.93. Significant distress over a person's gender identity is known clinically as gender ________________.

17.94. Nalaxone is a medication used by first responders to reverse the effects of a drug ________________.

17.95. Delusions and hallucinations can be symptoms of ________________, a disrupted thought pattern that makes it hard to determine what is real.

17.96. Previously known as dysthymia, ________________ depressive disorder is a low-grade chronic depression.

17.97. When people with similar issues meet together for support it is called ________________ therapy.

17.98. A validated ________________ tool can be used as a way of assessing for mental health issues in a variety of settings.

17.99. Pretending to have an illness to garner sympathy and attention is known as a ________________ disorder.

17.100. Repeated exposure to a fear in a controlled setting is a type of ________________ therapy.

The Human Touch

CRITICAL THINKING EXERCISE

The following story and questions are designed to stimulate critical thinking through class discussion or as a brief essay response. There are no right or wrong answers to these questions.

"So, why don't you tell me what brings you in today," said Dr. Shah with a warm, inviting smile. The psychologist's office had soft lighting, several decorative pillows, and a tasteful throw on the back of a small couch. Somehow this did little to put Ayana at ease. Lately it seemed like nothing could help her to relax; during the day she worried constantly about her grades and at night she lay awake with her mind racing as she wondered if she would be able to afford another semester of college.

Ayana didn't know where to begin describing her situation. Should she tell the therapist that several nights per week she drank to the point of blacking out, because it was the only thing that seemed to help her get some sleep? Did she need to tell the therapist about her Uncle Darren? She suspected he had died by suicide, but no one in the family ever really talked about it. And Ayana's grandmother often mentioned needing her pills to get through the day.

She took a deep breath, focused on the painting of lilies on the wall, and began to describe the experience she had recently during an organic chemistry exam. "Last week during a midterm, I thought maybe I was having a heart attack. My heart starting racing and I broke out in a cold sweat. It felt like there was nothing I could do to catch my breath. The doctor at the urgent care center did an EKG and told me that there is nothing wrong with my heart. He told me I had probably had a panic attack and gave me a list of names of therapists. Even though I know there's probably nothing wrong with me, I'd do anything to prevent that feeling from happening again... so that's why I'm here."

Dr. Shah began explaining what Ayana could expect from their weekly sessions together, using terms like anxiety disorder, CBT, and coping skills. She wanted to be open to receiving help, but wasn't sure she felt comfortable discussing her life with a stranger each week. Besides, compared to people with actual problems she was fine, wasn't she?

Suggested Discussion Topics

1. Ayana seems hesitant about seeking mental health care. Is there a stigma associated with seeing a therapist?
2. If cognitive behavioral therapy (CBT) with a psychologist doesn't help Ayana, what other options might she have for treatment of her anxiety?
3. Ayana alludes to self-medicating with alcohol. What concerns should she have about medications she could be prescribed for her anxiety combined with her history of substance abuse?
4. What factors of Ayana's life might make her more susceptible to mental illness?

CHAPTER 18

INFANT AND CHILD HEALTH

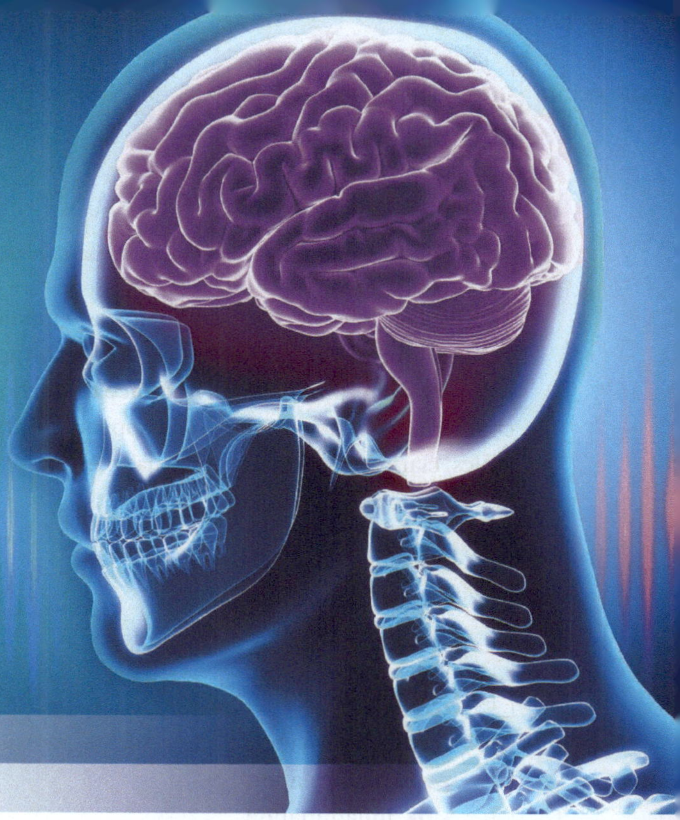

Overview of THE BASICS OF INFANT AND CHILD HEALTH

Infancy, which is the period from birth until age 2, is a time of rapid growth and change. From ages 2 to 20, as a child grows into adulthood, the body and mind undergo multiple processes of development including puberty. Nurturing and nutrition are essential for healthy growth during the childhood years. Children are also susceptible to a number of medical conditions and disorders specific to the young.

Vocabulary Related to **INFANT AND CHILD HEALTH**

This list contains essential word parts and medical terms for this chapter. These and the other important **primary terms** are shown in **boldface** throughout the chapter. *Secondary terms*, which appear in *orange* italics, clarify the meaning of primary terms.

Word Parts

- ☐ **-al** pertaining to
- ☐ **-arche** beginning
- ☐ **con-** together, with
- ☐ **dys-** bad
- ☐ **fet/o** unborn child, fetus
- ☐ **genit/o** formation
- ☐ **-itis** inflammation
- ☐ **men/o** menstruation
- ☐ **nat/o** born
- ☐ **neo-** new
- ☐ **-ologist** specialist
- ☐ **ped/o** child
- ☐ **pedicul/i** lice
- ☐ **-plasia** formation
- ☐ **umbilic/o** navel

Medical Terms

- ☐ **acne vulgaris** (**ACK**-nee vul-**GAY**-ris)
- ☐ **adolescence** (ah-doh-**LESS**-ance)
- ☐ **Apgar score**
- ☐ **asthma** (**AZ**-mah)
- ☐ **attention deficit/hyperactivity disorder**
- ☐ **birth defect**
- ☐ **birth weight**
- ☐ **bone age**
- ☐ **breast milk**
- ☐ **chickenpox**
- ☐ **childhood**
- ☐ **colic** (**KOL**-ick)
- ☐ **colostrum** (kuh-**LOS**-trum)
- ☐ **communicable disease** (kuh-**MEW**-nih-kuh-bul)
- ☐ **congenital disorders** (kon-**JEN**-ih-tahl)
- ☐ **congenital heart defects**
- ☐ **corrected age**
- ☐ **croup** (**KROOP**)
- ☐ **cradle cap**
- ☐ **developmental dysplasia of the hip**
- ☐ **DTaP vaccine**
- ☐ **fetal alcohol syndrome**
- ☐ **genetic disorder**
- ☐ **gestational age** (jess-**TAY**-shun-uhl)
- ☐ **growth chart**
- ☐ **growth spurt**
- ☐ **head circumference**
- ☐ **HPV vaccine**
- ☐ **human papillomavirus**
- ☐ **immunization schedule**
- ☐ **infancy** (**IN**-fan-see)
- ☐ **infectious mononucleosis** (**mon**-oh-**new**-klee-**OH**-sis)
- ☐ **isolette**
- ☐ **juvenile idiopathic arthritis**
- ☐ **MMR vaccine**
- ☐ **neonatologist** (**nee**-oh-nay-**TOL**-oh-jist)
- ☐ **newborn screening**
- ☐ **nocturnal enuresis** (nock-**TER**-nal **en**-you-**REE**-sis)
- ☐ **motor skills**
- ☐ **oral thrush**
- ☐ **pediatrician** (**pee**-dee-ah-**TRISH**-un)
- ☐ **pediatric intensive care unit**
- ☐ **pediculosis capitis** (pee-**dick**-you-**LOH**-sis)
- ☐ **permanent teeth**
- ☐ **premature birth**
- ☐ **primary teeth**
- ☐ **puberty** (**PYU**-ber-tee)
- ☐ **rectal thermometer**
- ☐ **roseola** (roe-zee-**OH**-la)
- ☐ **shaken baby syndrome**
- ☐ **strep throat**
- ☐ **sudden infant death syndrome** (SIDS)
- ☐ **Tanner staging**
- ☐ **tinea** (**TIN**-ee-ah)
- ☐ **tooth eruption**
- ☐ **umbilical hernia** (uhm-**BIL**-ic-al **HER**-nee-ah)
- ☐ **vaccine**
- ☐ **weaning** (**WEE**-ning)
- ☐ **well-child visits**
- ☐ **varicella vaccine** (**var**-ih-**SEL**-ah)

LEARNING OBJECTIVES

On completion of this chapter, you should be able to:

1. Describe the stages of infancy through adulthood.
2. Identify the standardized screening tools for child growth and development.
3. Identify the indicators of average physical child growth.
4. Define primary terms related to child health.
5. Identify common childhood immunizations and the recommended schedule for administering them to infants and children.
6. Identify the medical specialists who treat childhood disorders.
7. Identify the medical word parts related to child health.
8. Define the primary terms related to the pathology and the diagnostic and treatment procedures for common infant and childhood diseases, disorders, and injuries.
9. Spell the primary terms related to child health.
10. Pronounce the primary terms related to child health.
11. Define the common abbreviations related to child health.

STAGES OF GROWTH AND DEVELOPMENT

The journey from birth to adulthood can be divided into five main periods of development:

- Neonate
- Infant
- Toddler
- Child
- Adolescent

Prior to birth, an unborn baby is called a fetus. A newborn baby is known as a **neonate** (**NEE**-oh-nayt) during the first 4 weeks after birth. The next stage is called **infancy** (**IN**-fan-see) which lasts from 1 month to 1 year of age. Ages 1–3 is considered **toddlerhood**.

From age 3 on is **childhood**, sometimes referred to as ***preschool*** or ***school-aged***. This ends at *puberty* which happens around ages 11–14. **Adolescence** (ah-doh-**LESS**-ance), also known as ***young adulthood*** or the ***teenage years***, is considered to span ages 14–21.

HEALTHY GROWTH

Beginning at birth, a child's growth and development are routinely monitored to make sure that there are no underlying conditions impeding their natural course.

Newborn Assessment

An **Apgar score** is used to evaluate a newborn infant's physical status at 1 and 5 minutes after birth. The Apgar score is named for obstetrical anesthesiologist Virginia Apgar.

- The newborn is evaluated by assigning numerical values (0, 1, or 2) to each of five criteria: heart rate, respiratory effort, muscle tone, reflexes, and skin color.
- A total score of 8 to 10 indicates the best possible condition. If the score is less than 7, an additional score is given at 10 minutes after birth, and every 5 minutes thereafter for a maximum of 20 minutes.

In addition to Apgar scoring, a **newborn screening** is done prior to a newborn baby being discharged home from the hospital. Generally, this is a blood test using a few drops of blood taken from the heel to screen for numerous genetic diseases (Figure 18.11, later in this chapter, shows an example). A newborn will also have a **hearing test** and a **heart function test** using a pulse oximeter to screen for congenital heart defects.

Growth Charts

Throughout childhood, measurements will be taken by a pediatrician at regular **well-child visits** to assess a child's growth and development. The American Academy of

Pediatrics (AAP) suggests that well-child visits happen at the following ages:

- The first week visit (3 to 5 days old)
- 1 month old
- 2 months old
- 4 months old
- 6 months old
- 9 months old
- 12 months old
- 15 months old
- 18 months old
- 2 years old (24 months)
- 2½ years old (30 months)
- Yearly from 3 years old through 21 years old

The physical measurements taken at the exam are plotted on a **growth chart** (Figures 18.1 and 18.2), an age-based chart depicting lines called **growth curves**; these curved lines represent different *percentiles* (5th, 10th, 25th, 50th, 75th, 85th, and 95th) and can help alert a health care provider to a potential problem if the percentile changes drastically in a short period of time. A significant change in percentile, such as crossing a centile line for weight, height, or **body mass index** (BMI), a ratio of weight in kilograms to height in meters squared, could be cause for concern. Which growth chart is used will depend on the child's sex and age to ensure that the child is growing appropriately along their curve. There are two Centers for Disease Control and Prevention (CDC) growth charts for males and two for females by age range: birth–36 months and ages 2–20. From birth to 36 months, **weight**, **length** (as measured laying down in the recumbent position), **head circumference** (as measured with a measuring tape placed around the head), and **weight-for-length** are measured and plotted on the chart either digitally or by hand. From ages 2 through 20, a child should continue to follow their growth curve, with weight, stature, and BMI measurements plotted along the curve.

Many factors such as nutritional status, genetics, hormones, and a variety of medical conditions can affect growth. Some conditions which have expected growth patterns that are different from the general population have their own disease-specific growth charts, such as the genetic disorder Down syndrome.

Birth Through Age 2

In the first few days of life, a neonate is expected to lose 7–10% of their birth weight, which is largely fluid lost due to the transition from intrauterine to extrauterine life. The baby should regain the weight that has been lost within the first two weeks after birth. During the first month, approximately one ounce of weight gain is expected per day. By ages 3–5 months, an infant should have approximately doubled their birth weight, and by the first year they should have approximately tripled their birth weight. During this time, normal length will increase by approximately one inch per month for the first six months, and half an inch per month up until age 1. Head circumference is expected to increase by an average of 1 centimeter per month for the first year, with the rate slowing after that.

Skills being assessed during this period include **motor skills**, or ***movement milestones***. These include skills such as head and neck control, grip ability, smiling, connecting hands to mouth, and eventually rolling over.

If a mother chooses to breastfeed, food and nutrition during the neonatal period begins with **colostrum** (kuh-**LOS**-trum), the first form of milk produced immediately following delivery. This is a specialized form of breast milk that delivers essential nutrients and antibodies in a form that the newborn can digest during the first few days after being born.

- **Breast milk** is the optimal nutrition for a baby for at least the first 12 months of life, or as long as the mother chooses to breastfeed. Breast milk offers health benefits to both the infant and the mother.
- If breast milk is not an option or if a baby needs supplemental nutrition, **formula** (either mixed with breast milk or on its own) is the source of nutrition until solid foods are introduced into the diet. Formula is a manufactured liquid or powder made from iron-fortified cow's milk, soy, or another protein source with added vegetable oils, vitamins, minerals, and iron.
- **Weaning** (**WEE**-ning) is the process of discontinuing breastfeeding.

Most babies, whether exclusively breastfed or formula fed, will need to supplement with ***vitamin D*** for bone health.

Solid foods should begin to be introduced in addition to formula or breast milk between ages 4 and 6 months with the guidance of a health care provider. Iron-fortified infant cereal or other iron-rich foods such as pureed meat, poultry, or beans are important sources of nutrients at this stage. Cow's milk can be introduced in place of formula or breast milk at age 12 months. Children under the age of 12 months should never be given honey due to the risk of botulism, nor should they be given foods that could pose a choking hazard.

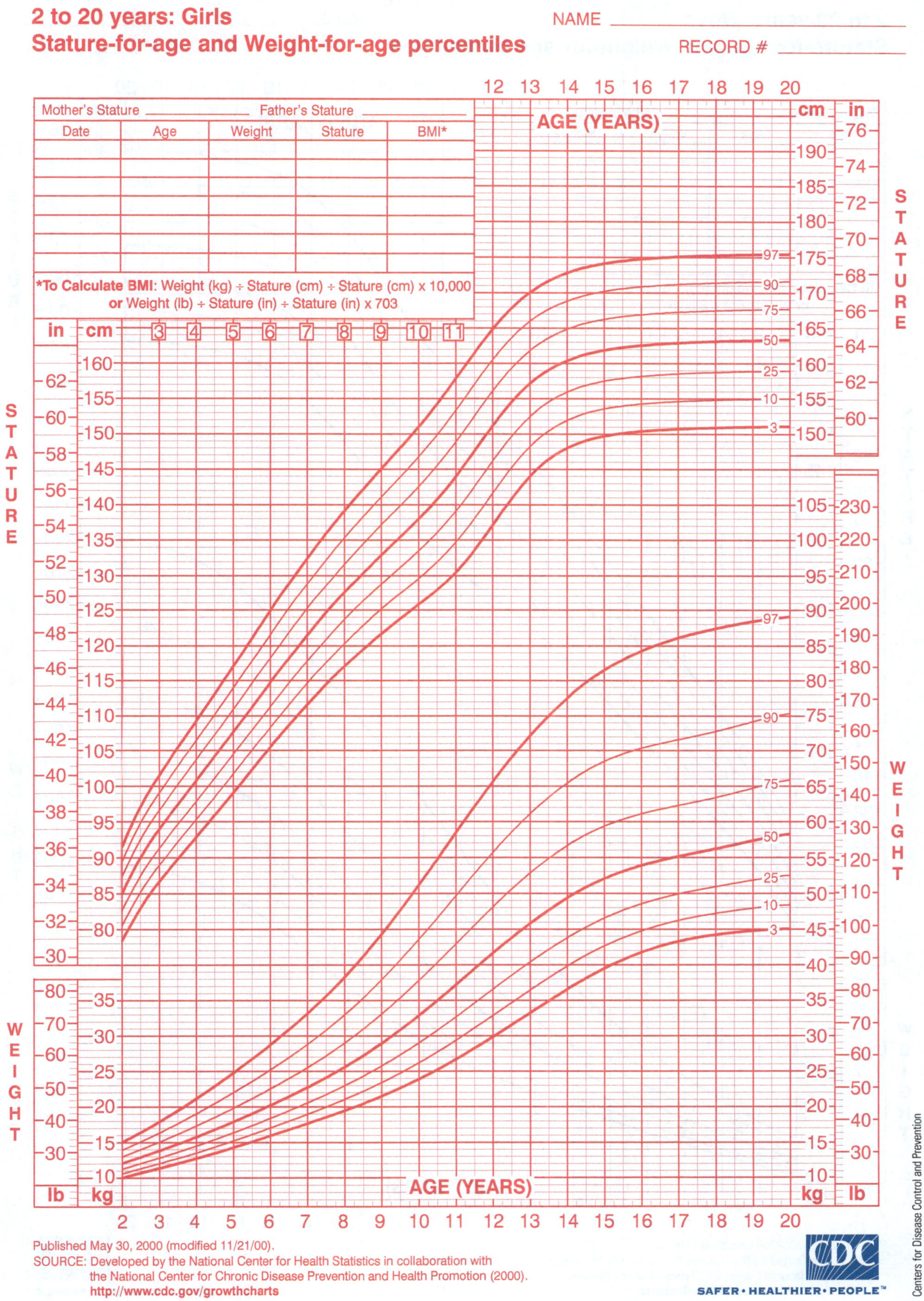

FIGURE 18.1 Girls ages 2–20 stature-for-age and weight-for-age growth chart.

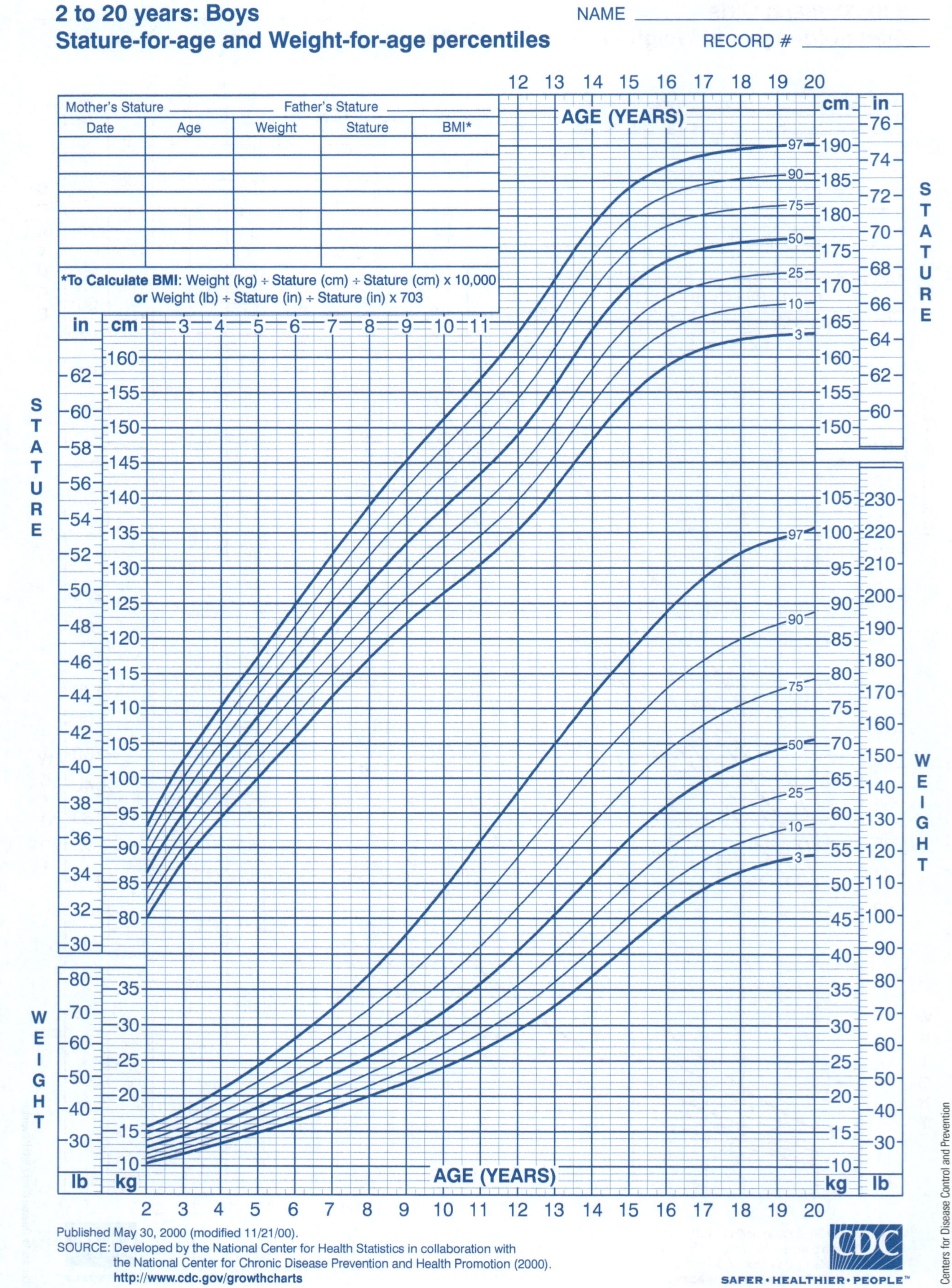

FIGURE 18.2 Boys ages 2–20 stature-for-age and weight-for-age growth chart.

Tooth eruption begins around age 6 months, normally with the lower and then upper central incisors. See Figure 18.3 for a chart of the **primary teeth** and their projected *eruption* (growing) and *shedding* (falling out) ages. Teething can cause discomfort for a baby or toddler and may cause symptoms such as irritability, drooling, inflammation of the gums, rash on the cheek, disrupted sleep, mild fever, and increased biting and chewing or gnawing.

Ages 2 Through 20

From age 2 onward, growth of 2.5 inches in height per year is expected until adolescence. During adolescence a **growth spurt** will occur for two to five years, after which time **physical maturity**, or peak height, is reached. To assess a child's adult height potential, a *midparental height* may be calculated, which takes into account the height of a child's birth mother and birth father.

Puberty (**PYU**-ber-tee) is the process of physical changes by which a child's body transitions into an adult body that is capable of reproducing (see Chapter 14). It is marked by the maturing of the genital organs, the development of secondary sex characteristics, and the first occurrence of **menstruation** in the female. *Precocious puberty* is the early onset of the changes of puberty, usually before age 8 in girls and age 9 in boys. *Precocious* means exceptionally early in development or occurrence. **Menarche** (**MEN**-ar-kee) is the beginning of menstruation (**men** means menstruation, and **-arche** means beginning). This begins after the maturation that occurs during puberty. In the United States the average age of menarche is 12½ years.

Tanner staging, also known as *sexual maturity rating*, is a tool used by health care providers to assess the current stage of *secondary sex characteristics*: pubic hair, female breast development, and male genitalia development during puberty (Figure 18.4). This can be useful to determine if there is an issue with development, in order to refer to a specialist (see Table 18.1). The **gonads** secrete the hormones that are responsible for the development and maintenance of the secondary sex characteristics that develop during puberty. Secondary sex characteristics are features that distinguish the two sexes but are not directly related to reproduction. The additional functions of the gonads are discussed in Chapter 14.

Nutrition during childhood and adolescence should focus on a balance of nutrient-rich foods. In order to consume a variety of macronutrients, vitamins, and minerals, each meal offered should contain a variety of carbohydrates, protein, and dietary fat, with plenty of fiber-containing foods such as fruits, vegetables, whole grains, and legumes.

Calcium and vitamin D are of particular importance to optimize bone health, and can be obtained from cow's milk and dairy products such as cheese or plant-based

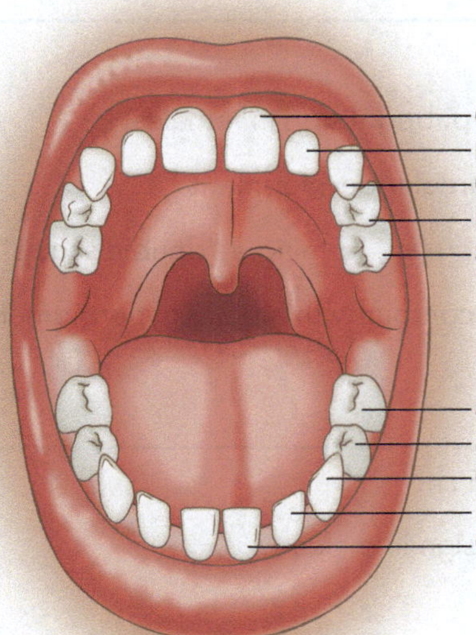

Primary Teeth

Upper teeth	Erupt	Shed
Central incisor	8–12 months	6–7 years
Lateral incisor	9–13 months	7–8 years
Canine (cuspid)	16–22 months	10–12 years
First molar	13–19 months	9–11 years
Second molar	25–33 months	10–12 years

Lower teeth	Erupt	Shed
Second molar	23–31 months	10–12 years
First molar	14–18 months	9–11 years
Canine (cuspid)	17–23 months	10–12 years
Lateral incisor	10–16 months	7–8 years
Central incisor	6–10 months	6–7 years

FIGURE 18.3 Tooth eruption chart for primary teeth.

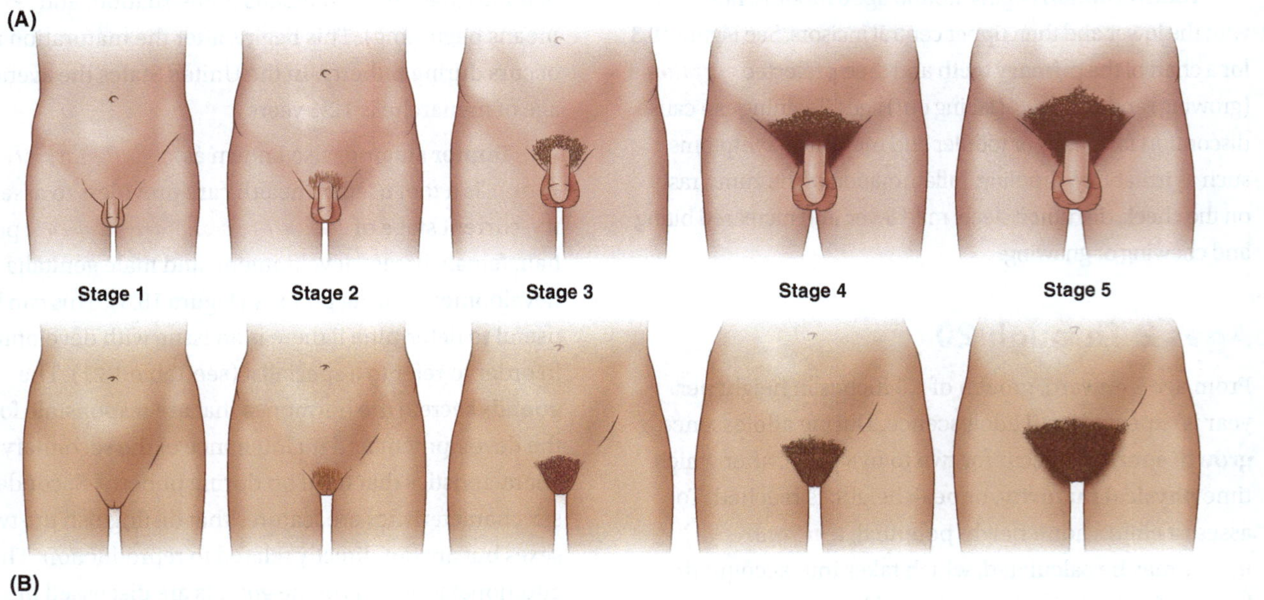

FIGURE 18.4 Pubic hair Tanner staging for (A) males and (B) females.

TABLE 18.1

Tanner Staging

Pubic Hair Scale (Both Males and Females)

- Stage 1: No hair
- Stage 2: Downy hair
- Stage 3: Scant terminal hair
- Stage 4: Terminal hair that fills the entire triangle overlying the pubic region
- Stage 5: Terminal hair that extends beyond the inguinal crease onto the thigh

Female Breast Development Scale

- Stage 1: No glandular breast tissue palpable
- Stage 2: Breast bud palpable under the areola (1st pubertal sign in females)
- Stage 3: Breast tissue palpable outside areola; no areolar development
- Stage 4: Areola elevated above the contour of the breast, forming a "double scoop" appearance
- Stage 5: Areolar mound recedes into single breast contour with areolar hyperpigmentation, papillae development, and nipple protrusion

Male External Genitalia Scale

- Stage 1: Testicular volume < 4 ml or long axis < 2.5 cm
- Stage 2: 4–8 ml (or 2.5–3.3 cm long); first pubertal sign in males
- Stage 3: 9–12 ml (or 3.4–4.0 cm long)
- Stage 4: 15–20 ml (or 4.1–4.5 cm long)
- Stage 5: >20 ml (or >4.5 cm long)

Source: https://www.ncbi.nlm.nih.gov/books/NBK470280/

dietary sources such as soy milk or supplements. The adolescent years are when peak bone mass is being built so calcium is especially important during this time. Iron remains an important nutrient during childhood and adolescence, with increased needs for females once they begin menstruating (due to cyclical blood loss).

The shedding of primary teeth and eruption of **permanent teeth** tends to happen between ages 6 and 12. See Chapter 9 for more information about dentition.

CHILDHOOD IMMUNIZATIONS

A **vaccine** can provide **immunity** against many diseases. **Natural immunity**, which is also known as ***passive immunity***, is resistance passed from mother to child at birth. Natural immunity is present without the administration of an antigen or exposure to a disease. **Active immunity** is obtained either by having had a contagious disease or being vaccinated against a contagious disease. Childhood vaccines are generally given before age 6. There is a suggested **immunization schedule** for delivering vaccinations at specific ages. Some vaccines need to be given at specific ages and intervals, and others have a range of acceptable ages, as shown in Table 18.2. After age 6 months, children should continue getting yearly influenza vaccinations. At ages 11–12 children should receive an additional tetanus, diphtheria, and pertussis (Tdap) vaccine (called DTaP when under age 6), human papillomavirus (HPV) vaccine, and meningococcal (MenACWY) vaccine (with a booster at age 16). Other vaccines, such as the COVID-19 vaccine, may be recommended at various ages throughout childhood for emerging contagious diseases. Additional vaccinations may be needed during childhood for situations such as high-risk health conditions or travel to countries with high rates of certain diseases such as yellow fever or malaria. An overview of diseases that can be prevented by vaccinations, as well as descriptions of those diseases and how they are spread, is shown in Table 18.3.

TABLE 18.2

Childhood Immunization Schedule

Birth	1 month	2 months	4 months	6 months	12 months	15 months	18 months	19–23 months	2–3 years	4–6 years
HepB	HepB			HepB						
		RV	RV	RV						
		DTaP	DTaP	DTaP		DTaP				DTaP
		Hib	Hib	Hib	Hib					
		PCV13	PCV13	PCV13	PCV13					
		IPV	IPV	IPV						IPV
				Influenza (yearly)*						
					MMR					MMR
					Varicella					Varicella
					HepA§					

* Two doses given at least four weeks apart are recommended for children ages 6 months through 8 years of age who are getting an influenza (flu) vaccine for the first time and for some other children in this age group.

§ Two doses of HepA vaccine are needed for lasting protection. The first dose of HepA vaccine should be given between 12 and 23 months of age. The second dose should be given 6 months after the first dose. All children and adolescents over 24 months of age who have not been vaccinated should also receive two doses of HepA vaccine.

This schedule is recommended by the Advisory Committee on Immunization Practices (ACIP) and approved by the Centers for Disease Control and Prevention (CDC).

Content source: National Center for Immunization and Respiratory Diseases

TABLE 18.3

Childhood Diseases Preventable by Vaccination

Disease	Vaccine	Disease spread by	Disease symptoms	Disease complications
Chickenpox	**Varicella vaccine** protects against chickenpox.	Air, direct contact	Rash, tiredness, headache, fever	Infected blisters, bleeding disorders, encephalitis (brain swelling), pneumonia (infection in the lungs)
Diphtheria	**DTaP* vaccine** protects against diphtheria (called Tdap when given after the age of 6).	Air, direct contact	Sore throat, mild fever, weakness, swollen glands in neck	Swelling of the heart muscle, heart failure, coma, paralysis, death
Hib	**Hib vaccine** protects against *Haemophilus influenzae* type b.	Air, direct contact	May be no symptoms unless bacteria enter the blood	Meningitis (infection of the covering around the brain and spinal cord), intellectual disability, epiglottitis (life-threatening infection that can block the windpipe and lead to serious breathing problems), pneumonia (infection in the lungs), death
Hepatitis A	**HepA vaccine** protects against hepatitis A.	Direct contact, contaminated food or water	May be no symptoms, fever, stomach pain, loss of appetite, fatigue, vomiting, jaundice (yellowing of skin and eyes), dark urine	Liver failure, arthralgia (joint pain), kidney, pancreatic, and blood disorders
Hepatitis B	**HepB vaccine** protects against hepatitis B.	Contact with blood or body fluids	May be no symptoms, fever, headache, weakness, vomiting, jaundice (yellowing of skin and eyes), joint pain	Chronic liver infection, liver failure, liver cancer
Human papillomavirus	**HPV vaccine** protects against human papillomavirus.	Direct skin contact	May be no symptoms, genital warts	Cervical, vaginal, vulvar, penile, anal, oropharyngeal cancers
Influenza (Flu)	**Flu vaccine** protects against influenza.	Air, direct contact	Fever, muscle pain, sore throat, cough, extreme fatigue	Pneumonia (infection in the lungs)
Measles	**MMR** vaccine** protects against measles.	Air, direct contact	Rash, fever, cough, runny nose, pink eye	Encephalitis (brain swelling), pneumonia (infection in the lungs), death

Meningococcal disease	**MenACWY and MenB vaccines** protect against meningococcal disease.	Air, direct contact	Sudden onset of fever, headache, and stiff neck, dark purple rash	Loss of limb, deafness, nervous system disorders, developmental disabilities, seizure disorder, stroke, death
Mumps	**MMR******vaccine** protects against mumps.	Air, direct contact	Swollen salivary glands (under the jaw), fever, headache, tiredness, muscle pain	Meningitis (infection of the covering around the brain and spinal cord), encephalitis (brain swelling), inflammation of testicles or ovaries, deafness
Pertussis	**DTaP* vaccine** protects against pertussis (whooping cough) (called Tdap when given after the age of 6).	Air, direct contact	Severe cough, runny nose, apnea (a pause in breathing in infants)	Pneumonia (infection in the lungs), death
Polio	**IPV vaccine** protects against polio.	Air, direct contact, through the mouth	May be no symptoms, sore throat, fever, nausea, headache	Paralysis, death
Pneumococcal	**PCV13 vaccine** protects against pneumococcus.	Air, direct contact	May be no symptoms, pneumonia (infection in the lungs)	Bacteremia (blood infection), meningitis (infection of the covering around the brain and spinal cord), death
Rotavirus	**RV vaccine** protects against rotavirus.	Through the mouth	Diarrhea, fever, vomiting	Severe diarrhea, dehydration
Rubella	**MMR** vaccine** protects against rubella.	Air, direct contact	Sometimes rash, fever, swollen lymph nodes	Very serious in pregnant women—can lead to miscarriage, stillbirth, premature delivery, birth defects
Tetanus	**DTaP* vaccine** protects against tetanus (called Tdap when given after the age of 6).	Exposure through cuts in skin	Stiffness in neck and abdominal muscles, difficulty swallowing, muscle spasms, fever	Broken bones, breathing difficulty, death

*DTaP combines protection against diphtheria, tetanus, and pertussis.

**MMR combines protection against measles, mumps, and rubella.

Content source: U.S. Department of Health and Human Services, Centers for Disease Control and Prevention, National Center for Immunization and Respiratory Diseases

MEDICAL SPECIALTIES RELATED TO INFANT AND CHILD HEALTH

- A **neonatologist** (**nee**-oh-nay-**TOL**-oh-jist) is a physician who specializes in diagnosing and treating disorders of the newborn (**neo-** means new, **nat** means born, and **-ologist** means specialist). The **neonatal intensive care unit** (NICU) is a nursery offering specialized care for premature or ill infants.
- A **pediatrician** (**pee**-dee-ah-**TRISH**-un) is a physician who specializes in diagnosing, treating, and preventing disorders and diseases of infants and children. This specialty is known as **pediatrics** (**ped** means child, and **-iatrics** means a field of medicine). A **pediatric intensive care unit** (PICU) is an area of a hospital offering specialized care for critically ill children. A **pediatric nurse practitioner** is an NP who has specialized advanced training in working with children and adolescents.
- An **adolescent medicine physician** is a primary care doctor who specializes in the care and treatment of teens and young adults.
- A **pediatric dentist** specializes in working with children's teeth.
- A **child psychiatrist** and a **child psychologist** have qualifications for working with children's mental health and behavioral issues, for example, diagnosing and managing ADHD.
- Many other medical specialties allow for specialization in pediatrics; for example, a ***pediatric endocrinologist*** works with children diagnosed with diseases of the endocrine system such as type 1 diabetes and growth disorders, and a ***pediatric oncologist*** works with children diagnosed with cancer.

PATHOLOGY OF INFANT AND CHILD HEALTH

Infants, children, and teens are susceptible to disease across all body systems. Some are specific to stage of life and others, like the common cold, are not. The conditions listed in this chapter either are dependent on stage of life or are common in childhood.

Premature Birth and Birth Injuries

Premature birth is a birth that occurs earlier than the 37th week of pregnancy. This can cause serious health problems because the baby's body systems have not finished developing. Breathing difficulties and heart problems are common in premature babies. Premature babies are sometimes referred to by their **gestational age** (jess-**TAY**-shun-uhl), which is the number of weeks since the first day of the birth mother's last menstrual period. **Chronologic age** is the age of an infant since birth, and **corrected age** or ***adjusted age*** is the age of an infant from birth minus the number of weeks they are premature. For example, a 12-week-old baby who was born 4 weeks premature has a corrected age of 8 weeks. Corrected age can be useful during the first two years of life for determining accurate nutritional needs as well as developmental goals that might not align with a premature baby's chronologic age.

- **Respiratory distress syndrome** (RDS), also called ***infant respiratory distress syndrome***, is a breathing disorder caused by underdeveloped lungs. A baby with RDS does not have enough ***surfactant***, the substance in the lungs that allows the air sacs to remain open.
- **Bronchopulmonary dysplasia** (BPD), also known as ***chronic lung disease of prematurity***, is a condition that most affects premature babies who require lung support for an extended period of time in order to breathe after birth. ***Dysplasia*** is the abnormal development or growth of cells, or the presence of abnormal cells within a type of tissue (**dys-** means bad, and **-plasia** means formation).

Birth injuries are disorders that occur as a result of trauma during labor or delivery. Most of these injuries, including fractures of the clavicle, heal quickly. **Meconium** (meh-**KOH**-nee-um) is the greenish material that collects in the intestines of a fetus and forms the first feces of a newborn. If a newborn passes meconium during labor or delivery, they can inhale it via the amniotic fluid, causing breathing problems.

Birth weight refers to a newborn infant's weight within hours of birth. There are subcategories based on specific weight:

- ***Small for gestational age*** (SGA) weight is less than the 10th percentile on the growth chart.
- ***Low birth weight*** (LBW) is less than 2,500 grams.
- ***Very low birth weight*** (VLBW) is less than 1,500 grams.
- ***Extremely low birth weight*** (ELBW) is less than 1,000 grams.

Low birth weight can be caused by a variety of factors including the birth mother's health and lack of access to prenatal care. Low birth weight can put a baby at risk for serious medical complications and is often treated in the NICU using enteral (feeding tube) or parenteral (intravenous) nutrition and hydration (see Chapter 9).

Pathology Specific to Infancy

- **Circumcision** (**ser**-kum-**SIZH**-un) is the surgical removal of the foreskin of the penis. This optional procedure is usually performed within a few days of birth, sometimes for religious reasons.
- **Colic** (**KOL**-ick) is a condition characterized by a generally healthy baby crying for more than three hours a day, more than three days a week for three or more weeks, and being difficult to soothe. The cause of colic is unknown. It usually starts when a baby is a couple of weeks old and resolves when they are a few months old.
- **Cradle cap**, a form of ***seborrheic dermatitis***, is a scalp rash in infants. This inflammation causes scaling and itching of the upper layers of the scalp.
- **Croup** (**KROOP**) is an acute respiratory infection in children and infants characterized by obstruction of the larynx, hoarseness, and swelling around the vocal cords, resulting in a barking cough and stridor. Stridor is a harsh, high-pitched sound caused by a blockage present when breathing in.
- **Failure to thrive** (FTT) is when an infant or child does not grow as expected due to any number of reasons including malabsorption, malnutrition, or environmental factors such as abuse or neglect. If the cause is nutritional, supplemental formula or additional foods may be recommended in order to increase caloric intake.
- A **hernia** is the protrusion of a part or structure through the tissues that normally contain it. In infants and children, it is a portion of the intestine that pushes through the abdominal muscles.
  - An **inguinal hernia** (**ING**-gwih-nal **HER**-nee-ah) is the protrusion of a small loop of the intestine through a weak place in the lower abdominal wall or groin (**inguin** means groin, and **-al** means pertaining to). This condition can cause pain when straining such as when coughing, lifting, or having a bowel movement.
  - An **umbilical hernia** (uhm-**BIL**-ic-al **HER**-nee-ah) is the protrusion of intestine in the area of the belly button, specifically the umbilical ring (**umbilic** means navel, and **-al** means pertaining to). About 20% of babies will have this, and it often resolves without medical treatment (Figure 18.5).
- Some babies have trouble turning their head, and due to the amount of time spent on their back can develop **flat head syndrome**, otherwise known as ***positional plagiocephaly***. This flattening on the back or side of the head is often caused by ***torticollis***, a twisting or tightening of the neck muscles resulting in the head tilting more to one side. It generally resolves on its own over time but may require treatment with a custom-made plagiocephaly helmet (Figure 18.6).
- **Developmental dysplasia of the hip** (DDH) (dis-**PLAY**-zhee-ah), also known as ***hip dysplasia***, is the dislocation of the thigh bone in the hip socket. It is caused by this joint not forming correctly. Pediatricians routinely screen infants for this condition shortly after birth and during well-child visits (Figure 18.7).

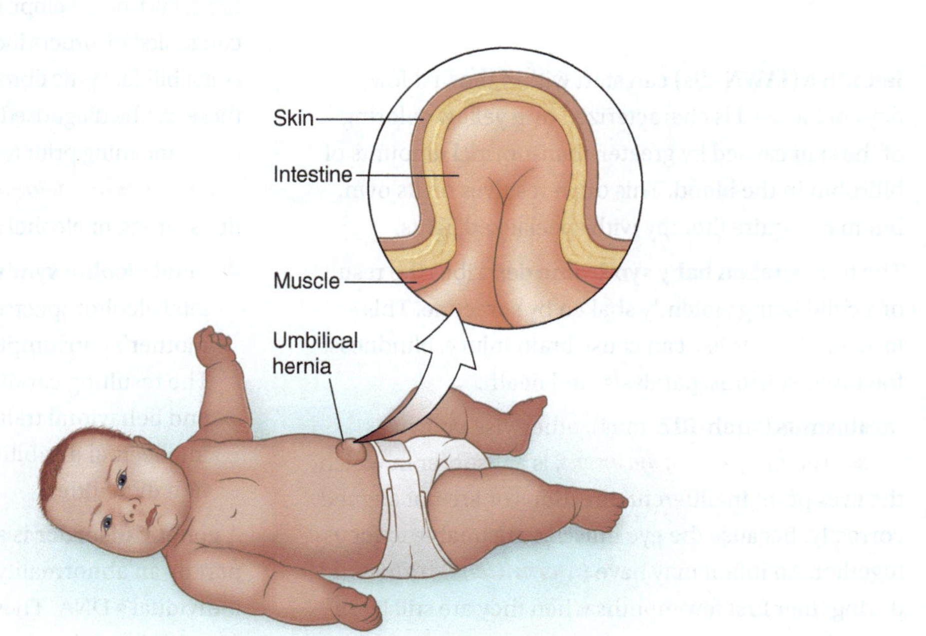

FIGURE 18.5 An umbilical hernia in a baby, forming a protrusion at the belly button.

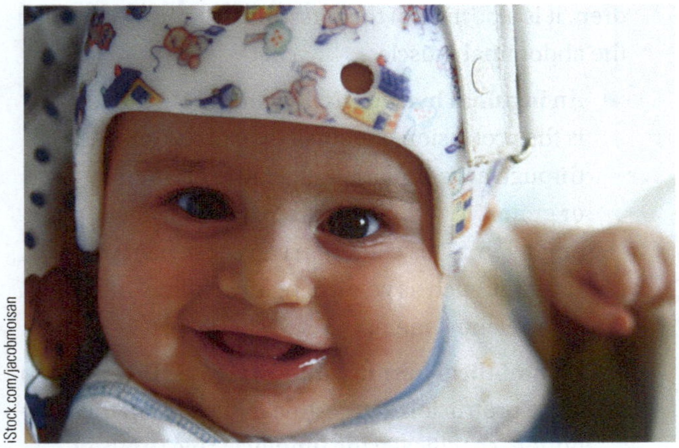

FIGURE 18.6 An infant wearing a plagiocephaly helmet to resolve flat head syndrome.

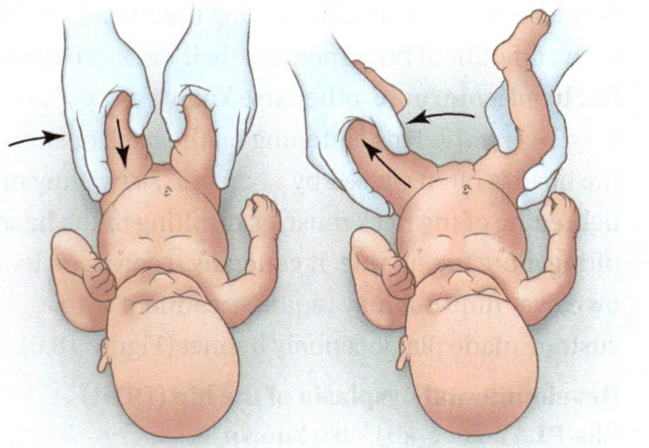

FIGURE 18.7 During a routine exam, the pediatrician will maneuver the baby's legs and hips in certain ways to detect hip instability when assessing for developmental dysplasia of the hip.

- **Jaundice** (**JAWN**-dis) can start within the first few days of life, and is characterized by a yellow coloring of the skin caused by greater-than-normal amounts of bilirubin in the blood. This often resolves on its own, but may require therapy with specialized lights.
- The term **shaken baby syndrome** describes the result of a child being violently shaken by someone. This form of ***child abuse*** can cause brain injury, blindness, fractures, seizures, paralysis, and death.
- **Strabismus** (strah-**BIZ**-mus), otherwise known as ***cross eyed*** or ***eye misalignment***, is a disorder in which the eyes point in different directions or are not aligned correctly, because the eye muscles are unable to focus together. An infant may have ***intermittent strabismus*** during their first few months when they are still learning to focus their eyes, or may have ***pseudostrabismus***, giving the false appearance of crossed eyes that goes away as the facial structure develops.
- **Sudden infant death syndrome** (SIDS) is the sudden and unexplainable death of an apparently healthy sleeping infant between the ages of 1 month to 1 year. Although the cause of SIDS is still unknown, the Safe to Sleep campaign recommending that infants sleep on their back (instead of facedown) with no blankets, pillows, or toys in the crib has significantly reduced the incidence of SIDS.
- **Oral thrush**, also known as ***oral candidiasis***, is a yeast infection in an infant's mouth that can occur when breastfeeding. It can cause white patches as well as soreness, though sometimes it is painless.
- A ***tongue-tie*** is caused by a tight or short membrane between the bottom of the tongue and the floor of the mouth. This can cause issues with breastfeeding and is treated with a simple procedure that is relatively painless to the infant.

Congenital Birth Defects and Genetic Disorders

Congenital disorders (kon-**JEN**-ih-tahl), also known as ***birth defects***, are abnormal conditions that exist at the time of birth and can be genetic; be inherited; have an environmental cause; or be ***multifactorial***, that is, caused by a combination of factors (**con-** means together, **genit** means formation, and **-al** means pertaining to).

Congenital disorders affect as many as 1 in every 33 babies and can cause infant death, physical malformations, and/or developmental issues. Some examples of congenital disorders include heart defects, cleft lip or palate, spina bifida, cystic fibrosis, and Down syndrome. Some of these can be diagnosed and even have treatments begin ***in utero***, meaning prior to the baby being born. Exposure to ***environmental factors*** such as infection, radiation, medications, drugs, or alcohol can cause birth defects.

- **Fetal alcohol syndrome** (FAS), the most severe type of fetal alcohol spectrum disorders, is the result of a birth mother's consumption of alcohol during pregnancy. The resulting condition is characterized by physical and behavioral traits, including growth abnormalities, intellectual disabilities, brain damage, and socialization difficulties.

A **genetic disorder** is a disease caused in whole or in part by an abnormality in the genetic makeup of an individual's DNA. These can be congenital (clearly present from birth) such as cystic fibrosis, sickle cell anemia, and

Down syndrome, or can present later in life such as colon cancer. Gene mutations can be inherited from one or both parents, or can happen during a person's lifetime.

- **Chromosomal congenital disorders** such as Down syndrome, trisomy 18, trisomy 13, and Turner's syndrome occur when there is an extra chromosome, or when a section of a chromosome is deleted or duplicated.

Congenital Anomalies

A **congenital anomaly** is an abnormality of a structure or function of the body that is prenatal in origin such as the absence of a limb or the presence of an extra toe. An ***anomaly*** is a deviation from what is regarded as normal.

- The term **atresia** (ah-**TREE**-zee-ah) describes the congenital absence or narrowing of a normal body opening or passage. ***Anal atresia*** is the congenital absence of the opening at the bottom end of the anus, and ***pulmonary atresia*** is the absence of a pulmonary valve.
- **Neural tube defects** (NTD) occur when the spinal canal fails to close completely around the spinal cord to protect it. The two most common NTDs are spina bifida and anencephaly.
    - **Spina bifida** (**SPY**-nah **BIF**-ih-dah) is a neural tube defect that occurs during early pregnancy, sometimes before a woman knows she is pregnant. ***Spina*** means pertaining to the spine. ***Bifida*** means split. Some cases of spina bifida are due to a lack of the nutrient folic acid in the mother's diet during the early stages of pregnancy.
    - **Anencephaly** (ah-nun-**SEF**-uh-lee) is characterized by the failure of the brain and skull to fully develop; most babies with this condition are stillborn or die within hours or days of being born. ***Stillborn*** means delivery of a baby who has died after the 20th week of pregnancy. If this happens prior to the 20th week of pregnancy, it is called a ***miscarriage***.
- **Congenital heart defects** (CHDs) are structural abnormalities caused by the failure of the heart to develop normally before birth and are the most common type of birth defect. Some congenital heart defects are apparent at birth, whereas others may not be detected until later in life.
    - A **ventricular septal defect** (ven-**TRICK**-you-lar) (VSD), which is characterized by a hole between the two ventricles of the heart, is the most prevalent CHD.
- A **cleft lip** is a birth defect in which there is a deep groove of the lip running upward to the nose as a result of the failure of this portion of the lip to close during prenatal development. A **cleft palate** is the failure of the palate to close during the early development of the fetus. This opening can involve the upper lip, hard palate, and/or soft palate. If not corrected, this opening between the nose and mouth makes it difficult for the child to eat and speak. Cleft lip and cleft palate can occur singly or together and usually can be corrected surgically (see Chapter 9, Figure 9.10).

Common Childhood Communicable Diseases

A **communicable disease** (kuh-**MEW**-nih-kuh-bul), also known as a ***contagious disease***, is any condition that is transmitted from one person to another either directly or by indirect contact with contaminated objects. ***Communicable*** means capable of being transmitted. Children are more susceptible to certain communicable diseases due to the sharing of germs by frequently putting their hands and other objects into their mouths, and being too young to use effective preventative measures such as covering a cough or sneeze or washing hands. Children attending daycare are more likely to experience frequent infections at a younger age and fewer infections once they start school. *Note:* Illnesses addressed in this section do not include those for which there is currently an effective vaccine. Those diseases are listed previously in the "Childhood Immunizations" section.

- **Upper respiratory infections** (URI) and ***acute nasopharyngitis*** are among the terms used to describe the ***common cold***. An upper respiratory infection can be caused by any one of 200 different viruses, the most common of which is the ***human rhinovirus***. Symptoms of URI include sneezing, cough, runny nose, and congestion. Children get an average of six URIs per year.
- **Erythema infectiosum** (**er**-ih-**THEE**-mah) (in-**FEKT**-shee-**oh**-sum), also known as ***fifth disease***, is a mildly contagious viral infection that is common in childhood. This infection produces a red, lace-like rash on the child's face that looks as if the child has been slapped. It is called fifth disease for its place on a list of six common childhood diseases that can cause a widespread rash. Others include measles and rubella. ***Erythema*** is redness of the skin due to capillary dilation (**erythem** means flushed, and **-a** is a noun ending). Dilation describes the expansion of the capillaries.

- **Roseola** (roe-zee-**OH**-la), also known as ***exanthem subitum*** or ***sixth disease***, is a common viral illness often occurring between ages 6 months and 3 years. It is characterized by several days of fever followed by a rash. A ***rash*** is a breaking out, or eruption, that changes the color or texture of the skin. ***Exanthem*** refers to a widespread rash, usually in children, and ***subitum*** is Latin for sudden.
- **Tinea** (**TIN**-ee-ah) is a fungal infection that can grow on the skin, hair, or nails. This condition is also known as ***ringworm***, not because a worm is involved, but because as the fungus grows on the skin, it spreads out in a worm-like circle. Tinea does not create this pattern when it grows on the nails. Warm, moist, unhygienic environments can foster fungal infections in children.
- **Otitis media** (oh-**TYE**-tis **MEE**-dee-ah), or ***ear infection***, is an inflammation of the middle ear. This common condition will affect five out of six children by the age of 3.
  - ***Acute otitis media*** is usually associated with an upper respiratory infection and is most commonly seen in young children. This condition can lead to a ruptured eardrum due to the buildup of pus or fluid in the middle ear.
  - ***Serous otitis media*** is a fluid buildup in the middle ear without symptoms of an infection. This condition can follow acute otitis media or can be caused by dysfunction of the eustachian tube. It is more common in infants and small children.
  - **Ear tubes**, formally known as ***tympanostomy tubes***, are tiny ventilating tubes placed through the eardrum of a child prone to repeated ear infections to provide ongoing drainage for fluids and to relieve pressure (see Chapter 12, Figure 12.16). Fluid buildup can lead to hearing problems and speech delays.
- **Hand, foot, and mouth disease** is a mild viral infection caused by and sometimes referred to as ***coxsackievirus***. It is common in children under 5 years of age. It is highly contagious and is characterized by sores in the mouth and throat, and a rash on the hands and feet. There is no treatment besides symptom management.
- **Impetigo** (**im**-peh-**TYE**-goh) is a highly contagious bacterial skin infection that commonly occurs in children. This condition is characterized by isolated pustules that become crusted and rupture. Topical or oral antibiotics may be used to treat impetigo.
- **Conjunctivitis** (kon-**junk**-tih-**VYE**-tis), also known as ***pinkeye***, is an inflammation of the conjunctiva that is caused by a viral or bacterial infection, allergy, or irritants (**conjunctiv** means conjunctiva, and **-itis** means inflammation). The ***conjunctiva*** (**kon**-junk-**TYE**-vah) is the transparent mucous membrane that lines the underside of each eyelid and continues to form a protective covering over the exposed surface of the eyeball. When caused by a virus or bacteria it is highly contagious. Symptoms include red, itchy, watery eyes that may feel gritty and produce discharge and/or crustiness (Figure 18.8).
- **Pediculosis** (pee-**dick**-you-**LOH**-sis) is an infestation with ***lice*** (**pedicul** means lice, and **-osis** means abnormal condition). An ***infestation*** is the dwelling of microscopic parasites on external surface tissue. Some parasites live temporarily on the skin. Others lay eggs and reproduce there. In order to get rid of the infestation, the lice eggs, which are known as nits, must be destroyed. **Pediculosis capitis** is an infestation with head lice. A medication called ***pediculicide*** is used to destroy the eggs (**pedicul/i** means lice, and **-cide** means causing death).
- **Scabies** (**SKAY**-beez) is a skin infection caused by an infestation of ***itch mites***. These tiny mites cause small, itchy bumps and blisters by burrowing into the top layer of human skin to lay their eggs. Medications applied to the skin kill the mites; however, itching may persist for several weeks.
- **Cold sores**, also known as ***herpes labialis*** or ***fever blisters***, are blister-like sores on the lips and adjacent facial tissue that are caused by the oral herpes simplex virus type 1 (HSV-1). This common condition in children will resolve on its own within a week or two.

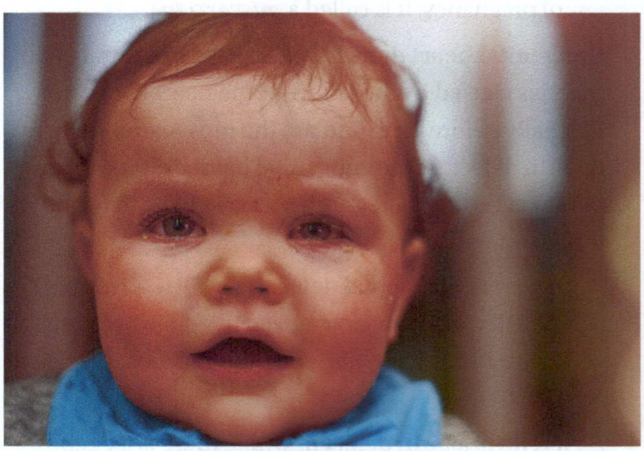

FIGURE 18.8 A small child suffering from conjunctivitis.

- **Infectious mononucleosis** (**mon**-oh-**new**-klee-**OH**-sis), also known as ***mono***, is caused by the *Epstein-Barr* virus, and is most common in adolescents and young adults. This condition is characterized by fever, a sore throat, and enlarged lymph nodes. Swelling of the spleen or liver involvement can also develop. This poses a serious risk for rupturing the spleen if the infected person plays contact sports.
- **Strep throat** is a sore throat caused by bacteria Group A *streptococci*. This common bacterial infection is characterized by swelling of the tonsils and neck glands (Figure 18.9). Diagnosis can be made with a ***rapid strep test*** using a culture taken from the back of the throat; this infection is treated with antibiotics.
- **Respiratory syncytial virus** (sin-**SIH**-shul), often referred to by its abbreviation ***RSV***, is a common, highly contagious viral infection spread by respiratory droplets. Most infections are mild and similar to the common cold. However, RSV can cause bronchiolitis in younger children and infants, which may require hospitalization. **Bronchiolitis** is inflammation of the bronchioles (**bronchiol** means bronchioles, and **-itis** means inflammation).
- **Gastroenteritis** (**gas**-troh-en-ter-**EYE**-tis) is an inflammation of the mucous membrane lining the stomach and intestines (**gastr/o** means stomach, **enter** means small intestine, and **-itis** means inflammation). Sometimes called ***stomach flu***, it is characterized by nausea, vomiting, diarrhea, and stomach cramping and can be caused by a virus such as *norovirus*, bacteria, or parasites. Treatment focuses on rest and preventing dehydration by providing plenty of fluids such as an oral electrolyte solution to help maintain electrolyte balance.
- **Pinworm** infection is caused by an infestation of parasitic worms in the intestines. It is common and is characterized by itchiness around the anus.
- **Sexually transmitted diseases** (STDs) are preventable diseases transmitted through sexual contact. Sexually active adolescents and young adults are more likely to contract an STD than are older adults. For descriptions and treatment of STDs, see Chapters 15 and 16.

Other Common Childhood Illnesses and Allergies

The following are other illnesses that children and teens are particularly susceptible to, as well as allergies, which have become an increasing issue over the past several decades.

Other Non-Communicable Childhood Illnesses

- **Acne vulgaris** (**ACK**-nee vul-**GAY**-ris), commonly known as ***acne***, is a chronic inflammatory disease characterized by pustular eruptions of the skin caused

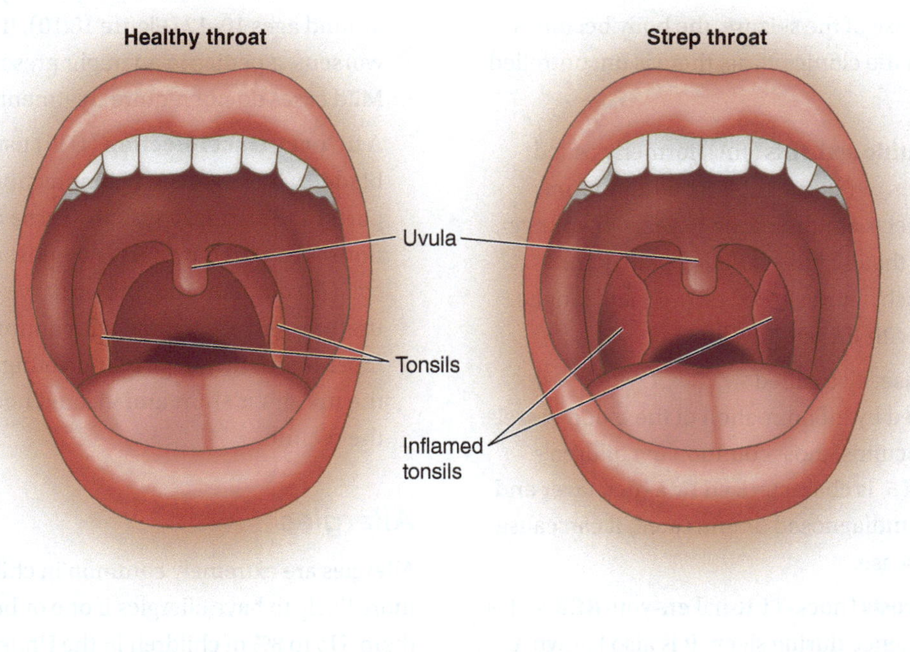

FIGURE 18.9 A healthy throat and strep throat with inflamed tonsils.

by an overproduction of sebum around the hair shaft. This condition is often triggered by hormones in puberty and adolescence. *Vulgaris* is a Latin term meaning common. A **pustule** (**PUS**-tyoul), also known as a *pimple*, is a small, circumscribed lesion containing pus.

- **Asthma** (**AZ**-mah) is a chronic inflammatory disease of the bronchial tubes, often triggered by an allergic reaction. An *asthma attack* is characterized by episodes of severe breathing difficulty, coughing, and wheezing. Wheezing is a breath sound caused by a partially obstructed airway. The frequency and severity of asthma attacks are influenced by a variety of factors, including allergens, environmental agents, exercise, and infection. It is estimated that 8.4% of children have asthma, which is more common in boys than in girls, is more common in African American children, and is the leading chronic childhood disease.
- **Epilepsy** (**EP**-ih-**lep**-see) is a chronic neurological condition characterized by recurrent episodes of seizures of varying severity. Also known as a *seizure disorder*, epilepsy can usually be controlled with medication. It is the most common neurological condition in children, and about two-thirds of children with epilepsy will outgrow the seizures by adolescence.
    - A **febrile seizure** is a tonic–clonic seizure that occurs in infants and young children in response to a fever. It is not indicative of a seizure disorder, and most children outgrow febrile seizures by age 5. A *tonic–clonic seizure* involves the entire body. In the tonic phase of the seizure, the body becomes rigid, and in the clonic phase, there is uncontrolled jerking.
- **Juvenile idiopathic arthritis** (JIA), formerly called *juvenile rheumatoid arthritis*, is an autoimmune disorder that affects children ages 16 years or younger, with symptoms that include stiffness, pain, joint swelling, skin rash, fever, slowed growth, and fatigue. Many children with JIA outgrow it.
- **Kawasaki disease**, also called *strawberry tongue disease*, is caused by inflammation of the blood vessels. This form of vasculitis, most common in children under the age of 5, is characterized by a high fever and peeling skin. If undiagnosed or untreated, it can cause lasting heart disease.
- **Nocturnal enuresis** (nock-**TER**-nal **en**-you-**REE**-sis) is urinary incontinence during sleep. It is also known as *bed-wetting* in a child that is otherwise potty trained. *Nocturnal* means pertaining to night. **Enuresis** (**en**-you-**REE**-sis) is the involuntary discharge of urine (**en-** means into, and **-uresis** means urination).
- **Type 1 diabetes**, formerly known as *juvenile diabetes*, is an autoimmune insulin deficiency disorder caused by the destruction of pancreatic islet beta cells. *Insulin deficiency* means that the pancreatic beta cells do not secrete enough insulin. This lifelong illness, which is usually diagnosed during childhood or adolescence, requires daily injections of insulin to control blood glucose levels.
- **Type 2 diabetes** is an insulin resistance disorder. *Insulin resistance* means that insulin is being produced, but the body does not use it effectively. In an attempt to compensate for this lack of response, the body secretes more insulin. With the rise of childhood obesity, type 2 diabetes is increasingly common in children and young adults. Symptom management includes lifestyle modifications through diet and exercise, and may also include medication.
- **Rickets** (**RICK**-ets) is a rare deficiency disease occurring in infants and very young children. This condition, which is characterized by defective bone growth resulting from a lack of vitamin D, has decreased due to the fortification of milk with vitamin D.
- **Scoliosis** (**skoh**-lee-**OH**-sis) is an abnormal lateral (sideways) curvature of the spine (**scoli** means curved, and **-osis** means abnormal condition or disease). *Idiopathic scoliosis* can occur at any age but most often occurs during the pre-puberty growth spurt around ages 10–12 (Figure 18.10). If the condition worsens, a pediatrician might prescribe a back brace. Mild cases do not require treatment.
- A **urinary tract infection** (UTI) usually begins in the bladder; however, such an infection can affect all parts of the urinary system. These common infections are caused by bacteria, most often *Escherichia coli* (*E. coli*), entering the urinary system through the urethra, and are treated with antibiotics. They occur more frequently in girls and young women because the urethra is short and located near the opening to the rectum.

Allergies

Allergies are extremely common in children, who are more likely to have allergies if one or both parents have them. Up to 8% of children in the United States have a food allergy.

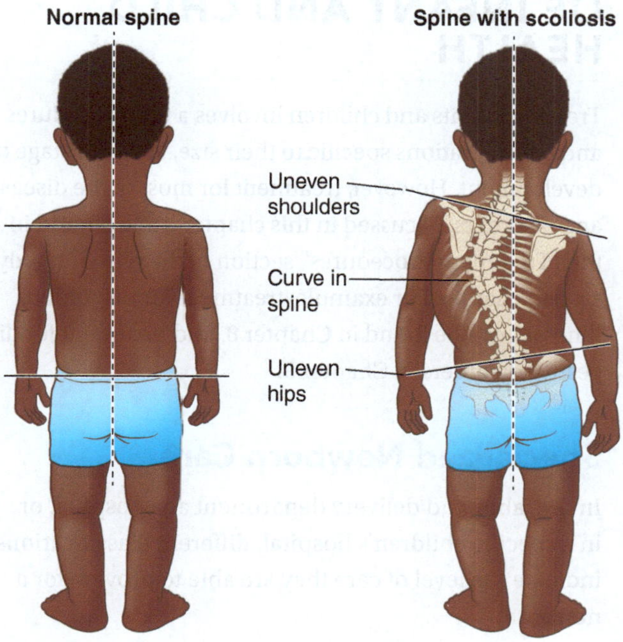

FIGURE 18.10 A normal spine and a spine with scoliosis.

- An **allergy**, also known as ***hypersensitivity***, is an overreaction by the body to a particular allergen.
- An **allergen** (**AL**-er-jen) is a substance that produces an allergic reaction in an individual. The most common airborne allergens are pollen, dust mites, mold, and pet dander. The most common food allergens are cow's milk, eggs, fish, shellfish, peanuts, tree nuts, soy, and wheat.
- An **allergic reaction** occurs when the body's immune system reacts to a harmless allergen such as pollen, food, or animal dander as if it were a dangerous invader.
- A **localized allergic response**, also known as a ***cellular response***, includes redness, itching, and burning where the skin has come into contact with an allergen. For example, contact with poison ivy can cause a localized allergic response in the form of an itchy rash (see Chapter 13). Although the body reacts mildly the first time it is exposed to the allergen, sensitivity is established, and future contacts can cause much more severe symptoms.
- A **systemic reaction** (sis-**TEH**-mik), which is also described as **anaphylaxis** (**an**-ah-fih-**LACK**-sis), is a severe response to an allergen. Without prompt medical aid, the patient can die within a few minutes.

Mental Health in Children and Adolescents

Diagnosable mental health disorders are common in children and adolescents. Some are more likely to have onset during childhood, whereas others such as anxiety or mood disorders can affect a person at any age, including during childhood.

Eating disorders such as **anorexia nervosa** and **bulimia nervosa** are commonly diagnosed between the ages of 12 and 25, with onset tending to occur during times of transition such as puberty or gaining the independence of leaving home. **Avoidant restrictive food intake disorder** (ARFID) is a feeding and eating disorder most often found in children and adolescents and characterized by extreme pickiness, often causing nutritional deficiencies, growth issues, or social issues.

An **attention deficit/hyperactivity disorder** (ADHD) is characterized by a short attention span and impulsive behavior that is inappropriate for the child's developmental age.

Other childhood-onset neurodevelopmental disorders include **autism spectrum disorder** (ASD) and **learning disabilities.**

For more in-depth information on these and other mental health disorders, see Chapter 17.

DIAGNOSTIC PROCEDURES OF INFANT AND CHILD HEALTH

Most diagnostic procedures performed on adults can also be performed on children, though sometimes with modifications due to size and age.

- A **capillary puncture** is the technique used when only a small amount of blood is needed as a specimen for a blood test. Named for where it is performed, a pediatric capillary puncture is usually known as a ***finger*** or ***heel stick*** (Figure 18.11).
- A **rectal thermometer** gives the most accurate reading of an infant's temperature (Figure 18.12). Fever in infants younger than 6 months should be reported to a pediatrician. For other methods of taking a child's temperature, see Chapter 21.
- A **bone age study** determines skeletal maturity by comparing an x-ray of a child's knee (under the age of 3) or hand and wrist (over the age of 3) with standards for their birth age. This is a diagnostic tool that can be helpful for determining nutritional, genetic, hormonal, and growth problems as well as disease states.

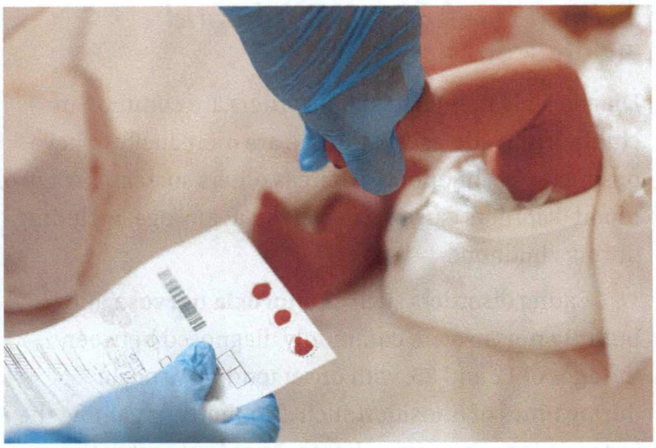

FIGURE 18.11 An infant having a heel stick capillary puncture during newborn screening.

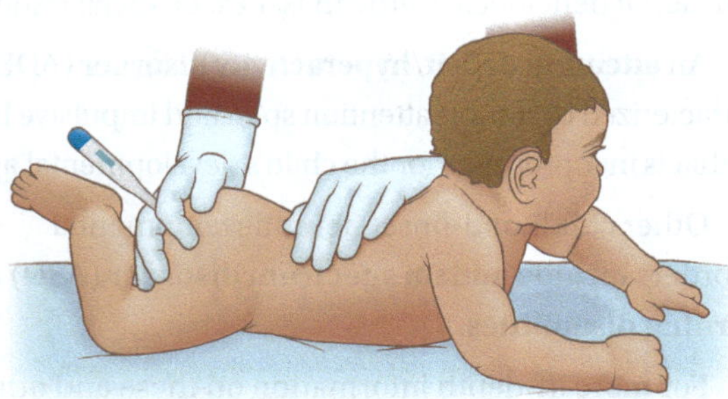

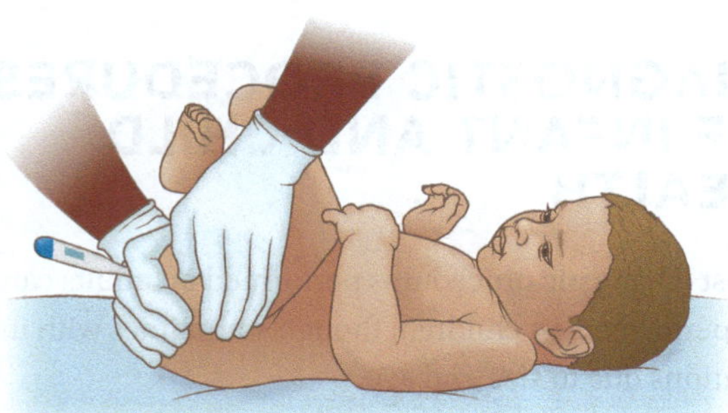

FIGURE 18.12 Different body positions for taking a rectal temperature reading.

- **Prenatal genetic testing** can be used to screen for some genetic diseases during pregnancy. These include screening for chromosomal abnormalities such as Down syndrome and gene mutations such as cystic fibrosis. The newborn screening performed shortly after birth tests for more than 30 genetic diseases including biotinidase deficiency, congenital adrenal hyperplasia, congenital hypothyroidism, cystic fibrosis, galactosemia, homocystinuria, maple syrup urine disease (MSUD), medium-chain acyl-CoA dehydrogenase deficiency, phenylketonuria (PKU), and sickle cell disease.

TREATMENT PROCEDURES OF INFANT AND CHILD HEALTH

Treating infants and children involves a few procedures and considerations specific to their size, age, and stage of development. However, treatment for most of the diseases and disorders discussed in this chapter can be found in the "Treatment Procedures" section of the relevant body system chapter. For example, treatment for respiratory illnesses can be found in Chapter 8, and treatment for digestive disorders in Chapter 9.

Specialized Newborn Care

In the labor and delivery department at a hospital, or in a specific children's hospital, different classifications indicate the level of care they are able to provide for a newborn:

- A ***level I well newborn nursery*** can provide care for infants born at 35 weeks or later, typically the lowest risk.
- A ***level II special care nursery*** can provide care for infants born at 32 weeks or later with associated complications. They do not provide subspecialty care.
- A ***level III NICU*** can provide constant access to subspecialty care for newborns in addition to providing life support.
- A ***level IV regional NICU*** can provide care for the most complex cases in addition to having subspecialists on staff and the ability to surgically care for complex patients.

An **isolette**, sometimes called an ***incubator***, is an apparatus for maintaining an environment of controlled temperature, humidity, and oxygen concentration for a premature or ill newborn (Figure 18.12).

Immediately after birth an infant is given an antibiotic ointment in their eyes to prevent infection. In the United States the infant will also be given an injection of vitamin K to help with blood coagulation and their first hepatitis B vaccination.

Pain Medication

Infants and children can be given ***liquid acetaminophen*** for pain or fever (the dosage is lower than that for adults and should be determined by a health care professional). After age 6 months, ***ibuprofen*** can also be used. No aspirin should ever be given to children under the age of 2,

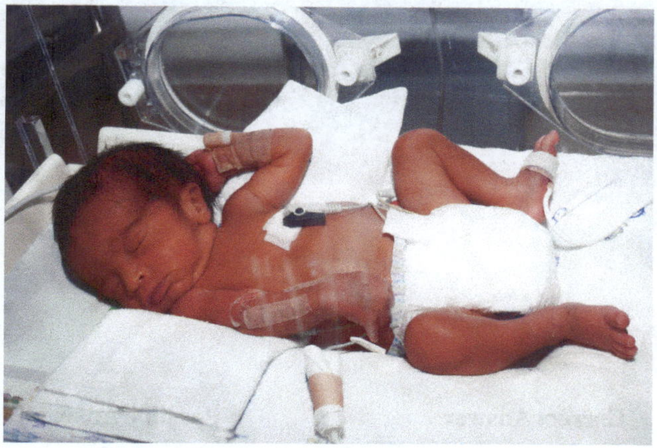

herjua/Shutterstock.com

FIGURE 18.13 An isolette provides a newborn infant with an environment of controlled temperature, humidity, and oxygen.

and aspirin is not recommended for those under the age of 18 due to risk of Reye's syndrome, a rare disorder that causes brain and liver damage.

ABBREVIATIONS RELATED TO INFANT AND CHILD HEALTH

Table 18.4 presents an overview of the abbreviations related to the terms introduced in this chapter. *Note:* To avoid errors or confusion, always be cautious when using abbreviations.

TABLE 18.4

Abbreviations Related to Infant and Child Health

developmental dysplasia of the hip = DDH	**DDH** = developmental dysplasia of the hip
diphtheria, tetanus, and pertussis = DTaP	**DTaP** = diphtheria, tetanus, and pertussis
human papillomavirus = HPV	**HPV** = human papillomavirus
low birth weight = LBW	**LBW** = low birth weight
measles, mumps, rubella = MMR	**MMR** = measles, mumps, rubella
neonatal intensive care unit = NICU	**NICU** = neonatal intensive care unit
pediatric intensive care unit = PICU	**PICU** = pediatric intensive care unit
respiratory syncytial virus = RSV	**RSV** = respiratory syncytial virus
sudden infant death syndrome = SIDS	**SIDS** = sudden infant death syndrome
tetanus, diphtheria, and pertussis = Tdap	**Tdap** = tetanus, diphtheria, and pertussis

LEARNING EXERCISES

Matching Word Parts 1

Write the correct answer in the middle column.

	Definition	Correct Answer	Possible Answers
18.1.	unborn child, fetus	______________	-arche
18.2.	together, with	______________	genit/o
18.3.	pertaining to	______________	con-
18.4.	beginning	______________	fet/o
18.5.	formation	______________	-al

Matching Word Parts 2

Write the correct answer in the middle column.

	Definition	Correct Answer	Possible Answers
18.6.	bad	______________	nat/o
18.7.	specialist	______________	dys-
18.8.	new	______________	men/o
18.9.	born	______________	neo-
18.10.	menstruation	______________	-ologist

Matching Word Parts 3

Write the correct answer in the middle column.

	Definition	Correct Answer	Possible Answers
18.11.	navel	___	-itis
18.12.	formation	___	ped/o
18.13.	lice	___	pedicul/i
18.14.	child	___	-plasia
18.15.	inflammation	___	umbilic/o

Definitions

Select the correct answer, and write it on the line provided.

18.16. The stage from age 3 through puberty is known as ___.

adolescence toddlerhood infancy childhood

18.17. Also known as sexual maturity rating, ___ staging is a tool to assess the development of secondary sex characteristics.

puberty Tanner menarche physical maturity

18.18. The process of discontinuing breastfeeding is called ___.

colostrum weaning menarche formula

18.19. An overreaction by the body to a substance such as pollen or pet dander is called a/an ___.

allergy allergen hypersensitivity insulin deficiency

18.20. The blood test to screen for numerous genetic diseases done prior to a newborn baby being discharged home from the hospital is called ___.

hearing test heart function test newborn screening Apgar score

18.21. Inflammation of the gums, drooling, increased biting, and mild fever are all potential signs of ___, which usually begins around age 6 months.

growth spurt tooth eruption puberty precocious puberty

18.22. A/An ______________________ works with children's mental health and behavioral issues.

pediatric nurse practitioner adolescent medicine physician child psychologist pediatric dentist

18.23. Birth that occurs earlier than the 37th week of pregnancy is known as ______________________.

premature birth gestational age corrected age birth defects

18.24. Screening for genetic diseases during pregnancy is known as ______________________.

newborn screening prenatal genetic testing Tanner staging bone age study

18.25. The stage from ages 14 to 21 is known as ______________________.

adolescence puberty menarche childhood

Matching Vaccines

Write the correct answer in the middle column.

	Definition	Correct Answer	Possible Answers
18.26.	protects against polio	______________	PCV13 vaccine
18.27.	protects against rubella	______________	MMR vaccine
18.28.	protects against rotavirus	______________	DTaP vaccine
18.29.	protects against tetanus	______________	IPV vaccine
18.30.	protects against pneumococcus	______________	RV vaccine

Which Word?

Select the correct answer, and write it on the line provided.

18.31. Baby Girl Singh was born at 36 weeks and needed to spend some time in the NICU being cared for by a ______________________ in order to gain enough weight and strength to be discharged home.

neonatologist pediatrician

18.32. An ______________________ is a substance that produces an allergic reaction in an individual.

allergen allergy

18.33. Formerly known as juvenile diabetes, ______________________ is an autoimmune insulin deficiency disorder.

type 1 diabetes type 2 diabetes

18.34. Passed from mother to child at birth, ______________ immunity is also called passive immunity.

active natural

18.35. A protrusion of intestine in the area of the belly button is called an ______________ hernia.

umbilical inguinal

Spelling Counts

Find the misspelled word in each sentence. Then write that word, spelled correctly, on the line provided.

18.36. A common childhood diagnosis, azmah is a chronic inflammatory disease of the bronchial tubes. ______________

18.37. The versela vaccine protects against chickenpox. ______________

18.38. The first breast milk a new mother produces is called calustrom. ______________

18.39. The suggested imunozation schedule for children determines specific ages and intervals for vaccines to be given. ______________

18.40. Anansefaly is a neural tube defect characterized by a failure of the brain and skull to fully develop. ______________

Abbreviation Identification 1

In the space provided, write the words that each abbreviation stands for.

18.41. **DDH** ______________

18.42. **LBW** ______________

18.43. **MMR** ______________

18.44. **SIDS** ______________

18.45. **Tdap** ______________

Term Selection

Select the correct answer, and write it on the line provided.

18.46. At his 2-month pediatrician appointment, Davante was given the RV, Hib, PCV13, IPV, and ______________ vaccines.

MMR HPV influenza DTaP

18.47. A ______________ disease is often preventable by abstaining or using a barrier such as a condom during sexual encounters.

communicable sexually transmitted Kawasaki congenital

18.48. A/An ______________ infection usually begins in the bladder and can be caused by improperly wiping after having a bowel movement.

urinary tract upper respiratory ear pinworm

18.49. The ______________ vaccine should be given yearly after the age of 6 months to protect against the flu, which can cause pneumonia.

Hib HepA MMR influenza

18.50. Also known as ringworm, ______________ is a contagious fungal infection.

pinworm tinea scabies pediculosis

Sentence Completion 1

Write the correct term or terms on the lines provided.

18.51. Malia brought her daughter to the pediatrician for her 2-month checkup, where she got several vaccines including the ______________ vaccine to help protect against pertussis.

18.52. Darnell's 12-year-old son, who has fear of needles, was upset to find out that at his yearly checkup he would need to get the ______________ vaccine to protect against the human papillomavirus.

18.53. Jamily was concerned when she used a ______________ thermometer to take her 4-month-old daughter's temperature and the reading displayed 102.4 degrees.

18.54. Kim and Frank Hu visited their son daily in the NICU, where he was being kept in a/an ______________ with a controlled environment.

18.55. Shantay's spine showed worsening curvature during her well-child checkup, so her doctor prescribed a back brace to help correct the ________________.

Word Surgery

Divide each term into its component word parts. Write these word parts, in sequence, on the lines provided. When necessary, use a slash (/) to indicate a combining vowel. (You may not need all of the lines provided.)

18.56. A **neonatologist** is a physician who specializes in diagnosing and treating disorders of the newborn.

__________ __________ __________ __________

18.57. **Congenital** disorders are abnormal conditions that exist at the time of birth and can be genetic, be inherited, have an environmental cause, or be multifactorial.

__________ __________ __________ __________

18.58. The medical specialty of diagnosing, treating, and preventing disorders and diseases of infants and children is known as **pediatrics**.

__________ __________ __________ __________

18.59. The involuntary discharge of urine is called **enuresis**.

__________ __________ __________ __________

18.60. Sometimes called the stomach flu, **gastroenteritis** is an inflammation in the stomach and intestines.

__________ __________ __________ __________

True/False 1

If the statement is true, write **True** on the line. If the statement is false, write **False** on the line.

18.61. ________ Prenatal genetic testing determines skeletal maturity by comparing an x-ray of a child's knee, hand, or wrist with standards for their birth age.

18.62. ________ It is cause for concern if a child's body mass index plots in a straight horizontal line for many years on their growth chart.

18.63. ________ Hand, foot, and mouth disease is a viral infection caused by the *coxsackievirus*.

18.64. ________ A lack of folic acid in a mother's diet can sometimes be the cause of cleft lip.

18.65. ________ A communicable disease cannot be transmitted from one person to another.

Clinical Conditions

Write the correct answer on the line provided.

18.66. Kumal attends daycare and came home complaining of a cough and runny nose. The doctor suggested he stay home and get some rest, since it sounds like he has the common cold, also known as a/an ________________ infection.

18.67. The condition in which a potty-trained child wets the bed at night is known clinically as ________________.

18.68. Grace noticed her son was itching his scalp excessively; at first she suspected dandruff but upon closer inspection her fears were confirmed—he had ________________ capitis, an infestation of head lice.

18.69. Precious Howard presented with a red, lace-like rash on her face and was diagnosed with ________________, also known as fifth disease.

18.70. Treyvon knew he couldn't take his son back to daycare that day when the doctor confirmed that the ________________, also known as pinkeye, was viral.

18.71. Luca complained to her mom of a sore throat; after doing a rapid test, the doctor confirmed she had ________________ and put her on antibiotics.

18.72. The Levinskys were concerned when Daniel developed a scaly rash on his head but the pediatrician said not to worry, because ________________ cap is common in infants.

18.73. Two-year-old Yolanda had chronic ear infections so her primary care provider suggested that she get ________________, formally known as tympanostomy tubes, to provide ongoing drainage.

18.74. Isla, a freshman in high school, went to see a dermatologist because of her ________________ vulgaris, a chronic inflammatory disease characterized by pimples.

18.75. Baby Myles had a fever for several days followed by a rash. During a telehealth visit the nurse practitioner suggested it appeared that he had ________________, also called sixth disease.

Which Is the Correct Medical Term?

Select the correct answer, and write it on the line provided.

18.76. A/An ________________________ is a physician who specializes in working with infants and children.

18.77. Madison was born when her mother was 34 weeks pregnant. Now that she is 12 weeks old, her ________________________ age is 6 weeks.

18.78. The optimal nutrition for babies for at least the first 12 months of life is ________________________.

18.79. A/An ________________________ score is used to determine an infant's physical status immediately after birth.

18.80. The stage of childhood from ages 1–3 is generally referred to as ________________________.

Abbreviation Identification 2

In the space provided, write the words that each abbreviation stands for.

18.81. **NICU** ________________________

18.82. **RSV** ________________________

18.83. **DTaP** ________________________

18.84. **URI** ________________________

18.85. **FAS** ________________________

True/False 2

If the statement is true, write **True** on the line. If the statement is false, write **False** on the line.

18.86. ________ Also known as hip dysplasia, pediatricians routinely screen for developmental dysplasia of the hip at routine exams.

18.87. ________ Croup is a condition characterized by a generally healthy baby crying for more than three hours a day, more than three days a week for three or more weeks, and being difficult to soothe.

18.88. ________ The first feces of a newborn, which can be inhaled if passed during labor, is called meconium.

18.89. ________ The MMR vaccine protects against the flu and is given yearly.

18.90. ________ Tooth eruption generally begins for the first time around age 2.

Sentence Completion 2

Write the correct term or terms on the lines provided.

18.91. Mumps, a disease which can cause meningitis and encephalitis, can be prevented by giving the ________________ vaccine at age 12 months and again between ages 4 and 6 years.

18.92. When an infant or child does not grow as expected, they are diagnosed with ________________ (FTT) and often need supplemental nutrition.

18.93. A/An ________________ disorder is a disease caused in whole or in part by an abnormality in the genetic makeup of an individual's DNA which may be present at birth (i.e., congenital) or may present later in life.

18.94. Abbreviated RSV, ________________ can cause bronchiolitis in young children and may require hospitalization.

18.95. Commonly referred to as an ear infection, ________________ will affect five out of six children by the age of 3.

18.96. The term used to describe the result of child abuse in the form of an infant being violently shaken is called ________________ syndrome.

18.97. Due to risk of rupture to the spleen, a person with infectious ________________ is recommended not to play contact sports.

18.98. Eating disorders such as ________________ and bulimia nervosa are often diagnosed between the ages of 12 and 25.

18.99. The most common type of birth defects are ________________ defects which are structural abnormalities caused by the failure of the heart to develop normally before birth.

18.100. The most prevalent congenital heart defect is a/an ________________ septal defect, in which there is a hole between the two ventricles of the heart.

The Human Touch

CRITICAL THINKING EXERCISE

The following story and questions are designed to stimulate critical thinking through class discussion or as a brief essay response. There are no right or wrong answers to these questions.

Nathalya woke up feeling groggy and disoriented to the sound of a baby crying. As her eyes slowly opened, she realized where she was: in the hospital room where she and her wife Willow had been moved late last night after she gave birth to their sweet little boy, Jasper. Based on how she felt, she was guessing that not many hours had passed since the big event. A nurse entered the room, picked Jasper up, and handed him to Nathalya, asking if she was feeling ready to try breastfeeding again. She knew how important the colostrum and eventually breast milk would be for her baby and was eager to provide him with what she'd heard called liquid gold.

Jasper's wailing only got louder as he struggled to latch onto her nipple. Nathalya remembered all the words she'd heard in the delivery room last night about Apgar scores and low birth weight. She closed her eyes, overwhelmed with anxiety as the baby continued to fail to latch.

"It's OK," the nurse said soothingly. "Why don't I take him for his newborn screening, heart function test, and hearing test. I'll have the lactation consultant come by in an hour and you can try again. Oh, and don't forget, we need to know what you've decided about circumcision by this afternoon."

Willow gave Nathalya's hand a squeeze to show her that she was sure they were up for the challenges. After all, they had read books on parenting and even taken a class on infant care and breastfeeding. Nevertheless, Nathalya felt the tears start to flow. What if they made the wrong decision about circumcision? What if Jasper couldn't nurse? She'd only been a mother for a few hours and already she felt overwhelmed.

Suggested Discussion Topics

1. What are the alternative sources of nutrition for Nathalya and Willow's baby boy if he is unable to breastfeed?
2. Nathalya seems to be putting a lot of pressure on herself, but breastfeeding is a partnership between mother and baby. What are some physical reasons her baby boy might be having a hard time breastfeeding?
3. The night nurse realizes that Jasper is having a hard time breastfeeding. She gathers a couple of cans of formula from the supply cabinet behind the nurse's station and offers them to Nathalya. Is it ethical for a hospital to provide samples of formula and coupons for formula to new parents?
4. Imagine you are a lactation consultant. What resources might you provide to Nathalya and Willow to use once they are discharged home tomorrow?

CHAPTER 19

GERONTOLOGY: CARE OF THE OLDER ADULT

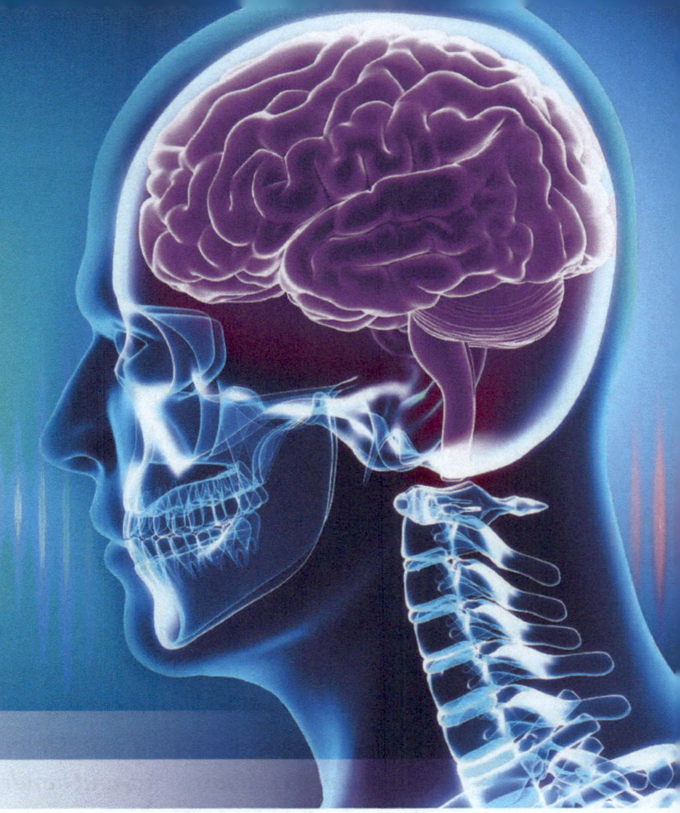

Overview of THE BASICS OF GERONTOLOGY

As adults grow older, their medical needs become increasingly complex and unique. Older adults are more likely to have chronic medical conditions which have progressed over years or even decades. Genetics, lifestyle, and environmental influences impact the health of older adults to a greater extent. The slowing of the immune response and other age-related changes make older adults more susceptible to disease. Eventually, whether from an acute or a chronic medical problem, every person reaches end of life.

Vocabulary Related to **GERONTOLOGY**

This list contains essential word parts and medical terms for this chapter. These and the other important **primary terms** are shown in **boldface** throughout the chapter. ***Secondary terms***, which appear in ***orange*** italics, clarify the meaning of primary terms.

Word Parts

- ☐ **a-**, **an-** without
- ☐ **de-** removal
- ☐ **dys-** painful, difficult
- ☐ **ger/i**, **geront/o** old age
- ☐ **-iatrics** field of medicine
- ☐ **-ology** the study of
- ☐ **-penia** deficiency
- ☐ **-phasia** speech
- ☐ **-phagia** swallowing
- ☐ **-pnea** breathing
- ☐ **post-** after
- ☐ **presby/o** old age
- ☐ **-sclerosis** abnormal hardening
- ☐ **-systole** contraction
- ☐ **xer/o** dry

Medical Terms

- ☐ **active dying**
- ☐ **activities of daily living**
- ☐ **advanced cirrhosis** (sih-**ROH**-sis)
- ☐ **agonal respirations** (**AH**-goh-nal)
- ☐ **air hunger**
- ☐ **Alzheimer's disease** (**ALTZ**-high-merz)
- ☐ **assisted living facility**
- ☐ **atherosclerosis** (**ah**-theh-roh-skleh-**ROH**-sis)
- ☐ **autopsy** (**AW**-top-see)
- ☐ **bone-on-bone**
- ☐ **bowel rest**
- ☐ **brain death**
- ☐ **bundle branch block**
- ☐ **cadaver** (kuh-**DAH**-vair)
- ☐ **cardiac arrest**
- ☐ **cerebrovascular accident** (**ser**-eh-broh-**VAS**-kyou-lar)
- ☐ **cognition** (kog-**NISH**-un)
- ☐ **death rattle**
- ☐ **death with dignity**
- ☐ **delirium** (deh-**LEER**-ee-um)
- ☐ **dementia** (dih-**MEN**-shah)
- ☐ **Do Not Resuscitate order**
- ☐ **dying process**
- ☐ **dyspnea on exertion** (**DISP**-nee-ah)
- ☐ **edentulous** (ee-**DEN**-too-lus)
- ☐ **end-stage COPD**
- ☐ **failure to thrive**
- ☐ **gastrointestinal bleeding**
- ☐ **geriatrics** (**jehr**-ee-**AH**-tricks)
- ☐ **gerontology** (**jehr**-un-**TOH**-luh-gee)
- ☐ **health care proxy**
- ☐ **heart valve disease**
- ☐ **hepatic encephalopathy** (en-**sef**-ah-**LOP**-ah-thee)
- ☐ **home health aide**
- ☐ **hospice care**
- ☐ **immunosenescence** (ih-**myoo**-noh-seh-**NEH**-sens)
- ☐ **inflamm-aging** (**in**-flah-**MAY**-jing)
- ☐ **lichen sclerosus** (**LYE**-ken skleh-**ROH**-sus)
- ☐ **living will**
- ☐ **manual disimpaction**
- ☐ **medication adherence**
- ☐ **memory care**
- ☐ **modified Rankin scale**
- ☐ **normal aging**
- ☐ **nursing home**
- ☐ **organ donation**
- ☐ **orientation**
- ☐ **osteoporosis** (**oss**-tee-oh-poh-**ROH**-sis)
- ☐ **osteoporotic hip fracture** (**oss**-tee-oh-pah-**ROT**-ick)
- ☐ **palliative care** (**PAH**-lee-ah-tiv)
- ☐ **polypharmacy** (**poh**-lee-**FAR**-mah-see)
- ☐ **postmenopause**
- ☐ **respiratory arrest**
- ☐ **sarcopenia** (**sar**-koh-**PEE**-nee-ah)
- ☐ **senile emphysema** (**SEE**-nye-ahl em-fih-**SEE**-mah)
- ☐ **skilled nursing facility**
- ☐ **small bowel obstruction**
- ☐ **stasis dermatitis** (**STAY**-sis **der**-mah-**TYE**-tis)
- ☐ **third-degree heart block**
- ☐ **venous stasis** (**VEE**-nus **STAY**-sis)

LEARNING OBJECTIVES

On completion of this chapter, you should be able to:

1. Describe the aging process.
2. Identify the medical specialists who treat the needs of the older adult.
3. Identify the medical word parts related to gerontology.
4. Define the primary terms related to gerontology.
5. Define the primary terms related to common geriatric pathology and the diagnostic and treatment procedures of gerontology.
6. Define the primary terms related to treatment considerations for older adults and assistive care.
7. Define the primary terms related to end of life and death and dying.
8. Spell the primary terms related to gerontology, end of life, and death and dying.
9. Pronounce the primary terms related to gerontology, end of life, and death and dying.
10. Define common abbreviations related to gerontology and end of life.

THE AGING PROCESS

Adults over 65 years of age are the largest growing population in the world. With more than 9% of the world's population over the age of 65 (16% in the United States), and the average person living to 78 years old, knowledge of how to care for the older adult is becoming increasingly important. According to a study by the CDC, people over 65 make up 16% of the visits to emergency rooms each year in the United States, and every health professional—unless they are specializing in pediatrics—is likely to encounter older adults in the course of their career.

- **Geriatrics** (**jehr**-ee-**AH**-tricks) is the branch of medicine relating to the health of older adults (**ger** means old age, and **-iatrics** means field of medicine). **Older adult** refers to a person over 65 years of age. ***Elderly*** is another term for older adults.
- **Gerontology** (**jehr**-un-**TOH**-loh-gee) is the study of the aging process (**geront** means old age, and **-ology** means the study of).

Normal aging, or ***senescence***, is the gradual progression of unavoidable physiologic changes that occur as a part of growing older. As people age, their bodies change in a number of common ways which can affect their health, mobility, and comfort (Table 19.1).

Medical needs change with age, and the progression of aging is determined by different factors, including a person's lifestyle, medical history, genetics, and environment. Because there are variables in the needs and age-related considerations of older adults, medical professionals differentiate between different geriatric age groups. Patients aged 65–74 are ***Young-Old***, patients 75–84 are ***Middle-Old***, and patients 85+ are ***Old-Old***.

Medical problems in older adults frequently affect multiple body systems, and there are often comorbidities. ***Comorbidity*** describes the presence of more than one disease or health condition in an individual at a given time.

MEDICAL SPECIALTIES RELATED TO GERONTOLOGY

- A **geriatrician** (**jer**-ee-ah-**TRISH**-un), or ***gerontologist***, is a physician who specializes in the care of older people.
- A **hospice nurse** is a registered nurse who specializes in end-of-life care to minimize pain and distress for patients who have a life expectancy of less than six months.
- A **home care provider** is a home health aide, certified nursing assistant, licensed practical or vocational nurse, or registered nurse who specializes in providing care in a patient's home (Figure 19.1). The responsibilities may include managing the organization of home medications for the patient, providing wound care and dressing changes, and assistance with toileting and other activities of daily living for an elderly or otherwise incapacitated individual.

TABLE 19.1

Physical Changes that Occur as Part of the Normal Aging Process

Body System	Common Age-Related Changes	Common Medical Problems
Muscular	decreased muscle mass (sarcopenia), difficulty with fine motor movements	weakness, falls
Skeletal	lower bone mineral content (osteopenia/osteoporosis), osteoarthritis	joint pain, falls, fractures
Heart	decreased elasticity of heart muscle, thickening of heart walls, increased likelihood of developing arrhythmias	increased risk of heart attack (myocardial infarction) and stroke (cerebrovascular accident)
Blood	narrowing/stiffening of the arteries	poor peripheral circulation, slower wound healing
Lymphatic and Immune	lymphatic: lymph vessels less flexible, more permeable	higher risk of secondary lymphedema as a result of surgery
	immune: more antibodies for specific diseases, but less robust immune system response to infection	increased difficulty fighting off new infections
Respiratory	decreased muscle strength makes coughing up mucus more difficult	increased risk of pneumonia from atelectasis, sedentary behavior, and aspiration increased likelihood of chronic respiratory problems such as chronic obstructive pulmonary disease and emphysema to progress to the later stages of illness
Digestive	outpouchings in the intestines (diverticulosis), decreased muscle strength cause an increased risk of constipation and bowel obstruction changes in smell and taste can cause changes in appetite or loss of appetite loss of teeth makes chewing difficult	risk of diverticulitis, increased risk of bleeding in gastrointestinal tract (due to blood-thinning medications), increased risk of constipation and bowel obstruction (due to narcotic pain medications)
Urinary	decreased ability to concentrate urine enlarged prostate common in men	increased likelihood of difficulty urinating due to neurologic problems or prostate problems in men increased likelihood that urinary tract infections will cause confusion, weakness, and falls
Neurological	normal changes in cognition associated with aging such as short-term memory problems, difficulty learning new skills, and increased time needed to understand and respond to questions	pathologic changes in cognition (dementia), short-term disorientation and confusion (delirium) when ill or hospitalized

Endocrine	increased insulin resistance	increased risk of diabetes, pre-existing poorly controlled diabetes causing damage and complications
Special Senses	normal loss of flexibility in the lens of the eye (presbyopia) normal loss of hearing (presbycusis)	changes in vision associated with cataracts, glaucoma, or macular degeneration, and increased hearing loss associated with noise-related damage over time
Integumentary	thin, fragile skin that heals slowly	increased risk of skin tears, higher likelihood of bruising (ecchymosis) and swelling from bruising (hematoma) due to blood-thinning medications
Male Reproductive	decrease in testosterone starting around age 40, erectile dysfunction and loss of libido, enlarged prostate	enlarged prostate, prostate cancer, difficulty urinating, and urinary retention
Female Reproductive	menopause often starts around age 50, decrease in estrogen can cause vaginal dryness	uterine bleeding after menopause is often a sign of cancer

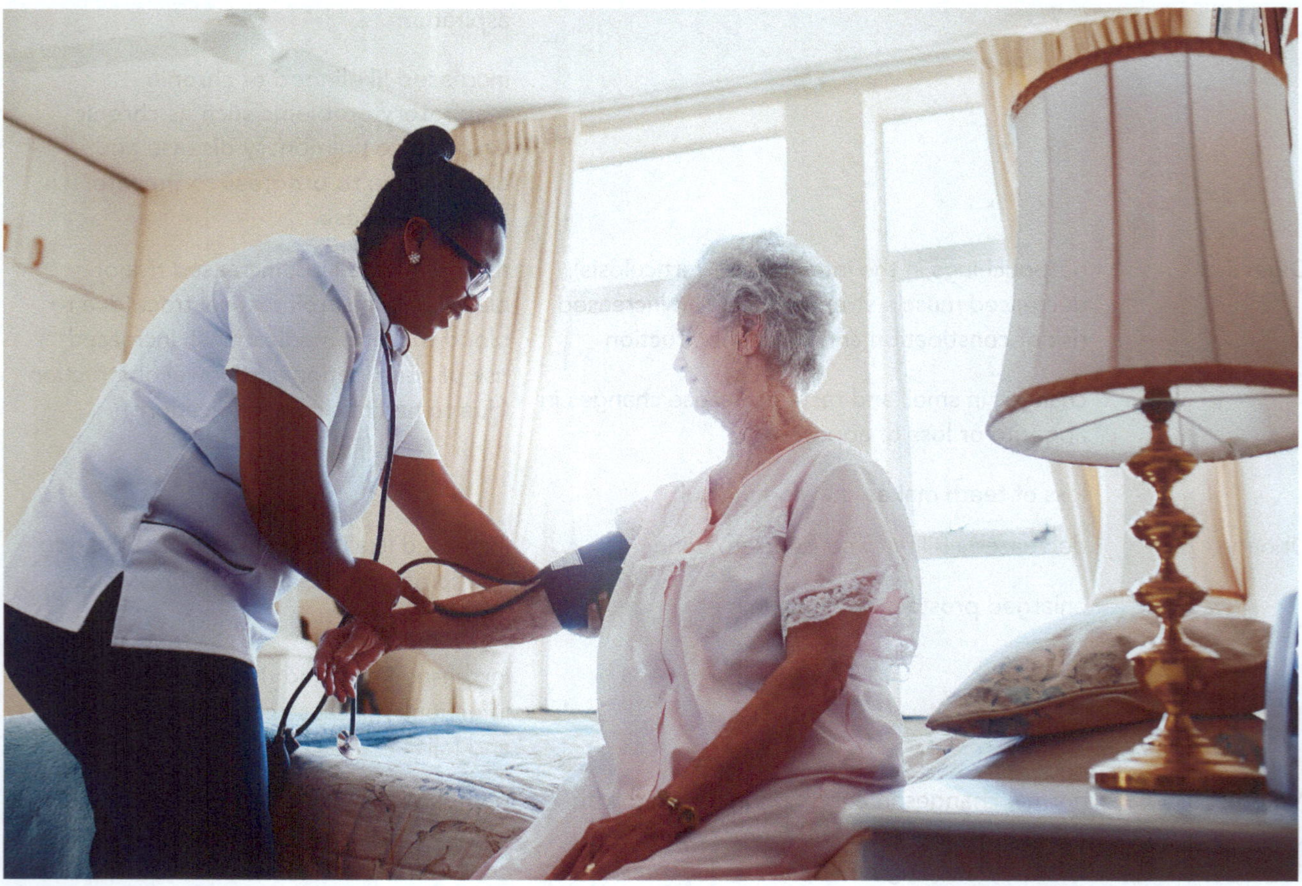

FIGURE 19.1 A home care provider is a healthcare professional who specializes in providing care in a patient's home.

GERIATRIC PATHOLOGY, DIAGNOSTIC AND TREATMENT PROCEDURES

The pathology of older adults varies depending on lifestyle, environmental factors, and chronic health problems. Many medical problems in older adults are the result of progressive chronic medical problems, and affect multiple body systems.

- Older adults are more likely to have been living with their medical conditions for years or even decades, and so may have progressed from the initial stages of disease—such as chronic kidney disease—to the later stages of disease—such as end-stage renal failure. Certain chronic medical problems also put older adults at higher risk of cardiac problems, cerebrovascular accident, and dementia.
- Diagnostic and treatment procedures for medical issues presenting in older adults are not necessarily different than those for patients of a younger age. For the sake of clarity, the most common diagnostic and treatment procedures have been included with each age-related issue. The diagnostic and treatment procedures that are commonly performed on older adults for the purpose of diagnosing, staging, and treating cancer can be found in Chapter 20. Other diagnostic and treatment procedures can be found in individual body system chapters.

Age-Related Mobility and Bone Problems and Falls

Older adults can develop mobility problems as part of the normal process of aging, and as a result of repetitive motions and damage to the body over a period of time. ***Mobility*** is the ability to move with ease and without restriction. Refer to Chapters 3 and 4 for more information.

- **Arthrosclerosis** (**ar**-throh-skleh-**ROH**-sis) is stiffness of the joints, especially in older adults (**arthr/o** means joint, and **-sclerosis** means abnormal hardening).
- **Sarcopenia** (**sar**-koh-**PEE**-nee-ah) is the loss of muscle mass, strength, and function that comes with aging (**sarc/o** means flesh, and **-penia** means deficiency). A weight or resistance training program can significantly improve muscle mass and slow, but not stop, this process.
- **Restless legs syndrome** (RLS) is a neurological disorder of unknown cause characterized by uncomfortable feelings in the legs, producing a strong urge to move them. The sensation is usually most noticeable at night or when trying to rest.

Arthritis

There are different types of arthritis which affect the bones and joints of the body.

Osteoarthritis (**oss**-tee-oh-ar-**THRIGH**-tis) (OA), also known as ***wear-and-tear arthritis***, is most commonly associated with aging (**oste/o** means bone, **arthr** means joint, and **-itis** means inflammation) (see Chapter 3, Figure 3.17).

- **Bone-on-bone** refers to osteoarthritis that has progressed to the point where the articular cartilage is gone, and the bones rub against each other with movement, causing intense pain.

Polymyalgia rheumatica (**pol**-ee-my-**AL**-jee-ah roo-**MA**-tih-kah) (PMR) is an inflammatory disorder of the muscles and joints characterized by pain and stiffness in the neck, shoulders, upper arms, and hips and thighs (**poly-** means many, **my** means muscle, and **-algia** means pain). PMR primarily affects adults over the age of 50.

Spondylosis (**spon**-dih-**LOH**-sis) is also known as ***spinal osteoarthritis***. This degenerative disorder can cause the loss of normal spinal structure and function (**spondyl** means vertebrae, and **-osis** means abnormal condition or disease).

Spinal Column Changes

Spinal stenosis (steh-**NOH**-sis) is a narrowing of the spaces within the spine, potentially putting pressure on the nerves and spinal cord that may cause *sciatica*.

- **Sciatica** (sigh-**AT**-ih-kah) is inflammation of the sciatic nerve (see Chapter 11, Figure 11.8A) caused by pressure on the nerve roots that results in pain, burning, and tingling along the course of the affected nerve through the thigh and leg, and sometimes into the foot.

A **compression fracture** occurs when the bone is pressed together (compressed) on itself. These fractures are sometimes caused by a *pathological fracture* or can be due to an injury. This results in pain and loss of height, and can lead to the development of the spinal curvature known as *kyphosis*.

- A **pathologic fracture** occurs when a bone breaks under normal strain. This is due to bones being weakened by osteoporosis or a disease process such as cancer.
- **Kyphosis** (kye-**FOH**-sis) is an abnormal increase in the outward curvature of the thoracic spine as viewed from the side (**kyph** means hump, and **-osis** means abnormal condition or disease). This condition, also known as ***hunchback***, is frequently associated with weakening of the spinal bones due to aging (see Chapter 3, Figure 3.19A).

Osteopenia and Osteoporosis

Osteopenia (**oss**-tee-oh-**PEE**-nee-ah) is thinner-than-average bone density (**oste/o** means bone, and **-penia** means deficiency). This term is used to describe the condition of someone who does not yet have osteoporosis but has a greater-than-average chance of developing it. More than 40% of all older adults have osteopenia.

Osteoporosis (**oss**-tee-oh-poh-**ROH**-sis) (OP) is a marked loss of bone density and an increase in bone porosity frequently associated with aging (**oste/o** means bone, **por** means small opening, and **-osis** means abnormal condition or disease). It is most common in women over 50 years old due to the decrease in estrogen after menopause.

Falls

Older adults are more likely to fall down, either from loss of balance or weakness. Due to underlying factors such as osteoporosis, they are also more likely to sustain serious damage from a fall.

- A **mechanical fall** occurs when a person slips, trips, or loses their balance.
- A **fall risk patient** is a person who is at higher risk of falling, and should be more closely monitored when they are moving around.

An **osteoporotic hip fracture** (**oss**-tee-oh-pah-**ROT**-ick), also known as a ***broken hip***, is usually caused by weakening of the bones due to osteoporosis and can occur either spontaneously or as the result of a fall (Figure 19.2). Complications from these fractures can result in the loss of function, mobility, and independence, or death. ***Osteoporotic*** means pertaining to or caused by the porous condition of bones.

An older person is more likely to sustain fall damage to their skin due to the decreased production of ***collagen*** and ***elastin***, the proteins that give skin its elasticity and resilience.

- A **skin tear** is an injury that occurs from shearing pressure, where a flap of epidermis is pulled away from the underlying tissue (Figure 19.3). ***Shearing*** refers to body tissues being moved forcefully in opposite directions.

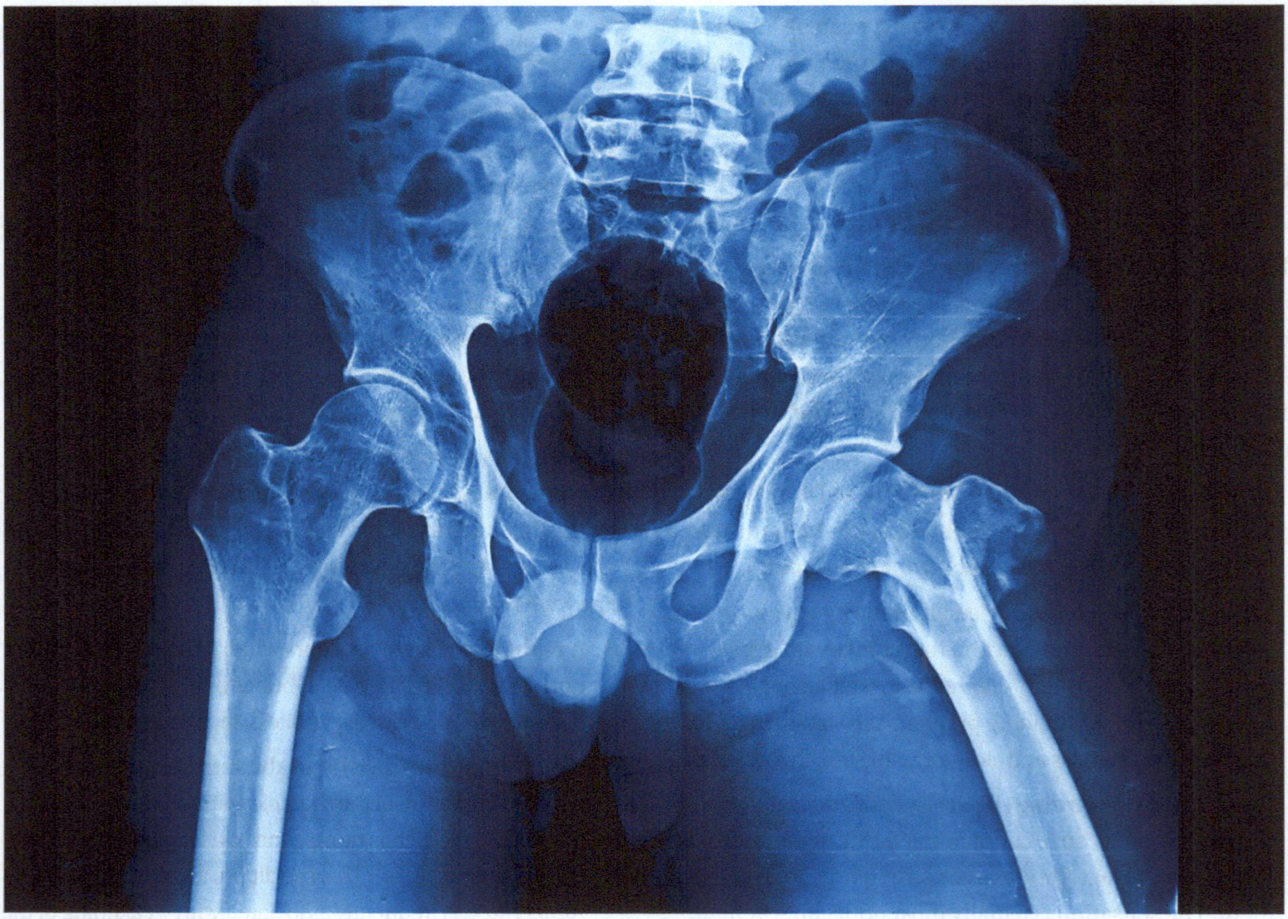

Yok_onepiece/Shutterstock.com

FIGURE 19.2 An osteoporotic hip fracture is caused by weakening of the bones due to osteoporosis.

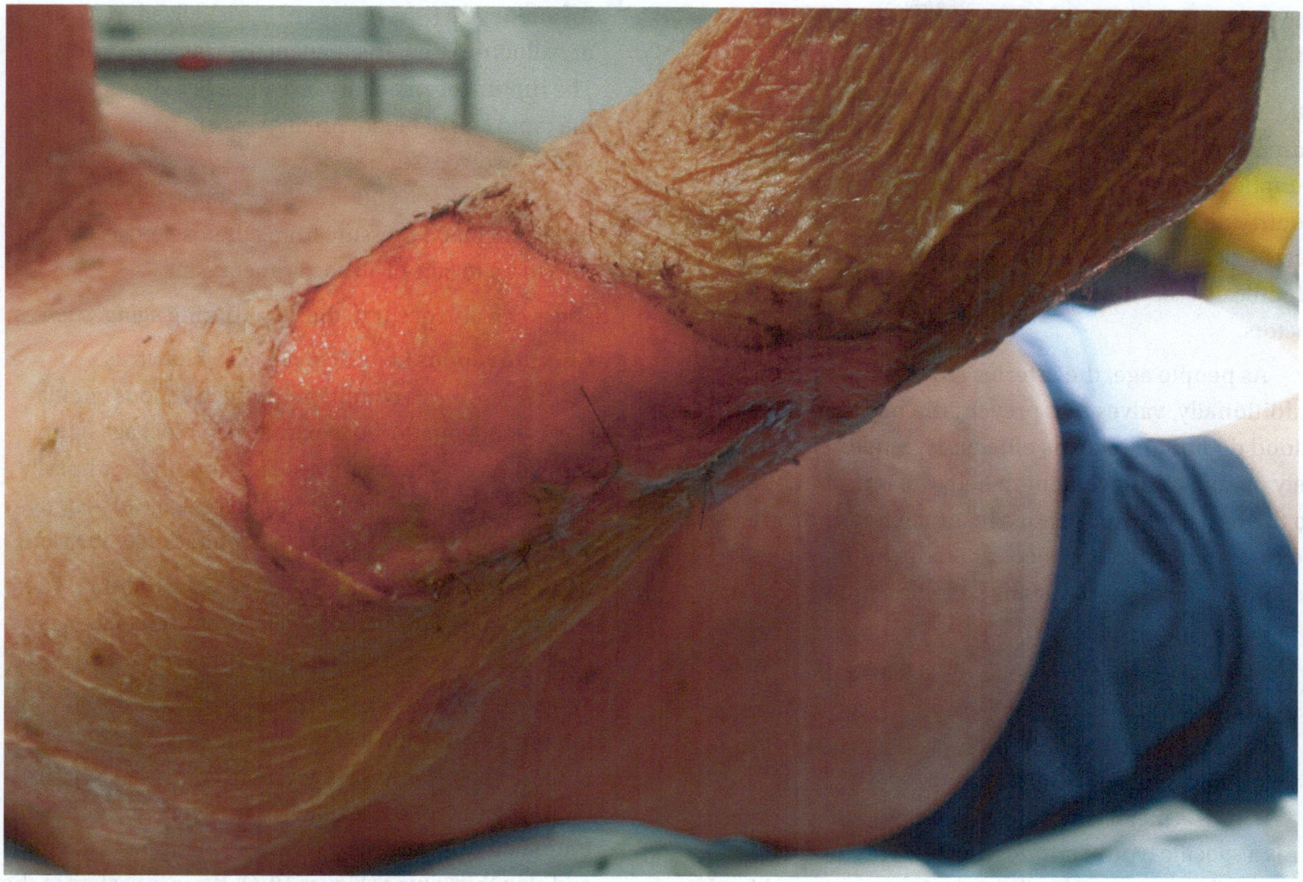
Wendy Townrow/Shutterstock.com

FIGURE 19.3 A skin tear is an injury that occurs when a flap of epidermis is pulled away from the underlying tissue.

- A **contusion** (kon-**TOO**-zhun) is an injury to underlying tissues without breaking the skin and is characterized by discoloration and pain (**contus** means bruise, and **-ion** means condition). This discoloration is caused by an accumulation of blood within the skin.
- An **ecchymosis** (**eck**-ih-**MOH**-sis), commonly known as a ***bruise***, is a large, irregular area of purplish discoloration due to bleeding under the skin (**ecchym** means pouring out of juice, and **-osis** means abnormal condition) (see Chapter 13, Figure 13.5). The plural form is *ecchymoses*.
- A **hematoma** (**hee**-mah-**TOH**-mah), which is usually caused by an injury, is a swelling of clotted blood trapped in the tissues (**hemat** means blood, and **-oma** means tumor). The body eventually reabsorbs this blood.

Diagnostic and Treatment Procedures Related to Mobility

Bone mineral density testing (BMD) is used to determine losses or changes in bone density. ***Bone density*** measures the amount of mineral in the bones, usually in the hip and spine, and compares the results with an established norm. In older adults, BMD is used to diagnose osteopenia or osteoporosis.

- **Dual energy x-ray absorptiometry** (ab-**sorp**-shee-**OM**-eh-tree) (DXA, DEXA) is a low-exposure x-ray measurement of the spine and hips to measure bone density. This test produces the most accurate results and can be repeated every few years to track bone density.
- **Corticosteroid injections** or ***cortisone shots*** can be made into the affected joint at a minimum of every six weeks for temporary relief of osteoarthritis pain. These have limited efficacy and may have side effects.
- A **total knee replacement** (TKR) means that all of the parts of the knee are replaced. This procedure, also known as a ***total knee arthroplasty*** (see Chapter 3, Figure 3.24), is usually necessitated by damage to the joint from arthritis.
- A **total hip replacement** (THR), also known as a ***total hip arthroplasty***, is performed to restore a damaged hip to full function (see Chapter 3, Figure 3.25). See Chapter 3 for more information.

Age-Related Heart and Blood Problems

Older adults are at higher risk of developing serious cardiovascular problems from difficulties with both central and peripheral blood flow. There are multiple factors which contribute to this risk, both unavoidable age-related physiological changes, and the consequences of ongoing chronic diseases, lifestyle, genetics, and environmental factors.

As people age, the arteries narrow and harden. Additionally, valves that prevent the backflow of venous blood do not function as efficiently. Since veins also rely on muscle movement to help the return of blood to the heart, chronic venous insufficiency and varicose veins are more likely to occur in older adults who are sedentary. **Sedentary** means spending most of the day seated.

- **Arteriosclerosis** (ar-**tee**-ree-oh-skleh-**ROH**-sis), also known as ***hardening of the arteries***, is any of a group of diseases characterized by thickening and the loss of elasticity of arterial walls (**arteri/o** means artery, and **-sclerosis** mean abnormal hardening). *Atherosclerosis* is a specific type of arteriosclerosis. This loss of elasticity makes it more difficult for the heart to pump blood. This increased strain on the heart can lead to *congestive heart failure*.
- **Atherosclerosis** (**ah**-theh-roh-skleh-**ROH**-sis) is the narrowing and stiffening of arteries due to the buildup of plaque. Nearly all older adults have some degree of atherosclerosis.

Complications of atherosclerosis include the following:

- **Carotid artery stenosis** is the abnormal narrowing of the carotid artery supplying blood to the brain, increasing the chance of blood clots that could cause an ischemic stroke. This condition is usually the result of atherosclerosis.
- **Peripheral artery disease** (PAD), also known as ***peripheral vascular disease***, is caused by atherosclerosis. This condition is a common and serious problem affecting 15–20% of adults over 70 years of age. In this case, ***peripheral*** means arteries that supply blood to parts of the body other than the heart or brain.
- **Intermittent claudication** (**klaw**-dih-**KAY**-shun) (IC) is pain in the leg muscles that occurs during exercise and is relieved by rest. ***Intermittent*** means coming and going at intervals, and ***claudication*** means limping. This condition, which is due to poor circulation, is associated with peripheral artery disease.
- An **aneurysm** (**AN**-you-rizm) is a localized weak spot or balloon-like enlargement of the wall of an artery. The rupture of an aneurysm can be fatal because of the rapid loss of blood. Aneurysms are named for the artery involved, such as ***aortic aneurysm***, ***abdominal aortic aneurysm***, and ***thoracic aortic aneurysm***. The increased blood pressure from atherosclerosis contributes to up to 80% of all aortic aneurysms.

Changes can also occur to the veins during aging, such as:

- **Chronic venous insufficiency**, also known as ***venous insufficiency***, is a condition in which venous circulation is inadequate due to partial vein blockage or to the leakage of venous valves. This condition primarily affects the feet and ankles, and the leakage of venous blood into the tissues causes discoloration of the skin.
- **Venous stasis** (**VEE**-nus **STAY**-sis) is a condition where venous blood flow in the lower extremities is sluggish, leading to an increased risk of *stasis dermatitis*.
- **Stasis dermatitis** (**STAY**-sis **der**-mah-**TYE**-tis) is inflammation in the lower extremities caused by chronic venous insufficiency and venous stasis. It initially causes redness, irritation, and weeping, and if untreated can cause venous ulcers, peripheral edema, and skin thickening (Figure 19.4). ***Weeping*** refers to the leakage of interstitial fluid through the skin. ***Skin thickening*** is the replacement of normal skin with fibrotic, thickened tissue.
- **Venous ulcers**, also known as ***venous stasis ulcers***, are irregular open pits in the skin that occur on the lower legs as a result of venous stasis (Figure 19.4).
- **Varicose veins** (**VAHR**-ih-**kohs VAYNS**) are abnormally swollen veins that usually occur in the superficial veins of the legs. This condition occurs when the valves in these veins do not function properly, so blood pools in the veins, causing them to enlarge.

Common Age-Related Cardiac Changes

Age-related changes to the heart include decreased elasticity of the heart muscle and thickening of the heart walls, which make it more difficult for the heart to pump blood effectively. The number of cells in the electrical pathways that cause the heart to contract decrease with age, increasing the risk of arrhythmias, particularly heart block. The heart valves can stop closing completely, allowing some blood to ***reflux***, or flow backward. Additionally, circulation to the heart can become compromised, causing ischemia and myocardial infarction. See Chapter 5 for more information.

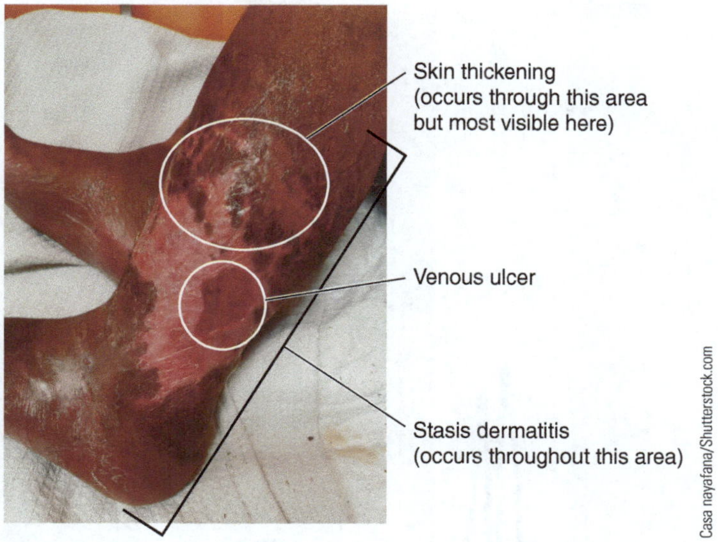

FIGURE 19.4 An older adult's leg with stasis dermatitis, skin thickening, and a venous ulcer.

An **arrhythmia** (ah-**RITH**-mee-ah) is the loss of the normal rhythm of the heartbeat. This can be a minor, severe, or fatal event. The severity of an episode depends on how much the heart's ability to pump blood is compromised. Rather than being a heart muscle problem, arrhythmias are usually caused by abnormalities in the electrical conduction system of the heart. Arrhythmias can cause either bradycardia or tachycardia (see Chapter 5).

- **Bundle branch block** (BBB) is a partial block in electrical conduction between the atrium and ventricle on one side of the heart at the bundle of His. BBB is named for the side it is located on, such as ***left bundle branch block*** (LBBB) or ***right bundle branch block*** (RBBB) and has a characteristic "bunny ears" appearance on an EKG (Figure 19.5). It may require treatment for the underlying condition.
- **Heart block**, also known as ***atrioventricular block*** (AV block), is a congenital or acquired arrhythmia caused by the electrical signal moving through the heart to the AV node being partially or completely blocked from reaching the ventricles. It is classified by degree (first through third). Heart block is more common in older adults, as a result of either age-related changes or damage to the heart.
- **First-degree heart block** is slowed electrical conduction between the atria and ventricles that causes a slight gap between atrial and ventricular contractions. It does not usually require treatment.
- **Second-degree heart block** is a partial block in electrical conduction between the atria and ventricles that stops the ventricles from contracting some of the time after the atria contract. It does not usually require treatment.
- **Third-degree heart block** is a complete block in electrical conduction between the atria and ventricles. The ventricles do not contract after any of the atrial contractions. A ***ventricular escape rhythm*** is a slow heart rate of 20–40 beats per minute that arises from the pacemaker cells in the ventricles. Without a ventricular escape rhythm, third-degree heart block causes sudden cardiac death. A person with third-degree heart block will need to have a *pacemaker* implanted.

Atrial fibrillation is the most common type of tachycardic arrhythmia, especially among people age 60 and older.

- **Atrial fibrillation** (**AY**-tree-al **fih**-brih-**LAY**-shun), also known as ***A-fib***, occurs when the normal rhythmic contractions of the atria are replaced by rapid, uncontrolled twitching of the muscular heart wall. Some of the increased electrical impulses reach the ventricles, producing an irregular rate of 80–180 beats per minute or more.

Heart valve disease is a medical condition where one or more of the four valves in the heart do not work well. In older adults, this most commonly involves regurgitation or stenosis.

- **Heart valve regurgitation**, also called ***insufficiency*** or ***incompetency***, occurs when a heart valve does not close tightly, thus allowing blood to leak back through the opening. The most common type is ***mitral valve prolapse***, where the flaps of the mitral

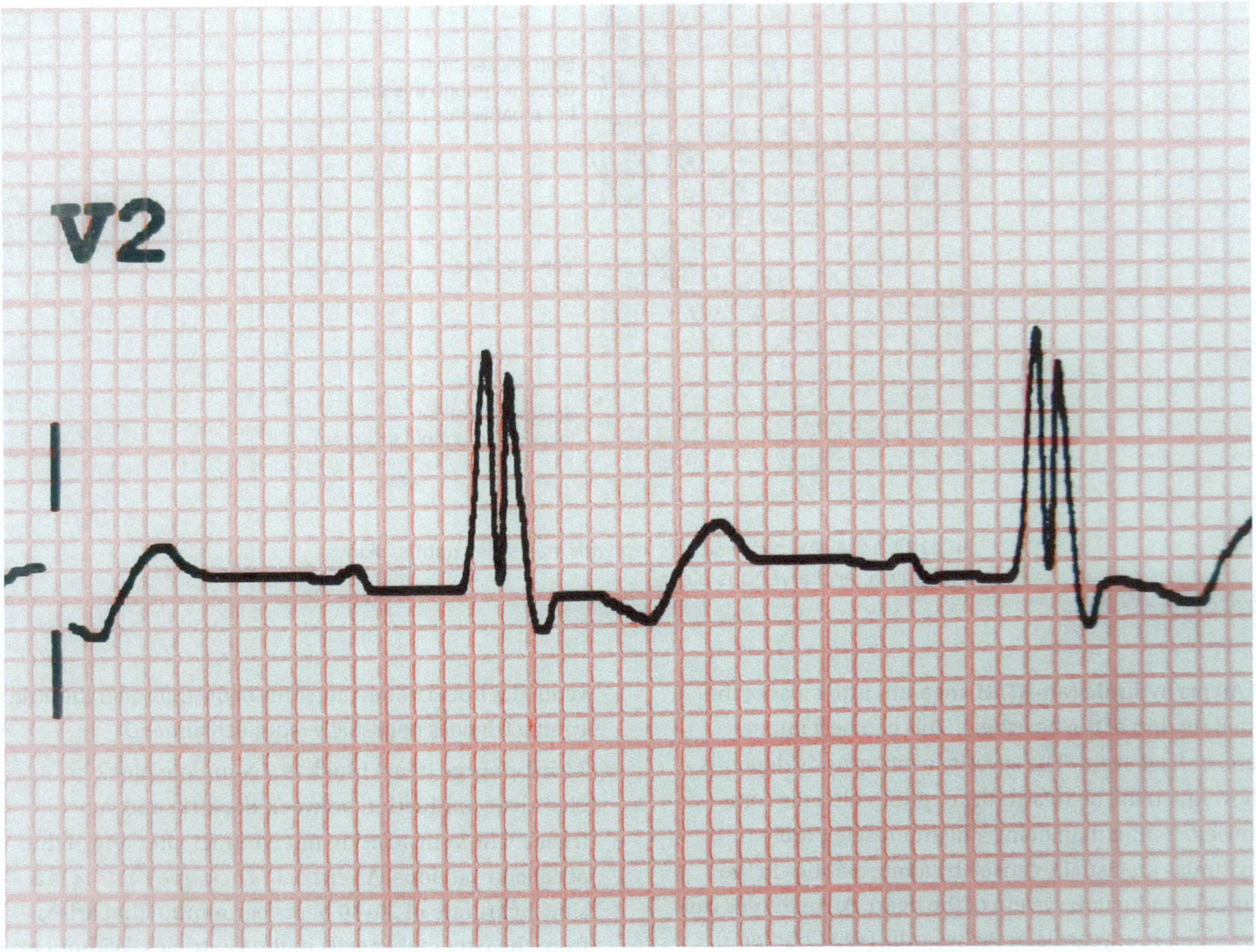

Thitiporn taingpan/Shutterstock.com

FIGURE 19.5 Bundle branch block has a characteristic "bunny ears" appearance on an EKG.

valve bulge upward into the left atrium rather than closing tightly.

- **Heart valve stenosis** is a condition where the flaps of a valve become stiff, thickened, or even fused together, limiting the amount of blood that can pass through.

Congestive heart failure (CHF) occurs most commonly in older adults, often after the heart has been weakened or damaged by other health problems. In this chronic condition, the heart is unable to pump out all of the blood that it receives. See Chapter 5 for more information.

- **Cardiomegaly** (**kar**-dee-oh-**MEG**-ah-lee) is the abnormal enlargement of the heart that is frequently associated with heart failure as the heart enlarges in an effort to compensate for its decreased pumping ability (**cardi/o** means heart, and **-megaly** means enlargement).
- **Pulmonary edema** (eh-**DEE**-mah) is an accumulation of fluid in lung tissues, especially the alveoli.
- **Dyspnea on exertion** (DOE) is shortness of breath that occurs with physical activity.

Treatment for CHF can include fluid restriction, medications (see Chapter 22), surgery to fix contributing factors such as heart valve disease, and more aggressive measures such as a ventricular assist device or heart transplant.

- **Fluid restriction** is a limit on the amount of water and other liquids a person drinks per day.
- A **ventricular assist device** is an implanted mechanical pump that helps the heart circulate blood. A ***left ventricular assist device*** (LVAD) is the most common type.

Diagnostic and Treatment Procedures Related to Circulation

Diagnostic procedures related to circulation include x-rays and computed tomography (see Chapter 21), electrocardiograms and stress tests (see Chapter 5), and blood tests (see Chapter 6).

Common treatment procedures for age-related heart and blood issues include:

- A **pacemaker** is used to treat third-degree heart block and other arrhythmias causing bradycardia. This battery-powered device can be attached externally or implanted temporarily or permanently under the skin with connections leading into the heart to regulate the heartbeat (Figure 19.6).
- **Synchronized cardioversion** is a procedure for restoring normal heart rhythm using a low-voltage electrical shock in a non-emergency situation.
- **Cardiac ablation** (ab-LAY-shun), also called ***catheter ablation***, is a procedure that uses radio-frequency energy (heat) or cryoablation (extreme cold) to scar or destroy the heart tissue triggering an abnormal heart rhythm.
- **Valvuloplasty** (**VAL**-view-loh-**plas**-tee) or ***balloon valvuloplasty*** is the surgical repair of a heart valve that has a narrowed opening (**valvul/o** means valve, and **-plasty** means surgical repair).
- **Heart valve replacement** is surgery to replace one of the heart's four valves, usually the aortic or mitral valve. The defective valve is replaced with either a mechanical valve or one made up of animal or human tissue.
- A **heart transplant** is a surgery to replace a person's heart with a healthy heart from an organ donor.

Age-Related Changes of the Lymphatic and Immune Systems

Lymph vessels become less flexible and more permeable with age, similar to blood vessels. Since lymph is moved upward through the body by muscle movement, similar to venous blood flow, older adults are more likely to experience gravity-induced edema in the legs and feet.

Lymphedema (**lim**-feh-**DEE**-mah) (LE) is swelling of the tissues due to an abnormal accumulation of lymph fluid within the tissues (**lymph** means lymph, and **-edema** means swelling). See Chapter 7 for more information.

- ***Secondary lymphedema*** is caused by damage to lymphatic vessels that is most frequently due to cancer treatment, surgery, trauma, or burns.
- **Peripheral edema**, also known as ***dependent edema***, is swelling in the legs that can occur as a result of multiple medical problems, including chronic venous insufficiency, congestive heart failure, kidney failure, and cirrhosis.

Herpes zoster (**HER**-peez **ZOS**-ter) (HZ), commonly known as ***shingles***, is an acute viral infection characterized by painful skin eruptions that follow the underlying route of an inflamed nerve (see Chapter 7, Figure 7.12). This inflammation occurs when the dormant varicella (chickenpox) virus is reactivated later in life. A vaccine is available to help prevent shingles and is recommended for adults 50 years and older.

- ***Postherpetic neuralgia*** is a complication that may follow herpes zoster if nerve fibers have been damaged during the outbreak. The resulting pain can be severe and persistent.

Immunosenescence (ih-**myoo**-noh-seh-**NEH**-sens) is the gradual, natural decline of the immune system as a result of aging.

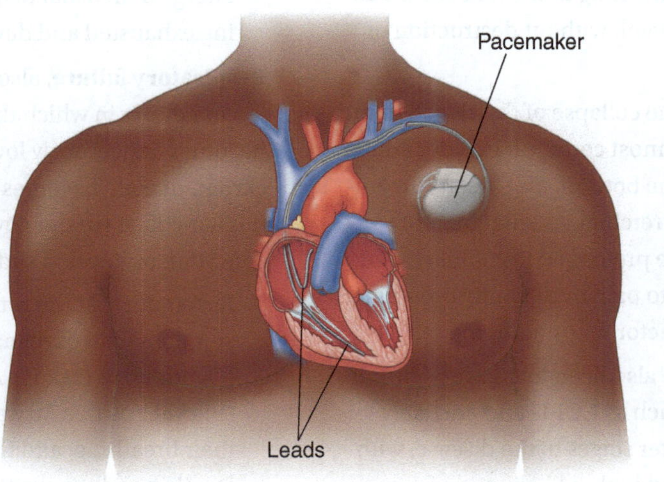

FIGURE 19.6 A permanent pacemaker implanted under the skin with connections leading into the heart to regulate the heartbeat.

- Older adults have more T and B cells which respond to specific antigens. However, in older adults there are fewer immune cells which can recognize new antigens. Because of this shift, older adults are less able to fight off new infections.

Inflamm-aging (**in**-flah-**MAY**-jing) is a recent term for age-related ongoing, low-grade systemic inflammation without apparent cause. It has been shown to increase the risk of developing or worsening Alzheimer's, cardiovascular disease, and diabetes.

Cancer

Cancer is a class of diseases characterized by the uncontrolled division of cells and the ability of these cells to invade other tissues, either through direct growth into adjacent tissue or by spreading into distant sites by metastasizing.

The risk of cancer increases with age, and people in their 80s are at the highest risk of developing cancer, according to the American Cancer Society. See Chapter 20 for more information.

Age-Related Respiratory Problems

Older adults are prone to respiratory problems, including increased risk of pneumonia. The loss of muscle strength associated with aging makes it more difficult to take a deep breath or cough, and loss of intervertebral space from compression fractures also shrinks the space available for the lungs to expand, contributing to atelectasis.

Senile emphysema (**SEE**-nye-ahl **em**-fih-**SEE**-mah) is an age-related change in the lung tissue that causes an increase in the size of the alveoli without destruction of the alveolar walls.

Basilar atelectasis is the collapse of the alveoli in the bases of the lungs, which is most common in older adults (**basilar** means located at the bottom, **atel** means incomplete, and **-ectasis** means stretching or enlargement). Contributing factors include prolonged immobility, and taking shallow breaths due to pain or difficulty breathing. Basilar atelectasis is a risk factor for pneumonia.

Many older adults have also been living with chronic, progressive lung diseases such as COPD and are likely to have progressed to the later stages of the disease, with more difficulty breathing and higher likelihood of complications. See Chapter 8 for more information on COPD. Lung cancer is the most common type of cancer in older adults, and is discussed in Chapter 20.

COPD

A **COPD exacerbation** is an acute episode of worsening chronic obstructive pulmonary disease symptoms, causing increased dyspnea. Older adults are at higher risk for COPD exacerbation, which may be triggered by pneumonia, or may not have an obvious cause.

- **Dyspnea** (**DISP**-nee-ah), also known as ***shortness of breath*** (SOB), is difficult or labored breathing (**dys-** means painful, and **-pnea** means breathing). Shortness of breath can be caused by strenuous physical exertion or can be due to lung damage or heart failure.
- **Pneumonia** (new-**MOH**-nee-ah) (PNA) is a serious inflammation of the lungs in which the alveoli and air passages fill with pus and other fluids (**pneumon** means lung, and **-ia** means abnormal condition). Pneumonia is most commonly caused by an infection and often follows a cold, flu, chronic illness, or other condition, especially in older adults that weakens the immune system and its ability to stave off infection.

End-stage COPD is the final stage of COPD. It is characterized by severe dyspnea at rest and frequent COPD exacerbations, and patients frequently require supplemental oxygen at home (***home O2***).

Treatment of COPD exacerbation includes antibiotics for pneumonia, bronchodilator inhalers and nebulizers to open the airway, and steroids to reduce airway swelling. For patients who have increased work of breathing, more aggressive airway support measures can also be used.

- **Work of breathing** refers to the amount of energy required to inhale and exhale. Patients who are experiencing ***increased work of breathing*** require more energy than usual to breathe, and are at risk of becoming exhausted and developing *respiratory failure.*

Respiratory failure, also known as ***respiratory acidosis***, is a condition in which the level of oxygen in the blood becomes dangerously low (hypoxemia) or the level of carbon dioxide becomes dangerously high (hypercapnia). It is a medical emergency that can result from a chronic condition or develop suddenly.

- Respiratory failure is treated by first administering supplemental oxygen; placing the patient on a CPAP (Continuous Positive Airway Pressure) or BiPAP (Bilevel Positive Airway Pressure) machine to support their breathing; and finally sedating the patient, performing endotracheal intubation, and placing them on a ventilator if they are unable to effectively breathe on their own. However, older adults with severe COPD are often unable to successfully breathe independently after spending time on a ventilator, and are unable to be weaned from the ventilator.

- **Weaning** is the gradual process of decreasing the amount of work of breathing done by the ventilator, to measure whether a patient can breathe spontaneously before extubation.
- **Extubation** is the removal of an endotracheal tube and the removal of a patient from a ventilator. This is done either for patients who have regained the ability to breathe spontaneously, or at end-of-life for patients who are being removed from life-sustaining measures.

See Chapter 8 for more information on these interventions.

Age-Related Digestive Problems

Older adults can experience numerous age-related changes of the digestive system that can cause problems. The loss of some or all teeth due to periodontal disease is common. Decreased muscle mass and strength also lead to slowed peristalsis and can contribute to constipation and bowel obstruction. Additionally, changes in smell and taste from aging, illness, or medication side effects can contribute to a loss of appetite.

Xerostomia (**zeer**-oh-**STOH**-mee-ah), also known as ***dry mouth***, is the lack of adequate saliva due to diminished secretions by the salivary glands (**xer/o** means dry, **stom** means mouth or oral cavity, and **-ia** means pertaining to). This condition can be due to medications or radiation of the salivary glands, and can cause discomfort, difficulty in swallowing, changes in the taste of food, and dental decay.

Dentures are a removable set of artificial teeth that replace either some or all of a person's teeth. They are often referred to as ***uppers*** and ***lowers***, depending on which set of teeth they replace. ***Partials*** are dentures that replace some of a person's teeth.

- **Edentulous** (ee-**DEN**-too-lus) means without teeth. This term describes the situation after the natural permanent teeth have been lost.
- Missing teeth and poorly fitting dentures may limit a person's ability to effectively chew and safely swallow food, and can contribute to malnutrition and a higher risk of aspiration.

Older adults who are unable to take in adequate nutrition due to loss of appetite, difficulty absorbing nutrients, inability to prepare appropriate meals for themselves, or persistent diarrhea are at higher risk of poor outcomes and slowed healing.

Failure to thrive (FTT) in older adults is characterized by weight loss, anorexia, dehydration, malnutrition, and a decrease in physical activity. It is often a symptom of an underlying illness or depression, and can have multiple causes.

- **Anorexia** (**an**-oh-**RECK**-see-ah) is the loss of appetite for food, especially when caused by disease (**an-** means without, and **-orexia** means appetite).
- **Dehydration** is a condition in which fluid loss exceeds fluid intake and disrupts the body's normal electrolyte balance (**de-** means removal, **hydr/a** means water, and **-tion** means the process of). This can be caused by decreased intake of fluid, or persistent diarrhea.
- **Malnutrition** is a lack of proper food or nutrients in the body due to a shortage of food; poor eating habits; or the inability of the body to digest, absorb, and distribute these nutrients. **Mal-** is a prefix meaning bad or poor.

Treatment for FTT include treating the underlying illness or depression, providing appetite stimulants and nutritional supplements, and loosening dietary restrictions.

Gastrointestinal Bleeding

Gastrointestinal bleeding (GI bleed) is the loss of blood from the digestive tract. The risk of GI bleed increases with age. The anemia caused by a GI bleed can also cause shortness of breath, confusion, and weakness before the GI bleed itself is discovered. See Chapter 6 for more information on anemia.

- An **upper GI bleed** (UGIB) is blood loss from the esophagus, stomach, or duodenum. This can be caused by a peptic ulcer, frequent use of NSAIDs, or esophageal varices from alcoholism. The symptoms can include vomiting of either bright red blood (***hematemesis***) or black, granular digested blood (***coffee ground emesis***), or passing of black, tarry stools (***melena***).
- A **lower GI bleed** (LGIB) is blood loss from below the jejunum to the rectum, most frequently from the colon. It is less common than UGIB, and can be caused by diverticulosis, colorectal cancer, frequent use of NSAIDs, or clotting problems due to blood-thinning medications. The symptoms can include passing of black, tarry stools containing digested blood (melena), which indicates a LGIB relatively high in the intestines, or passing of large quantities of clots and dark red blood (***hematochezia***), which indicates a LGIB closer to the rectum.

- Treatment of GI bleed usually involves reversal of any blood-thinning medications, blood transfusion, and endoscopy or surgery to locate and stop the bleeding. See Chapter 20 for more information about colorectal cancer.

Constipation

Constipation is defined as having a bowel movement fewer than three times per week. Constipation can cause severe abdominal pain and urinary retention. Older adults have multiple contributing factors for developing constipation, including medication side effects, loss of appetite, dehydration, and decreased physical activity.

- A **laxative** is an oral medication such as magnesium citrate that is given to prevent or relieve constipation.
- **Manual disimpaction** is the physical removal of stool from the rectal vault with a gloved finger.
- An **enema** (**EH**-neh-ma) is the placement of a solution into the rectum and colon to empty the lower intestine through bowel activity.

Diverticulosis (**dye**-ver-tick-you-**LOH**-sis) is the chronic presence of an abnormal number of diverticula, or sacs, formed in weak spots of the colon wall (**diverticul** means diverticulum, and **-osis** means abnormal condition or disease). Over half of all adults over age 60 in the U.S. have diverticulosis. While many people have no symptoms, diverticulosis can be a cause of constipation. See Chapter 9 for more information.

Small Bowel Obstruction

As muscle movement in the intestines slows, older adults are also at higher risk of developing an intestinal obstruction.

A **small bowel obstruction** (SBO) is a partial or complete blockage of the small intestine. Symptoms include abdominal pain, distention, vomiting of dark green bile, and inability to pass gas or stool. SBO is the most common type of intestinal obstruction in older adults.

Initial conservative treatment for SBO includes placing an NG tube, bowel rest, and IV fluids. If this treatment is unsuccessful, surgery is then required to remove the blocked section of intestine.

- **Nasogastric intubation** (**nay**-zoh-**GAS**-trick **in**-too-**BAY**-shun) is the placement of a flexible nasogastric (NG) tube through the nose and into the stomach (**nas/o** means nose, **gastr** means stomach, and **-ic** means pertaining to). This temporary tube suctions out gastric contents for patients with SBO, which can alleviate some of the discomfort from the obstruction.
- **Bowel rest** involves not giving a person anything to eat or drink by mouth, and instead providing hydration and nutrition intravenously, usually for one to two days. This gives the digestive tract a chance to recover and return to normal function.

Progression of Chronic Liver Disease

Chronic liver disease can be caused by several different diseases, including alcoholism, viral hepatitis B or C, or cancer such as hepatocellular carcinoma. It is a slowly progressing disease characterized by destruction of the liver tissue and cirrhosis (see Chapter 9, Figure 9.17).

Cirrhosis (sih-**ROH**-sis) is a chronic degenerative disease of the liver characterized by scarring (**cirrh** means yellow or orange, and **-osis** means abnormal condition or disease).

Advanced cirrhosis, also known as *advanced chronic liver failure*, is often marked by hepatic encephalopathy, ascites, jaundice, and increased risk of bleeding due to failure of the liver to make clotting factors.

- **Hepatic encephalopathy** (en-**sef**-ah-**LOP**-ah-thee) is an altered level of consciousness caused by elevated blood ammonia levels, which is usually characterized by lethargy, confusion, and short-term memory problems.
- **Ascites** (ah-**SIGH**-teez) is an abnormal accumulation of serous fluid in the peritoneal cavity which causes shortness of breath.
- **Jaundice** (**JAWN**-dis) is a yellow discoloration of the skin, mucous membranes, and eyes. This condition is caused by greater-than-normal amounts of bilirubin in the blood.

Age-Related Changes in Cognition

Normal changes in cognition associated with aging include short-term memory problems, difficulty learning new skills, and increased time needed to understand and respond to questions.

- The term **cognition** (kog-**NISH**-un) describes the mental activities associated with thinking, learning, and memory.
- **Mild cognitive impairment** is decline from normal function characterized by short-term memory loss, which may be an early predictor of dementia. Some decline in cognition is a normal part of the aging process.

There are multiple specialized diagnostic tests available to assess a person's level of cognitive function or impairment. The most basic initial assessment is to check orientation.

- **Orientation** is the awareness of different aspects of one's environment.
- **Alert and oriented** (A&O) refers to someone who is spontaneously awake (alert), and aware of who they are (oriented to person), where they are (oriented to place), what day/month it is (oriented to time), and what is going on (oriented to event). Someone who is able to answer all of those questions correctly is considered A&O × 4.

Dementia

Dementia (dih-**MEN**-shah) is a slowly progressive decline in mental abilities, including memory, thinking, and judgment, that is often accompanied by personality changes. ***Senile dementia*** is dementia of the aged. ***Sundowning*** refers to a state of confusion that can happen toward the late afternoon and into the night in patients with dementia.

- **Alzheimer's disease** (**ALTZ**-high-merz) (AD) is a group of disorders involving the parts of the brain that control thought, memory, and language. It is the leading form of dementia and is marked by progressive deterioration that affects both the memory and reasoning capabilities of an individual.
- ***Lewy body dementia***, which is the second most common type of dementia, occurs when abnormal proteins interfere with cell function in the brain. It is named after neurologist Frederic Lewy. ***Parkinson's disease dementia*** is a type of Lewy body dementia.
- **Vascular dementia** is a form of dementia caused by a stroke or other restriction of the flow of blood to the brain. Although Alzheimer's disease is the primary cause of dementia, vascular dementia accounts for about 10–20% of all cases.

Delirium

Older adults are at high risk of developing delirium when hospitalized.

- **Delirium** (deh-**LEER**-ee-um) is an acute condition of confusion, disorientation, disordered thinking and memory, agitation, and hallucinations.

Risk factors for delirium in older adults include dementia or cognitive impairment, decreased vision or hearing, electrolyte abnormalities, and the use of sedative medications such as benzodiazepines.

- This condition is usually caused by a treatable physical condition, such as a high fever. An individual suffering from this condition is described as being ***delirious***.

Delirium in older adults is associated with a decline in cognitive function even after the delirium has resolved.

Age-Related Nervous System Problems

Older adults are at higher risk of experiencing both chronic problems, such as Parkinson's disease, and acute problems, such as cerebrovascular accident.

Parkinson's disease (PD) is a chronic, degenerative central nervous disorder characterized by fine muscle tremors, rigidity, and a slow or shuffling gait. As Parkinson's disease progresses, additional symptoms are common, including dementia, depression, insomnia, orthostatic hypotension, and balance problems. See Chapter 11 for more information.

Cerebrovascular Accidents

A ***stroke*** is properly known as a **cerebrovascular accident** (**ser**-eh-broh-**VAS**-kyou-lar) (CVA). A CVA is brain damage that occurs when blood flow to the brain is disrupted because a blood vessel either is blocked or has ruptured. Strokes are currently the third-leading cause of death and the primary cause of long-term disability. See Chapter 11 for more information.

An **ischemic stroke** (iss-**KEE**-mick), which is the most common type of stroke in older adults, occurs when the flow of blood to the brain is blocked by the narrowing or blockage of an artery.

- **Carotid ultrasonography** (kah-**ROT**-id **ul**-trah-son-**OG**-rah-fee) is an ultrasound study of the carotid artery (**ultra-** means beyond, **son/o** means sound, and **-graphy** means the process of producing a picture or record). This diagnostic test is performed to detect plaque buildup in the artery to predict or diagnose an ischemic stroke.
- A **carotid endarterectomy** (kah-**ROT**-id **end**-ar-ter-**ECK**-toh-mee) is the surgical removal of the lining of a portion of a clogged carotid artery leading to the brain. This procedure is performed to reduce the risk of a stroke due to blood clots.
- **Tissue plasminogen activator** (plaz-**MIN**-oh-jen) (tPA), also known as ***alteplase***, is a thrombolytic that is administered to some patients having a stroke. If administered within a few hours after symptoms begin, this medication can dissolve the damaging blood clots. *Note:* Use caution with the abbreviation tPA, which can be confused with other drug abbreviations.

A **hemorrhagic stroke** (**hem**-oh-**RAJ**-ick), also known as a ***bleed***, occurs when a blood vessel in the brain leaks. This type of stroke is less common than ischemic strokes, accounting for only about 20% of strokes in older adults, and is often fatal, especially in older adults on blood-thinning medications.

- A **cranial hematoma** (**hee**-mah-**TOH**-mah) is a collection of blood trapped in the tissues of the brain (**hemat** means blood, and **-oma** means tumor). Cranial hematomas may be caused by a major or minor head injury, particularly by falls in older adults (see Chapter 11, Figure 11.10).

Management of Cerebrovascular Accidents

Long-term complications from a cerebrovascular accident depend on the severity of the damage to the brain, and the location of the damage. The effects of an ischemic stroke can be reduced by prompt administration of a clot-busting medication or neurosurgery to retrieve the clot and restore blood flow. The effects of a hemorrhagic stroke can be reduced by neurovascular surgery to stop the bleeding, or administration of a reversal agent or platelets to promote clotting if the patient is on blood thinners.

Immediately after a CVA, whether or not interventions have been given, the primary concerns are to assess the patient's cognition, coordination, and muscle tone. Different hospitals vary in their use of neurological assessment tools, but one common tool is the NIHSS.

The **National Institutes of Health Stroke Scale** (NIHSS) is an 11-item tool for measuring the severity of neurological deficit after a stroke. Items tested include level of consciousness, orientation, ability to follow basic commands, eye movement, muscle movement (hemiparesis/hemiplegia) and coordination (ataxia), facial droop, sense of touch, and the ability to speak clearly and coherently (aphasia).

- **Hemiparesis** (**hem**-ee-pah-**REE**-sis) is a weakness or slight paralysis affecting one side of the body (**hemi-** means half, and **-paresis** means partial or incomplete paralysis). It is one of the most common effects of a stroke, with damage to one side of the brain causing paralysis on the opposite side of the body.
- **Hemiplegia** (**hem**-ee-**PLEE**-jee-ah) (HEMI) is total paralysis affecting only one side of the body (**hemi-** means half, and **-plegia** means paralysis).
- **Ataxia** (ah-**TACK**-see-ah) is the lack of muscle coordination during voluntary movement (**a-** means without, **tax** means coordination, and **-ia** means condition). These movements, which are often shaky and unsteady, are most frequently caused by abnormal activity in the cerebellum (see Chapter 11).
- **Aphasia** (ah-**FAY**-zee-ah), which is often caused by brain damage associated with a stroke, is the loss of the ability to speak, write, and/or comprehend the written or spoken word (**a-** means without, and **-phasia** means speech).

In addition to the NIHSS or a similar neurological assessment, a **swallow evaluation** is done to assess the stroke patient's ability to swallow safely, as the muscles involved in swallowing can be weakened by the stroke, putting the patient at higher risk of dysphagia and aspiration.

- **Dysphagia** (dis-**FAY**-jee-ah) is difficulty in swallowing (**dys-** means difficult, and **-phagia** means swallowing).
- **Aspiration** (ass-pih-**RAY**-shun) means inhaling or drawing a foreign substance into the upper respiratory tract.

Older adults with dysphagia may require a modified diet, such as thickened liquids and soft ground, or pureed food, to decrease their risk of aspiration. If they are unable to safely take any food or liquid by mouth, then a gastrostomy tube can be placed (see Chapter 9 for more information).

Disability After Cerebrovascular Accident

Worldwide, up to 50% of people who have a CVA become permanently disabled. The **modified Rankin scale** (mRS) is an assessment tool to measure level of disability after a CVA (Table 19.2).

A person with an mRS score of 0–3 is likely to be able to return home either independently or with some caregiver assistance. A person with an mRS score of 4 is likely to be placed in an assisted living facility, and a person with an mRS score of 5 is likely to be placed in a skilled nursing facility if there is a likelihood of recovery of function with rehabilitation, or a nursing home if they are likely to require constant caregiver assistance. See the section "Assistive Care" for more information on long-term care facilities.

Bedbound, also known as ***bedridden***, refers to someone who is unable to independently get out of bed due to weakness, paralysis, or injury. A bedbound person who is unable to independently reposition themselves in the bed is at high risk of developing a pressure ulcer, especially if they have urinary or fecal incontinence.

TABLE 19.2

Modified Rankin Scale to Measure Level of Disability After a CVA

0	no symptoms
1	no significant disability; able to carry out all usual duties and activities
2	slight disability; unable to carry out all previous activities, but able to look after own affairs without assistance
3	moderate disability; requiring some help, but able to walk without assistance
4	moderately severe disability; unable to walk and attend to bodily needs without assistance
5	severe disability; bedridden, incontinent, and requiring constant nursing care and attention
6	dead

- A **pressure ulcer**, also known as a ***decubitus ulcer*** or ***bedsore***, is an open ulcerated wound that is caused by prolonged pressure on an area of skin over a bony prominence, such as heels, elbows, sacrum, hips, and spine (Figure 19.7). Without proper care, these sores quickly become seriously infected and can result in tissue death. A pressure ulcer often starts as a ***deep tissue injury***, or damage to the tissues under intact skin, which looks like an area of redness or bruising that does not change color when touched.

Prolonged immobilization after CVA increases the likelihood of atrophy and contractures. The goal of physical therapy and rehabilitation after CVA is to assist with a return to function and independence.

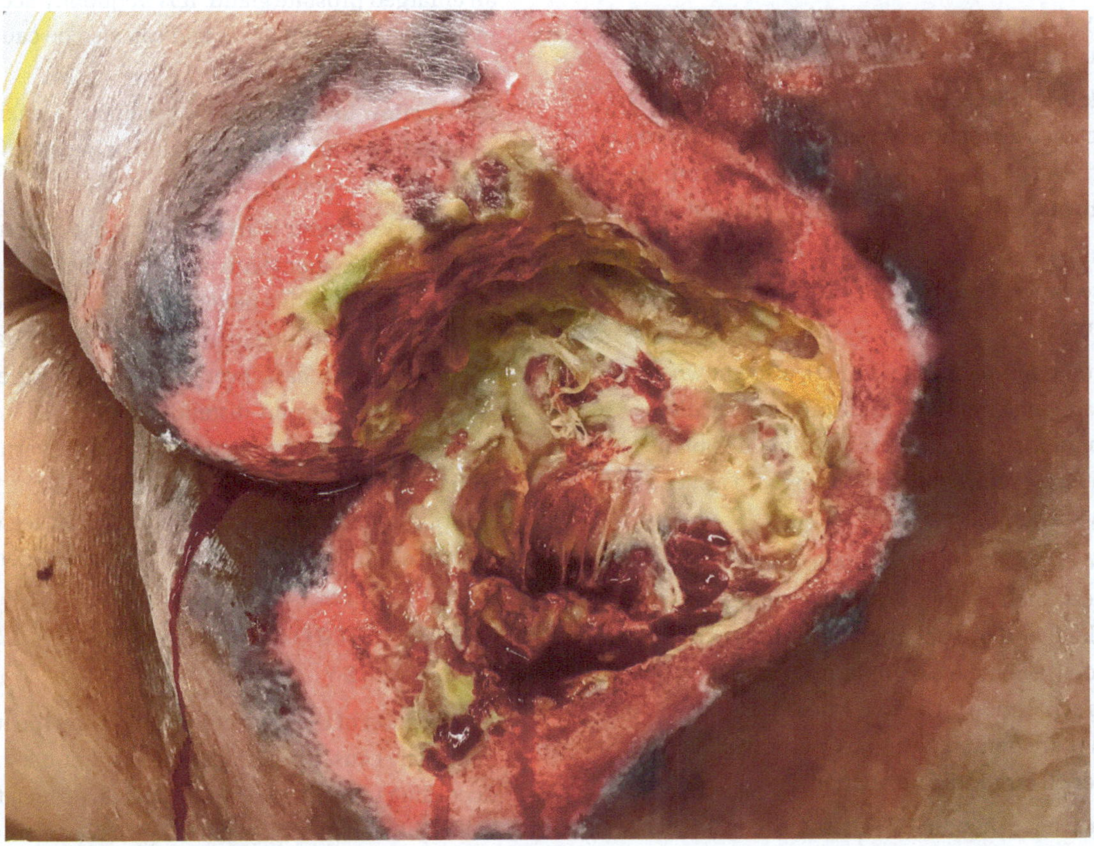

Chinnabanchon9Job/Shutterstock.com

FIGURE 19.7 A pressure ulcer is an open ulcerated wound caused by prolonged pressure on an area of skin over a bony prominence, such as the sacrum.

- **Atrophy** (**AT**-roh-fee) means weakness or wearing away of body tissues and structures. Atrophy of a muscle or muscles can be caused by pathology or by disuse of the muscle over a long period of time.
- A **contracture** (kon-**TRACK**-chur) is the permanent tightening of fascia, muscles, tendons, ligaments, or skin that occurs when normally elastic connective tissues are replaced with nonelastic fibrous tissues. The most common causes of contractures are scarring or the lack of use due to immobilization or inactivity.

Age-Related Kidney and Urinary Problems

Renal failure, also known as ***kidney failure***, is the inability of one or both of the kidneys to perform their functions. The body cannot replace damaged nephrons, and when too many nephrons have been destroyed, the result is kidney failure.

- **Acute renal failure** (ARF) has sudden onset and can be fatal if not reversed promptly. This condition can be caused by the kidneys not receiving enough blood to filter due to dehydration or a sudden drop in blood volume or blood pressure from injury, burns, or a severe infection. ARF is treated by treating the cause and usually administering IV fluids or blood transfusions to restore the lost blood volume.

Chronic kidney disease (CKD) is the progressive loss of renal function over months or years. This common condition, which can be life-threatening, may result from diabetes mellitus, hypertension, or a family history of kidney disease.

- The buildup of waste in the blood from chronic kidney disease can be a contributing factor in heart attacks and strokes.
- **End-stage renal disease** (ESRD), also known as ***kidney failure***, is the final stage of chronic kidney disease, and this condition is fatal unless the functions of the failed kidneys are replaced by dialysis, or with a successful kidney transplant.
- **Dialysis** (dye-**AL**-ih-sis) is a procedure to remove waste products, such as urea, creatinine, and excess water, from the blood of a patient whose kidneys no longer function (**dia-** means complete or through, and **-lysis** means separation). The two types of dialysis in common use are hemodialysis and peritoneal dialysis. See Chapter 10 for more information.

A **urinary tract infection** (UTI) usually begins in the bladder; however, such an infection can affect all parts of the urinary system. In older adults, a UTI often causes weakness, confusion, and increased risk of falls rather than urinary symptoms, and can cause urosepsis.

- **Urosepsis** (you-roh-**SEP**-sis) is a life-threatening systemic bacterial infection that can occur when a urinary tract infection spreads to the kidneys.

Older women are more prone to UTIs if they have urinary incontinence, as the use of absorbent incontinence pads traps urine close to the skin and provides an environment for bacteria to grow (Figure 19.8).

Urinary incontinence (in-**KON**-tih-nents) is the inability to control the voiding of urine.

- **Stress incontinence** is the inability to control the voiding of urine under physical stress such as running, sneezing, laughing, or coughing. This common condition occurs more often in women than in men.
- **Overactive bladder** (OAB), also known as ***urge incontinence***, occurs when the muscles of the bladder contract involuntarily even though the bladder is not actually full enough to indicate the need to urinate. See Chapter 10 for more information.

Urinary retention is the inability to completely empty the bladder when attempting to urinate. This condition is more common in men and is frequently associated with an enlarged prostate gland. It is frequently accompanied by overflow incontinence, and can also be caused by constipation.

- **Overflow incontinence** is continuous leaking from the bladder either because it is full or because it does not empty completely.
- A **Foley catheter** is an indwelling catheter used to drain urine for a patient with urinary retention. It is made of a flexible tube with a balloon that inflates inside the bladder to hold the tube in place. The Foley usually remains in place for at least several days, to allow the bladder to adjust to being non-distended. A ***bedside bag*** is a large urine collection bag that is often used overnight or for patients who are not able to walk. A ***leg bag*** is a small urine collection bag that attaches to the leg with elastic straps, and is emptied directly into the toilet.

Age-Related Male Genitourinary Problems

The location of the prostate, surrounding the urethra, frequently causes problems with urination for older men. According to the American Urological Association, over half of all men over 51 years of age have an enlarged prostate, and the incidence increases with age. See Chapter 10 for more information.

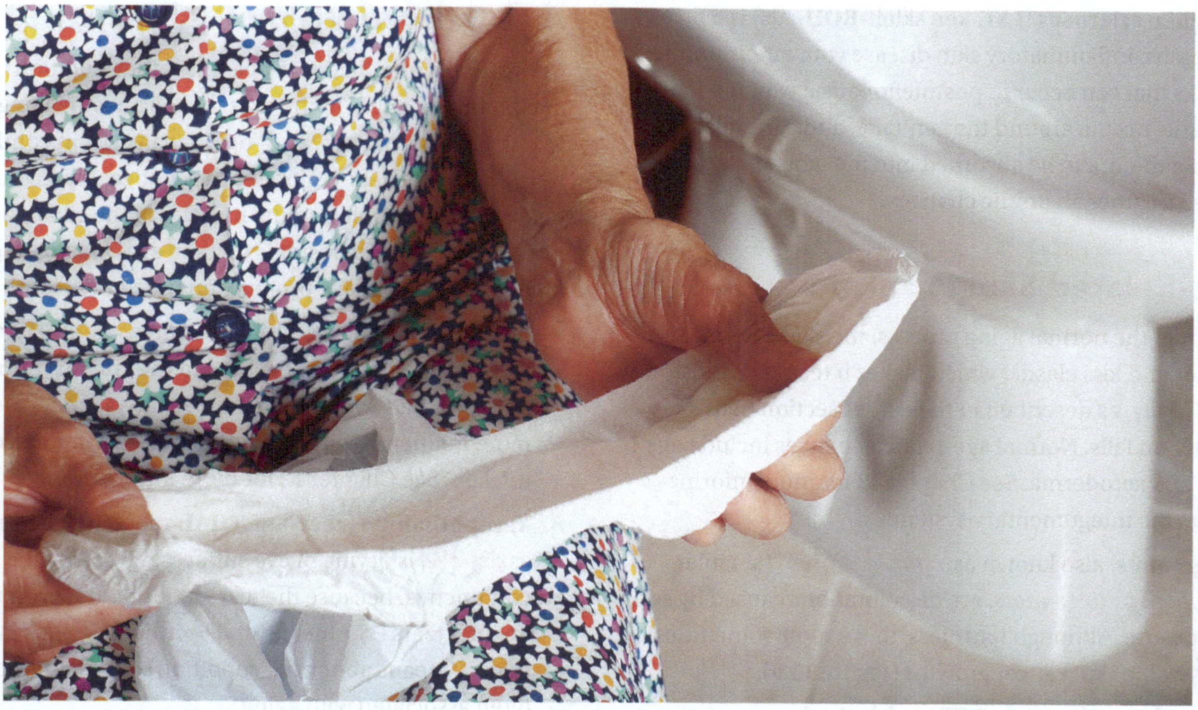

FIGURE 19.8 The use of absorbent incontinence pads increases the risk of a UTI.

- **Benign prostatic hyperplasia** (bee-**NINE** pros-**TAT**-ick **high**-per-**PLAY**-zee-ah) (BPH), also known as ***benign prostatic hypertrophy*** or ***enlarged prostate***, is an enlargement of the prostate gland that most often occurs in men older than age 50 (see Chapter 10, Figure 10.9). This condition can make urination difficult and causes other urinary tract problems for men.
- **Prostatism** (**PROS**-tah-tizm) is a disorder resulting from the compression or obstruction of the urethra due to benign prostatic hyperplasia (**prostat** means prostate gland, and **-ism** means condition of). This can produce difficulties with urination, including urinary retention.
- **Urinary hesitancy** is difficulty in starting a urinary stream. This condition is most common in older men with enlarged prostate glands.

Erectile dysfunction (ED), also known as ***impotence***, is the inability of the male to achieve or maintain a penile erection. A penis that is not erect is referred to as being ***flaccid***, or limp. Some medications may interfere with the ability to maintain an erection. See Chapter 15 for more information.

Age-Related Female Reproductive Problems

The average woman in the United States experiences menopause around 51 years old, and by age 65 most women are likely to be *postmenopausal*.

Postmenopause is the period of life after experiencing menopause, or the cessation of periods for at least 12 months. A person experiencing postmenopause is ***postmenopausal***. The hormonal changes associated with postmenopause include a decreased level of estrogen, which contributes to a higher risk of developing osteoporosis and heart disease.

- A **uterine prolapse** (**YOU**-ter-ihn proh-**LAPS**), also known as a ***pelvic floor hernia***, is a condition in which the weakening of pelvic muscles and supportive tissues allows the uterus to slide from its normal position in the pelvic cavity and sag into the vagina. ***Prolapse*** (also pronounced *PROH-laps*) means the falling or dropping down of an organ or internal part.
- A **pessary** is a soft, flexible rubber ring that fits into the vagina to help hold the uterus in place.
- **Vaginal atrophy**, also known as ***genitourinary syndrome of menopause*** (GSM), is thinning, drying, and inflammation of the vaginal walls caused by hormonal changes. It affects about half of all postmenopausal women and can be treated with vaginal moisturizers, lubricants, or estrogen therapy.
- **Postmenopausal labial fusion** is a severe version of vaginal atrophy in which the labia minora fuse together at least partially, obstructing access to the vagina and urethral meatus.

- **Lichen sclerosus** (**LYE**-ken skleh-**ROH**-sus) is a progressive inflammatory skin disease with autoimmune links that can occur in postmenopausal women. It primarily occurs around the genitalia, and can cause the labia minora to be absorbed into the labia majora, as well as other anatomic changes.

Age-Related Skin Problems

As part of the normal aging process, the skin becomes thinner and less elastic, which makes it tear and bruise more easily, as described in the earlier section in this chapter on falls. Normal age-related changes include age spots and xeroderma. See Chapter 13 for more information on the integumentary system.

- **Age spots**, also known as ***solar lentigines*** (singular, *lentigo*) or ***liver spots***, are discolorations caused by sun exposure. Although harmless, these spots sometimes resemble skin cancer growths (Figure 19.9).
- **Xeroderma** (zee-roh-**DER**-mah), also known as ***xerosis***, is excessively dry skin (**xer/o** means dry, and **-derma** means skin).

Age-Related Vision Problems

Presbyopia (**pres**-bee-**OH**-pee-ah) is the condition of common changes in the eyes that occur with aging (**presby** means old age, and **-opia** means vision condition). With age, near vision declines noticeably as the lens becomes less flexible and the muscles of the ciliary body become weaker. The result is that the eyes are no longer able to focus the image properly on the retina.

- **Floaters**, also known as ***vitreous floaters***, are particles of cellular debris that float in the vitreous humor and cast shadows on the retina. Floaters tend to occur more frequently with age as parts of the vitreous humor thicken. See Chapter 12 for more information.
- **Xerophthalmia** (**zeer**-ahf-**THAL**-mee-ah), also known as ***dry eye***, is drying of eye surfaces, including the conjunctiva, because the tear glands do not produce enough tears (**xer** means dry, **ophthalm** means eye, and **-ia** means abnormal condition). This condition is often associated with aging.
- **Ptosis** (**TOH**-sis) is the drooping of the upper eyelid that is usually due to muscle weakness or paralysis (**ptosis**

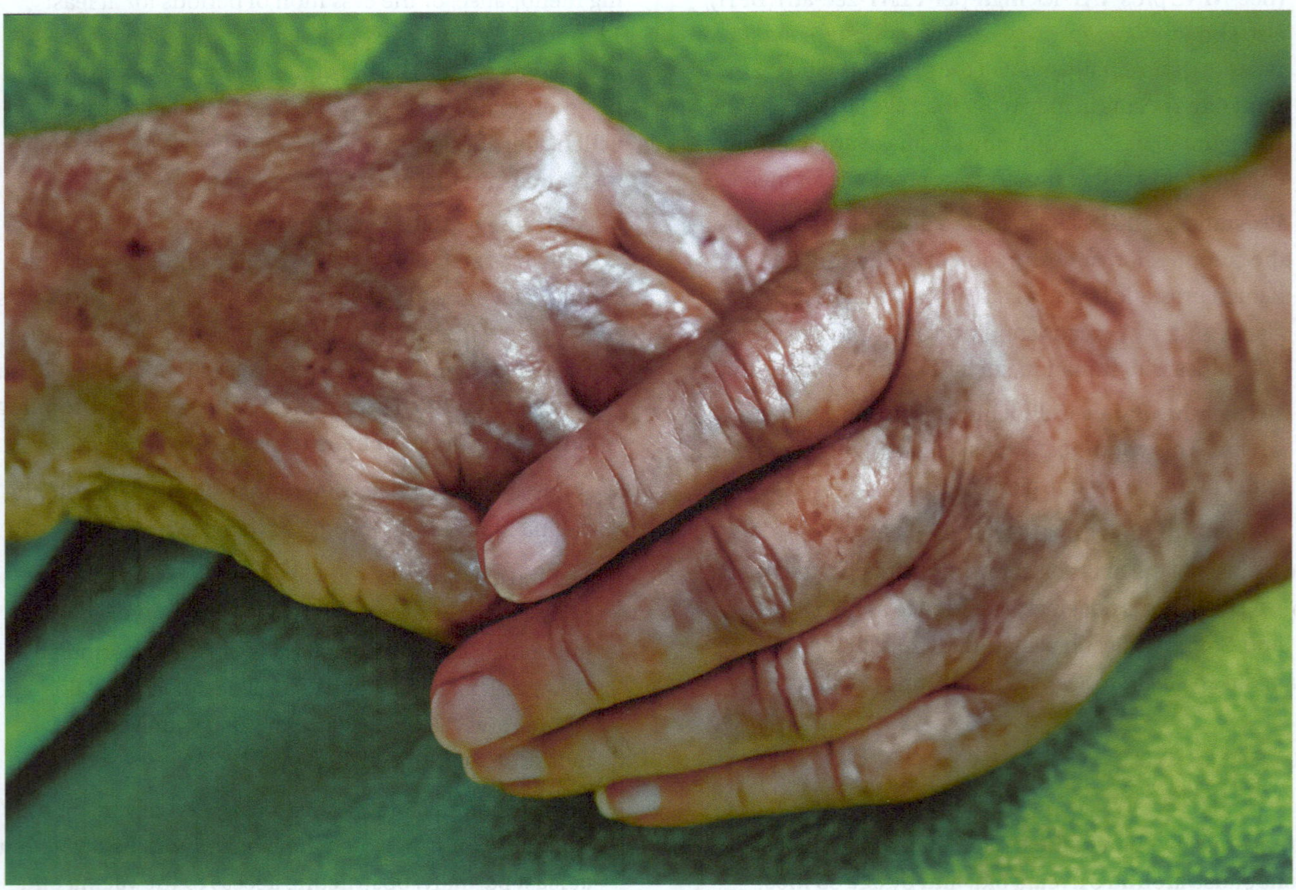

iStock.com/HAYKIRDI

FIGURE 19.9 Age spots are discolorations caused by sun exposure.

means drooping or sagging). The term *blepharoptosis* has the same meaning.

- **Involutional ectropion** (**in**-voh-**LOO**-shuh-nal eck-**TROH**-pee-on) is the eversion of the edge of an eyelid (**ec-** means out, **trop** means turn, and **-ion** means condition). *Eversion* means turning outward. This usually affects the lower lid, thereby exposing the inner surface of the eyelid to irritation and preventing tears from draining properly. Involutional ectropion is most common in older adults, and occurs as a result of the collagen fibers in the eyelid weakening with age, allowing the lower lid to sag with gravity. See Chapter 12 for more information.

A **cataract** (**KAT**-ah-rakt) is the loss of transparency of the lens that causes a progressive loss of visual clarity. The formation of most cataracts is associated with aging. Cataracts are treated with surgery. See Chapter 12 for more information.

Glaucoma (glaw-**KOH**-mah) is a group of diseases characterized by increased intraocular pressure that causes damage to the retinal nerve fibers and the optic nerve (see Chapter 12, Figure 12.8C). This increase in pressure is caused by a blockage in the flow of fluid out of the eye. If untreated, this pressure can cause the loss of peripheral vision and eventually blindness. Glaucoma is most common in adults over the age of 60. See Chapter 12 for more information.

- **Tonometry** (toh-**NOM**-eh-tree) is the measurement of intraocular pressure (**ton/o** means tension, and **-metry** means to measure). Abnormally high pressure can be an indication of glaucoma.
- A **laser trabeculoplasty** (trah-**BECK**-you-loh-**plas**-tee) is used to treat open-angle glaucoma by creating openings in the trabecular meshwork to allow the fluid to drain properly.

Age-related macular degeneration (AMD) occurs most frequently in older people and is the leading cause of severe vision loss in those over 60. While the symptoms often start in one eye, there is a high risk that AMD will also develop in the other eye. **Macular degeneration** (**MACK**-you-lar) (MD) is a gradually progressive condition in which the macula at the center of the retina is damaged, resulting in the loss of central vision but not in total blindness (**macul** means spot, and **-ar** mean pertaining to). See Chapter 12 for more information.

Age-Related Hearing Problems

At least 30% of adults over 65 years of age have some hearing loss, and hearing loss becomes more common and severe with age.

Presbycusis (pres-beh-**KOO**-sis) is a gradual loss of sensorineural hearing that occurs as the body ages (**presby** means old age, and **-cusis** means hearing). The amount of hearing loss varies, and may be affected by a person's genetics, environment, and exposure to loud noises.

- **Impacted cerumen** is an accumulation of earwax that forms a solid mass by adhering to the walls of the external auditory canal. *Impacted* means lodged or wedged firmly in place. Impacted cerumen can cause otalgia, tinnitus, and temporary hearing loss. Impacted cerumen is more common in older adults, and removal of the earwax can help improve hearing.
- **Vertigo** (**VER**-tih-goh) is a sense of whirling, dizziness, and loss of balance that is often combined with nausea and vomiting. Vertigo occurs more frequently with age, and can also occur after a stroke. See Chapter 12 for more information.

Sensorineural hearing loss (sen-suh-ree-**NOOR**-al), also known as *nerve deafness*, develops when the auditory nerve or hair cells in the inner ear are damaged. This is usually due to age, noise exposure, or an acoustic neuroma. The source of this hearing loss can be located in the inner ear, in the nerve from the inner ear to the brain, or in the brain.

- **Deafness** is the complete or partial loss of the ability to hear. It can range from the inability to hear sounds of a certain pitch or intensity, to a complete loss of hearing. See Chapter 12 for more information.

Hearing Aids

Hearing aids are electronic devices that are worn to correct a hearing loss. See Chapter 12 for more information.

- Hearing aids are worn *behind the ear* (BTE), *in the ear* (ITE), *in the canal* (ITC), or *completely in the canal* (CIC).
- ITC and CIC hearing aids are best for adults with mild to moderate hearing loss.
- ITE and BTE hearing aids are best for adults with mild to severe hearing loss.
- An **assistive listening device** (ALD) transmits, processes, or amplifies sound and can be used with or without a hearing aid. An ALD can be helpful in eliminating distracting background noise. The Americans with Disabilities Act (ADA) requires that many public places provide assisted listening devices.
- *Lip reading* is another way for adults with hearing loss to understand speech, although the technique can be difficult to master and not fully reliable.

Age-Related Endocrine Problems

Metabolic syndrome is a common medical condition that is present in up to 40% of people over the age of 60. Metabolic syndrome is characterized by risk factors for developing heart disease, stroke, and type 2 diabetes. These factors may include hypertension, hyperlipidemia, obesity with central adiposity (excessive fat in the abdomen), and high insulin levels in the blood.

- **Hypertension** (HTN), commonly known as ***high blood pressure***, is the elevation of arterial blood pressure to a level that is likely to cause damage to the cardiovascular system.
- **Hyperlipidemia** (**high**-per-**lip**-ih-**DEE**-mee-ah) is the general term used to describe elevated levels of cholesterol and other fatty substances in the blood (**hyper-** means excessive, **lipid** means fat, and **-emia** means blood condition). Excessively high levels of certain types of cholesterol can lead to heart disease.
- **Obesity** (oh-**BEE**-sih-tee) is a weight classification based on BMI that is higher than 30. Obesity is frequently present as a comorbidity with conditions such as metabolic syndrome, hypertension, and diabetes.
- **Type 2 diabetes mellitus** (**dye**-ah-**BEE**-teez **MEL**-ih-tus) (DM) is an insulin resistance disorder characterized by hyperglycemia resulting from defects in the body's ability to use insulin properly.

Complications of Poorly Controlled Diabetes

- **Diabetic retinopathy** (**ret**-ih-**NOP**-ah-thee) occurs when diabetes damages the tiny blood vessels in the retina. This causes blood to leak into the posterior segment of the eyeball and produces the damage that causes the loss of vision. The risk of diabetic retinopathy continues to increase over time, especially in poorly controlled diabetes.
- **Diabetic neuropathy** (new-**ROP**-ah-thee) is peripheral neuropathy caused by poorly controlled diabetes. The loss of sensation, especially coupled with poor peripheral circulation, increases the likelihood of developing a wound on the foot from an unnoticed blister. Hyperglycemia and poor circulation cause slow wound healing, and gangrene is a serious risk.
- **Gangrene** is tissue death caused by a severe shortage of blood supply due to illness, injury, and/or infection (Figure 19.10). This condition usually affects fingers, toes, or limbs, and untreated can lead to *sepsis*. If circulation cannot be restored, the affected limb is amputated.
- **Sepsis** (**SEP**-sis), also known as ***septicemia***, is a potentially life-threatening infection that results from bacteria or other infectious organisms entering the bloodstream.

TREATMENT CONSIDERATIONS FOR OLDER ADULTS

While the treatment procedures for older adults are not necessarily different than those for other patients, the medical care of older adults can present multiple challenges. In addition to age-related physiologic changes, there is also a higher likelihood of comorbidities that may complicate care and result in medication interactions. The risk of a treatment to an older adult must be weighed against the benefit, including quality of life. The psychosocial aspects of treatment cannot be overlooked, including the challenges of ensuring adherence to medical recommendations, recognizing the risk of isolation and depression, and eventually documenting the patient's preferences for life-sustaining treatment and end-of-life care.

Medication Considerations

Polypharmacy (**poh**-lee-**FAR**-mah-see) is the use of multiple medications by a single person, often for different conditions. A 2010 study by the NIH found that older adults take an average of four different daily medications, and nearly 40% of all older adults take six or more daily medications.

Each medication added to an older adult's daily regimen adds a risk of interaction between medications, as well as side effects of each individual medication.

- Older adults with impaired kidney function or kidney failure experience diminished ***renal clearance***, or the excretion of a medication into the urine by the kidneys.
- **Renal dosing** is the adjustment of a medication dose to compensate for decreased kidney function. Medications that may require renal dosing include lithium, digoxin, gabapentin, and multiple antibiotics including cephalexin and ciprofloxacin.
- Older adults with impaired liver function experience diminished ***hepatic clearance***, or the removal of a medication from the blood by the liver.
- **Hepatic dosing** is the adjustment of a medication dose to compensate for decreased liver function. Medications that may require hepatic dosing include heparin, hydralazine, morphine, and multiple antibiotics including clindamycin and doxycycline.

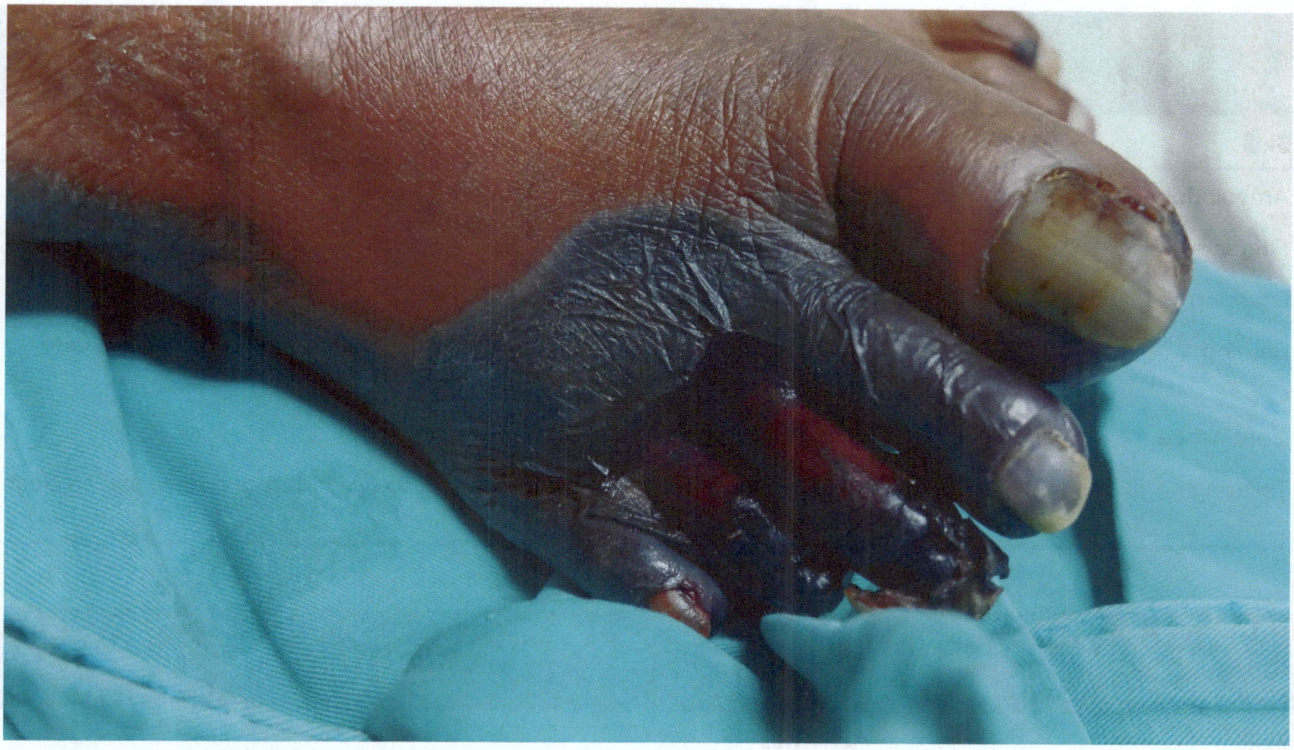

Casa nayafana/Shutterstock.com

FIGURE 19.10 Gangrene is tissue death caused by a severe shortage of blood supply.

Medication adherence is the extent to which a person is taking their medications as prescribed by their doctor. Several studies have shown that medication adherence is less common in older adults who have been prescribed a large number of daily medications than for older adults who only have one daily medication.

Factors in medication adherence, particularly for older adults, include:

- Financial burden of buying multiple medications, especially for older adults on a fixed income
- Difficulty understanding dosage instructions
- Difficulty remembering to take the medications
- Lack of understanding of why the medication is important, or belief that it is unnecessary
- Concern about potential or actual side effects
- Inconvenience of dosage schedules requiring more than one daily dose

Assistive Care

As aging progresses, older adults who had been living independently may benefit from caregiver assistance, either part time or full time. Older adults often want to remain in their home as long as possible, and caregiver assistance can help achieve that goal. In order to ensure that older adults have the level of help that they need to live independently, health care providers use assessment measures such as the ***Katz Index of Independence in Activities of Daily Living*** (Katz ADL) and ***Lawton-Brody Instrumental Activities of Daily Living*** scales.

Activities of daily living (ADLs) are the basic skills needed to independently care for one's self (Table 19.3).

Instrumental ADLs (IADLs) are more complex activities needed to live independently (Table 19.4).

For older adults who only need assistance with some IADLs or ADLs, a **home health aide** is a caregiver who can help with errands, tasks around the house, daily activities, preparing food, and organizing home medications.

Long-Term Care Facilities

Older adults who are no longer able to continue living at home have several options for alternative living environments, also known as ***long-term care facilities***, depending on the level of assistance they require. These facilities include board and care, assisted living, and nursing homes. Each care facility has caregivers available around the clock, and provides assistance with housekeeping, laundry, and food preparation. Some facilities offer different levels of care so that residents can remain in the same place even as their needs change.

TABLE 19.3

Activities of Daily Living

Skill	Activities
Ambulation/Transferring	ability to walk or move from bed to a wheelchair
Feeding	ability to feed oneself
Dressing	ability to select appropriate clothing and put it on
Bathing	ability to wash and groom oneself and maintain dental hygiene, nail care, and hair care
Continence	ability to control bladder and bowel function
Toileting	ability to reach the toilet when needed, to use it appropriately, and to clean oneself

TABLE 19.4

Instrumental Activities of Daily Living

Skill	Activities
Ability to Use Phone	ability to use telephone
Shopping	ability to manage shopping for clothing and other necessities
Food Preparation	ability to manage grocery shopping and meal preparation
Housecleaning	ability to manage home maintenance needs, clean the kitchen after meals, maintain living areas reasonably well
Laundry	ability to do laundry independently
Transportation	ability to manage transport needs, either by driving or arranging alternative transportation
Responsibility for Own Medications	ability to obtain medications and take them as directed
Ability to Handle Finances	ability to pay bills, budget, and manage assets

- A **board and care** (B&C) is a small assisted living facility, usually based in someone's personal home. A board and care is ideal for an older adult who wants a home-like environment and may spend part of their day independently.
- A traditional **assisted living facility** (ALF) is a hotel-like residential facility with caregivers; some maintain medical staff on the property. Most assisted living facilities have small, individual rooms for residents and large communal areas that are shared, including dining rooms. There are often group activities for residents, including fitness classes, concerts, bingo, and trivia.

Older adults who require more medical assistance on a short-term basis to recover from a specific problem, such as a broken bone, can go to a skilled nursing facility, while older adults who require medical assistance for an extended length of time can go to a nursing home.

- A **skilled nursing facility** (SNF), also known as a ***rehab***, is a medical facility that offers all of the same amenities as an assisted living facility, but also includes specialty medical care, such as skilled nursing care, speech-language pathology, and physical and occupational therapy. Patients who are not sick enough to require continued hospitalization but still need specialized medical assistance for their recovery can go to a SNF.

- A **nursing home** is a long-term care facility that has medical staff and caregivers on site. Patients who require 24-hour monitoring and assistance, either for medical or behavioral reasons, often live in a nursing home. Many nursing homes also have memory care units.
- **Memory care** is a specific unit in an assisted living facility or nursing home for older adults with dementia. The staff is specially trained in management of dementia patients, and the units are locked to keep patients from leaving the premises.

END OF LIFE, DEATH AND DYING

As they age, older adults become increasingly at risk of developing health problems that are eventually fatal. Death is the end of life, and is inevitable. It is important to discuss priorities with the patient. ***Quantity of life*** means trying every treatment despite potential side effects, to prolong one's life for as long as possible. ***Quality of life*** means focusing treatment on remaining comfortable and maximizing the quality of one's remaining life.

Advance Directives

Advance directives are documents used to provide guidance about what types of treatment a person may or may not want to receive in case of a future medical emergency. They can also state who is authorized to make health care decisions if a person cannot do so themselves.

- A **health care proxy** (HCP), also referred to as a ***durable power of attorney for health care***, is an advance directive allowing the patient to appoint a trusted individual, such as a family member or close friend, to make treatment decisions should the patient be unable make them.
- A **living will**, also known as ***Physician's Orders for Life-Sustaining Treatment*** (POLST), is a document that allows a person to state their wishes for end-of-life medical care, in case they become unable to communicate their decisions.
- A **Do Not Resuscitate order** (DNR), also known as ***no code*** or ***allow natural death***, is a legal document stating that a person does not wish to receive cardiopulmonary resuscitation (CPR) if their heart or breathing stops. This advance directive is sometimes put in place near the end of life, or when a patient has a terminal illness with no possibility of a cure.
- An advance directive specifying that a person wishes everything possible done to save their life, including CPR and intubation, is called a ***full code***.

End-of-Life Care

Palliative care (**PAH**-lee-ah-**tiv**) is medical care given to a patient with a medical condition that cannot be cured, such as cancer. Palliative treatment focuses on quality of life and may still involve interventions such as chemotherapy and radiation.

Hospice care is medical care given to a patient with a life expectancy of six months or less. Hospice treatment is designed to maximize the patient's comfort and quality of life, and often involves medication to minimize distressing symptoms associated with the dying process.

- **Death with dignity**, also known as ***physician-assisted death***, is an end-of-life option that allows terminally ill adults to obtain medications from their doctor in order to have the choice of ending their own life. This is only legal in certain states and countries, and there are strict restrictions and a waiting period before the medications are dispensed.

Dying Process

The **dying process** is a period of time that may occur leading up to death when a person's body begins to shut down. People who die from cancer and other chronic illnesses are more likely to experience a dying process rather than a sudden death. There are two recognizable stages in the dying process, pre-active dying and active dying, although not every person will experience every symptom.

- **Pre-active dying** is the first stage of the dying process. Pre-active dying usually lasts two weeks, and is characterized by restlessness/agitation/confusion, increased lethargy, decreased appetite, slow wound healing, generalized edema, episodes of apnea, and a recognition of dying paired with a desire to ensure affairs are in order.
- **Active dying** is the last stage of the dying process before death. Active dying usually lasts three days and is characterized by hypotension, periods of unresponsiveness, Cheyne-Stokes respiration, mottled skin, decreased urine output, terminal agitation, severe respiratory congestion, and labored, noisy breathing through a wide-open mouth.
- **Cheyne-Stokes respiration** (**CHAYN STOHKS**) is an irregular pattern of breathing characterized by

alternating rapid or shallow respiration followed by slower respiration or apnea. This pattern sometimes occurs in comatose patients or those nearing death.

The person going through the dying process can also experience some distressing signs and symptoms.

- **Terminal agitation** is a form of delirium that occurs at end-of-life. It is characterized by restlessness, agitation, anxiety, and confusion.
- **Air hunger** is a persistent, distressing feeling of shortness of breath and inability to fully catch one's breath that often occurs at end-of-life. ***Morphine*** is used to help ease air hunger, as it decreases respiratory drive, which is the normal bodily mechanism to keep blood oxygen levels normal.
- **Death rattle**, also known as ***terminal respiratory secretions***, refers to the labored, noisy breathing that can occur at end-of-life from retained respiratory secretions and inability to swallow. ***Atropine*** is used to dry respiratory secretions.

Death

Medically speaking, **death** is the irreversible end of all brain, heart, and lung activity. Depending on the cause of death, one may happen before the others (Figure 19.11).

Cardiac arrest is an event in which the heart abruptly stops beating or develops an arrhythmia that prevents it from pumping blood effectively. ***Sudden cardiac death*** results when treatment of cardiac arrest is not provided within a few minutes.

- **Asystole** (ay-**SIS**-toh-lee), known as a ***flat line***, is the complete lack of electrical activity in the heart (**a-** means without, and **systole** means contraction). The resulting lack of heart contractions, with no blood pumping from the heart and no blood flow through the body, is one of the conditions required for a medical practitioner to certify death.
- **Cardiopulmonary resuscitation**, commonly known as ***CPR***, is an emergency procedure for life support consisting of artificial respiration (mouth-to-mouth breathing)

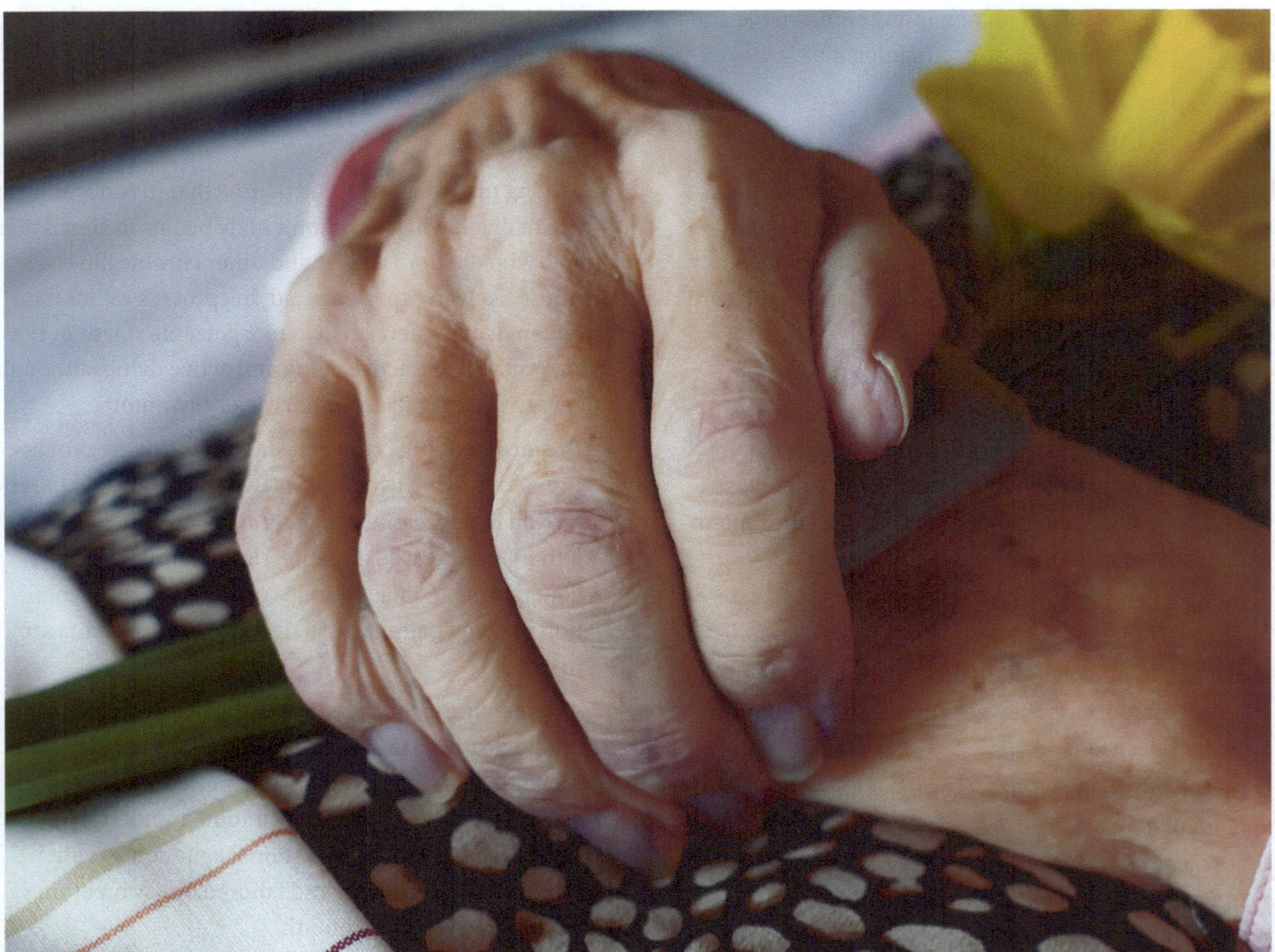

iStock.com/Kliim

FIGURE 19.11 Death is the irreversible end of all brain, heart, and lung activity.

and manual external chest compression. *Cardiopulmonary* means pertaining to the heart and lungs.

Respiratory arrest is the absence of breathing and can manifest as apnea or agonal respirations.

- **Apnea** (**AP**-nee-ah) is the absence of spontaneous respiration (**a-** means without, and **-pnea** means breathing).
- **Agonal respirations** (**AH**-goh-nal), also known as *guppy breathing*, are ineffective breaths that frequently accompany cardiac arrest. They should not be mistaken for effective breaths and are a form of respiratory failure.

Brain death is the complete loss of brain function. Brain death can be difficult to diagnose, and criteria for certifying brain death usually include physical exam with absence of reflexes, and no detectable activity on electroencephalography (EEG). A person who is brain dead can be temporarily kept alive by mechanical ventilation if they are donating their organs.

After Death

Postmortem means after death. A postmortem examination is also known as an autopsy.

- An **autopsy** (**AW**-top-see) is a surgical examination of a cadaver usually conducted to determine the cause of death. However, it is also a way of evaluating the presence of disease and the effectiveness of treatment.
    - A **cadaver** (kuh-**DAH**-vair), also known as a *corpse*, is a dead human body.
- **Organ donation** is the process through which a person volunteers to have their organs removed and transplanted into another person. Most organ donation occurs after death, but some organs such as the kidneys and liver can be donated while the donor is alive.
- A **medical examiner** (ME) is an official who performs autopsies to determine the cause of death, most commonly on people who died unexpectedly or in suspicious circumstances.
- A **morgue** is a refrigerated area in the hospital where cadavers are kept temporarily until they are released for autopsy, cremation, or burial (Figure 19.12).

ABBREVIATIONS RELATED TO GERONTOLOGY

Table 19.5 presents an overview of the abbreviations related to the terms introduced in this chapter. *Note:* To avoid errors or confusion, always be cautious when using abbreviations.

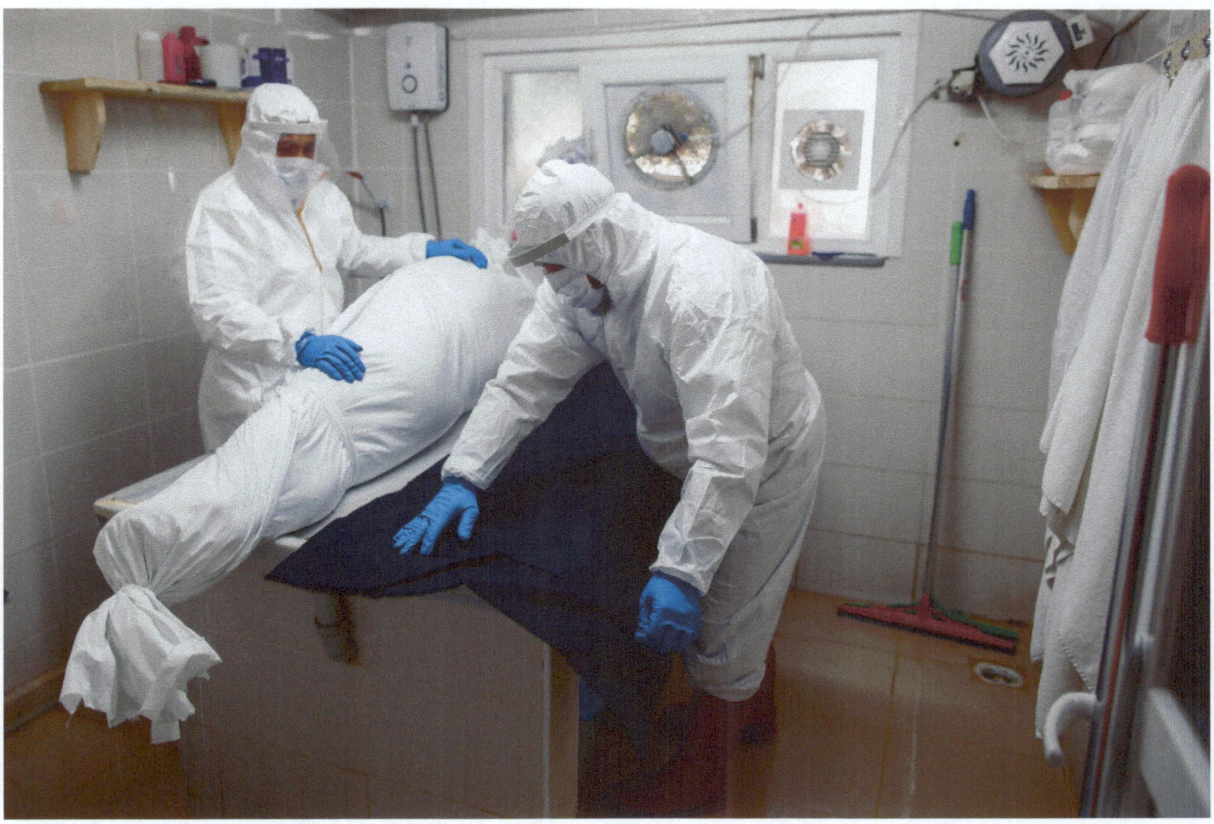

Huseyin Aldemir/Shutterstock.com

FIGURE 19.12 Morgue workers prepare a cadaver to be transferred for burial.

TABLE 19.5

Abbreviations Related to Gerontology

Activities of Daily Living = ADLs	**ADLs** = Activities of Daily Living
alert and oriented = A&O	**A&O** = alert and oriented
assisted living facility = ALF	**ALF** = assisted living facility
board and care = B&C	**B&C** = board and care
bundle branch block = BBB	**BBB** = bundle branch block
congestive heart failure = CHF	**CHF** = congestive heart failure
do not resuscitate order = DNR	**DNR** = do not resuscitate order
dyspnea on exertion = DOE	**DOE** = dyspnea on exertion
failure to thrive = FTT	**FTT** = failure to thrive
instrumental ADLs = IADLs	**IADLs** = instrumental ADLs
skilled nursing facility = SNF	**SNF** = skilled nursing facility

CHAPTER 19

LEARNING EXERCISES

Matching Word Parts 1

Write the correct answer in the middle column.

	Definition	Correct Answer	Possible Answers
19.1.	old age	______________	xer/o
19.2.	without	______________	-penia
19.3.	deficiency	______________	geront/o
19.4.	breathing	______________	an-
19.5.	dry	______________	-pnea

Matching Word Parts 2

Write the correct answer in the middle column.

	Definition	Correct Answer	Possible Answers
19.6.	removal	______________	presby/o
19.7.	speech	______________	dys-
19.8.	painful, difficult	______________	-phagia
19.9.	old age	______________	de-
19.10.	swallowing	______________	-phasia

Matching Word Parts 3

Write the correct answer in the middle column.

	Definition	Correct Answer	Possible Answers
19.11.	after	______________	-ology
19.12.	the study of	______________	-systole

19.13. abnormal hardening ______________________ **post-**

19.14. field of medicine ______________________ **-sclerosis**

19.15. contraction ______________________ **-iatrics**

Definitions

Select the correct answer, and write it on the line provided.

19.16. A ______________________ is a physician who specializes in the care of older people.

gerontologist primary care provider geriatrician hospice nurse

19.17. ______________________ dying is the first stage of the dying process and is characterized by a recognition of dying paired with a desire to ensure affairs are in order.

Pre-active Active Terminal Hospice

19.18. ______________________ dosing is the adjustment of a medication dose to compensate for decreased liver function.

Cardiac Adherence Renal Hepatic

19.19. A ______________________ is an implanted mechanical pump that helps the heart circulate blood.

pacemaker ventricular assist device heart transplant heart valve replacement

19.20. A/An ______________________ is the permanent tightening of muscles and ligaments that occurs when connective tissues are replaced with fibrous tissues.

contracture pressure ulcer atrophy cataract

19.21. A/An ______________________ is also known as a durable power of attorney for health care.

advance directive living will health care proxy Do Not Resuscitate order

19.22. A form of delirium that occurs at end-of-life, characterized by restlessness, agitation, anxiety, and confusion is known as ______________________.

agonal respirations Cheyne–Stokes active dying terminal agitation

19.23. The surgical examination of a cadaver usually conducted to determine the cause of death is called a/an ______________________.

autopsy morgue postmortem organ donation

19.24. ________________ is an end-of-life option that allows terminally ill adults to have the choice of ending their own life.

Active dying   Death with dignity   Do Not Resuscitate order   Hospice care

19.25. The gradual progression of unavoidable physiologic changes that occur as a part of growing older are known as ________________.

normal aging   senescence   inflamm-aging   gerontology

Matching Facilities

Write the correct answer in the middle column.

	Definition	Correct Answer	Possible Answers
19.26.	a small assisted living facility based in a personal home	________________	memory care
19.27.	a medical facility that offers specialty medical care	________________	board and care
19.28.	a locked unit for older adults with dementia	________________	skilled nursing facility
19.29.	a hotel-like residential facility with caregivers	________________	nursing home
19.30.	a long-term care facility with medical staff on site	________________	assisted living facility

Which Word? 1

Select the correct answer, and write it on the line provided.

19.31. ________________ care is quality of life-focused medical care given to a patient with a medical condition that cannot be cured, such as cancer, and may still involve interventions such as chemotherapy and radiation.

Hospice   Palliative

19.32. ________________ is an acute condition of confusion, disorientation, disordered thinking and memory, agitation, and hallucinations.

Delirium   Dementia

19.33. The gradual process of decreasing the amount of work of breathing done by the ventilator is known as

______________________.

weaning extubation

19.34. A limit on the amount of water and other liquids a person drinks per day is known as

______________________.

bowel rest fluid restriction

19.35. Ineffective breaths that frequently accompany cardiac arrest are called ______________________.

agonal respirations respiratory arrest

Spelling Counts

Find the misspelled word in each sentence. Then write that word, spelled correctly, on the line provided.

19.36. Lichen schlerosis is a progressive inflammatory skin disease that can occur in postmenopausal women.

____

19.37. Assites is an abnormal accumulation of serous fluid in the peritoneal cavity which causes shortness of breath. ______________________

19.38. Someone who has lost all of their teeth is edentaluss. ______________________

19.39. Immunosinesince is the gradual, natural decline of the immune system as a result of aging.

____

19.40. An eckimosis is commonly known as a bruise. ______________________

Abbreviation Identification 1

In the space provided, write the words that each abbreviation stands for.

19.41. **SNF** ______________________

19.42. **BBB** ______________________

19.43. **B&C** ______________________

19.44. **CHF** ______________________

19.45. **FTT** ______________________

Term Selection

Select the correct answer, and write it on the line provided.

19.46. A complete block in electrical conduction between the atria and ventricles is known as ______________________ heart block.

first-degree | third-degree | second-degree | bundle branch

19.47. The amount of energy required to inhale and exhale is known as ______________________.

work of breathing | air hunger | respiratory failure | dyspnea

19.48. ______________________ is the narrowing and stiffening of arteries due to the buildup of plaque.

Chronic venous insufficiency | Carotid artery stenosis | Atherosclerosis | Aneurysm

19.49. The branch of medicine relating to the health of older adults is known as ______________________.

palliative care | geriatrics | hospice | gerontology

19.50. The term *heart valve* ______________________ means a condition when a heart valve does not close tightly, allowing blood to leak back through the opening.

stenosis | disease | reflux | regurgitation

Sentence Completion 1

Write the correct term on the line provided.

19.51. The term ______________________ describes the mental activities associated with thinking, learning, and memory.

19.52. The term ______________________ describes the progressive loss of renal function over months or years.

19.53. The ______________________ is a period of time that may occur leading up to death when a person's body begins to shut down.

19.54. The term ______________________ describes a persistent, distressing feeling of shortness of breath and inability to fully catch one's breath that often occurs at end-of-life.

19.55. ______________________ involves not giving a person anything to eat or drink by mouth for one to two days to give the digestive tract a chance to return to normal function.

Word Surgery

Divide each term into its component word parts. Write these word parts, in sequence, on the lines provided. When necessary, use a slash (/) to indicate a combining vowel. (You may not need all of the lines provided.)

19.56. **Xerostomia** is the lack of adequate saliva due to diminished secretions by the salivary glands.

__________ __________ __________ __________

19.57. **Valvuloplasty** is the surgical repair of a heart valve that has a narrowed opening.

__________ __________ __________ __________

19.58. **Osteoporosis** is a marked loss of bone density and an increase in bone porosity frequently associated with aging.

__________ __________ __________ __________

19.59. **Sarcopenia** is the loss of muscle mass, strength, and function that comes with aging.

__________ __________ __________ __________

19.60. **Nasogastric intubation** is the placement of a flexible tube through the nose and into the stomach.

__________ __________ __________ __________

True/False

If the statement is true, write **True** on the line. If the statement is false, write **False** on the line.

19.61. ________ Death is the irreversible end of all brain, heart, and lung activity.

19.62. ________ Diabetic neuropathy occurs when diabetes damages the tiny blood vessels in the retina.

19.63. ________ Xerophthalmia is excessively dry skin.

19.64. ________ Lack of muscle coordination during voluntary movements is known as ataxia.

19.65. ________ The physical removal of stool from the rectal vault is called manual disimpaction.

Clinical Conditions

Write the correct answer on the line provided.

19.66. After weeks of passing clots and dark red blood in his stools, Mr. Panlasigui was diagnosed with bleeding from the colon. His doctor referred to this as a/an ____________________ GI bleed.

19.67. Dr. Nguyen looked at the persistent atrial fibrillation on her patient's EKG. Since it hadn't responded to treatment, it was time to consider ______________________, using heat or extreme cold to destroy the heart tissue triggering the abnormal heart rhythm.

19.68. When Mr. Yang's family decided to stop treatment and let him die naturally, the ICU staff removed him from the ventilator and took the endotracheal tube out. This is known as ______________________.

19.69. After Barry White's second fall at home, the nurse in the ER put a yellow band on his wrist to mark him as a/an ______________________ patient, indicating that he should be closely monitored when moving around.

19.70. After his stroke, Jerome Braceros was unable to get out of bed independently, and developed an open ulcerated wound on his sacrum. This is known as a/an ______________________.

19.71. In the days leading up to her death, Mrs. Lipkin developed labored, noisy breathing. Although her daughters were concerned, the hospice nurse said it was a/an ______________________, which can occur normally at end-of-life from retained respiratory secretions.

19.72. After his death in the hospital, Mr. Dimengo's body was taken to the ______________________, a refrigerated area where cadavers are temporarily kept until they are released for autopsy, cremation, or burial.

19.73. The term for the drooping of the upper eyelid that is usually due to muscle weakness or paralysis is ______________________.

19.74. While Prateek Ambhalal was being assessed for a potential stroke, the nurse performed a/an ______________________. This is a test to assess the patient's risk of dysphagia and aspiration.

19.75. Dr. Fong warned Mrs. Rodriguez's family that while she currently only had ______________________, this condition, characterized by short-term memory loss, may be an early predictor of dementia.

Which Is the Correct Medical Term?

Select the correct answer, and write it on the line provided.

19.76. A ______________________ is a registered nurse who specializes in end-of-life care.

home care provider hospice nurse home health aide palliative care nurse

19.77. Inflammation in the lower extremities caused by chronic venous insufficiency and venous stasis is called ______________________.

stasis dermatitis venous ulcer chronic venous insufficiency varicose veins

19.78. Ongoing, low-grade, age-related systemic inflammation without apparent cause is known as ______________________.

presbyopia immunosenescence inflamm-aging presbycusis

19.79. ______________________ is a slowly progressive decline in mental abilities that is often accompanied by personality changes.

Delirium Dementia Mild cognitive impairment Cognition

19.80. The study of the aging process is known as ______________________.

normal aging geriatrics senescence gerontology

Abbreviation Identification 2

In the space provided, write the words that each abbreviation stands for.

19.81. **ADLs** ______________________

19.82. **A&O** ______________________

19.83. **DNR** ______________________

19.84. **ALF** ______________________

19.85. **DOE** ______________________

Sentence Completion 2

Write the correct term on the line provided.

19.86. The term ______________________ *dementia* describes a form of dementia caused by a stroke or other restriction of the flow of blood to the brain.

19.87. The term ______________________ describes osteoarthritis that has progressed to the point where the articular cartilage is gone.

19.88. A/An ______________________ *fall* occurs when a person slips, trips, or loses their balance.

19.89. A/An ______________________ is a caregiver who can help with errands, tasks around the house, and daily activities.

19.90. ______________________ is the period of life after experiencing the cessation of periods for at least 12 months.

Which Word? 2

Select the correct answer, and write it on the line provided.

19.91. A/An ______________________________ GI bleed is blood loss from the esophagus, stomach, or duodenum.

upper lower

19.92. ______________________________ care is medical care given to a patient with a life expectancy of six months or less.

Palliative Hospice

19.93. The loss of the normal rhythm of the heartbeat is known as a/an ______________________________.

arrhythmia heart block

19.94. Irregular open pits in the skin that occur as a result of venous stasis are called ______________________________.

venous ulcers stasis dermatitis

19.95. A ______________________________ is an injury that occurs from shearing pressure, where a flap of epidermis is pulled away from the underlying tissue.

pressure ulcer skin tear

Abbreviation Identification 3

In the space provided, write the words that each abbreviation stands for.

19.96. **HCP** ______________________________

19.97. **IADLs** ______________________________

19.98. **ME** ______________________________

19.99. **SBO** ______________________________

19.100. **NIHSS** ______________________________

The Human Touch

CRITICAL THINKING EXERCISE

The following story and questions are designed to stimulate critical thinking through class discussion or as a brief essay response. There are no right or wrong answers to these questions.

Corazon Pamintuan barely held back a sigh as her mother, Regina, pushed her plate to the floor after just a few bites of lunch in the memory care unit of Serene Care Assisted Living Facility. Mrs. Pamintuan had been living in Serene Care for five years, moving in shortly after her 70th birthday, when the demands of managing her type 2 diabetes, diabetic neuropathy, and dementia had become too difficult for Corazon to manage at home.

During that time, she had been fairly communicative and compliant with treatment, despite her advancing dementia. Her appetite had always been good. However, over the last few months, she seemed to be noticeably declining. Much of her communication had been limited to "Yes" or "No" to direct questions, and sometimes she refused to speak at all. Additionally, she no longer seemed to care as much about food.

Corazon leaned forward and took one of her mother's hands, trying to get her to make eye contact, her eyes filling with tears. "Mom, please don't do that. Are you hungry? Do you want some different food? What can I get for you?" Mrs. Pamintuan just shook her head and wandered over to take a seat in front of the TV instead, her daughter's presence apparently already forgotten.

Alfred Black, Serene Care's registered dietitian, waited a moment, until Corazon seemed to have her emotions under control, before he started talking. "This has become a pretty common pattern at mealtimes, unfortunately. She doesn't tend to eat more than half of her food at best, even the things she used to eat every week. As I mentioned on the phone, we've noticed that she's losing weight. Does Mrs. Pamintuan have any favorite foods that you think we could try?"

Corazon nodded and pulled a list of foods from her purse. "My mom used to eat a lot of traditional Filipino foods, and she always had a sweet tooth—senorita bread, leche flan, turon—you know, all the things that aren't good for her diabetes. But maybe if we tried something closer to what she used to eat back home, she might want more of it, without it having to be sweets? I can bring some adobo and see if she'll eat that the next time I come."

Alfred took the list and looked it over. "Of course, and we can also try some calorie supplement drinks. I know you'd previously said that you didn't want to consider a feeding tube, so I just wanted to check and see if you still feel the same way about that."

"No, absolutely not!" Corazon's answer was immediate and emphatic, and she brushed away tears angrily. "She told me before she came in here that she didn't want anything like that, and I promised her we'd never do it. I'm not going to break my promise to her!"

Suggested Discussion Topics

1. Loss of appetite often accompanies advancing dementia and is one of the signs that someone is approaching end-of-life. How aggressively do you think this should be treated?
2. Would your answer be different if Mrs. Pamintuan were only 56 years old? What if she were 96?
3. With increased life expectancy and an aging population, what do you think geriatric and end-of-life care are going to look like in the future?
4. What additional challenges would arise for Mrs. Pamintuan's care if her family lived far away or were not actively involved in her care?

CHAPTER 20

ONCOLOGY

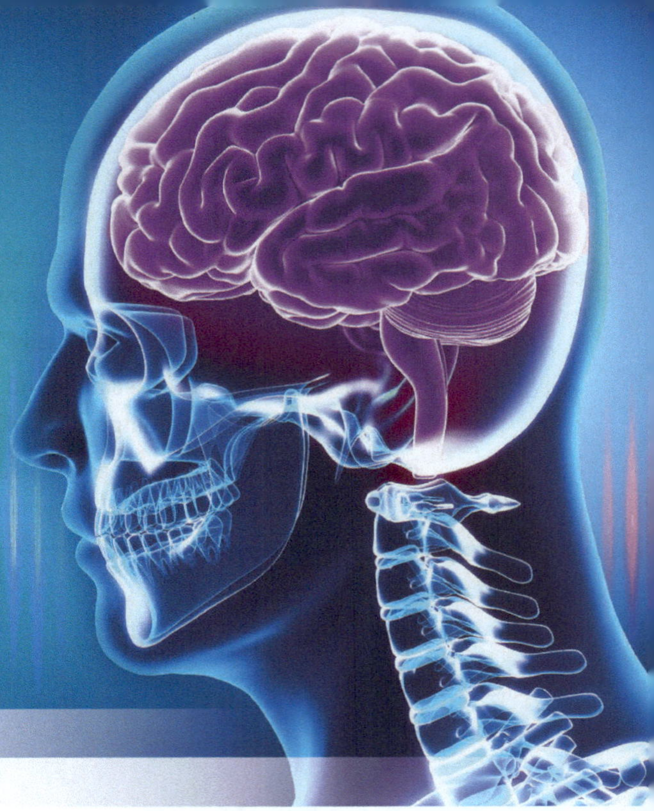

Overview of THE BASICS OF CANCER

Cancer can affect cells in any body system and can spread to other body systems. Genetics, lifestyle, and environmental influences affect each person's risk of developing cancer. Once cancer has been identified, there are multiple treatment options, including radiation, surgery, and chemotherapy. These treatment options increase the likelihood of surviving cancer.

Vocabulary Related to **ONCOLOGY**

This list contains essential word parts and medical terms for this chapter. These and the other important **primary terms** are shown in **boldface** throughout the chapter. *Secondary terms*, which appear in *orange* italics, clarify the meaning of primary terms.

Word Parts

- ☐ **aden/o** gland
- ☐ **angi/o** blood vessel
- ☐ **bi/o** life
- ☐ **carcin/o** cancerous
- ☐ **-genesis** reproduction
- ☐ **melan/o** black
- ☐ **neo-**, **ne/o** new, strange
- ☐ **-occult** hidden
- ☐ **-oma** tumor, neoplasm
- ☐ **onc/o** tumor
- ☐ **-opsy** a view of
- ☐ **path/o** disease
- ☐ **-plasm** formation
- ☐ **proto-** first, original
- ☐ **sarc/o** flesh

Medical Terms

- ☐ **abdominocentesis** (ab-**dom**-ih-noh-sen-**TEE**-sis)
- ☐ **acral lentiginous melanoma** (**ACK**-rahl len-**TIH**-jih-nuhs mel-ah-**NOH**-mah)
- ☐ **adenocarcinoma** (**ad**-eh-noh-**kar**-sih-**NOH**-mah)
- ☐ **adjuvant therapy** (**AD**-jeh-vant)
- ☐ **anaplasia** (**ah**-nah-**PLAY**-zhee-ah)
- ☐ **angiogenesis** (**an**-jee-oh-**JEN**-eh-sis)
- ☐ **antineoplastic** (**an**-tih-nee-oh-**PLAS**-tick)
- ☐ **antioxidants** (**an**-tee-**OCK**-sih-dantz)
- ☐ **benign** (bee-**NINE**)
- ☐ **biopsy** (**BYE**-op-see)
- ☐ **blastoma** (blas-**TOH**-ma)
- ☐ **Bowen disease** (**BOH**-wan)
- ☐ **brachytherapy** (**brack**-ee-**THER**-ah-pee)
- ☐ **cancer**
- ☐ **carcinogen** (kar-**SIH**-noh-jen)
- ☐ **carcinogenesis** (kar-**sih**-noh-**JEH**-neh-sis)
- ☐ **carcinoma** (**kar**-sih-**NOH**-mah)
- ☐ **carcinoma in situ** (**kar**-sih-**NOH**-mah in **SIGH**-too)
- ☐ **chemotherapy** (**kee**-moh-**THEH**-ruh-pee)
- ☐ **chemotherapy nurse** (**kee**-moh-**THEH**-ruh-pee)
- ☐ **colonoscopy** (**koh**-lun-**OSS**-koh-pee)
- ☐ **complete remission** (ree-**MIH**-shun)
- ☐ **core needle biopsy**
- ☐ **dysplasia** (dis-**PLAY**-zhee-ah)
- ☐ **hereditary cancer syndromes**
- ☐ **hormone therapy**
- ☐ **hyperplasia** (**high**-per-**PLAY**-zhee-ah)
- ☐ **immunotherapy** (ih-**myoo**-noh-**THEH**-rah-pee)
- ☐ **infiltrating ductal carcinoma** (in-**FILL**-tray-ting **DUK**-tal)
- ☐ **ionizing radiation** (**EYE**-oh-**nye**-zing **ray**-dee-**AY**-shun)
- ☐ **leukemia** (loo-**KEE**-mee-ah)
- ☐ **lymphoma** (lim-**FOH**-mah)
- ☐ **malignant** (mah-**LIG**-nant)
- ☐ **malignant melanoma** (mah-**LIG**-nant mel-ah-**NOH**-mah)
- ☐ **metastasis** (meh-**TAS**-tah-sis)
- ☐ **metastasize** (meh-**TAS**-tah-sighz)
- ☐ **Mohs surgery** (**MOZE**)
- ☐ **monoclonal antibodies** (**maw**-noh-**KLOH**-null **AN**-tih-**bod**-eez)
- ☐ **multiple myeloma** (**my**-eh-**LOH**-mah)
- ☐ **myelodysplastic syndrome** (**my**-eh-loh-dis-**PLAS**-tick **SIN**-drohm)
- ☐ **neoplasm**
- ☐ **normal cell growth**
- ☐ **oncogene** (**ON**-koh-jeen)
- ☐ **oncologist** (ong-**KOL**-oh-jist)
- ☐ **oncology** (ong-**KOL**-oh-jee)
- ☐ **partial remission** (ree-**MIH**-shun)
- ☐ **pathologist** (pah-**THOL**-oh-jist)
- ☐ **photodynamic therapy** (**foh**-toh-dye-**NAH**-mik)
- ☐ **positron emission tomography** (**PAW**-zih-tron ee-**MIH**-shun tuh-**MAW**-gruh-fee)
- ☐ **prostatic intraepithelial neoplasia** (praw-**STAH**-tik **in**-trah-ep-ih-**THEE**-lee-al **nee**-uh-**PLAY**-zhuh)
- ☐ **proto-oncogene** (**proh**-toh-**ON**-koh-jeen)
- ☐ **radiation therapy**
- ☐ **remission** (ree-**MIH**-shun)
- ☐ **sarcoma** (sar-**KOH**-mah)
- ☐ **targeted therapy**
- ☐ **teletherapy** (**tel**-eh-**THER**-ah-pee)
- ☐ **thoracentesis** (**thoh**-rah-sen-**TEE**-sis)
- ☐ **TNM staging**
- ☐ **tomotherapy**
- ☐ **tumor**

LEARNING OBJECTIVES

On completion of this chapter, you should be able to:

1. Differentiate benign and malignant tumors.
2. Define the primary terms related to tumor growth.
3. Identify the three classes of risk factors for developing cancer.
4. Identify the medical specialists who treat oncological disorders.
5. Identify the medical word parts related to oncology.
6. Describe the classification of tumors.
7. Describe the staging and grading of tumors.
8. Define the primary terms related to common diagnostic tools used in oncology.
9. Define the primary terms related to common cancer treatment options.
10. Define the primary terms related to remission.
11. Spell the primary terms related to oncology.
12. Pronounce the primary terms related to oncology.
13. Identify common abbreviations related to oncology.

CANCER AND ONCOLOGY

Cancer (CA) is a class of diseases characterized by the uncontrolled division of cells and the ability of these cells to invade other tissues, either by direct growth into adjacent tissue or by spreading into distant sites by metastasizing. Cancer in its initial location is known as a **primary cancer**, or ***primary site***.

- For example, ***primary bone cancer*** is a relatively rare malignant tumor that originates in a bone.

To **metastasize** (meh-**TAS**-tah-sighz) means to spread from one place to another. Cancer sometimes moves from its primary site and metastasizes to a secondary site, often through the circulatory or lymphatic system. The most common sites of ***metastatic tumors*** are the bones, liver, lungs, and brain.

Metastasis (meh-**TAS**-tah-sis) describes the process by which cancer is spread to a new site, and can also describe the tumor itself (plural, *metastases*). A metastasis can be in the same body system or within another body system at a distance from the primary site. *Metastasis* is a Latin word meaning transition. A metastasis is known as a **secondary cancer**.

- Following the example above, ***secondary bone cancer***, or ***bone metastasis***, occurs when cancer cells metastasize to the bones from other organs such as the breast, prostate, or lung.

Cancer can attack any and all body systems and is the second leading cause of death in the United States after heart disease. There are over 200 different types of cancers that affect humans. Most cancers are named for the part of the body where the cancer originated, such as lung cancer.

Oncology (ong-**KOL**-oh-jee) is the study of the prevention, causes, and treatment of tumors and cancer (**onc** means tumor, and **-ology** means study of). The terms *cancer* and *tumor* are sometimes treated as synonyms; however, this is not accurate because not all tumors are cancerous.

Tumors

A **tumor**, which is also known as a **neoplasm** (**NEE**-oh-plazm) (**neo-** means new or strange, and **-plasm** means formation), is an abnormal growth of body tissue creating a mass. Within this mass, the multiplication of cells is uncontrolled, abnormal, rapid, and progressive.

A **benign tumor** is *not* a form of cancer, and it is not life-threatening. **Benign** (bee-**NINE**) means not life-threatening, although this type of tumor can cause damage as it grows and places pressure on adjacent structures. Benign tumors tend to grow more slowly than malignant tumors, and do not metastasize.

- A ***myoma*** (my-**OH**-mah) is an example of a benign tumor made up of muscle tissue (**my** means muscle, and **-oma** means tumor).

A **malignant tumor** is a form of cancer. It is capable of spreading to distant body sites, including to other body systems, and is potentially life-threatening. **Malignant** (mah-**LIG**-nant) means harmful, capable of spreading, and potentially life-threatening.

- A ***myosarcoma*** (my-oh-sahr-**KOH**-mah) is an example of a malignant tumor derived from muscle tissue (**my/o** means muscle, **sarc** means flesh, and **-oma** means tumor).

Tumor Growth

The growth of a tumor begins as the normal reproduction and function of cells becomes progressively altered. **Carcinogenesis** (kar-**sih**-noh-**JEH**-neh-sis) is the process through which normal cells become cancer cells (**carcin/o** means cancerous, and **-genesis** means creation).

Normal cell growth is the regular process in which cells divide and become differentiated in an orderly fashion according to the needs of the body, fulfill their specialized roles in the body, and die off after a standard life span or after sustaining damage (Figure 20.1A). ***Differentiation*** is the maturation of an immature cell into a specific type of cell in a body tissue or organ, such as an epithelial or muscle cell. ***Apoptosis*** is cell death that is triggered in normal cells once they have reached the end of their expected life span or sustained damage.

- Every time a cell divides, there is the possibility of an error being introduced into the genes stored within the cell's chromosomes. As this would suggest, the cells that are replaced the most frequently have the highest likelihood of developing errors over time.
- A **proto-oncogene** (**proh**-toh-**ON**-koh-jeen) is a normal gene within a cell that controls one of the normal processes of the cell, such as cell growth, division, or apoptosis (**proto-** means first or original, **onc/o** means tumor, and **-gene** means gene). If an error in the cell's reproduction causes a mutation in a proto-oncogene, it can become an *oncogene*.
- An **oncogene** (**ON**-koh-jeen) is a mutated gene within a cell that causes that cell to function abnormally, either by excessive growth, uncontrolled division, or not producing the signal for apoptosis (**onc/o** means tumor, and **-gene** means gene). The oncogene lacks the controls that allow normal gene functions to be turned on and off.

Hyperplasia (**high**-per-**PLAY**-zhee-ah) is an increase in the number of cells in a tissue or organ (**hyper-** means excessive, and **-plasia** means formation). Some hyperplasia, such as the increase in breast tissue caused by the hormones released during pregnancy, is normal. In other types of hyperplasia, the cells may be precancerous (Figure 20.1B). ***Precancerous*** describes a growth that is not yet malignant; however, if not treated, it may become malignant. Hyperplasia does not always progress to dysplasia.

Dysplasia (dis-**PLAY**-zhee-ah) is the abnormal development or growth of cells, or the presence of abnormal cells within a type of tissue (**dys** means bad, and **-plasia** means formation) (Figure 20.1C). *Cervical dysplasia*, for example, refers to abnormal cells lining the cervix which increase the risk of cervical cancer (see the section "Diagnostic Procedures Related to Oncology").

- Dysplasia is classified as mild, moderate, or severe. ***Severe dysplasia*** is a precancerous condition, and may be surgically removed or closely monitored for development into anaplasia.

Anaplasia (**ah**-nah-**PLAY**-zhee-ah) is the uncontrolled growth of abnormal, poorly differentiated cells commonly seen in most malignant tumors (Figure 20.1D). These cells may contain significant variation even within the same mass, and often include more errors and mutations in the genes than normal cells do.

- These cells may form into abnormal shapes, multiply more frequently than normal, and live longer than normal cells by ignoring the signal for apoptosis.
- Additionally, many malignant tumors support their own growth through angiogenesis.

Angiogenesis (**an**-jee-oh-**JEN**-eh-sis) is the process through which a tumor supports its growth by creating its own blood supply (**angi/o** means vessel, and **-genesis** means reproduction). Angiogenesis is the opposite of *antiangiogenesis* (see the section "Targeted Therapy").

Risk Factors for Cancer

There are several classes of risk factors that increase the likelihood of developing cancer. These include genetics, lifestyle, and environmental exposure to carcinogens.

Genetic Risk Factors

Hereditary cancers account for 5–10% of all cancers. These are caused by mutations in genes that are passed down from one family member to another. The mutated gene does not guarantee that the person will develop cancer, but it does increase their risk of developing it.

Hereditary cancer syndromes are known mutations in certain genes that can be passed down from parent

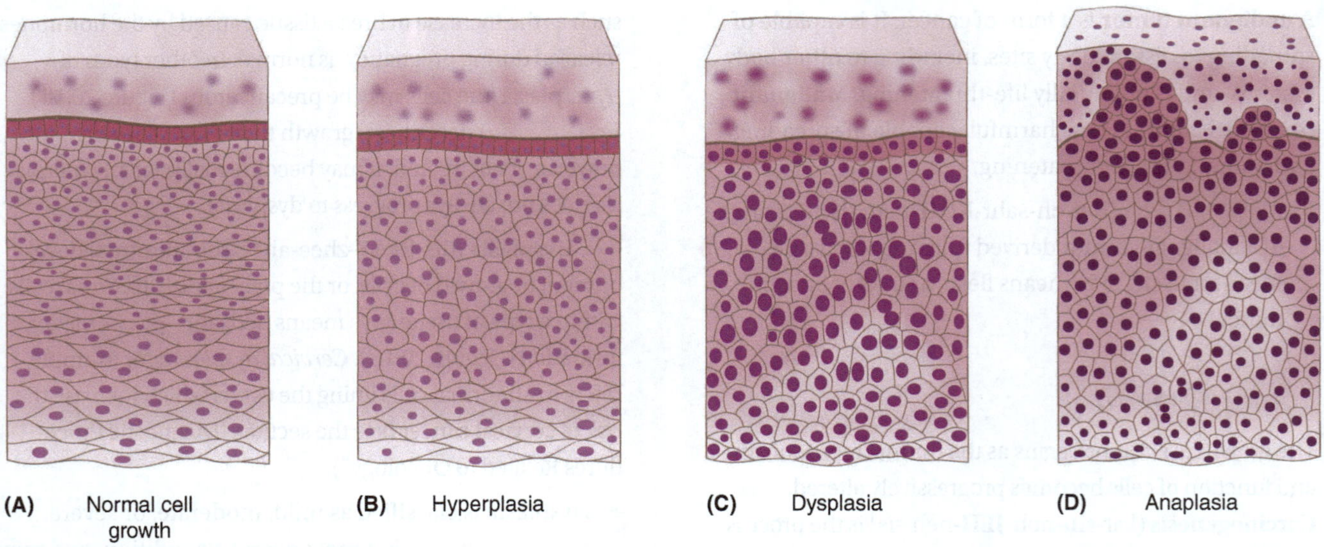

FIGURE 20.1 Comparing different types of cell growth. (A) Normal cell growth, (B) hyperplasia, (C) dysplasia, (D) anaplasia.

to child, and are linked with an increased risk of cancer. ***Hereditary breast & ovarian cancer syndrome*** (HBOC) is the most common type of hereditary cancer syndrome. HBOC is caused by mutations in ***BRCA1*** and ***BRCA2 genes*** (**BR**east **CA**ncer **1** and **2**), and causes an increased risk of developing breast, ovarian, or prostate cancer.

Lifestyle Risk Factors

Some cancers may seem to have a hereditary factor because they affect multiple members of the same family, but are actually the result of sharing a similar lifestyle. While some lifestyle risks are obvious, others are less straightforward.

- **Smoking tobacco** increases the risk of developing lung cancer, and is a causative factor in 90% of lung cancer cases in the United States. However, smoking or chewing tobacco is also associated with an increased risk of developing cancer of the mouth, larynx, trachea, esophagus, stomach, pancreas, liver, kidney, bladder, cervix, and colon/rectum.
- **Alcohol consumption** increases the risk of developing cancer of the mouth, larynx, esophagus, breast, liver, and colon/rectum. The risk of cancer increases with the total amount of alcohol consumed.
- **Human papillomavirus infection** (HPV) can be sexually transmitted, and certain types of HPV increase the risk of developing cancer of the mouth, pharynx, cervix, vagina, penis, and anus.
  - **Cervical cancer** is a slow-growing squamous cell cancer caused by HPV. An ***HPV vaccine*** is now available to help protect males and females against the types of HPV that cause most cancer, and works most effectively when administered at age 11 or 12 (see Chapter 18).
- Obesity, sedentary lifestyle, and a poor diet are associated with increased risk of cancer of the esophagus, breast, uterus, prostate, and colon/rectum. *Note:* Obesity is not exclusively a lifestyle factor, and has environmental and genetic components.
  - **Antioxidants** (**an**-tee-**OCK**-sih-dantz) are substances found in many fruits and vegetables which may help decrease the risk of cancer (**anti-** means against, **oxid** means oxidation, and **-ant** means a thing that promotes) (Figure 20.2).
  - Regular exercise is important to reduce the risk of many cancers.

Environmental Risk Factors

Environmental risk factors include accidental and deliberate exposure to carcinogens, such as secondhand smoke and air pollution. A **carcinogen** (kar-**SIH**-noh-jen) is a substance known to cause cancer.

- **Chemical exposure** increases the risk of certain types of cancer, particularly in the case of repeated exposure linked to a person's profession. For example, benzene is used in the manufacture of rubber and gasoline, so people whose work exposes them to these products may experience greater exposure to the chemical. Inhalation of benzene increases the risk of developing leukemia.

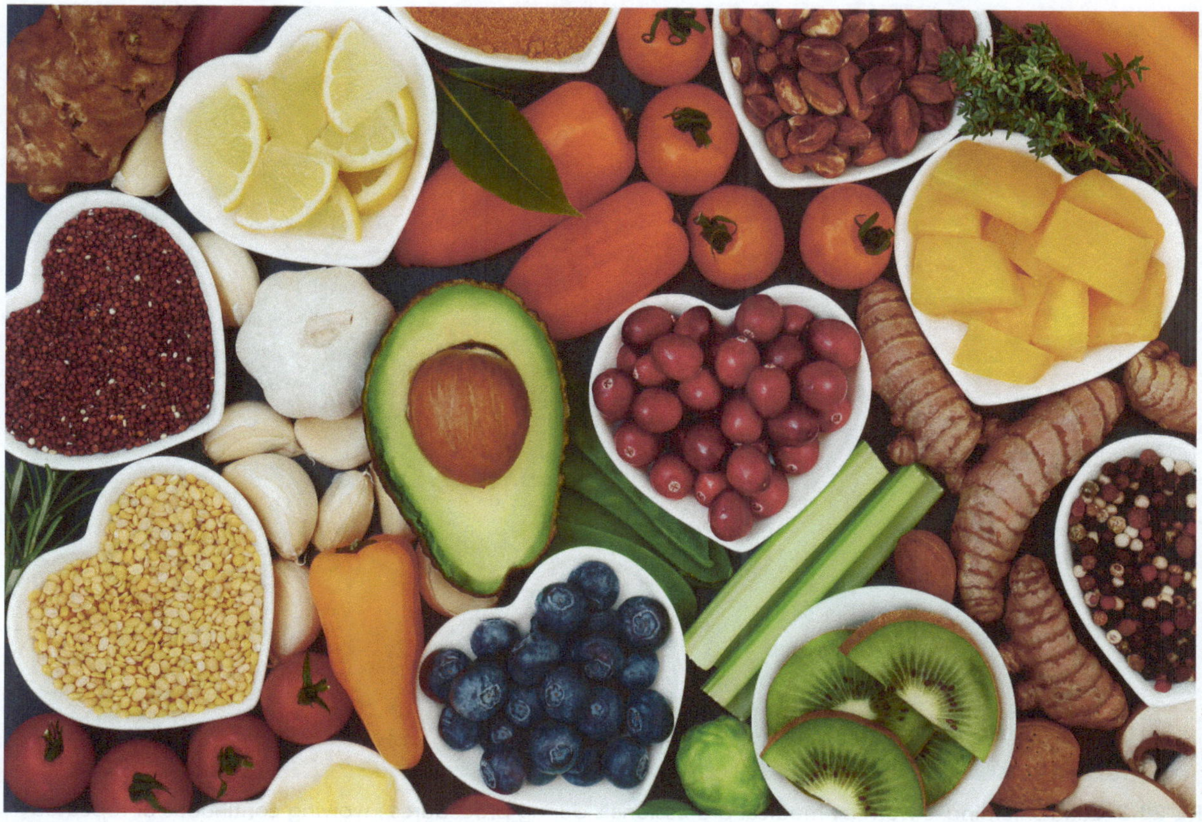

FIGURE 20.2 Antioxidants are substances found in many fruits and vegetables which may help decrease the risk of cancer.

- **Air pollution** includes byproducts of combustion engines, such as automobiles, wood smoke, and industrial waste, and increases the risk of lung cancer.
    - *Secondhand smoke* is the inhalation of tobacco smoke by people other than the tobacco user.
- **Water pollution** includes chemical runoff from fertilizers, pesticides, detergents, and industrial waste, and increases the risk of cancer of the esophagus, breast, stomach, and bladder.
- **Ionizing radiation** (**EYE**-oh-**nye**-zing **ray**-dee-**AY**-shun) is present in x-rays and other medical imaging procedures such as CT scans, PET scans, and nuclear medicine. *Ionizing* means that the radiation can remove electrons from the body tissue they pass through, potentially altering the cells. Ionizing radiation is also produced by the sun, and plane travel is another activity that involves exposure to low levels of ionizing radiation. Repeated exposure to ionizing radiation increases the risk of damage to the body's cells, and the cumulative exposure risk is an important consideration when ordering medical imaging.
    - **Lead shielding** is used to protect body parts that do not need to be included in medical imaging from exposure to ionizing radiation. Lead is also worn by imaging technicians and other medical professionals during procedures involving continuous or repeated imaging, such as fluoroscopy (Figure 20.3).
    - A *radiation dosimetry badge* is worn by medical professionals who are repeatedly exposed to ionizing radiation. The badge is not protective, but measures the amount of radiation to which the person has been exposed.
- **Ultraviolet rays** (UV) are present in sunlight and indoor tanning machines. Exposure to UV rays causes the skin to produce more *melanin*, the pigment that darkens skin, in an attempt to prevent damage to the skin cells. Repeated exposure to UV rays increases the risk of developing skin cancer.
    - **Sunscreen** that blocks out the harmful ultraviolet B (UVB) rays is sometimes measured in terms of the strength of the *sun protection factor* (SPF). Some sunscreens also give protection against ultraviolet A (UVA) rays.

MEDICAL SPECIALTIES RELATED TO ONCOLOGY

- A **pathologist** (pah-**THOL**-oh-jist) is a physician who specializes in the laboratory analysis of diseased tissue

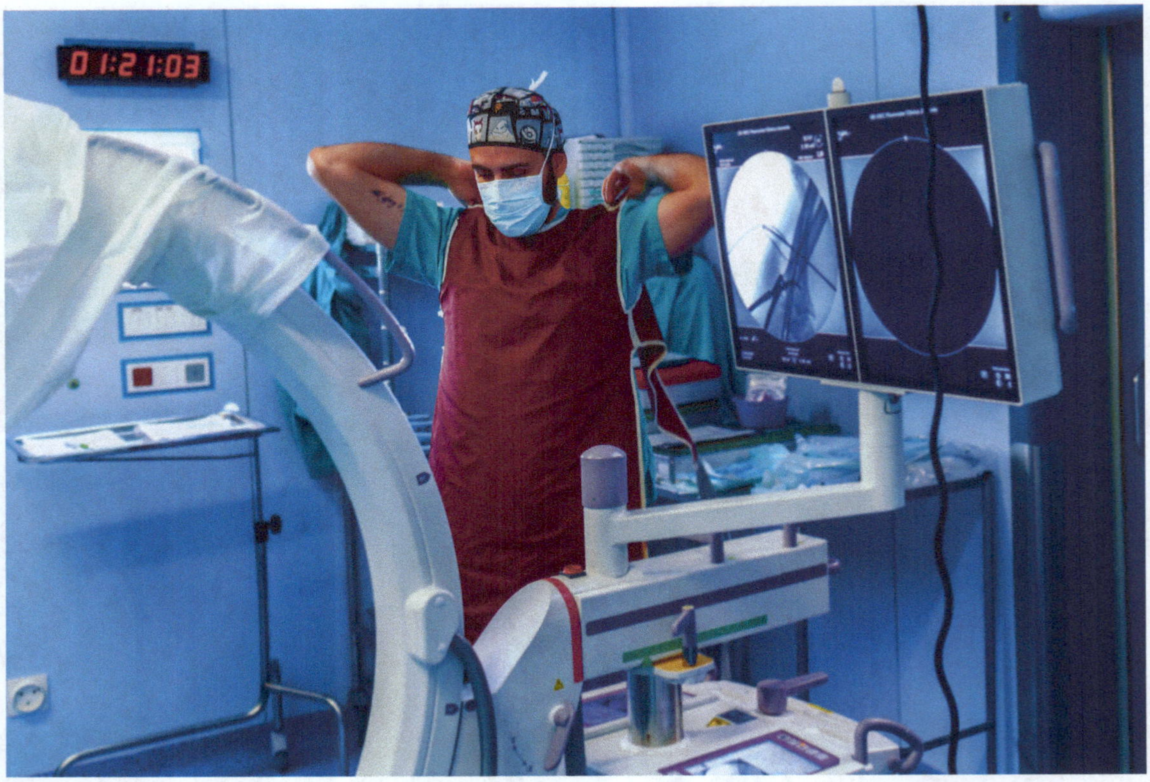

Juan Miguel Aparicio/Shutterstock.com

FIGURE 20.3 Lead shielding is worn by medical professionals during procedures involving continuous or repeated imaging, such as fluoroscopy.

samples to confirm or establish a diagnosis (**path** means disease, and **-ologist** means specialist). These tissue specimens can be removed in biopsies, during operations, or in postmortem examinations. The role of a pathologist in oncology is to provide an accurate diagnosis as quickly as possible, so that treatment can be started for the patient.

- An **oncologist** (ong-**KOL**-oh-jist) is a physician who studies the prevention, causes, and treatment of cancer. Oncologists and pathologists play different roles on the care team of a patient with cancer. Once a pathologist uses laboratory analysis to identify the type of cancer, an oncologist develops a treatment plan based on that information, and remains involved in the patient's case throughout treatment. A ***medical oncologist*** specializes in cancer treatment using chemotherapy and other agents. A ***radiation oncologist*** specializes in designing care plans for radiation therapy. Medical and radiation oncologists work together closely to plan and deliver patient care.
- A **radiation therapist** is a medical professional who specializes in the delivery of radiation treatment for cancer patients. The radiation therapist is responsible for correctly administering the treatment, monitoring and assessing the patient throughout the treatment period, and communicating with the oncologist about any side effects.
- A **chemotherapy nurse** (**kee**-moh-**THEH**-ruh-pee) is a registered nurse who specializes in the administration of intravenous (IV) chemotherapeutic agents and monitoring patients during treatment. Most chemotherapy nurses work in infusion centers. An **infusion center** is an outpatient clinic for patients who need IV medications or transfusions on a planned, ongoing basis rather than in an emergency or temporary inpatient setting.

CLASSIFICATION OF CANCER

Cancer is classified based on the type of cell it arises from, its location in the body, and how far its development has progressed.

Cancers Classified by Type

Some types of cancer are named for the different cells and body tissues from which they form. These histological types of cancers include carcinoma, sarcoma, leukemia, lymphoma, and blastoma. ***Histological*** means having to do with tissues and cells.

Carcinoma

A **carcinoma** (**kar**-sih-**NOH**-mah) is a type of cancer that occurs in epithelial tissue (**carcin** means cancer, and **-oma** means tumor). Epithelial tissue forms the protective covering for all of the internal and external surfaces of the body, including the skin and organs.

Carcinomas tend to infiltrate and produce metastases that can affect any organ or part of the body. ***Infiltrate*** means to gain access to.

- An **adenocarcinoma** (**ad**-eh-noh-**kar**-sih-**NOH**-mah) is any one of a large group of carcinomas derived from glandular tissue (**aden/o** means gland, **carcin** means cancer, and **-oma** means tumor).
- **Thyroid carcinoma** is the most common cancer of the endocrine system and is the most rapidly increasing cancer in the United States. Thyroid carcinoma, which has a high survival rate, affects significantly more women than men and is commonly diagnosed between ages 20 and 55.
- A **carcinoma in situ** (**kar**-sih-**NOH**-mah in **SIGH**-too) is a malignant tumor in its original position that has not yet disturbed or invaded the surrounding tissues. ***In situ*** means in the place where the cancer first occurred.

Sarcoma

A **sarcoma** (sar-**KOH**-mah) is a type of cancer that arises from connective tissues, including hard and, more commonly, soft tissues (**sarc** means flesh, and **-oma** means tumor) (plural, ***sarcomas*** or ***sarcomata***).

- **Hard-tissue sarcomas** arise from bone or cartilage (see Chapter 3). For example, an **osteosarcoma** (**oss**-tee-oh-sar-**KOH**-mah) is a hard-tissue sarcoma that usually involves the upper shaft of the long bones, pelvis, or knee (**oste/o** means bone, **sarc** means flesh, and **-oma** means tumor).
- **Soft-tissue sarcomas** are cancers of the muscle, fat, fibrous tissue, blood and lymphatic vessels, or other supporting tissue, including the synovial tissues that line the cavities of joints. For example, a **synovial sarcoma** is a tumor of the tissues surrounding a synovial joint such as the knees or elbows.

Leukemia

Leukemia (loo-**KEE**-mee-ah) is a type of cancer characterized by a progressive increase in the number of abnormal leukocytes (white blood cells) found in blood-forming tissues, other organs, and the circulating blood (**leuk** means white, and **-emia** means blood condition). Types of leukemia are named based on how quickly they progress and the type of white blood cells involved. The four most common types of leukemia are *acute* or *chronic myeloid leukemia* and *acute* or *chronic lymphocytic leukemia*.

- **Acute myeloid leukemia** (AML) is a type of cancer characterized by a sudden increase in abnormal immature leukocytes in place of normal blood cells. AML has a rapid progression leading to death within weeks or months if not treated. Risk factors for AML include previous chemotherapy, exposure to ionizing radiation, and myelodysplastic syndrome.
- **Chronic myeloid leukemia** (CML) is a type of cancer characterized by a slow buildup of partly mature leukocytes. CML has a slow progression and may not immediately cause symptoms. CML most often occurs in older adults over the age of 65, and is commonly treated with oral chemotherapy.
- **Acute lymphocytic leukemia** (ALL) is a type of cancer characterized by a sudden increase in abnormal immature lymphocytes. ALL has a rapid progression leading to death within weeks or months if not treated. ALL is the most common type of cancer in children, and has a 90% survival rate. Risk factors for ALL include previous chemotherapy, exposure to ionizing radiation, and Down syndrome.
- **Chronic lymphocytic leukemia** (CLL) is a type of cancer characterized by a slow buildup of partly mature lymphocytes. CLL has a slow progression and does not immediately cause symptoms, although patients may eventually experience ongoing weight loss, fatigue, and fever. CLL most often occurs in adults over the age of 50, and affects twice as many men as women.
- **Myelodysplastic syndrome** (**my**-eh-loh-dis-**PLAS**-tick **SIN**-drohm) is a type of cancer in which there is insufficient production of one or more types of blood cells due to dysfunction of the bone marrow. Some patients later develop acute myeloid leukemia.

Lymphoma

Lymphoma (lim-**FOH**-mah) is a general term applied to malignancies affecting lymphoid tissues (**lymph** means lymph, and **-oma** means tumor). Lymphoid tissue is found in lymph nodes, the spleen, the liver, and bone marrow. The two most common types of lymphomas are Hodgkin's lymphoma and non-Hodgkin's lymphoma.

- **Hodgkin's lymphoma** (**HODJ**-kinz lim-**FOH**-mah) (HL), also known as ***Hodgkin's*** (or ***Hodgkin***) ***disease***, is a cancer of the immune system distinguished by the presence of large, cancerous lymphocytes known as ***Reed-Sternberg cells***. The spread of these cells compromises the body's ability to fight infection.
- **Non-Hodgkin's lymphoma** (NHL), which is the more common type, refers to all lymphomas other than Hodgkin's lymphoma. There are many different types of non-Hodgkin's lymphomas, all of which originate in the lymphocytes. Some are ***aggressive*** (fast growing) and some are ***indolent*** (slow growing).

Myeloma

Multiple myeloma (**my**-eh-**LOH**-mah) is a type of cancer that occurs in blood-making plasma cells found in the red bone marrow (**myel** means bone marrow, and **-oma** means tumor). This condition, which is more common in African Americans, weakens the bones and can impact other body systems such as the kidneys.

Blastoma

A **blastoma** (blas-**TOH**-ma) is a cancer that develops from immature undifferentiated cells, occurring most frequently in children. Two common types of blastomas are hepatoblastoma and Wilms tumor.

- **Hepatoblastoma** (heh-**pah**-toh-blas-**TOH**-ma) is a rare type of malignant liver cancer that occurs in children under age 3. While rare, it is the most common type of blastoma.
- A **Wilms tumor**, also known as a ***nephroblastoma***, is a rare type of malignant tumor of the kidney that occurs in young children. There is a high cure rate for this condition when treated promptly.

Cancers Classified by Location

Some cancers are named by the body organ in which they are found. The most common types of cancer identified by location are lung, breast, prostate, colorectal, and skin cancer.

Lung Cancer

Lung cancer, which is the leading cause of cancer death in the United States, is a condition in which cancer cells form in the tissues of the lung. There are two general types of lung cancer: small cell and non-small cell.

- **Small cell lung cancer** is a fast-growing cancer that occurs most often in smokers. Most small cell lung cancers are ***small cell carcinoma***, also known as ***oat cell cancer*** due to the appearance of the cells. Chemotherapy and radiation therapy are most commonly used to treat this type of cancer.
- **Non-small cell lung cancer** is the most common type of lung cancer. Most non-small cell lung cancers are ***adenocarcinoma of the lung***, which begins in the glands in the outer layer of the lung. Surgery is most commonly used to treat this type of cancer if it has not yet spread outside the lung.

Breast Cancer

Breast cancer is a carcinoma that develops from the cells of the breast and can spread to adjacent lymph nodes and other body sites (Figure 20.4).

- **Ductal carcinoma in situ** (DCIS) is breast cancer at its earliest stage before the abnormal cells have broken through the wall of the milk ducts. These cells may or may not become cancerous and spread. At this stage, the cure rate is nearly 100%.
- **Infiltrating ductal carcinoma** (in-**FILL**-tray-ting **DUK**-tal) (IDC) starts in the milk duct and invades the fatty breast tissue outside the duct. This is the most common form of breast cancer.

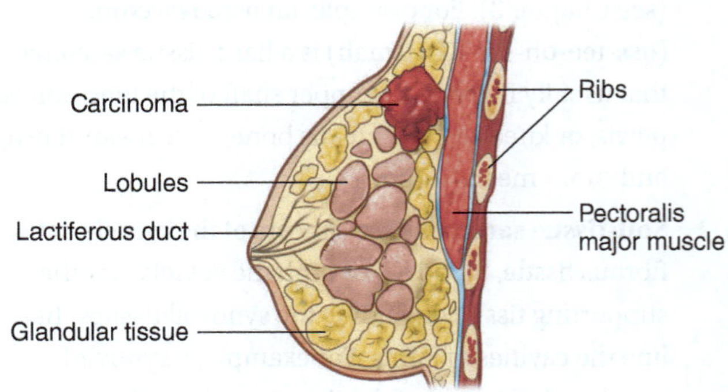

FIGURE 20.4 Most breast cancers are initially detected as a lump. When this lump is malignant, it is a form of carcinoma.

- **Inflammatory breast cancer** (IBC) is a rare but aggressive form of breast cancer in which the cancer cells block the lymphatic vessels in the skin of the breast. IBC grows rapidly, and the symptoms include pain, rapid increase in breast size, redness or a rash on the breast, and swelling of nearby lymph nodes.
- ***Male breast cancer*** can occur in the small amount of breast tissue that is normally present in men. The types of cancers are similar to those occurring in women.

Breast cancers are classified based on the presence or absence of specific hormone receptors.

- ***ER-positive breast cancer*** (ER+) has estrogen receptors, and grows in response to estrogen.
- ***PR-positive breast cancer*** (PR+) has progesterone receptors, and grows in response to progesterone.
- ***HER2-positive breast cancer*** (HER2+) has high levels of *HER2* protein, which promotes growth.
- **Triple-negative breast cancer** does not have receptors for estrogen or progesterone, and has low levels of HER2. Hormone therapy cannot be used to treat triple-negative breast cancer. 10–20% of breast cancers are triple-negative, and it is aggressive and difficult to treat.
- **Triple-positive breast cancer** has receptors for estrogen and progesterone, and has high levels of HER2.

Prostate Cancer

Prostate cancer is one of the most common cancers among men, second only to skin cancer. Adenocarcinoma starts in the glands that produce prostate fluid, and is the most common type of prostate cancer. The disease can grow slowly with no symptoms, or it can grow aggressively and spread throughout the body. Prostate cancer is most commonly diagnosed when a person starts having urinary symptoms, which leads to a medical exam and blood work.

- **Prostatic intraepithelial neoplasia** (praw-**STAH**-tik **in**-trah-ep-ih-**THEE**-lee-al **nee**-uh-**PLAY**-zhuh) (PIN) is a precancerous change to prostate gland cells that can be mildly abnormal (***low-grade PIN***), or moderately abnormal (***high-grade PIN***).
- **Proliferative inflammatory atrophy** (PIA) is a potentially precancerous change to prostate cells in which the cells are smaller than usual and surrounded by inflammation. This may progress to high-grade PIN or prostate cancer.
- The **prostate-specific antigen** (PSA) **blood test** is used to screen for prostate cancer. This test measures the amount of prostate-specific antigen that is present in a blood specimen. The ***prostate-specific antigen*** is a protein produced by the cells of the prostate gland to help liquefy semen. The higher a man's PSA level, the more likely it is that cancer is present.

Colorectal Cancer

Colorectal cancer often first manifests itself in polyps in the colon or rectum (Figure 20.5). Nearly all cases of colorectal cancer are caused by adenocarcinoma. Risk factors for colorectal cancer include age above 50 years old, obesity, smoking, alcohol consumption, diabetes, and sedentary lifestyle.

- A **polyp** (**POL**-up) is a mushroom-like growth from the surface of a mucous membrane. ***Non-neoplastic polyps*** have no risk of developing into cancer. ***Neoplastic polyps*** are potentially precancerous.
  - An **adenomatous polyp**, also known as an ***adenoma***, is the most common type of precancerous neoplastic polyp.

Skin Cancer

Skin cancer is a malignant growth on the skin which can have many causes, including repeated severe sunburns or long-term exposure to the sun. Skin cancer often begins as a mole or small patch of skin with a different color or texture than the surrounding skin. Skin cancer is the most common cancer in the U.S., affecting about one in five Americans in their lifetime. There are three main types of skin cancer: basal cell carcinoma, squamous cell carcinoma, and malignant melanoma. See Chapter 13 for more information on these types of skin cancer.

- **Basal cell carcinoma** (**BAYS**-al) (BCC) is a malignant tumor of the basal cell layer of the epidermis.
- **Squamous cell carcinoma** (**SKWAY**-mus) (SCC) is a malignant tumor of the squamous cells of the epithelium.
  - **Bowen disease** (**BOH**-wan) (alternative spelling, *Bowen's disease*) is squamous cell carcinoma in situ. Bowen disease usually consists of a single red, scaly patch 10–15 mm in diameter on an area with repeated sun exposure, such as the head, neck, arms or legs. Bowen disease is named for American dermatologist John Templeton Bowen.

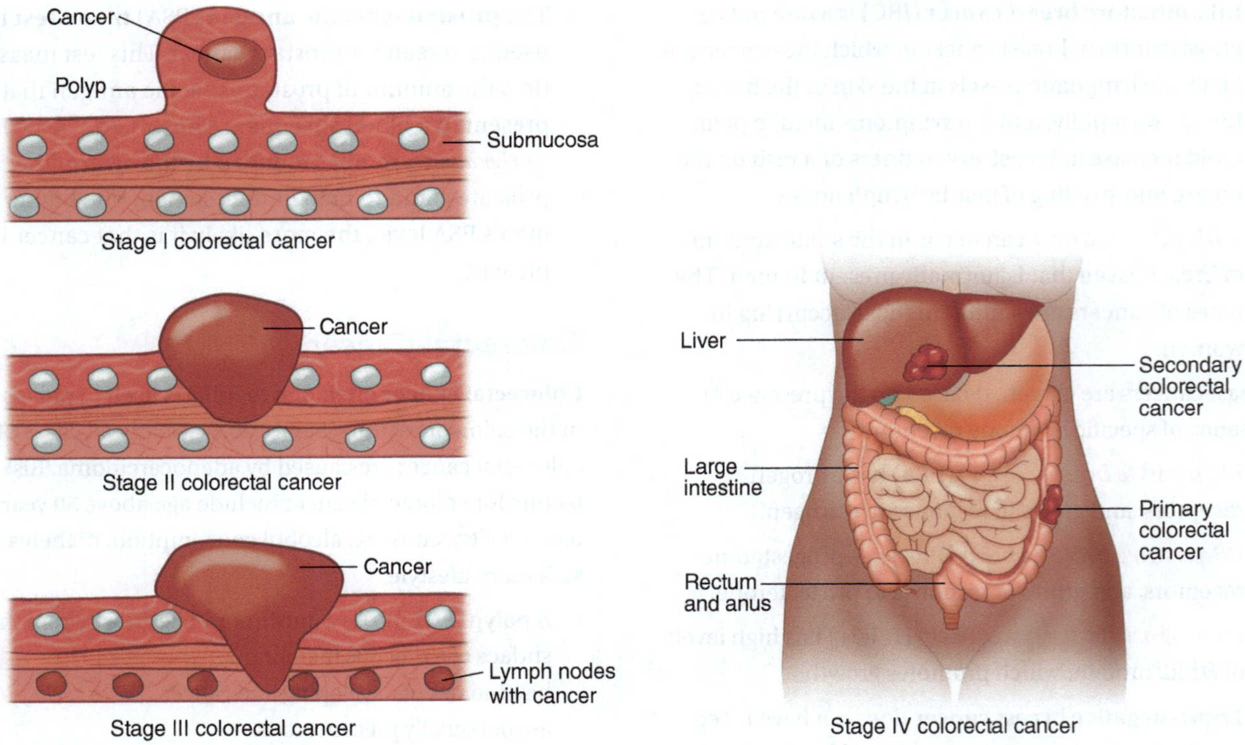

FIGURE 20.5 Stages of colorectal cancer. *Stage I*: The cancerous tumor has formed within a polyp inside the colon but has not yet invaded the surrounding tissue. *Stage II*: The cancer has invaded the underlying tissue. *Stage III*: The cancer has spread to the underlying tissues and nearby lymph nodes. *Stage IV*: The cancer has spread to other tissues throughout the body, most commonly the liver.

- **Malignant melanoma** (mah-**LIG**-nant mel-ah-**NOH**-mah) (MM), also known as ***melanoma***, is a type of skin cancer that occurs in the melanocytes (**melan** means black, and **-oma** means tumor). Malignant melanoma accounts for about 1% of all skin cancers, but is the cause of most skin cancer deaths.
  - **Acral lentiginous melanoma** (**ACK**-rahl len-**TIH**-jih-nuhs mel-ah-**NOH**-mah) (ALM) is the most common form of skin cancer in African Americans (Figure 20.6). ALM occurs on the palms of the hands, soles of the feet, and skin under the nails, and is not linked to sun exposure.

Staging and Grading Cancer

Staging is the process of classifying tumors by how far the disease has progressed, the potential for its responding to therapy, and the patient's prognosis. Stages can be indicated by letters, numbers, or Roman numerals. Specific staging systems are used for different types of cancer (Figure 20.5).

TNM staging is one of the most commonly used cancer staging systems for detailed discussion of cancer progression, and is usually used for pathology reports (Table 20.1). ***Pathology reports*** are medical documents written by pathologists presenting their findings.

Cancer staging can also be discussed in more general terms, based on the size and spread of the cancer.

- **Stage 0** means cancer cells are found in one location, such as carcinoma in situ.
  - *Note:* Not all cancers use a Stage 0 designation. Some begin with Stage 1.

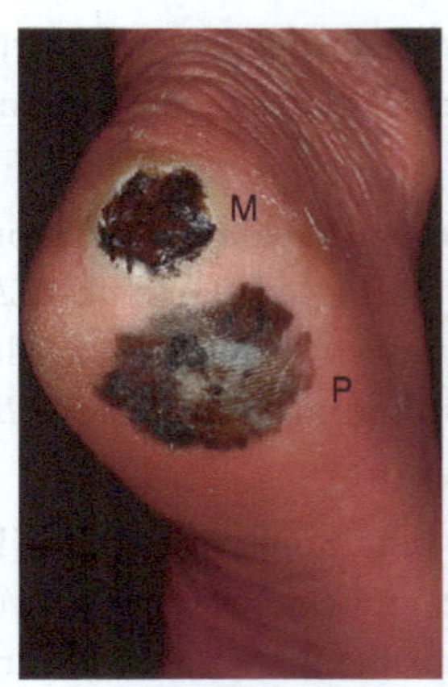

FIGURE 20.6 Acral lentiginous melanoma on the sole of the foot.

TABLE 20.1

TNM Staging Systems

Characteristic being measured	Abbreviation	Meaning
T is the size or spread of the main tumor.	TX	Main tumor cannot be measured.
	T0	Main tumor cannot be found.
	T1	Main tumor size and intrusion into surrounding tissues.
	T2 T3 T4	The higher the number, the larger the tumor.
N is the number of nearby lymph nodes with cancer.	NX	Cancer in nearby lymph nodes cannot be measured.
	N0	No cancer in nearby lymph nodes.
	N1	Cancer in nearby lymph nodes.
	N2 N3	The higher the number, the larger the number of nearby lymph nodes with cancer.
M is the presence of metastases.	MX	Metastases cannot be measured.
	M0	There are no metastases.
	M1	Metastases are present.

- **Stage 1** means cancer has begun to grow into nearby tissues but not yet reached lymph nodes.
- **Stage 2** means cancer has increased in size and/or reached nearby lymph nodes.
- **Stage 3** means cancer has increased in size, spread to nearby lymph nodes, and/or broken through into surrounding tissues.
- **Stage 4** means cancer has spread to other organs, most commonly the brain, lungs, liver, or bones.
  - This stage is also known as ***advanced*** or ***metastatic cancer***.

Tumors can also be **graded** by a pathologist based on the amount of abnormality in the cell structure at a microscopic level.

- **Grade 1** means the cancer is well differentiated, and appears mostly normal (***low grade***).
- **Grade 2** means the cancer is moderately differentiated (***intermediate grade***).
- **Grade 3** means the cancer is poorly differentiated (***high grade***).
- **Grade 4** means the cancer is undifferentiated (***high grade***).

DIAGNOSTIC PROCEDURES RELATED TO ONCOLOGY

Screening for early detection of cancer and precancerous changes is an important part of cancer prevention and treatment. Much screening can be done at home or during regular doctor's visits.

Non-Invasive Diagnostic Procedures

Physical examination by a medical professional or home self-examination is an important cancer screening tool. Regular screening is recommended for cancer of the breast, cervix, and testicle, and older adults are also screened for cancer of the prostate and colon.

Home Screening

Self-examination and home screening kits are easy ways to screen for common types of cancer among adults in high-risk populations.

- **Testicular self-examination** is a self-help step in the early detection of testicular cancer by detecting lumps, swelling, or changes in the skin of the scrotum.

- **Breast self-examination** is a self-care procedure for the early detection of breast cancer. The focus of self-examination is checking for a new lump or for changes in an existing lump, the shape of the nipple, or the skin covering the breast.
- A **Hemoccult® test** (**HEE**-moh-kult), also known as a ***fecal occult blood test***, is a laboratory test for hidden blood in stool (**hem** means blood, and **-occult** means hidden), which may be an early sign of colorectal cancer. The test kit is used to obtain the specimens at home, and the results are then evaluated in a laboratory.
- ***Cologuard®*** is a noninvasive, collect-at-home stool test that uses DNA testing along with screening for hidden blood to determine the potential presence of colorectal cancer.

Medical Office Screening

Physical examination by a trained health care provider is regularly performed to screen for cancer in high-risk populations. This includes regular physical examination techniques such as palpation and auscultation (see Chapter 21), as well as specialty examinations to screen for specific types of cancer.

- **Palpation of the breast** is a test performed by a trained health care provider to check the texture, size, and consistency of the breast as well as the lymph nodes in the armpit.
- **Exfoliative cytology** (ecks-**FOH**-lee-**ay**-tiv sigh-**TOL**-oh-jee), also referred to as ***skin scraping***, is a technique in which cells are scraped from the tissue and examined under a microscope. ***Exfoliation*** is the removal of dead epidermal cells.

Diagnostic Imaging Procedures

Because cancer can spread throughout the body, accurate diagnostic imaging is an important part of cancer screening, diagnosis, and treatment monitoring.

Radiography and MRI

- **Mammography** (mam-**OG**-rah-fee) is an x-ray examination of the breasts to detect the presence of tumors or precancerous cells (**mamm/o** means breast, and **-graphy** means the process of producing a picture or record) (Figure 20.7). The resulting record is a ***mammogram*** (Figure 20.8).
- **Computed tomography** (CT), also known as a ***CT scan***, uses a rotating x-ray beam to form multiple cross-section images of the soft tissues of the body. CT can be used to diagnose and monitor cancer.
- **Magnetic resonance imaging** (MRI) uses magnets and radio waves, and the insertion of a contrast medium via IV, to get more detailed information for those already diagnosed with cancer or to look for signs of cancer in patients at high risk. An MRI can show areas in more

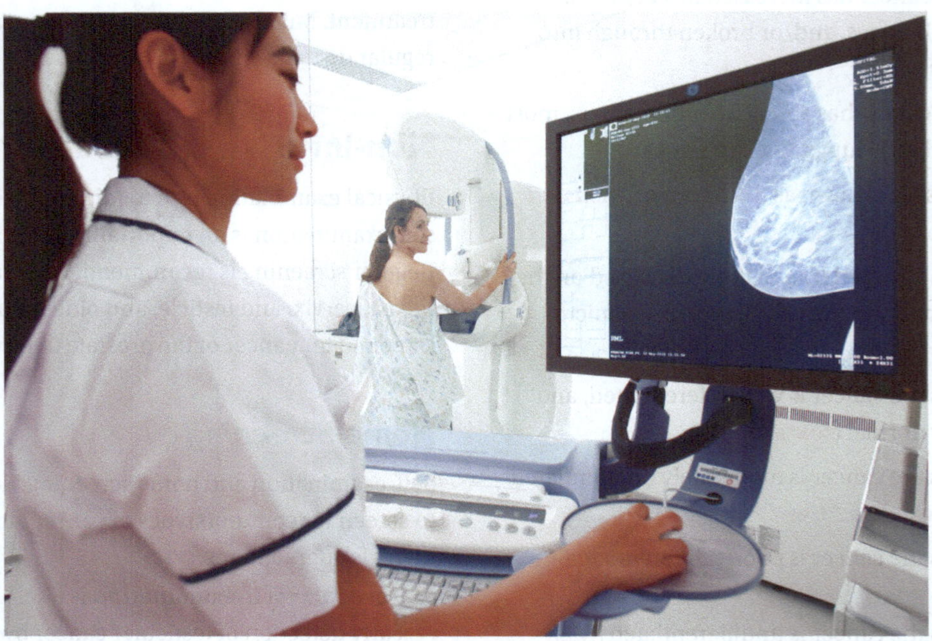

Echo/GettyImages

FIGURE 20.7 In mammography, the breast is gently flattened and x-rayed from various angles.

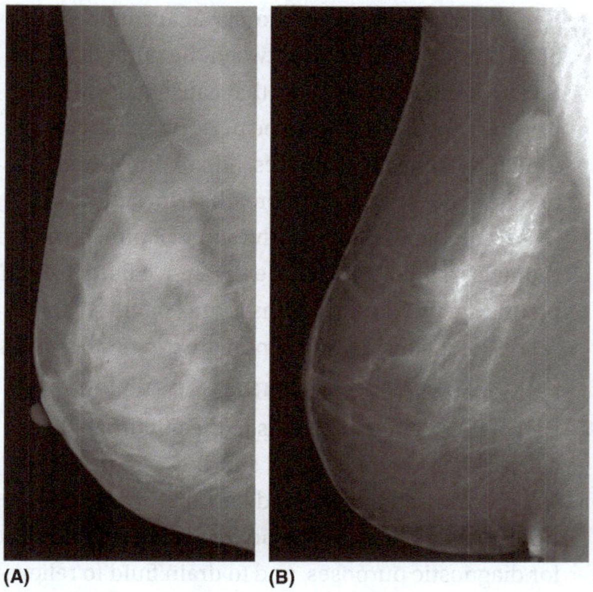

FIGURE 20.8 (A) A normal mammogram in which no abnormal mass is visible. (B) A mammogram in which breast cancer is visible.

detail than a CT, and is often performed after a CT shows an abnormal finding.

Nuclear Medicine

A **nuclear scan** is a diagnostic procedure that uses nuclear medicine technology to gather information about the structure and function of organs or body systems that cannot be seen on conventional x-rays.

- **Positron emission tomography** (**PAW**-zih-tron ee-**MIH**-shun tuh-**MAW**-gruh-fee) (PET), also known as ***PET scans***, combines computed tomography with radionuclide tracers, usually inserted into a vein, to produce enhanced images of selected body organs or areas. Damaged tissues have reduced metabolic activity, so the gamma radiation from these areas is reduced or absent. Cancer cells have increased metabolic activity, and show as bright areas on PET scans.
  - PET scans of the whole body are often used to detect cancer and to monitor the effects of cancer treatment.
- A **bone scan** is a nuclear scanning test similar to a PET scan that identifies new areas of bone growth or breakdown. The results are obtained after a radionuclide tracer is injected into the bloodstream, and the patient then waits while the material travels through the body tissues (see Chapter 21, Figure 21.20). This is different than ***bone density testing***, which is discussed in Chapter 3.
  - This testing can be done to evaluate damage to the bones, detect cancer that has metastasized (spread) to the bones, and monitor conditions that can affect the bones. See Chapter 21 for more information.
- **Molecular breast imaging** (MBI) is a nuclear medicine technique (see Chapter 21) that uses gamma radiation to detect potential tumors in particularly dense breast tissue.

Identifying Cancer

Since cancer involves the abnormal growth of cells, which may not occur in normal or recognizable patterns or forms, laboratory analysis is important to gain as much information as possible about the tissue sample.

- By examining a tissue sample under a microscope, a pathologist can differentiate between benign and malignant tumors. A pathologist can also gain more information about the cancer based on the type of cells examined. For example, epithelial cells found in a malignant bone tumor can suggest that the primary location of the cancer is actually in the lung. This can help identify other locations of cancer and help determine the best methods of treatment.

Invasive Diagnostic Procedures

In addition to blood tests, which are discussed in Chapter 6, some diagnostic procedures are invasive and may involve endoscopy or surgery to directly access the potential cancer in order to test for abnormal cells. An ***invasive*** procedure involves placing medical instruments inside the body, either through an incision or an orifice such as the mouth.

- **Pap smear** screening is routinely performed to detect and treat precancerous changes in the cervix to prevent the development of cervical cancer (see Chapter 16, Figure 16.11).
- A **digital rectal examination** (DRE) is performed on men by using a lubricated, gloved finger placed in the rectum to palpate the prostate gland to detect prostate enlargement and to look for indications of prostate cancer or tumors of the rectum. In this context, the term ***digital*** means using a finger. ***Palpate*** means the use of touch to examine a body part.

Endoscopy

An **endoscopy** is the direct visual examination of the interior of a body cavity. The gastrointestinal tract is the part of the body where endoscopy is most frequently done, and the procedure can be used to diagnose cancer of the stomach.

- An **esophagogastroduodenoscopy** (EGD), also known as an ***upper endoscopy***, is the direct visual examination of the inner surface of the gastrointestinal tract down to the duodenum with an endoscope. An EGD can be used to diagnose cancer of the esophagus or stomach, and to remove samples for biopsy.
- A **colonoscopy** (**koh**-lun-**OSS**-koh-pee) is the direct visual examination of the inner surface of the entire colon from the rectum to the cecum using a colonoscope (**colon/o** means colon, and **-scopy** means visual examination). A colonoscopy can be used to diagnose cancer of the colon or rectum, and to remove samples for biopsy (see the section "Colorectal Cancer Surgery").
  - In a ***virtual colonoscopy***, a small, flexible tube is inserted into the rectum, and an MRI or a CT machine is used to produce two- and three-dimensional images of the colon. The preparation, which requires that the bowels be completely emptied, is the same for both a virtual and regular colonoscopy.

Centesis

Centesis (sen-**TEE**-sis) is a surgical puncture to remove excess fluid or to remove fluid for diagnostic purposes. *Note: Centesis* is used alone as a noun or as a suffix in conjunction with the combining form describing the body part being treated.

- A **malignant pleural effusion** is an accumulation of fluid and cancer cells between the outer layer of the lung and the chest wall that causes shortness of breath. Thoracentesis can be performed to remove fluid for diagnostic purposes, and to drain fluid to relieve the shortness of breath. **Thoracentesis** (**thoh**-rah-sen-**TEE**-sis) is the surgical puncture of the thoracic cavity with a needle to remove fluid from the pleural cavity (**thor/a** means thorax or chest, and **-centesis** means a surgical puncture to remove fluid).
- **Malignant ascites** (ah-**SIGH**-teez) is an accumulation of fluid and cancer cells in the abdomen that causes abdominal swelling, shortness of breath, weight gain, fatigue, and indigestion (Figure 20.9). Abdominocentesis can be performed to remove fluid for diagnostic purposes, and to drain fluid to relieve the symptoms of malignant ascites. **Abdominocentesis** (ab-**dom**-ih-noh-sen-**TEE**-sis) is the surgical puncture of the abdominal cavity to remove fluid (**abdomin/o** means abdomen, and **-centesis** means a surgical puncture to remove fluid).

Biopsy

A **biopsy** (**BYE**-op-see) is the removal of a small piece of living tissue for examination to confirm or establish a diagnosis (**bi** means pertaining to life, and **-opsy** means

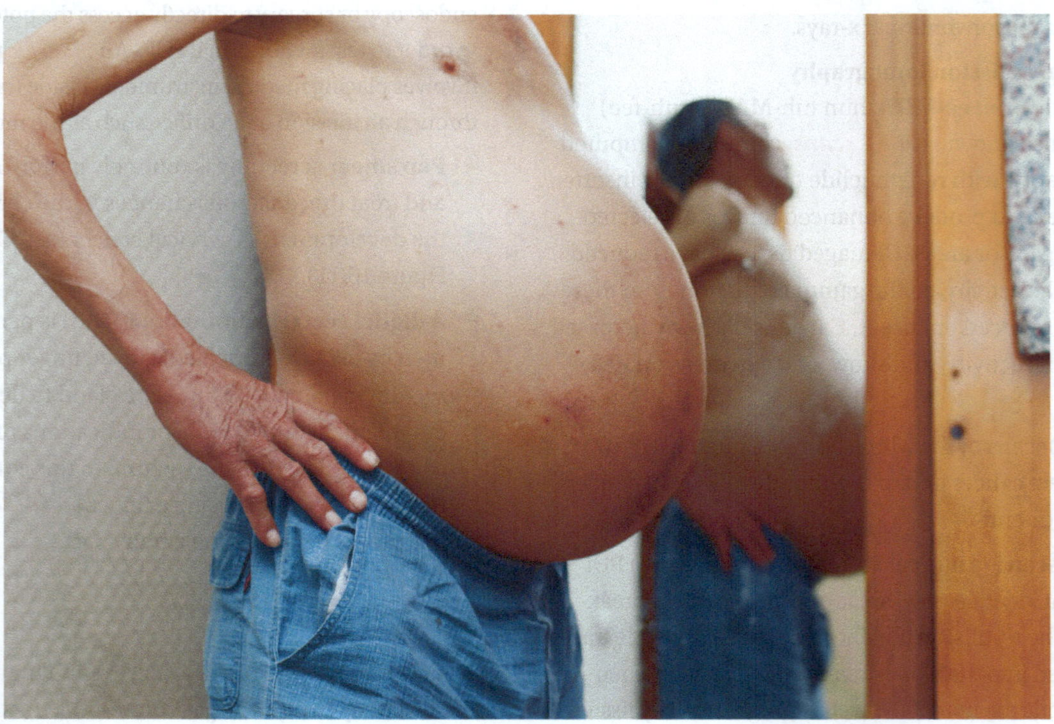

donikz/Shutterstock.com

FIGURE 20.9 Malignant ascites is an accumulation of fluid and cancer cells in the abdomen that causes abdominal swelling.

view of). After a biopsy the sample is sent to a laboratory for testing by a pathologist.

- A **core needle biopsy**, also known as a *needle biopsy*, is a technique in which a hollow needle is used with or without imaging such as ultrasound to remove small samples of tissue for diagnosis and the planning of treatment. It is less painful and disfiguring than a surgical biopsy.
- A **surgical biopsy** is the removal of a larger piece of tissue for examination to confirm a diagnosis. The entire mass may be removed at this time, prior to the biopsy results confirming diagnosis.
  - In an *incisional biopsy*, a piece, but not all, of the tumor or lesion is removed.
  - In an *excisional biopsy*, the entire tumor or lesion and a margin of surrounding tissue are removed. *Excision* means the complete removal of a lesion or organ.
- A **sentinel node biopsy** is a biopsy of the first lymph node to come into contact with cancer cells as they leave the organ of origination and start spreading into the rest of the body. After the sentinel lymph node has been identified, only this and the other affected nodes are removed for dissection.
  - **Lymph node dissection** is a surgical procedure in which all of the lymph nodes in a major group are removed to determine or slow the spread of cancer in this area. For example, an *axillary lymph node dissection* is sometimes performed as part of the surgical treatment of breast cancer.
- **Conization** (**kon**-ih-**ZAY**-shun), also known as a *cone biopsy*, is the surgical removal of a cone-shaped specimen of tissue from the cervix. This is performed as a diagnostic procedure or to remove abnormal tissue.

TREATMENT PROCEDURES RELATED TO ONCOLOGY

The most common forms of treatment for all types of cancer are surgery, radiation therapy, and chemotherapy.

- **Adjuvant therapy** (**AD**-jeh-vant) is sometimes used after the primary cancer treatments have been completed to decrease the chance that a cancer will recur. The term *adjuvant* refers to an agent intended to increase the effectiveness of a drug; however, adjuvant treatments for cancer can also include chemotherapy, hormone therapy, radiation, immunotherapy, or targeted therapy.
- **Neoadjuvant therapy** (**nee**-oh-**AD**-jeh-vant) is when systemic treatment, such as chemotherapy or radiation, is used to reduce the size of the cancer before surgery is performed.
- **Clinical trials** involve testing new and promising cancer treatments that have not yet received Food and Drug Administration (FDA) approval on patients who agree to be part of the research.

Cancer Surgery

Most commonly, cancer surgery involves removing the malignancy plus a margin of normal surrounding tissue. It may also involve the removal of one or more nearby lymph nodes to detect whether the cancer has started to spread. Other types of cancer surgery include:

- *Laser surgery*, which uses targeted beams of light to destroy cancer cells
- *Cryosurgery*, in which cancerous cells are frozen and destroyed using a substance such as liquid nitrogen

Most types of surgery are named for the object being removed, while some are named for the person who invented the surgery.

Lung Cancer Surgery

- A **pneumonectomy** (**new**-moh-**NECK**-toh-mee) is the surgical removal of all or part of a lung (**pneumon** means lung, and **-ectomy** means surgical removal).
- A **lobectomy** (loh-**BECK**-toh-mee) is the surgical removal of a lobe of an organ, usually the lung, brain, liver, or thyroid gland (**lob** means lobe, and **-ectomy** means surgical removal).
- **Wedge resection** is a surgery in which a small wedge-shaped piece of cancerous lung tissue is removed, along with a margin of healthy tissue around the cancer. A wedge resection removes less tissue than a lobectomy.

Breast Cancer Surgery

- A **lumpectomy**, also called *partial mastectomy* or *breast-conserving surgery*, is the surgical removal of only the cancerous tissue with the surrounding margin of normal tissue (Figure 20.10). The remainder of the tissue of the affected breast is not removed.
- A **mastectomy** (mas-**TECK**-toh-mee) is the surgical removal of the entire breast and nipple (**mast** means breast, and **-ectomy** means surgical removal).

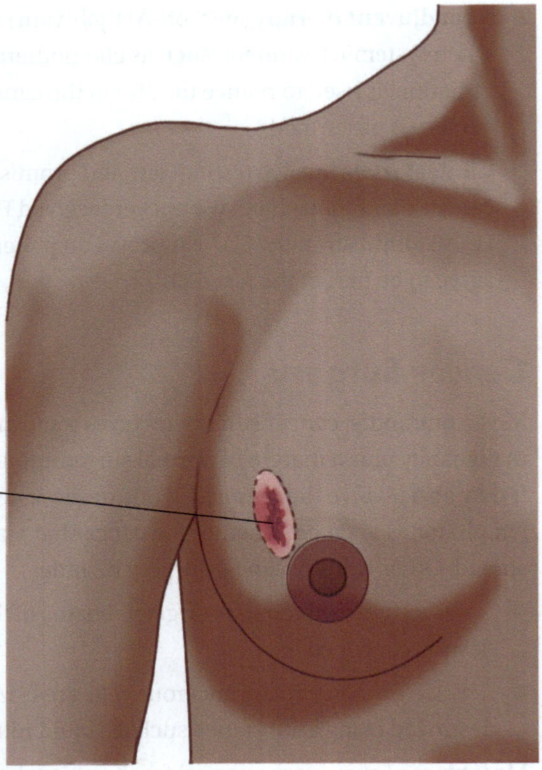

FIGURE 20.10 A lumpectomy is the removal of the cancerous tissue plus a margin of healthy tissue.

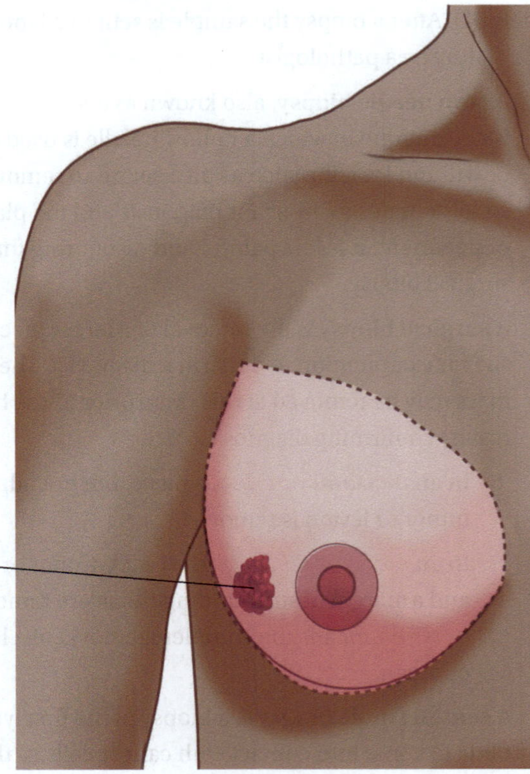

FIGURE 20.11 A modified radical mastectomy is the removal of the entire breast and the adjacent lymph nodes.

Although described as a mastectomy, this procedure, also referred to as a *simple* or *total mastectomy*, may include the removal of some axillary lymph nodes under the adjacent arm. A *double mastectomy* refers to the surgical removal of both breasts. A mastectomy can be referred to as *skin-sparing* or *nipple-sparing* in order to preserve some tissue to aid in reconstruction.

- A **modified radical mastectomy** is the surgical removal of the entire breast and all of the axillary lymph nodes under the adjacent arm (Figure 20.11).

Skin Cancer Surgery

- **Mohs surgery** (**MOZE**) is a technique used to treat various types of skin cancer. Individual layers of cancerous tissue are removed and examined under a microscope one at a time until a margin that is clear of all cancerous tissue has been achieved (Figure 20.12).

Prostate Cancer Surgery

- **Ablation** (ab-**LAY**-shun) is the term used to describe some types of treatment of prostate cancer. This treatment involves the removal of a body part or the destruction of its function through the use of surgery, hormones, drugs, heat, chemicals, electrocautery, or other methods. *Electrocautery* is the use of high-frequency electrical current to destroy tissue.
- A **prostatectomy** (**pros**-tah-**TECK**-toh-mee) is the surgical removal of part or all of the prostate gland (**prostat** means prostate, and **-ectomy** means surgical removal). This procedure is performed to treat prostate cancer or to reduce an enlarged prostate gland; however, this treatment can lead to erectile difficulties. A *radical prostatectomy* is the surgical removal of the entire prostate gland in cases where it is extremely enlarged or when cancer is suspected.
- A **transurethral prostatectomy** (TURP) is the removal of excess tissue from an enlarged prostate gland with the use of a resectoscope. A *resectoscope* is a specialized endoscopic instrument that resembles a cystoscope (see Chapter 10, Figure 10.18).

Colorectal Cancer Surgery

- A **polypectomy** (**poh**-lih-**PECK**-toh-mee) is the surgical removal of a polyp from the lining of the colon or rectum. This is often performed during a colonoscopy.

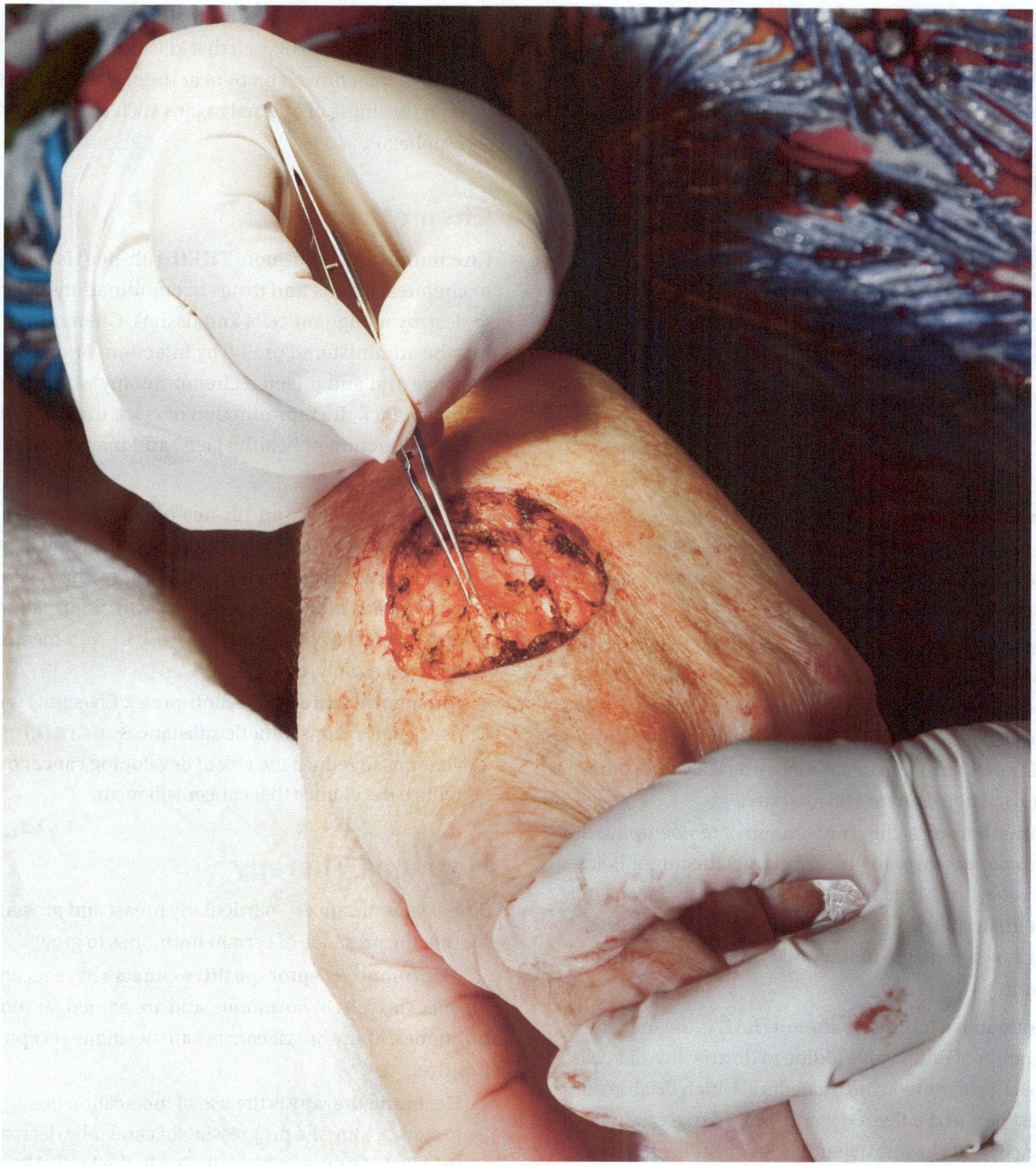

FIGURE 20.12 Mohs surgery in the process of removing a melanoma.

- A **partial colectomy** (koh-**LECK**-toh-mee), also known as a ***hemicolectomy***, is the surgical removal of part of the colon (**col** means colon, and **-ectomy** means surgical removal). Once part of the colon is removed, the remaining sections of colon may be reattached to each other, or a *colostomy* may be placed at the end of the remaining intestine.
  - A **colostomy** (koh-**LAHS**-toh-mee) is the surgical creation of an artificial excretory opening between the colon and the body surface (**col** means colon, and **-ostomy** means surgically creating an opening). The fecal matter flows through the stoma into a disposable bag.

Radiation Therapy

Radiation therapy is used in the treatment of some cancers, with the goal of destroying only the cancerous tissues while sparing healthy tissues (Figure 20.13).

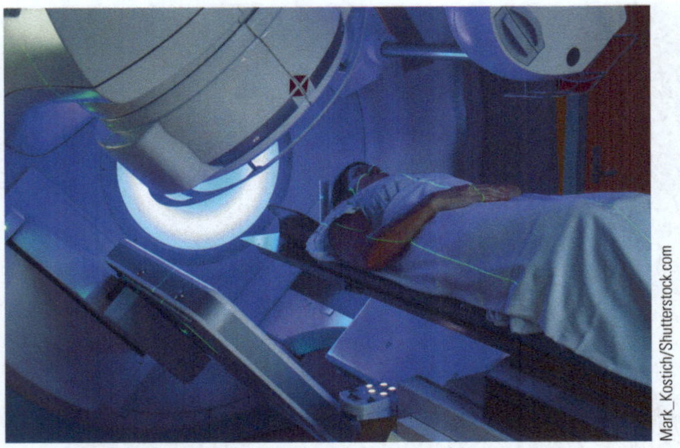

FIGURE 20.13 Radiation therapy destroys cancerous cells while sparing healthy tissues.

- **Brachytherapy** (**brack**-ee-**THER**-ah-pee) is the use of radioactive materials in contact with or implanted into the tissues to be treated (**brachy-** means short, and **-therapy** means treatment).
- **Teletherapy** (**tel**-eh-**THER**-ah-pee) is radiation therapy administered at a distance from the body (**tele-** means distant, and **-therapy** means treatment). With the assistance of three-dimensional computer imaging, it is possible to aim doses more precisely than other kinds of non-targeted teletherapy.
- **Tomotherapy** is the combination of *tomography* with *radiation therapy* to precisely target the tumor being treated (**tom/o** means slice, and **-therapy** means treatment). In this type of therapy, radiation is delivered slice by slice to the tumor and is able to avoid healthy tissue.
- **Radioactive iodine treatment** (RAI) is the oral administration of radioactive iodine to destroy thyroid cells. This nuclear medicine procedure, which disables at least part of the thyroid gland, is used to treat thyroid cancer and chronic hyperthyroid disorders such as Graves' disease. For more information on nuclear medicine, see Chapter 21.

Photodynamic Therapy

Photodynamic therapy (**foh**-toh-dye-**NAH**-mik) (PDT), also known as ***blue-light therapy***, is a technique used to treat damaged and precancerous skin, as well as various types of cancer.

- A ***photosensitizing drug*** is administered topically or by injection. An incubation period is followed by exposure to a specific wavelength of light, administered either externally or endoscopically.
- When the photosensitizers are thus activated, they produce a form of oxygen that kills nearby cells. PDT is used to treat tumors on or near the surface of the skin, or in the lining of internal organs such as the lungs and esophagus.

Chemotherapy

Chemotherapy (**kee**-moh-**THEH**-ruh-pee) is the use of chemical agents and drugs in combinations selected to destroy malignant cells and tissues. Chemotherapy may be administered orally, by injection, or topically. Because oral and injected chemotherapy work systemically to block the reproduction of cells, they also affect the reproduction of healthy cells, and may cause severe side effects.

- An **antineoplastic** (**an**-tih-nee-oh-**PLAS**-tick) is a medication that blocks the development, growth, or proliferation of malignant cells (**anti-** means against, **ne/o** means new, **plast** means growth or formation, and **-ic** means pertaining to). ***Proliferation*** means to increase rapidly.
- **Chemoprevention** (**kee**-moh-pree-**VEN**-shun) is the use of natural or synthetic substances such as drugs or vitamins to reduce the risk of developing cancer or to reduce the chance that cancer will recur.

Hormone Therapy

Some types of cancer—particularly breast and prostate—require the presence of certain hormones to grow.

Hormone receptor–positive cancers have receptors for specific types of hormones, and are named for those hormones. Many breast cancers are hormone receptor–positive.

- **Hormone therapy** is the use of medication or surgery to slow or stop the progression of cancer by decreasing the level of hormones circulating in the body. Hormone therapy may work by preventing the hormone from binding with cancer cells, changing the way the hormone functions, or stopping the body from producing the hormone.

Targeted Therapy

Targeted therapy is a form of anticancer drug therapy that uses drugs or other substances to identify and attack specific cancer cells without harming normal cells. Targeted therapy drugs may be given by mouth or by injection, depending on the medication.

- **Monoclonal antibodies** (**maw**-noh-**KLOH**-null **AN**-tih-**bod**-eez) are molecules designed to locate and attack specific proteins on cancer cells. These molecules can either function like antibodies to destroy the protein, or can be used to deliver doses of chemotherapy or radiation directly to cancer cells.
- **Immunotherapy** (ih-**myoo**-noh-**THEH**-rah-pee) boosts the ability of the immune system to recognize and fight cancer. An ***immune checkpoint inhibitor***, which prevents cancer cells from passing immune system checkpoints by pretending to be normal cells, is one example of immunotherapy.
- **Angiogenesis inhibitors** are medications that interfere with the ability of the tumor to create new blood vessels.
    - **Antiangiogenesis** (**an**-tih-an-jee-oh-**JEN**-eh-sis) is a form of treatment that disrupts the blood supply to the tumor (**anti-** means against, **angi/o** means vessel, and **-genesis** means reproduction). Antiangiogenesis is the opposite of *angiogenesis.*

REMISSION

Remission (ree-**MIH**-shun) is the complete or partial end of cancer signs and symptoms for at least one month. Remission does not necessarily mean that the cancer has been cured. It is not always permanent, and does not ensure that the cancer will not recur with time.

- **Partial remission** is the reduction of cancer in response to treatment, most often by at least 50%.
- **Complete remission** is the absence of cancer in response to treatment. This is also referred to as *No Evidence of Disease* (NED). Complete remission for at least five years may be considered a sign that the patient is *cured* or *cancer-free*. However, there is still a possibility of cancer recurring after that time.
- A **cancer survivor** is a person who is living with or after cancer. A cancer survivor may be in remission, or their cancer may now be a chronic condition managed with ongoing treatments. Cancer survivors are often anxious that any new physical symptoms are a sign of cancer recurrence, and may either request additional testing or postpone routine screening exams.

ABBREVIATIONS RELATED TO ONCOLOGY

Table 20.2 presents an overview of the abbreviations related to the terms introduced in this chapter. *Note:* To avoid errors or confusion, always be cautious when using abbreviations.

TABLE 20.2

Abbreviations Related to Oncology

acute myeloid leukemia = AML	**AML** = acute myeloid leukemia
basal cell carcinoma = BCC	**BCC** = basal cell carcinoma
cancer = CA	**CA** = cancer
chronic myeloid leukemia = CML	**CML** = chronic myeloid leukemia
ductal carcinoma in situ = DCIS	**DCIS** = ductal carcinoma in situ
Hodgkin's lymphoma = HL	**HL** = Hodgkin's lymphoma
malignant melanoma = MM	**MM** = malignant melanoma
non-Hodgkin's lymphoma = NHL	**NHL** = non-Hodgkin's lymphoma

CHAPTER 20

LEARNING EXERCISES

Matching Word Parts 1

Write the correct answer in the middle column.

	Definition	Correct Answer	Possible Answers
20.1.	tumor	________________	**carcin/o**
20.2.	flesh	________________	**path/o**
20.3.	cancerous	________________	**proto-**
20.4.	disease	________________	**sarc/o**
20.5.	first, original	________________	**onc/o**

Matching Word Parts 2

Write the correct answer in the middle column.

	Definition	Correct Answer	Possible Answers
20.6.	life	________________	**angi/o**
20.7.	hidden	________________	**-occult**
20.8.	a view of	________________	**aden/o**
20.9.	gland	________________	**-opsy**
20.10.	blood vessel	________________	**bi/o**

Matching Word Parts 3

Write the correct answer in the middle column.

	Definition	Correct Answer	Possible Answers
20.11.	tumor, neoplasm	________________	**-plasm**
20.12.	formation	________________	**melan/o**
20.13.	reproduction	________________	**neo-**

20.14. new, strange ________________ -genesis

20.15. black ________________ -oma

Definitions

Select the correct answer, and write it on the line provided.

20.16. A ________________ is a cancer that develops from immature undifferentiated cells.

lymphoma | blastoma | carcinoma | leukemia

20.17. ________________ leukemia is characterized by a slow buildup of partly mature leukocytes.

Acute myeloid | Acute lymphocytic | Chronic myeloid | Chroniclymphocytic

20.18. A/An ________________ is a physician who studies the prevention, causes, and treatment of cancer.

chemotherapist | pathologist | radiation therapist | oncologist

20.19. The use of drugs or other substances to identify and attack specific cancer cells without harming normal cells is known as ________________.

neoadjuvant therapy | hormone therapy | immunotherapy | targeted therapy

20.20. Abdominocentesis is performed to treat ________________, an accumulation of fluid and cancer cells in the abdomen.

lymphoma | malignant ascites | thoracentesis | malignant pleural effusion

20.21. A ________________ is a nuclear scanning test that identifies new areas of bone growth or breakdown.

bone scan | bone density test | Pap smear | CT scan

20.22. The process of classifying tumors by how far the disease has progressed, the potential for its responding to therapy, and the patient's prognosis is known as ________________.

adjuvant therapy | staging | partial remission | immunotherapy

20.23. A mutated gene within a cell that causes that cell to function abnormally is called a/an ________________.

oncogene | proto-oncogene | carcinogen | metastasis

20.24. A/An ________________ is a mushroom-like growth from the surface of a mucous membrane.

lymphoma | adenoma | polyp | neoplasm

20.25. A medical professional who specializes in the delivery of radiation treatment is known as a

________________.

radiation oncologist pathologist chemotherapy nurse radiation therapist

Matching Techniques

Write the correct answer in the middle column.

	Definition	Correct Answer	Possible Answers
20.26.	removal of a small piece of living tissue for examination	________________	neoadjuvant therapy
20.27.	surgical removal of the entire breast and all axillary lymph nodes	________________	biopsy
20.28.	systemic treatment used to reduce the size of cancer before surgery	________________	modified radicalmastectomy
20.29.	surgical removal of the entire breast and nipple	________________	sentinel node biopsy
20.30.	biopsy of the first lymph node to come into contact with cancer	________________	mastectomy

Which Word? 1

Select the correct answer, and write it on the line provided.

20.31. ________________ is the use of radioactive materials in contact with or implanted into the tissues to be treated.

Brachytherapy Teletherapy

20.32. ________________ is the complete or partial end of cancer signs and symptoms for at least one month.

Metastasis Remission

20.33. A technique in which cells are scraped from the tissue and examined under a microscope is known as ________________.

exfoliative cytology ablation

20.34. A rare type of malignant liver cancer that occurs in children under age 3 is known as a

________________________.

hepatoblastoma Wilms tumor

20.35. Substances found in many fruits and vegetables which may help decrease the risk of cancer are called

________________________.

carcinogens antioxidants

Spelling Counts

Find the misspelled word in each sentence. Then write that word, spelled correctly, on the line provided.

20.36. Inizing radiation is present in x-rays and other medical imaging procedures. ________________________

20.37. A carcenoma is a type of cancer that occurs in epithelial tissue. ________________________

20.38. Squamous cell carcinoma in situ is also known as Bowan disease. ________________________

20.39. A surgical puncture to remove fluid for diagnostic purposes is called sentesis. ________________________

20.40. Angiogenisis inhibitors are medications that interfere with the ability of the tumor to create new blood vessels. ________________________

Abbreviation Identification 1

In the space provided, write the words in English that each abbreviation stands for.

20.41. **CML** ________________________

20.42. **HL** ________________________

20.43. **CA** ________________________

20.44. **DCIS** ________________________

20.45. **MM** ________________________

Term Selection

Select the correct answer, and write it on the line provided.

20.46. Breast cancer that does not have receptors for estrogen or progesterone, and has low levels of HER2 is known as ______________ breast cancer.

triple-negative triple-positive inflammatory infiltrating ductal

20.47. The blood test used to screen for prostate cancer is known as the ______________ blood test.

conization Mohs prostate-specific antigen Hemoccult

20.48. ______________ is an x-ray examination of the breasts to detect the presence of tumors or precancerous cells.

Mammography Palpation of the breast Breast self-examination Mastectomy

20.49. Treatment sometimes used after primary cancer treatments have been completed to decrease the chance that a cancer will recur is known as ______________.

neoadjuvant therapy adjuvant therapy clinical trials chemoprevention

20.50. Treatment that boosts the ability of the immune system to recognize and fight cancer is known as ______________.

radiation chemotherapy monoclonal antibodies immunotherapy

Sentence Completion 1

Write the correct term on the line provided.

20.51. The term ______________ describes the process through which normal cells become cancer cells.

20.52. The term ______________ describes a type of cancer characterized by a sudden increase in abnormal immature lymphocytes.

20.53. A/An ______________ is a registered nurse who specializes in the administration of intravenous chemotherapeutic agents and monitoring patients during treatment.

20.54. The term ______________ describes the uncontrolled growth of abnormal, poorly differentiated cells commonly seen in most malignant tumors.

20.55. ________________________ is breast cancer at its earliest stage before the abnormal cells have broken through the wall of the milk ducts.

Word Surgery

Divide each term into its component word parts. Write these word parts, in sequence, on the lines provided. When necessary use a slash (/) to indicate a combining vowel. (You may not need all of the lines provided.)

20.56. An **antineoplastic** is a medication that blocks the development, growth, or proliferation of malignant cells.

________ ________ ________ ________

20.57. **Osteosarcoma** is a hard-tissue sarcoma that usually involves the upper shaft of the long bones, pelvis, or knee.

________ ________ ________ ________

20.58. **Antiangiogenesis** is a form of cancer treatment that disrupts the blood supply to the tumor.

________ ________ ________ ________

20.59. A **proto-oncogene** is a normal gene within a cell that controls one of the normal processes of the cell.

________ ________ ________ ________

20.60. **Tomotherapy** is the combination of tomography with radiation therapy to precisely target the tumor being treated.

________ ________ ________ ________

True/False

If the statement is true, write **True** on the line. If the statement is false, write **False** on the line.

20.61. ________ Inflammatory breast cancer is a rare but aggressive form of breast cancer.

20.62. ________ Partial remission is the absence of cancer in response to treatment.

20.63. ________ A colectomy is the surgical creation of an artificial excretory opening between the colon and the skin.

20.64. ________ Reed-Sternberg cells are present in Hodgkin's lymphoma.

20.65. ________ Teletherapy is radiation therapy administered at a distance from the body.

Clinical Conditions

Write the correct answer on the line provided.

20.66. As part of the diagnosis of Juanita Phillips's cancer, a/an ______________________ biopsy was performed using a hollow, ultrasound-guided needle.

20.67. Dorothy Peterson was diagnosed with breast cancer. She and her doctor agreed upon treating this surgically with a/an ______________________. This is a procedure in which the cancerous tissue and a margin of normal tissue are removed.

20.68. John Fogelman was diagnosed with having a/an ______________________. This is a type of cancer that arises from connective tissues, including hard and soft tissues.

20.69. After Elias Fowler's colonoscopy, his doctor told him they had also surgically removed several polyps from the lining of his colon. This procedure is known as a/an ______________________.

20.70. Jenys Shoemaker's doctor suggested treating her squamous cell carcinoma with ______________________, also known as blue-light therapy.

20.71. Dr. Eusebio was concerned about the abnormal growth of body tissue creating a mass. She told Mr. Herder that they would closely examine his ______________________, also known as a neoplasm.

20.72. It came as a shock to Mrs. Oguntala to be diagnosed with ______________________, a type of cancer that occurs in blood-making plasma cells found in the red bone marrow.

20.73. Betsy Wong was 3 years old when she was diagnosed with a/an ______________, also known as a nephroblastoma.

20.74. Mr. Galves was diagnosed with ______________________ leukemia. This is a type of cancer characterized by a slow buildup of partly mature lymphocytes.

20.75. Angie Hoskin's breast cancer had receptors for both estrogen and progesterone, in addition to high levels of HER2. This is called ______________________ breast cancer.

Which Is the Correct Medical Term?

Select the correct answer, and write it on the line provided.

20.76. A/An ______________________ is any one of a large group of carcinomas derived from glandular tissue.

adenocarcinoma lymphoma myosarcoma myoma

20.77. The abnormal development or growth of cells, or the presence of abnormal cells within a type of tissue, is called ______________________.

normal cell growth | hyperplasia | anaplasia | dysplasia

20.78. A person who is living with or after cancer is known as a ______________________.

partial remission | complete remission | cancer survivor | clinical trial

20.79. A ______________________ *tumor* is not a form of cancer, and is not life-threatening.

malignant | benign | neoplasm | primary site

20.80. The use of natural or synthetic substances such as drugs or vitamins to reduce the risk of developing cancer or to reduce the chance that cancer will recur is known as ______________________.

chemoprevention | antioxidants | chemotherapy | proto-oncogenes

Abbreviation Identification 2

In the space provided, write the words in English that each abbreviation stands for.

20.81. **PIN** ______________________

20.82. **ALL** ______________________

20.83. **IDC** ______________________

20.84. **PIA** ______________________

20.85. **DRE** ______________________

Sentence Completion 2

Write the correct term on the line provided.

20.86. The term ______________________ describes molecules designed to locate and attack specific proteins on cancer cells.

20.87. The term ______________________ describes the surgical removal of a cone-shaped specimen of tissue from the cervix.

20.88. ______________________ *imaging* is a nuclear medicine technique using gamma radiation to detect potential tumors in dense breast tissue.

20.89. ______________________ are known mutations in certain genes that can be passed down from parent to child, and are linked with an increased risk of cancer.

20.90. ______________________ is the study of the prevention, causes, and treatments of tumors and cancer.

Which Word? 2

Select the correct answer, and write it on the line provided.

20.91. A/An ______________________ polyp is the most common type of precancerous neoplastic polyp.

adenomatous colorectal

20.92. ______________________ melanoma is the most common form of skin cancer in African Americans, and is not linked to sun exposure.

Malignant Acral lentiginous

20.93. Cancer in its initial location is known as a ______________________ cancer.

secondary primary

20.94. The process by which cancer is spread to a new site is called ______________________.

metastasis metastasize

20.95. ______________________ lung cancer is a fast-growing cancer that occurs most often in smokers.

Small cell Non-small cell

Matching Staging and Grading

Write the correct answer in the middle column.

	Definition	Correct Answer	Possible Answers
20.96.	Cancer is undifferentiated.	______________________	Stage 2
20.97.	Cancer cells are found in one location.	______________________	Grade 2
20.98.	Cancer has spread to other organs.	______________________	Grade 4
20.99.	Cancer is moderately differentiated.	______________________	Stage 4
20.100.	Cancer has increased in size and/or reached nearby lymph nodes.	______________________	Stage 0

The Human Touch

CRITICAL THINKING EXERCISE

The following story and questions are designed to stimulate critical thinking through class discussion or as a brief essay response. There are no right or wrong answers to these questions.

Matthew Montgomery, a 37-year-old father of two, had been rushed to the emergency room two months ago when he'd felt sudden chest pains while lifting boxes at his warehouse job. Although he'd been relieved when the ER doctor determined he wasn't having a heart attack, the chest x-ray did reveal a suspicious mass in one lung. His primary care doctor had ordered a biopsy and further imaging, and referred him to oncologist Shauni Jacobs. Matthew was terrified of the possibility of cancer, and had been dreading the results, but he knew he owed it to his family to figure out what was going on.

Dr. Jacobs glanced down at her computer, and then back at Matthew sitting nervously across the desk from her. "I'm afraid the pathology results confirm that you do have cancer," Dr. Jacobs began. "It's what we call non-small cell lung cancer, or to be more specific, a stage 1 adenocarcinoma. That means that it hasn't spread to any of the lymph nodes nearby, and there aren't signs of cancer anywhere else in your body. The tumor is about 4 centimeters in size, and there's no sign that it's intruding into your airway at all."

She paused for a moment to give Matthew a chance to speak, but he seemed to be focused on something happening outside the office window. After a moment, she continued. "I'm optimistic that we can do surgery to remove the entire mass, especially since we found the cancer at such an early stage. I think that surgery has a high probability of being successful. Another possibility would be to try some radiation to shrink the mass before surgery, or if you aren't comfortable with any interventions right now, we could monitor it for another few months."

Dr. Jacobs cleared her throat to get Matthew's attention. "I know that a cancer diagnosis can be upsetting, Mr. Montgomery. Would you like to tell me what you're thinking?"

Matthew tossed his pen down on the desk and shook his head. "It's just not fair—I quit smoking five years ago, and I still get lung cancer. And all of my coworkers still smoke right outside the loading dock on their breaks. I might as well start back up smoking again. It's not like quitting has done me any good!"

While Dr. Jacobs knew that if Mr. Montgomery started smoking again, it would impede his healing and recovery, she sensed that he was expressing his anger and grief at the cancer diagnosis. She was also concerned that he might put off making choices about treatment options while he was upset. Glancing back at her computer, she wondered how best to proceed with the conversation.

Suggested Discussion Topics

1. Who can Mr. Montgomery turn to for help in making a decision about treatment?
2. How would your own feelings about a patient's cancer treatment change if you felt he had "brought it upon himself?" Would those feelings change if Mr. Montgomery were still smoking?

3. What is Dr. Jacobs's responsibility if she cannot get Mr. Montgomery to decide on a treatment plan and there is a risk of the tumor becoming larger or metastasizing? What is her responsibility regarding the emotional side of a cancer diagnosis?
4. There is a direct link between smoking and lung cancer. Why do you think people continue to smoke despite knowing this? Are there new ways this fact can be used to discourage smoking?

CHAPTER 21

DIAGNOSTIC PROCEDURES, NUCLEAR MEDICINE, AND COMPLEMENTARY MEDICINE

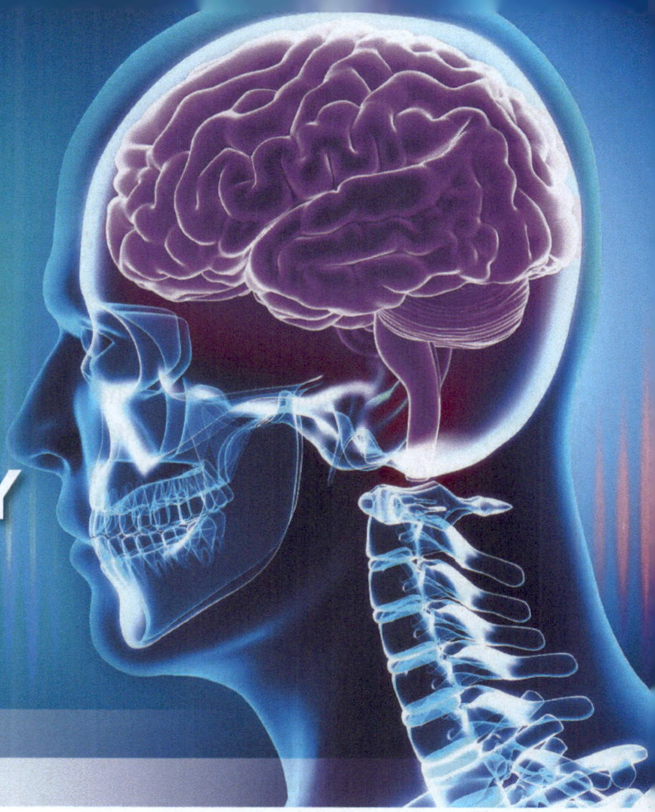

Overview of

DIAGNOSTIC PROCEDURES, NUCLEAR MEDICINE, AND COMPLEMENTARY MEDICINE

Major Headings	Including
Basic Diagnostic Procedures	Vital signs Auscultation Palpation and percussion Basic examination instruments
Examination Positions	Recumbent positions Sims' position Knee–chest position Lithotomy position
Laboratory Tests	Blood tests Urinalysis Stool analysis
Endoscopy	Endoscopes
Centesis	Diagnostic procedures involving the removal of body fluids
Imaging Techniques	Radiography Computed tomography Magnetic resonance imaging Fluoroscopy Ultrasonography
Nuclear Medicine	Nuclear medicine
Complementary and Alternative Therapies	Alternative medicine Complementary medicine

Vocabulary Related to DIAGNOSTIC PROCEDURES, NUCLEAR MEDICINE, AND COMPLEMENTARY MEDICINE

This list contains essential word parts and medical terms for this chapter. These and the other important **primary terms** are shown in **boldface** throughout the chapter. *Secondary terms*, which appear in *orange* italics, clarify the meaning of primary terms.

Word Parts

- ☐ **albumin/o** albumin, protein
- ☐ **calc/i** calcium, lime, the heel
- ☐ **-centesis** surgical puncture to remove fluid
- ☐ **creatin/o** creatinine
- ☐ **fluor/o** glowing
- ☐ **glycos/o** glucose, sugar
- ☐ **lapar/o** abdomen, abdominal wall
- ☐ **-otomy** cutting, surgical incision
- ☐ **radi/o** radiation, x-rays
- ☐ **-scope** instrument for visual examination
- ☐ **-scopy** visual examination
- ☐ **son/o** sound
- ☐ **steth/o** chest
- ☐ **therm/o** heat
- ☐ **ultra-** beyond

Medical Terms

- ☐ **acupuncture** (**AK**-you-**punk**-cher)
- ☐ **albuminuria** (**al**-byou-mih-**NEW**-ree-ah)
- ☐ **alternative medicine**
- ☐ **arthrocentesis** (**ar**-throh-sen-**TEE**-sis)
- ☐ **auscultation** (**aws**-kul-**TAY**-shun)
- ☐ **bacteriuria** (back-**tee**-ree-**YOU**-ree-ah)
- ☐ **basic metabolic panel**
- ☐ **biofeedback**
- ☐ **bruit** (**BREW**-ee)
- ☐ **calciuria** (**kal**-sih-**YOU**-ree-ah)
- ☐ **complementary medicine**
- ☐ **complete blood count**
- ☐ **computed tomography** (toh-**MOG**-rah-fee)
- ☐ **craniosacral therapy** (**kray**-nee-oh-**SAK**-ral)
- ☐ **creatinuria** (**kree**-at-ih-**NEW**-ree-ah)
- ☐ **echocardiography** (**eck**-oh-**kar**-dee-**OG**-rah-fee)
- ☐ **endoscope** (**EN**-doh-**skope**)
- ☐ **fluoroscopy** (floo-**ROS**-koh-pee)
- ☐ **glycosuria** (**glye**-koh-**SOO**-ree-ah)
- ☐ **guided imagery**
- ☐ **hematocrit** (hee-**MAT**-oh-krit)
- ☐ **hematuria** (**hee**-mah-**TOO**-ree-ah)
- ☐ **homeopathy** (**hoh**-mee-**OP**-ah-thee)
- ☐ **hyperthermia** (**high**-per-**THER**-mee-ah)
- ☐ **hypothermia** (**high**-poh-**THER**-mee-ah)
- ☐ **integrative medicine**
- ☐ **interventional radiology**
- ☐ **ketonuria** (**kee**-toh-**NEW**-ree-ah)
- ☐ **laparoscopy** (**lap**-ah-**ROS**-koh-pee)
- ☐ **lithotomy position** (lih-**THOT**-oh-mee)
- ☐ **magnetic resonance imaging**
- ☐ **mindfulness meditation**
- ☐ **naturopathy** (**nay**-cher-**AH**-pah-thee)
- ☐ **neuromuscular therapy**
- ☐ **nuclear imaging**
- ☐ **ophthalmoscope** (ahf-**THAL**-moh-skope)
- ☐ **otoscope** (**OH**-toh-skope)
- ☐ **palpation** (pal-**PAY**-shun)
- ☐ **percussion** (per-**KUSH**-un)
- ☐ **perfusion** (per-**FYOU**-zhun)
- ☐ **pericardiocentesis** (**pehr**-ih-**kar**-dee-oh-sen-**TEE**-sis)
- ☐ **phlebotomy** (fleh-**BOT**-oh-mee)
- ☐ **positron emission tomography**
- ☐ **prone position**
- ☐ **proteinuria** (**proh**-teen-**UHR**-ree-ah)
- ☐ **pyuria** (pye-**YOU**-ree-ah)
- ☐ **radiolucent** (**ray**-dee-oh-**LOO**-sent)
- ☐ **radiopaque** (**ray**-dee-oh-**PAYK**)
- ☐ **rales** (**RAHLZ**)
- ☐ **recumbent** (ree-**KUM**-bent)
- ☐ **rhonchi** (**RONG**-kye)
- ☐ **Sims' position**
- ☐ **single photon emission computed tomography**
- ☐ **speculum** (**SPECK**-you-lum)
- ☐ **sphygmomanometer** (**sfig**-moh-mah-**NOM**-eh-ter)
- ☐ **stethoscope** (**STETH**-oh-skope)
- ☐ **stridor** (**STRYE**-dor)
- ☐ **transesophageal echocardiography** (**trans**-eh-**sof**-ah-**JEE**-al eck-oh-**kar**-dee-**OG**-rah-fee)
- ☐ **ultrasonography** (**ul**-trah-son-**OG**-rah-fee)
- ☐ **urinalysis** (**you**-rih-**NAL**-ih-sis)

LEARNING OBJECTIVES

On completion of this chapter, you should be able to:

1. Define the primary terms associated with basic examination procedures and positions.
2. Define the primary terms associated with frequently performed blood, stool, and urinalysis tests.
3. Define the primary terms associated with endoscopy, centesis, and biopsy.
4. Define the primary terms associated with radiography and other imaging techniques.
5. Describe the uses of nuclear medicine in diagnosis and treatment.
6. Describe the most common types of complementary and alternative therapies and their uses.
7. Identify the medical specialists related to diagnostic procedures, nuclear medicine, and complementary medicine.
8. Identify the medical word parts related to diagnostic procedures and nuclear medicine.
9. Spell the primary terms used for diagnostic procedures.
10. Pronounce the primary terms used for diagnostic procedures.
11. Identify common abbreviations related to diagnostic procedures.

DIAGNOSTIC PROCEDURES

A wide range of diagnostic tools are used to determine the patient's general state of health and to look for specific medical conditions.

Basic Examination Procedures

Basic examination procedures are performed during the assessment of the patient's condition. As used in medicine, the term **assessment** means the evaluation or appraisal of the patient's condition. This information is used in reaching a diagnosis and in formulating a plan of care.

Observation

The first step in a physical assessment is to observe the patient's overall appearance, emotional affect, and ambulation.

- *Overall appearance* includes a number of factors: how appropriately the patient is dressed, whether there is any body odor, or if there are signs of possible difficulties with self-care.
- *Emotional affect* refers to the patient's expression, tone of voice, mood, and emotions. *Affect* means the outward expression of emotion.
- *Ambulation* means the way the patient walks, including gait, any unsteadiness, or possible difficulty.

Vital Signs

Vital signs are the four key indications that the body systems are functioning. These signs, which are recorded for most patient visits, are *temperature*, *pulse*, *respiration*, and *blood pressure*. The abbreviation *VSS* stands for vital signs stable.

Temperature

An average normal body **temperature** is around 98.6°F (Fahrenheit) or 37.0°C (Celsius).

- An oral body temperature of higher than approximately 100°F is a **fever**.
- A fever is most commonly caused by an infection, an injury, or medications.
- Temperature readings are named for the location in which they are taken: *oral* (in the mouth), *aural* (in the ear), *axillary* (in the armpit), and *rectal* (in the rectum). A *temporal artery* (forehead) scanner may also be used. *Caution: Oral* and *aural* sound alike; however, they require different styles of thermometers and are taken in different locations.
- Temperature readings vary slightly depending upon the location in which they are taken.
- **Hyperthermia** (**high**-per-**THER**-mee-ah) is an extremely high body temperature, usually caused by prolonged exposure to environmental heat (**hyper-** means excessive, **therm** means heat, and **-ia** means pertaining to).

- **Hypothermia** (**high**-poh-**THER**-mee-ah) is an abnormally low body temperature (**hypo-** means deficient, **therm** means heat, and **-ia** means pertaining to).

Pulse

The **pulse** is the rhythmic pressure against the walls of an artery that is caused by the beating of the heart. The **heart rate** reflects the number of times the heart beats each minute and is recorded as ***bpm*** (beats per minute). The pulse can be measured at different points on the body, called **pulse points** (Figure 21.1).

- The *normal resting heart rate* differs by age group. In adults, a normal resting heart rate is 60–100 bpm. Generally heart rates are higher in children, and for a newborn the resting heart rate is 100–160 bpm. Athletes, however, can have a normal resting heart rate of 40–60 bpm.
- Among the pulse points of the body, four main points where the pulse is assessed are the **carotid pulse point** (on either side of the front of the neck), **radial pulse point** (at the wrist), **femoral pulse point** (at the inner thigh), and **dorsalis pedis pulse point** (on the top of the foot, in line with the second toe). When assessing a person's pulse, it is important to palpate for at least 15 seconds, and to avoid palpating with your thumb, which has its own palpable pulse.

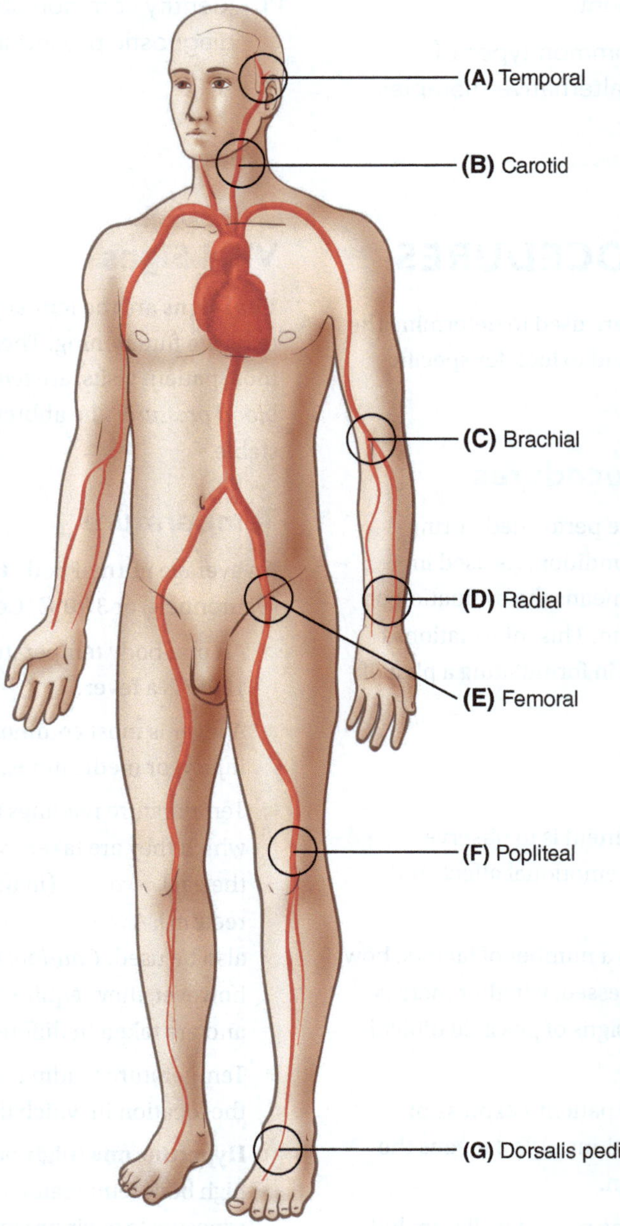

FIGURE 21.1 Pulse points of the body.

Respiration

Respiration, which is also known as the **respiratory rate** (RR), is the number of complete breaths per minute. A single respiration consists of one inhalation and one exhalation (see Chapter 8). The normal respiratory rate for adults ranges from 12 to 20 respirations per minute.

Blood Pressure

Blood pressure (BP) is the force of the blood against the walls of the arteries. This force is measured using a **sphygmomanometer** (**sfig**-moh-mah-**NOM**-eh-ter). When using a manual style, as shown in Figure 21.2, a stethoscope is required to listen to the blood sounds. A digital sphygmomanometer is automated and does not require the use of a stethoscope.

Blood pressure is recorded as a ratio with the **systolic** (sis-**TOL**-ick) over the **diastolic** (dye-ah-**STOL**-ick) reading. The systolic is the first beat heard. The diastolic is the last beat heard. Memory aid: *SSSS-systolic* as in going up to the *sky*. *DDDD-diastolic* as in going *down* (Figure 21.3). Blood pressure ranges are explained in Table 5.3 of Chapter 5.

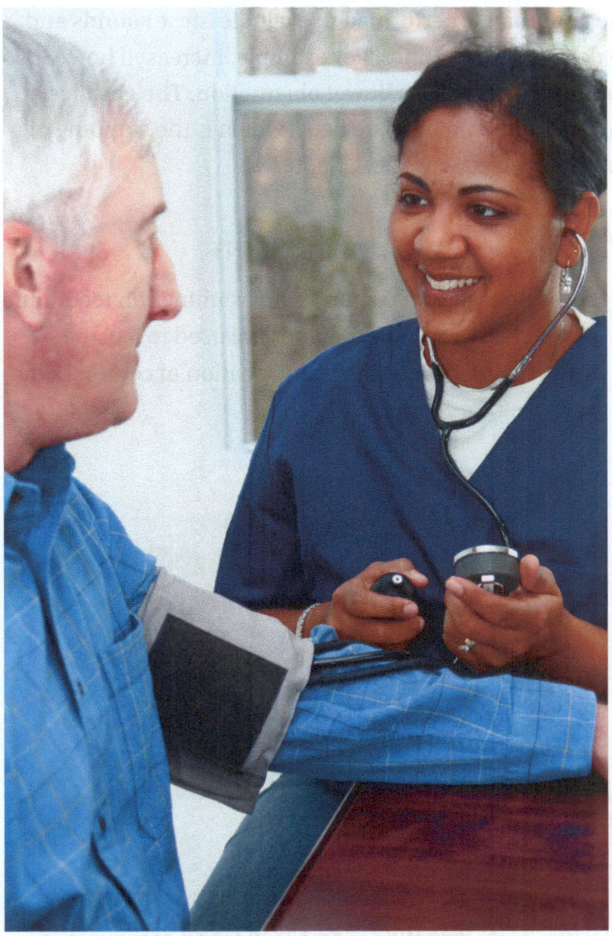

Rob Marmion/Shutterstock.com

FIGURE 21.2 A manual sphygmomanometer being used with a stethoscope to measure blood pressure.

Pain

In certain settings, such as a hospital, **pain** is considered to be the fifth vital sign. Since this is a subjective symptom that cannot be measured objectively, it must be reported by the patient.

- Using a ***pain rating scale***, the patient is asked to describe his or her level of pain from 0 (no pain) to 10 (severe pain) (Figure 21.4).
- ***Acute pain***, which comes on quickly, can be severe and lasts only a relatively short time. It can be caused by disease, inflammation, or injury. When the cause of the pain is diagnosed and treated, the pain goes away.
- ***Chronic pain***, which can be mild to severe, persists over a longer period of time than acute pain and is resistant to most medical treatments.

Auscultation

The term **auscultation** (**aws**-kul-**TAY**-shun) means listening for sounds within the body and is usually performed through a stethoscope (**auscult/a** means to listen, and **-tion** means the process of) (Figure 21.5).

Respiratory Sounds

Respiratory sounds heard through a stethoscope provide information about the condition of the lungs and pleura as the patient breathes (see Chapter 8).

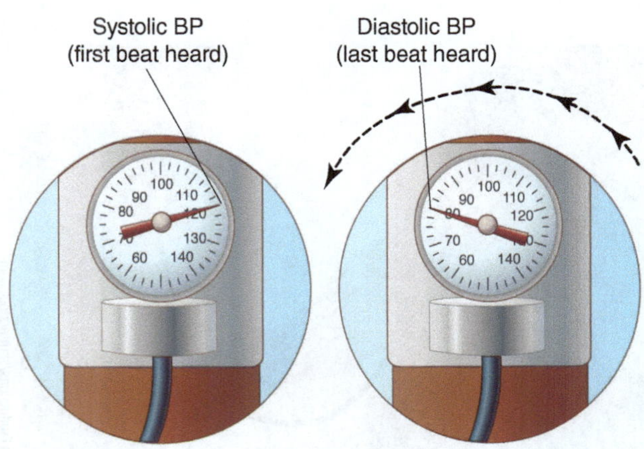

FIGURE 21.3 Using a stethoscope, the systolic pressure is the first sound heard, and the diastolic pressure is the last beat heard.

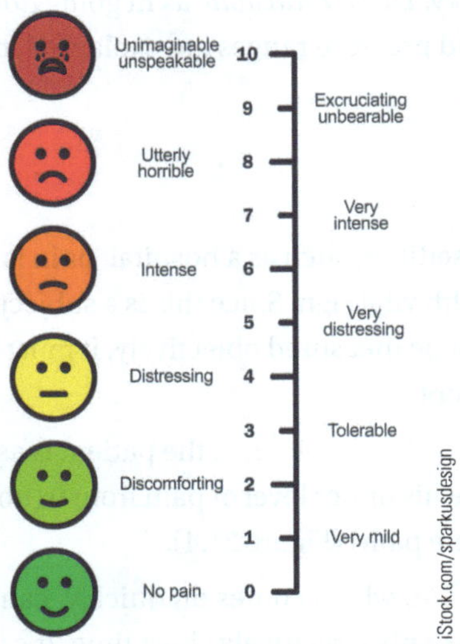

FIGURE 21.4 A pediatric pain scale uses facial expressions instead of numbers.

- **Rales** (**RAHLZ**), also known as ***crackles***, are abnormal crackle-like lung sounds heard through a stethoscope during inspiration (breathing in).
- **Rhonchi** (**RONG**-kye) are coarse rattling sounds that are somewhat like snoring. These sounds are usually caused by secretions in the bronchial airways (singular, *rhonchus*).
- **Stridor** (**STRYE**-dor) is an abnormal, high-pitched, musical breathing sound caused by a blockage in the throat or in the larynx (voice box).

Heart Sounds

The heartbeat heard through a stethoscope has two distinct sounds. These are known as the "lubb dupp" or "lub dub" sounds.

- The ***lubb sound*** is heard first. It is caused by the tricuspid and mitral valves closing between the atria and the ventricles.
- The ***dupp sound***, which is shorter and higher pitched, is heard next. It is caused by the closing of the valves in the aorta and pulmonary arteries as blood is pumped out of the heart.
- A **bruit** (**BREW**-ee) is an abnormal sound or murmur heard during auscultation of an artery. These sounds are usually due to a partially blocked, narrowed, or diseased artery. A ***thrill*** is an abnormal rhythmic vibration felt when palpating an artery. (*Note:* The term *bruit* is sometimes pronounced **BROOT**.)
- A **heart murmur** is an abnormal heart sound that is most commonly a sign of defective heart valves. Heart murmurs are described by volume and the stage of the heartbeat when the murmur is heard.

Abdominal Sounds

Abdominal sounds, also known as ***bowel sounds***, are normal noises made by the intestines. Auscultation of the abdomen is performed to evaluate these sounds and to detect abnormalities. For example, increased bowel sounds can indicate a bowel obstruction. The absence of these sounds can indicate ileus, which is the stopping of intestinal peristalsis (see Chapter 9).

Palpation and Percussion

- **Palpation** (pal-**PAY**-shun) is an examination technique in which the examiner's hands are used to feel the texture, size, consistency, and location of certain body parts (Figure 21.6).

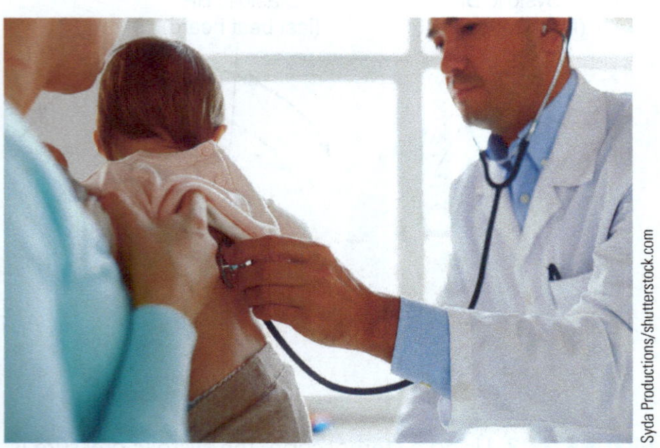

FIGURE 21.5 Auscultation is listening through a stethoscope to sounds within the body.

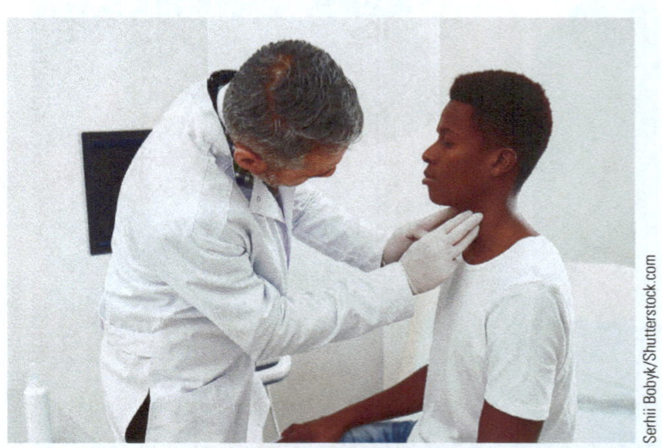

FIGURE 21.6 Palpation is an examination technique in which the examiner's hands are used to feel the texture, size, consistency, and location of certain body parts.

- **Percussion** (per-**KUSH**-un) is a diagnostic procedure designed to determine the density of a body part by the sound produced by tapping the surface with the fingers (Figure 21.7).

Basic Examination Instruments

- An **ophthalmoscope** (ahf-**THAL**-moh-skope) is an instrument used to examine the interior of the eye (**ophthalm/o** means eye, and **-scope** means instrument for visual examination) (Figure 21.8).
- An **otoscope** (**OH**-toh-skope) is an instrument used to visually examine the external ear canal and tympanic membrane (**ot/o** means ear, and **-scope** means instrument for visual examination) (see Chapter 12, Figure 12.15).
- A **speculum** (**SPECK**-you-lum) is an instrument used to enlarge the opening of any canal or cavity, especially the vagina, to facilitate inspection of its interior (see Chapter 16, Figure 16.11A).
- A **stethoscope** (**STETH**-oh-skope) is an instrument used to listen to sounds within the body (**steth/o** means chest, and **-scope** means instrument for examination) (Figures 21.2 and 21.5).

RECUMBENT EXAMINATION POSITIONS

Specific basic examination positions are used to examine different areas of the body. The term **recumbent** (ree-**KUM**-bent) describes any position in which the patient is lying down. This can be on the back, front, or side. In radiography, the term ***decubitus*** describes the patient lying in a recumbent position.

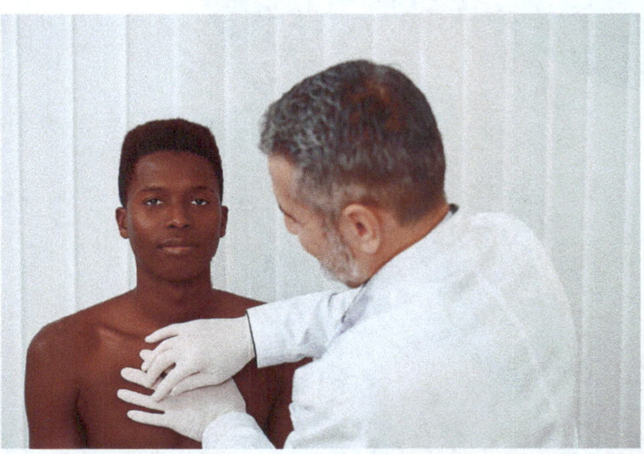

Serhii Bobyk/Shutterstock.com

FIGURE 21.7 Percussion is a diagnostic procedure in which the examiner's hands are used to determine the density of a body area by tapping the surface with the fingers.

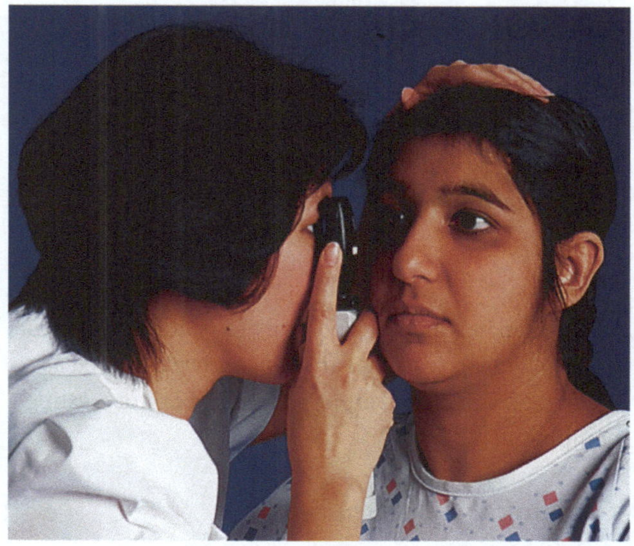

FIGURE 21.8 An ophthalmoscope is used to examine the interior of the eye.

These are positions in which the patient is *face up*:

- In the **horizontal recumbent position**, also known as the ***supine position***, the patient is lying on the back, face up. This position is used for examination and treatment of the anterior surface of the body and for x-rays.
- In the **dorsal recumbent position**, the patient is lying on the back, face up, with the knees bent. This position is used for the examination and treatment of the abdominal area and for vaginal or rectal examinations.
- In the **lithotomy position** (lih-**THOT**-oh-mee) the patient is lying on the back, face up, with the feet and legs raised and supported in stirrups. This position is used for vaginal and rectal examinations and during childbirth. See Chapter 1 for another meaning of lithotomy.

These are positions in which the patient is *face down* or *on his or her side*:

- In a **prone position**, the patient is lying on the abdomen face down. The arms may be placed under the head for comfort. This position is used for the examination and treatment of the back and buttocks.
- In **Sims' position**, the patient is lying on the left side with the right knee and thigh drawn up with the left arm placed along the back. This position is used in the examination and treatment of the rectal area.
- In the **knee-chest position**, the patient is lying face down with the hips bent so that the knees and chest rest on the table. This position is also used for rectal examinations.

LABORATORY TESTS

When a laboratory test is ordered **stat**, the results are needed immediately, and the test has top priority in the laboratory. *Stat* comes from the Latin word meaning immediately.

Blood Tests

When used in regard to laboratory tests, the term ***profile*** or ***panel*** means tests that are frequently performed as a group on automated multi-channel laboratory testing equipment.

Obtaining Specimens

- **Phlebotomy** (fleh-**BOT**-oh-mee), also known as ***venipuncture***, is the puncture of a vein for the purpose of drawing blood (**phleb** means vein, and **-otomy** means a surgical incision) (Figure 21.9).
- An **arterial stick** is the puncture of an artery, usually on the inside of the wrist, to obtain arterial blood. Arterial blood differs from venous blood mostly in the concentration of dissolved gases it contains.
- A ***capillary puncture*** is the technique used when only a small amount of blood is needed as a specimen for a blood test. Named for where it is performed, a capillary puncture is usually known as a ***finger***, ***heel***, or ***earlobe stick***.

Complete Blood Counts

A **complete blood count** (CBC) is a series of tests performed as a group to evaluate several blood conditions. Blood disorders are discussed in Chapter 6.

- **Erythrocyte sedimentation rate** (eh-**RITH**-roh-site) (ESR), also known as a ***sed rate***, is a test based on the speed with which the red blood cells separate from the plasma and fall to the bottom of a specialized test tube. An elevated sed rate indicates the presence of inflammation in the body.
- The term **hematocrit** (hee-**MAT**-oh-krit) (Hct) describes the percentage, by volume, of a blood sample occupied by red cells (**hemat/o** means blood, and **-crit** means to separate). This test is used to diagnose abnormal states of ***hydration*** (fluid levels in the body), ***polycythemia*** (excess red blood cells), and ***anemia*** (deficient red blood cells).
- A **platelet count** measures the number of platelets in a specified amount of blood and is a screening test to evaluate platelet function. It is also used to monitor changes in the blood associated with chemotherapy and radiation therapy. These changes include ***thrombocytosis*** (an abnormal increase in the number of platelets) and ***thrombocytopenia*** (an abnormal decrease in the number of platelets).
- A **red blood cell count** (RBC) is a determination of the number of erythrocytes in the blood. A

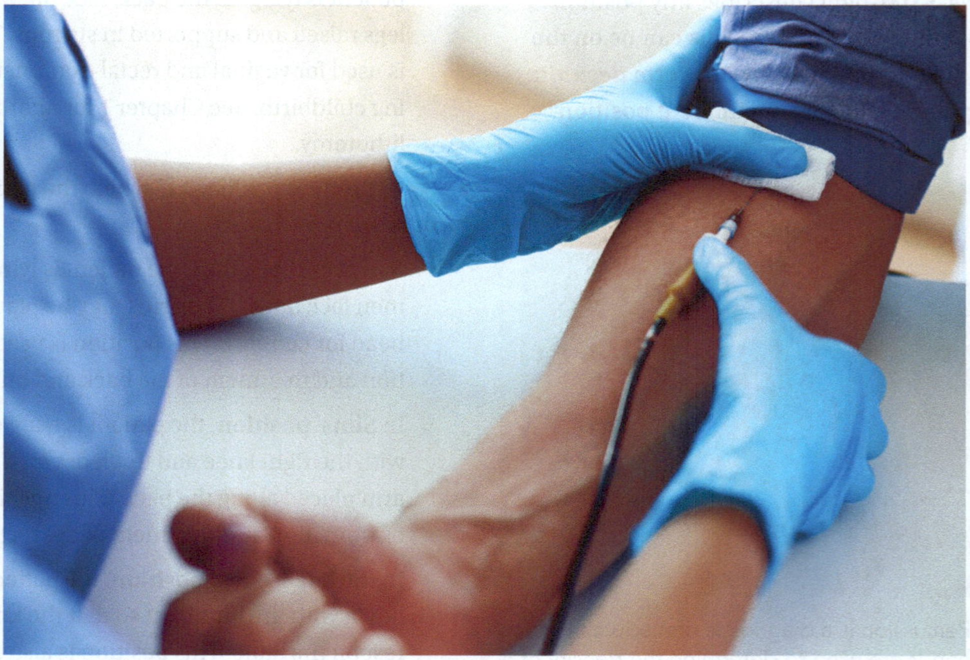

iStock.com/mediaphotos

FIGURE 21.9 A phlebotomist draws a blood sample from a patient for testing.

depressed count can indicate anemia or an acute hemorrhage.

- A **total hemoglobin test** (Hb) is usually part of a complete blood count (**hem/o** means blood, and **-globin** means protein). Elevated Hb levels indicate a higher-than-normal hemoglobin concentration in the plasma due to polycythemia or dehydration. Low Hb indicates lower-than-normal hemoglobin concentration due to anemia, recent hemorrhage, or fluid retention.
- A **white blood cell count** (WBC) is a determination of the number of leukocytes in the blood. An elevated count can be an indication of infection or inflammation.
- A **white blood cell differential count** tests to see what percentage of the total white blood cell count is composed of each of the five types of leukocytes. This provides information about the patient's immune system, detects certain types of leukemia, and determines the severity of infection.

Additional Blood Tests

- A **basic metabolic panel** (BMP, or Profile 8) is a group of eight specific blood tests that provide important information about the current status of the patient's kidneys, electrolyte balance, blood sugar, and calcium levels. Significant changes in these test results can indicate acute problems such as kidney failure, diabetes-related complications, or respiratory problems.
- A **blood urea nitrogen test** (BUN) measures the amount of nitrogen in the blood due to the waste product urea. This test is performed to obtain an indication of kidney function. **Urea** (you-**REE**-ah) is the major end product of protein metabolism found in urine and blood (see Chapter 10).
- **Crossmatch tests** are performed to determine the compatibility of donor blood and the recipient before a blood transfusion. Agglutination is a positive reaction that indicates the donor unit is not a suitable match. *Agglutination* is the clumping together of red blood cells.
- A **C-reactive protein test** (CRP) is performed to identify high levels of inflammation within the body. The C-reactive protein is produced by the liver only during episodes of acute inflammation. Although this test does not identify the specific cause of the inflammation, an elevated level can indicate a heart attack, coronary artery disease, or an autoimmune disorder.
- A **lipid panel**, also called a *lipid profile*, measures the amounts of total cholesterol, high-density lipoprotein (HDL), low-density lipoprotein (LDL), and triglycerides in a blood sample (see Chapter 6).
- **Prothrombin time** (proh-**THROM**-bin) (PT), also known as *pro time*, is a coagulation test used to diagnose conditions associated with abnormalities of clotting time and to monitor anticoagulant therapy. A longer prothrombin time can be caused by serious liver disease, bleeding disorders, blood-thinning medicines, or a lack of vitamin K.
- A **serum bilirubin test** measures the ability of the liver to take up, process, and secrete bilirubin into the bile. This test is useful in determining whether a patient has a condition such as liver disease or a blocked bile duct.
- A **thyroid-stimulating hormone assay** measures the circulating blood level of thyroid-stimulating hormone (TSH) that can indicate abnormal thyroid activity (see Chapter 14).
- An **arterial blood gas analysis** (ABG) measures the pH, oxygen, and carbon dioxide levels of arterial blood. This test is used to evaluate lung and kidney function and overall metabolism.

Genetic Tests

Genetic tests are done using blood, saliva, hair, amniotic fluid, or other tissue to look at a single gene in a person's DNA.

- **Genome testing** or *genomic testing* is whole genome screening that uses DNA to identify genetic variants that may increase the risk of certain diseases or disorders. It can also be used to pinpoint unexplained conditions suspected to be genetic in origin.
- A few examples of genetic testing include newborn screening for congenital disorders, testing for the BRCA gene to determine the risk of breast and ovarian cancer, and a test to confirm a diagnosis of cystic fibrosis or Huntington's disease.

Urinalysis

Urinalysis (**you**-rih-**NAL**-ih-sis) is the examination of the physical and chemical properties of urine to determine the presence of abnormal elements.

- *Routine urinalysis* is performed to screen for urinary and systemic disorders. This test uses a dipstick. This is a plastic strip impregnated with chemicals that react with substances in the urine and change color when abnormalities are present (Figure 21.10).

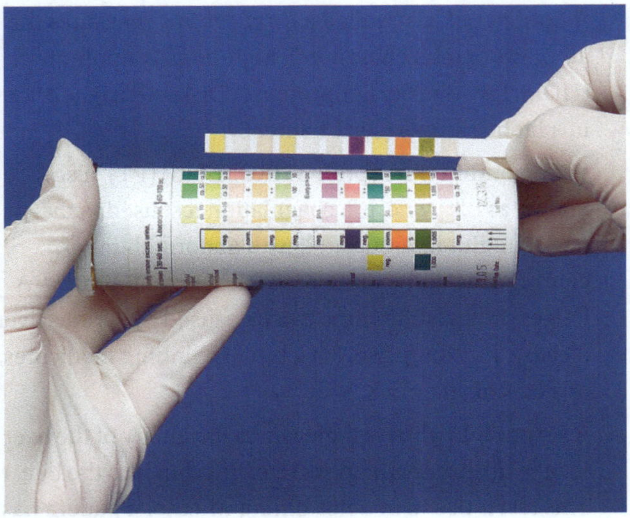

FIGURE 21.10 A dipstick is used for routine urinalysis.

- *Microscopic examination* of the specimen is performed when more detailed testing of the specimen is necessary, for example, to identify casts. **Casts** are fibrous or protein materials, such as pus and fats, that are thrown off into the urine in kidney disease. (*Note:* The term *cast* is also used to describe a rigid dressing, traditionally made of gauze and plaster, used to immobilize a bone that has been fractured.)

pH Values of Urine

The average normal pH range of urine is from 4.5 to 8.0. The abbreviation *pH* describes the degree of acidity or alkalinity of a substance.

- A pH value *below* 7 indicates acid urine and is an indication of acidosis. **Acidosis** (ass-eh-**DOH**-sis) is excessive acid in the body fluids. The opposite of acidosis is ***alkalosis***. (*Note:* You can remember that alkalosis has a *l* for elevated, and acidosis has a *d* for down.)
- A pH value *above* 7 indicates alkaline urine and can indicate conditions such as a urinary tract infection.

Specific Gravity

The specific gravity of urine reflects the amount of wastes, minerals, and solids that are present.

- *Low specific gravity* (dilute urine) is characteristic of diabetes insipidus, which is discussed in Chapter 14.
- *High specific gravity* (concentrated urine) occurs in conditions such as dehydration, liver failure, or shock.

Conditions and Drug Use Identified Through Urinalysis

- **Albuminuria** (**al**-byou-mih-**NEW**-ree-ah) is the presence of the protein albumin in the urine (**albumin** means albumin or protein, and **-uria** means urine). High test levels are a sign of impaired kidney function. ***Albumin*** is a form of protein found in most body tissues.
- **Bacteriuria** (back-**tee**-ree-**YOU**-ree-ah) is the presence of bacteria in the urine (**bacteri** means bacteria, and **-uria** means urine).
- **Calciuria** (**kal**-sih-**YOU**-ree-ah) is the presence of calcium in the urine (**calci** means calcium, and **-uria** means urine). Abnormally high levels can be diagnostic for hyperparathyroidism as described in Chapter 14. Lower-than-normal levels can indicate osteomalacia, which is discussed in Chapter 3.
- **Creatinuria** (**kree**-at-ih-**NEW**-ree-ah) is an increased concentration of creatinine in the urine (**creatin** means creatinine, and **-uria** means urine). ***Creatinine*** is a waste product of muscle metabolism that is normally removed by the kidneys. The presence of excess creatinine is an indication of increased muscle breakdown or a disruption of kidney function.
- A **drug-screening urine test** is a rapid method of identifying the presence in the body of one or more drugs such as cocaine, heroin, or marijuana. These tests are also used to detect performance-enhancing drugs in athletes.
- **Glycosuria** (**glye**-koh-**SOO**-ree-ah) is the presence of glucose in the urine (**glycos** means glucose, and **-uria** means urine). This condition is most commonly caused by untreated diabetes mellitus.
- **Hematuria** (**hee**-mah-**TOO**-ree-ah) is the presence of blood in the urine (**hemat** means blood, and **-uria** means urine). This condition can be caused by kidney stones, infection, kidney damage, or bladder cancer.
- **Ketonuria** (**kee**-toh-**NEW**-ree-ah) is the presence of ketones in the urine (**keton** means ketones, and **-uria** means urine). ***Ketones*** are formed when the body breaks down fat, and their presence in urine can indicate starvation or uncontrolled diabetes.
- **Proteinuria** (**proh**-teen-**UHR**-ree-ah) is the presence of an abnormal amount of protein in the urine (**protein** means protein, and **-uria** means urine). This condition is usually a sign of kidney disease.

- **Pyuria** (pye-**YOU**-ree-ah) is the presence of pus in the urine (**py** means pus, and **-uria** means urine). When pus is present, the urine is turbid in appearance. *Turbid* means having a cloudy or smoky appearance.
- A **urine culture and sensitivity test**, also known as a *urine C and S*, is a laboratory test that is used to identify the cause of a urinary tract infection and to determine which antibiotic would be the most effective treatment.

Stool Analysis

Stool analysis is the examination of the physical and chemical properties of stool to determine the presence of abnormal elements such as bacteria, blood, enzymes, bile, fat, and undigested nutrients. These tests can help to diagnose malabsorption, cancer, and infection.

- A *stool gram stain* tests for which bacteria are present in a sample.
- A *stool guaiac test* looks for blood in the stool.
- A *fecal fat test* analyzes how much fat is contained in the sample to determine how well the body is digesting fat and whether the necessary functions in fat absorption by the pancreas and gallbladder are working.

ENDOSCOPY

Endoscopy (en-**DOS**-koh-pee) is the visual examination of the interior of a body cavity (**endo** means within, and **-scopy** means visual examination). These procedures are usually named for the organs or body systems involved such as an upper GI endoscopy.

Endoscopic surgery is a surgical procedure that is performed through very small incisions with the use of an endoscope and specialized instruments. These procedures are named for the body parts involved, for example arthroscopic surgery, which is discussed in Chapter 3.

Endoscopes

An **endoscope** (**EN**-doh-**skope**) is a small, flexible tube with a light and a lens on the end (**endo** means within, and **-scope** means an instrument for visual examination). These fiber optic instruments are named for the body parts they are designed to examine. For example, a hysteroscope is used to examine the interior of the uterus, while a laparoscope is used to examine the interior of the abdomen (Figure 21.11).

Laparoscopic Procedures

Laparoscopy (**lap**-ah-**ROS**-koh-pee) is the visual examination of the interior of the abdomen with the use of a laparoscope that is passed through a small incision in the abdominal wall (**lapar/o** means abdomen, and **-scopy** means visual examination).

Laparoscopic surgery involves the use of a laparoscope plus specialized instruments inserted into the abdomen through small incisions (Figure 21.11). A laparoscope is used for several purposes:

- Explore and examine the interior of the abdomen.
- Take specimens to be biopsied.
- Perform surgical procedures such as the endoscopic removal of a diseased gallbladder (see Chapter 9).

CENTESIS

Centesis (sen-**TEE**-sis) is a surgical puncture to remove excess fluid or to remove fluid for diagnostic purposes. *Note:* Centesis is used alone as a noun or as a suffix in conjunction with the combining form describing the body part being treated.

- **Abdominocentesis** (ab-**dom**-ih-noh-sen-**TEE**-sis) is the surgical puncture of the abdominal cavity to remove fluid (**abdomin/o** means abdomen, and **-centesis** means a surgical puncture to remove fluid).
- *Amniocentesis*, which is a diagnostic test performed during pregnancy, is discussed in Chapter 16.
- **Arthrocentesis** (**ar**-throh-sen-**TEE**-sis) is a surgical puncture of the joint space to remove synovial fluid for analysis to determine the cause of pain or swelling in a joint (**arthr/o** means joint, and **-centesis** means a surgical puncture to remove fluid).
- **Cardiocentesis** (**kar**-dee-oh-sen-**TEE**-sis), also known as *cardiopuncture*, is the puncture of a chamber of the heart for diagnosis or therapy (**cardi/o** means heart, and **-centesis** means a surgical puncture to remove fluid).
- **Pericardiocentesis** (**pehr**-ih-**kar**-dee-oh-sen-**TEE**-sis) is the puncture of the pericardial sac for the purpose of removing fluid (**peri-** means surrounding, **cardi/o** means heart, and **-centesis** means a surgical puncture to remove fluid). This procedure is performed to treat pericarditis (see Chapter 5).

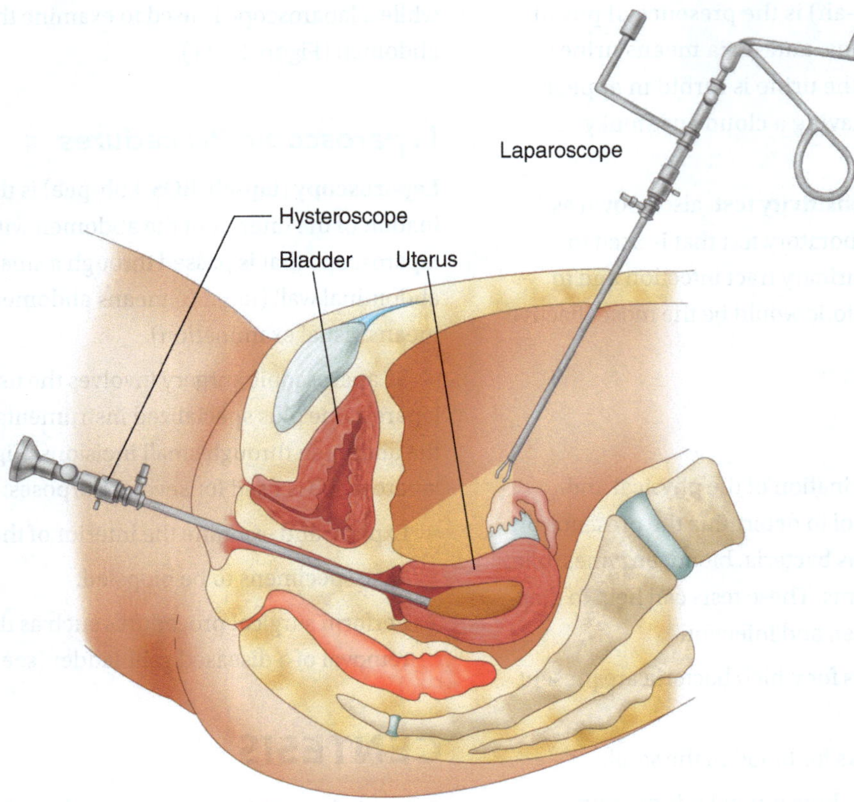

FIGURE 21.11 A laparoscope is used to examine the interior of the abdomen. A hysteroscope is used to examine the interior of the uterus.

BIOPSY

A **biopsy** (**BYE**-op-see) is the removal of a small piece of living tissue for examination to confirm or establish a diagnosis (**bi** means pertaining to life, and **-opsy** means view of). Biopsy can be done with a tissue or fluid sample from skin (see Chapter 13), muscle (see Chapter 4), bone, and other organs such as the liver or lungs. After a biopsy the sample is sent to a laboratory for testing.

- *Fine-needle aspiration* (FNA) uses a very thin needle inserted through the skin and into the intended fluid or tissue.
- *Core needle biopsy* uses a larger needle to collect more of the fluid or tissue.

IMAGING TECHNIQUES

Imaging techniques are used to visualize and examine internal body structures. The three most commonly used techniques are compared in Table 21.1.

Contrast Medium

A **contrast medium** is administered by swallowing, via an enema, or intravenously to make specific body structures visible. Specialized substances are used depending on the imaging systems and the body parts to be enhanced. These media are either radiopaque or radiolucent.

- **Radiopaque** (**ray**-dee-oh-**PAYK**) means that the substance *does not allow x-rays to pass through* and appears white or light gray on the resulting film. Radiopaque is the opposite of *radiolucent*.
- **Radiolucent** (**ray**-dee-oh-**LOO**-sent) means that the substance, such as air or nitrogen gas, *allows x-rays to pass through* and appears black or dark gray on the resulting film. Radiolucent is the opposite of *radiopaque*.
- An **intravenous contrast medium** is injected into a vein to make the flow of blood through blood vessels and organs visible (**intra-** means within, **ven** means vein, and **-ous** means pertaining to).

Barium (chemical symbol Ba) is a radiopaque barium-sulfate compound contrast medium used primarily to visualize the gastrointestinal tract (Figure 21.12). It is administered orally as a ***barium swallow*** for an upper GI study. It is administered rectally as a ***barium enema*** for a lower GI study. Radiography and fluoroscopy are used to trace the flow of the barium.

TABLE 21.1

Imaging Systems Compared

Method	How It Works
X-ray (radiography)	Uses x-rays passing through the patient to expose a film or create a digital image that shows the body in profile. In the resulting film, hard tissues are light, soft tissues are shades of gray, and air is black.
Computed tomography (CT)	Uses an x-ray beam with computer assistance to produce multiple cross-sectional views of the body. Hard tissues are light, and soft tissues appear as shades of gray.
Magnetic resonance imaging (MRI)	Uses a combination of radio waves and a strong magnetic field to produce images. Hard tissues are dark, and soft tissues appear as shades of gray.

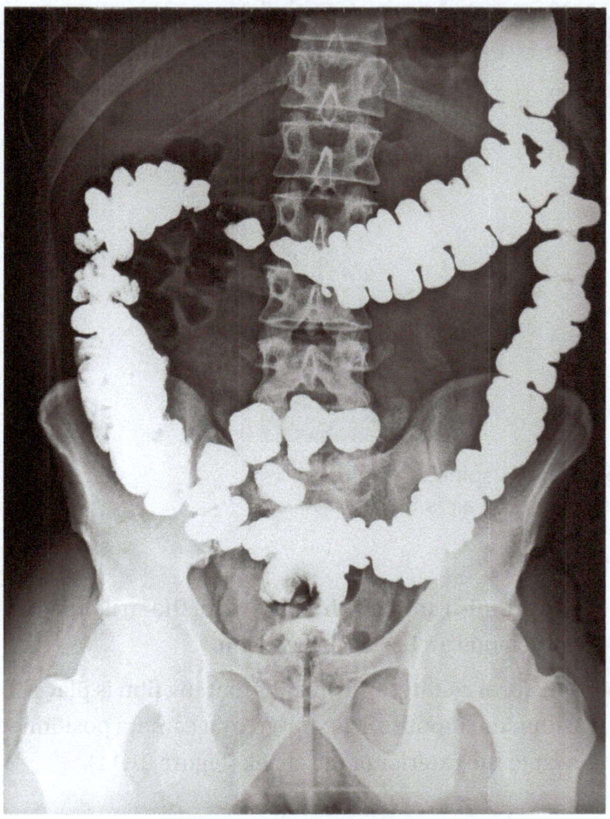

Danilo Ascione/Shutterstock.com

FIGURE 21.12 An x-ray (radiograph) of the abdomen using barium, a radiopaque contrast medium.

Radiology

Conventional **radiology** creates an image of hard-tissue internal structures by the exposure of sensitized film to x-radiation (**radi** means radiation, and **-ology** means study of). The resulting film is known as an **x-ray** or ***radiograph***. Advances in technology have made ***computed radiology*** and ***digital radiology*** more convenient formats for storing and sharing x-ray data without the use of film.

- X-radiation, which is also referred to as ***ionizing radiation***, is beneficial in producing diagnostic images and in treating cancer; however, excess exposure to this radiation is dangerous, and the effects are cumulative. Because x-radiation is invisible, has no odor, and cannot be felt, appropriate precautions must always be taken to protect the technician and the patient. The science of measuring radiation exposure is called ***dosimetry***.
- ***Radiopaque hard tissues***, such as bone and tooth enamel, appear white or light gray on the radiograph.
- ***Radiolucent soft tissues***, such as muscles and skin, appear as shades of gray to black on the radiograph (Figure 21.13).
- **Interventional radiology** is the use of radiographic imaging to guide a procedure such as a biopsy. It is also used to confirm the placement of an inserted object such as a stent or feeding tube.

Radiographic Positioning

The term **radiographic positioning** describes the placement of the patient's body and the part of the body that is closest to the x-ray film. For example, in a *left lateral position*, the left side of the patient's body is placed nearest the film.

Radiographic Projections

The term **radiographic projection** describes the path that the x-ray beam follows through the patient's body from the entrance to the exit.

- When the name of the projection combines two terms into a single word, the term listed first is the one that the x-ray penetrates first.

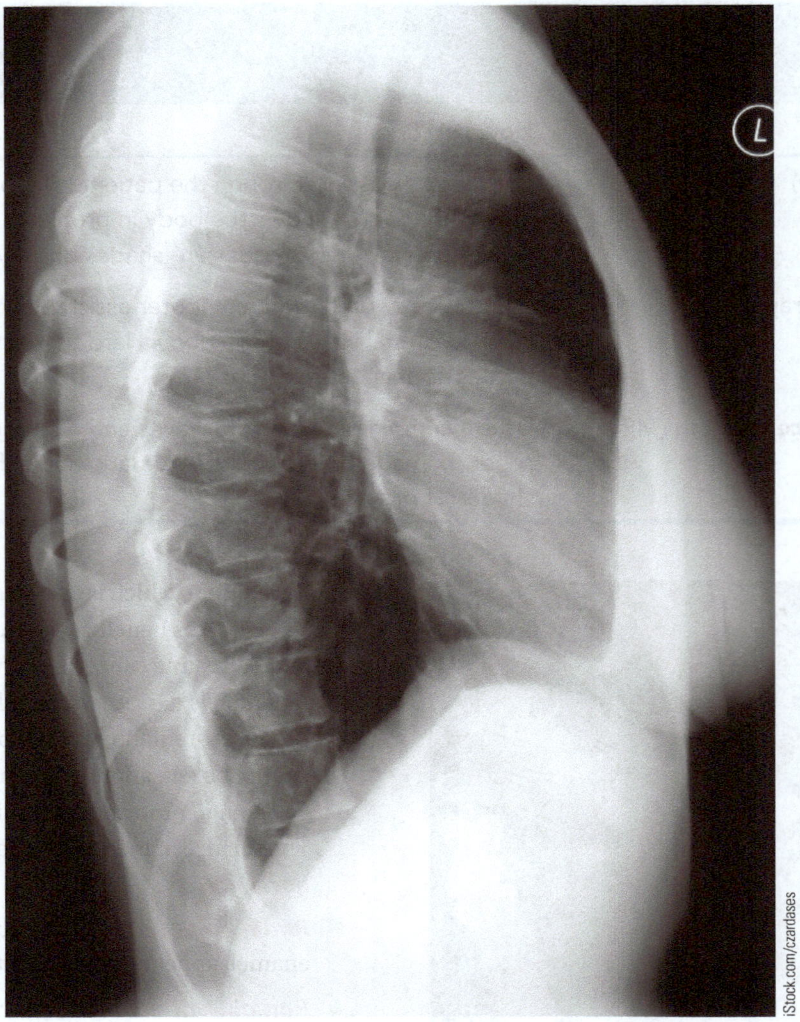

FIGURE 21.13 A lateral chest x-ray. Bones of the spine are white, and the soft tissues are shades of gray. The surrounding air is black.

Dental Radiography

Specialized techniques and equipment are used in obtaining dental x-rays.

- The term **extraoral radiography** means that the film is placed and exposed outside of the mouth. A **panoramic radiograph** shows all of the structures in both dental arches in a single film.
- **Intraoral radiography** means that the film is placed within the mouth and exposed by a camera positioned next to the exterior of the cheek (Figure 21.14).

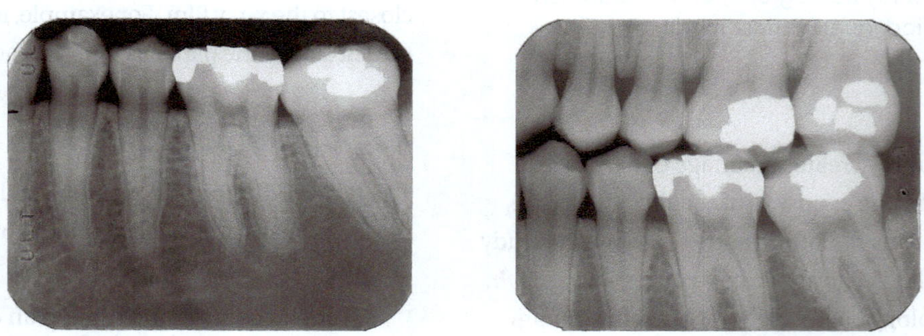

FIGURE 21.14 Intraoral dental radiographs. The white areas are fillings that restore decayed teeth.

Computed Tomography

- **Computed tomography** (toh-**MOG**-rah-fee) (CT), sometimes referred to as ***computerized axial tomography*** (CAT), is a scan that uses a thin, fan-shaped x-ray beam that rotates around the patient to produce multiple cross-sectional views of the body (Figure 21.15). **Tomography** (toh-**MOG**-rah-fee) is the imaging of cross-sections of a part of the body (**tom/o** means to slice, and **-graphy** means the process of recording a picture or record).
- Information gathered by radiation detectors is downloaded to a computer, analyzed, and converted into gray-scale images corresponding to anatomic slices of the body (Figure 21.16). These images are viewed on a monitor, stored as digital files, or printed as films.
- Computed tomography is more effective than MRI at imaging compact bone and is frequently preferred for patients with head injuries or strokes.
- Computed tomography scans can be performed with or without contrast dye. The contrast dye contains iodine, which can trigger a reaction in patients with iodine sensitivity.
- The use of tomography in the cancer treatment method ***tomotherapy*** is discussed in Chapter 20.

Magnetic Resonance Imaging

Magnetic resonance imaging (MRI) uses a combination of radio waves and a strong magnetic field to create signals that are sent to a computer and converted into images of any plane through the body. These images are used to construct images of internal organs and tissues that often do not show up well in x-rays. An MRI is a noninvasive means of examining soft tissues such as those of the heart, blood vessels, brain, spinal cord, joints, muscles, and internal organs (Figure 21.17).

- MRI images can be produced in *coronal, sagittal*, or *oblique* planes (see Chapter 2) and are created without the use of x-radiation.
- Because of the use of powerful magnets, the presence of metal implants such as a knee replacement, an artificial pacemaker, or metal stents or aneurysm clips can be contraindications for using an MRI on a patient.
- A ***closed MRI***, which is the most commonly used type of equipment, produces the most accurate images; however, patients may be uncomfortable because of the loud noise and the feeling of being closed in. In addition, some patients may not fit into the narrow tube of a closed MRI machine.
- As an alternative, an ***open MRI*** is designed to be less confining and is more comfortable for some people, especially large patients and those suffering from claustrophobia (see Chapter 17). However, the open MRI has a lower field strength, which limits its uses in certain situations.
- Some MRI exams use gadolinium contrast. Unlike CT scan contrast dye, this does not use iodine, which is an allergy risk for those who have an iodine sensitivity. ***Gadolinium*** is a natural chemical element.
- **Magnetic resonance angiography** (MRA), also known as ***magnetic resonance angio***, helps locate problems within blood vessels throughout the body. This diagnostic imaging, which sometimes includes the use of a contrast dye, is frequently used as an alternative to the conventional angiography discussed in Chapter 5 (**angi/o** means blood vessel, and **-graphy** means the process of recording).

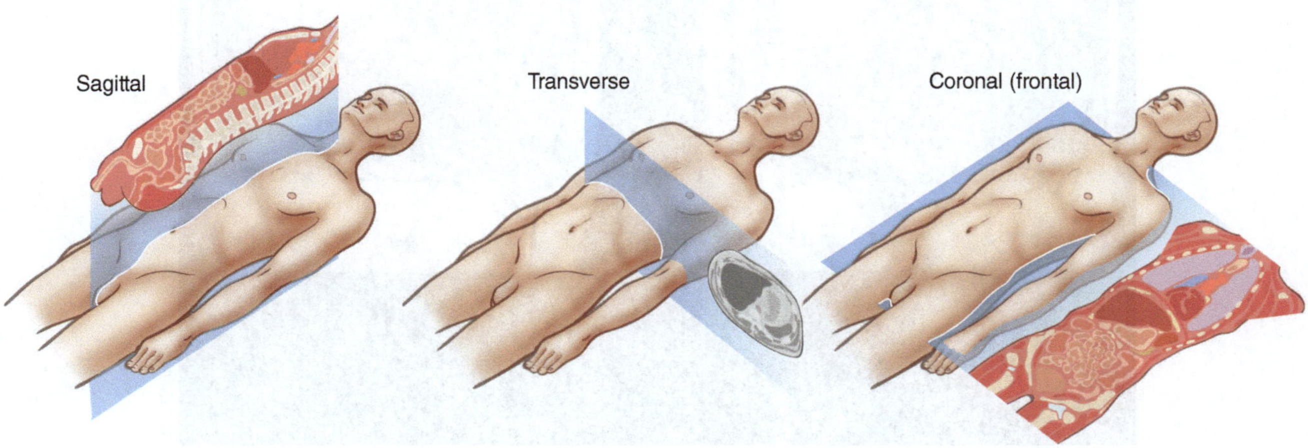

FIGURE 21.15 Computed tomography (CT scan) provides cross-sectional views of different body planes.

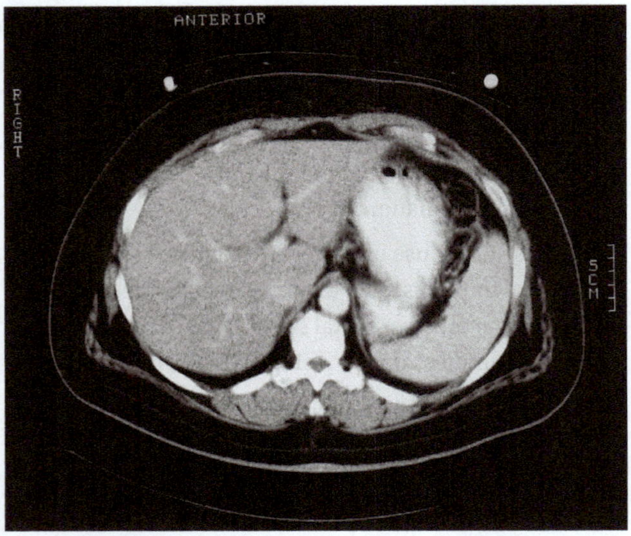

FIGURE 21.16 An abdominal computed tomography scan in which the liver is predominant in the upper left and the stomach is visible in the upper right.

Fluoroscopy

Fluoroscopy (floo-**ROS**-koh-pee) is the visualization of body parts in motion by projecting x-ray images on a luminous fluorescent screen (**fluor/o** means glowing, and **-scopy** means visual examination). ***Luminous*** means glowing. Fluoroscopy is used with or without a contrast medium to see movement in a particular area of the body such as the intestines, joints, or flow of blood through veins and arteries. It can be viewed normally or in slow motion.

Ultrasonography

Ultrasonography (**ul**-trah-son-**OG**-rah-fee), commonly referred to as ***ultrasound*** or ***diagnostic ultrasound***, is imaging of deep body structures by recording the echoes of sound wave pulses that are above the range of human hearing (**ultra-** means beyond, **son/o** means sound, and **-graphy** means the process of recording a picture or record). Unlike CT and x-rays, ultrasonography does not involve radiation.

A **sonogram** (**SOH**-noh-gram) is the image created by ultrasonography (**son/o** means sound, and **-gram** means a picture or record).

- This technique is most effective for viewing solid organs of the abdomen and soft tissues where the signal is not stopped by intervening bone or air. Common uses of ultrasound include evaluating fetal development; detecting the presence of gallstones or a blood clot; identifying tears in tendons, muscles, or ligaments; or confirming the presence of a mass found on a mammogram.

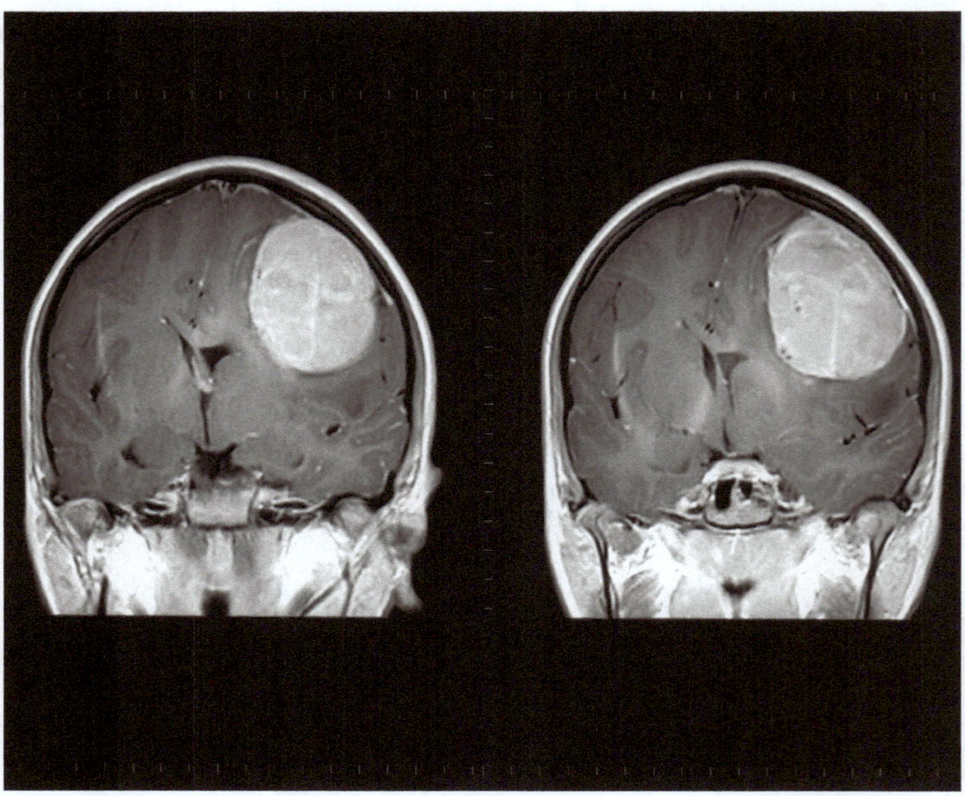

FIGURE 21.17 An MRI of the brain with a tumor visible in the upper right.

- Ultrasound can also be used to guide interventional procedures such as injections of anti-inflammatory drugs, the removal of fluid, and needle placement for a biopsy.
- *Carotid ultrasonography* is the use of sound waves to image the carotid artery to detect an obstruction that could cause an ischemic stroke (see Chapter 11).
- **Echocardiography** (**eck**-oh-**kar**-dee-**OG**-rah-fee) is an ultrasonic diagnostic procedure used to evaluate the structures and motion of the heart (**ech/o** means sound, **cardi/o** means heart, and **-graphy** means the process of recording a picture or record). The resulting record is an *echocardiogram*. *Note:* not to be confused with an *electrocardiogram* (EKG), discussed in Chapter 5.
- A **Doppler echocardiogram** is performed in the same way as an echocardiogram; however, this procedure measures the speed and direction of the blood flow within the heart.
- A **Doppler ultrasound** uses sound waves to measure blood flow within the veins and arteries, and is used to look for problems such as decreased or absent blood flow.
- **Fetal ultrasound** is a noninvasive procedure used to image and evaluate fetal development during pregnancy (Figures 21.18 and 21.19). *3D/4D ultrasound* is a technique that uses specialized equipment to create photograph-like images of the developing child.
- **Transesophageal echocardiography** (**trans**-eh-**sof**-ah-**JEE**-al **eck**-oh-**kar**-dee-**OG**-rah-fee) (TEE) is an ultrasonic imaging technique used to evaluate heart structures. This diagnostic test is performed from inside the esophagus, and because the esophagus is so close to the heart, this technique produces clearer images than those obtained with echocardiography.

NUCLEAR MEDICINE

In **nuclear medicine**, drugs known as **radiopharmaceuticals** are used for either diagnostic or treatment purposes. Radiopharmaceuticals contain radioactive materials called *radioisotopes* that produce a powerful form of energy called radiation. They can be inserted into a vein, taken by mouth, or placed inside the body. See Chapters 14 and 20 for examples of *radiation therapy* in which nuclear medicine is used for the treatment of thyroid disease and cancer.

- **Nuclear imaging** is the use of radiopharmaceuticals for diagnostic purposes. These images document the structure and function of the organ or organs being examined. Unlike x-ray technology, in which the

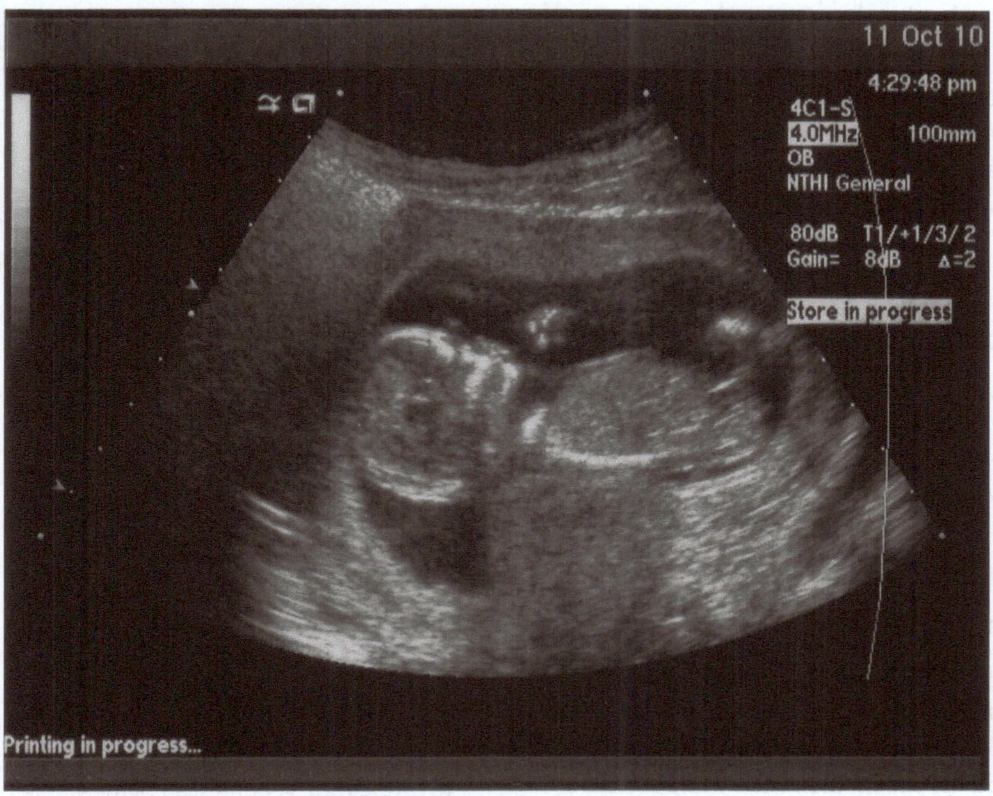

FIGURE 21.18 Fetal ultrasound at about 15 weeks gestation.

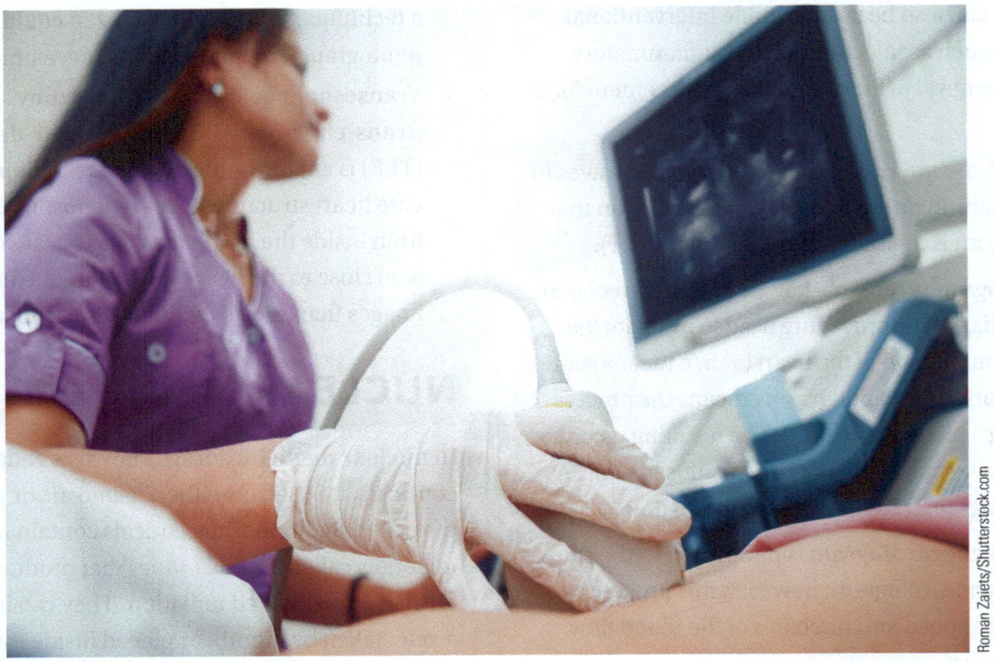

FIGURE 21.19 Fetal ultrasound is a noninvasive procedure used to image and evaluate fetal development before birth.

radiation is external, nuclear imaging involves a low dose of radiopharmaceuticals taken internally.

- Each radiopharmaceutical contains a ***radionuclide tracer***, also known as a ***radioactive tracer***, which is specific to the body system being examined. The short-lived tracer can be given by mouth or inserted into a vein.
- Radiopharmaceuticals emit ***gamma rays*** that are detected by a special camera attached to a computer. The data is used to generate an image showing the pattern of absorption that can be indicative of pathology.

Nuclear Scans

A **nuclear scan**, also known as a ***scintigram***, is a diagnostic procedure that uses nuclear medicine technology to gather information about the structure and function of organs or body systems that cannot be seen on conventional x-rays.

Bone Scans

A **bone scan** is a nuclear scanning test that identifies new areas of bone growth or breakdown. The results are obtained after a radionuclide tracer is injected into the bloodstream, and the patient then waits while the material travels through the body tissues (Figure 21.20). This is

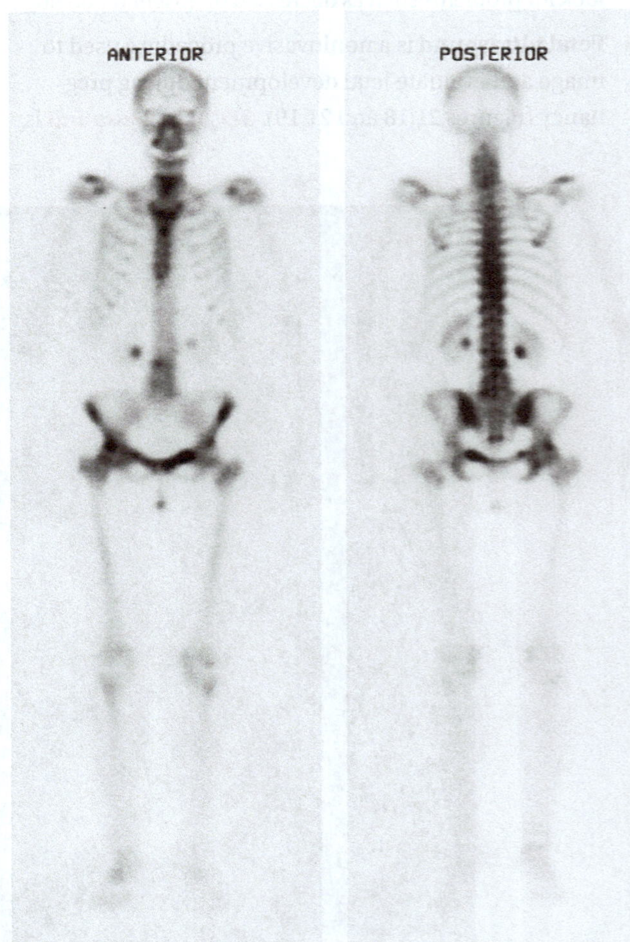

FIGURE 21.20 A bone scan of the whole body showing the anterior and posterior views.

different than *bone density testing,* which is discussed in Chapter 3.

This testing can be done to evaluate damage to the bones, detect cancer that has metastasized (spread) to the bones, and monitor conditions that can affect the bones. A bone scan can often detect a problem days to months earlier than a regular x-ray. Only pathology in the bones absorbs the radionuclide, and these are visible as dark areas. Areas of the bones where cells and tissues are actively repairing themselves take up the largest amounts of tracer.

Thyroid Scans

A **thyroid scan** provides information about the size, shape, location, and relative activity of different parts of the thyroid gland. For a thyroid scan, a radiopharmaceutical containing radioactive iodine is administered. This scan makes use of the thyroid gland's ability to concentrate certain radioactive isotopes to generate images of it.

Single Photon Emission Computed Tomography

Single photon emission computed tomography (SPECT) is a type of nuclear imaging test that produces 3D computer-reconstructed images showing perfusion through tissues and organs. **Perfusion** (per-**FYOU**-zhun) means the flow of blood through an organ. A *photon* is a particle that travels at the speed of light.

- SPECT scanning is used primarily to view the flow of blood through arteries and veins in the brain. It is useful in diagnosing blood-deprived areas of brain following a stroke, dementia, epileptic seizures or a head injury, and tumors. In addition, SPECT is used to monitor some heart problems such as clogged coronary arteries or reduced pumping efficiency as well as hidden bone fractures.

Positron Emission Tomography

Positron emission tomography (PET), also known as *PET imaging*, combines computed tomography with radionuclide tracers, usually inserted into a vein, to produce enhanced images of selected body organs or areas. Damaged tissues have reduced metabolic activity, so the gamma radiation from these areas is reduced or absent.

- PET scans of the whole body are often used to detect cancer and to examine the effects of cancer therapy.
- PET scans of the heart are used to determine blood flow to the heart muscle. This procedure helps evaluate signs of coronary artery disease or to differentiate nonfunctional heart muscle from tissue that would benefit from a procedure such as angioplasty or coronary artery bypass surgery.
- PET scans of the brain are used to evaluate patients who have memory disorders of an undetermined cause, suspected or proven brain tumors, or seizure disorders that are not responsive to medical therapy and are therefore candidates for surgery.

COMPLEMENTARY AND ALTERNATIVE MEDICINE

There is a wide range of **complementary and alternative medicine** (CAM) available to patients today. Some have been researched and proven effective, while others have little research to support their claims. These therapies can be used to supplement or replace allopathic medicine.

- **Allopathic medicine** (**ah**-low-**PAH**-thick) is another term for conventional, or Western, medical practices and systems of health care.
- **Alternative medicine** is a general term for practices and systems of health care other than allopathic approaches used *in place of* these treatments.
- **Complementary medicine** is a general term for practices and systems of health care other than allopathic approaches used to *supplement* these treatments.
- **Integrative medicine** is a model of health care based on both allopathic and alternative medicine.
- The term **holistic** (**hoe**-**LISS**-tick) refers to a treatment approach that takes into consideration the whole body and its environment, including the mind, body, and spirit.
- **Wellness** is a general term that means actively working toward a state of being in good physical and mental health. Factors contributing to wellness include a healthy diet, exercise, stress reduction, and the avoidance of risky behavior such as smoking or not wearing a seatbelt.

Alternative Medicine

Some forms of alternative medicine are rooted in traditional systems, such as Ayurvedic medicine and traditional Chinese medicine, while others have been developed more recently, such as homeopathy. It is important to be aware of any herbal supplements or remedies that patients may be taking, as some can interact negatively with other medications or have potentially dangerous side effects.

- **Ayurvedic medicine** (ay-uhr-**VEH**-dick) is the traditional Hindu system of medicine, emphasizing a holistic approach to preventive treatment through hygiene, exercise, herbal preparations, and yoga, and the treatment of illnesses with herbal medicines, physiotherapy, and diet.
- **Traditional Chinese medicine** is a system of ancient Chinese medicinal treatments including acupuncture, diet, herbal therapy, meditation, physical exercise, and massage to prevent, diagnose, and treat disease. Parts of traditional Chinese medicine, such as acupuncture, are also used as complementary medicine.
- **Kinesiology** (kih-**NEES**-ee-**ol**-oh-jee) is the study of body movements and physical activity. This science should not be confused with ***applied kinesiology***, an alternative therapy that combines muscle monitoring with the principles of Chinese medicine.
- **Naturopathy** (**nay**-cher-**AH**-pah-thee), also known as ***naturopathic medicine***, is a combination of nutrition, medicinal supplements and herbs, water therapy, homeopathy, and lifestyle modifications used to identify and treat the root causes of symptoms and diseases. It emphasizes supporting the body's own innate healing ability and the healing power of nature over surgery and medications.
- ***Herbal medicine*** or ***phytotherapy*** is the use of plants as a dietary supplement. Supplements are considered food, not medicine, and are not regulated in the same way by the FDA. In contrast, some medications are made from plant products and are regulated by the FDA.
- **Homeopathy** (**hoh**-mee-**OP**-ah-thee) involves the use of substances created from plant or mineral products diluted a thousand-fold in water or alcohol to treat symptoms and diseases. Homeopaths believe that the body can stimulate its own healing responses when the right trigger is given in minute doses, producing symptoms similar to the disease being treated.

Complementary Medicine

Types of complementary medicine can be broken down into three categories: mind–body therapies, hands-on therapies, and energy therapies.

Mind–Body Therapies

Mind–body therapies try to reduce stress and prevent its negative effects on the body. They can be used for stress reduction, pain management, lifestyle changes, and depression. These therapies are based on the belief that emotions, such as stress, trigger physiological responses. By becoming aware of and reducing stressful emotions and thoughts, it is possible to decrease physical stress and its negative effects.

- **Biofeedback** is a patient-guided treatment that teaches individuals to control muscle tension, pain, body temperature, brain waves, and other bodily functions through relaxation, visualization, and other cognitive control techniques.
- **Guided imagery**, or ***visualization***, is a type of treatment in which a patient follows verbal prompts to envision a specific, peaceful location in detail, distancing him- or herself from any pain or stress the patient is currently experiencing.
- **Hypnosis** is a type of therapy in which a patient is placed in a state of focused concentration and narrowed attention that makes him or her more susceptible to suggestions, and then given suggestions directed toward the patient's treatment goal.
- **Mindfulness meditation** focuses on becoming aware of thoughts and emotions and their physiological responses, as well as accepting them and maintaining a calm, constant awareness.

Energy Therapies

Energy therapies try to improve or maintain health by manipulating the body's energy flow, or qi. ***Qi*** is believed to be the fundamental life energy responsible for health and vitality. These therapies are based on the belief that illness is linked to blocked or insufficient energy levels.

- **Acupressure** (**AK**-que-**presh**-ur) is a traditional Chinese touch therapy involving finger pressure applied to specific areas of the body to restore the flow of qi.
- **Acupuncture** (**AK**-you-**punk**-cher) is a traditional Chinese medical practice using very thin acupuncture needles inserted into specific points of the body to restore the flow of qi (Figure 21.21).
- **Qi Gong** (**CHEE**-gong) is a Chinese system of movement, breathing techniques, and meditation designed to improve and enhance the flow of qi.

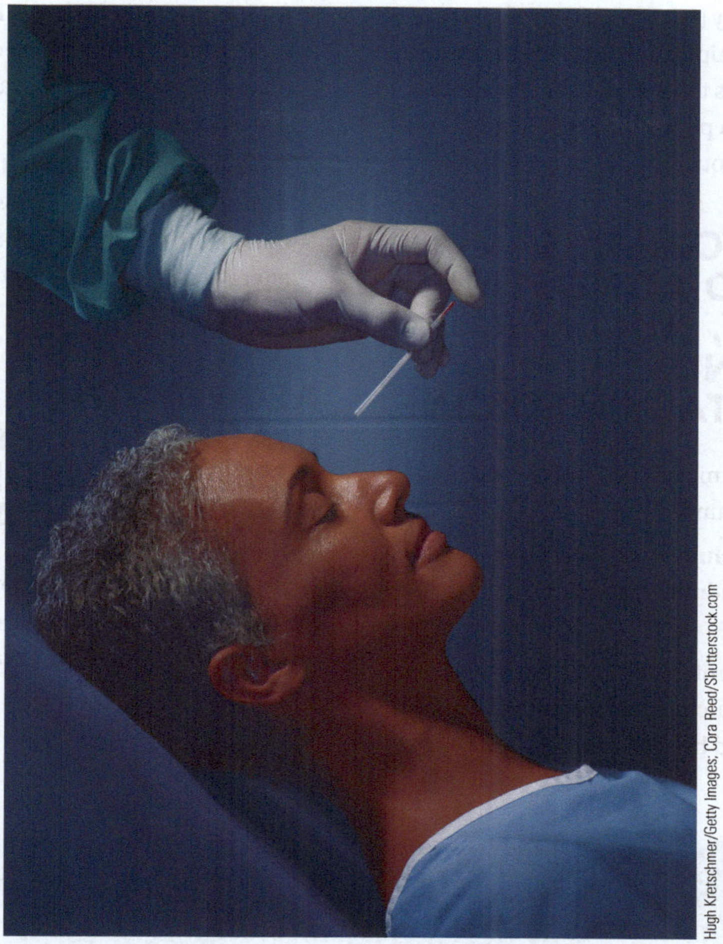

FIGURE 21.21 Acupuncture uses thin needles inserted into specific body points.

- **Reiki** (**RAY**-kee) is a Japanese technique in which the practitioner transfers healing energy to the patient by means of visualization or gentle touch.

Hands-on Therapies

Hands-on therapies try to improve body function by physically manipulating or massaging the body. They can be used for neck or back pain, relaxation, and increased range of motion. This therapy is based on the belief that the body functions more efficiently when it is in proper alignment, and that it is possible to identify and correct poor movement and posture habits.

- **Chiropractic manipulative therapy** is a system of mechanical spinal adjustments made by a chiropractor to correct biomechanical problems in the skeletal framework of the body (see Chapter 3).
- **Osteopathic manipulative therapy** is mechanical spinal adjustment used in conjunction with conventional medical therapies by an osteopath (see Chapter 3).
- **Therapeutic massage** is the use of touch and pressure to relieve pain.
  - **Craniosacral therapy** (**kray**-nee-oh-**SAK**-ral) is the use of gentle touch to help the body release tension, stress, and trauma to correct restrictions resulting from stress on the central nervous system (**crani/o** means skull, and **sacral** means referring to the sacrum).
  - **Myofascial release** (**my**-oh-**FASH**-ee-ahl) is a specialized soft-tissue manipulation technique used to ease the pain of conditions such as fibromyalgia, myofascial pain syndrome, movement restrictions, temporomandibular joint disorders (TMJ), and carpal tunnel syndrome (**my/o** means muscle, and **fascial** refers to the fascia) (see Chapter 4).

- **Neuromuscular therapy** (NMT) is a form of massage that uses soft-tissue manipulation focusing on applying pressure to trigger points to treat injuries and alleviate pain. A ***trigger point*** is a particularly taut band of muscle that is tender to the touch.

MEDICAL SPECIALTIES RELATED TO DIAGNOSTIC PROCEDURES, NUCLEAR MEDICINE, AND COMPLEMENTARY MEDICINE

- A **sonographer** is a technician specifically trained in the technique of ultrasound.
- A **nuclear medicine technologist** specializes in the preparation and administration of radiopharmaceuticals.
- An **acupuncturist** is a professional who has had extensive education in acupuncture and traditional Chinese medicine and is licensed by each state.
- A **phlebotomist** (fleh-**BOT**-oh-mist) is a medical professional who is trained to draw blood from patients for various laboratory tests and other procedures.
- A **radiologist** (**ray**-dee-**OL**-oh-jist) is a physician who specializes in diagnosing and treating diseases and disorders with x-rays and other forms of radiant energy (**radi** means radiation, and **-ologist** means specialist).

ABBREVIATIONS RELATED TO DIAGNOSTIC PROCEDURES, NUCLEAR MEDICINE, AND COMPLEMENTARY MEDICINE

Table 21.2 presents an overview of the abbreviations related to the terms introduced in this chapter. *Note:* To avoid errors or confusion, always be cautious when using abbreviations.

TABLE 21.2

Abbreviations Related to Diagnostic Procedures, Nuclear Medicine, and Complementary Medicine

beats per minute = bpm	**bpm** = beats per minute
blood pressure = BP	**BP** = blood pressure
blood urea nitrogen = BUN	**BUN** = blood urea nitrogen
complete blood count = CBC	**CBC** = complete blood count
computed tomography scan = CT scan	**CT scan** = computed tomography scan
erythrocyte sedimentation rate = ESR	**ESR** = erythrocyte sedimentation rate
hematocrit = Hct	**Hct** = hematocrit
magnetic resonance imaging = MRI	**MRI** = magnetic resonance imaging
red blood cell count = RBC	**RBC** = red blood cell count
respiratory rate = RR	**RR** = respiratory rate
white blood cell count = WBC	**WBC** = white blood cell count

CHAPTER 21

LEARNING EXERCISES

Matching Word Parts 1

Write the correct answer in the middle column.

	Definition	Correct Answer	Possible Answers
21.1.	abdomen	____________	lapar/o
21.2.	albumin, protein	____________	glycos/o
21.3.	calcium	____________	creatin/o
21.4.	creatinine	____________	calc/i
21.5.	sugar	____________	albumin/o

Matching Word Parts 2

Write the correct answer in the middle column.

	Definition	Correct Answer	Possible Answers
21.6.	surgical puncture to remove fluid	____________	son/o
21.7.	blood	____________	-otomy
21.8.	surgical incision	____________	hemat/o
21.9.	process of producing a picture or record	____________	-graphy
21.10.	sound	____________	-centesis

Matching Word Parts 3

Write the correct answer in the middle column.

	Definition	Correct Answer	Possible Answers
21.11.	direct visual examination	____________	-uria
21.12.	radiation	____________	-scopy

21.13. urine ______________________ **-scope**

21.14. vein ______________________ **radi/o**

21.15. visual examination instrument ______________________ **phleb/o**

Definitions

Select the correct answer, and write it on the line provided.

21.16. The type of therapy in which a patient is placed in a state of focused concentration and narrowed attention that makes him or her more susceptible to suggestions and then given suggestions directed toward the treatment goal is called ______________________.

mindfulness meditation | hypnosis | biofeedback | guided imagery

21.17. A/An ______________________ is used to enlarge the opening of any body canal or cavity to facilitate inspection of its interior.

endoscope | otoscope | speculum | sphygmomanometer

21.18. The imaging technique that produces multiple cross-sectional images using x-radiation is ______________________.

computed tomography | fluoroscopy | magnetic resonance imaging | radiography

21.19. ______________________ medicine is the traditional Hindu system of medicine, emphasizing a holistic approach to preventive treatment through hygiene, exercise, herbal preparations, and yoga, and the treatment of illnesses with herbal medicines, physiotherapy, and diet.

Ayurvedic | Traditional Chinese | Alternative | Allopathic

21.20. The diagnostic technique ______________________ creates images of deep body structures by recording the echoes of pulses of sound waves that are above the range of human hearing.

positron emission tomography | extraoral radiography | fluoroscopy | ultrasonography

21.21. The presence of calcium in the urine is known as ______________________.

albuminuria | calciuria | creatinuria | glycosuria

21.22. A/An ______________________ test is used to identify high levels of inflammation within the body.

blood urea nitrogen | C-reactive protein | erythrocyte sedimentation | serum bilirubin

21.23. In the ______________ position, the patient is lying on the back with the knees bent.

dorsal recumbent   horizontal recumbent   knee-chest   supine

21.24. A ______________ is an abnormal sound heard during auscultation of an artery.

bruit   rale   rhonchi   stridor

21.25. The presence of pus in the urine, which causes the urine to be cloudy or smoky in appearance, is called ______________.

glycosuria   ketonuria   hematuria   pyuria

Matching Techniques

Write the correct answer in the middle column.

	Definition	Correct Answer	Possible Answers
21.26.	produces cross-sectional views	______________	x-ray
21.27.	produces views in only one direction	______________	MRI
21.28.	the removal of fluid for diagnostic purposes	______________	fluoroscopy
21.29.	uses a luminous fluorescent screen	______________	centesis
21.30.	uses radio waves and a magnetic field	______________	CT

Which Word?

Select the correct answer, and write it on the line provided.

21.31. A/An ______________ is the image created by ultrasonography.

sonogram   x-ray

21.32. ______________ tomography combines tomography with radionuclide tracers to produce enhanced images of selected body organs or areas.

Positron emission   Single photon emission computed

21.33. A substance that does not allow x-rays to pass through is described as being ______________.

radiolucent   radiopaque

21.34. When film is placed within the mouth and exposed by a camera positioned next to the cheek, this is called ______________________ radiography.

extraoral intraoral

21.35. ______________________ involves the use of substances created from plant or mineral products diluted a thousand-fold in water or alcohol to treat symptoms and diseases.

Homeopathy Reiki

Spelling Counts

Find the misspelled word in each sentence. Then write that word, spelled correctly, on the line provided.

21.36. Listening through a stethoscope for sounds within the body to determine the condition of the lungs, pleura, heart, and abdomen is known as asultation. ______________________

21.37. A sphygnomanometer is used to measure blood pressure. ______________________

21.38. Fluroscopy is the visualization of body parts in motion by projecting x-ray images on a luminous fluorescent screen. ______________________

21.39. Raki is a Japanese technique in which the practitioner transfers healing energy to the patient by means of visualization or gentle touch. ______________________

21.40. An opthalmoscope is used to examine the interior of the eye. ______________________

Abbreviation Identification

In the space provided, write the words in English that each abbreviation stands for.

21.41. **ESR** ______________________

21.42. **bpm** ______________________

21.43. **CBC** ______________________

21.44. **NMT** ______________________

21.45. **WBC** ______________________

Term Selection

Select the correct answer, and write it on the line provided.

21.46. Drawing fluid from the sac surrounding the heart is known as ______________________.

abdominocentesis cardiocentesis pericardiocentesis arthrocentesis

21.47. The presence of blood in the urine is known as ______________________.

albuminuria creatinuria hematuria ketonuria

21.48. ______________________ is a combination of nutrition, medicinal supplements and herbs, water therapy, homeopathy, and lifestyle modifications used to identify and treat the root causes of symptoms and disease.

Naturopathy Homeopathy Qi Gong Biofeedback

21.49. A ______________________ is the examination of the physical and chemical properties of stool to determine the presence of abnormal elements.

stool guaiac test genome test stool analysis urinalysis

21.50. The term ______________________ refers to a treatment approach that takes into consideration the whole body and its environment, including the mind, body, and spirit.

wellness holistic naturopathy hypnosis

Sentence Completion

Write the correct term on the line provided.

21.51. The term *radiographic* ______________________ describes the path that the x-ray beam follows through the body from entrance to exit.

21.52. The term ______________________ describes an abnormal, high-pitched, musical breathing sound that is heard during inspiration.

21.53. A/An ______________________ is a medical professional trained to draw blood from patients for laboratory tests and other procedures.

21.54. A/An ______________________ is an instrument used to visually examine the external ear and tympanic membrane.

21.55. ______________________ is a traditional Chinese touch therapy involving finger pressure applied to specific areas of the body to restore the flow of qi.

Word Surgery

Divide each term into its component word parts. Write these word parts, in sequence, on the lines provided. When necessary use a slash (/) to indicate a combining vowel. (You may not need all of the lines provided.)

21.56. **Arthrocentesis** is a surgical puncture of the joint space to remove synovial fluid for analysis to determine the cause of pain or swelling in a joint.

__________ __________ __________ __________

21.57. **Ultrasonography** is the imaging of deep body structures by recording the echoes of sound wave pulses.

__________ __________ __________ __________

21.58. **Echocardiography** is an ultrasonic diagnostic procedure used to evaluate the structures and motion of the heart.

__________ __________ __________ __________

21.59. **Bacteriuria** is the presence of bacteria in the urine.

__________ __________ __________ __________

21.60. **Hyperthermia** is an is an extremely high body temperature.

__________ __________ __________ __________

True/False

If the statement is true, write **True** on the line. If the statement is false, write **False** on the line.

21.61. __________ Neuromuscular therapy is a form of massage that uses soft-tissue manipulation focusing on applying pressure to trigger points.

21.62. __________ Casts are fibrous or protein materials, such as pus and fats, that are thrown off into the urine in kidney disease.

21.63. __________ A sphygmomanometer is used to measure the respiratory rate.

21.64. __________ An MRI creates images by combining sound wave pulses and strong magnets.

21.65. __________ Wellness is a general term that means actively working toward a state of being in good physical and mental health.

Clinical Conditions

Write the correct answer on the line provided.

21.66. The urinalysis for Sophia O'Keefe showed the presence of ketones. The medical term for this condition is ________________.

21.67. Dr. Jamison suspected her patient had an infection. An elevated count in the patient's ________________ cell count test would confirm her diagnosis.

21.68. Kelly Harrison was extremely cold after being stranded in a snowstorm. When rescued, the paramedics said she was suffering from ________________.

21.69. During his examination of the patient, Dr. Wong used ________________ to feel the texture, size, consistency, and location of certain body parts.

21.70. Dr. McDowell ordered a blood transfusion. Before the transfusion, ________________ tests were required to determine the compatibility of donor's and recipient's blood.

21.71. In preparation for his upper GI series, Dwight Oshone swallowed a liquid containing the contrast medium ________________.

21.72. Maria Martinez required ________________ echocardiography to evaluate the structures of her heart.

21.73. Another term for conventional, or Western, medical practices is ________________.

21.74. The urinalysis for Kathleen McCaffee showed ________________. This is the presence of glucose in the urine.

21.75. Dr. Roberts used ________________ during the examination. This technique involves tapping the surface of the body with a finger or instrument.

Which Is The Correct Medical Term?

Select the correct answer, and write it on the line provided.

21.76. A/An ________________ is the removal of a small piece of living tissue for examination to confirm or establish a diagnosis.

biopsy endoscopy laparoscopy centesis

21.77. The urinalysis indicated ______________. This is an increased concentration of creatinine in the urine.

creatinuria glycosuria ketonuria proteinuria

21.78. The energy therapy where finger pressure is applied to specific areas of the body is called ______________.

Qi Gong acupuncture acupressure hypnosis

21.79. During a/an ______________ examination, some patients feel uncomfortable because of the noise generated by the machine and the feeling of being closed in.

CT MRI PET x-ray

21.80. The examination position that has the patient lying on the back with the feet and legs raised and supported in stirrups is the ______________ position.

dorsal recumbent lithotomy prone Sims'

Challenge Word Building

These terms are *not* primary terms in the chapter; however, they are made up of the following familiar word parts. If you need help in creating the term, refer to your medical dictionary.

hyper-	**albumin/o**	**-centesis**
hypo-	**calc/i**	**-emia**
	cyst/o	**-gram**
	glycos/o	**-scope**
	protein/o	**-uria**
	pleur/o	
	py/o	

21.81. The term meaning the presence of abnormally low concentrations of protein in the blood is ______________.

21.82. The term meaning abnormally high levels of albumin in the blood is ______________.

21.83. The term meaning unusually large amounts of sugar in the urine is ______________.

21.84. The instrument used to visually examine the interior of the urinary bladder is a/an ______________.

21.85. The term meaning a surgical puncture of the chest wall with a needle to obtain fluid from the pleural cavity is ______________. This procedure is also known as thoracentesis.

21.86. An x-ray examination of the bladder is called a/an ______________________.

21.87. The term meaning an abnormally low level of calcium in the circulating blood is

______________________.

21.88. The term meaning abnormally large amounts of calcium in the urine is ______________________.

21.89. The term meaning the presence of pus-forming organisms in the blood is ______________________.

21.90. The term meaning the presence of excess protein in the urine is ______________________.

Labeling Exercises

Identify the numbered items on the accompanying figures.

21.91. This is the ______________________ position.

21.92. This is the ______________________ recumbent position.

21.93. This is the ______________________ position.

21.94. This is the ______________________ recumbent position.

21.95. This is the ______________________ position.

21.96. This is the ______________________ position.

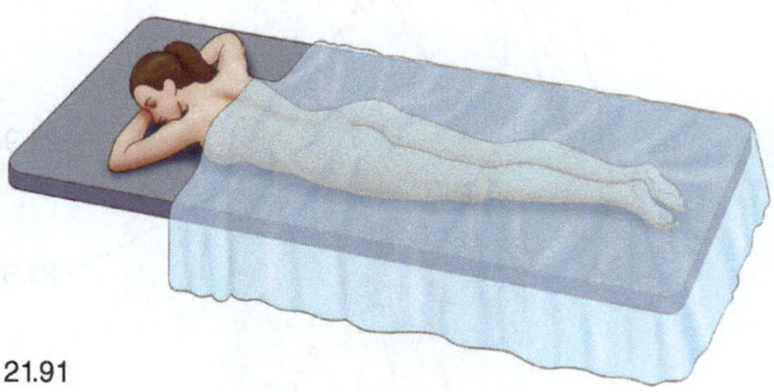

21.91

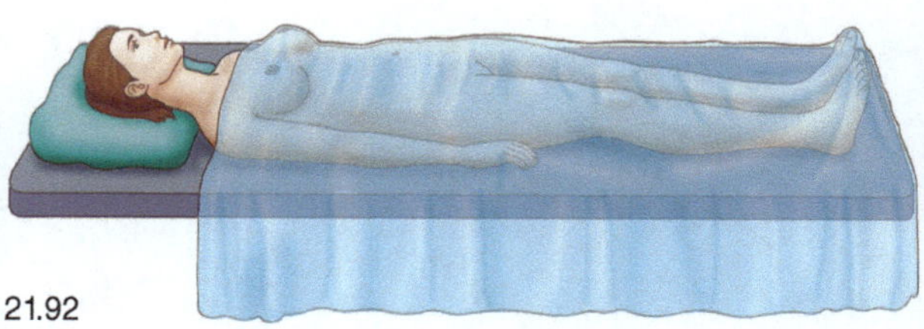

21.92

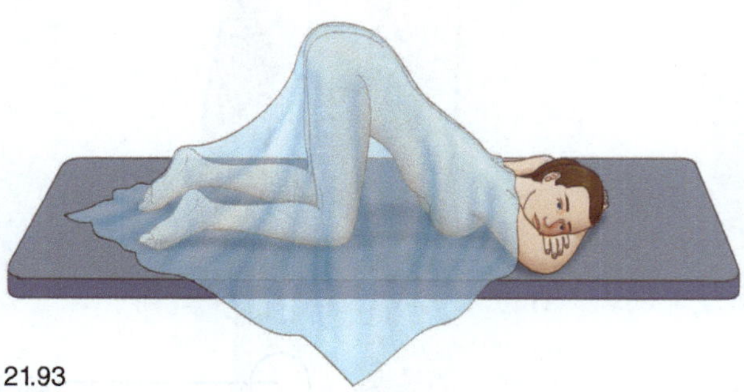

21.93

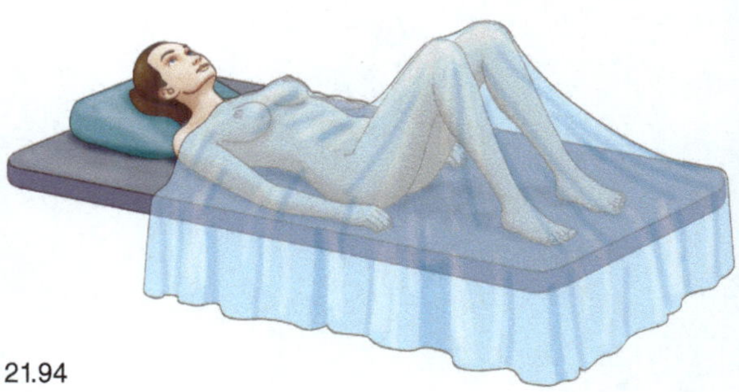

21.94

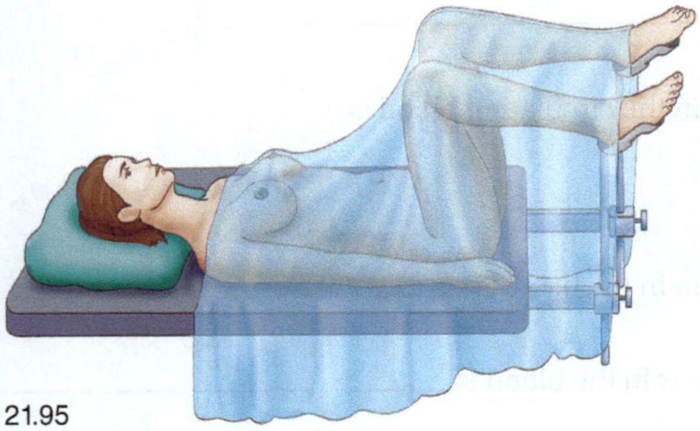

21.95

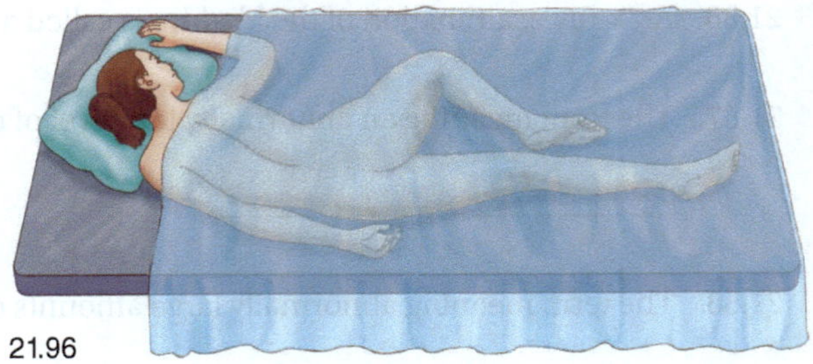

21.96

21.97. This is the ______________________ pulse point.

21.98. This is the ______________________ pulse point.

21.99. This is the ______________________ pulse point.

21.100. This is the ______________________ pulse point.

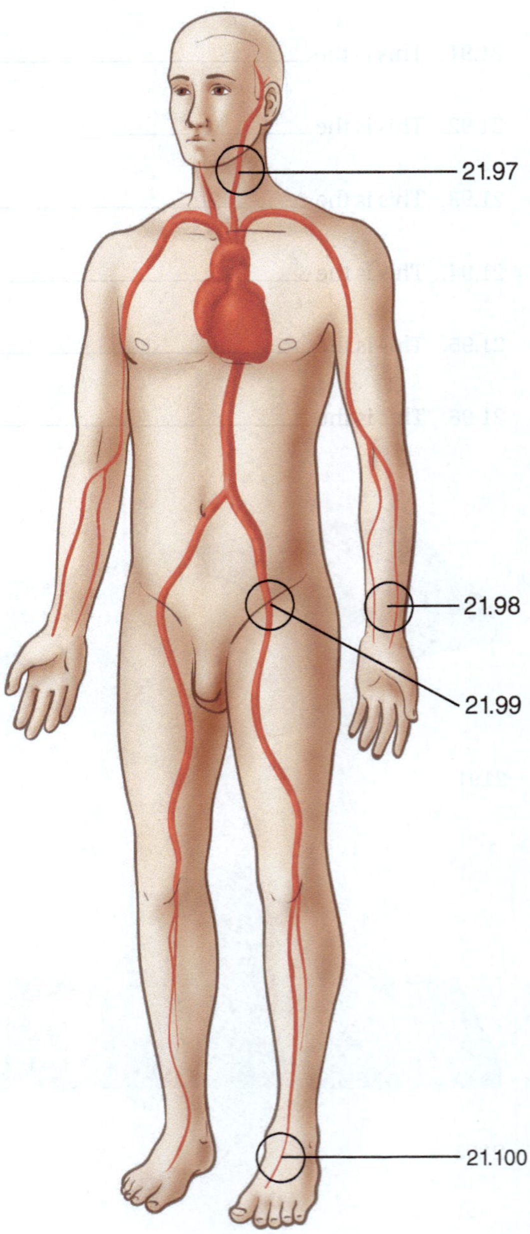

The Human Touch

CRITICAL THINKING EXERCISE

The following story and questions are designed to stimulate critical thinking through class discussion or as a brief essay response. There are no right or wrong answers to these questions.

"Elena Kwon?" Priya picked up the paperwork for her next patient and looked out into the waiting room. A slender young woman stood up and paused for a moment to shake her head in response to a question from the man sitting with her before saying, "That's me."

"Hi there, Mrs. Kwon. My name is Priya Jankar. I'm Dr. Skerry's medical assistant. I'll be checking your vital signs today before your visit with Dr. Skerry. Just come with me, please." Priya stepped back from the door to let the patient enter, and indicated a chair next to the computer and portable vital blood pressure machine. "Go ahead and have a seat right there, and please pull your sleeve up for me so I can check your blood pressure."

Priya picked the proper size blood pressure cuff, and leaned down to wrap it around Mrs. Kwon's arm. She immediately noticed a number of small oval bruises on the patient's upper arm that almost looked like finger marks. She glanced over at Mrs. Kwon again, realizing that Mrs. Kwon was wearing a long-sleeved shirt even though it was a hot day.

After Priya placed the blood pressure cuff and pulse oximeter, and started the automatic sphygmomanometer, she smiled down at Mrs. Kwon and picked up her pen, trying to sound casual. "I just have a few basic questions for you that we routinely ask all of our patients. Do you feel safe at home? Is anyone hurting you? Do you want to hurt yourself or anyone else?"

Elena Kwon shook her head, but she wouldn't quite meet Priya's gaze. "No, no, I'm fine. Everything's fine at home."

Priya suspected that she might not be telling the truth, but she didn't want to call the patient a liar, or make a big deal out of what might just be some random bruises. She wondered what she should tell Dr. Skerry—or if she should just hope that he noticed the bruises on his own.

Suggested Discussion Topics

1. Health care professionals are required to report suspected or confirmed domestic violence. If Mrs. Kwon denies any problems, what do you think Priya's next steps can be?
2. What do you think Priya could consider doing differently if Mrs. Kwon had a family member sitting next to her?
3. What factors in this story are suspicious for possible domestic violence? How would you document this in a patient's chart?
4. How do you think health care professionals can best offer resources for potential victims of domestic violence?

CHAPTER 22

PHARMACOLOGY

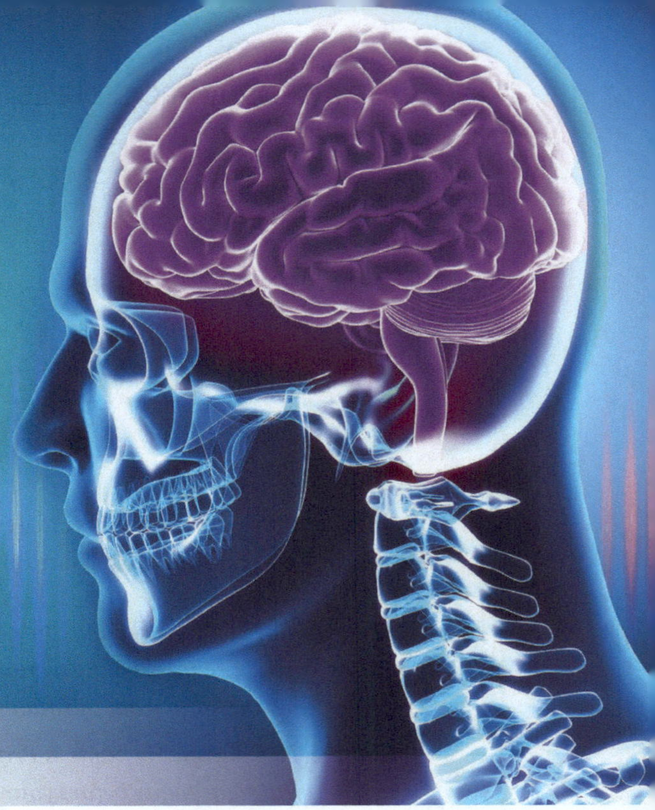

Overview of THE BASICS OF PHARMACOLOGY

Pharmacology plays a crucial role in human health, examining the interaction of drugs with the living body. For medical professionals, this branch of medicine requires familiarity with commonly encountered classes of drugs and their corresponding routes of administration. Accuracy in medical terminology is particularly important in pharmacology, where a mistake in drug name, dosage, or route of administration can have serious and even fatal consequences.

Vocabulary Related to **PHARMACOLOGY**

This list contains essential word parts and medical terms for this chapter. These and the other important **primary terms** are shown in **boldface** throughout the chapter. *Secondary terms*, which appear in *orange* italics, clarify the meaning of primary terms.

Word Parts

- ☐ **-al** pertaining to
- ☐ **derm/o** skin
- ☐ **enter/o** digestive tract, small intestine
- ☐ **intra-** within
- ☐ **lingu/o** tongue
- ☐ **muscul/o** muscle
- ☐ **-ous** pertaining to
- ☐ **par-** outside
- ☐ **pharmac/o** drug
- ☐ **pyret/o** fever
- ☐ **sub-** under
- ☐ **thec/o** sheath
- ☐ **toxic/o** poison
- ☐ **trans-** through, across
- ☐ **ven/o** vein

Medical Terms

- ☐ **ACE inhibitors**
- ☐ **addiction**
- ☐ **adherence**
- ☐ **adverse drug reaction**
- ☐ **analgesic**
- ☐ **antacid**
- ☐ **antibiotics** (**an**-tih-bye-**AH**-tiks)
- ☐ **anticoagulants**
- ☐ **anticonvulsant** (**an**-tih-kon-**VUL**-sant)
- ☐ **antiemetic** (**an**-tee-eh-**MEH**-tik)
- ☐ **antitussive**
- ☐ **antipyretic**
- ☐ **beta-blockers**
- ☐ **bisphosphonates** (bis-**FOS**-foh-nayts)
- ☐ **bolus** (**BOH**-lus)
- ☐ **brand name drug**
- ☐ **bronchodilator** (**brawn**-koh-**DYE**-lay-tor)
- ☐ **calcium channel blockers**
- ☐ **contraindication** (**kon**-trah-inn-dih-**KAY**-shun)
- ☐ **conscious sedation**
- ☐ **controlled substances**
- ☐ **corticosteroid** (**kor**-tih-koh-**STAY**-royd)
- ☐ **dependence**
- ☐ **dietary supplements**
- ☐ **diuretics** (**dye**-you-**REH**-tiks)
- ☐ **drug**
- ☐ **drug tolerance**
- ☐ **formulary**
- ☐ **generic drug**
- ☐ **insulin**
- ☐ **intradermal injection**
- ☐ **intramuscular injection**
- ☐ **intravenous injection** (**in**-trah-**VEE**-nus)
- ☐ **laxative** (**LACK**-sah-tiv)
- ☐ **loading dose**
- ☐ **maintenance dose**
- ☐ **medication**
- ☐ **opioids** (**OH**-pee-oydz)
- ☐ **overdose**
- ☐ **over-the-counter drug**
- ☐ **palliative** (**PAL**-ee-**ay**-tiv)
- ☐ **paralytic** (**pair**-ah-**LIH**-tik)
- ☐ **pharmacology** (**far**-mah-**KAH**-loh-gee)
- ☐ **prescription drug**
- ☐ **proton pump inhibitor**
- ☐ **reversal agent**
- ☐ **sedative**
- ☐ **side effect**
- ☐ **stimulant**
- ☐ **subcutaneous injection** (**sub**-kyoo-**TAY**-nee-yus)
- ☐ **sublingual administration** (sub-**LING**-gwal)
- ☐ **suppository** (suh-**PAW**-zih-toh-ree)
- ☐ **synergism** (**SIN**-er-jizm)
- ☐ **therapeutic dose**
- ☐ **tissue plasminogen activator** (plaz-**MIN**-oh-jen)
- ☐ **topical application**
- ☐ **topical retinoids**
- ☐ **toxicity**
- ☐ **toxicology**
- ☐ **transdermal** (tranz-**DUR**-mahl)

LEARNING OBJECTIVES

On completion of this chapter, you should be able to:

1. Identify terminology related to the study of pharmacology.
2. Identify the role of federal agencies in the regulation of drugs.
3. List the three names associated with a given drug.
4. Identify the three ways of classifying drugs.
5. Identify the medical specialists within the pharmacology field.
6. Describe the routes of drug administration and administration methods used.
7. Identify terminology related to medication dosing.
8. Identify terminology related to the actions and interactions of drugs.
9. Identify the commonly used medications for each body system and specialty area, and their drug classifications.
10. Identify the medical word parts related to pharmacology.
11. Spell the primary terms related to pharmacology.
12. Pronounce the primary terms related to pharmacology.
13. Identify abbreviations related to drug administration and pharmacology.

PHARMACOLOGY

Pharmacology (far-mah-**KAH**-loh-gee) is the study of the nature, uses, and effects of drugs for medical purposes (**pharmac** means drug, and **-ology** means study of). The two subspecialties of pharmacology are pharmacodynamics and pharmacokinetics.

- **Pharmacodynamics** is the study of the effects of drugs on the human body.
- **Pharmacokinetics** is the study of how drugs move through the human body from the time of administration to the time of elimination from the body.

Toxicology is the study of the nature, effects, and treatments of poisons and harmful substances (**toxic** means toxin or poison, and **-ology** means study of).

A **drug** is any substance that has a psychological or physiological effect on the human body.

A **medication** is a drug with proven benefit that is used for medical treatment.

FEDERAL REGULATION OF DRUGS

The **Food and Drug Administration** (FDA) is the federal agency responsible for ensuring the quality and safety of all prescription drugs, over-the-counter drugs, vitamins, minerals, and other dietary supplements sold in the United States.

- The **United States Pharmacopeia-National Formulary** (USP-NF) is a continuously updated set of quality standards for prescription drugs, over-the-counter drugs, and dietary supplements. The USP-NF is primarily used by drug manufacturers.

The **Drug Enforcement Administration** (DEA) is a federal law enforcement agency responsible for fighting the distribution of illegal and illicit drugs by licensing and tracking the prescription and dispensing of controlled substances.

- **Controlled substances** are addictive prescription medicines and illicit drugs whose manufacture, possession, and use are highly regulated by the government.
- The **Controlled Substances Act** is a law regulating the manufacture, possession, distribution, and use of drugs by classifying them into five groups called ***schedules*** according to their potential for abuse (Table 22.1).

Illicit Drugs

Illicit drugs, also known as ***street drugs***, are controlled substances without known medical benefit (or with

TABLE 22.1

Drug Enforcement Administration Drug Schedules

	Accepted Medical Use?	Potential for Abuse and Addiction	Examples
Schedule I	No	High	Heroin, lysergic acid diethylamide (commonly known as LSD), 3-4 methylenedioxymethamphetamine (commonly known as ecstasy), methaqualone, peyote
Schedule II	Yes, but considered dangerous	High	Combination products with less than 15 mg of hydrocodone per dosage unit, hydrocodone/acetaminophen (Vicodin®), oxycodone (OxyContin®), fentanyl (Sublimaze®), hydromorphone (Dilaudid®), meperidine (Demerol®), methadone (Dolophine®), cocaine, methamphetamine, dextroamphetamine (Dexedrine®), racemic amphetamine/dextroamphetamine (Adderall®), methylphenidate (Ritalin®)
Schedule III	Yes	Moderate	Products with less than 90 mg of codeine per dosage unit, acetaminophen with codeine (Tylenol #3®), ketamine (Ketalar®), anabolic steroids, testosterone
Schedule IV	Yes	Low	Alprazolam (Xanax®), diazepam (Valium®), lorazepam (Ativan®), zolpidem (Ambien®), carisoprodol (Soma®), propoxyphene (Darvon®), propoxyphene/acetaminophen (Darvocet®), pentazocine/naloxone (Talwin®), tramadol (Ultram®)
Schedule V	Yes	Lowest	Cough syrup with less than 200 mg of codeine (Robitussin AC®), pregabalin (Lyrica®), diphenoxylate/atropine (Lomotil®), difenoxin/atropine (Motofen®)

Credit: https://www.dea.gov/drug-scheduling

side effects that outweigh any medical benefit) that are obtained illegally and are usually addictive. While any drug is considered illicit if it is obtained illegally, all Schedule I drugs are illicit drugs.

- An **addiction** is compulsive, uncontrollable dependence on a drug, alcohol, or other substance. It can also be a habit or practice that cannot be stopped without causing severe emotional, mental, or physiologic reactions (see Chapter 17).
- ***Marijuana*** is a Schedule I drug that is legal to grow, purchase, and possess in certain quantities in some states without a prescription; legal in some states with a prescription (***medical marijuana***); and illegal in other states.

Prescription Drugs

A **prescription drug** is a medication that can legally only be dispensed by a licensed pharmacist with an order from a licensed prescriber such as a physician or dentist. For example, Schedule II–V drugs are prescription drugs.

- A **prescription** is a written order from a licensed medical professional such as a physician or dentist that specifies a medication or product to be dispensed to a patient.
- A **pharmacy** is a place where medications are prepared and sold (Figure 22.1). A pharmacy can sell medications through a brick-and-mortar store, an online store, or both, and may also offer mail order service.

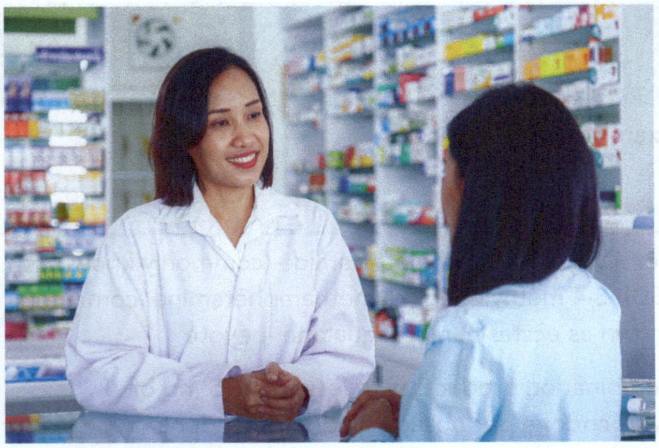

FIGURE 22.1 A pharmacy is a place where medications are prepared and sold.

- A **formulary** (**FOR**-myoo-**lah**-ree) is a list of prescription drugs covered by a specific health care plan. The term originally referred to a book listing ingredients and formulas for making medicines.
- The **Prescriber's Digital Reference** (PDR) is the most commonly used drug information guide. It is an online resource that is updated monthly.
- **Durable medical equipment** (DME) refers to products prescribed by a physician that are not medications. These include things like wheelchairs, walkers, crutches, CPAP devices, blood sugar monitors, home oxygen equipment and nebulizers. These may or may not be covered by insurance.

Over-the-Counter Drugs

An **over-the-counter drug**, also known as an *OTC*, is a medication that can be purchased without a prescription.

A **dietary supplement** is a product containing nutrients intended to be beneficial for health. All dietary supplements are considered to be foods and are regulated differently than medications by the FDA. Some dietary supplements can interact with prescription medications. In order to provide the best care, medical providers must always obtain an accurate list of all illicit, prescription, and over-the-counter drugs—as well as dietary supplements—a patient is taking.

- A **vitamin** or **mineral** is a dietary supplement containing one or more substances that are beneficial for humans and can be obtained from food or in supplement (pill, liquid, beverage) form.
- An **herbal supplement** is a dietary supplement containing one or more substances derived from plants.
- The FDA is not required to confirm the safety of dietary supplements before they are offered for sale. It is illegal to market dietary supplements as treatments or cures for specific diseases or symptoms.

DRUG NAMES

Every medication has three different names.

- A **brand name drug** is sold under the name given the drug by the manufacturer. A brand name is always spelled with a capital letter. For example, Valium® is a brand name for the generic drug diazepam.
  - Some brand names hint at the purpose of the drug. For example, ProAir® is a brand name for inhaled albuterol.
  - Some drugs may have more than one brand name. For example, ibuprofen is sold under the brand names Advil® and Motrin®, among others.
  - *Note:* In this chapter, brand names are shown in parentheses following the generic name.
- A **generic drug** is usually named for its chemical structure and is not protected by a brand name or trademark. For example, diazepam is the generic name of a drug frequently used as a skeletal muscle relaxant, sedative, and anti-anxiety agent.
- A **chemical name** is the specific name for a chemical compound, created according to international guidelines to avoid confusion. For example, the chemical name of diazepam is *7-chloro-1,3-dihydro-1-methyl-5-phenyl-2H-1,4-benzodiazepin-2-one*. The chemical name is rarely used in medical terminology.

Many medications have a brand name and generic name that sound alike. For example, Buspar® is a brand name for buspirone.

How Drugs Are Classified

A **drug class**, also known as a *drug category*, is a group of drugs with similar features. Drugs can be classified based on their mechanisms of action, physiological effects on the body, or similar chemical structures.

- Drugs may fall into more than one class. For example, metoprolol (Lopressor®) is classified as a beta-blocker, antihypertensive, and anti-arrhythmic.
- The **Anatomical Therapeutic Chemical Classification system** (ATC) is a five-level drug classification system developed by the World Health Organization (WHO).

The levels become increasingly specific from the first level, which indicates the body system upon which the drug works, down to the fifth level, which indicates the chemical structure of the drug.

   - For example, the ATC code for metoprolol is C07AB02. The ATC code is rarely used in medical terminology.

- The **United States Pharmacopeia** (USP) classifies drugs by therapeutic category, pharmacologic class, and subgroup.
   - For example, metoprolol is in the cardiovascular agent category, beta-adrenergic blocking agent class, and cardioselective beta-adrenergic blocking agent subgroup.

MEDICAL SPECIALTIES RELATED TO PHARMACOLOGY

- A **pharmacist** is a medical professional with a doctor of pharmacy (PharmD) degree who formulates and dispenses prescribed medications at a pharmacy (Figure 22.2).
- A **pharmacy technician** is a licensed professional who helps run a pharmacy under the supervision of a pharmacist. Their duties may include medication preparation and maintaining inventory and patient medical records.
- A **medical toxicologist** is a physician who specializes in the care of patients who have been exposed to toxic levels of drugs or other substances, either by overdose or accidental exposure.

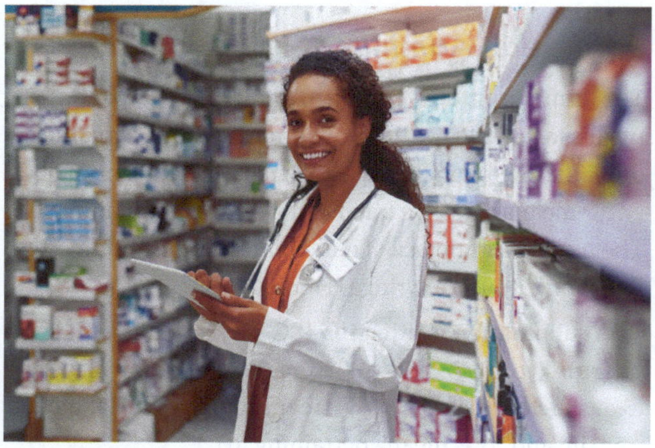

iStock.com/Ridofranz

FIGURE 22.2 A pharmacist is a medical professional who prepares and dispenses prescribed medications at a pharmacy.

TERMINOLOGY RELATED TO PHARMACOLOGY

Accuracy in medical terminology is particularly important in pharmacology, where a mistake in drug name, dosage, or route of administration can have serious and even fatal consequences.

Terminology Related to Drug Administration

- A **syringe** (suh-**RINJ**), also known as a ***hypodermic syringe***, is a plastic tube with markings along the side, which is used to measure and administer liquid medication, either by mouth or by injection (Figure 22.3).
- A **tablet**, also known as a ***pill***, is a round or oval object containing medication in solid form which is designed to be swallowed or dissolved under the tongue (Figure 22.4).
- A **capsule** (**KAP**-suhl) is a round or oval object containing medication in solid or liquid form covered in a dissolvable gelatin or starch casing which is designed to be swallowed (Figure 22.4).
- A **suppository** (suh-**PAW**-zih-toh-ree) is medication in a semisolid form that is placed in the rectum, vagina, or urethra (Figure 22.5).
- An **enema** (**EH**-neh-ma) is liquid medication placed in the rectum.
- A **placebo** (plah-**SEE**-boh) is an inactive substance, such as a sugar pill or liquid, that is administered only for its suggestive effects. In medical research, a placebo

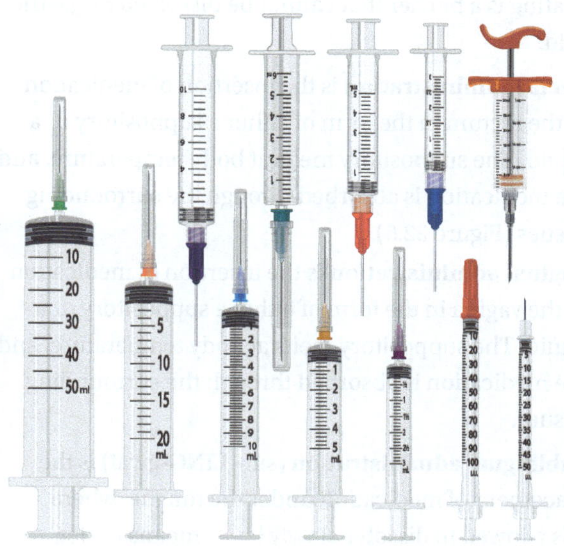

Elzloy/Shutterstock.com

FIGURE 22.3 Different types of syringes.

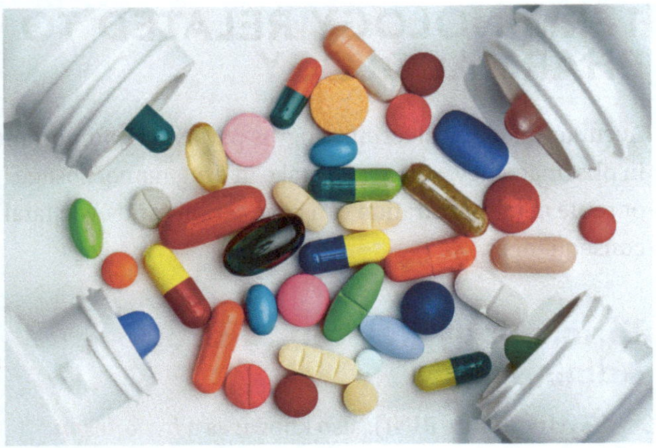

iStock.com/apomares

FIGURE 22.4 Examples of tablets and capsules.

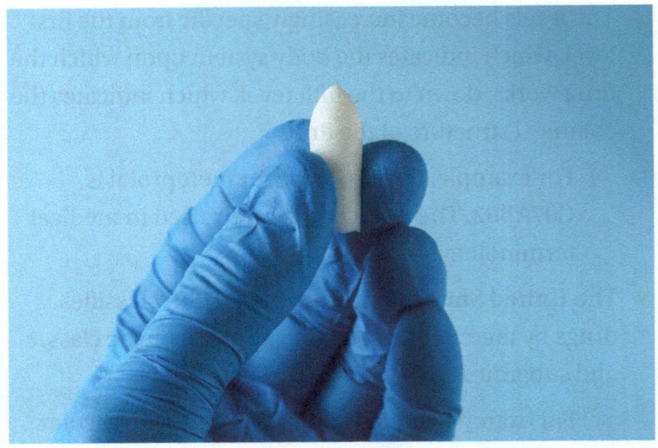

iStock.com/Adragan

FIGURE 22.5 Example of a suppository.

is sometimes administered to a control group, while the drug being studied is administered to the other group in order to determine whether the drug is effective or not.

Routes of Medication Administration

- **Inhalation administration** describes vapors, gases, or powders taken in through the nose or mouth and absorbed into the bloodstream through the lungs. One example is the use of a metered-dose inhaler to treat asthma (see Chapter 8) or the gases used for general anesthesia (see Chapter 11).
- **Oral administration** refers to medications taken by mouth to be absorbed through the walls of the stomach or small intestine. These drugs can be in the form of liquids, tablets, or capsules. Medications designed to be released in the small intestine are covered with an *enteric coating* to prevent them from being absorbed as they pass through the stomach. An enteric coating is a barrier that cannot be dissolved by gastric acid.
- **Rectal administration** is the insertion of medication in the rectum in the form of either a suppository or a liquid. The suppository melts at body temperature, and the medication is absorbed through the surrounding tissues (Figure 22.5).
- **Vaginal administration** is the insertion of medication in the vagina in the form of either a suppository or a liquid. The suppository melts at body temperature, and the medication is absorbed through the surrounding tissues.
- **Sublingual administration** (sub-**LING**-gwal) is the placement of medication under the tongue, where it is allowed to dissolve slowly (**sub-** means under, **lingu** means tongue, and **-al** means pertaining to). Because the sublingual tissues are highly vascular, the medication is quickly absorbed directly into the bloodstream. *Highly vascular* means containing many blood vessels. *Buccal administration* allows the drug to dissolve between the gums and cheek.
- **Topical application** is a method for applying liquid or ointment by rubbing it into the skin on the area to be treated. For example, *cortisone ointment* is applied topically to relieve itching and to speed healing; *antibiotic ointments* are applied over minor wounds to prevent and treat infection.
- A **transdermal** (tranz-**DUR**-mahl) medication is administered from a patch that is applied to unbroken skin (**trans-** means through or across, **derm** means skin, and **-al** means pertaining to). The medication, which is continuously released by the patch, is absorbed through the skin and transmitted to the bloodstream so that it can produce a systemic effect. These multilayered patches are used to convey medications, such as nitroglycerin for angina or hormones for hormone replacement therapy.

Parenteral Administration

The term **parenteral administration** (pah-**REN**-ter-al) means taken into the body or administered in a manner other than through the digestive tract (**par-** means outside, **enter** means digestive tract, and **-al** means pertaining to). The most common use of parenteral administration is by injection through a syringe (Figure 22.6).

- A **subcutaneous injection** (SC, SQ) (**sub**-kyoo-**TAY**-nee-yus) is made into the fatty layer just below the skin (**sub-** means under, **cutan/e** means skin, and **-ous** means pertaining to).
- An **intradermal injection** is made into the middle layers of the skin (**intra-** means within, **derm** means skin, and **-al** means pertaining to).

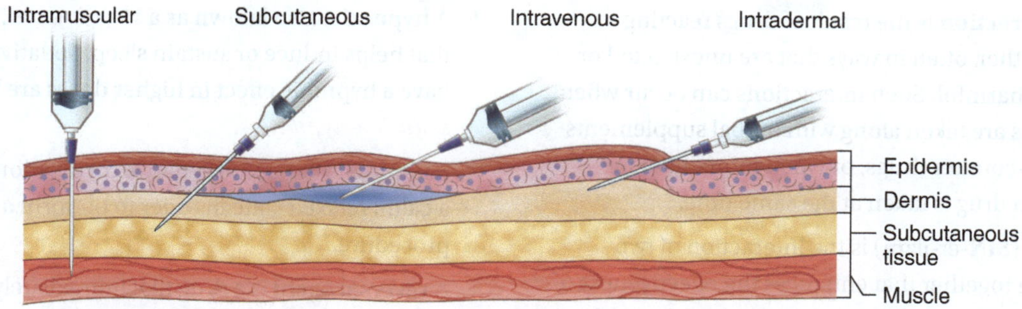

FIGURE 22.6 Types of injections.

- An **intramuscular injection** (IM) is made directly into muscle tissue (**intra-** means within, **muscul** means muscle, and **-ar** means pertaining to).
- An **intravenous injection** (IV) (**in**-trah-**VEE**-nus) is made directly into a vein (**intra-** means within, **ven** means vein, and **-ous** means pertaining to). An ***IV infusion*** is administered into a vein over a period of time.
- A **PICC line**, PICC being an acronym for ***peripherally inserted central catheter***, is frequently used for a patient who will need IV therapy for more than seven days.
- A **bolus** (**BOH**-lus), also known as a ***bolus infusion***, is a single, concentrated dose of a drug usually injected into a blood vessel over a short period of time. The term *bolus* is also used in relation to the digestive system (see Chapter 9).
- **Intrathecal administration** (**in**-trah-**THEE**-kahl) is the injection of medication directly into the cerebrospinal fluid (**intra-** means within, **thec** means sheath, and **-al** means pertaining to).

Medication Dosing

A **dose** is a measured quantity of a medication ordered to be given at one time.

- A **therapeutic dose** is the amount of medication necessary to achieve the desired outcome. ***Therapeutic*** means relating to the treatment or curing of a disorder or disease.
- A **therapeutic level** is a blood test showing whether the amount of medication circulating in the blood is sufficient to achieve the desired outcome.
- A **loading dose** is an initial, higher dose of medication given to achieve therapeutic levels when a patient is started on a medication. This is used for medications that have a long ***half-life***, meaning that they are cleared slowly from the body, or for medications such as anti-convulsants, where it is important to achieve therapeutic levels immediately.
- A **maintenance dose** is the regular dose of medication given on an ongoing basis to maintain therapeutic levels.
- A **medication regimen** is a course of treatment involving taking certain medications on a regular basis as instructed by a physician or other health care professional.
- **Adherence** or ***compliance*** is the patient's consistency and accuracy in following the regimen prescribed by a physician or other health care professional.
- An **overdose** (OD) is a deliberate or accidental ingestion of more medication than has been prescribed or is safe.

Terminology Related to the Actions and Interactions of Drugs

- An **adverse drug reaction** (ADR) is an undesirable reaction that accompanies the principal response for which the drug was taken. ADRs can include side effects, idiosyncratic reactions, and drug toxicity.
  - A **side effect** is a secondary response that accompanies the principal response for which the drug was taken. Side effects can be beneficial or undesirable.
  - An **idiosyncratic reaction** (**id**-ee-oh-sin-**KRAT**-ick) is an unexpected reaction to a drug that is particular to the individual.
  - Drug **toxicity** occurs when a harmful dose of a drug builds up in the body, either because of overdose or slowed removal of the drug from the body.
- A **contraindication** (**kon**-trah-inn-dih-**KAY**-shun) is a factor of the patient's condition that makes the use of a medication or specific treatment dangerous or ill advised. For example, a patient with a history of bleeding from stomach ulcers should not take blood thinners or other medications that will increase their risk of bleeding.

- A **drug interaction** is the result of drugs reacting with each other, often in ways that are unexpected or potentially harmful. Such interactions can occur when medications are taken along with herbal supplements or over-the-counter drugs, or when more than one prescription drug is taken at the same time.
- **Synergism** (**SIN**-er-jizm) is the interaction of two drugs taken together that enhances the effectiveness of both. The term comes from the Greek term for working together.
- A **paradoxical reaction** is the result of medical treatment that yields the opposite of normally expected results. ***Paradoxical*** means not being normal or the usual kind.
- **Drug tolerance** is when the body has become accustomed to a medication after taking it for a length of time, and higher doses are required to achieve the desired effect.
- **Dependence** is when the body has become accustomed to a medication or substance after repeated use, and experiences physical and/or psychological withdrawal symptoms if its use is stopped.

COMMON DRUG CLASSES AND MEDICATIONS

While individual medications used will vary between regions and facilities, there are common drug classes that every medical professional is likely to encounter. Many drugs work on specific body systems, and are discussed in the "Common Drug Classes and Medications by Body System" section. Other drug classes, such as sedatives and pain medications, include medications that work in different ways to produce a similar effect on the body.

Sedatives and Levels of Sedation

Sedative is a blanket term for controlled substances that relax the body by suppressing neurotransmitters in the central nervous system. Many sedatives are Schedule IV drugs.

- Classes of sedatives include benzodiazepines such as lorazepam (Ativan®), and barbiturates such as phenobarbital (Luminal®). Other medications, such as opioids, can also have a sedative effect.
- In low doses, sedatives have a relaxing, ***anxiolytic*** (anxiety-reducing) effect. In higher doses, they induce sleep and can lead to unconsciousness and death in cases of overdose.
- A **hypnotic**, also known as a ***sleeping pill***, is a drug that helps induce or sustain sleep. Sedatives that have a hypnotic effect in higher doses are known as ***sedative-hypnotics***.
- **Sedation** is the use of sedative medication to induce a calm, relaxed state in order to perform a medical procedure.
- A **reversal agent** is a drug that immediately reverses the effect of another drug, such as a sedative or opioid. Reversal agents are used in the case of overdose. The reversal agent for opioid overdose is naloxone (Narcan®), which is given intravenously or intranasally (squirted up the nose) (Figure 22.7). The reversal agent for benzodiazepine overdose is flumazenil (Romazicon®), which is given intravenously.

Levels of Sedation

- **Conscious sedation**, also known as ***procedural sedation***, is a state of light to moderate sedation where the patient is calm, relaxed, and less responsive to stimuli. The patient is still able to support their own breathing, and can respond to some basic commands, but experiences less anxiety, pain, and discomfort, and does not remember the procedure afterward. Conscious sedation is often used for brief procedures such as re-aligning a broken bone. Commonly used sedatives for conscious sedation include midazolam (Versed®), fentanyl, dexmedetomidine (Precedex®), and ketamine (Ketalar®).

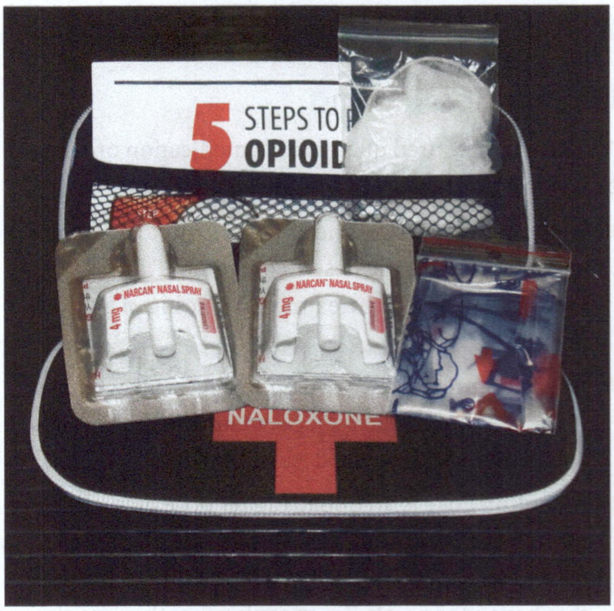

New2me86/Shutterstock.com

FIGURE 22.7 A Narcan kit. Narcan kits are available by prescription and over-the-counter for anyone who may be at risk for opioid overdose.

- **General anesthesia** is a state of *deep sedation* where the patient is unresponsive even to painful stimuli. In general anesthesia, the patient is given both sedative and paralytic drugs, and must be intubated and placed on a ventilator to support their breathing. Commonly used sedatives for general anesthesia include propofol (Diprivan®), ketamine (Ketalar®), and etomidate (Amidate®).
  - ***Anesthesia*** is the absence of normal sensation, especially sensitivity to pain, that is induced by the administration of an anesthetic agent (**an-** means without, and **-esthesia** means feeling). See Chapter 11 for more information on types of anesthesia.
  - A **paralytic** (**pair**-ah-**LIH**-tik) is a drug class containing medications that relax all muscles and are used to make intubation easier. Commonly used paralytics are succinylcholine (Anectine®), rocuronium (Zemuron®), and vecuronium (Norcuron®).

Common Drug Classes and Medications for Pain Management

The term **analgesic** (**an**-al-**JEE**-zick) refers to the class of drugs that relieves pain without affecting consciousness. These include such drugs as aspirin, acetaminophen, and ibuprofen.

- *Non-narcotic analgesics*, such as aspirin, are a class of drugs sold over the counter for relief of mild to moderate pain. Prescription pain relievers, sold through a pharmacy under the direction of a physician, are used for moderate to severe pain.
- **Opioids** (**OH**-pee-oydz), also called *narcotics*, such as morphine, hydrocodone, oxycodone, and codeine, are controlled substances available by prescription only to relieve severe pain. Medications in this drug class also have a sedative effect; however, prolonged use can cause physical dependence and addiction. There is currently an epidemic of opioid-related overdoses, many involving fentanyl, with tens of thousands of people dying annually.
- **Nonsteroidal anti-inflammatory drugs** (NSAIDs) (**EN**-saids) are a drug class of non-narcotic analgesics administered to control pain by reducing inflammation and swelling. Some NSAIDs, such as aspirin and ibuprofen, are available over the counter. Stronger NSAIDs are available by prescription. Side effects of regular use of NSAIDs can include stomach ulcers and increased risk of bleeding.
  - An **anti-inflammatory** medication relieves inflammation and pain without affecting consciousness.
- **Aspirin** (ASA) is an NSAID that works as an antipyretic and interferes with the normal production of platelets. At low levels, also known as *baby aspirin*, it is taken daily to prevent heart attack or stroke. Aspirin can be abbreviated as *ASA*, which refers to its chemical name, *acetylsalicylic acid*.
- **Ibuprofen** (eye-byoo-**PRO**-fen) is an NSAID that is sold over the counter under the brand names of Advil® and Motrin®, among others. Ibuprofen is also an antipyretic.
  - An **antipyretic** (**an**-tih-pye-**RET**-ick) is a class of medications administered to prevent or reduce fever (**anti-** means against, **pyret** means fever, and **-ic** means pertaining to). These medications act by lowering a raised body temperature; however, they do not affect a normal body temperature when a fever is not present.
- **Acetaminophen** (ah-**seet**-ah-**MIN**-oh-fen) is an analgesic that reduces pain but does not relieve inflammation; however, it does not have the negative side effects of NSAIDs. This substance is the basic ingredient found in Tylenol® and its generic equivalents. Acetaminophen is also an antipyretic. Acetaminophen can be abbreviated as *APAP*, which refers to its chemical name, *N-acetyl-para-aminophenol*.

Common Drug Classes and Medications by Body System

There are thousands of different medications available, many of which can be used for multiple medical problems. This section provides a brief overview of the most commonly encountered medication classes for each body system, with examples of each.

Skeletal System

- **Bisphosphonates** (bis-**FOS**-foh-nayts) are a class of drugs that slow the loss of bone density in osteoporosis. Common examples include alendronate (Fosamax®) and zoledronic acid (Reclast®).
- ***Parathyroid hormone analogs*** are a drug class of synthetic forms of parathyroid hormone that can help rebuild bone but come with an increased risk of bone cancer. A common example is teriparatide (Forteo®).

Muscular System

- **Muscle relaxants**, also known as *skeletal muscle relaxants*, are a class of drugs that treat muscle spasms by reducing muscle tension. Common examples include cyclobenzaprine (Flexeril®), tizanidine (Zanaflex®), and baclofen (Lioresal®). Some sedatives are also used as muscle relaxants.

Cardiovascular System

Anti-arrhythmics are a broad class of drugs that work to stop or prevent arrhythmias. Common examples include beta-blockers, calcium channel blockers, digoxin (Lanoxin®), and amiodarone (Pacerone®).

Antihypertensives (**an**-tih-high-per-**TEN**-sivs) are a class of drugs that work to lower blood pressure in various ways. Some of these drugs are also used to treat other heart conditions.

- **Beta-blockers** are a class of drugs that have both anti-arrhythmic and antihypertensive properties and work by blocking the release of the stress hormones epinephrine and norepinephrine to slow the heart rate. Common examples of beta-blockers include metoprolol (Lopressor®), atenolol (Tenormin®), and propranolol (Inderal®). Beta-blockers are commonly used to treat hypertension, heart failure, and angina.
- **ACE** (angiotensin-converting-enzyme) **inhibitors** are a class of drugs that have antihypertensive properties and work by blocking the action of the enzyme that causes blood vessels to contract. Common examples of ACE inhibitors include benazepril (Lotensin®), enalapril (Vasotec®), and lisinopril (Prinivil®, Zestril®). ACE inhibitors are primarily used to treat hypertension and heart failure.
- **Angiotensin-II receptor blockers** (ARBs) are a class of drugs that have antihypertensive properties and work by relaxing blood vessels. Common examples of ARBs include losartan (Cozaar®), irbesartan (Avapro®), and valsartan (Diovan®).
- **Calcium channel blockers** are a class of drugs that have antihypertensive and anti-arrhythmic properties and work by decreasing the movement of calcium ions into the cells of the heart and arteries, causing the arteries to relax and slowing the heart rate. Common examples of calcium channel blockers include amlodipine (Norvasc®), nicardipine (Cardene®), nifedipine (Procardia®), and diltiazem (Cardizem®). Calcium channel blockers are used to treat hypertension, angina, and tachycardic arrhythmias.
- **Nitroglycerin** (NTG) (**nye**-troh-**GLIH**-seh-rin) is a medication with antihypertensive properties that works by dilating veins, reducing the workload of the heart. It is sold under multiple brand names, including Nitrostat®, and can be administered sublingually, transdermally, or intravenously. Nitroglycerin is used to treat hypertensive emergencies, angina, and myocardial infarction.
- **Diuretics** (**dye**-you-**REH**-tiks) are a class of drugs that work to lower blood pressure by increasing the amount of urine output to rid the body of excess sodium and water. Common examples of diuretics include furosemide (Lasix®), torsemide (Demadex®), spironolactone (Aldactone®), and hydrochlorothiazide, which is often abbreviated HCTZ. Common side effects of diuretics include dehydration, low potassium, dizziness, and muscle cramps. Diuretics are used to treat hypertension and heart failure.

Blood System

- **Cholesterol-lowering** medications are a class of drugs that work to decrease high cholesterol levels. Common examples include gemfibrozil (Lopid®), atorvastatin (Lipitor®), lovastatin (Mevacor®), and simvastatin (Zocor®). ***Statin*** is a commonly used general term for cholesterol-lowering medications whose names end in *-statin*.
- **Anticoagulants**, also known as ***blood thinners***, are a class of drugs that slow the clotting of blood to either prevent or treat blood clots. Common examples include aspirin, warfarin (Coumadin®), heparin, enoxaparin (Lovenox®), dabigatran (Pradaxa®), and rivaroxaban (Xarelto®). The most common side effect from anticoagulants is bleeding. Some types of anticoagulants have reversal agents. For example, ***vitamin K*** is a reversal agent for warfarin.

Immune System

- **Antibiotics** (**an**-tih-bye-**AH**-tiks) are a class of drugs capable of killing bacteria (**anti-** means against, **bio** means life, and **-tic** means pertaining to). There are a broad range of antibiotics available, and the specific antibiotic prescribed is based on the type of bacterial infection and desired route of administration. Commonly prescribed antibiotics include azithromycin (Zithromax®, Z-Pak®), ciprofloxacin (Cipro®), metronidazole (Flagyl®), penicillin (Pen VK®), and sulfamethoxazole/trimethoprim (Bactrim®).
- An **antifungal** (**an**-tih-**FUNG**-gul) is one of a class of drugs that destroys or inhibits the growth of fungi (**anti-** means against, **fung** means fungus, and **-al** means pertaining to). This type of medication is also

known as an *antimycotic*. Common examples include fluconazole (Diflucan®), clotrimazole (Lotrimin-AF®), and amphotericin B (Fungizone®).

- An **antiviral drug** (**an**-tih-**VYE**-ral) is one of a class of drugs used to treat viral infections or to provide temporary immunity (**anti-** means against, **vir** means virus, and **-al** means pertaining to). Common examples include oseltamivir (Tamiflu®), acyclovir (Zovirax®), abacavir (Ziagen®), and emtricitabine/tenofovir (Truvada®).
- **Antihistamines** (**an**-tee-**HISS**-tah-meens) are a class of drugs that decrease the body's response to an allergen by blocking the histamine receptors. Common examples include diphenhydramine (Benadryl®), cetirizine (Zyrtec®), and fexofenadine (Allegra®).
- An **immunosuppressant** is one of a class of medications that reduces the immune system's response. Immunosuppressants are often used to prevent rejection after organ transplant, or in response to an autoimmune condition. Common examples include tacrolimus (Prograf®), mycophenolate (CellCept®), prednisone (Deltasone®), and rituximab (Rituxin®).

Respiratory System

- A **bronchodilator** (**brawn**-koh-**DYE**-lay-tor) is one of several classes of drugs that help relieve shortness of breath by relaxing the bronchi. Bronchodilators are mostly administered as inhalers.
  - Short-acting bronchodilators, also known as *rescue inhalers*, include albuterol (ProAir®, Ventolin®) and levalbuterol (Xopenex®).
  - Long-acting bronchodilators, also known as *maintenance inhalers*, include fluticasone/salmeterol (Advair Diskus®), tiotropium (Spiriva®), and ipratropium bromide (Atrovent®).
  - A *nebulizer* uses compressed air or oxygen to turn liquid medication into an aerosol for inhalation (see Chapter 8). An **aerosol** is a mist of tiny particles suspended in air. Commonly aerosolized bronchodilators include albuterol (Accuneb®) and ipratropium bromide (Atrovent®).
- A **corticosteroid** (**kor**-tih-koh-**STAY**-royd) is one of a class of medications used to reduce inflammation. Corticosteroids are frequently used in the treatment of asthma and COPD exacerbation, and can be administered orally, intravenously, or via inhalation. Common examples include prednisone (Deltasone®), methylprednisolone (Solu-Medrol®), fluticasone (Flovent®), and beclomethasone (QVAR®).
- An **antitussive** is one of a class of medications that helps decrease the frequency of coughs. Common examples are dextromethorpan (Robitussin DM®, Delsym®, and Dimetapp® among others) and benzonatate (Tessalon®).
- A **decongestant** is one of a class of drugs that reduces nasal congestion. Common examples are pseudoephedrine (Sudafed®) and oxymetazoline (Afrin®).

Digestive System

- *Oral analgesics* are a class of drugs that help relieve pain in and near the mouth such as a toothache or cold sore. Some common examples are benzocaine (Kanka®, Orajel®) and camphor/phenol (Campho-Phenique®). An *analgesic lozenge* is used to ease the pain of a sore throat, as is a *throat spray*. One common example is benzocaine/menthol (Chloraseptic®, Cepacol®).
- An **antacid** is one of a class of drugs that temporarily relieves indigestion by decreasing or neutralizing stomach acid. Common examples include calcium carbonate (Alka-Seltzer®, Tums®), magnesium hydroxide (Milk of Magnesia®), and aluminum hydroxide/magnesium hydroxide/simethicone (Maalox®).
- A **proton pump inhibitor** (PPI) is a class of medication that prevents ulcers and treats GERD by reducing the production of stomach acid. Common examples include pantoprazole (Protonix®), omeprazole (Prilosec®), and esomeprazole (Nexium®).
- A **histamine-2 blocker** (H2 blocker) is a class of medication that, similarly to a PPI, reduces the production of stomach acid and is used to prevent ulcers and treat GERD. The most common example is famotidine (Pepcid®).
- An **antiemetic** (**an**-tee-eh-**MEH**-tik) is one of several classes of medications that work in different ways to prevent or relieve nausea and vomiting. Antiemetics can be administered orally, sublingually, intramuscularly, intravenously, or rectally. Common examples include ondansetron (Zofran®), prochlorperazine (Compazine®), meclizine (Antivert®, Bonine®), and promethazine (Phenergan®).
- A **laxative** (**LACK**-sah-tiv) is one of several classes of medications that prevent or treat constipation by increasing bowel movements. Laxatives can be administered orally or rectally. Common examples include psyllium husk (Metamucil®), docusate sodium (Colace®), sennosides (Senokot®), polyethylene glycol (Miralax®), and bisacodyl (Dulcolax®).

- An **antidiarrheal** is one of a class of medications that temporarily relieves diarrhea. Common examples are loperamide (Imodium®), atropine/diphenoxylate (Lomotil®), and bismuth subsalicylate (Kaopectate®, Pepto-Bismol®).

Urinary System

- **Alpha blockers** are a class of drugs that improve urination in men with benign prostatic hyperplasia by relaxing the muscles in the prostate. Common examples include tamsulosin (Flomax®), terazosin (Hytrin®), and prazosin (Minipres®).
- An **anticholinergic** (**an**-tye-**koh**-lih-**NER**-jik) is one of a class of medications that can be used to treat overactive bladder by relaxing the smooth muscle of the bladder. However, their action is not limited to the bladder. Anticholinergics have a number of side effects, including dry mouth, hyperthermia, hallucinations, and blurry vision. Common examples of anticholinergics include trospium (Sanctura®) and oxybutynin (Ditropan®).

Nervous System

- An **anticonvulsant** (**an**-tih-kon-**VUL**-sant), also known as an *antiepileptic*, is one of several classes of drugs that prevent or stop seizures. Benzodiazepines such as lorazepam (Ativan®) are given intravenously, intramuscularly, or intranasally to stop a seizure, and other anticonvulsants are used to prevent further seizures. Commonly used examples of anticonvulsants include phenytoin (Dilantin®), fosphenytoin (Cerebyx®), levetiracetam (Keppra®), and lamotrigine (Lamictal®). Chlordiazepoxide (Librium®) is a benzodiazepine used as an anticonvulsant to prevent alcohol withdrawal–induced seizures.
- **Dopaminergic drugs** (**doh**-pah-mih-**NER**-jik) are a class of medications that treat the symptoms of Parkinson's disease by increasing dopamine activity in the brain. Commonly used examples include carbidopa/levodopa (Sinemet®), pramipexole (Mirapex®), and ropinirole (Requip®).
- An **acetylcholinesterase inhibitor** (ah-**see**-tihl-**koh**-lin-**ESS**-ter-ayz) is one of a class of medications that treat the symptoms of Alzheimer's disease by increasing the levels of acetylcholine in the brain. They do not slow or prevent the progression of Alzheimer's, but can improve cognitive function in people with mild to moderate dementia. A commonly used acetylcholinesterase inhibitor is donepezil (Aricept®).
- **Tissue plasminogen activator** (plaz-**MIN**-oh-jen) (tPA) is a drug class of powerful thrombolytics used in treatment of acute ischemic stroke. Commonly used tissue plasminogen activators include alteplase (Activase®) and tenecteplase (TNKase®).
- A **stimulant** is one of several classes of drugs that increases the activity of the central nervous system. Stimulants include controlled substances such as amphetamines, cocaine, and methylphenidate (Ritalin®), as well as commonly available substances such as caffeine and nicotine.

Special Senses: Eyes and Ears

Eye drops are liquid medications administered onto the cornea. Eye drops are used to treat dry eyes, bacterial infection, glaucoma, or other medical conditions of the eye.

- *Artificial tears* are eye drops that temporarily treat the symptoms of dry eyes by adding moisture to the cornea. Common examples include carboxymethylcellulose sodium (Refresh®, Retaine®) and polyethylene glycol (Systane®, Blink®).
- **Prostaglandin analogs** are a class of medicated eye drops used to treat glaucoma by increasing the amount of fluid leaving the eye. A commonly used prostaglandin analog is latanoprost (Xalatan®).
- *Beta-blockers* are also used in eye drop form to treat glaucoma by decreasing the amount of fluid produced in the eye. One commonly used beta-blocker is timolol (Timoptic®).

Ear drops are liquid medication administered into the ear. Ear drops are used to treat earwax buildup or bacterial infection in the outer ear. A commonly used antibiotic ear drop is ofloxacin (Floxin Otic®).

- *Earwax removal drops* are ear drops used to remove built-up earwax by softening and loosening it. A common example is carbamide peroxide (Debrox®).

Integumentary System

- **Topical corticosteroids** are a class of drugs used to temporarily treat the redness and itching from rashes and allergic reactions by reducing inflammation. Common examples include triamcinolone acetonide (Kenalog®), fluocinolone (Vanos®), and hydrocortisone.
- **Burn creams** are a class of medicated creams used to treat burns by preventing loss of moisture through the missing skin, covering nerve endings to decrease pain,

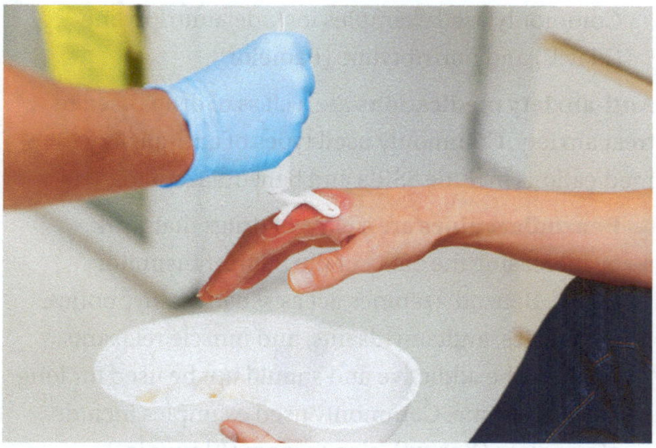

iStock.com/choja

FIGURE 22.8 Silver sulfadiazine cream being applied to a burn.

and preventing bacterial infection. **Silver sulfadiazine** (Silvadene®) is the most commonly used burn cream, and contains both antibiotics and silver to prevent infection (Figure 22.8).

- **Topical retinoids** are a class of drugs used to treat acne by increasing the rate at which skin cells grow. One common example is tretinoin (Retin-A®).
- **Topical analgesics** are a class of pain-relieving creams applied to the skin to relieve pain due to conditions such as osteoarthritis, rheumatoid arthritis, back pain, or burns. One primary active ingredient in these ointments is ***capsaicin***, a chemical found in chili peppers. Another is ***lidocaine***, a numbing agent.

Endocrine System

- ***Thyroid replacement*** drugs are a class of synthetic forms of thyroid hormones used to treat hypothyroidism. A common example is **levothyroxine** (Synthroid®).
- **Insulin** is a medication used in the treatment of type 1 and type 2 diabetes. There are multiple different forms of insulin with different times of onset.
  - ***Rapid-acting insulin*** takes effect 15 minutes after injection and can last up to 5 hours. Types of rapid-acting insulin include insulin aspart (Novolog®) and insulin lispro (Humalog®).
  - ***Short-acting insulin*** takes effect 30–60 minutes after injection and can last up to 8 hours. A common short-acting insulin is regular insulin (Humulin®, Novolin®).
  - ***Intermediate-acting insulin*** takes effect 1–2 hours after injection and can last more than 12 hours. A common intermediate-acting insulin is NPH insulin (Humulin N®, Novolin N®).
  - ***Long-acting insulin*** takes effect 1–2 hours after injection and lasts for up to 24 hours. Types of long-acting insulin include insulin glargine (Lantus®) and insulin detemir (Levemir®).
- **Metformin** (Glucophage®) is an oral medication that increases the body's sensitivity to insulin. Metformin is used for people with insulin resistance and diabetes.
- **Dipeptidyl peptidase-4** (DPP-4) **inhibitors**, also known as ***gliptins***, are a class of oral diabetes medications that work by increasing the amount of insulin released by the pancreas and slowing the absorption of food. Some common examples are sitagliptin (Januvia®), and linagliptin (Tradjenta®). The combination of sitagliptin and metformin is marketed as Janumet®.
- **Sulfonylureas** (sull-**fah**-nee-**LOU**-ree-ahz) are a class of oral diabetes medications that work by increasing the amount of insulin released by the pancreas. Common examples are glipizide (Glucotrol®) and glimepiride (Amaryl®).
- **Thiazolidinediones** (TZD), also known as ***glitazones***, are a class of oral diabetes medications that work by increasing the metabolism of glucose by the body. Common examples are pioglitazone (Actos®) and rosiglitazone (Avandia®).

Male Reproductive System

- A **phosphodiesterase** (PDE5) **inhibitor** is one of a class of drugs used to treat erectile dysfunction by increasing blood flow to the penis. Common examples are sildenafil (Viagra®) and tadalafil (Cialis®). PDE5 inhibitors are also used to treat pulmonary hypertension by relaxing the smooth muscles in the lungs.

Female Reproductive System

- **Birth control pills**, also known as ***oral contraceptives***, are pills taken daily by women to regulate hormones and prevent pregnancy. Common examples include drospirenone/ethinyl estradiol (Ocella®, Yasmin®) and norethindrone (Nora-BE®, Aygestin®).
- A **contraceptive implant** is a form of long-term birth control placed under the skin of the upper arm to prevent pregnancy. A common example is etonogestrel (Nexplanon®).
- An **intrauterine device** (IUD) is a form of long-term birth control placed into the uterus to prevent pregnancy (Figure 22.9). Common examples include copper wire (ParaGard®) and levonorgestrel (Mirena®).

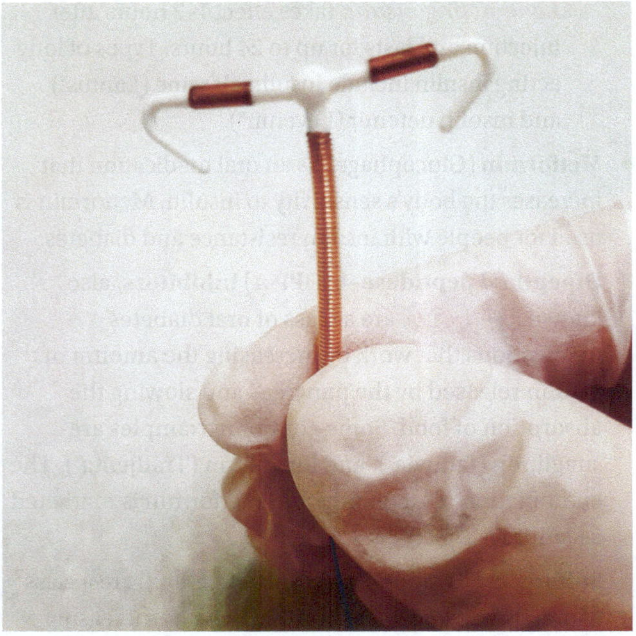

lauramntg/Shutterstock.com

FIGURE 22.9 An intrauterine device (IUD).

Common Drug Classes and Medications by Specialty Area

Mental Health

Psychotropic drugs (**sigh**-koh-**TROP**-ick) are a class of drugs which act primarily on the central nervous system.

Antidepressants are drugs administered to prevent or relieve depression.

- **SSRIs** (**S**elective **S**erotonin **R**euptake **I**nhibitors) are a class of popular antidepressants, and are commonly used as a first-line treatment against depression. Common examples include citalopram (Celexa®), fluoxetine (Prozac®), sertraline (Zoloft®), and escitalopram oxalate (Lexapro®). SSRIs are also used as anti-anxiety medications.
- **SNRIs** (**S**erotonin and **N**orepinephrine **R**euptake **I**nhibitors) are a class of drugs used to treat depression and anxiety. Commonly used SNRIs include duloxetine (Cymbalta®) and venlafaxine (Effexor®).
- **MAOIs** (**M**ono**a**mine **O**xidase **I**nhibitors) are a class of drugs mainly used to treat treatment-resistant depression. Examples include selegiline (Emsam®), phenelzine (Nardil®), and tranylcypromine (Parnate®).
- **Tricyclic antidepressants** (TCAs) are a class of drugs that work by increasing the levels of serotonin and norepinephrine. TCAs are also used to treat chronic nerve pain, anxiety, panic attacks, PTSD, and OCD. Commonly used examples include amitriptyline (Elavil®) and nortriptyline (Pamelor®).

Anti-anxiety medications are a class of drugs used to treat anxiety. Commonly used types of anti-anxiety medications include SSRIs and benzodiazepines.

- **Benzodiazepines** are a class of drugs that work by increasing the effect of the neurotransmitter GABA. Benzodiazepines act as sedatives, hypnotics, anxiolytics, anticonvulsants, and muscle relaxants. They can be addictive and should not be used for long periods of time. Commonly used examples include alprazolam (Xanax®), clonazepam (Klonopin®), diazepam (Valium®), and lorazepam (Ativan®).

Antipsychotic drugs (**an**-tih-sigh-**KOT**-ick) are a class of medications administered to treat symptoms of severe disorders of thinking and mood. Commonly used examples include aripiprazole (Abilify®), lurasidone (Latuda®), olanzapine (Zyprexa®), quetiapine (Seroquel®), risperidone (Risperdal®), haloperidol (Haldol®), and ziprasidone (Geodon®).

Mood stabilizers are a class of medications used to treat mood instability and bipolar disorders. Commonly used examples include carbamazepine (Tegretol®), divalproex sodium (Depakote®), lithium, and lamotrigine (Lamictal®).

Some stimulants are used to treat attention deficit/hyperactivity disorder by increasing dopamine levels in the brain. Commonly used examples include racemic amphetamine/dextroamphetamine (Adderall®) and methylphenidate (Ritalin®).

Oncology

- **Chemotherapy**, also known as a ***chemotherapeutic agent***, is a class of drugs that stop or slow the growth of cancer cells (Figure 22.10). There are many types of chemotherapy drugs which target weaknesses of specific types of cancer. Common examples include methotrexate (Trexall®), hydroxyurea (Hydrea®), tamoxifen (Nolvadex®), and vincristine (Oncovin®).
  - Chemotherapy medications have special handling guidelines, including special ***personal protective equipment*** (PPE) recommendations, for the safety of the medical professionals preparing and administering the chemotherapy.
  - The PPE worn for handling chemotherapy should include an impermeable gown, face mask, eye protection, and chemotherapy-qualified gloves, which are heavier weight than regular exam gloves.

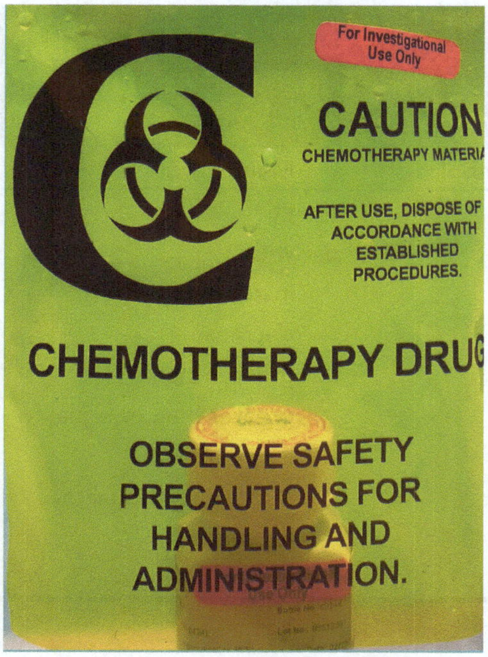
For Investigational Use Only
CAUTION
CHEMOTHERAPY MATERI
AFTER USE, DISPOSE OF
ACCORDANCE WITH
ESTABLISHED
PROCEDURES.
CHEMOTHERAPY DRUG
OBSERVE SAFETY
PRECAUTIONS FOR
HANDLING AND
ADMINISTRATION.

Grace Thoma/Shutterstock.com

FIGURE 22.10 Chemotherapy medications are indicated by a biohazard symbol on a yellow background.

- Chemotherapy drugs and waste from administration are indicated by a biohazard symbol on a yellow background.
- An **aromatase inhibitor** (ah-**ROH**-mah-tayz) is one of a class of drugs that prevents hormone-positive breast cancer growth by blocking estrogen in the body. A common example is anastrozole (Arimidex®).
- An **angiogenesis inhibitor** is one of a class of drugs that slows tumor growth by blocking the development of new blood vessels. A common example is bevacizumab (Avastin®).
- A **palliative** (**PAL**-ee-ay-tiv) is a substance that eases the pain or severity of the symptoms of a disease but does not cure it. For example, opioids such as morphine are considered palliatives, because they relieve pain without treating the underlying problem. ***Palliative care*** is treatment that focuses on alleviating pain and relieving symptoms rather than curing the disease.

FREQUENTLY USED DRUG ADMINISTRATION ABBREVIATIONS AND SYMBOLS

Many abbreviations used in prescriptions and drug administration come from Latin terms. It may be helpful to look at the original words to remember their meaning and common abbreviations (Table 22.2).

TABLE 22.2
Frequently Used Drug Administration Abbreviations

Abbreviation	Meaning	Latin Origin
ac	before meals	*ante cibum*
ad lib	as desired	*ad libitum*
amt	amount	
bid	twice a day	*bis in die*
gtt	drops, drip	*guttae*
hs	at bedtime (hour of sleep)	
NPO	nothing by mouth	*nil per os*
pc	after meals	*post cibum*
po	by mouth	*per os*
prn	as needed	*pro re nata*
qh	every hour	*quaque hora*
qid	four times a day	*quater in die*
Rx	prescription	*recipe (to take)*
sig	to be labeled accordingly	*signa (to write)*
tid	three times a day	*ter in die*

The Joint Commission has released a list of "Do Not Use" abbreviations designed to reduce medication errors by eliminating some frequently confused abbreviations (see Chapter 1). When in doubt, write it out!

Many of the symbols used in prescriptions are similar to those used in mathematics (Table 22.3).

Measurements of medication dosage strength have standard abbreviations, some of which are used in mathematics (Table 22.4).

ABBREVIATIONS RELATED TO PHARMACOLOGY

Table 22.5 presents an overview of the abbreviations related to the terms introduced in this chapter. *Note:* To avoid errors or confusion, always be cautious when using abbreviations.

TABLE 22.3

Frequently Used Drug Administration Symbols

Symbol	Meaning
@	at
c	with
↑	increase
↓	decrease
>	greater than
≥	greater than or equal to
<	less than
≤	less than or equal to
♀	female
♂	male

TABLE 22.4

Frequently Used Drug Dosage Abbreviations

Abbreviation	Measurement	Meaning
G, g	gram	1,000 milligrams
mg	milligram	one thousandth of a gram
mcg	microgram	one millionth of a gram
IU	international unit	an internationally standardized quantity of a particular drug
U	unit	a standardized quantity of a particular drug
L	liter	1,000 milliliters
ml, mL	milliliter	one thousandth of a liter (same as cc)
cc	cubic centimeter	one thousandth of a liter (same as mL)
fl oz	fluid ounce	30 milliliters
C, c	cup	8 fluid ounces 250 milliliters
Tbsp, tbsp	tablespoon	15 milliliters
tsp	teaspoon	5 milliliters

TABLE 22.5

Abbreviations Related to Pharmacology

adverse drug reaction = ADR	**ADR** = adverse drug reaction
angiotensin-II receptor blockers = ARBs	**ARB**s = angiotensin-II receptor blockers
intramuscular injection = IM	**IM** = intramuscular injection
intrauterine device = IUD	**IUD** = intrauterine device
intravenous injection = IV	**IV** = intravenous injection
nitroglycerin = NTG	**NTG** = nitroglycerin
nonsteroidal anti-inflammatory drugs = NSAIDs	**NSAID**s = nonsteroidal anti-inflammatory drugs
proton pump inhibitor = PPI	**PPI** = proton pump inhibitor
subcutaneous injection = SC or SQ	**SC** or **SQ** = subcutaneous injection
tissue plasminogen activator = tPA	**tPA** = tissue plasminogen activator

LEARNING EXERCISES

Matching Word Parts 1

Write the correct answer in the middle column.

	Definition	Correct Answer	Possible Answers
22.1.	skin	________________	**lingu/o**
22.2.	under	________________	**par-**
22.3.	within	________________	**derm/o**
22.4.	tongue	________________	**intra-**
22.5.	outside	________________	**sub-**

Matching Word Parts 2

Write the correct answer in the middle column.

	Definition	Correct Answer	Possible Answers
22.6.	fever	________________	**pharmac/o**
22.7.	digestive tract	________________	**pyret/o**
22.8.	drug	________________	**muscul/o**
22.9.	vein	________________	**enter/o**
22.10.	muscle	________________	**ven/o**

Matching Word Parts 3

Write the correct answer in the middle column.

	Definition	Correct Answer	Possible Answers
22.11.	sheath	________________	**-ous**
22.12.	poison	________________	**thec/o**
22.13.	through, across	________________	**trans-**

22.14. skin	______________	toxic/o
22.15. pertaining to	______________	cutane/o

Definitions

Select the correct answer, and write it on the line provided.

22.16. Drug ______________ is when the body has become accustomed to a medication after being on it for a length of time, and higher doses are required to achieve the desired effect.

tolerance	compliance	side effect	paradoxical reaction

22.17. A/An ______________, also known as a sleeping pill, is a drug that helps induce or sustain sleep.

barbiturate	hypnotic	analgesic	enema

22.18. A/An ______________ is one of several types of drugs that help relieve shortness of breath by relaxing the bronchi.

nebulizer	bronchodilator	antacid	immunosuppressant

22.19. ______________ is one of a class of medications that stop or slow the growth of cancer cells.

Metformin	Nitroglycerin	Chemotherapy	Insulin

22.20. A/An ______________ is one of a class of medications that can be used to treat overactive bladder by relaxing the smooth muscle of the bladder.

antitussive	anticholinergic	alpha blocker	corticosteroid

22.21. A/An ______________ is one of several classes of medication that work to prevent or relieve nausea and vomiting.

antiemetic	antipyretic	antidiarrheal	antacid

22.22. A/An ______________ is a form of long-term birth control placed under the skin of the upper arm to prevent pregnancy.

birth control pill	intrauterine device	proton pump inhibitor	contraceptive implant

22.23. ______________ are a class of drugs that work to lower blood pressure by increasing the amount of urine output.

Diuretics	Anticoagulants	Nitroglycerin	Calcium channel blockers

22.24. A/An ______________________ is one of several classes of drugs that prevent or stop seizures.

stimulant sedative anticonvulsant antiepileptic

22.25. Topical ______________________ are a class of drugs used to treat acne by increasing the rate at which skin cells grow.

analgesics burn creams corticosteroids retinoids

Matching Medication Dosing

Write the correct answer in the middle column.

Definition	Correct Answer	Possible Answers
22.26. a course of treatment involving taking certain medications on a regular basis	______________________	therapeutic dose
22.27. the amount of medication necessary to achieve the desired outcome	______________________	loading dose
22.28. a measured quantity of a medication ordered to be given at a time	______________________	maintenance dose
22.29. an initial, higher dose of medication given	______________________	medication regimen
22.30. the regular dose of medication given on an ongoing basis	______________________	dose

Which Word?

Select the correct answer, and write it on the line provided.

22.31. An ______________________ reaction is an unexpected reaction to a drug that is peculiar to the individual.

idiosyncratic adverse drug

22.32. ______________________ are a class of medicated eye drops used to treat glaucoma by increasing the amount of fluid leaving the eye.

Histamine-2 blockers Prostaglandin analogs

22.33. One of several classes of medication that prevent or treat constipation by increasing bowel movements is known as a ______________________.

laxative palliative

22.34. Also known as SSRIs, ____________ reuptake inhibitors are commonly used as a first-line treatment for depression.

selective serotonin   serotonin and norepinephrine

22.35. A ____________ drug is sold under the name given by the manufacturer. These drug names are always spelled with a capital letter.

brand name   generic

Spelling Counts

Find the misspelled word in each sentence. Then write that word, spelled correctly, on the line provided.

22.36. Sinergism is the interaction of two drugs taken together that enhances the effectiveness of both.

____

22.37. An antitussif is one of a class of medications that helps decrease the frequency of coughs.

____

22.38. Sulfonilurees are a class of oral diabetes medications that work by increasing the amount of insulin released by the pancreas. ____________

22.39. A conterindication is a factor in the patient's condition that makes the use of a medication or specific treatment dangerous or ill advised. ____________

22.40. An airosol is a mist of tiny particles suspended in air. ____________

Drug Administration Abbreviation Identification

In the space provided, write the words that each abbreviation stands for.

22.41. **Rx** ____________

22.42. **NPO** ____________

22.43. **prn** ____________

22.44. **hs** ____________

22.45. **ac** ____________

Term Selection

Select the correct answer, and write it on the line provided.

22.46. A single, concentrated dose of a drug usually injected into a blood vessel is known as a/an ______________.

infusion   bolus   suppository   PICC line

22.47. The patient's consistency and accuracy in following the regimen prescribed by a health care professional is known as ______________.

adherence   therapeutic level   compliance   drug tolerance

22.48. ______________ is when the body has become accustomed to a medication or substance after repeated use, and experiences physical and/or psychological withdrawal symptoms if its use is stopped.

Dependence   Synergism   Addiction   Drug interaction

22.49. A/An ______________ relieves inflammation and pain without affecting consciousness.

opioid   analgesic   anti-inflammatory   palliative

22.50. A/An ______________ is a secondary response that accompanies the principal response for which the drug was taken.

paradoxical reaction   drug interaction   side effect   overdose

Sentence Completion

Write the correct term on the line provided.

22.51. The term ______________ *sedation* describes a state of light to moderate sedation where the patient is calm, relaxed, and less responsive to stimuli.

22.52. The term ______________ refers to a blood test showing whether the amount of medication circulating in the blood is sufficient to achieve the desired outcome.

22.53. The term ______________ is the study of how drugs move through the human body.

22.54. A/An ______________ is any substance that has a psychological or physiological effect on the human body.

22.55. The ________________________ Administration is the federal agency responsible for ensuring the quality and safety of all drugs and dietary supplements sold in the United States.

Word Surgery

Divide each term into its component word parts. Write these word parts, in sequence, on the lines provided. When necessary, use a slash (/) to indicate a combining vowel. (You may not need all of the lines provided.)

22.56. An **antipyretic** is medication administered to prevent or reduce fever.

__________ __________ __________ __________

22.57. **Intrathecal** administration is the injection of medication directly into the cerebrospinal fluid.

__________ __________ __________ __________

22.58. **Parenteral** administration means taken into the body or administered in a manner other than through the digestive tract.

__________ __________ __________ __________

22.59. A **transdermal** medication is administered from a patch that is applied to unbroken skin.

__________ __________ __________ __________

22.60. **Sublingual** administration is the placement of medication under the tongue, where it is allowed to dissolve slowly.

__________ __________ __________ __________

True/False

If the statement is true, write **True** on the line. If the statement is false, write **False** on the line.

22.61. ________ Illicit drugs are controlled substances without known medical benefit that are obtained illegally.

22.62. ________ A formulary is a list of prescription drugs covered by a specific health care plan.

22.63. ________ A placebo contains medication and has the potential to cure a disease.

22.64. ________ An over-the-counter drug requires a written prescription.

22.65. ________ An enema is medication in a semisolid form that is placed in the rectum, vagina, or urethra.

Pharmacology Terminology

Write the correct answer on the line provided.

22.66. The specific name for a chemical compound created according to international guidelines is a/an

__________________________.

22.67. A physician who specializes in the care of patients who have been exposed to toxic levels of drugs or other substances is a/an __________________________.

22.68. A plastic tube used to measure and administer liquid medication is known as a/an

__________________________.

22.69. The deliberate or accidental ingestion of more medication than has been prescribed or is safe is known as a/an __________________________.

22.70. The paramedics gave Narcan to the unresponsive man who was suspected of overdosing on fentanyl, and watched as he suddenly took a deep breath and started groaning. Narcan is an example of a/an

__________________________.

22.71. In preparation for surgery, Ubaldo Melendez was given medication to make him unresponsive even to painful stimuli, and then intubated. This state of deep sedation is known as __________________________.

22.72. The Tong baby was given Tylenol in a semisolid form placed into his rectum. This is called a/an

__________________________.

22.73. Prasan Durairaj was started on medication to treat the symptoms of Parkinson's. This class of medications are called __________________________.

22.74. When Arthur Callaghan experienced angina, he knew to take __________________________. This medication works by dilating veins, thus reducing the workload of the heart.

22.75. Mrs. Chon was diagnosed with osteoporosis and prescribed __________________________. This class of drugs slow the loss of bone density.

22.76. After ending up in the ER for hypertension and atrial fibrillation, Mr. Champsi was started on __________________________. This class of drugs work by blocking the release of the stress hormones epinephrine and norepinephrine to slow the heart rate.

22.77. Dr. Conlon decided to treat the patient's hormone-positive breast cancer growth by starting her on a/an ______________________, which blocks estrogen in the body.

22.78. When Fernando Cruz's chronic nerve pain wasn't being adequately controlled with pain medication, his doctor prescribed ______________________ antidepressants, which work by increasing the levels of serotonin and norepinephrine.

22.79. Amandiu Cabral's doctor recommended a new type of medication to better control his diabetes by increasing the metabolism of glucose by the body. This class of medications, ______________________, are also known as *glitazones*.

22.80. Mr. Jacobsen's family decided to try a/an ______________________ to treat the symptoms of his Alzheimer's by increasing the levels of acetylcholine in the brain.

Which Is The Correct Medical Term?

Select the correct answer, and write it on the line provided.

22.81. A/An ______________________ drug reaction is an undesirable reaction that accompanies the principal response for which the drug was taken.

adverse   idiosyncratic   placebo   synergism

22.82. The term meaning a drug that relaxes all muscles is a/an ______________________.

sedative   paralytic   muscle relaxant   benzodiazepine

22.83. The term for one of a class of medications administered to treat symptoms of severe disorders of thinking and mood is a/an ______________________.

mood stabilizer   antidepressant   antipsychotic drug   psychotropic drug

22.84. One of a class of drugs used to treat erectile dysfunction by increasing blood flow to the penis is a/an ______________________ inhibitor.

phosphodiesterase   aromatase   dipeptidyl peptidase-4   acetylcholinesterase

22.85. The term for pain-relieving cream applied to the skin is ______________________.

burn cream   topical analgesic   topical corticosteroid   antibiotic

22.86. Controlled substances available by prescription only to relieve severe pain are known as

________________________.

opioids muscle relaxants ibuprofen analgesics

22.87. The term for a class of antihypertensive, anti-arrhythmic drugs that work by decreasing the movement of calcium ions into the cells is ________________________.

beta-blockers ACE inhibitors calcium channel blockers nitroglycerin

22.88. The term meaning a drug with proven benefit that is used for medical treatment is

________________________.

drug class medication tablet drug

22.89. The term meaning the study of the nature, uses, and effects of drugs for medical purposes is

________________________.

pharmacodynamics toxicology pharmacokinetics pharmacology

22.90. The term meaning a group of drugs with similar features is a/an ________________________.

drug class Schedule 1 controlled substances drug category

Drug Dosage Abbreviation Identification

In the space provided, write the words that each abbreviation stands for.

22.91. **IU** ________________________

22.92. **mL** ________________________

22.93. **fl oz** ________________________

22.94. **mcg** ________________________

22.95. **cc** ________________________

22.96. **G** ________________________

Labeling Exercises

Identify the numbered items on the accompanying figure.

22.97. This is a/an ______________________ injection.

22.98. This is a/an ______________________ injection.

22.99. This is a/an ______________________ injection.

22.100. This is a/an ______________________ injection.

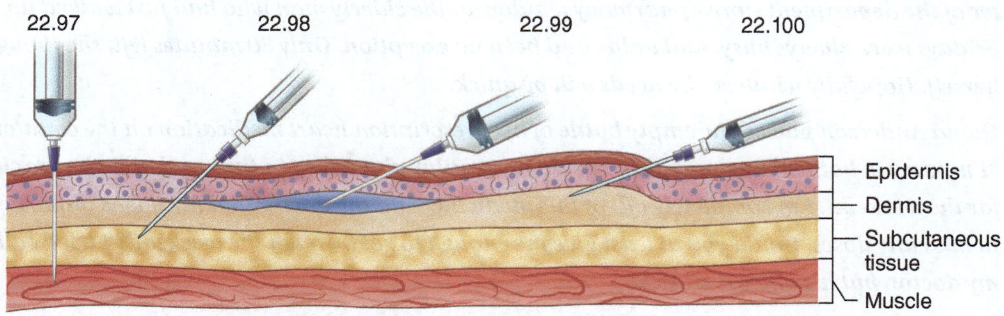

The Human Touch

CRITICAL THINKING EXERCISE

The following story and questions are designed to stimulate critical thinking through class discussion or as a brief essay response. There are no right or wrong answers to these questions.

"Good evening, sir, what can I do for you today?" Helen Edison, PharmD, looked over the counter of the department store's pharmacy window at the elderly man who had just walked up. Fridays were always busy, and today had been no exception. Only 30 minutes left, she thought to herself. Hopefully whatever he needs will be quick.

David Anderson placed the empty bottle of his prescription heart medication on the counter. "I'm sorry to bother you, but I didn't get to my regular pharmacy in time and now they're closed for the weekend. I'm completely out of this medicine, and the doctor told me it was important not to miss any doses. Could you at least give me enough to get through the weekend? I tried calling my doctor, but his office is closed."

Helen picked up the bottle and read the prescription information on the label. Metoprolol tartrate, generic for Lopressor, 50 mg, to be taken twice daily. Zero refills left. Dr. Venkman's office. I know that name, she thought. I must have sent them 20 faxes about refills last week, and they always take forever to respond. "I'll see what I can do for you, sir. May I please see your photo ID and insurance card?"

She stepped over to her desk and quickly sent a fax through to Dr. Venkman's office with a refill request, even though she doubted anyone would still be there. Just 25 minutes left in my shift, too, and I still have to finish prepping those other medications for pickup tomorrow, Helen thought to herself. She looked at the label of the empty bottle, reviewing the options in her head, none of them ideal.

Suggested Discussion Topics

1. What do you think the pharmacist should do if she cannot get a response from the prescribing doctor's office before the pharmacy closes?
2. Would your advice be different if the medication were prescribed for a different issue, such as pain?
3. Some doctors will not refill medications unless a patient has an appointment first. Do you think Mr. Anderson should be given more metoprolol before he sees his doctor? Why or why not?
4. Does the pharmacy have any responsibility if missing some doses causes harm to Mr. Anderson?

COMPREHENSIVE MEDICAL TERMINOLOGY REVIEW

Overview of
COMPREHENSIVE MEDICAL TERMINOLOGY REVIEW: BODY SYSTEMS AND MEDICAL SPECIALTY CHAPTERS

Study Tips	Hints to help you review more effectively.
Answer Sheets	Write the letter of the correct answer for the questions in the review tests. Although only one set of answer sheets is included, you can take these tests as often as you want.
Review Sessions	A 100-multiple-choice-question Body System Review Session (BRS) covering Chapters 1 and 2 and the body system chapters, and a 50-multiple-choice-question Medical Specialty Chapters Review Session (SRS) covering the specialty chapters to help you determine where you need more study emphasis. However, be aware that none of these questions are from the actual final exam.
Simulated Medical Terminology Final Tests	A 100-multiple-choice-question "mock" Body System Final Test (BFT) covering Chapters 1 and 2 and the body system chapters, and a 50-multiple-choice-question Medical Specialty Chapters (SFT) "mock" Final Test to help you evaluate your progress. However, be aware that none of these questions are from the actual final exam.
Answer Keys	The answer keys for self-grading these practice tests are at the end of the respective review sections.

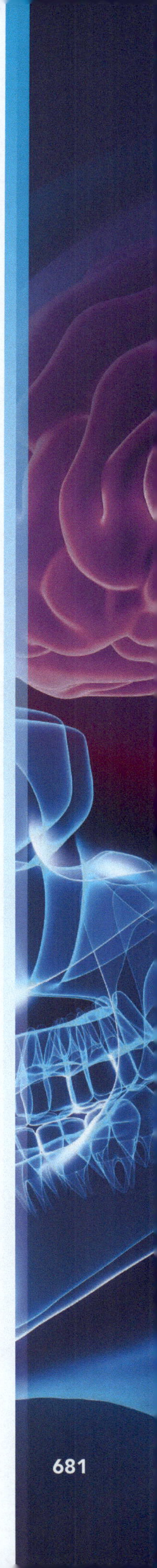

STUDY TIPS

Use Your Vocabulary Lists

- Photocopy or scan and print the vocabulary list for each chapter from your textbook, and add any terms suggested by your instructor. This creates a study aid that is easy to carry with you for additional review whenever you have a free minute.
- Review the terms on each list. When you have mastered a term, put a check in the box next to it. If you cannot spell and define a term, highlight it for further study.
- Look up the meanings of the highlighted terms in the textbook, and work on mastering them.
- *Caution*: Do not limit your studying to these lists. Although they contain important terms, there are many additional important words in each chapter that you need to know.

Make Your Own Study List

- By now you should have greatly reduced the number of terms still to be mastered. Make a list of these terms and word parts and concentrate on them.

Review Your Learning Exercises

At review time go through the Learning Exercises and note where you made mistakes. Ask yourself, "Do I know the correct answer now?" If not, add the term or word part to your study list.

For the True/False questions in the Learning Exercises, you can challenge yourself to change all the "false" answers into true ones. For example, "Cholangiography is an endoscopic diagnostic procedure" is false. Ask yourself: "What is the correct definition of cholangiography?"

Help Someone Else

One of the greatest ways to really learn something is to teach it! If a classmate is having trouble, tutoring that person will help both of you learn the material.

Use the Practice Sessions

Use the answer sheets with the Review Sessions and Simulated Medical Terminology Final Tests. The answer keys for self-grading these tests are at the end of the respective sections.

BODY SYSTEMS REVIEW SESSION ANSWER SHEET

Write the **letter** of the correct answer on the line next to the question number.

Name ______________________________

BRS.1. ________	BRS.26. ________	BRS.51. ________	BRS.76. ________
BRS.2. ________	BRS.27. ________	BRS.52. ________	BRS.77. ________
BRS.3. ________	BRS.28. ________	BRS.53. ________	BRS.78. ________
BRS.4. ________	BRS.29. ________	BRS.54. ________	BRS.79. ________
BRS.5. ________	BRS.30. ________	BRS.55. ________	BRS.80. ________
BRS.6. ________	BRS.31. ________	BRS.56. ________	BRS.81. ________
BRS.7. ________	BRS.32. ________	BRS.57. ________	BRS.82. ________
BRS.8. ________	BRS.33. ________	BRS.58. ________	BRS.83. ________
BRS.9. ________	BRS.34. ________	BRS.59. ________	BRS.84. ________
BRS.10. ________	BRS.35. ________	BRS.60. ________	BRS.85. ________
BRS.11. ________	BRS.36. ________	BRS.61. ________	BRS.86. ________
BRS.12. ________	BRS.37. ________	BRS.62. ________	BRS.87. ________
BRS.13. ________	BRS.38. ________	BRS.63. ________	BRS.88. ________
BRS.14. ________	BRS.39. ________	BRS.64. ________	BRS.89. ________
BRS.15. ________	BRS.40. ________	BRS.65. ________	BRS.90. ________
BRS.16. ________	BRS.41. ________	BRS.66. ________	BRS.91. ________
BRS.17. ________	BRS.42. ________	BRS.67. ________	BRS.92. ________
BRS.18. ________	BRS.43. ________	BRS.68. ________	BRS.93. ________
BRS.19. ________	BRS.44. ________	BRS.69. ________	BRS.94. ________
BRS.20. ________	BRS.45. ________	BRS.70. ________	BRS.95. ________
BRS.21. ________	BRS.46. ________	BRS.71. ________	BRS.96. ________
BRS.22. ________	BRS.47. ________	BRS.72. ________	BRS.97. ________
BRS.23. ________	BRS.48. ________	BRS.73. ________	BRS.98. ________
BRS.24. ________	BRS.49. ________	BRS.74. ________	BRS.99. ________
BRS.25. ________	BRS.50. ________	BRS.75. ________	BRS.100. ________

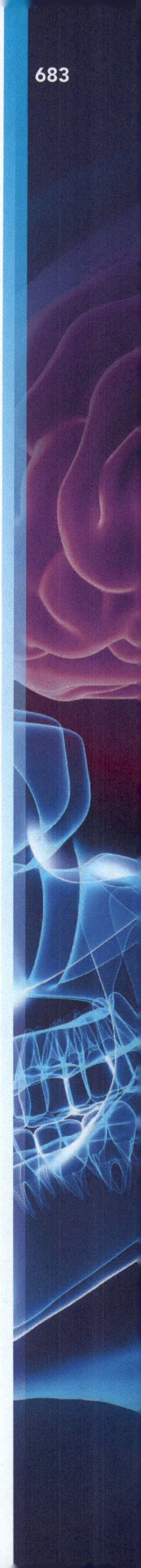

BODY SYSTEMS SIMULATED FINAL TEST ANSWER SHEET

Write the **letter** of the correct answer on the line next to the question number.

Name ____

BFT.1. ________	BFT.26. ________	BFT.51. ________	BFT.76. ________
BFT.2. ________	BFT.27. ________	BFT.52. ________	BFT.77. ________
BFT.3. ________	BFT.28. ________	BFT.53. ________	BFT.78. ________
BFT.4. ________	BFT.29. ________	BFT.54. ________	BFT.79. ________
BFT.5. ________	BFT.30. ________	BFT.55. ________	BFT.80. ________
BFT.6. ________	BFT.31. ________	BFT.56. ________	BFT.81. ________
BFT.7. ________	BFT.32. ________	BFT.57. ________	BFT.82. ________
BFT.8. ________	BFT.33. ________	BFT.58. ________	BFT.83. ________
BFT.9. ________	BFT.34. ________	BFT.59. ________	BFT.84. ________
BFT.10. ________	BFT.35. ________	BFT.60. ________	BFT.85. ________
BFT.11. ________	BFT.36. ________	BFT.61. ________	BFT.86. ________
BFT.12. ________	BFT.37. ________	BFT.62. ________	BFT.87. ________
BFT.13. ________	BFT.38. ________	BFT.63. ________	BFT.88. ________
BFT.14. ________	BFT.39. ________	BFT.64. ________	BFT.89. ________
BFT.15. ________	BFT.40. ________	BFT.65. ________	BFT.90. ________
BFT.16. ________	BFT.41. ________	BFT.66. ________	BFT.91. ________
BFT.17. ________	BFT.42. ________	BFT.67. ________	BFT.92. ________
BFT.18. ________	BFT.43. ________	BFT.68. ________	BFT.93. ________
BFT.19. ________	BFT.44. ________	BFT.69. ________	BFT.94. ________
BFT.20. ________	BFT.45. ________	BFT.70. ________	BFT.95. ________
BFT.21. ________	BFT.46. ________	BFT.71. ________	BFT.96. ________
BFT.22. ________	BFT.47. ________	BFT.72. ________	BFT.97. ________
BFT.23. ________	BFT.48. ________	BFT.73. ________	BFT.98. ________
BFT.24. ________	BFT.49. ________	BFT.74. ________	BFT.99. ________
BFT.25. ________	BFT.50. ________	BFT.75. ________	BFT.100. ________

MEDICAL SPECIALTY CHAPTERS REVIEW SESSION ANSWER SHEET

Write the **letter** of the correct answer on the line next to the question number.

Name ____________________

SRS.1. ________

SRS.2. ________

SRS.3. ________

SRS.4. ________

SRS.5. ________

SRS.6. ________

SRS.7. ________

SRS.8. ________

SRS.9. ________

SRS.10. ________

SRS.11. ________

SRS.12. ________

SRS.13. ________

SRS.14. ________

SRS.15. ________

SRS.16. ________

SRS.17. ________

SRS.18. ________

SRS.19. ________

SRS.20. ________

SRS.21. ________

SRS.22. ________

SRS.23. ________

SRS.24. ________

SRS.25. ________

SRS.26. ________

SRS.27. ________

SRS.28. ________

SRS.29. ________

SRS.30. ________

SRS.31. ________

SRS.32. ________

SRS.33. ________

SRS.34. ________

SRS.35. ________

SRS.36. ________

SRS.37. ________

SRS.38. ________

SRS.39. ________

SRS.40. ________

SRS.41. ________

SRS.42. ________

SRS.43. ________

SRS.44. ________

SRS.45. ________

SRS.46. ________

SRS.47. ________

SRS.48. ________

SRS.49. ________

SRS.50. ________

MEDICAL SPECIALTY CHAPTERS SIMULATED FINAL TEST ANSWER SHEET

Write the **letter** of the correct answer on the line next to the question number.

Name ______________________________

SFT.1. ________

SFT.2. ________

SFT.3. ________

SFT.4. ________

SFT.5. ________

SFT.6. ________

SFT.7. ________

SFT.8. ________

SFT.9. ________

SFT.10. ________

SFT.11. ________

SFT.12. ________

SFT.13. ________

SFT.14. ________

SFT.15. ________

SFT.16. ________

SFT.17. ________

SFT.18. ________

SFT.19. ________

SFT.20. ________

SFT.21. ________

SFT.22. ________

SFT.23. ________

SFT.24. ________

SFT.25. ________

SFT.26. ________

SFT.27. ________

SFT.28. ________

SFT.29. ________

SFT.30. ________

SFT.31. ________

SFT.32. ________

SFT.33. ________

SFT.34. ________

SFT.35. ________

SFT.36. ________

SFT.37. ________

SFT.38. ________

SFT.39. ________

SFT.40. ________

SFT.41. ________

SFT.42. ________

SFT.43. ________

SFT.44. ________

SFT.45. ________

SFT.46. ________

SFT.47. ________

SFT.48. ________

SFT.49. ________

SFT.50. ________

BODY SYSTEMS REVIEW SESSION

BRS.1. An abnormally rapid rate of respiration usually of more than 20 breaths per minute is known as ______________________.

a. bradypnea

b. eupnea

c. hyperventilation

d. tachypnea

BRS.2. An abnormally slow heart rate of less than 60 beats per minute is known as ______________________.

a. atrial fibrillation

b. bradycardia

c. palpitation

d. tachycardia

BRS.3. The ability to distinguish object details at a distance is called ______________________.

a. refraction

b. convergence

c. visual acuity

d. emmetropia

BRS.4. A highly contagious viral respiratory infection that usually occurs in seasonal epidemics is known as ______________________.

a. influenza

b. West Nile virus

c. measles

d. COVID-19

BRS.5. A collection of pus within a body cavity is known as a/an ______________________.

a. cyst

b. empyema

c. hernia

d. tumor

BRS.6. The grating sound heard when the ends of a broken bone move together is known as ______________________.

a. closed reduction

b. amputation

c. callus

d. crepitation

BRS.7. The abnormal development or growth of cells is known as ______________________.

a. anaplasia

b. dysplasia

c. hyperplasia

d. hypertrophy

BRS.8. Which form of anemia is a genetic disorder?

a. aplastic

b. hemolytic

c. megaloblastic

d. sickle cell

BRS.9. The processes through which the body maintains a constant internal environment are known as ______________________.

a. hemothorax

b. homeostasis

c. hypophysis

d. metabolism

BRS.10. An inflammation of the myelin sheath of peripheral nerves characterized by rapidly worsening muscle weakness that can lead to temporary paralysis is known as ______________________.

a. Bell's palsy

b. Guillain–Barré syndrome

c. Lou Gehrig's disease

d. Raynaud's disease

BRS.11. The term that describes weakness or wearing away of body tissues and structures caused by pathology or by disuse of the muscle over a long period of time is ______________________.

a. adhesion

b. ankylosis

c. atrophy

d. contracture

BRS.12. The term that refers to a blood coagulation test used to diagnose conditions associated with abnormalities of clotting time is ______________________.

a. blood clotting test

b. blood differential test

c. total protein test

d. prothrombin time

BRS.13. The procedure in which an anastomosis is created between the upper portion of the stomach and the duodenum is a/an ______________________.

a. esophagogastroduodenoscopy

b. gastroparesis

c. gastroduodenostomy

d. gastrostomy

BRS.14. Another term for iron overload disease is ______________________.

a. hemochromatosis

b. hematopoiesis

c. polycythemia

d. pancytopenia

BRS.15. The term that means abnormal enlargement of the liver is ______________________.

a. hepatitis

b. hepatomalacia

c. hepatomegaly

d. hepatorrhexis

BRS.16. The term describing the suppuration of a kidney is ______________________.

a. hydronephrosis

b. pyonephrosis

c. polycystic kidney disease

d. renal colic

BRS.17. Which of these conditions is commonly known as a bruise?

a. ecchymosis

b. epistaxis

c. hematoma

d. lesion

BRS.18. The acute respiratory infection characterized by obstruction of the larynx, hoarseness, and a barking cough in children and infants is known as ______________________.

a. asthma

b. croup

c. bronchiectasis

d. pneumonia

BRS.19. An autoimmune disease in which the body's own antibodies attack and destroy the cells of the thyroid gland is ______________________.

a. Addison's disease

b. Hashimoto's disease

c. Lou Gehrig's disease

d. Graves' disease

BRS.20. Which sexually transmitted disease is passed from person to person through direct contact with a chancre?

a. chlamydia

b. gonorrhea

c. syphilis

d. trichomoniasis

BRS.21. A blood clot attached to the interior wall of a vein or artery is known as a/an ______________________.

a. embolism

b. embolus

c. thrombosis

d. thrombus

BRS.22. The term that describes the removal of a body part or the destruction of its function through the use of surgery, hormones, drugs, heat, chemicals, electrocautery, or other methods is ______________________.

a. ablation

b. abrasion

c. cryosurgery

d. exfoliative cytology

BRS.23. The term that describes a condition in which gastric motility slows down, causing delayed gastric emptying, is _______________.

a. gastritis

b. cachexia

c. malabsorption

d. gastroparesis

BRS.24. A woman who has borne one viable child is referred to as a _______________.

a. nulligravida

b. nullipara

c. primigravida

d. primipara

BRS.25. The term that means inflammation of the pancreas is _______________.

a. insulinoma

b. diabetic ketoacidosis

c. pancreatitis

d. myasthenia gravis

BRS.26. The condition in which excess cerebrospinal fluid accumulates in the ventricles of the brain is known as _______________.

a. encephalitis

b. hydrocephalus

c. hydronephrosis

d. vascular dementia

BRS.27. The surgical removal of one or both testicles is known as a/an _______________.

a. orchiectomy

b. orchiopexy

c. circumcision

d. vasovasostomy

BRS.28. An involuntary spasm of the pelvic floor muscles is called _______________.

a. vaginitis

b. vaginismus

c. vulvodynia

d. eclampsia

BRS.29. Which statement is accurate regarding cystic fibrosis (CF)?

a. CF is a congenital disorder in which red blood cells take on a sickle shape.

b. CF is also known as iron overload disease.

c. CF is a genetic disorder that affects the lungs and digestive system.

d. CF is characterized by short-lived red blood cells.

BRS.30. Which condition, which is thinner-than-average bone density, causes the patient to be at an increased risk of developing osteoporosis?

a. osteochondroma

b. osteopenia

c. osteosclerosis

d. rickets

BRS.31. A fluid-filled sac in the scrotum along the spermatic cord leading from the testicles is a/an _______________.

a. varicocele

b. inguinal hernia

c. cystocele

d. hydrocele

BRS.32. Which of the following is characterized by exophthalmos?

a. Conn's syndrome

b. Graves' disease

c. Hashimoto's disease

d. Huntington's disease

BRS.33. Which hormone stimulates uterine contractions during childbirth?

a. estrogen

b. oxytocin

c. progesterone

d. testosterone

BRS.34. An unfavorable response due to prescribed medical treatment is known as _______________.

a. idiopathic disorder

b. nosocomial infection

c. functional disorder

d. iatrogenic illness

BRS.35. The surgical freeing of a kidney from adhesions is known as ______________________.

a. nephrolithiasis

b. nephrolysis

c. pyonephrosis

d. pyelotomy

BRS.36. Which term means tissue death of an artery or arteries?

a. arterionecrosis

b. aortic stenosis

c. atherosclerosis

d. arthrosclerosis

BRS.37. The plane that divides the body vertically into unequal left and right portions is the ______________________ plane.

a. frontal

b. midsagittal

c. sagittal

d. transverse

BRS.38. Which term means toward or nearer the midline?

a. distal

b. dorsal

c. medial

d. ventral

BRS.39. A definitive test was performed to determine if Alice Wilkinson has osteoporosis. This test is known as a ______________________.

a. bone marrow biopsy

b. dual x-ray absorptiometry

c. MRI

d. nuclear scan

BRS.40. Which term means movement of a limb away from the midline of the body?

a. abduction

b. adduction

c. extension

d. flexion

BRS.41. When he fell, Manuel tore the posterior femoral muscles in his left leg. This injury is known as a/an ______________________ injury.

a. Achilles tendon

b. hamstring

c. myofascial

d. shin splint

BRS.42. Mrs. Valladares has a bacterial infection of the lining of her heart. This condition is known as infective ______________________.

a. endocarditis

b. myocarditis

c. pericarditis

d. valvulitis

BRS.43. Tooth decay is commonly known as which of the following?

a. dental caries

b. dental plaque

c. gingivitis

d. periodontal disease

BRS.44. Henry was diagnosed as having an inflammation of the bone marrow and adjacent bone. Which term describes this condition?

a. Encephalitis

b. Meningitis

c. Osteomyelitis

d. Myelosis

BRS.45. The term for an inflammation of the sheath surrounding a tendon is ______________________.

a. bursitis

b. tendinitis

c. fasciitis

d. tenosynovitis

BRS.46. Which term describes drooping of the upper eyelid that is usually due to paralysis?

a. ptosis

b. dacryocystitis

c. scleritis

d. dacryoadenitis

BRS.47. The medical term for an earache is ________________.

a. otitis

b. otalgia

c. otomycosis

d. barotrauma

BRS.48. Mr. Ramirez had a heart attack. His physician recorded this as ________________.

a. angina

b. a myocardial infarction

c. congestive heart failure

d. coronary artery disease

BRS.49. A decrease in the number of disease-fighting leukocytes circulating in the blood is known as ________________.

a. anemia

b. leukemia

c. leukopenia

d. myelodysplastic syndrome

BRS.50. Which common skin disorder is characterized by flare-ups in which red papules covered with silvery scales occur on the elbows, knees, scalp, back, or buttocks?

a. ichthyosis

b. systemic lupus erythematosus

c. psoriasis

d. rosacea

BRS.51. The medical term for a group of disorders involving the parts of the brain that control thought, memory, and language is ________________.

a. Alzheimer's disease

b. amyotrophic lateral sclerosis

c. radiculitis

d. Reye's syndrome

BRS.52. Which term refers to the act of raising or lifting a body part?

a. circumduction

b. flexion

c. elevation

d. pronation

BRS.53. Which term describes an abnormal softening of bones in adults?

a. costochondritis

b. osteomalacia

c. osteomyelitis

d. periostitis

BRS.54. Slight paralysis of one side of the body is known as ________________.

a. hemiparesis

b. hemiplegia

c. myoparesis

d. quadriplegia

BRS.55. The specialized cells that play an important role in blood clotting are ________________.

a. basophils

b. erythrocytes

c. leukocytes

d. thrombocytes

BRS.56. Which term means located behind the peritoneum?

a. retroperitoneal

b. parietal peritoneum

c. inguinal

d. caudal

BRS.57. Which structure receives the sound vibrations and relays them to the auditory nerve fibers?

a. cochlea

b. eustachian tube

c. organ of Corti

d. semicircular canal

BRS.58. Which of the following patrol the body, searching for antigens that produce infections? When one is found, these cells grab, swallow, and internally break apart the captured antigen.

a. B cells

b. Dendritic cells

c. Interleukins

d. T cells

BRS.59. The medical term for the large, proximal tip of the ulna commonly known as the funny bone is the ____________________.

a. hallux valgus

b. acromion

c. torticollis

d. olecranon

BRS.60. A normal scar resulting from the healing of a wound is a/an ____________________.

a. callus

b. cicatrix

c. crepitus

d. keloid

BRS.61. Which bone is commonly known as the collar bone?

a. clavicle

b. xiphoid process

c. patella

d. sternum

BRS.62. Which of the following are long, slender, spiral-shaped bacteria that have flexible walls and are capable of movement?

a. Bacilli

b. Spirochetes

c. Staphylococci

d. Streptococci

BRS.63. A fluid such as pus leaking out of an open wound is called ____________________.

a. emesis

b. exudate

c. enucleation

d. exanthem

BRS.64. Which of these diseases is transmitted to humans by the bite of an infected blacklegged tick?

a. cytomegalovirus

b. human immunodeficiency virus

c. Lyme disease

d. West Nile virus

BRS.65. Which of the following involves compression of nerves and blood vessels due to swelling within the enclosed space created by the fascia that separates groups of muscles?

a. chronic fatigue syndrome

b. compartment syndrome

c. fibromyalgia

d. myofascial pain syndrome

BRS.66. A large, tender, swollen area caused by a staphylococcal infection around a hair follicle or sebaceous gland, also known as a *boil,* is a/an ____________________.

a. abscess

b. carbuncle

c. furuncle

d. pustule

BRS.67. Resistance to a disease present without the administration of an antigen or exposure to the disease is known as ____________________.

a. passive immunity

b. acquired immunity

c. vaccination

d. natural immunity

BRS.68. Fine muscle tremors, rigidity, and a slow or shuffling gait are all symptoms of the progressive condition known as ____________________.

a. multiple sclerosis

b. muscular dystrophy

c. myasthenia gravis

d. Parkinson's disease

BRS.69. A form of vasculitis that can cause headaches, visual impairment, jaw pain, and other symptoms, and is diagnosed when a biopsy shows the presence of abnormally large cells, is called ____________________.

a. temporal arteritis

b. hemangioma

c. migraine

d. peripheral vascular disease

BRS.70. During her pregnancy, Ruth had a skin condition commonly known as the mask of pregnancy. The medical term for this condition is ________________.

a. melasma

b. albinism

c. exanthem

d. vitiligo

BRS.71. Which of the following is caused by the failure of the bones of the limbs to grow to an appropriate length?

a. acromegaly

b. gigantism

c. hyperpituitarism

d. short stature

BRS.72. A bone is splintered or crushed in which type of fracture?

a. comminuted

b. compound

c. compression

d. spiral

BRS.73. In which surgery is bone cement injected to stabilize compression fractures within the spinal column?

a. percutaneous diskectomy

b. percutaneous vertebroplasty

c. laminectomy

d. spinal fusion

BRS.74. Which heart chamber receives oxygen-poor blood from all tissues except the lungs?

a. left atrium

b. left ventricle

c. right atrium

d. right ventricle

BRS.75. Which substance is commonly known as good cholesterol?

a. high-density lipoprotein cholesterol

b. homocysteine

c. low-density lipoprotein cholesterol

d. triglycerides

BRS.76. Which term means the grapelike clusters in the lungs where the exchange of oxygen and carbon dioxide takes place?

a. alveoli

b. bronchioles

c. bronchi

d. mediastinum

BRS.77. When there is less amniotic fluid than usual, this condition is known as ________________.

a. molar pregnancy

b. oligohydramnios

c. preeclampsia

d. hyperemesis gravidarum

BRS.78. The medical term for the viral infection known as chickenpox is ________________.

a. herpes zoster

b. cytomegalovirus

c. varicella

d. rubella

BRS.79. Which term describes a feeling of general discomfort or uneasiness that is often the first indication of an infection or other disease?

a. inflammation

b. symptom

c. trauma

d. malaise

BRS.80. An autoimmune disorder characterized by a severe reaction to ingesting gluten is known as ________________.

a. irritable bowel syndrome

b. diverticulosis

c. dyspepsia

d. celiac disease

BRS.81. Which term describes inflammation of the gallbladder?

a. cholecystectomy

b. cholecystitis

c. cholecystotomy

d. cholelithiasis

BRS.82. Which term means vomiting?

a. emesis

b. epistaxis

c. reflux

d. singultus

BRS.83. The bluish discoloration of the skin caused by a lack of adequate oxygen is known as ________________.

a. cyanosis

b. erythema

c. jaundice

d. pallor

BRS.84. A disorder of the adrenal glands due to excessive production of aldosterone is ________________.

a. Conn's syndrome

b. Crohn's disease

c. Cushing's syndrome

d. Raynaud's disease

BRS.85. Any substance that the body regards as being foreign is known as an ________________.

a. allergen

b. antibody

c. antigen

d. immunoglobulin

BRS.86. Which condition has purple discolorations on the skin due to bleeding underneath the skin?

a. dermatosis

b. pruritus

c. purpura

d. suppuration

BRS.87. A brief disturbance in brain function in which there is a loss of awareness, often described as a staring episode, is known as a/an ________________ seizure.

a. narcolepsy

b. tonic-clonic

c. absence

d. grand mal

BRS.88. A band of fibrous tissue that holds structures together abnormally is a/an ________________.

a. adhesion

b. ankylosis

c. contracture

d. ligation

BRS.89. Which procedure is performed to treat spider veins?

a. blepharoplasty

b. Botox

c. liposuction

d. sclerotherapy

BRS.90. The instrument used to examine the external ear canal is known as a/an ________________.

a. anoscope

b. ophthalmoscope

c. otoscope

d. speculum

BRS.91. Which is the outer region of the kidney?

a. medulla

b. renal cortex

c. nephron

d. glomerulus

BRS.92. Enlarged and swollen veins at the lower end of the esophagus are known as ________________.

a. esophageal aneurysms

b. esophageal varices

c. hemorrhoids

d. varicose veins

BRS.93. A progressive autoimmune disorder characterized by inflammation that causes demyelination of the myelin sheath is ________________.

a. systemic lupus erythematosus

b. multiple sclerosis

c. muscular dystrophy

d. spina bifida

BRS.94. The abdominal region located below the stomach is known as which region?

a. epigastric

b. hypogastric

c. left hypochondriac

d. umbilical

BRS.95. Which of the following sexually transmitted diseases is a bacterial infection?

a. acquired immunodeficiency syndrome

b. gonorrhea

c. genital herpes

d. trichomoniasis

BRS.96. Narrowing of the opening of the foreskin so that it cannot be retracted to expose the glans penis is known as ______________________.

a. balanitis

b. Peyronie's disease

c. phimosis

d. priapism

BRS.97. An exfoliative screening biopsy for the detection and diagnosis of conditions of the cervix and surrounding tissues is a/an ______________________.

a. endometrial biopsy

b. lymph node dissection

c. Pap smear

d. sentinel node biopsy

BRS.98. Which term is used to describe a narrow tube that transports urine from the kidney to the bladder?

a. ureter

b. renal pelvis

c. urethra

d. urethral meatus

BRS.99. Which term describes turning the palm upward or forward?

a. circumduction

b. pronation

c. rotation

d. supination

BRS.100. Which term describes the inflammation of a vein?

a. vasculitis

b. arteritis

c. phlebitis

d. phlebostenosis

BODY SYSTEMS REVIEW SESSION ANSWER KEY

BRS.1. D
BRS.2. B
BRS.3. C
BRS.4. A
BRS.5. B
BRS.6. D
BRS.7. B
BRS.8. D
BRS.9. B
BRS.10. B
BRS.11. C
BRS.12. D
BRS.13. C
BRS.14. A
BRS.15. C
BRS.16. B
BRS.17. A
BRS.18. B
BRS.19. B
BRS.20. C
BRS.21. D
BRS.22. A
BRS.23. D
BRS.24. D
BRS.25. C
BRS.26. B
BRS.27. A
BRS.28. B
BRS.29. C
BRS.30. B
BRS.31. D
BRS.32. B
BRS.33. B
BRS.34. D
BRS.35. B
BRS.36. A
BRS.37. C
BRS.38. C
BRS.39. B
BRS.40. A
BRS.41. B
BRS.42. A
BRS.43. A
BRS.44. C
BRS.45. D
BRS.46. A
BRS.47. B
BRS.48. B
BRS.49. C
BRS.50. C
BRS.51. A
BRS.52. C
BRS.53. B
BRS.54. A
BRS.55. D
BRS.56. A
BRS.57. C
BRS.58. B
BRS.59. D
BRS.60. B
BRS.61. A
BRS.62. B
BRS.63. B
BRS.64. C
BRS.65. B
BRS.66. C
BRS.67. D
BRS.68. D
BRS.69. A
BRS.70. A
BRS.71. D
BRS.72. A
BRS.73. B
BRS.74. C
BRS.75. A
BRS.76. A
BRS.77. B
BRS.78. C
BRS.79. D
BRS.80. D
BRS.81. B
BRS.82. A
BRS.83. A
BRS.84. A
BRS.85. C
BRS.86. C
BRS.87. C
BRS.88. A
BRS.89. D
BRS.90. C
BRS.91. B
BRS.92. B
BRS.93. B
BRS.94. B
BRS.95. B
BRS.96. C
BRS.97. C
BRS.98. A
BRS.99. D
BRS.100. C

BODY SYSTEMS SIMULATED FINAL TEST

BFT.1. Which term describes a torn or jagged wound?

a. fissure

b. fistula

c. laceration

d. lesion

BFT.2. The bone and soft tissues that surround and support the teeth are known as the ________________.

a. dentition

b. rugae

c. gingiva

d. periodontium

BFT.3. A chronic condition in which the heart is unable to pump out all of the blood that it receives is known as ________________.

a. atrial fibrillation

b. heart failure

c. tachycardia

d. ventricular fibrillation

BFT.4. Inflammation of the connective tissues that enclose the spinal cord and brain is known as ________________.

a. encephalitis

b. encephalopathy

c. meningitis

d. myelopathy

BFT.5. The partial or complete blockage of the small and/or large intestine that is caused by the stopping of normal intestinal peristalsis is ________________.

a. Crohn's disease

b. ileus

c. cheilitis

d. intestinal obstruction

BFT.6. Which term describes a condition in which the eye does not focus properly because of uneven curvatures of the cornea?

a. ametropia

b. astigmatism

c. ectropion

d. entropion

BFT.7. A procedure in which pressurized fluid is used to clean out wound debris is known as ________________.

a. irrigation and debridement

b. dilation and curettage

c. incision and drainage

d. dermabrasion

BFT.8. Which term describes persistent severe burning pain that usually follows an injury to a sensory nerve?

a. causalgia

b. hyperesthesia

c. paresthesia

d. peripheral neuropathy

BFT.9. Which of the following procedures is performed to reduce the risk of a stroke caused by a disruption of the blood flow to the brain?

a. aneurysm clipping

b. cardiac ablation

c. carotid endarterectomy

d. coronary artery bypass graft

BFT.10. Which term means bleeding from the ear?

a. barotrauma

b. otomycosis

c. otopyorrhea

d. otorrhagia

BFT.11. The medical term meaning itching is ________________.

a. perfusion
b. pruritus
c. purpura
d. suppuration

BFT.12. A condition characterized by episodes of severe chest pain due to inadequate blood flow to the myocardium is ________________.

a. angina
b. claudication
c. cyanosis
d. myocardial infarction

BFT.13. The condition of excessive mammary development in the male is called ________________.

a. Cushing's syndrome
b. hypergonadism
c. hypogonadism
d. gynecomastia

BFT.14. The genetic disorder caused by changes in the MR1 gene that usually makes a protein needed for normal brain development is called ________________.

a. Marfan syndrome
b. fragile X syndrome
c. metabolic syndrome
d. phenylketonuria

BFT.15. A prediction of the probable course and outcome of a disease or disorder is ________________.

a. differential diagnosis
b. diagnosis
c. prognosis
d. syndrome

BFT.16. Yellow discoloration of the skin, mucous membranes, and eyes is ________________.

a. vitiligo
b. jaundice
c. erythema
d. albinism

BFT.17. Which fracture occurs at the lower end of the radius when a person tries to break a fall by landing on his or her hand?

a. Colles fracture
b. comminuted fracture
c. greenstick fracture
d. spiral fracture

BFT.18. Which term describes excessive urination during the night?

a. nocturia
b. polydipsia
c. polyuria
d. urinary retention

BFT.19. A closed sac associated with a sebaceous gland that contains yellow, fatty material is known as a/an ________________.

a. comedo
b. epidermoid cyst
c. seborrheic dermatitis
d. seborrheic keratosis

BFT.20. Which term describes the condition commonly known as swollen glands?

a. adenoiditis
b. vasculitis
c. lymphadenitis
d. lymphangioma

BFT.21. A sudden, involuntary contraction of one or more muscles is called a/an ________________.

a. adhesion
b. contracture
c. spasm
d. sprain

BFT.22. The respiratory disease commonly known as whooping cough is also known as ________________.

a. croup
b. pharyngitis
c. emphysema
d. pertussis

BFT.23. The lymphocytes that play an important role in the killing of cancer cells and cells infected by viruses are known as ________________.

a. cytokines

b. natural killer cells

c. B cells

d. T cells

BFT.24. An abnormal lateral curvature of the spine is known as ________________.

a. kyphosis

b. lordosis

c. lumbago

d. scoliosis

BFT.25. The surgical creation of an artificial excretory opening between the ileum and the outside of the abdominal wall is a/an ________________.

a. colostomy

b. pyelotomy

c. gastroparesis

d. ileostomy

BFT.26. An x-ray examination of the uterus and fallopian tubes is called a ________________.

a. colposcopy

b. hysteroscopy

c. hysterosalpingography

d. colporrhaphy

BFT.27. As the condition known as ________________ progresses, the chest sometimes assumes an enlarged barrel shape.

a. asthma

b. epistaxis

c. emphysema

d. bronchiectasis

BFT.28. Which term means to stop or control bleeding?

a. hemorrhage

b. hemostasis

c. homeostasis

d. sepsis

BFT.29. An accumulation of pus in the fallopian tube is known as ________________.

a. leukorrhea

b. otopyorrhea

c. pyosalpinx

d. salpingitis

BFT.30. The bruising of brain tissue as a result of a head injury is known as a ________________.

a. cerebral contusion

b. concussion

c. hydrocele

d. meningocele

BFT.31. Which term means vomiting blood?

a. epistaxis

b. hemarthrosis

c. hematemesis

d. hyperemesis

BFT.32. A blood clot that originates in a vein is a/an ________________.

a. venous thromboembolism

b. coronary thrombosis

c. embolus

d. thrombus

BFT.33. Abnormally rapid, deep breathing resulting in decreased levels of carbon dioxide in the blood is known as ________________.

a. apnea

b. dyspnea

c. hyperventilation

d. hypoventilation

BFT.34. Which term describes difficult or painful urination?

a. dyspepsia

b. dysphagia

c. dystrophy

d. dysuria

BFT.35. The treatment using injections of hyaluronic acid into the knee to provide temporary relief from arthritis pain is called __________.

a. platelet-rich plasma therapy
b. viscosupplementation
c. cortisone injections
d. sclerotherapy

BFT.36. The normal rhythmic contractions of the atria are replaced by rapid irregular twitching of the muscular heart wall in which of the following?

a. atrial fibrillation
b. bradycardia
c. tachycardia
d. ventricular fibrillation

BFT.37. The eye condition characterized by increased intraocular pressure is known as __________.

a. cataracts
b. glaucoma
c. macular degeneration
d. monochromatism

BFT.38. The presence of blood in the seminal fluid is known as __________.

a. azoospermia
b. hematuria
c. hematospermia
d. prostatitis

BFT.39. The condition of common changes in the eyes that occur with aging is known as __________.

a. hyperopia
b. presbycusis
c. presbyopia
d. strabismus

BFT.40. Which body cavity protects the brain?

a. Anterior
b. Cranial
c. Caudal
d. Ventral

BFT.41. A hernia of the bladder through the vaginal wall is known as a __________.

a. cystocele
b. cystopexy
c. vaginocele
d. vesicovaginal fistula

BFT.42. Which disease is caused by a parasite most commonly transmitted to humans by contact with contaminated animal feces?

a. giardiasis
b. malaria
c. toxoplasmosis
d. candidiasis

BFT.43. A ringing, buzzing, or roaring sound in one or both ears is known as __________.

a. labyrinthitis
b. syncope
c. tinnitus
d. vertigo

BFT.44. An outbreak of a disease occurring over a large geographic area that is possibly worldwide is known as a/an __________.

a. endemic
b. epidemic
c. pandemic
d. syndrome

BFT.45. An abnormal accumulation of serous fluid in the peritoneal cavity is called __________.

a. ascites
b. aerophagia
c. melena
d. bolus

BFT.46. A discolored flat spot that is less than 1 cm in diameter, such as a freckle, is known as a __________.

a. macule
b. papule
c. plaque
d. vesicle

BFT.47. The ELISA test is used to screen for the presence of ______________.

a. HIV antibodies

b. hepatitis C

c. Kaposi's sarcoma

d. tuberculosis

BFT.48. Which term describes excessive uterine bleeding both at the usual time of menstrual periods and at other irregular intervals?

a. dysmenorrhea

b. polymenorrhea

c. menometrorrhagia

d. oligomenorrhea

BFT.49. Which of the following is a form of sexual dysfunction in which the penis is bent or curved during erection?

a. erectile dysfunction

b. Peyronie's disease

c. phimosis

d. priapism

BFT.50. The excess accumulation of fluid in the pleural space is called ______________.

a. pulmonary edema

b. a pyothorax

c. pleurisy

d. a pleural effusion

BFT.51. The condition commonly known as wear-and-tear arthritis is ______________.

a. gout

b. osteoarthritis

c. rheumatoid arthritis

d. spondylosis

BFT.52. Which term means to free a tendon from adhesions?

a. tenodesis

b. tenolysis

c. myorrhaphy

d. insertion

BFT.53. An inflammation of the lips characterized by crack-like sores at the corners of the mouth is called ______________.

a. cheilitis

b. gingivitis

c. cholangitis

d. ulcerative colitis

BFT.54. The chronic, degenerative disease characterized by scarring that causes disturbance of the structure and function of the liver is ______________.

a. cirrhosis

b. hepatitis

c. hepatomegaly

d. jaundice

BFT.55. The procedure that removes waste products directly from the bloodstream of patients whose kidneys no longer function is known as ______________.

a. diuresis

b. epispadias

c. hemodialysis

d. peritoneal dialysis

BFT.56. The medical term for the condition commonly known as fainting is ______________.

a. delirium

b. singultus

c. stupor

d. syncope

BFT.57. A condition in which there is an insufficient supply of oxygen in the tissues due to a restricted blood flow to a part of the body is known as ______________.

a. angina

b. infarction

c. ischemia

d. perfusion

BFT.58. A collection of blood in the pleural cavity is known as a ________________.

a. hemophilia
b. hemoptysis
c. hemostasis
d. hemothorax

BFT.59. The return of swallowed food into the mouth is known as ________________.

a. dysphagia
b. emesis
c. pyrosis
d. regurgitation

BFT.60. An inflammation of the lacrimal gland that can be a bacterial, viral, or fungal infection is known as ________________.

a. anisocoria
b. dacryoadenitis
c. exophthalmos
d. hordeolum

BFT.61. The contraction of the pupil, normally in response to exposure to light, but also possibly due to the use of prescription or illegal drugs, is known as ________________.

a. nystagmus
b. mydriasis
c. miosis
d. mycosis

BFT.62. Which term means excessive urination?

a. enuresis
b. oliguria
c. overactive bladder
d. polyuria

BFT.63. The surgical removal of the gallbladder is known as a ________________.

a. cholecystectomy
b. cholecystostomy
c. cholecystotomy
d. hepatectomy

BFT.64. Castration is another name for a bilateral ________________, which is the surgical removal of both testicles.

a. vasectomy
b. varicocelectomy
c. orchiopexy
d. orchiectomy

BFT.65. A groove or crack-like break in the skin is known as a/an ________________.

a. abrasion
b. fissure
c. laceration
d. ulcer

BFT.66. An inflammation of both the renal pelvis and kidney is called ________________.

a. renal colic
b. pyelonephritis
c. hydronephrosis
d. urosepsis

BFT.67. Which structure has roles in both the immune and endocrine systems?

a. pancreas
b. pituitary gland
c. spleen
d. thymus

BFT.68. Which term describes an inflammation of the brain?

a. encephalitis
b. mastitis
c. meningitis
d. myelitis

BFT.69. The hormone secreted by fat cells is known as ________________.

a. interstitial cell-stimulating hormone
b. growth hormone
c. leptin
d. neurohormone

BFT.70. A type of catheter made of a flexible tube with a balloon filled with sterile water at the end to hold it in place in the bladder is known as a/an ________________ catheter.

a. Foley
b. indwelling
c. suprapubic
d. intermittent

BFT.71. Which of the following is acquired in a hospital or clinic setting?

a. functional disorder
b. iatrogenic illness
c. idiopathic disorder
d. nosocomial infection

BFT.72. Which term describes a group of lung diseases in which the bronchial airflow is obstructed, making it difficult to breathe out?

a. chronic obstructive pulmonary disease
b. emphysema
c. tuberculosis
d. pneumonia

BFT.73. Which term describes an eye disorder that can develop as a complication of diabetes?

a. diabetic neuropathy
b. diabetic retinopathy
c. papilledema
d. retinal detachment

BFT.74. The physical wasting with the loss of weight and muscle mass due to diseases such as advanced cancer is known as ________________.

a. cachexia
b. anorexia nervosa
c. bulimia nervosa
d. malnutrition

BFT.75. Which term means difficulty in swallowing?

a. aerophagia
b. dyspepsia
c. dysphagia
d. eructation

BFT.76. Which of the following occurs when a blood vessel in the brain leaks or ruptures?

a. cerebral hematoma
b. embolism
c. hemorrhagic stroke
d. ischemic stroke

BFT.77. Which hormonal disorder results from the pituitary gland producing too much growth hormone in adults?

a. acromegaly
b. cretinism
c. gigantism
d. pituitarism

BFT.78. Which term describes the condition commonly known an ingrown toenail?

a. cryptorchidism
b. onychocryptosis
c. onychomycosis
d. priapism

BFT.79. The instrument used to examine the interior of the eye is called an ________________.

a. ophtalmoscope
b. ophthalmoscope
c. opthalmoscope
d. opthlmoscope

BFT.80. A protrusion of part of the stomach upward into the chest through an opening in the diaphragm is a/an ________________.

a. esophageal hernia
b. esophageal varices
c. hiatal hernia
d. hiatal varices

BFT.81. A surgical incision made to enlarge the vaginal orifice to facilitate childbirth is a/an ________________.

a. sacrocolpopexy
b. episiotomy
c. epispadias
d. epistaxis

BFT.82. Severe itching of the external female genitalia is known as ________________.

a. colpitis

b. leukorrhea

c. pruritus vulvae

d. vaginal candidiasis

BFT.83. A urinary problem caused by interference with the normal nerve pathways associated with urination is ________________.

a. neurogenic bladder

b. overactive bladder

c. polyuria

d. overflow incontinence

BFT.84. A general term for sleep disorders is ________________.

a. narcolepsy

b. insomnia

c. sleep deprivation

d. parasomnia

BFT.85. The medical term for a collection of dried serum and cellular debris, also known as a *scab*, is a ________________.

a. crust

b. nodule

c. plaque

d. scale

BFT.86. Dermatitis caused by the friction of skin rubbing together in skin folds is called ________________.

a. pruritus

b. melasma

c. contact dermatitis

d. intertrigo

BFT.87. Which of the following can occur when a foreign substance, such as vomit, is inhaled into the lungs?

a. aspiration pneumonia

b. bacterial pneumonia

c. mycoplasma pneumonia

d. pneumocystis pneumonia

BFT.88. Ankylosis of the bones of the middle ear that causes a conductive hearing loss is known as ________________.

a. labyrinthitis

b. mastoiditis

c. osteosclerosis

d. otosclerosis

BFT.89. Which procedure is the surgical fusion of two bones to stiffen a joint?

a. arthrodesis

b. arthrolysis

c. synovectomy

d. tenodesis

BFT.90. Inflammation of the tissues surrounding the elbow is known as ________________.

a. impingement syndrome

b. epicondylitis

c. Morton's neuroma

d. overuse tendinitis

BFT.91. A contagious inflammation that causes painful blisters on the eardrum is called ________________.

a. infectious myringitis

b. otitis media

c. otomycosis

d. infectious meningitis

BFT.92. The distortion or impairment of voluntary movement such as in a tic or spasm is ________________.

a. bradykinesia

b. dyskinesia

c. hyperkinesia

d. myoclonus

BFT.93. Which structure secretes bile?

a. gallbladder

b. liver

c. pancreas

d. spleen

BFT.94. The process of recording the electrical activity of the brain through the use of electrodes attached to the scalp is ________________.

a. myelography

b. electroencephalography

c. electromyography

d. magnetic resonance imaging

BFT.95. What small bacterium that lives in lice, fleas, ticks, and mites causes Rocky Mountain spotted fever?

a. spirochetes

b. anthrax

c. rickettsia

d. bacilli

BFT.96. The eye condition that causes the loss of central vision, but not total blindness, is known as ________________.

a. cataracts

b. glaucoma

c. macular degeneration

d. presbyopia

BFT.97. Which procedure is performed to remove excess skin and fat for the elimination of wrinkles?

a. ablation

b. blepharoplasty

c. rhytidectomy

d. sclerotherapy

BFT.98. Which condition describes total paralysis affecting only one side of the body?

a. hemiparesis

b. hemiplegia

c. paraplegia

d. quadriplegia

BFT.99. Which term describes the congenital absence of a normal body opening or passage?

a. atresia

b. hypoplasia

c. aplasia

d. anaplasia

BFT.100. Which of these hormones is produced by the pituitary gland?

a. adrenocorticotropic hormone

b. calcitonin

c. cortisol

d. epinephrine

BODY SYSTEMS SIMULATED FINAL TEST ANSWER KEY

BFT.1. C
BFT.2. D
BFT.3. B
BFT.4. C
BFT.5. B
BFT.6. B
BFT.7. A
BFT.8. A
BFT.9. C
BFT.10. D
BFT.11. B
BFT.12. A
BFT.13. D
BFT.14. B
BFT.15. C
BFT.16. B
BFT.17. A
BFT.18. A
BFT.19. B
BFT.20. C
BFT.21. C
BFT.22. D
BFT.23. B
BFT.24. D
BFT.25. D
BFT.26. C
BFT.27. C
BFT.28. B
BFT.29. C
BFT.30. A
BFT.31. C
BFT.32. A
BFT.33. C
BFT.34. D
BFT.35. B
BFT.36. A
BFT.37. B
BFT.38. C
BFT.39. C
BFT.40. B
BFT.41. A
BFT.42. C
BFT.43. C
BFT.44. C
BFT.45. A
BFT.46. A
BFT.47. A
BFT.48. C
BFT.49. B
BFT.50. D
BFT.51. B
BFT.52. B
BFT.53. A
BFT.54. A
BFT.55. C
BFT.56. D
BFT.57. C
BFT.58. D
BFT.59. D
BFT.60. B
BFT.61. C
BFT.62. D
BFT.63. A
BFT.64. D
BFT.65. B
BFT.66. B
BFT.67. D
BFT.68. A
BFT.69. C
BFT.70. A
BFT.71. D
BFT.72. A
BFT.73. B
BFT.74. A
BFT.75. C
BFT.76. C
BFT.77. A
BFT.78. B
BFT.79. B
BFT.80. C
BFT.81. B
BFT.82. C
BFT.83. A
BFT.84. C
BFT.85. A
BFT.86. D
BFT.87. A
BFT.88. D
BFT.89. A
BFT.90. B
BFT.91. A
BFT.92. B
BFT.93. B
BFT.94. B
BFT.95. C
BFT.96. C
BFT.97. C
BFT.98. B
BFT.99. A
BFT.100. A

MEDICAL SPECIALTY CHAPTERS REVIEW SESSION

SRS.1. The presence of glucose in the urine is known as ____________________.

a. albuminuria
b. calciuria
c. glycosuria
d. hematuria

SRS.2. Which term describes blood in the urine?

a. hemangioma
b. hematemesis
c. hematoma
d. hematuria

SRS.3. Which term refers to a class of drugs that relieves pain without affecting consciousness?

a. analgesic
b. barbiturate
c. hypnotic
d. sedative

SRS.4. A malignant tumor usually involving the upper shaft of long bones, the pelvis, or knee is known as ____________________.

a. an adenocarcinoma
b. Hodgkin's lymphoma
c. an osteochondroma
d. an osteosarcoma

SRS.5. Another term for conventional, or Western, medical practices and systems of health care is ____________________ medicine.

a. alternative
b. complementary
c. allopathic
d. integrative

SRS.6. Which symbol means less than?

a. >
b. ≥
c. <
d. 1

SRS.7. When medication is placed under the tongue and allowed to dissolve slowly, this is known as ____________________ administration.

a. oral
b. parenteral
c. sublingual
d. topical

SRS.8. A sonogram is the image created by ____________________.

a. computerized tomography
b. fluoroscopy
c. magnetic resonance imaging (MRI)
d. ultrasonography

SRS.9. Which condition is breast cancer at its earliest stage before the cancer has broken through the wall of the milk duct?

a. ductal carcinoma in situ
b. infiltrating lobular carcinoma
c. inflammatory breast cancer
d. invasive lobular carcinoma

SRS.10. Which term is used to describe practices and systems of health care used to supplement traditional Western medicine?

a. allopathic medicine
b. complementary medicine
c. alternative medicine
d. homeopathy

SRS.11. A deliberate or accidental ingestion of more medication than has been prescribed or is safe is known as a/an ____________________.

a. adverse drug reaction
b. adherence
c. overdose
d. loading dose

SRS.12. A specific unit in an assisted living facility or nursing home for older adults with dementia is known as ____________________.

a. rehab

b. home health

c. board & care

d. memory care

SRS.13. Which of the following are a class of drugs that slow the loss of bone density in osteoporosis?

a. prostaglandin analogs

b. bisphosphonates

c. beta-blockers

d. dopaminergic drugs

SRS.14. Irregular open pits in the skin that occur on the lower legs as a result of venous stasis are known as ____________________.

a. chronic venous insufficiency

b. stasis dermatitis

c. varicose veins

d. venous ulcers

SRS.15. Which lifestyle risk factor increases the risk of developing cancer of the mouth, larynx, esophagus, breast, liver, and colon/rectum?

a. smoking tobacco

b. chemical exposure

c. alcohol consumption

d. hereditary cancer syndromes

SRS.16. Which eating disorder is characterized by frequent episodes of binge eating followed by compensatory behaviors to purge the food?

a. binge eating disorder

b. bulimia nervosa

c. anorexia nervosa

d. avoidant restrictive food intake disorder

SRS.17. An infant breathing disorder caused by underdeveloped lungs is called ____________________.

a. bronchopulmonary dysplasia

b. respiratory distress syndrome

c. croup

d. oral thrush

SRS.18. A complete block in electrical conduction between the atria and ventricles is known as a ____________________ heart block.

a. first-degree

b. second-degree

c. third-degree

d. bundle branch

SRS.19. The personality disorder characterized by a pattern of disregard for and violation of the rights of others is called ____________________.

a. antisocial personality disorder

b. borderline personality disorder

c. narcissistic personality disorder

d. schizoaffective disorder

SRS.20. A written order from a licensed medical professional that specifies a medication or product to be dispensed to a patient is known as a ____________________.

a. pharmacy

b. controlled substance

c. prescription

d. formulary

SRS.21. Which term describes the congenital absence or narrowing of a normal body opening or passage?

a. atresia

b. strabismus

c. hernia

d. anencephaly

SRS.22. Uncontrollable physical and/or verbal "tics" such as shrugging shoulders, blinking eyes, or yelling offensive words are characteristics of ________________.

a. autism spectrum disorder
b. impulse control disorders
c. Tourette syndrome
d. oppositional defiant disorder

SRS.23. Which environmental risk factor is present in x-rays and other medical imaging procedures?

a. nuclear medicine
b. ultraviolet rays
c. chemical exposure
d. ionizing radiation

SRS.24. The failure of the brain and skull to fully develop in a fetus is called ________________.

a. spina bifida
b. atresia
c. anencephaly
d. congenital disorder

SRS.25. A low-grade, chronic depression with symptoms milder than severe depression is called ________________.

a. bipolar disorder
b. anhedonia
c. seasonal affective disorder
d. persistent depressive disorder

SRS.26. Apgar scoring of a newborn evaluates the infant's ________________ 1 and 5 minutes after birth.

a. weight
b. height
c. hearing
d. physical status

SRS.27. Osteoarthritis that has progressed to the point where the articular cartilage is gone is known as ________________ arthritis.

a. bone-on-bone
b. rheumatoid
c. spinal
d. ankylosing

SRS.28. A traditional Chinese medical practice using thin needles inserted into specific points of the body to restore the flow of qi is known as ________________.

a. acupressure
b. acupuncture
c. Qi Gong
d. reiki

SRS.29. An excessive fear of environments where the person fears a panic attack might occur is known as ________________.

a. acrophobia
b. agoraphobia
c. claustrophobia
d. social anxiety disorder

SRS.30. Tanner staging is a tool used to assess ________________.

a. secondary sex characteristics
b. growth curves
c. body mass index
d. active immunity

SRS.31. The form of massage that uses soft-tissue manipulation focusing on applying pressure to trigger points to treat injuries and alleviate pain is known as ________________.

a. chiropractic manipulative therapy
b. myofascial release
c. craniosacral therapy
d. neuromuscular therapy

SRS.32. Which term refers to a person whose gender identity does not match their sex assigned at birth?

a. transgender
b. cisgender
c. non-binary
d. dissociative identity disorder

SRS.33. A birth is considered premature if it occurs earlier than the ________________ week of pregnancy.

a. 40th
b. 39th
c. 38th
d. 37th

SRS.34. The disorder characterized by a child or adolescent's persistent disruptive behavior toward authority figures is ______________________.

a. kleptomania

b. impulse control disorder

c. oppositional defiant disorder

d. manic behavior

SRS.35. A common viral illness between ages 6 months and 3 years that is characterized by several days of fever followed by a rash is known as ______________________.

a. tinea

b. roseola

c. erythema infectiosum

d. hand, foot, and mouth disease

SRS.36. Which of the following is a class of oral diabetes medications that work by increasing the amount of insulin released by the pancreas?

a. Metformin

b. Insulin

c. Thiazolidinediones

d. Sulfonylureas

SRS.37. An anxiety disorder in which a child capable of speech is unable to speak in certain settings is called ______________________.

a. agoraphobia

b. panic disorder

c. impulse control disorder

d. selective mutism

SRS.38. Which of the following is a highly contagious bacterial skin infection that commonly occurs in children?

a. conjunctivitis

b. scabies

c. impetigo

d. pediculosis

SRS.39. A cancer that develops from immature undifferentiated cells and occurs most frequently in children is ______________________.

a. lymphoma

b. blastoma

c. leukemia

d. sarcoma

SRS.40. A condition where the flaps of a valve become stiff, thickened, or even fused together, limiting the amount of blood that can pass through, is known as heart valve ______________________.

a. stenosis

b. regurgitation

c. disease

d. insufficiency

SRS.41. A mutated gene within a cell that causes that cell to function abnormally is known as a/an ______________________.

a. oncogene

b. proto-oncogene

c. carcinogen

d. metastasis

SRS.42. The physical removal of stool from the rectal vault with a gloved finger is known as ______________________.

a. digital rectal exam

b. nasogastric intubation

c. manual disimpaction

d. bowel rest

SRS.43. Which term refers to a surgical puncture to remove excess fluid or to remove fluid for diagnostic purposes?

a. centesis

b. biopsy

c. laparoscopy

d. interventional radiology

SRS.44. What is the gradual process of decreasing the amount of work of breathing done by the ventilator, to measure whether a patient can breathe spontaneously before extubation?

a. intubation

b. weaning

c. respiratory failure

d. senile emphysema

SRS.45. Any substance that has a psychological or physiological effect on the human body is known as a ____________________.

a. drug

b. placebo

c. medication

d. tablet

SRS.46. The disorder characterized by the overaccumulation of belongings in a way that interferes with daily living is ____________________.

a. obsessive-compulsive disorder

b. posttraumatic stress disorder

c. adjustment disorder

d. hoarding disorder

SRS.47. The complete or partial end of cancer signs and symptoms for at least one month is known as ____________________.

a. partial remission

b. remission

c. complete remission

d. cancer survivorship

SRS.48. The correct term for the mildly contagious childhood viral infection known as fifth disease is ____________________.

a. roseola

b. infectious mononucleosis

c. strep throat

d. erythema infectiosum

SRS.49. Breast cancer that has receptors for estrogen and progesterone and has high levels of HER2 is known as ____________________ breast cancer.

a. inflammatory

b. triple-negative

c. triple-positive

d. HER2-positive

SRS.50. An acute condition of confusion, disorientation, disordered thinking and memory, agitation, and hallucinations is known as ____________________.

a. delirium

b. dementia

c. sundowning

d. vascular dementia

MEDICAL SPECIALTY CHAPTERS REVIEW SESSION ANSWER KEY

SRS.1. C
SRS.2. D
SRS.3. A
SRS.4. D
SRS.5. C
SRS.6. C
SRS.7. C
SRS.8. D
SRS.9. A
SRS.10. B
SRS.11. C
SRS.12. D
SRS.13. B
SRS.14. D
SRS.15. C
SRS.16. B
SRS.17. B
SRS.18. C
SRS.19. A
SRS.20. C
SRS.21. A
SRS.22. C
SRS.23. D
SRS.24. C
SRS.25. D
SRS.26. D
SRS.27. A
SRS.28. B
SRS.29. B
SRS.30. A
SRS.31. D
SRS.32. A
SRS.33. D
SRS.34. B
SRS.35. B
SRS.36. D
SRS.37. D
SRS.38. C
SRS.39. B
SRS.40. A
SRS.41. A
SRS.42. C
SRS.43. A
SRS.44. B
SRS.45. A
SRS.46. D
SRS.47. B
SRS.48. D
SRS.49. C
SRS.50. A

MEDICAL SPECIALTY CHAPTERS SIMULATED FINAL TEST

SFT.1. A new cancer site that results from the spreading process is known as ________________.

a. in situ

b. metabolism

c. metastasis

d. metastasize

SFT.2. An abnormal fear of being in small or enclosed spaces is known as ________________.

a. acrophobia

b. agoraphobia

c. social phobia

d. claustrophobia

SFT.3. A type of cancer that occurs in blood-making cells found in the red bone marrow is ________________.

a. carcinoma

b. multiple myeloma

c. osteochondroma

d. sarcoma

SFT.4. An instrument used to enlarge the opening of any canal or cavity to facilitate inspection of its interior is known as a/an ________________.

a. endoscope

b. speculum

c. sphygmomanometer

d. stethoscope

SFT.5. Which of the following injections is made into the fatty layer just below the skin?

a. intradermal

b. intramuscular

c. intravenous

d. subcutaneous

SFT.6. An elevated ________________ indicates the presence of inflammation in the body.

a. complete blood cell count

b. erythrocyte sedimentation rate

c. platelet count

d. total hemoglobin test

SFT.7. Which malignant condition is distinguished by the presence of Reed–Sternberg cells?

a. Hodgkin's lymphoma

b. leukemia

c. Non-Hodgkin's lymphoma

d. osteosarcoma

SFT.8. An abnormal sound or murmur heard during auscultation of an artery is known as a/an ________________.

a. auscultation

b. bruit

c. rhonchi

d. stridor

SFT.9. Which neurodevelopmental disorder is characterized by difficulty developing normal social relationships and communication skills?

a. autism spectrum disorder

b. attention deficit disorder

c. dyslexia

d. intellectual disability

SFT.10. A diagnostic procedure designed to determine the density of a body part by the sound produced by tapping the surface with the fingers is known as ________________.

a. auscultation

b. palpation

c. percussion

d. range of motion

SFT.11. Which of the following is the result of medical treatment that yields the exact opposite of normally expected results?

a. drug interaction

b. paradoxical reaction

c. placebo

d. idiosyncratic reaction

SFT.12. Which examination technique is the visualization of body parts in motion by projecting x-ray images on a luminous fluorescent screen?

a. computed tomography

b. fluoroscopy

c. magnetic resonance imaging

d. positron emission tomography

SFT.13. The greenish material that forms the first stools of a newborn is known as ________________.

a. colostrum

b. lochia

c. meconium

d. vernix

SFT.14. A false personal belief that is maintained despite obvious proof or evidence to the contrary is known as a ________________.

a. delusion

b. dementia

c. mania

d. phobia

SFT.15. A technique in which a hollow needle is used to remove small samples of tissue for diagnosis and the planning of treatment is a ________________ biopsy.

a. surgical

b. sentinel node

c. core needle

d. lymph node

SFT.16. The gradual, natural decline of the immune system as a result of aging is known as ________________.

a. inflamm-aging

b. immunosenescence

c. sarcopenia

d. presbycusis

SFT.17. A secondary response—either beneficial or undesirable—that accompanies the principal response for which a drug was taken is known as a/an ________________.

a. adverse drug reaction

b. side effect

c. contraindication

d. idiosyncratic reaction

SFT.18. An altered level of consciousness caused by elevated blood ammonia levels is known as ________________.

a. delirium

b. dementia

c. hepatic encephalopathy

d. vascular dementia

SFT.19. A greater-than-normal amount of bilirubin in the blood can cause ________________ in a newborn.

a. strabismus

b. colic

c. jaundice

d. oral thrush

SFT.20. The 11-item tool for measuring the severity of neurological deficit after a stroke is known as the ________________ scale.

a. orientation

b. Cincinnati Prehospital Stroke

c. modified Rankin

d. National Institutes of Health Stroke

SFT.21. A type of medicine that acts primarily on the central nervous system, producing temporary changes affecting the mind, emotions, and behavior is known as a/an ________________.

a. antipsychotic drug

b. psychotropic drug

c. tranquilizer

d. anxiolytic drug

SFT.22. Spina bifida is an example of a ________________.

a. neural tube defect

b. genetic disorder

c. chromosomal congenital disorder

d. systemic reaction

SFT.23. The medication mainly used to treat depression that has proven resistant to treatment is an ________________.

a. SSRI

b. SNRI

c. MAOI

d. EMDR

SFT.24. An accumulation of fluid and cancer cells between the outer layer of the lung and chest wall that causes shortness of breath is known as a/an ________________.

a. malignant ascites

b. thoracentesis

c. malignant pleural effusion

d. abdominocentesis

SFT.25. A patient-guided treatment to control bodily functions through relaxation, visualization, and other cognitive control techniques is known as ________________.

a. biofeedback

b. guided imagery

c. hypnosis

d. mindfulness meditation

SFT.26. The childhood illness characterized by inflammation of the blood vessels is ________________.

a. Kawasaki disease

b. asthma

c. epilepsy

d. anaphylaxis

SFT.27. A severe version of vaginal atrophy in which the labia minora fuse together at least partially is known as ________________.

a. vaginal atrophy

b. postmenopausal labial fusion

c. lichen sclerosus

d. genitourinary syndrome of menopause

SFT.28. The use of multiple medications by a single person, often for different conditions, is known as ________________.

a. medication adherence

b. polypharmacy

c. formulary

d. hepatic dosing

SFT.29. Therapy that focuses on changing thoughts and behaviors affecting a person's emotions and functioning is known as ________________.

a. cognitive behavioral therapy

b. psychoanalysis

c. biofeedback

d. exposure therapy

SFT.30. A substance that eases the pain or severity of the symptoms of a disease but does not cure it is known as a/an ________________.

a. palliative

b. opioid

c. sedative

d. placebo

SFT.31. Which term refers to a persistent, distressing feeling of shortness of breath and an inability to fully catch one's breath that often occurs at end-of-life?

a. death rattle

b. terminal agitation

c. agonal respirations

d. air hunger

SFT.32. The vaccine that protects against mumps is known as ________.

a. IPV

b. DTaP

c. RV

d. MMR

SFT.33. A class of medications administered to treat symptoms of severe disorders of thinking and mood are ________.

a. benzodiazepines

b. antipsychotic drugs

c. tricyclic antidepressants

d. mood stabilizers

SFT.34. The use of systemic treatment to reduce the size of a cancer before surgery is performed is known as ________.

a. adjuvant therapy

b. clinical trial

c. ablation

d. neoadjuvant therapy

SFT.35. An initial, higher dose of medication given when a patient is first started on a medication is known as a ________.

a. therapeutic dose

b. loading dose

c. maintenance dose

d. bolus

SFT.36. Which condition can be caused by a peptic ulcer, frequent use of NSAIDs, or esophageal varices?

a. upper GI bleed

b. lower GI bleed

c. small bowel obstruction

d. hematemesis

SFT.37. The treatment using brief, powerful, repetitive electromagnetic pulses to alter electrical pathways in the brain is called ________.

a. electroconvulsive therapy

b. biofeedback

c. transcranial magnetic stimulation

d. EMDR

SFT.38. Which of the following is one of several classes of medication that work in different ways to prevent or relieve nausea and vomiting?

a. antacid

b. antitussive

c. laxative

d. antiemetic

SFT.39. Premature infants requiring lung support for an extended period after birth are often diagnosed as having ________.

a. asthma

b. respiratory distress syndrome

c. bronchopulmonary dysplasia

d. croup

SFT.40. The sleep disorder characterized by sudden and uncontrollable brief episodes of falling asleep during the day is known as ________.

a. insomnia

b. parasomnia

c. sleep deprivation

d. narcolepsy

SFT.41. A partial block in electrical conduction between the atrium and ventricle on one side of the heart at the bundle of His is known as ________ block.

a. first-degree heart

b. second-degree heart

c. third-degree heart

d. bundle branch

SFT.42. A nuclear scanning test that identifies new areas of bone growth or breakdown is a ________.

a. sonogram

b. scintigram

c. bone scan

d. bone density test

SFT.43. A medication that blocks the development, growth, or proliferation of malignant cells is known as a/an ________________.

a. antineoplastic

b. monoclonal antibody

c. angiogenesis inhibitor

d. clinical trial

SFT.44. Which of the following viral infections is a common, highly contagious disease spread by respiratory droplets?

a. Infectious mononucleosis

b. Respiratory syncytial virus

c. Strep throat

d. Respiratory distress syndrome

SFT.45. A class of drugs that have both anti-arrhythmic and antihypertensive properties and work by blocking the release of epinephrine and norepinephrine to slow the heart rate is known as ________________.

a. beta-blockers

b. alpha blockers

c. calcium channel blockers

d. diuretics

SFT.46. A ventral septal defect is an example of a ________________.

a. neural tube defect

b. chromosomal congenital disorder

c. congenital heart defect

d. birth injury

SFT.47. The traditional Hindu system of medicine, emphasizing a holistic approach to preventive treatment, is called ________________medicine.

a. allopathic

b. Ayurvedic

c. traditional Chinese

d. integrative

SFT.48. An injury that occurs from shearing pressure, where a flap of epidermis is pulled away from the underlying tissue, is known as a/an ________________.

a. skin tear

b. contusion

c. ecchymosis

d. hematoma

SFT.49. A form of treatment that disrupts blood supply to a tumor is known as ________________.

a. angiogenesis

b. antiangiogenesis

c. immunotherapy

d. hormone therapy

SFT.50. A drug that helps induce or sustain sleep is called a/an ________________.

a. sedative

b. opioid

c. hypnotic

d. analgesic

MEDICAL SPECIALTY CHAPTERS SIMULATED FINAL TEST ANSWER KEY

SFT.1. C
SFT.2. D
SFT.3. B
SFT.4. B
SFT.5. D
SFT.6. B
SFT.7. A
SFT.8. B
SFT.9. A
SFT.10. C
SFT.11. B
SFT.12. B
SFT.13. C
SFT.14. A
SFT.15. C
SFT.16. B
SFT.17. B
SFT.18. C
SFT.19. C
SFT.20. D
SFT.21. B
SFT.22. A
SFT.23. C
SFT.24. C
SFT.25. A
SFT.26. A
SFT.27. B
SFT.28. B
SFT.29. A
SFT.30. A
SFT.31. D
SFT.32. D
SFT.33. B
SFT.34. D
SFT.35. B
SFT.36. A
SFT.37. C
SFT.38. D
SFT.39. C
SFT.40. D
SFT.41. D
SFT.42. C
SFT.43. A
SFT.44. B
SFT.45. A
SFT.46. C
SFT.47. B
SFT.48. A
SFT.49. B
SFT.50. C

Appendix A

PREFIXES, COMBINING FORMS, AND SUFFIXES

Pertaining to

-ac pertaining to
-al pertaining to
-ar pertaining to
-ary pertaining to
-eal pertaining to
-ial pertaining to
-ical pertaining to
-ic pertaining to
-ine pertaining to
-ior pertaining to
-ory pertaining to
-ous pertaining to
-tic pertaining to

Abnormal Conditions

-ago abnormal condition, disease
-esis abnormal condition, disease
-ia abnormal condition, disease
-iasis abnormal condition, disease
-ion condition
-ism condition, state of
-nic pertaining to
-osis abnormal condition, disease

Noun Endings

-a noun ending
-ae plural noun ending
-e noun ending
-i plural noun ending
-um singular noun ending
-us singular noun ending
-y noun ending

A

a-	no, not, without, away from, negative
-a	noun ending
ab-	away from, negative, absent
abdomin/o	abdomen
-able	capable of, able to
abrad/o, **abras/o**	rub or scrape off
abrupt/o	broken away from
abs-	away from
abscess/o	collection of pus
-ac	pertaining to
-acious	characterized by
acous/o, **acoust/o**	hearing, sound
acr/o	extremities (hands and feet), top, extreme point
actin/o	light
acu/o	sharp, severe, sudden
ad-	toward, to, in the direction of
aden/o	gland
adenoid/o	adenoids
adhes/o	stick to, cling to
adip/o	fat
adnex/o	bound to
adren/o, **adrenal/o**	adrenal glands
aer/o	air, gas
af-	toward, to
affect/o	exert influence on
-ago	abnormal condition, disease
agor/a	marketplace
-agra	excessive pain, seizure
-aise	comfort, ease
-al	pertaining to
alb/o, **albin/o**	white
albumin/o	albumin, protein
alg/o, **alges/o**	pain, relationship to pain
-algia	pain, suffering, painful condition
align/o	bring into line or correct position
aliment/o	to nourish
all/o, **all-**	other, different from normal, reversal
alopec/o	baldness
alveol/o	alveolus, air sac, small sac
ambi-	both sides, around or about, double
ambly/o	dull, dim
ambulat/o	walking
-amine	nitrogen compound
amni/o	amnion, amniotic sac
amput/o	cut away, cut off a part of the body
amyl/o	starch, carbohydrate
an-	not, without
ana-	up, apart, excessive
an/o	anus, ring
-an	characteristic of, pertaining to
-ancy	state of
andr/o	male, masculine
aneurysm/o	aneurysm
angi/o	relating to blood or lymph vessels
anis/o	unequal
ankyl/o	crooked, bent, stiff
anomal/o	irregularity
ante-	before, in front of, forward
anter/o	before, front
anti-	against
anxi/o	anxiety, anxious, uneasy
aort/o	aorta
ap-	toward, to
-apheresis	removal
aphth/o	ulcer
apic/o	apex, tip
ap-, **apo-**	separation, away from, opposed, detached
append/o, **appendic/o**	appendix
aque/o	water
-ar	pertaining to
-arche	beginning
areat/o	occurring in patches or circumscribed areas
areol/o	little open space, space around the nipple
-aria	connected with
arter/o, **arteri/o**	artery
arthr/o	joint
articul/o	joint
-ary	pertaining to
as-	toward, to
asbest/o	asbestos
-ase	enzyme
aspir/o, **aspirat/o**	to breathe in
-asthenia	weakness, lack of strength
asthm/o	asthma
astr/o	star, star-shaped
at-	toward, to
atel/o	incomplete, imperfect
ather/o	plaque, fatty substance
-ation	state or action
atri/o	atrium (of the heart)
attenu/o	diluted, weakened
audi/o, **audit/o**	ear, hearing, the sense of hearing

aur/i	ear, hearing
auscult/a, auscult/o	listen
aut/o	self
axill/o	armpit

B

bacteri/o	bacteria (singular, bacterium)
balan/o	glans penis
bar/o	pressure, weight
bas/o	base, opposite of acid (alkaline)
bi-	twice, double, two
bi/o	life
bifid/o	split, divided into two parts
bil/i	bile, gall
bilirubin/o	bilirubin
bin-	two
-blast	embryonic, immature, formative element
blephar/o	eyelid
brachi/o	arm
brachy-	short
brady-	slow
bronchi/o, bronch/o	bronchial tube, bronchus
bronchiol/o	bronchiole, bronchioles
brux/o	grind
bucc/o	cheek
burs/o	bursa, sac of fluid near joint

C

calcane/o	calcaneus, heel bone
calc/i	calcium, lime, the heel
calci-, calc/o	calcium
calcul/o	stone, little stone
cali/o, calic/o	cup-like structure, calyx
calor/i	heat
canth/o	corner of the eye
capill/o	capillary, resembling a hair
capit/o	head
capn/o	carbon dioxide, sooty or smoky appearance
capsul/o	little box
carb/o	carbon
carcin/o	cancerous
cardi/o, card/o	heart
cari/o	caries, tooth decay
carp/o	wrist bones
catabol/o	a breaking down
caud/o	lower part of body, tail
caus/o	burning, burn
cav/o	hollow, cave
cec/o	cecum
-cele	hernia, tumor, swelling
celi/o	abdomen, belly
-centesis	surgical puncture to remove fluid
cephal/o	head
cerebell/o	cerebellum
cerebr/o	cerebrum, brain
cervic/o	neck, cervix (neck of uterus)
cheil/o	lip or lips
chem/o	drug, chemical
chir/o	hand
chol/e	bile, gall
cholangi/o	bile duct
cholecyst/o	gallbladder
choledoch/o	common bile duct
cholesterol/o	cholesterol
chondr/i, chondr/o	cartilage
chori/o, chorion/o	chorion, membrane
choroid/o	choroid layer of eye
chrom/o, chromat/o	color
chron/o	time
-cide	causing death
cili/o	eyelashes
cine-	movement
circulat/o	circulate, go around in a circle
cirrh/o	orange-yellow, tawny
cis/o	to cut
-clasis	break down
claudicat/o	to limp
claustr/o	barrier, enclosed space
clavicul/o, cleid/o	clavicle, collar bone
clon/o	violent action
co-	together, with
coagul/o	clotting, coagulation
coarct/o, coarctat/o	press together, narrow
cocc/o, -cocci	spherical bacteria
coccyg/o	coccyx, tailbone
cochle/o	spiral, snail, snail shell
coit/o	a coming together
col/o	colon, large intestine

coll/a glue
colon/o colon, large intestine
colp/o vagina
com- together, with
comat/o deep sleep
comminut/o break into pieces
communic/o share, to make common
con- together, with
concav/o hollow
concept/o become pregnant
concuss/o shaken together, violently agitated
coni/o dust
constrict/o draw tightly together
contin/o hold together
contra- against, counter, opposite
contus/o bruise
convex/o arched, vaulted
convuls/o pull together
cor/o pupil
cordi/o heart
coron/o coronary, crown
corpor/o body
cortic/o cortex, outer region
cost/o rib
crani/o skull
-crasia a mixture or blending
creatin/o creatinine
crin/o, -crine to secrete
-crit to separate
cry/o cold
crypt/o hidden
cubit/o elbow
culd/o cul-de-sac, blind pouch
-cusis hearing
cusp/o point
cutane/o skin
cyan/o blue
cycl/o ciliary body of eye, cycle
cyst/o urinary bladder, cyst, sac of fluid
cyt/o, -cyte cell

D

dacry/o tear, lacrimal duct (tear duct)
dacryocyst/o lacrimal sac (tear sac)
dactyl/o finger, toe
de- down, lack of, from, not, removal
deci- ten, tenth
decidu/o shedding, falling off
delt/o Greek letter delta, a triangular shape
delus/o delude, cheat
dem/o people, population
demi- half
dendr/o branching, resembling a tree
dent/i, dent/o tooth, teeth
depress/o press down, lower, pressed or sunk down
-derma, dermat/o, derm/o skin
desicc/o drying, to dry
-desis to bind, tie together
dextr/o right side
di- twice, twofold, double
dia-, di- through, between, apart, complete
diaphor/o sweat
diaphragmat/o diaphragm
didym/o testes, twins
digest/o digest, break down (food)
digit/o digit, finger or toe
dilat/o spread out, widen
dipl/o double
dips/o, -dipsia thirst
dis- negative, apart, absence of
dissect/o cutting apart
dist/o far, away from the point of origin
distend/o stretch apart, expand
diverticul/o diverticulum
dors/o back of body
-dote what is given
-drome to run, running
-duct opening
duct/o to lead, carry
duoden/o duodenum, first part of small intestine
dur/o dura mater
-dynia pain
dys- bad, difficult, painful

E

e- out of, from
-e noun ending
-eal pertaining to
ec- out, outside
ecchym/o pouring out of juice or blood
ech/o sound wave, echo
-ectasis stretching, dilation, enlargement
ecto- out, outside
-ectomy surgical removal, cutting out, excision
-ectopy displacement

-edema	swelling
edentul/o	without teeth
ef-	out
effus/o	pouring out
ejaculat/o	throw or hurl out
electr/o	electricity, electric
em-	in
embol/o	something inserted or thrown
embry/o	fertilized ovum, embryo
-emesis	vomiting
emet/o	vomit
-emia	blood, blood condition
en-	in, within, into
encephal/o	brain
end-, endo-	in, within, inside
enter/o	small intestine, digestive tract
ento-	within
epi-	above, upon, on
epididym/o	epididymis
epiglott/o	epiglottis
episi/o	vulva
-er	one who
erect/o	upright
erg/o	work
erupt/o	break out, burst forth
erythem/o, erythemat/o	flushed, redness
erythr/o	red
es-	out of, outside, away from
-esis	abnormal condition, disease
eso-	inward
esophag/o	esophagus
-esthesia	sensation, feeling
esthet/o	feeling, nervous sensation, sense of perception
estr/o	female
ethm/o	sieve, ethmoid bone
eti/o	cause of disease
eu-	good, normal, well, easy
-eurysm	widening
ex-	out of, outside, away from
exacerb/o	aggravate, irritate
excori/o	abrade or scratch
excret/o	separate, discharge
exo-	out of, outside, away from
extern/o	outside, outer
extra-	on the outside, beyond, outside
extrins/o	from the outside, contained outside
exud/o	to sweat, exude fluid

F

faci/o	face, form
fasci/o	fascia, fibrous band
fec/a, fec/o	dregs, sediment, waste
femor/o	femur, thigh bone
fenestr/a	window, small opening
fer/o	to bear, carry
fertil/o	fertile, able to conceive
fet/o	fetus, unborn child
fibr/o	fibrous tissue, fiber
fibrin/o	fibrin, fibers, threads of a clot
fibul/o	fibula
-fic	making, producing, forming
-fication	process of making
-fida	split
filtr/o, filtrat/o	filter, to strain through
fiss/o	crack, split, cleft
flatul/o	flatus, rectal gas
flex/o	bend
fluor/o	glowing, luminous
foc/o	focus, point
follicul/o	follicle, small sac
foramin/o	opening, foramen
fore-	before, in front of
-form, form/o	resembling, in the shape of
fove/o	small pit, depressed area
fract/o	break
front/o	front, forehead
fund/o	bottom, base, fundus
fung/o	fungus
-fusion	to come together

G

galact/o	milk
ganglion/o	ganglion, cluster of nerve cell bodies
gangren/o	tissue death, gangrene
gastr/o	stomach
gemin/o	twin, double, group
gen-, gen/o, -gen	producing, forming
-gene	production, origin, gene
-genic, -genesis	creation, reproduction
genit/o	reproduction, formation
-genous	producing
ger/i, geront/o	old age
germin/o	bud, sprout, embryonic tissue
geront/o	old age
gest/o, gestat/o	pregnancy, gestation to birth

gigant/o	giant, very large
gingiv/o	gingival tissue, gums
glauc/o	gray
glen/o	socket of a joint
gli/o	neurologic cells, supportive tissue of nervous system
-globin	protein
globul/o	shaped like a ball
glomerul/o	glomerulus
glott/o	pertaining to the tongue
gluc/o	glucose, sugar
glyc/o, **glycos/o**	glucose, sugar
glycer/o	sweet
gon/o	seed
gonad/o	gonad, sex glands
goni/o	angle
-gram	a picture or record
granul/o	granule(s), granular
-graph	a picture or record, machine for producing a record
-graphy	the process of producing a picture or record
-gravida	pregnant
gynec/o	woman, female

H

hal/o, **halit/o**	breath
hallucin/o	hallucination
hem/o, **hemat/o**	blood, relating to the blood
hemi-	half
hemoglobin/o	hemoglobin
hepat/o	liver
hered/o, **heredit/o**	inherited, hereditary
herni/o	hernia
hiat/o	opening, gap
hidr/o	sweat
hirsut/o	hairy, rough
hist/o	tissue
hom/o	same, like, alike
home/o	sameness, unchanging, constant
hormon/o	hormone
humer/o	humerus (upper arm bone)
hydr/o	relating to water
hygien/o	health
hyper-	excessive, increased
hypn/o	sleep
hypo-	deficient, decreased
hyster/o	uterus

I

-ia	abnormal condition, disease, also the plural of a singular noun ending -ium
-ial	pertaining to
-iasis	abnormal condition, disease
-iatrics	field of medicine, healing
-iatrist	specialist
-iatry	field of medicine
-ible	capable of, able to
-ic	pertaining to
-ical	pertaining to
-ician	specialist
icter/o	jaundice
idi/o	peculiar to one individual or organ, unknown
-iferous	bearing, carrying, producing
-ific	making, producing
-iform	shaped or formed like, resembling
-ile	capable of
ile/o	ileum, small intestine
ili/o	ilium, hip bone
im-	not
immun/o	immune, protection, safe
impact/o	pushed against, wedged against, packed
in-	in, into, not, without
-in	a substance or chemical
incis/o	cutting into
-ine	pertaining to, or a substance or chemical
infarct/o	filled in, stuffed
infect/o	infected, tainted
infer/o	below, beneath
inflammat/o	flame within, set on fire
infra-	below, beneath, inferior to
inguin/o	groin
inject/o	to force or put in, insert
insul/o	island
insulin/o	insulin
inter-	between, among
intern/o	within, inside
intestin/o	intestine
intra-	within, inside
intrins/o	contained within, on the inside
intro-	within, into, inside
intussuscept/o	take up or receive within
iod/o	iodine
-ion	condition, action, process, state
ion/o	ion, to wander

-ior	pertaining to
-is	noun ending
ir/i, **ir/o**, **irid/o**, **irit/o**	iris, colored part of eye
isch	to hold back
ischi/o	ischium (hip bone)
-ismus	spasm, contraction
-ism	condition, state of
iso-	equal, same
-ist	a person who practices, specialist
-isy	noun ending
-itis	inflammation
-ium	structure, tissue
-ive	performs, tends toward
-ize	to make, to treat

J

jejun/o	jejunum
jugul/o	throat
juxta-	beside, near, nearby

K

kary/o	nucleus, nut
kel/o	growth, tumor
kerat/o	horny, hard, cornea
ket/o, **keton/o**	ketones, acetones
kines/o, **kinesi/o**	movement
-kinesis	movement
klept/o	to steal
kyph/o	bent, hump

L

labi/o	lip, labium
labyrinth/o	maze, labyrinth, the inner ear
lacer/o	torn, mangled
lacrim/o	tears, tear duct
lact/i, **lact/o**	milk
lamin/o	lamina, posterior portion of a vertebra
lapar/o	abdomen, abdominal wall
laryng/o	larynx, throat
later/o	side
lei/o	smooth
lent/o	the lens of the eye
lenticul/o	lens, shaped like a lens
-lepsy	seizure
-leptic	to seize, take hold of
leuk/o	white
lev/o	raise, lift
lex/o, **-lexia**	word, phrase
ligament/o	ligament
ligat/o	binding or tying off
lingu/o	tongue
lipid/o, **lip/o**	fat, lipid
-listhesis	slipping
lith/o, **-lith**	stone, calculus
-lithiasis	presence of stones
lob/o	lobe, well-defined part of an organ
loc/o	place
loch	childbirth
-logy, **-log**	study of
lord/o	curve, swayback, bent
lumb/o	lumbar, lower back, loin
lumin/o	light, lumen
lun/o	moon
lymph/o	lymph, lymphatic tissue, lymphatic system
lymphaden/o	lymph node or gland
lymphangi/o	lymph vessel
-lysis	set free, breakdown, decomposition, destruction, loosening
-lyst	agent that causes lysis or loosening
-lytic	to reduce, destroy

M

macro-	large, abnormal size or length, long
macul/o	spot
mal-	bad, abnormal
-malacia	abnormal softening
malign/o	bad, harmful
malle/o	malleus, hammer
malleol/o	malleolus, little hammer
mamm/o	breast
manu/o	hand
mandibul/o	mandible, lower jaw
-mania	obsessive preoccupation, madness
mast/o	breast, mastoid process
mastic/o	chew
mastoid/o	mastoid process
matur/o	ripe, mature
maxill/o	maxilla (upper jaw)
meat/o	urethral meatus
medi/o	middle
mediastin/o	mediastinum, middle
medic/o	medicine, physician, healing
medull/o	medulla (inner section), middle, marrow
mega-, **megal/o**	large, great
-megaly	enlargement

melan/o black, dark
men/o menstruation, month
mening/o, meningi/o membranes, meninges
menisc/o meniscus, crescent-shaped
menstru/o menstruation
ment/o mind, chin
mesenter/o mesentery
mesi/o middle, median plane
meso- middle
meta- change, beyond, subsequent to, behind, after
metabol/o change
-meter measure, instrument used to measure
metr/o, metri/o uterus
-metrist one who measures
-metry to measure
micr/o, micro- small
mictur/o urinate
mid- middle
milli- one-thousandth
mineral/o mineral
mio- smaller, less
-mission to send
mit/o thread, thread-like
mitr/o like a miter, i.e. having two points on top
-mnesia memory
mobil/o capable of moving, movement
mono- one, single
morbid/o disease, sickness
morph/o shape, form
mort/o death, dead
mot/o, motil/o motion, movement
muc/o, mucos/o mucus
multi- many, much
muscul/o muscle
mutat/o to change
my/o muscle
myc/o fungus
mydr/o widening
myel/o spinal cord, bone marrow
myos/o muscle
myring/o tympanic membrane, eardrum
myx/o mucus

N

narc/o numbness, stupor, sleep
nas/o nose
nat/o birth, born
necr/o death
-necrosis tissue death
neo-, ne/o new, strange
nephr/o kidney
nerv/o, neur/i, neur/o nerve, nerve tissue
neutr/o neither, neutral
-nic pertaining to
nitro- nitrogen
noct/o night
nod/o knot, swelling, node
nodul/o little knot or node
non- no, not
nor- chemical compound
norm/o normal or usual
nucle/o nucleus
nucleol/o little nucleus, nucleolus
nulli- none
nutri/o nourishment, food, nourish, feed

O

ob- against
obes/o obese, extremely fat
obstetr/o pregnancy, birth
occipit/o back of the skull, occiput
-occult hidden
ocul/o eye
odont/o tooth
-oid like, resembling
olfact/o smell, sense of smell
olig/o scanty, few
-ologist specialist
-ology the science or study of
-oma tumor, neoplasm
omphal/o umbilicus, the navel
onc/o tumor
-one hormone
onych/o fingernail or toenail
o/o egg
oophor/o ovary
-opaque obscure, not transparent
operat/o perform, operate
ophthalm/o eye, vision
-opia vision condition
-opsia vision, view of
-opsy a view of
opt/i, opt/o, optic/o eye, vision
or/o mouth, oral cavity

orch/o, **orchid/o**, **orchi/o** testicles, testis, testes
-orexia appetite
organ/o organ
orth/o straight, normal, correct
-ory pertaining to
os- mouth, bone
-ose full of, pertaining to, sugar
-osis abnormal condition, disease
-osmia smell, odor
oss/e, **oss/i** bone
ossicul/o ossicle (small bone)
oste/o, **ost/o** bone
-ostomy the surgical creation of an artificial opening to the body surface
ot/o ear, hearing
-otomy cutting, surgical incision
-ous pertaining to
ov/i, **ov/o** egg, ovum
ovari/o ovary
ovul/o egg, ovum
ox/i, **ox/o**, **ox/y** oxygen

P

palat/o palate, roof of mouth
palpat/o touch, feel, stroke
palpit/o throbbing, quivering
pan- all, entire, every
pancreat/o pancreas
papill/o nipple-like, optic disc
par-, **para-** beside, near, beyond, abnormal, apart from, opposite, along side of, outside, around
par/o birth
-para to give birth
parathyroid/o parathyroid glands
-paresis partial or incomplete paralysis
-pareunia coitus, sexual intercourse
-parous having borne one or more children
paroxysm/o sudden attack
-partum childbirth, labor
patell/o patella, kneecap
path/o, **-pathy** disease, suffering, feeling, emotion
-pause stopping
pector/o chest
ped/o child, foot
pedicul/o louse (singular), lice (plural)
pelv/i, **pelv/o** pelvic bone, pelvic cavity, hip
pen/i penis
-penia deficiency, lack, too few
-pepsia, **pept/o** to digest, digestion
per- completely, through
percuss/o strike, tap, beat
peri- surrounding, around
perine/o perineum
peritone/o peritoneum
perme/o to pass or go through
perone/o fibula
-pexy surgical fixation
phac/o, **phak/o** lens of eye
phag/o eat, swallow
-phage a cell that destroys, eat, swallow
-phagia eating, swallowing
phalang/o phalanges, finger, toe
phall/i penis
pharmac/o, **pharmaceut/o** drug
pharyng/o throat, pharynx
phas/o speech
-phasia speak, speech
phe/o dusky, gray
-pheresis removal
-philia, **phil/o** attraction to, like, love
phleb/o vein
-phobia abnormal fear
phon/o sound, voice
phor/o carry, bear, movement
-phoresis carrying, transmission
-phoria to bear, carry, feeling, mental state
phot/o light
phren/o diaphragm, mind
-phylactic protective, preventive
-phylaxis protection
physi/o nature, physical
-physis to grow
pigment/o pigment, color
pil/i, **pil/o** hair
pineal/o pineal gland
pinn/i external ear, auricle
pituit/o, **pituitar/o** pituitary gland
placent/o placenta
plak/o, **-plakia** plaque, plate, thin flat layer or scale
plant/i, **plant/o** sole of foot
plas/i, **plas/o**, **-plasia** development, growth, formation
-plasm formative material of cells, formation
plasm/o something molded or formed
plasma, **plasm/o** something molded or formed, plasma
-plastic pertaining to formation
-plasty surgical repair

-plegia	paralysis, stroke
-plegic	one affected with paralysis
pleur/o	pleura, side of the body
pne/o	breath, breathing
-pnea	breathing
pneum/o, pneumon/o	lung, air
pod/o	foot
-poiesis	to make
poli/o	gray matter of brain and spinal cord
poly-	many
polyp/o	polyp, small growth
poplite/o	back of the knee
por/o	pore, small opening
-porosis	lessening in density, porous condition
port/o	gate, door
post-	after, behind
poster/o	behind, toward the back
potent/o	powerful, capable
pract/o	practice, pursue an occupation
pre-	before, in front of
pregn/o	pregnant, full of
presby/o	old age
primi-	first
pro-	before, on behalf of, supporting
proct/o	anus and rectum
product/o	lead forward, yield, produce
pronat/o	bent forward, face down
pros-	before, forward
prostat/o	prostate gland
prosthet/o	addition, appendage
prot/o, proto-	first, original
protein/o	protein
proxim/o	near
prurit/o	itching
pseud/o	false
psor/o	itch, itching
psych/o	mind
-ptosis	droop, sag, prolapse, fall
-ptysis	spitting, coughing up
pub/o	pubis, part of hip bone
pulm/o, pulmon/o	lung
pulsat/o	beat, beating, striking
punct/o	hole, prick, puncture
pupill/o	pupil (of the eye)
purul/o	pus, pus-filled
py/o	pus
pyel/o	renal pelvis, bowl of kidney
pyr/o, pyret/o	fever, fire

Q

quadr/i, quadr/o	four

R

radi/o	radiation, x-rays, radius (lateral lower arm bone)
radicul/o	root, nerve root
re-	back, again
recept/o	receive, receiver
rect/o	rectum, straight
reduct/o	bring back together
refract/o	bend back, turn aside
remiss/o	give up, send back, relax
ren/o	kidney
resuscit/o	to revive
retent/o	hold back
reticul/o	network
retin/o	retina (of the eye), net
retro-	behind, backward, back of
rhabdomy/o	striated (skeletal) muscle
rheumat/o	watery flow, subject to flow
rhin/o	nose
rhiz/o	root, spinal nerve root
rhythm/o	rhythm
rhytid/o	wrinkle
-rrhage, -rrhagia	abnormal excessive fluid discharge
-rrhaphy	surgical suturing
-rrhea	flow, discharge
-rrhexis	rupture
rug/o	wrinkle, fold, ruga

S

sacchar/o	sugar
sacr/o	sacrum
saliv/o	saliva
salping/o	fallopian (uterine) tube, auditory (eustachian) tube
-salpinx	fallopian (uterine) tube
saphen/o	clear, apparent, manifest
sarc/o	flesh, connective tissue
schiz/o	division, to split
scler/o	sclera (white of the of eye), hard
-sclerosis	abnormal hardening
scoli/o	curved, bent
-scope	instrument for visual examination
-scopic	pertaining to visual examination
-scopy	visual examination

script/o	write
scrot/o	bag or pouch, scrotum
seb/o	sebum
secret/o	produce, separate out
sect/o	cut, cutting
semi-	half
semin/i	semen, seed, sperm
sen/o	old age
sens/o	feeling, sensation
sensitiv/o	sensitive to, affected by
sept/o	infection, partition, septum
ser/o	serum
sigmoid/o	sigmoid colon
silic/o	glass
sin/o	hollow, sinus
sinistr/o	left, left side
sinus/o	sinus
-sis	abnormal condition, disease
sit/u	place
soci/o	companion, fellow being
-sol	solution
somat/o	body
somn/o	sleep
son/o	sound
-spasm, **spasmod/o**	sudden involuntary contraction, tightening, cramping
sperm/o, **spermat/o**	sperm, spermatozoa, seed
sphen/o	sphenoid bone, wedge-shaped
spher/o	round, sphere, ball
sphincter/o	tight band, sphincter
sphygm/o	pulse
spin/o	spine, backbone
spir/o	to breathe, coil
splen/o	spleen
spondyl/o	vertebrae, vertebral column, backbone
squam/o	scale, scale-like cell
-stalsis	contraction, constriction
staped/o	stapes (middle ear bone)
staphyl/o	clusters, bunch of grapes
-stasis, **-static**	control, maintenance of a constant level
steat/o	fat, lipid, sebum
sten/o	narrowing, contracted
-stenosis	abnormal narrowing, tightening
stere/o	solid, three-dimensional
stern/o	sternum (breast bone)
steth/o	chest
-sthenia	strength
stigmat/o	point, spot
stimul/o	goad, prick, incite
stom/o, **stomat/o**	mouth, oral cavity
-stomosis, **-stomy**	furnish with a mouth or outlet, new opening
strept/o	twisted chain, curved
styl/o	pen, pointed instrument, stake
sub-	under, less, below
sucr/o	sugar
sud/o, **sudor/i**	sweat
super-	above, excessive, higher than
supinat/o	bent backward, lying on the back
suppress/o	press down
suppur/o	to form pus
supra-	above, upper, excessive
-surgery	operative procedure
sym-	with, together, joined together
symptomat/o	falling together, symptom(s)
syn-	together, with, union, association
syncop/o	to cut short, cut off, faint
synovi/o, **synov/o**	synovial membrane, synovial fluid
system/o	body system, body as a whole
systol/o, **-systole**	contraction, contracting

T

tachy-	fast, rapid
tars/o	tarsus (ankle bone), tarsal plate (on the edge of the eyelid)
tax/o	coordination, order
techn/o	skill
tel/e	distant, remote
tempor/o	temporal bone, temple (on head)
ten/o, **tend/o**	tendon, stretch out, extend, strain
tendin/o	tendon
tens/o	stretch out, extend, tension
termin/o	end, limit
test/i	testicle, testis
tetra-	four
thalam/o	thalamus
thanat/o	death
thec/o	sheath, case
therapeut/o	treatment
-therapy	treatment
therm/o	heat
thor/a, **thorac/o**	chest, thorax
-thorax	chest, pleural cavity
thromb/o	clot, thrombus
thym/o	thymus gland
-thymia	a state of mind
thyr/o, **thyroid/o**	thyroid gland

tibi/o	tibia (shin bone)
-tic	pertaining to
till/o	hair
-tion	process, state or quality of
toc/o, -tocin	labor, birth
tom/o	cut, section, slice
-tomy	process of cutting
ton/o	tension, tone, stretching
tonsill/o	tonsil, throat
tort/i	twisted
tox/o, toxic/o	poison, poisonous, toxin
trabecul/o	little beam or cross bar, mesh
trache/o	trachea, windpipe
tract/o	draw, pull, path, bundle of nerve fibers
tranquil/o	quiet, calm, tranquil
trans-	across, through
traumat/o	injury
tremul/o	fine tremor, shaking
tri-	three
trich/o	hair
-tripsy	to crush
trop/o	to turn, change
troph/o, -trophy	development, nourishment
-tropia	to turn
-tropic	affinity for
-tropin	to stimulate, act on
tub/o	tube, pipe
tubercul/o	little knot, swelling, tuberculosis
tuss/o	cough
tympan/o	tympanic membrane, eardrum
-type	classification, picture

U

-ula	small, little
-ule	small one, little
uln/o	ulna (medial lower arm bone)
ultra-	beyond, excess
-um	singular noun ending
umbilic/o	navel
un-	not
ungu/o	nail
uni-	one
ur/o	urine, urinary tract
-uresis	urination
ureter/o	ureter
urethr/o	urethra
-uria	urination, urine
urin/o	urine or urinary organs
urtic/o	nettle, rash, hives
-us	thing, singular noun ending
uter/o	uterus
uve/o	iris, choroid, ciliary body (of the eye)

V

vaccin/o	vaccine
vag/o	vagus nerve, wandering
vagin/o	vagina
valv/o, valvul/o	valve
varic/o	varicose veins, swollen or dilated vein
vas/o	vas deferens, blood vessel
vascul/o	blood vessel, little vessel
ven/o	vein
ventilat/o	expose to air, oxygenate
ventr/o	in front, abdomen side of body
ventricul/o	ventricle of brain or heart, small chamber
vener/o, venere/o	venereal, sexual intercourse
-verse, -version	to turn
vers/o, vert/o	turn, travel
vertebr/o	vertebra, backbone
vertig/o	whirling round
vesic/o	urinary bladder
vesicul/o	seminal vesicle, blister, little bladder
vestibul/o	entrance, vestibule (of the inner ear)
vir/o	virus, poison
viril/o	masculine, manly
vis/o	seeing, sight, vision
viscer/o	viscera, internal organ
viscos/o	sticky, thickness
vit/a	life
vitre/o	glassy, vitreous humor (of the eye)
vulv/o	vulva, covering

X

xanth/o	yellow
xen/o	strange, foreign
xer/o	dry
xiph/o	sword-shaped

Y

-y	noun ending

Z

zoo, zo/o	(animal) life
zygomat/o	cheek bone

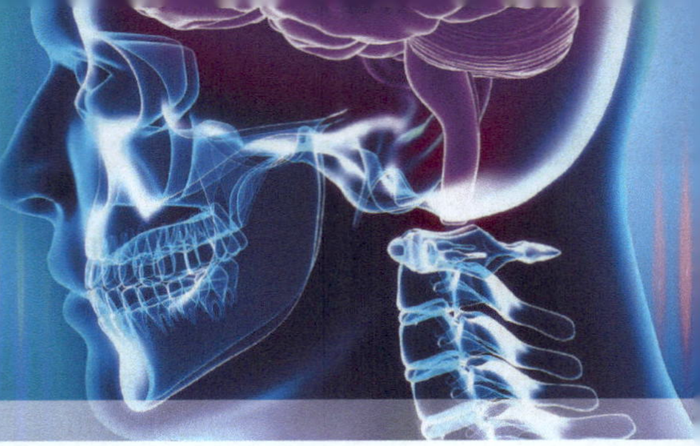

Appendix B

ABBREVIATIONS AND THEIR MEANINGS

Reminder about abbreviations: An abbreviation can have several meanings, and a term can have several abbreviations. When in doubt, always verify the meaning of the abbreviation!

A

Abbreviation	Meaning
A	abnormal; allergy; anterior
a	accommodation; acid; artery
ā	before
aa	amino acid
AA	alopecia areata; asthma; asthmatic
AAA	abdominal aortic aneurysm
AAP	American Academy of Pediatrics
AB	abortion
Ab	antibody
ABC	aspiration, biopsy, and cytology; airway, breathing, and circulation
Abd	abdomen
ABG	arterial blood gas [analysis]
ABP	arterial blood pressure
abx	antibiotics
AC	anticoagulant; adrenal cortex; air conduction; antecubital
ac, a.c.	before meals (Latin *ante cibum*) (*use with caution* due to possible confusion with other meanings of **AC**)
acc.	accommodation
ACE	angiotensin-converting enzyme
ACG	angle closure glaucoma
ACH	adrenocortical hormone
ACL	anterior cruciate ligament
ACLS	advanced cardiac life support
ACT	anticoagulant therapy; acceptance and commitment therapy
ACTH	adrenocorticotropic hormone
ACU	acute care unit; ambulatory care unit
ACVD	acute cardiovascular disease
AD	atopic dermatitis; advance directive; Alzheimer's disease; right ear (*use with caution* due to possible confusion with **OD**, right eye)
ad.	add, let there be added (Latin *addatur*)
ADAM	androgen decline in the aging male
ADD	attention deficit disorder
ADH	adhesion; antidiuretic hormone
ADHD	attention deficit/hyperactivity disorder
ADL	activities of daily life, activities of daily living
ad lib.	as desired (Latin *ad libitum*)
adm	admission, admitted
ADR	adverse drug reaction
ADT	admission, discharges, and transfers
AE	above elbow; adverse event; acute exacerbation
AED	automated external defibrillator
AF	acid-fast; amniotic fluid; atrial flutter
A-Fib, AF	atrial fibrillation
Ag	antigen
AH	abdominal hysterectomy
AI	aortic insufficiency; artificial insemination
AICD	automated implantable cardioverter-defibrillator
AIDS	acquired immunodeficiency syndrome
AK	above knee; actinic keratosis
alb	albumin
ALD	aldosterone; assistive listening device

ALF assisted living facility
alk alkaline
ALL acute lymphoblastic leukemia; acute lymphocytic leukemia
ALLO allogeneic (transplant)
ALM acral lentiginous melanoma
ALND axillary lymph node dissection
ALOC altered level of consciousness
ALS amyotrophic lateral sclerosis; advanced life support
alt. dieb. every other day (Latin *alternis diebus*)
alt. hor. every other hour (Latin *alternis horis*)
alt. noc. every other night (Latin *alternis noctibus*)
a.m. morning (Latin *ante meridiem*)
AMA advanced maternal age; American Medical Association; against medical advice
amb ambulance; ambulatory
AMD age-related macular degeneration
AMI acute myocardial infarction
AML acute myeloid leukemia
AMN amniocentesis
amp ampule; amputation
AMS altered mental status
amt amount
AN aneurysm; anorexia nervosa
ANA anaphylaxis
anat anatomy; anatomic
anes anesthesia; anesthetic
ANS autonomic nervous system
ant. anterior
Anti-VEGF anti-vascular endothelial growth factor [therapy]
ANUG acute necrotizing ulcerative gingivitis
A & O alert and oriented
AOM acute otitis media
A & P anatomy and physiology; auscultation and percussion
AP abruptio placenta; angina pectoris; anterior-posterior
a.p. before a meal (Latin *ante prandium*)
APAP acetaminophen (chemical name *N-acetyl-para-aminophenol*); automatic positive airway pressure [machine]
APD automated peritoneal dialysis
Aph aphasia
app, appx appendix
appy appendectomy
aq aqueous; water
AR abnormal record; artificial respiration; acoustic reflectometry
ARB angiotensin-II receptor blocker
ARDS acute respiratory distress syndrome
ARF acute renal failure; acute respiratory failure
ARFID avoidant restrictive food intake disorder
ARI acute renal insufficiency
ART antiretroviral therapy; arthritis; assisted reproductive technology; androgen replacement therapy
AS ankylosing spondylitis; aortic stenosis; astigmatism; left ear (Latin *auris sinistra*) (*use with caution* due to possible confusion with **OS** left eye)
ASA aspirin (acetylsalicylic acid)
ASCVD atherosclerotic cardiovascular disease
ASD autism spectrum disorder; atrial septal defect
ASHD atherosclerotic heart disease, coronary artery disease
AT Achilles tendon; alopecia totalis
ATC around the clock; Anatomical Therapeutic Chemical [classification system]
AU both ears (Latin *aures unitas*); alopecia universalis
AUSC auscultation
AUTO autologous (transplant)
AV aortic valve; artificial ventilation; atrioventricular [node]
AVM arteriovenous malformation
A & W alive and well
Ax axillary

B

b. bone
BA bronchial asthma
Ba barium
BAC blood alcohol concentration
BACT, bact bacteria, bacterium
BAE barium enema
BAHA bone-anchored hearing aid
bas basophils
BBB bundle branch block
B & C board and care [facility]
BC bone conduction
BCC basal cell carcinoma
BD bronchodilator; bipolar disorder
BDT bone density testing
BE barium enema; below elbow
BED binge eating disorder
BG blood glucose

bid, b.i.d.	twice a day (Latin *bis in die*)
B, bil	bilateral
BiPAP	bilevel positive airway pressure [machine]
BK	below the knee
Bld	blood
BM	bone marrow; bowel movement; breast milk
BMB, BMBx	bone marrow biopsy
BMD	Becker muscular dystrophy; bone mineral density [testing]
BMI	body mass index
BMP	basic metabolic panel
BMR	basal metabolic rate
BMT	bone marrow transplant
BOM	bilateral otitis media
BP	blood pressure; Bell's palsy
BPD	borderline personality disorder; bronchopulmonary dysplasia
BPH	benign prostatic hyperplasia
bpm	beats per minute
BPP	biophysical profile test
BPPV	benign paroxysmal positional vertigo
BRBPR	bright red blood per rectum
BRCA1	**BR**east **CA**ncer **1** [genes]
BRCA2	**BR**east **CA**ncer **2** [genes]
BS	blood sugar; bowel sounds; breath sounds
BSE	breast self-examination
BSO	bilateral salpingo-oophorectomy
BTE	behind the ear [hearing aid]
BUN	blood urea nitrogen [test]
BV	bacterial vaginosis; blood volume
BVM	bag valve mask
BW	birth weight; blood work [tests]
Bx	biopsy

C

C1 through C7	cervical vertebrae
C	centigrade; cholesterol; convergence; cyanosis; chlamydia; cup
c	centimeter; circa
$\bar{c}$	with
Ca	calcium
CA, Ca	cancer; cardiac arrest; carcinoma; chronological age
CAB	coronary artery bypass
CABG	coronary artery bypass graft
CAD	coronary artery disease
cal	calorie
CAM	complementary and alternative medicine
CAP	community-acquired pneumonia
cap	capsule
CAPD	continuous ambulatory peritoneal dialysis
CAT scan	computed axial tomography
cath	catheter; catheterization; catheterize
caut	cauterization
CBC, cbc	complete blood count
CBI	continuous bladder irrigation
CBR	complete bed rest
CBT	cognitive behavioral therapy
CC	chief complaint; cardiac catheterization
cc	cubic centimeter (1/1,000 liter)
CCPD	continuous cycling peritoneal dialysis
CCT	computed cranial tomography; critical care transport
CCU	coronary care unit
CD	communicable disease; contact dermatitis; Crohn's disease
CDC	Centers for Disease Control and Prevention
CDE	certified diabetes educator
C. diff	*Clostridium difficile* infection
CEA	carotid endarterectomy
CEPH	cephalic
CF	cystic fibrosis
CFS	chronic fatigue syndrome
CGM	continuous glucose monitoring
CH	chromosome
CHD	coronary heart disease
CHDs	congenital heart defects
CHF	congestive heart failure
CHO	carbohydrate
chol	cholesterol
chole	cholecystectomy
chr	chromosome; chronic
CI	conjunctivitis; coronary insufficiency
cib	food (Latin *cibus*)
CIC	completely in the canal [hearing aid]
CIRC, circum	circumcision
CIS	carcinoma in situ
ck	check
CKD	chronic kidney disease
Cl, cl	clinic; chloride; chlorine
CL	cholelithiasis; chronic leukemia; cirrhosis of the liver; corpus luteum

CLL chronic lymphocytic leukemia
cl liq clear liquid
CMP comprehensive metabolic panel
cm centimeter
CM certified midwife
CMA certified medical assistant
CML chronic myeloid leukemia
CMT certified medication technician
CMV cytomegalovirus
CNA certified nursing assistant
CNM certified nurse midwife
CNS central nervous system
c/o complaining of; in care of
CO carbon monoxide; cardiac output
CO_2 carbon dioxide
COD cause of death
COH carbohydrate
comp compound; compounded of
cond condition
cong. congenital
cont. continue
contra against
COPD chronic obstructive pulmonary disease
CP cerebral palsy; cleft palate
CPAP continuous positive airway pressure [machine]
CPB cardiopulmonary bypass
CPR cardiopulmonary resuscitation
CPS cycles per second
CPSS Cincinnati Prehospital Stroke Scale
CR closed reduction; complete response; conditioned reflex
CRC colorectal cancer
CRD chronic respiratory disease; chronic renal disease
CRF chronic renal failure
CRN creatinine
CRP C-reactive protein [test]
CRPS complex regional pain syndrome
CRYO cryosurgery
CS Cushing's syndrome; cesarean section
CSB Cheyne–Stokes breathing
C-section cesarean section
CSF cerebrospinal fluid
CSR Cheyne–Stokes respiration
CST contraction stress test
CT computed tomography; calcitonin
CTA computed tomography angiography
CTG cardiotocography
CTR carpal tunnel release
CTS carpal tunnel syndrome
CV cardiovascular
CVA cerebrovascular accident
CVD cardiovascular disease
CVI chronic venous insufficiency
CVP central venous pressure
CVS chorionic villus sampling; cardiovascular system
Cx cervix
CXR chest x-ray
cysto cystoscopy

D

D diopter; dorsal; density; dose (Latin *dosis*)
DASH diet Dietary Approaches to Stop Hypertension diet
dB decibel
DBP diastolic blood pressure
DBS deep brain stimulation
DBT dialectical behavior therapy
D & C dilation and curettage
DC Doctor of Chiropractic
D/C, dc discharge; discontinue (*use with caution* due to possible confusion between the two meanings)
DCIS ductal carcinoma in situ
DD, DDx differential diagnosis
DDH developmental dysplasia of the hip
DDS Doctor of Dental Surgery, dentist
debr debridement
del delivery
DEXA dual energy x-ray absorptiometry (see also **DXA**)
Dg, dg, DG diagnosis (see also **DX**)
DGE delayed gastric emptying
DI diabetes insipidus
DID dissociative identity disorder
disch discharge
DJD degenerative joint disease
DKA diabetic ketoacidosis
dl deciliter
DM diabetes mellitus
DMD Duchenne muscular dystrophy; Doctor of Medical Dentistry
DMDD disruptive mood dysregulation disorder
DME durable medical equipment
DNA deoxyribonucleic acid

DNC	dermatology nurse certified
DNR	do not resuscitate
DNS	deviated nasal septum
DO	Doctor of Osteopathy
DOA	dead on arrival
DOB	date of birth
DOC	date of conception
DOE	dyspnea on exertion
DP	Doctor of Podiatry
DPT	Doctor of Physical Therapy
DQ	developmental quotient
DR	diabetic retinopathy; digital radiography; doctor
dr.	dram
DRE	digital rectal exam
DSA	digital subtraction angiography
dsg	dressing
DSM, DSM-5	*The Diagnostic and Statistical Manual of Mental Disorders, 5th Edition*
DT	diphtheria/tetanus [vaccine]
DTaP	diphtheria/tetanus/acellular pertussis [vaccine] (see also **Tdap**)
DTR	deep tendon reflex
DTs	delirium tremens
du	decubitus ulcer
DUB	dysfunctional uterine bleeding
DVT	deep vein thrombosis
D/W	dextrose in water
Dx	diagnosis
DXA	dual x-ray absorptiometry (see also **DEXA**)

E

E	enema; etiology; estrogen; eye
EBL	estimated blood loss
EBV	Epstein-Barr virus
ECG, EKG	electrocardiogram; electrocardiography
ECHO	echocardiogram; echocardiography
E. coli	*Escherichia coli* bacteria
ECT	electroconvulsive therapy
Ecz	eczema
ED	effective dose; emergency department; erectile dysfunction
EDA	epidural anesthesia
EDB	epidural block
EDC	electrodesiccation and curettage
EDD	estimated date of delivery
EECG, EEG	electroencephalography
EENT	eye, ear, nose, and throat
EFM	electronic fetal monitoring
EGD	esophagogastroduodenoscopy, upper GI endoscopy
EIA	enzyme immunosorbent assay
EKG, ECG	electrocardiogram; electrocardiography
ELBW	extremely low birth weight
ELISA	enzyme-linked immunosorbent assay
EM, em	electron microscope; emmetropia; erythema multiforme
emb	embolism
EMDR	eye movement desensitization and reprocessing
EMG	electromyogram; electromyography
EMP	emphysema
EMR	electronic medical record
EMS	emergency medical services
EMT	emergency medical technician
EN	enteral nutrition
Endo	endometriosis; endocrine
ENT	ear, nose, and throat [specialist]
EOM	extraocular muscles
EOS	eosinophils
EP	ectopic pregnancy
Epi, EPI	epinephrine
epi, epil	epilepsy
epid	epidemic
epis	episiotomy
ER	emergency room
ER+	estrogen receptor-positive [breast cancer]
ERCP	endoscopic retrograde cholangiopancreatography
ERPF	effective renal plasma flow
ERT	estrogen replacement therapy; external radiation therapy
ESPF	end-stage pulmonary fibrosis
ESR	erythrocyte sedimentation rate
ESRD	end-stage renal disease
ESWL	extracorporeal shockwave lithotripsy
ET	embryo transfer; eustachian tube
ETI	endotracheal intubation
ETT	endotracheal tube; exercise tolerance testing; exercise treadmill test
EU	emergency unit
EV	esophageal varices
ex	excision; exercise
exam	examination
exp	expiration
ext	extraction; external
Ez, Ecz	eczema

F

F	Fahrenheit; female
FA	fluorescein angiography
FAS	fetal alcohol syndrome
FB	foreign body
FBD	fibrocystic breast disease
FBS	fasting blood sugar [test]
FESS	functional endoscopic sinus surgery
fet	fetus
FH	family history
fld.	fluid
FHR	fetal heart rate
fl oz	fluid ounce
Fluor	fluoroscopy
fMRI	functional magnetic resonance imaging
FMT	fecal microbiota transplantation
FNA	fine-needle aspiration
FOBT	fecal occult blood test
FP	family practice; family practitioner
FPG	fasting plasma glucose
Fr	French (gauge for catheter size)
FROM	full range of motion
FS	frozen section; fluoroscopy
FSH	follicle-stimulating hormone
FT	family therapy; foot
FTT	failure to thrive
FU, f/u	follow up
FUO	fever of unknown origin
Fx	fracture

G

G	gingiva; glycogen; gravida (pregnant)
g	gram (see also **gm**)
GA	general anesthesia; gestational age
GABA	gamma-aminobutryic acid
GAD	generalized anxiety disorder
GB	gallbladder
GBS	Guillain–Barré syndrome
GBS test	group B strep test
GC	gonorrhea
GCG	glucagon
GCs	glucocorticoids
GCS	Glasgow coma scale
GD	Graves' disease; gender dysphoria
GDM	gestational diabetes mellitus
GE	gastroenteritis
GER	gastroesophageal reflux
GERD	gastroesophageal reflux disease
GFR	glomerular filtration rate
GH	growth hormone
GI	gastrointestinal [tract]
GLTT	glucose tolerance test
gm	gram (see also **g**)
GN	glomerulonephritis
GP	general practitioner
gr	grain
grav	gravida (pregnant)
GS	general surgery
GT	glucose tolerance [test]
gtt	drops, drip (Latin *guttae*)
GU	genitourinary
GVHD	graft-versus-host disease
GYN, Gyn	gynecology; gynecologist

H

H	hydrogen; hypodermic; hyperopia
h, hr	hour
H & H	hemoglobin and hematocrit [test]
H & P	history and physical [examination]
HA	hemolytic anemia; histamine
halluc	hallucination
HAV	hepatitis virus
HB	heart block; hepatitis B
Hb	hemoglobin
HBOC	hereditary breast & ovarian cancer syndrome
HBO, HBOT	hyperbaric oxygen therapy
HBP	high blood pressure
HBV	hepatitis B virus
HCG	human chorionic gonadotropin
HCl	hydrochloric acid
HCP	health care proxy [legal document]
HCT	hematocrit
HCV	hepatitis C virus
HD	heart disease; hemodialysis; Huntington's disease
HDL	high-density lipoprotein
HE	hyperextension
He	helium; hemorrhage
HEENT	head, eyes, ears, nose, throat
HELLP	hemolysis, elevated liver enzymes, low platelet count [syndrome]
HEM, hemo	hemophilia; hemodialysis
hemi	hemiplegia

HepA hepatitis A [vaccine]
HepB hepatitis B [vaccine]
HER2+ HER2 protein positive [breast cancer]
HF heart failure
Hg chemical element mercury
Hgb hemoglobin
HH hiatal hernia
Hi, his histamine
Hib haemophilus influenzae type b [vaccine]
HIS histology
HIV human immunodeficiency virus
HL Hodgkin's lymphoma
HM hand motion; Holter monitor
HMO health maintenance organization
HO hyperbaric oxygen
HOB head of bed
HP hyperparathyroidism
HPN hypertension
HPV human papillomavirus
HR heart rate; hazard ratio
hr hour
HRT hormone replacement therapy
HS hamstring; herpes simplex; hospital stay
hs at bedtime; hour of sleep (*use with caution* due to confusion with *half strength*)
HSCT hematopoietic stem cell transplant
HSG hysterosalpingogram; hysterosalpingography
HSV herpes simplex virus
HT Hashimoto's thyroiditis; hormone therapy
ht height; hematocrit
HTN hypertension
HV hallux valgus
HVD hypertensive vascular disease
HVT hyperventilation
Hx history [of]
hypo hypodermic
HYS hysteroscopy
HZ herpes zoster
Hz hertz

I

I iodine
IADH inappropriate antidiuretic hormone [secretion]
IADLs instrumental activities of daily living
IBC inflammatory breast cancer
IBD inflammatory bowel disease
IBS irritable bowel syndrome
IC intermittent claudication; interstitial cystitis
ICCU intensive coronary care unit
ICD implantable cardioverter defibrillator
ICS ileocecal sphincter; intercostal space
ICSI intracytoplasmic sperm injection
ICU intensive care unit
I & D incision and drainage; irrigation and debridement
ID infectious disease; intradermal
id. the same (Latin *idem*)
IDC infiltrating ductal carcinoma; invasive ductal carcinoma
IF interstitial fluid; intrinsic factor
IFN interferon
Ig, IG immunoglobulin
IgA immunoglobulin A
IgD immunoglobulin D
IgE immunoglobulin E
IgG immunoglobulin G
IgM immunoglobulin M
IH infectious hepatitis; inguinal hernia
IL interleukin
ILC infiltrating lobular carcinoma; invasive lobular carcinoma
ILD interstitial lung diseases
ILR implantable loop recorder
IM infectious mononucleosis; intramuscular
IN intranasal (*use with caution* due to possible confusion with **IM** and **IV**)
inf inferior; infusion; inflammation
I & O intake and output
IO intestinal obstruction; intraocular, intraosseous
IOD iron-overload disease (hemochromatosis)
IOL intraocular lens
IOP intraocular pressure; intensive outpatient program
IPV inactivated polio vaccine
IQ intelligence quotient
irrig irrigation
IS impingement syndrome; intercostal space
ISG immune serum globulin
ISO, isol isolation
IT immunotherapy
ITBS iliotibial band syndrome
ITC in the canal [hearing aid]
ITE in the ear [hearing aid]
IU international unit, on The Joint Commission's *Do Not Use* list because it can be mistaken for the number **10** or the abbreviation **IV** for intravenous
IUD intrauterine device

IUI	intrauterine insemination
IV	intravenous; intravenously
IVC	inferior vena cava
IVD	intervertebral disk
IVDA	intravenous drug abuse
IVF	in vitro fertilization
IVP	intravenous pyelogram

J

JIA	juvenile idiopathic arthritis
JRA	juvenile rheumatoid arthritis
jt	joint

K

K	potassium
KCF	key clinical findings
KDU	kidney dialysis unit
kg	kilogram
kj	knee jerk
KS	Kaposi's sarcoma
KUB	kidneys, ureters, bladder
KVO	keep vein open

L

L	liter; left
L1 through L5	lumbar vertebrae
LA	left atrium
lab	laboratory
lac	laceration
LAGB	lap-band adjustable gastric banding
LAP	laparoscopy
LARC	long-acting, reversible contraception
laryn	laryngitis; laryngoscopy
laser	light amplification by stimulated emission of radiation
LASIK	laser-assisted in situ keratomileusis [eye surgery]
lat	lateral
LB	large bowel; low back; lower body
lb	pound
LBP	low back pain
LBW	low birth weight
LCSW	licensed clinical social worker
L & D	labor and delivery
LD	learning disabilities
LDL	low-density lipoprotein
LE	left eye; life expectancy; lower extremity; lymphedema
LES	lower esophageal sphincter
lg	large
LGIB	lower GI bleed
LH	luteinizing hormone; left hand
LICSW	licensed independent clinical social worker
lig	ligament
liq	liquid
litho	lithotripsy
LLE	left lower extremity
LLL	left lower lobe
LLQ	left lower quadrant
LMFT	licensed marriage and family therapist
LMHC	licensed mental health counselor
LMP	last menstrual period
LOC	levels of consciousness; loss of consciousness
LOM	limitation of motion; loss of motion
LOS	length of stay
LP	light perception; lumbar puncture
LPC	licensed professional counselor
LPN	licensed practical nurse
LQTS	long QT syndrome
LR	light reaction
LRT	lower respiratory tract
LSHF	left-sided heart failure
LTC	long-term care
LTH	lactogenic hormone
LUE	left upper extremity
LUL	left upper lobe
LUQ	left upper quadrant
LV	left ventricle
LVN	licensed vocational nurse
LYMP	lymphocyte

M

M	meter; heart murmur; myopia; male
MAb	monoclonal antibodies
MAOI	monoamine oxidase inhibitor
MAR	medication administration record
MBI	molecular breast imaging
mcg	microgram
MD	macular degeneration; medical doctor; muscular dystrophy
MDI	metered-dose inhaler
MDS	myelodysplastic syndrome
ME	middle ear; medical examiner
MED	minimal effective dose; medial

meds medicines, drugs
med/surg hospital medical/surgical unit
men meningitis; menstruation
MenACWY, MenB meningococcal disease [vaccine]
MET medical emergency team; to metastasize
met metastasis
mg milligram; magnesium
MG myasthenia gravis
MHC mental health care
MI myocardial infarction
MICU medical intensive care unit; mobile intensive care unit
ml, mL milliliter
MM multiple myeloma; malignant melanoma
mm millimeter
mm Hg millimeters of mercury [blood pressure measurement]
MMR measles, mumps, and rubella [vaccine]
MO morbid obesity
MPS myofascial pain syndrome
MRA magnetic resonance angiography
MRI magnetic resonance imaging
mRS modified Rankin scale
MRSA methicillin-resistant or multidrug-resistant *Staphylococcus aureus* infection
MS multiple sclerosis; musculoskeletal; morphine sulfate (is on The Joint Commission's *Do Not Use* list due to confusion with magnesium sulfate)
MSH melanocyte-stimulating hormone
MSUD maple syrup urine disease
MSW Master of Social Work
MV mitral valve
MVP mitral valve prolapse
MYOP myopia

N

NA, n/a not applicable
Na sodium
NaCl sodium chloride (saline)
NAD no abnormality detected; no apparent distress
NAFLD nonalcoholic fatty liver disease
NB newborn
NC nasal cannula
NED no evidence of disease
neg negative
Neph nephron
neuro neurology
NG nasogastric [tube]
NHL non-Hodgkin's lymphoma
NI nuclear imaging
NICU neonatal intensive care unit
NIH National Institutes of Health
NIHL noise-induced hearing loss
NIHSS National Institutes of Health Stroke Scale
NK cell natural killer cell
NKA no known allergies
NKDA no known drug allergies
NM nuclear medicine
NMT neuromuscular therapy
no. number
noc, noct night (nocturnal); in the night
norm normal
NOS not otherwise specified
NP nurse practitioner
NP-MBU nurse practitioner, mother-baby unit
NPO nothing by mouth (Latin *nil per os*)
NR no response; not reported
NRB non-rebreather [mask]
NS nephrotic syndrome; normal saline; not stated; not sufficient
NSA no significant abnormality
NSAIDs nonsteroidal anti-inflammatory drugs
NSR normal sinus rhythm
NSSI non-suicidal self-injury
nst nystagmus
Nt neutralization
NTD neural tube defects
NTG nitroglycerin
N/V nausea and vomiting
NVD nausea, vomiting, diarrhea
ny nystagmus
NYD not yet diagnosed

O

OA osteoarthritis
OAB overactive bladder
OB, Obs obstetrics; obstetrician
OB-GYN obstetrics and gynecology
obl oblique
OC office call; oral contraceptive
OCD obsessive–compulsive disorder

OCT oral contraceptive therapy
OD overdose; right eye (Latin *oculus dexter*) (*use with caution* due to possible confusion with **AD**, right ear)
ODD oppositional defiant disorder
OGN obstetric-gynecologic-neonatal
OGTT oral glucose tolerance test
oint ointment
OM otitis media
OME otitis media with effusion
OP osteoporosis; outpatient; oropharynx
OPD outpatient department
Ophth ophthalmic
OR operating room
ORIF open reduction internal fixation
ORT oral rehydration therapy
Orth orthopedics
OS left eye (Latin *oculus sinister*) (*use with caution* due to possible confusion with **AS**, left ear and **os**, per mouth)
os mouth (Latin *os*), per os (by mouth) (*use with caution* due to possible confusion with **OS**, left eye)
OSA obstructive sleep apnea
OSHA Occupational Safety and Health Administration
OT occupational therapy/therapist
OTC over-the-counter
OU each eye (Latin *oculus unitas*) (*use with caution* due to possible confusion with **AU**, each ear)
o.u. both eyes (Latin *oculus uterque*)
OXT oxytocin
oz ounce

P

P percussion; physiology; posterior; presbyopia; pulse
P & A percussion and auscultation [examination]
PA physician's assistant
PAD peripheral artery disease
PAOD peripheral artery occlusive disease
Pap Pap smear
PARA paraplegic
paren parenteral
Path pathology
Pb presbyopia
PC, PCA prostate cancer
pc, p.c. after meals (Latin *post cibum*)
PCNL percutaneous nephrolithotomy
PCOS polycystic ovary syndrome
PCP primary care provider; pneumocystis pneumonia (see also **PJP**)
PCU progressive care unit
PCV13 pneumococcal conjugate vaccine
PD Parkinson's disease; peritoneal dialysis; Peyronie's disease; personality disorder
PDD persistent depressive disorder
PDR Prescribers' Digital Reference
PDT photodynamic therapy
PE pulmonary embolism; pulmonary edema; physical examination
PEA pulseless electrical activity
Peds pediatrics
PEEP positive end-expiratory pressure
PEF peak expiratory flow rate
PEP post-exposure prophylaxis
per by; through
PERRLA pupils equal, round, reactive (respond) to light and accommodation
PET positron emission tomography [scan]
PFT pulmonary function tests
PG pregnant; prostaglandin
PGH pituitary growth hormone
PH past history; personal history; public health
pH acidity; hydrogen ion concentration
PHN postherpetic neuralgia
PHP partial hospitalization program
PI present illness
PIA proliferative inflammatory atrophy
PICC peripherally inserted central catheter [line]
PICU pulmonary intensive care unit; pediatric intensive care unit
PID pelvic inflammatory disease
PIF peak inspiratory flow
PIH pregnancy-induced hypertension
PIN prostatic intraepithelial neoplasia
PJP pneumocystis pneumonia (see also **PCP**)
PK pyruvate kinase (enzyme); pyruvate kinase deficiency
PKD polycystic kidney disease, also **PCKD**
PKR partial knee replacement
PKU phenylketonuria
PL light perception
pl placenta
PLC platelet count
PLE pleural effusion
PLTS platelets

PM postmortem
p.m. evening or afternoon (Latin *post meridiem*)
PMDD premenstrual dysphoric disorder
PMH past medical history
PMP past menstrual period; previous menstrual period
PMR polymyalgia rheumatica
PMS premenstrual syndrome
PN peripheral neuropathy; postnatal; parenteral nutrition
PNA pneumonia
Pno pneumothorax
PNP peripheral neuropathy
PNS peripheral nervous system
PNT [ultrasound-guided] percutaneous needle tenotomy
PO, p.o. by mouth, orally (Latin *per os*); phone order; postoperative
POI primary ovarian insufficiency
POLST Physician's Orders for Life-Sustaining Treatment, living will
POS polycystic ovary syndrome
pos positive
Post. posterior
post-op post-operatively
PP placenta previa; postprandial (after meals); pulse pressure
PPD postpartum depression
PPE personal protective equipment
PPI proton pump inhibitors
PPS post-polio syndrome
PPT partial prothrombin time
PPV positive-pressure ventilation
PR peripheral resistance; pulse rate
Pr presbyopia; prism
pr by rectum, rectally
PR+ progesterone receptor-positive [breast cancer]
preg pregnant
preop preoperative
prep prepare
PrEP pre-exposure prophylaxis
PRK photorefractive keratectomy
prn, p.r.n. as needed (Latin *pro re nata*)
PRO protein
Proct proctology
prog, progn prognosis
PROM passive range of motion; premature rupture of membranes
pro time prothrombin time (see also **PT**)
PRP platelet-rich plasma [treatment]
Prx prognosis
Ps psoriasis
PSA prostate-specific antigen [blood test]
PSNS parasympathetic nervous system
psych psychiatry
PT physical therapy/therapist; prothrombin time
pt patient; pint
PTA physical therapy assistant
PTCA percutaneous transluminal coronary angioplasty
PTD permanent and total disability
PTH parathyroid hormone
PTSD posttraumatic stress disorder
PU peptic ulcer; prostatic urethra
PUD peptic ulcer disease; pulmonary disease
pul pulmonary
PVD peripheral vascular disease
PVS persistent vegetative state
pvt private
PWB partial weight-bearing
PX prognosis

Q

q every, each (Latin *quaque*)
q2h every 2 hours
QD, q.d. daily, every day (Latin *quaque die*), on The Joint Commission's *Do Not Use* list due to confusion with **QID** (four times every day) and **QOD** (every other day)
q.d.s. four times every day (Latin *quater die sumendus*)
q.h. every hour (Latin *quaque hora*)
QID, q.i.d. four times every day (Latin *quater in die*), on The Joint Commission's *Do Not Use* list due to confusion with **QD** (daily) and **QOD** (every other day)
qm every morning
qn every night
qns quantity not sufficient
QOD, q.o.d. every other day (Latin *quaque altera die qua*), on The Joint Commission's *Do Not Use* list due to confusion with **QD** (daily) and **QID** (four times every day)
qoh every other hour
QOL quality of life
qp as much as desired
q.s. quantity sufficient, i.e., as much as needed (Latin *quantum sufficit*)

qt	quart; quiet
q.q.	each (Latin *quaque*)
QUAD	quadriplegic

R

R	rectal; respiration; right
RA	rheumatoid arthritis; right arm; right atrium
RAI	radioactive iodine [treatment]
RAIU	radioactive iodine uptake [test]
RAT	radiation therapy
RBC	red blood cell; red blood count
RBCV	red blood cell volume
RCA	right coronary artery
RD	respiratory distress; retinal detachment; Registered Dietitian
RDA	recommended daily allowance
RDS	respiratory distress syndrome
RE	right eye
reg	regular
rehab	rehabilitation
REM	rapid eye movement [sleep]
resp	respiration
RF	rheumatoid factor; rheumatic fever
RFA	radiofrequency ablation
RH	right hand
RHD	rheumatic heart disease
Rh neg	Rhesus factor negative
Rh pos	Rhesus factor positive
RIA	radioimmunoassay
RICE	rest, ice, compression, elevation
RIFLE	risk factors and life expectancy
RK	radial keratotomy
RL	right leg
RLD	related living donor
RLE	right lower extremity
RLL	right lower lobe
RLQ	right lower quadrant
RLS	restless legs syndrome
RMD	repetitive motion disorder
RML	right mediolateral; right middle lobe of lung
RN	Registered Nurse
R/O	rule out
ROA	radiopaque agents
ROM	range-of-motion [testing]
RP	radiopharmaceuticals; retrograde pyelogram
RPG	retrograde pyelogram
RPM	revolutions per minute
RPO	right posterior oblique
RPR	rapid plasma reagin [test]
RR	recovery room; respiratory rate
RS	Reye's syndrome
RSD	repetitive stress disorder
RSHF	right-sided heart failure
RSI	repetitive stress injuries; rapid sequence intubation
RSR	regular sinus rhythm
RSV	respiratory syncytial virus; right subclavian vein
RT	radiation therapy; respiratory therapist
rt	right; routine
R/T	related to
rt lat	right lateral
RTT	respiratory therapy technician
RU	routine urinalysis
RUE	right upper extremity
RUL	right upper lobe
RUQ	right upper quadrant
RV	residual volume; right ventricle; rotavirus [vaccine]
Rx	prescription; treatment (Latin *recipere*)

S

s̄	without (Latin *sine*)
SA	salicylic acid; sinoatrial [node]; sperm analysis
SAB	spontaneous abortion
SAD	seasonal affective disorder
SAL	sensorineural activity level; suction-assisted lipectomy
Sal, Salm	salmonella
SAM	self-administered medication [program]
SARS	severe acute respiratory syndrome
SAS	sleep apnea syndrome; social adjustment scale
SB	small bowel; spina bifida; stillbirth; suction biopsy
SBO	small bowel obstruction
SBP	systolic blood pressure
SC	Snellen chart; spinal cord; subcutaneous(ly) (*use with caution* due to possible confusion with **SL**, sublingual; see also **SQ**)
SCA	sickle cell anemia; sudden cardiac arrest
SCC	squamous cell carcinoma
SCD	sudden cardiac death; scleroderma; social communication disorder
schiz	schizophrenia
SCI	spinal cord injury

SCID severe combined immunodeficiency
SD spontaneous delivery; standard deviation; sudden death
SDM standard deviation of the mean
SDS sudden death syndrome
sec second [measure of time]; secretion
sed rate sedimentation rate
semi half
sev sever; severed
SF spinal fluid
SG serum globulin; skin graft
SGA small for gestational age
SH serum hepatitis; sex hormone; social history
sh shoulder
SI suicidal ideation
SIADH syndrome of inappropriate antidiuretic hormone [secretion]
SICU surgical intensive care unit
s.i.d. once a day (Latin *semel in die*)
SIDS sudden infant death syndrome
sig. write, let it be labeled (Latin *signa*)
SIRS systemic inflammatory response syndrome
SL sublingual
SLE slit-lamp examination; systemic lupus erythematosus
SLP speech–language pathologist
sm small
SNF skilled nursing facility
SNRI serotonin/norepinephrine reuptake inhibitor
SNS sensory nervous system; sympathetic nervous system
SO salpingo-oophorectomy
SOAP medical notation format: subjective, objective, assessment, plan
SOB shortness of breath
sol solution
SOM serous otitis media
SONO sonography
SOP standard operating procedure
sp gr specific gravity
spec specimen
SPECT single-photon emission computed tomography
SPF sun protective factor
SQ, s.q., SubQ subcutaneous(ly) (*use* **SQ** *with caution* due to possible confusion with **5Q,** five every dose; see also **SC**)
SR sedimentation rate; stimulus response; system review
ss half (Latin *semis*)
s/s signs and symptoms
SSD somatic symptom disorder
SSRI selective serotonin reuptake inhibitor
SSU sterile supply unit
ST esotropia; sclerotherapy
st. let it stand (Latin *stet*)
staph *Staphylococcus* bacteria
stat immediately (Latin *statim*)
STDs sexually transmitted diseases
STH somatotropic hormone
STIs sexually transmitted infections
strab strabismus
strep *streptococcus* bacteria
SUDEP sudden unexpected death in epilepsy
SUI stress urinary incontinence
supp suppository
surg surgical; surgery
SVC superior vena cava
SVG saphenous vein graft
SVT supraventricular tachycardia
Sx symptoms
Sz seizure

T

T temperature; thrombosis
T1 through T12 thoracic vertebrae
T_3 triiodothyronine thyroid hormone
T_4 thyroxine thyroid hormone
TA, TAB therapeutic abortion
tab tablet
tachy tachycardia
TAH total abdominal hysterectomy
TAVR transcatheter aortic valve replacement
TB tuberculosis; tuberculin
TBF total body fat
TBI traumatic brain injury
Tbsp, tbsp tablespoon
TBW total body weight
TCA tricyclic antidepressant
TD total disability; transdermal
Tdap tetanus/diphtheria/acellular pertussis [vaccine] (see also **DTaP**)
TDM therapeutic drug monitoring
TE tetanus; tonsillectomy
TEE transesophageal echocardiography
temp temperature; temporary

TENS	transcutaneous electrical nerve stimulation
THR	total hip replacement
TIA	transient ischemic attack
TID, t.i.d.	three times a day (Latin *ter in die*)
tinct	tincture
TKO	to keep open
TKR	total knee replacement
TLC	tender loving care; total lung capacity
TM	temporomandibular; tympanic membrane
TMJ	temporomandibular joint
TMS	transcranial magnetic stimulation
TMT	treadmill test
TNM	tumor, nodes, metastases [cancer staging system]
top	topically, topical
tPA	tissue plasminogen activator (*use with caution* due to possible confusion with other drug abbreviations)
TPE	therapeutic plasma exchange
TPN	total parenteral nutrition
TPR	temperature, pulse, respiration
trach	trachea; tracheostomy
TRBF	total renal blood flow
TRH	thyrotropin-releasing hormone
trich	trichomoniasis
TS	Tourette syndrome
TSE	testicular self-examination
TSH	thyroid stimulating hormone
TSP	total serum protein
tsp	teaspoon
TSS	toxic shock syndrome
TST	thallium stress test; tuberculin skin test
TT	thrombin time
TURP	transurethral resection of prostate
TVH	total vaginal hysterectomy
TVS	transvaginal ultrasound
Tx	treatment

U

U, u	unit, on The Joint Commission's *Do Not Use* list because letter **U** can be mistaken for **0** (zero), the number **4**, or cc
UA	urinalysis
UB	urinary bladder
UC	ulcerative colitis; urine culture; uterine contractions
UE	upper extremity
UGI	upper gastrointestinal
UGIB	upper GI bleed
UHF	ultrahigh frequency
UK	unknown
UL	upper lobe
ULQ	upper left quadrant
umb	umbilical; umbilicus
ung.	ointment (Latin *unguentum*)
UOQ	upper outer quadrant
ur	urine
URI, URTI	upper respiratory infection; upper respiratory tract infection
urol	urology
URQ	upper right quadrant
URT	upper respiratory tract
US	ultrasonic; ultrasonography
USG	ultrasound guided
USP	United States Pharmacopeia
ut dict.	as directed (Latin *ut dictum*)
UTI	urinary tract infection
UVA	ultraviolet A
UVB	ultraviolet B
UV	ultraviolet

V

v	vein
VA	vacuum aspiration; visual acuity
vag	vaginal
VAS	vasectomy
VATS	video-assisted thoracic surgery
VB	viable birth
VBAC	vaginal birth after cesarean
VBG	venous blood gases
VC	vena cava; vital capacity
VCUG	voiding cystourethrography
VD	venereal disease
VDRL	venereal disease research laboratory [blood test]
VDS	venereal disease, syphilis
Vent, ventr	ventral
Vf	field of vision
V-fib, VF	ventricular fibrillation
VH	vaginal hysterectomy
VHD	valvular heart disease; ventricular heart disease
VI	volume index
vit.	vitamin
VLBW	very low birth weight

vol.	volume
VP	venipuncture; venous pressure
VRT	vestibular rehabilitation therapy
VS, vs	vesicular sound; vital signs
VSD	ventricular septal defect
VSS	vital signs stable
V-tach, VT	ventricular tachycardia
VTE	venous thromboembolism
VUR	vesicoureteral reflux
VV	varicose veins; veins
VVF	vesicovaginal fistula
VZV	varicella zoster virus (chickenpox)

W

W	water; white
w/	with
WA	while awake
WB	weight-bearing; whole blood
WBC	white blood cell; white blood count
W/C, WC	wheelchair
wd	wound
w/f	with food
WH	well-hydrated
WIC	Women, Infants, and Children (federal nutrition program)
WN	well-nourished
WNL	within normal limits
w/o	without
wt.	weight

X

X	xerophthalmia
x	multiplied by, times
xfer	transfer
XR	x-ray, radiograph
XT	exotropia
XU	excretory urography

Y

y/o, yo	year(s) old
YOB	year of birth
yr	year
YTD	year to date

Z

Z	no effect; zero

Appendix C

TERMS RELATED TO DIAGNOSIS, PATHOLOGY, AND PROCEDURES

A

abdominal computed tomography: a radiographic procedure that produces a detailed cross-section of the tissue structure within the abdomen.

abdominal ultrasound: a noninvasive test used to visualize internal organs by using very high-frequency sound waves.

abdominocentesis (ab-**dom**-ih-noh-sen-**TEE**-sis): surgical puncture of the abdominal cavity to remove fluid.

ablation (ab-**LAY**-shun): the removal of a body part or the destruction of its function.

abnormal uterine bleeding: a condition characterized by abnormal bleeding during or outside of the menstrual period.

abortion (ah-**BOR**-shun): the interruption or termination of pregnancy before the fetus is viable.

abrasion (ah-**BRAY**-zhun): an injury in which superficial layers of skin are scraped or rubbed away.

abruptio placentae (ab-**RUP**-shee-oh plah-**SEN**-tee): a disorder in which the placenta separates from the uterine wall before the birth of the fetus.

abscess (**AB**-sess): a closed pocket containing pus caused by a bacterial infection.

absence seizure: a brief disturbance in brain function in which there is a loss of awareness, often described as a staring episode.

acanthosis nigricans (ak-an-**THO**-sis **NIG**-rih-kans): a condition where one or more areas of the skin develop dark, velvety areas of discoloration, usually in skin folds.

ACE inhibitor: antihypertensive medication that works by relaxing blood vessels.

acetaminophen (ah-**seet**-ah-**MIN**-oh-fen): analgesic that reduces pain and fever but does not relieve inflammation.

acetylcholinesterase inhibitor (ah-**SEH**-tul-koh-leh-**neh**-sta-rayz): medication that treats the symptoms of Alzheimer's disease.

Achilles tendinitis (ah-**KIH**-leez **ten**-dih-**NIGH**-tis): inflammation of the Achilles tendon caused by excessive stress being placed on that tendon.

acidosis (ass-eh-**DOH**-sis): excessive acid in the body fluids.

acne vulgaris (**ACK**-nee vul-**GAY**-ris): a chronic inflammatory disease that is characterized by pustular eruptions of the skin caused by an overproduction of sebum around the hair shaft.

acoustic neuroma (new-**ROH**-mah): a benign brain tumor that develops adjacent to the cranial nerve running from the brain to the inner ear.

acoustic reflectometry: measures how much sound is reflected back from the eardrum.

acquired immunity: immunity obtained by having had a contagious disease.

acquired immunodeficiency syndrome (AIDS): the advanced stage of an HIV infection.

acral lentiginous melanoma: a form of melanoma that occurs on the palms, soles, and under the nails.

acromegaly (**ack**-roh-**MEG**-ah-lee): abnormal enlargement of the extremities caused by excessive secretion of growth hormone after puberty.

acrophobia (**ack**-roh-**FOH**-bee-ah): an excessive fear of heights.

actinic keratosis (ack-**TIN**-ick **kerr**-ah-**TOH**-sis): a precancerous skin growth that occurs on sun-damaged skin.

active dying: the last stage of the dying process before death.

acupressure (**AK**-que-**presh**-ur): a traditional Chinese touch therapy involving finger pressure applied to specific areas of the body.

acupuncture (**AK**-que-**punk**-cher): a traditional Chinese medical practice using very thin acupuncture needles inserted into specific points of the body.

acute bronchitis: inflammation of the bronchi usually caused by a viral infection; also known as a chest cold.

acute lymphocytic leukemia: a blood cancer characterized by a sudden increase in abnormal lymphocytes.

acute myeloid leukemia: a blood cancer characterized by a sudden increase in abnormal leukocytes.

acute necrotizing ulcerative gingivitis: an abnormal growth of bacteria in the mouth.

acute renal failure: sudden onset of kidney failure that may be caused by the kidneys not receiving enough blood.

acute respiratory distress syndrome: a life-threatening condition in which inflammation in the lungs and fluid in the alveoli lead to low levels of oxygen in the blood.

addiction: compulsive, uncontrollable dependence on a substance, habit, or practice.

Addison's disease (**AD**-ih-sonz): a condition that occurs when the adrenal glands do not produce enough cortisol or aldosterone.

adenitis (ad-eh-**NIGH**-tis): inflammation of a gland.

adenocarcinoma (**ad**-eh-noh-**kar**-sih-**NOH**-mah): carcinoma derived from glandular tissue.

adenoma (**ad**-eh-**NOH**-mah): benign tumor that starts in the epithelial tissue of a gland or gland-like structure.

adenomatous polyp: most common type of pre-cancerous neoplastic polyp.

adenosis (**ad**-eh-**NOH**-sis): any disease or condition of a gland.

adherence: a patient's consistency and accuracy in following the instructions given by their physician.

adhesion (ad-**HEE**-zhun): a band of fibrous tissue that holds structures together abnormally.

adhesive capsulitis (ad-**HEE**-siv **kap**-suh-**LIE**-tis): painful ankylosis of the shoulder caused by adhesions forming in the synovial capsule surrounding the shoulder.

adjuvant therapy (**AD**-jeh-vant): cancer treatment sometimes used after the primary treatments have been completed to decrease the chance that a cancer will recur.

adrenalitis (ah-**dree**-nal-**EYE**-tis): inflammation of the adrenal glands.

advanced cirrhosis: advanced chronic liver failure marked by ascites, hepatic encephalopathy and jaundice.

adverse drug reaction: an undesirable reaction that accompanies the principal response for which the drug was taken.

aerophagia (**ay**-er-oh-**FAY**-jee-ah): excessive swallowing of air while eating or drinking.

aerosol: a mist of tiny particles suspended in air.

age spots: skin discolorations caused by sun exposure.

agonal respirations (**AH**-goh-nal): ineffective breaths that are a form of respiratory failure.

agoraphobia (**ag**-oh-rah-**FOH**-bee-ah): an excessive fear of environments where the person fears a panic attack might occur.

airborne transmission: disease transmission that occurs through contact with germs floating in the air.

air hunger: a persistent, distressing feeling of shortness of breath that occurs at end of life.

airway inflammation: swelling and clogging of the bronchial tubes with mucus.

airway obstruction: occurs when food or a foreign object partially or completely blocks the airway and prevents air from entering or leaving the lungs.

albinism (**AL**-bih-niz-um): a genetic condition characterized by a deficiency or absence of pigment in the skin, hair, and irises.

albuminuria (**al**-byou-mih-**NEW**-ree-ah): the presence of the protein albumin in the urine.

alcoholism (**AL**-koh-hol-izm): chronic alcohol dependence with specific signs and symptoms upon withdrawal.

aldosteronism (al-**DOSS**-teh-roh-**niz**-em): an abnormality of electrolyte balance caused by the excessive secretion of aldosterone.

alert and oriented: someone who is spontaneously awake, aware of who they are, and what is going on.

allergen (**AL**-er-jen): a substance that produces an allergic reaction in an individual.

allergic reaction: occurs when the body's immune system reacts to a harmless allergen as if it were a dangerous invader.

allergic rhinitis (rye-**NIGH**-tis): an allergic reaction to airborne allergens that causes an increased flow of mucus.

allergy: an overreaction by the body to a particular antigen.

allogeneic transfusion (**al**-loh-jen-**EEH**-ick): transfusion using donated blood of a compatible type.

allogeneic transplant: a transplant in which the recipient receives tissues, cells, or organs from a compatible donor.

allopathic medicine (**ah**-low-**PAH**-thick): conventional Western medical practices and systems of health care.

alopecia (**al**-oh-**PEE**-shee-ah): the partial or complete loss of hair, most commonly on the scalp.

alopecia areata: an autoimmune disorder that attacks the hair follicles, causing well-defined bald areas on the scalp or elsewhere on the body.

alopecia totalis: an uncommon condition characterized by the loss of all the hair on the scalp.

alopecia universalis: the total loss of hair on all parts of the body.

alpha blocker: medication that improves urination in men with benign prostatic hyperplasia.

alternative medicine: a general term for practices and systems of health care used in place of allopathic medicine.

Alzheimer's disease (**ALTZ**-high-merz): a group of disorders involving the parts of the brain that control thought, memory, and language.

amblyopia (**am**-blee-**OH**-pee-ah): dimness of vision or the partial loss of sight, especially in one eye, without detectable disease of the eye.

Ambu® bag: emergency resuscitator used to assist ventilation, also called a BVM (Bag Valve Mask).

amenorrhea (ah-**men**-oh-**REE**-ah): the abnormal absence of menstrual periods for 90 days or more.

ametropia (**am**-eh-**TROH**-pee-ah): any error of refraction in which images do not focus properly on the retina.

amnesia (am-**NEE**-zee-ah): a memory disturbance marked by a total or partial inability to recall past experiences.

amniocentesis (**am**-nee-oh-sen-**TEE**-sis): surgical puncture with a needle to obtain a specimen of amniotic fluid to evaluate fetal health and to diagnose certain congenital disorders.

amputation: surgical or accidental removal of a limb.

amyotrophic lateral sclerosis (ah-**my**-oh-**TROH**-fick): a rapidly progressive neurological disease that attacks the nerve cells responsible for controlling voluntary muscles.

anal fissure: a small crack-like sore in the skin of the anus that can cause severe pain during a bowel movement.

analgesic (**an**-al-**JEE**-zick): medication that relieves pain without affecting consciousness.

anaphylaxis (**an**-ah-fih-**LACK**-sis): a severe, systemic response to an allergen.

anaplasia (**an**-ah-**PLAY**-zhee-ah): the uncontrolled growth of abnormal, poorly differentiated cells commonly seen in cancer.

anastomosis (ah-**nas**-toh-**MOH**-sis): a surgical or natural connection between two hollow or tubular structures such as blood vessels or loops of intestines.

androgen replacement therapy: therapy used to treat conditions related to testosterone loss.

androgenic alopecia (an-**DROH**-jen-ik **al**-oh-**PEE**-shee-ah): the most common type of hair loss, called male pattern baldness in men and female pattern baldness in women.

andropause (**AN**-droh-pawz): marked by the decrease of the male hormone testosterone, gradually beginning in the late 40s and progressing very gradually over several decades.

anemia (ah-**NEE**-mee-ah): a disorder characterized by lower-than-normal levels of red blood cells in the blood.

anencephaly (ah-nun-**SEF**-uh-lee): a neural tube defect characterized by the failure of the brain and skull to fully develop.

anesthesia (**an**-es-**THEE**-zee-ah): the absence of normal sensation, especially sensitivity to pain.

anesthetic (**an**-es-**THET**-ick): medication used to induce anesthesia.

aneurysm (**AN**-you-rizm): a localized weak spot or balloon-like enlargement of the wall of an artery.

aneurysm clipping: a surgical method to isolate an aneurysm from the rest of the circulatory system by placing a small clip across its neck.

angina (an-**JIGH**-nah): episodes of severe chest pain due to inadequate blood flow to the myocardium.

angiogenesis (**an**-jee-oh-**JEN**-eh-sis): the process through which the tumor supports its growth by creating its own blood supply.

angiogenesis inhibitor: medication that interferes with the ability of a tumor to create new blood vessels.

angiogram (**AN**-jee-oh-**gram**): the film produced by angiography.

angiography (**an**-jee-**OG**-rah-fee): a radiographic study of the blood vessels after the injection of a contrast medium.

angioplasty (**AN**-jee-oh-**plas**-tee): mechanically widening a narrowed or obstructed blood vessel.

angiotensin-II receptor blocker: antihypertensive medication that blocks the action of the enzyme that causes the blood vessels to contract.

anhidrosis (**an**-high-**DROH**-sis): the abnormal condition of lacking sweat in response to heat.

anisocoria (**an**-ih-so-**KOH**-ree-ah): a condition in which the pupils are unequal in size.

ankylosing spondylitis (**ang**-kih-**LOH**-sing **spon**-dih-**LYE**-tis): a form of rheumatoid arthritis that primarily causes inflammation of the joints between the vertebrae.

ankylosis (**ang**-kih-**LOH**-sis): the loss or absence of mobility in a joint due to disease, injury, or a surgical procedure.

anomaly (ah-**NOM**-ah-lee): a deviation from what is regarded as normal.

anorexia (**an**-oh-**RECK**-see-ah): the loss of appetite for food, especially when caused by disease.

anorexia nervosa (ner-**VOH**-sah): an eating disorder characterized by a false perception of body appearance that leads to a fear of weight gain and inability to maintain a healthy body weight.

anoscopy (ah-**NOS**-koh-pee): the visual examination of the anal canal and lower rectum.

anovulation (**an**-ov-you-**LAY**-shun): the absence of ovulation when it would normally be expected.

anoxia (ah-**NOCK**-see-ah): the absence of oxygen from the body's tissues or organs despite adequate flow of blood.

antacid: medication to relieve indigestion or help peptic ulcers heal by neutralizing stomach acids.

anthrax (**AN**-thraks): a contagious disease that can be transmitted through livestock.

antiangiogenesis: cancer treatment that disrupts the blood supply to the tumor.

anti-anxiety medication: drug used to treat anxiety.

anti-arrhythmic (**an**-tih-ah-**RITH**-mick): medication that stops or prevents irregularities of the heartbeat.

antibiotic-resistant bacteria: bacteria that are resistant to a particular drug.

antibiotic: medication capable of inhibiting the growth of or killing pathogenic bacteria.

antibody (**AN**-tih-**bod**-ee): a disease-fighting protein created by the immune system in response to the presence of a specific antigen.

anticholinergic: medication used to treat overactive bladder by relaxing the smooth muscle of the bladder.

anticoagulant (**an**-tih-koh-**AG**-you-lant): medication that slows clotting and prevents new clots from forming.

anticonvulsant (**an**-tih-kon-**VUL**-sant): medication that prevents or stops seizures.

antidepressant: medication administered to prevent or relieve depression.

antidiarrheal: medication that temporarily relieves diarrhea.

antiemetic (**an**-tee-eh-**MET**-ick): medication administered to prevent or relieve nausea and vomiting.

antifungal (**an**-tih-**FUNG**-gul): medication that destroys or inhibits the growth of fungi.

antigen (**AN**-tih-jen): any substance that the body regards as being foreign.

antihistamine: medication administered to relieve or prevent the symptoms of allergic reactions.

antihypertensive (**an**-tih-**high**-per-**TEN**-siv): medication administered to lower blood pressure.

anti-inflammatory: medication administered to relieve inflammation and pain.

antineoplastic (**an**-tih-nee-oh-**PLAS**-tick): medication that blocks the development, growth, or proliferation of malignant cells.

antioxidants (**an**-tee-**OCK**-sih-dantz): chemicals such as vitamins A, C, and E; carotene; and lutein that may prevent or delay cell damage.

antiplatelet agent: medication such as low-dose aspirin that reduces the ability of platelets to form clots.

antipsychotic drug (**an**-tih-sigh-**KOT**-ick): medication administered to treat symptoms of severe disorders of thinking and mood.

antipyretic (**an**-tih-pye-**RET**-ick): medication administered to prevent or reduce fever.

antisocial personality disorder: a pattern of disregard for and violation of the rights of others which can include aggression.

antispasmodic: medication administered to suppress smooth muscle contractions.

antithyroid drug: medication administered to slow the ability of the thyroid gland to produce thyroid hormones.

antitussive (**an**-tih-**TUSS**-iv): medication administered to prevent or relieve coughing.

anti-VEGF injections: intravitreal injections used to treat wet macular degeneration by slowing the growth of abnormal blood vessels in the eye.

antiviral drug (**an**-tih-**VYE**-ral): medication administered to treat viral infections or to provide temporary immunity.

anuria (ah-**NEW**-ree-ah): the absence of urine formation by the kidneys.

anxiety disorder: mental condition characterized by excessive, irrational dread of everyday situations, or fear that is out of proportion to the real danger in a situation.

anxiolytic drug (**ang**-zee-oh-**LIT**-ick): medication administered to temporarily relieve anxiety and reduce tension.

aortic stenosis: a buildup of calcium and fat deposits in the aortic valve, which causes narrowing that prevents the valve from opening fully.

Apgar score: an evaluation of a newborn infant's physical status.

aphasia (ah-**FAY**-zee-ah): loss of the ability to speak, write, and/or comprehend the written or spoken word.

aphonia (ah-**FOH**-nee-ah): the loss of the ability of the larynx to produce normal speech sounds.

aplasia (ah-**PLAY**-zhee-ah): the defective development or congenital absence of an organ or tissue.

aplastic anemia (ay-**PLAS**-tick ah-**NEE**-mee-ah): a condition marked by the absence of all formed blood elements.

apnea (**AP**-nee-ah): the absence of spontaneous respiration.

appendectomy (**ap**-en-**DECK**-toh-mee): surgical removal of the appendix.

appendicitis (ah-**pen**-dih-**SIGH**-tis): inflammation of the appendix.

aromatase inhibitor (ah-**ROH**-mah-tase): medication that blocks the growth of hormone-positive breast cancer.

arrhythmia (ah-**RITH**-mee-ah): a loss of the normal rhythm of the heartbeat.

arterial blood gas analysis: a test to measure the oxygen and carbon dioxide levels of arterial blood.

arterial stick: the puncture of an artery to obtain arterial blood.

arteriomalacia (ar-**tee**-ree-oh-mah-**LAY**-shee-ah): abnormal softening of the walls of an artery or arteries.

arterionecrosis (ar-**tee**-ree-oh-neh-**KROH**-sis): tissue death of an artery or arteries.

arteriosclerosis (ar-**tee**-ree-oh-skleh-**ROH**-sis): abnormal hardening of the walls of an artery or arteries.

arteriostenosis (ar-**tee**-ree-oh-steh-**NOH**-sis): abnormal narrowing of an artery or arteries.

arteriovenous malformation (ar-**tee**-ree-oh-**VEE**-nus): an abnormal connection between the arteries and veins in the brain; may cause a hemorrhagic stroke.

arthralgia (ar-**THRAL**-jee-ah): pain in one or more joints.

arthritis (ar-**THRIGH**-tis): an inflammatory condition of one or more joints.

arthrocentesis (**ar**-throh-sen-**TEE**-sis): surgical puncture of the joint space to remove synovial fluid for analysis.

arthrodesis (**ar**-throh-**DEE**-sis): a surgical procedure to stiffen a joint.

arthroplasty (**AR**-throh-**plas**-tee): surgical repair of a damaged joint; also the surgical replacement of a joint with an artificial joint.

arthrosclerosis (**ar**-throh-skleh-**ROH**-sis): stiffness of the joints, especially in the elderly.

arthroscopic surgery (**ar**-throh-**SKOP**-ick): a minimally invasive procedure for the treatment of the interior of a joint.

arthroscopy (ar-**THROS**-koh-pee): visual examination of the internal structure of a joint using an arthroscope.

artificial insemination: a technique in which sperm from a woman's partner or a donor are introduced into the vagina or uterus during the ovulatory phase of her menstrual cycle.

asbestosis (**ass**-beh-**STOH**-sis): the form of pneumoconiosis caused by asbestos particles in the lungs.

ascites (ah-**SIGH**-teez): an abnormal accumulation of serous fluid in the peritoneal cavity.

asphyxia (ass-**FICK**-see-ah): the loss of consciousness that occurs when the body cannot get the oxygen it needs to function.

aspiration (**ass**-pih-**RAY**-shun): inhaling or drawing a foreign substance into the upper respiratory tract.

aspiration pneumonia: pneumonia caused by a foreign substance, such as vomit, being inhaled into the lungs.

aspirin: medication that may be recommended in a very small daily dose to reduce the risk of a heart attack or stroke by slightly reducing the ability of the blood to clot.

assisted reproductive technology: techniques used to aid an infertile couple in achieving a viable pregnancy.

assistive listening device: a device that transmits, processes, or amplifies sound and can be used with or without a hearing aid.

asthma (**AZ**-mah): a chronic inflammatory disease of the bronchial tubes.

astigmatism (ah-**STIG**-mah-tizm): a condition in which the eye does not focus properly because of uneven curvatures of the cornea.

asystole (ay-**SIS**-toh-lee): complete lack of electrical activity in the heart.

ataxia (ah-**TACK**-see-ah): the lack of muscle coordination during voluntary movement.

atelectasis (**at**-ee-**LEK**-tah-sis): incomplete expansion of part or all of the lung.

atherectomy (**ath**-er-**ECK**-toh-mee): surgical removal of plaque buildup from the interior of an artery.

atheroma (**ath**-er-**OH**-mah): a deposit of fatty plaque within the wall of an artery.

atherosclerosis (**ah**-theh-roh-skleh-**ROH**-sis): narrowing and stiffening of arteries due to a buildup of cholesterol plaque.

atonic (ah-**TON**-ick): lacking normal muscle tone or strength.
atresia (at-**TREE**-zee-ah): describes the congenital absence or narrowing of a normal opening or passage.
atrial fibrillation: rapid uncontrolled twitching of the muscular wall of the atria.
atrophy (**AT**-roh-fee): weakness or wearing away of body tissues and structures.
attention deficit/hyperactivity disorder: a condition characterized by a short attention span and impulsive behavior inappropriate for the child's developmental age.
audiological evaluation: the measurement of the ability to hear and understand speech sounds based on their pitch and loudness.
audiometry (**aw**-dee-**OM**-eh-tree): the use of an audiometer to measure hearing acuity.
auscultation (**aws**-kul-**TAY**-shun): listening for sounds within the body, usually done with a stethoscope.
autism spectrum disorder (**AW**-tizm): a condition with different levels of symptom severity in which a person has difficulty developing normal social relationships and communication skills, may compulsively follow repetitive routines, and has narrowly focused, intense interests.
autoimmune disorder (**aw**-toh-ih-**MYOUN**): a disease in which the immune system produces antibodies against the body's own tissues.
autologous stem cell transplant (aw-**TOL**-uh-guss): a transplant utilizing stem cells from the patient's own bone marrow that were harvested before treatment began.
autologous transfusion: transfusion using the patient's own blood that has been stored.
automated external defibrillator (dee-**fib**-rih-**LAY**-ter): electronic equipment that externally shocks the heart to restore a normal cardiac rhythm.
autopsy (**AW**-top-see): postmortem examination.
avascular necrosis: an area of bone tissue death caused by insufficient blood flow.
avoidant restrictive food intake disorder: a feeding and eating disorder of extreme pickiness that can interfere with adequate nutrition, appropriate growth, and social functioning.
Ayurvedic medicine (**ay**-uhr-**VEH**-dick): traditional Hindu system of medicine.
azoospermia (ay-**zoh**-oh-**SPER**-mee-ah): the absence of sperm in the semen.
azotemia (**ay**-zoh-**TEE**-mee-ah): an elevation of the blood urea nitrogen (BUN) caused by a lack of blood flow to each kidney.

B

bacilli (bah-**SILL**-eye): rod-shaped, spore-forming bacteria.
bacteria (back-**TEE**-ree-ah): one-celled microscopic organisms.
bacterial pneumonia: pneumonia most commonly caused by *Streptococcus pneumoniae*.
bacterial vaginosis (vaj-ih-**NOH**-sis): a condition in which there is an abnormal overgrowth of certain bacteria in the vagina.
bactericide (back-**TEER**-ih-side): a substance that causes the death of bacteria.
bacteriostatic: a substance that slows or stops the growth of bacteria.
bacteriuria (back-**tee**-ree-**YOU**-ree-ah): the presence of bacteria in the urine.
Baker's cyst: a fluid-filled sac behind the knee that usually results from a condition such as rheumatoid arthritis triggering the production of excess synovial fluid.
balanitis (bal-ah-**NIGH**-tis): inflammation of the glans penis.
balloon angioplasty: a treatment procedure to open a partially blocked coronary artery by flattening the plaque deposit and stretching the lumen.
barbiturates (bar-**BIT**-you-raytz): a class of medications whose major action is a calming or depressed effect on the central nervous system.
bariatric surgery: performed to treat severe obesity by restricting the amount of food that can enter the stomach and be digested.
bariatrics (bayr-ee-**AT**-ricks): the branch of medicine for the prevention and management of obesity and associated diseases.
barium: a radiopaque contrast medium used primarily to visualize the gastrointestinal tract.
barium swallow study: a test using barium-coated foods or barium-containing liquids to assess for aspiration risk.
barotrauma (bar-oh-**TRAW**-mah): pressure-related ear condition.
Barrett's esophagus: a condition that occurs when the cells in the epithelial tissue of the esophagus are damaged by chronic acid exposure.

basal cell carcinoma: a malignant tumor of the basal cell layer of the epidermis.

basic metabolic panel: a group of specific blood tests that provide important information about the patient's kidney function and electrolyte levels.

basilar atelectasis: collapse of the alveoli in the lung bases.

bedbound: the state of being unable to independently get out of bed due to weakness, paralysis, or injury.

behavioral therapy: therapy that focuses on changing behavior by identifying problem behaviors, replacing them with appropriate behaviors, and using rewards or other consequences to make the changes.

Bell's palsy: temporary paralysis of the seventh cranial nerve that causes paralysis only on the affected side of the face.

benign: something that is not life-threatening.

benign paroxysmal positional vertigo: vertigo resulting from a shift in the location of small crystals in the semicircular canals of the ears.

benign prostatic hyperplasia (high-per-**PLAY**-zhee-ah): abnormal enlargement of the prostate gland often found in men over age 50.

benign tumor: a non-cancerous abnormal growth of body tissue creating a mass.

benzodiazepine: a drug that has sedative, hypnotic, anticonvulsant and muscle relaxant properties.

beta-blocker: antihypertensive, anti-arrhythmic medication that slows the heart rate by blocking the release of stress hormones.

bilateral orchiectomy: surgical removal or destruction of both testicles.

binaural testing (bye-**NAW**-rul *or* bin-**AW**-rahl): hearing testing that involves both ears.

binge eating disorder: frequent episodes of eating large quantities of food, accompanied by a sense of loss of control and feelings of guilt or shame afterward.

biofeedback: treatment that teaches a person to control bodily functions through cognitive control techniques.

bioimpedance spectroscopy (**BYE**-oh-im-**pee**-dens): a noninvasive method of diagnosing lymphedema by measuring the limb's resistance to an electrical current.

biophysical profile test: a noninvasive test to measure the health of the fetus.

biopsy (**BYE**-op-see): the removal of a small piece of living tissue for examination to confirm or establish a diagnosis.

BiPAP machine: noninvasive ventilation device that can be set at a higher pressure for inhaling and a lower pressure for exhaling.

bipolar disorder: a mental condition characterized by cycles of severe mood changes shifting from highs and severe lows.

birth control pill: daily pill taken by women to regulate hormones and prevent pregnancy.

bisphosphonates: a class of medications used to slow the loss of bone density due to osteoporosis.

bladder retraining: behavioral training in which the patient learns to urinate on a schedule with increasingly longer time intervals between scheduled urination.

bladder ultrasound: the use of a handheld ultrasound transducer to measure the amount of urine remaining in the bladder after urination.

blastoma (blas-**TOH**-ma): cancer that develops from immature undifferentiated cells, most commonly in children.

blepharitis (**BLEF**-ar-**eye**-tis): swelling of the eyelid.

blepharoplasty (**BLEF**-ah-roh-**plas**-tee): surgical reduction of the upper and lower eyelids.

blindness: the inability to see.

blood clotting test: a coagulation blood test used to check for suspected blood clotting disorders.

blood dyscrasia (dis-**KRAY**-zhee-ah): any pathologic condition of the cellular elements of the blood.

blood differential test: a blood test that measures the percentage of each type of leukocyte present in the blood.

blood enzyme test: a blood test used to diagnose a targeted health issue by measuring the level of specific enzymes.

blood gas analysis: measures the amount of oxygen and carbon dioxide in the blood.

blood glucose test: measures the level of glucose, a type of simple sugar, in the blood.

blood urea nitrogen (you-**REE**-ah): a blood test performed to determine the amount of urea nitrogen present in the blood.

bloodborne transmission: the spread of a disease through contact with infected blood or other body fluids that are contaminated with infected blood.

body dysmorphic disorder: a preoccupation with perceived flaws in a person's own appearance.

body mass index: a number that shows body weight adjusted for height.

bolus (**BOH**-lus): a single dose of a drug usually injected into a blood vessel over a short period of time.

bone age study: a diagnostic procedure to determine skeletal maturity in a child.

bone density testing: a diagnostic test to determine losses or changes in bone density.
bone grafting: a surgical procedure using transplanted bone to repair and rebuild bones damaged by injury or disease.
bone marrow aspiration: the procedure used to procure a sample of the aspirate of the bone marrow.
bone marrow biopsy (**BYE**-op-see): a diagnostic test to determine why blood cells are abnormal or to find a donor match for a bone marrow transplant.
bone marrow transplant: cancer treatment in which abnormal bone marrow is destroyed and replaced with new stem cells.
bone mineral density testing: test to determine losses or changes in bone density.
bone-on-bone: osteoarthritis that has progressed to the point where the articular cartilage is gone.
bone scan: a specialized nuclear scan that identifies new areas of bone growth or breakdown.
borborygmus (**bor**-boh-**RIG**-mus): the rumbling noise caused by the movement of gas in the intestine.
borderline personality disorder: impulsive actions, often with the potential for self-harm, as well as mood instability and chaotic relationships.
Botox®: a formulation of botulinum toxin that is administered by injection to temporarily improve the appearance of frown lines between the eyebrows.
bowel rest: not giving a person anything to eat or drink by mouth to allow the digestive tract to recover and return to normal function.
Bowen disease (**BOH**-wan): squamous cell carcinoma in situ.
brachytherapy (**brack**-ee-**THER**-ah-pee): the use of radioactive materials in contact with or implanted into the tissues to be treated.
bradycardia (**brad**-ee-**KAR**-dee-ah): an abnormally slow resting heart rate, usually at a rate of less than 60 beats per minute.
bradykinesia (**brad**-ee-kih-**NEE**-zee-ah): extreme slowness in movement.
bradypnea (**brad**-ihp-**NEE**-ah): an abnormally slow rate of respiration, usually of less than 10 breaths per minute.
brain death: the complete loss of brain function.
brain tumor: an abnormal growth located inside the skull.
Braxton Hicks contractions: intermittent painless uterine contractions that are not true labor pains.
breast augmentation: mammoplasty performed to increase breast size.
breast cancer: carcinoma that develops from the cells of the breast and can spread to adjacent lymph nodes and other body sites.
breast reconstruction surgery: the creation of the shape a missing breast after a mastectomy.
breast reduction: mammoplasty performed to decrease and reshape excessively large, heavy breasts.
breast self-examination: a self-care procedure for the early detection of breast cancer.
breath test: a test used to diagnose certain intestinal disorders, which is named for the gas being tested.
breech presentation: a birth complication in which the buttocks or feet of the fetus are positioned to enter the birth canal first instead of the head.
bronchiectasis (**brong**-kee-**ECK**-tah-sis): permanent thickening of the walls of the bronchi caused by chronic infection and inflammation.
bronchiolitis: inflammation of the bronchioles.
bronchodilator (**brong**-koh-**DYE**-lay-tor): an inhaled medication that relaxes and expands the bronchial passages into the lungs.
bronchopneumonia (**brong**-koh-new-**MOH**-nee-ah): a localized form of pneumonia that often affects the bronchioles.
bronchopulmonary dysplasia (**brong**-koh-**PUL**-mon-eh-ree dis-**PLAY**-zhee-ah): condition affecting premature babies who require lung support for an extended period of time in order to breathe after birth.
bronchorrhea (**brong**-koh-**REE**-ah): an excessive discharge of mucus from the bronchi.
bronchoscopy (brong-**KOS**-koh-pee): the visual examination of the bronchi using a bronchoscope.
bronchospasm (**BRONG**-koh-spazm): a contraction of the smooth muscle in the walls of the bronchi and bronchioles that tighten and squeeze the airway shut.
bruit (**BREW**-ee): an abnormal sound or murmur heard during auscultation of an artery.
bruxism (**BRUCK**-sizm): involuntary grinding of the teeth that usually occurs during sleep.
bulimia nervosa (byou-**LIM**-ee-ah *or* boo-**LEE**-mee-ah): an eating disorder characterized by frequent episodes of binge eating followed by compensatory behaviors, such as self-induced vomiting.
bulla (**BULL**-ah): a large blister that is usually more than 0.5 cm in diameter.
bundle branch block: partial block in electrical conduction between the atrium and ventricle on one side of the heart.

burn: an injury to body tissues caused by heat, flame, electricity, sun, chemicals, or radiation.

burn cream: topical medication used to treat burns by preventing moisture loss and bacterial infection.

burn, first-degree: a burn in which there are no blisters and only superficial damage to the epidermis.

burn, second-degree: a burn in which there are blisters and damage to both the epidermis and the dermis.

burn, third-degree: a burn in which there is damage to the epidermis, dermis, subcutaneous layers, and possibly also the muscle below.

bursitis (ber-**SIGH**-tis): inflammation of a bursa.

C

cachexia (kah-**KEKS**-eeh-ah): physical wasting away due to the loss of weight and muscle mass that occurs in patients with diseases such as advanced cancer or AIDS.

cadaver (kuh-**DAH**-vair): a dead human body.

calcium channel blocker: antihypertensive, anti-arrhythmic medication that decreases the movement of calcium ions into the cells of the heart and arteries, causing the arteries to relax and slowing the heart rate.

calciuria (**kal**-sih-**YOU**-ree-ah): the presence of calcium in the urine.

callus (**KAL**-us): a bulging deposit that forms around the area of the break in a bone; also a thickening of the skin that is caused by repeated rubbing.

cancer: a class of diseases characterized by the uncontrolled division of cells and the ability of these cells to invade other tissues.

cancer survivor: a person living with or after cancer.

candidiasis (**kan**-dih-**DYE**-ah-sis): a yeast infection.

canker sores: gray-white pits (aphthous ulcers) with a red border in the soft tissues lining the mouth.

capillary hemangioma (**KAP**-uh-**ler**-ee hee-**man**-jee-**OH**-mah): a soft, raised, pink or red vascular birthmark.

capillary puncture: technique for obtaining a small about of blood.

capsule: a round or oval object containing liquid or solid medication covered in a dissolvable coating designed to be swallowed.

carbon monoxide poisoning: a potentially fatal condition in which exposure to carbon monoxide causes high concentrations of carbon monoxide in the bloodstream, interfering with the body's ability to utilize oxygen.

carbuncle (**KAR**-bung-kul): a cluster of connected furuncles (boils).

carcinogen (kar-**SIH**-noh-jen): a substance known to cause cancer.

carcinogenesis (kar-**sih**-noh-**JEH**-neh-sis): the process through which normal cells become cancer cells.

carcinoma (**kar**-sih-**NOH**-mah): a malignant tumor that occurs in epithelial tissue.

carcinoma in situ: a malignant tumor in its original position that has not yet disturbed or invaded the surrounding tissues.

cardiac ablation (ab-**LAY**-shun): a procedure using heat or extreme cold to scar or destroy the heart tissue triggering an abnormal heart rhythm.

cardiac arrest: an event in which the heart abruptly stops beating or develops an arrhythmia that prevents it from pumping blood effectively.

cardiac catheterization (**KAR**-dee-ack **kath**-eh-ter-eye-**ZAY**-shun): a diagnostic and treatment procedure in which a catheter is passed into a vein or artery and guided into the heart.

cardiocentesis (**kar**-dee-oh-sen-**TEE**-sis): the puncture of a chamber of the heart for diagnosis or therapy.

cardiomegaly (**kar**-dee-oh-**MEG**-ah-lee): abnormal enlargement of the heart.

cardiomyopathy (**kar**-dee-oh-my-**OP**-pah-thee): all diseases of the heart muscle.

cardiopulmonary resuscitation: an emergency procedure for life support consisting of artificial respiration and manual external cardiac compression.

carditis (kar-**DYE**-tis): an inflammation of the heart.

carotid artery stenosis: abnormal narrowing of the carotid artery supplying blood to the brain.

carotid endarterectomy (**end**-ar-ter-**ECK**-toh-mee): surgical removal of the lining of a portion of a clogged carotid artery.

carotid ultrasonography: an ultrasound study of the carotid artery performed to predict or diagnose an ischemic stroke.

carpal tunnel release: surgical enlargement of the carpal tunnel or cutting of the carpal ligament to relieve pressure on the median nerve.

carpal tunnel syndrome: swelling that creates pressure on the median nerve as it passes through the carpal tunnel.

casts: protein or fibrous material found in the urine in kidney disease.

cataract (**KAT**-ah-rakt): the loss of transparency of the lens of the eye.

cataract surgery: general term to describe the surgical removal of a cataract-clouded lens and its replacement with an artificial intraocular lens.

catatonic behavior (**kat**-ah-**TON**-ick): behavior marked by a lack of responsiveness, stupor, and a tendency to remain in a fixed posture.

causalgia (kaw-**ZAL**-jee-ah): persistent, severe, burning pain that usually follows an injury to a sensory nerve.

cauterization (**kaw**-ter-eye-**ZAY**-shun): the destruction of tissue by burning.

celiac disease (**SEE**-lee-ak): an autoimmune disorder characterized by a severe reaction to ingesting gluten.

cellulitis (**sell**-you-**LYE**-tis): an acute, rapidly spreading bacterial infection within the connective tissues of the skin.

centesis (sen-**TEE**-sis): a surgical puncture to remove fluid for diagnostic purposes or to remove excess fluid.

cephalalgia (**sef**-ah-**LAL**-jee-ah): headache.

cephalic presentation: when a baby is born head first.

cerebral contusion (**SER**-eh-bral kon-**TOO**-zhun): bruising of brain tissue as the result of a head injury that causes the brain to bounce against the skull.

cerebral palsy (**SER**-eh-bral *or* **seh-REE**-bral **PAWL**-zee): a group of disorders characterized by poor muscle control, spasticity, and other neurologic deficiencies.

cerebrovascular accident (**ser**-eh-broh-**VAS**-kyou-lar): brain damage that occurs when blood flow to the brain is disrupted.

cervical cancer: slow-growing squamous cell cancer that develops in the cervix.

cervical cerclage (sir-**KLAZH**): procedure in which sutures or a type of synthetic tape are used to reinforce the cervix in order to prevent premature birth.

cervical dysplasia (**SER**-vih-kal dis-**PLAY**-zhee-ah): the presence of precancerous changes in the cells that make up the inner lining of the cervix.

cervical insufficiency: weakened tissue in the cervix.

cervical radiculopathy (rah-**dick**-you-**LOP**-ah-thee): nerve pain caused by pressure on the spinal nerve roots in the neck region.

cervicitis (**ser**-vih-**SIGH**-tis): inflammation of the cervix.

cesarean section (seh-**ZEHR**-ee-un **SECK**-shun): the delivery of a baby through an incision in the maternal abdominal and uterine walls.

chalazion (kah-**LAY**-zee-on): a nodule or cyst, usually on the upper eyelid, caused by obstruction of a sebaceous gland.

chancre (**SHANK**-er): a sore caused by syphilis.

cheilitis (kye-**LIGH**-tis): inflammation of the lips characterized by crack-like sores at the corners of the mouth.

chemabrasion (keem-ah-**BRAY**-shun): the use of chemicals to remove the outer layers of skin.

chemoprevention: the use of natural or synthetic substances such as drugs or vitamins to reduce the risk of developing cancer or to reduce the chance that cancer will recur.

chemotherapy (**kee**-moh-**THEH**-ruh-pee): medication that stops or slows the growth of cancer cells.

chest x-ray: radiographic view of the chest, used to diagnose disorders of the lungs and heart.

Cheyne–Stokes respiration (**CHAYN STOHKS**): an irregular pattern of breathing characterized by alternating rapid or shallow respiration followed by slow respiration or apnea.

Chiari malformation (kee-**AR**-ee): a congenital condition in which part of the cerebellum extends down into the spinal canal.

chiropractic manipulative therapy: a system of mechanical spinal adjustments made by a chiropractor to correct biomechanical problems in the skeleton.

chlamydia (klah-**MID**-ee-ah): a sexually transmitted disease caused by the bacteria *Chlamydia trachomatis.*

chloasma (kloh-**AZ**-mah): melasma, a pigmentation disorder characterized by brownish spots on the face.

cholangiography (koh-**LAN**-jee-**og**-rah-fee): radiographic examination of the bile ducts with the use of a contrast medium.

cholangitis (**koh**-lan-**JIGH**-tis): acute inflammation of the bile duct characterized by pain in the right upper quadrant of the abdomen, fever, and jaundice.

cholecystectomy (**koh**-luh-sis-**TECK**-toh-mee): surgical removal of the gallbladder.

cholecystitis (**koh**-luh-sis-**TYE**-tis): inflammation of the gallbladder usually associated with gallstones.

cholelithiasis (**koh**-lee-luh-**THIGH**-ah-sis): the presence of gallstones in the gallbladder or bile ducts.

cholesteatoma (koh-**les**-tee-ah-**TOH**-mah): destructive epidermal cyst in the middle ear made up of epithelial cells and cholesterol.

cholesterol (koh-**LES**-ter-ol): a fatty substance that travels through the blood and is found in all parts of the body.

cholesterol-lowering drug: medication that is administered to reduce the undesirable cholesterol levels in the blood.

chondromalacia (**kon**-droh-mah-**LAY**-shee-ah): abnormal softening of cartilage.

chorionic villus sampling (**kor**-ee-**ON**-ick **VIL**-us): examination of cells retrieved from the chorionic villi between the 11th and 14th weeks of pregnancy.

chromosomal congenital disorders: occur when there is an extra chromosome, or when a section of a chromosome is deleted or duplicated.

chronic bronchitis: a disease in which the airways have become inflamed due to recurrent exposure to an inhaled irritant.

chronic fatigue syndrome: a disorder of unknown cause that affects many body systems, with symptoms similar to those of fibromyalgia.

chronic kidney disease: the progressive loss of renal function over months or years.

chronic lymphocytic leukemia: a blood cancer characterized by a slow buildup of abnormal lymphocytes.

chronic myeloid leukemia: a blood cancer characterized by a slow buildup of abnormal leukocytes.

chronic obstructive pulmonary disease: a group of lung diseases in which the bronchial airflow is obstructed, making it difficult to breathe out.

chronic venous insufficiency: a condition in which venous circulation is inadequate due to partial vein blockage or leakage of venous valves.

cicatrix (sick-**AY**-tricks): a normal scar resulting from the healing of a wound.

circumcision (**ser**-kum-**SIZH**-un): surgical removal of the foreskin of the penis.

cirrhosis (sih-**ROH**-sis): a chronic degenerative disease of the liver characterized by scarring.

claustrophobia (**klaws**-troh-**FOH**-bee-ah): abnormal fear of being in small or enclosed spaces.

cleft lip: a birth defect resulting in a deep groove of the lip running upward to the nose.

cleft palate: failure of the palate to close during the early development of the fetus that involves the upper lip, hard palate, and/or soft palate.

clinical trials: testing new treatments that have not yet received FDA approval on patients who agree to be part of the research.

closed-angle glaucoma: a type of glaucoma in which the opening between the cornea and iris narrows so that fluid cannot reach the trabecular meshwork.

closed fracture: a fracture in which the bone is broken but there is no open wound in the skin.

closed reduction: the attempted non-surgical realignment of the bone involved in a fracture or joint dislocation.

Clostridium difficile (klos-**TRID**-ee-um dif-us-**SEEL**): a bacterial infection common to older adults in hospitals or long-term care facilities.

clubbing: abnormal curving of the nails that is often accompanied by enlargement of the fingertips.

clubfoot: any congenital deformity of the foot involving the ankle bones.

cluster headaches: intensely painful headaches that affect one side of the head and often occur in groups or clusters.

coagulopathy (koh-**ag**-you-**LOP**-ah-thee): a bleeding disorder that occurs when the blood's ability to coagulate is impaired.

cochlear implant (**KOCK**-lee-ar): an electronic device that bypasses the damaged portions of the ear and directly stimulates the auditory nerve.

cognition (kog-**NISH**-un): the mental activities associated with thinking, learning, and memory.

cognitive behavioral therapy: treatment that focuses on changing thoughts that are affecting a person's emotions and actions.

cold sores: blister-like sores on the lips caused by the herpes simplex virus (HSV) type 1.

colectomy (koh-**LECK**-toh-mee): surgical removal of all or part of the colon.

colic: a condition of a generally healthy baby crying for more than three hours a day, more than three days a week for three or more weeks, and being difficult to soothe.

collagen replacement therapy: a form of soft-tissue augmentation used to soften facial lines or scars, or to make lips appear fuller.

Colles fracture (**KAHL**-es): a fracture at the lower end of the radius that occurs when a person tries to break a fall by landing on his or her hands.

colonoscopy (**koh**-lun-**OSS**-koh-pee): direct visual examination of the inner surface of the colon from the rectum to the cecum.

color blindness: the inability to distinguish certain colors in a normal manner.

colorectal cancer: a common form of cancer that often first manifests itself in polyps in the colon.

colostomy (koh-**LAHS**-toh-mee): surgical creation of an artificial excretory opening between the colon and the body surface.

colporrhaphy (kol-**POR**-ah-fee): surgical suturing of a tear in the vagina.

colposcopy (kol-**POS**-koh-pee): direct visual examination of the tissues of the cervix, vagina, and vulva.

coma (**KOH**-mah): a deep state of unconsciousness marked by the absence of spontaneous eye movements, no response to painful stimuli, and no vocalization.

comedo (**KOM**-eh-doh): a noninfected lesion formed by the buildup of sebum and keratin in a hair follicle.

comminuted fracture (**KOM**-ih-**newt**-ed): a fracture in which the bone is splintered or crushed.

communicable disease (kuh-**MEW**-nih-kuh-bul): any condition that is transmitted from one person to another by either direct or indirect contact with contaminated objects.

communication disorders: difficulty either comprehending or communicating with others.

community-acquired pneumonia: any pneumonia that results from contagious infection outside of a hospital or clinic.

compartment syndrome: the compression of nerves and blood vessels due to swelling within the enclosed space created by the fascia that separates groups of muscles.

complementary medicine: practices and systems of health care used to supplement allopathic medicine.

complete blood count: tests that measure various components of the blood in order to identify blood disorders and diseases.

complete remission (ree-**MIH**-shun): absence of cancer in response to treatment.

complex regional pain syndrome: chronic nerve pain affecting one limb usually following an injury.

comprehensive metabolic panel: a screening tool used to provide information about the state of the body's metabolism by measuring different substances in the blood.

compression fracture: a fracture in which the bone is pressed together on itself.

computed tomography (toh-**MOG**-rah-fee): an imaging technique that uses a thin, fan-shaped x-ray beam to produce multiple cross-sectional views of the body.

concussion (kon-**KUSH**-un): a violent shaking up or jarring of the brain.

conductive hearing loss: a hearing loss in which sound waves are prevented from passing from the air to the fluid-filled inner ear.

congenital anomaly: abnormality of a structure or function of the body that is prenatal in origin.

congenital disorder (kon-**JEN**-ih-tahl): an abnormal condition that exists at the time of birth.

congenital heart defects: structural abnormalities caused by the failure of the heart to develop normally before birth.

congestive heart failure: chronic condition in which the heart is unable to pump out all of the blood it receives.

conization (**kon**-ih-**ZAY**-shun *or* **koh**-nih-**ZAY**-shun): surgical removal of a cone-shaped section of tissue from the cervix.

conjunctivitis (kon-**junk**-tih-**VYE**-tis): inflammation of the conjunctiva, usually caused by an infection or allergy.

conscious: the state of being awake, alert, aware, and responding appropriately.

conscious sedation: a state of light to moderate sedation where the patient is calm, relaxed, and less responsive to stimuli.

constipation: having a bowel movement fewer than three times per week.

contact dermatitis: a localized rash caused by repeated contact with an irritant or allergen.

continuous glucose monitoring: a method of constantly tracking blood glucose levels through a tiny sensor inserted under the skin.

contraceptive: a measure taken to lessen the likelihood of pregnancy.

contraceptive implant: a form of long-term birth control placed under the skin of the upper arm.

contracture (kon-**TRACK**-chur): the permanent tightening of fascia, muscles, tendons, ligaments, or skin that occurs when normally elastic connective tissues are replaced with nonelastic fibrous tissues.

contraindication (**kon**-trah-inn-dih-**KAY**-shun): a factor in the patient's condition that makes the use of a medication or specific treatment dangerous or ill advised.

contrast medium: a substance used to make visible structures that are otherwise hard to see.

controlled substances: addictive prescription medicines and illegal drugs whose manufacture, possession, and use are regulated by the government.

contusion (kon-**TOO**-zhun): an injury to underlying tissues without breaking the skin, characterized by discoloration and pain.

COPD exacerbation: acute episode of worsening chronic obstructive pulmonary disease symptoms.

core needle biopsy: a technique in which a hollow needle is used to remove small samples of tissue from the breast for diagnosis and the planning of treatment.

corneal abrasion: an injury, such as a scratch or irritation, to the outer layers of the cornea.

corneal transplant: surgical replacement of a scarred or diseased cornea with clear corneal tissue from a donor.

corneal ulcer: an open sore on the cornea caused by an infection or injury.

coronary artery bypass graft: a surgical procedure in which a piece of vein from the leg is implanted on the heart to replace a blocked coronary artery.

coronary artery disease: atherosclerosis of the coronary arteries that reduces the blood supply to the heart muscle.

coronary thrombosis (**KOR**-uh-**nehr**-ee throm-**BOH**-sis): damage to the heart muscle caused by a thrombus blocking a coronary artery.

corticosteroid drug: synthetic hormone that closely resembles the cortisol secreted by the adrenal glands, used to reduce inflammation.

corticosteroid injection: injections of cortisone into an affected joint for temporary relief of osteoarthritis pain.

cortisone (**KOR**-tih-sohn): the synthetic equivalent of natural corticosteroids that are administered to suppress inflammation and to act as an immunosuppressant.

costochondritis (**kos**-toh-kon-**DRIGH**-tis): inflammation of the cartilage that connects a rib to the sternum.

cover test: an exam of how the two eyes work together, used to assess binocular vision.

COVID-19 (**KOH**-vid): a highly contagious viral infection caused by the SARS-CoV-2 virus.

CPAP machine: a noninvasive ventilation device used in the treatment of sleep apnea.

cradle cap: scalp rash in an infant.

cramp: a painful localized muscle spasm.

cranial hematoma (**hee**-mah-**TOH**-mah): a collection of blood trapped in the tissues of the brain.

craniosacral therapy (**kray**-nee-oh-**SAK**-ral): the use of gentle touch to help the body release tension in order to correct restrictions resulting from stress on the central nervous system.

craniotomy (**kray**-nee-**OT**-oh-mee): a surgical incision or opening into the skull.

C-reactive protein: a blood test that detects high levels of inflammation within the body.

creatinuria (kree-**at**-ih-**NEW**-ree-ah): an increased concentration of creatinine in the urine.

crepitation (**krep**-ih-**TAY**-shun): the grating sound heard when the ends of a broken bone move together.

cretinism (**CREE**-tin-izm): a congenital form of hypothyroidism.

Crohn's disease: a chronic autoimmune disorder that can occur anywhere in the digestive tract; however, it is most often found in the ileum and in the colon.

crossmatch tests: blood tests performed to determine the compatibility of blood donor and recipient before a transfusion.

croup (**KROOP**): an acute respiratory infection in children and infants characterized by obstruction of the larynx, hoarseness, and swelling around the vocal cords resulting in a barking cough and stridor.

crust: a collection of dried serum and cellular debris that forms as a barrier over a partial-thickness wound.

cryopreservation: the freezing of sperm, tissue, or organs for later use.

cryosurgery: the destruction or elimination of abnormal tissue cells through the application of extreme cold by using liquid nitrogen.

cryptorchidism (krip-**TOR**-kih-dizm): a developmental defect seen in newborns in which one or both testicles fail to descend into the scrotum.

curettage (**kyou**-reh-**TAHZH**): the removal of material from the surface by scraping.

Cushing's syndrome (**KUSH**-ingz): a condition caused by prolonged exposure to high levels of cortisol.

cyanosis (**sigh**-ah-**NOH**-sis): bluish discoloration of the skin and mucous membranes caused by a lack of adequate oxygen in the blood.

cyst: an abnormal sac containing fluid, gas, or a semisolid material.

cystalgia (sis-**TAL**-jee-ah): pain in the urinary bladder.

cystectomy (sis-**TECK**-toh-mee): surgical removal of all or part of the urinary bladder.

cystic fibrosis (**SIS**-tick figh-**BROH**-sis): a life-threatening genetic disorder in which the lungs and pancreas are clogged with large quantities of abnormally thick mucus.

cystitis (sis-**TYE**-tis): inflammation of the bladder.

cystocele (**SIS**-toh-seel): a hernia of the bladder through the vaginal wall.

cystography (sis-**TOG**-rah-fee): an x-ray or fluoroscopy examination of the bladder after instillation of a contrast medium via a urethral catheter.

cystolith (**SIS**-toh-lith): a stone located within the urinary bladder.

cystorrhaphy (sis-**TOR**-ah-fee): surgical suturing of a wound or defect in the bladder.

cystoscopy (sis-**TOS**-koh-pee): the visual examination of the urinary bladder using a cystoscope.

cytomegalovirus (**sigh**-toh-**meg**-ah-loh-**VYE**-rus): a type of herpes virus found in most body fluids.

cytotoxic drug (**sigh**-toh-**TOK**-sick): medication that kills or damages cells.

D

dacryoadenitis (**dack**-ree-oh-ad-eh-**NIGH**-tis): an inflammation of the lacrimal gland caused by a bacterial, viral, or fungal infection.

dacryocystitis (**dack**-ree-oh-sis-**TYE**-tis): an inflammation of the lacrimal sac usually caused by blockage of the lacrimal duct.

deafness: the complete or partial loss of the ability to hear.

death: the irreversible end of all brain, heart, and lung activity.

death rattle: the labored, noisy breathing that can occur at end of life.

debridement (dah-**BREED**-ment): the removal of dirt, foreign objects, damaged tissue, and cellular debris from a wound to prevent infection and to promote healing.

decibel: commonly used as the measurement of the loudness of sound.

decompression sickness: accumulated nitrogen damaging blood vessels and tissue or triggering small blood clots.

decompressive craniectomy (**kray**-nee-**ECK**-toh-mee): surgical removal of a portion of the skull.

decongestant: an oral or intranasal medication administered to relieve nasal congestion from allergies or illness.

deep brain stimulation: a neurosurgical procedure used in the treatment of dystonia, tremors, and Parkinson's disease.

deep tendon reflexes: testing of reflexes to diagnose disruptions of the nerve supply to the involved muscles.

deep vein thrombosis: the condition of having a thrombus attached to the interior wall of a deep vein.

defibrillation (dee-**fib**-rih-**LAY**-shun): the emergency use of electrical shock to restore the heart's normal rhythm.

dehydration: a condition in which fluid loss exceeds fluid intake and disrupts the body's normal electrolyte balance.

delirium (deh-**LEER**-ee-um): an acute condition of confusion, disorientation, disordered thinking and memory, agitation, and hallucinations.

delirium tremens (**TREE**-mens): a disorder involving sudden and severe mental changes or seizures caused by abruptly stopping the use of alcohol.

delusion (dih-**LOO**-zhun): a false personal belief that is maintained despite obvious proof or evidence to the contrary.

dementia (dih-**MEN**-shee-ah): a slowly progressive decline in mental abilities including memory, thinking, and judgment that is often accompanied by personality changes.

dental calculus (**KAL**-kyou-luhs): hardened dental plaque on the teeth.

dental caries (**KAYR**-eez): an infectious disease that destroys the enamel and dentin of the tooth.

dental implant: the anchoring of a crown, bridge, or denture to the bone of the jaw.

dental plaque (**PLACK**): a soft deposit consisting of bacteria and bacterial by-products that builds up on the teeth.

dental prophylaxis (**proh**-fih-**LACK**-sis): the professional cleaning of the teeth to remove plaque and calculus.

dentures: a removable set of artificial teeth that replace some or all of a person's teeth.

dependence: when the body becomes accustomed to a medication or substance after repeated use, and experiences physical and/or psychological withdrawal symptoms if it is stopped.

depression: a common mood disorder characterized by sadness, changes in sleep, energy, and concentration and may be accompanied by lack of interest in formerly pleasurable activities, or inability to enjoy oneself.

dermabrasion (**der**-mah-**BRAY**-zhun): a form of abrasion involving the use of a revolving wire brush or sandpaper.

dermatitis (**der**-mah-**TYE**-tis): inflammation of the skin.

dermatosis (**der**-mah-**TOH**-sis): a general term used to denote skin lesions or eruptions of any type that are not associated with inflammation.

dermoid cyst: benign tumor containing various tissues such as teeth, bone, skin glands, or hair.

developmental disorder: disorder that can result in an anomaly or malformation such as the absence of a limb or the presence of an extra toe.

developmental dysplasia of the hip: dislocation of the thigh bone in the hip socket found in children.

diabetes insipidus (**dye**-ah-**BEE**-teez in-**SIP**-ih-dus): a condition caused by insufficient production of the antidiuretic hormone or by the inability of the kidneys to respond to this hormone.

diabetes mellitus (**dye**-ah-**BEE**-teez **MEL**-ih-tus): a group of metabolic disorders characterized by hyperglycemia resulting from defects in the body's production of insulin (type 1) or its ability to use it properly (type 2).

diabetic coma: a diabetic emergency caused by very high or very low blood glucose resulting in unconsciousness.

diabetic ketoacidosis: a life-threatening complication of uncontrolled diabetes caused by a buildup of acids in the blood.

diabetic neuropathy (new-**ROP**-ah-thee): peripheral neuropathy caused by poorly controlled diabetes.

diabetic retinopathy (**ret**-ih-**NOP**-ah-thee): damage to the retina as a complication of uncontrolled diabetes.

dialysis (dye-**AL**-ih-sis): a procedure to remove waste products from the blood of patients whose kidneys no longer function.

diaphoresis: profuse sweating.

diaphragm: a barrier contraceptive inserted into the vagina to cover the cervix.

diarrhea (**dye**-ah-**REE**-ah): the frequent flow of loose or watery stools.

dietary supplement: a product containing nutrients believed to be beneficial for health.

digital rectal examination: an examination performed on men to palpate the prostate gland.

digitalis (**dij**-ih-**TAL**-is): medication that strengthens the heart muscle contractions, slows the heart rate, and helps eliminate fluid from body tissues.

dilation and curettage (dye-**LAY**-shun and **kyou**-reh-**TAHZH**): a surgical procedure in which the cervix is dilated and the endometrium of the uterus is scraped away.

diopter (dye-**OP**-ter): the unit of measurement of a lens's refractive power.

diphtheria: infection characterized by sore throat, mild fever, weakness, swollen glands in neck. DTap and Tdap vaccine protect against it.

diplopia (dih-**PLOH**-pee-ah): the perception of two images of a single object.

direct antiglobulin test: a blood test used to investigate possible hemolytic transfusion reaction or hemolytic disease.

dislocation: the total displacement of a bone from its joint.

dissociative disorders: conditions that occur when normal thought is separated from consciousness.

dissociative identity disorder: a mental illness characterized by the presence of two or more distinct personalities, each with its own characteristics, which appear to exist within the same individual.

diuresis (**dye**-you-**REE**-sis): the increased output of urine.

diuretic (**dye**-you-**RET**-ick): antihypertensive medication administered to increase urine output to rid the body of excess sodium and water.

diverticulectomy (**dye**-ver-**tick**-you-**LECK**-toh-mee): surgical removal of a diverticulum.

diverticulitis (**dye**-ver-tick-you-**LYE**-tis): inflammation or infection of one or more diverticula in the wall of the colon.

diverticulosis (**dye**-ver-**tick**-you-**LOH**-sis): the chronic presence of an abnormal number of diverticula in the wall of the colon.

diverticulum (**dye**-ver-**TICK**-you-lum): a small pouch or sac occurring in the lining or wall of a tubular organ.

dopaminergic drug: medication that treats the symptoms of Parkinson's by increasing brain dopamine activity.

Doppler echocardiogram: an ultrasonic diagnostic procedure that measures the speed and direction of the blood flow within the heart.

dorsal recumbent position: position in which the patient is lying on the back, face up, with the knees bent.

dose: a measured quantity of a medication ordered to be given at one time.

Down syndrome: a genetic variation that is associated with characteristic facial appearance, learning disabilities, and physical abnormalities such as heart valve disease.

droplet transmission: the spread of diseases such as measles, cold, and flu through large respiratory droplets sprayed by coughing or sneezing onto a nearby person or object.

drug abuse: the excessive use of illegal drugs or the misuse of prescription drugs.

drug interaction: the result of drugs reacting with each other, often in ways that are unexpected or potentially harmful.

drug-screening urine test: a urine test to identify the presence of one or more drugs of abuse in the body.

drug overdose: potentially fatal, accidental, or intentional use of an illegal drug or prescription medicine in an amount higher than what is safe or normal.

drug tolerance: when the body has been accustomed to a medication after taking it for a length of time and higher doses are required to achieve the desired effect.

dual x-ray absorptiometry (ab-**sorp**-shee-**OM**-eh-tree): a low-exposure x-ray measurement of the spine and hips to measure bone density.

ductal carcinoma in situ: breast cancer at its earliest stage before the cancer has broken through the wall of the milk duct.

duplex ultrasound: a diagnostic procedure to image the structures of the blood vessels and the flow of blood through these vessels.

dying process: the period of time that may occur leading up to death when a person's body begins to shut down.

dysentery (**DIS**-en-**ter**-ee): a bacterial infection spread through food or water contaminated by human feces.

dyskinesia (**dis**-kih-**NEE**-zee-ah): distortion or impairment of voluntary movement.

dyslexia (dis-**LECK**-see-ah): a learning disability characterized by substandard reading achievement due to the inability of the brain to process symbols correctly.

dysmenorrhea (**dis**-men-oh-**REE**-ah): pain caused by uterine contractions during a menstrual period.

dyspareunia (**dis**-pah-**ROO**-nee-ah): pain during sexual intercourse.

dyspepsia (dis-**PEP**-see-ah): pain or discomfort in digestion.

dysphagia (dis-**FAY**-jee-ah): difficulty in swallowing.

dysphonia (dis-**FOH**-nee-ah): difficulty in speaking, which may include any impairment in vocal quality.

dysplasia (dis-**PLAY**-zhee-ah): abnormal development or growth of cells, tissues, or organs, or the presence of abnormal cells within a type of tissue.

dysplastic nevi (dis-**PLAS**-tick **NEE**-vye): atypical moles that can develop into skin cancer.

dyspnea (**DISP**-nee-ah): difficult or labored breathing.

dyspnea on exertion: shortness of breath that occurs with physical activity.

dystonia (dis-**TOH**-nee-ah): a movement disorder characterized by the involuntary and sometimes repetitive contraction of certain muscles.

dysuria (dis-**YOU**-ree-ah): difficult or painful urination.

E

ear drop: liquid medication administered into the ear.

ear tubes: tiny ventilating tubes placed through the eardrum to provide ongoing drainage for fluids and to relieve pressure that can build up after childhood ear infections.

Ebola (ee-**BOH**-lah): a rare and generally fatal disease transmitted by contact with any bodily fluids infected with the *Ebola* virus.

ecchymosis (**eck**-ih-**MOH**-sis): a large, irregular area of purplish discoloration due to bleeding under the skin.

echocardiography (**eck**-oh-**kar**-dee-**OG**-rah-fee): an ultrasonic diagnostic procedure used to evaluate the structures and motion of the heart.

eclampsia (eh-**KLAMP**-see-ah): a serious condition characterized by seizures and coma that can develop during or after pregnancy from uncontrolled preeclampsia.

E. coli: infection caused by the bacteria *Escherichia coli,* transmitted through improperly cooked, contaminated foods.

ectopic kidney: congenital condition in which one kidney is located in an abnormal position or has fused with the other kidney.

ectopic pregnancy (eck-**TOP**-ick): a condition in which a fertilized egg is implanted and begins to develop outside of the uterus.

eczema (**ECK**-zeh-mah): a form of recurring dermatitis characterized by itching, redness, and dryness.

edema (eh-**DEE**-mah): swelling caused by an abnormal accumulation of fluid in cells, tissues, or cavities of the body.

edentulous: a person without teeth, after the natural permanent teeth have been lost.

electrophysiologist: a doctor specializing in the diagnosis and treatment of heart arrhythmias.

electrocardiogram (ee-**leck**-troh-**KAR**-dee-oh-**gram**): a record of the electrical activity of the myocardium.

electrocardiography (ee-**leck**-troh-kar-dee-**OG**-rah-fee): the noninvasive process of recording the electrical activity of the myocardium.

electroconvulsive therapy (ee-**leck**-troh-kon-**VUL**-siv): a procedure in which small amounts of electric current are passed through the brain, deliberately triggering a brief seizure in order to reverse symptoms of certain mental illnesses.

electrodesiccation (ee-**leck**-troh-des-ih-**KAY**-shun): a surgical technique in which tissue is destroyed using an electric spark.

electroencephalography (ee-**leck**-troh-en-**sef**-ah-**LOG**-rah-fee): the process of recording the electrical activity of the brain through the use of electrodes attached to the scalp.

electrolysis: the use of electric current to destroy hair follicles for the removal of undesired hair.

electromyography (ee-**leck**-troh-my-**OG**-rah-fee): a diagnostic test that measures the electrical activity within muscle fibers in response to nerve stimulation.

electronic fetal monitoring: the recording of the heartbeat of the fetus and the contractions of the woman's uterus.

ELISA: the acronym for enzyme-linked immunosorbent assay, a blood test that is used to screen for the presence of HIV antibodies.

embolism (**EM**-boh-lizm): the sudden blockage of a blood vessel by an embolus.

embolus (**EM**-boh-lus): a foreign object, such as a blood clot, a quantity of air or gas, or a bit of tissue or tumor, that is circulating in the blood.

EMDR: an evidence-based treatment for PTSD that involves revisiting traumatic memories while simultaneously focusing on specific bilateral physical stimuli.

emesis (**EM**-eh-sis): the reflex ejection of the stomach contents outward through the mouth (vomiting).

emphysema (**em**-fih-**SEE**-mah): the progressive, long-term loss of lung function, usually due to smoking.

empyema (**em**-pye-**EE**-mah): an accumulation of pus in a body cavity.

encephalitis (**en**-sef-ah-**LYE**-tis): inflammation of the brain.

encephalocele (en-**SEF**-ah-loh-**seel**): a congenital herniation of brain tissue through a gap in the skull.

endemic (en-**DEM**-ick): refers to the ongoing presence of a disease within a population, group, or area.
endocarditis (**en**-doh-kar-**DYE**-tis): inflammation of the inner lining of the heart.
endometrial biopsy (**en**-doh-**MEE**-tree-al **BYE**-op-see): a diagnostic test in which a small amount of the tissue lining the uterus is removed for microscopic examination.
endometrial cancer: a cancerous growth that begins in the lining of the uterus.
endometriosis (**en**-doh-**mee**-tree-**OH**-sis): a condition in which patches of endometrial tissue escape the uterus and become attached to other structures in the pelvic cavity.
endophthalmitis (**end**-op-thahl-**MYE**-tis): inflammation of the intraocular fluids.
endoscope (**EN**-doh-**skope**): a small, flexible tube with a light and lens on the end.
endoscopic surgery: a surgical procedure performed through very small incisions with the use of an endoscope and specialized instruments.
endoscopy (en-**DOS**-koh-pee): the visual examination of the interior of a body cavity or organ.
endotracheal intubation (**en**-doh-**TRAY**-kee-al **in**-too-**BAY**-shun): the passage of a tube through the mouth into the trachea to establish or maintain an open airway.
end-stage COPD: the final stage of chronic obstructive pulmonary disease.
end-stage renal disease: the final stage of chronic kidney disease.
enema (**EN**-eh-ma): liquid medication placed in the rectum.
enteral nutrition: feeding using the digestive system either through normal eating by mouth or via tube feeding.
enteritis (**en**-ter-**EYE**-tis): inflammation of the small intestine caused by ingesting substances contaminated with pathogens.
entropion (en-**TROH**-pee-on): the inversion of the edge of an eyelid.
enucleation (ee-**new**-klee-**AY**-shun): the removal of the eyeball, leaving the eye muscles intact.
enuresis (**en**-you-**REE**-sis): the involuntary discharge of urine.
eosinophilic esophagitis (**ee**-oh-sin-ah-**FIL**-ik eh-**sof**-ah-**JEYE**-tis): a chronic immune system disease in which a type of white blood cell builds up in the esophagus, usually as the result of an allergy to certain foods.
epicondylitis (**ep**-ih-**kon**-dih-**LYE**-tis): inflammation of the tissues surrounding the elbow.
epidemic (**ep**-ih-**DEM**-ick): a sudden and widespread outbreak of a disease within a specific population group or area.
epidermoid cyst (**ep**-ih-**DER**-moyd **SIST**): a closed sac that is found just under the skin.
epididymitis (**ep**-ih-did-ih-**MY**-tis): inflammation of the epididymis resulting from a bacterial infection.
epidural anesthesia (**ep**-ih-**DOO**-ral **an**-es-**THEE**-zee-ah): regional anesthesia produced by injecting medication into the epidural space of the lumbar or sacral region of the spine.
epidural block: anesthesia that blocks the nerve impulses to the lower half of the body during labor and childbirth, or surgery in the lower body.
epilepsy (**EP**-ih-**lep**-see): a chronic neurologic condition characterized by recurrent episodes of seizures of varying severity.
episiotomy (eh-**piz**-ee-**OT**-oh-mee): a surgical incision made into the perineum to enlarge the vaginal orifice to prevent tearing of the tissues as the infant moves out of the birth canal.
epispadias (**ep**-ih-**SPAY**-dee-as): a congenital abnormality of the urethral opening. In the male this opening is located on the upper surface of the penis; in the female the urethral opening is in the region of the clitoris.
epistaxis (**ep**-ih-**STACK**-sis): bleeding from the nose.
erectile dysfunction: the inability of the male to achieve or maintain a penile erection.
ergonomics (er-goh-**NOM**-icks): the study of the human factors that affect the design and operation of tools and the work environment.
erosion (eh-**ROH**-zhun): the wearing away of a surface.
eructation (eh-ruk-**TAY**-shun): the act of belching or raising gas orally from the stomach.
erythema (**er**-ih-**THEE**-mah): redness of the skin due to capillary dilation.
erythema infectiosum: mildly contagious viral infection common in childhood.
erythema multiforme: a skin disorder resulting from a generalized allergic reaction, characterized by a diffuse rash.
erythrocyte sedimentation rate (eh-**RITH**-roh-sight): a blood test for inflammation based on the speed with which red blood cells separate from plasma.
erythroderma (eh-**rith**-roh-**DER**-mah): abnormal redness of the entire skin surface.
eschar: dead crust-like tissue found in a full-thickness wound.

esophageal varices (eh-**sof**-ah-**JEE**-al **VAYR**-ih-seez): enlarged and swollen veins at the lower end of the esophagus.

esophagogastroduodenoscopy (eh-**sof**-ah-goh-**gas**-troh-**dew**-oh-deh-**NOS**-koh-pee): the endoscopic examination of the upper GI tract.

esotropia (**es**-oh-**TROH**-pee-ah): strabismus characterized by an inward deviation of one or both eyes.

etiology (**ee**-tee-**OL**-oh-jee): the study of the causes of diseases.

eupnea (youp-**NEE**-ah): easy or normal breathing.

exanthem (eck-**ZAN**-thum): a widespread rash, usually in children.

exfoliative cytology (ecks-**FOH**-lee-**ay**-tiv sigh-**TOL**-oh-jee): a biopsy technique in which cells are scraped from the tissue and examined under a microscope.

exfoliative dermatitis (ecks-**FOH**-lee-**ay**-tiv **der**-mah-**TYE**-tis): a condition in which there is widespread scaling of the skin.

exophthalmos (**eck**-sof-**THAL**-mos): an abnormal protrusion of the eyeball out of the orbit.

exotropia (**eck**-soh-**TROH**-pee-ah): strabismus characterized by the outward deviation of one eye relative to the other.

expectorant: an oral medication that makes it easier to cough up mucus by making it thinner and less viscous.

expectoration (eck-**SPEK**-toh-**ray**-shun): the act of coughing up and spitting out saliva, mucus, or other body fluid.

exposure therapy: treatment for anxiety disorders, including phobias, by repeated exposure to a fear in a safe and controlled setting.

external fixation: a fracture treatment procedure in which pins are placed through the soft tissues and bone so that an external appliance can be used to hold the pieces of bone firmly in place during healing.

extracorporeal shockwave lithotripsy: the destruction of kidney stones using high-energy ultrasonic waves traveling through water or gel.

extraoral radiography: dental x-ray in which the film is placed and exposed outside of the mouth.

extubation: the removal of an endotracheal tube and removal of a patient from the ventilator.

exudate (**ECKS**-you-dayt): fluid, such as pus, that leaks out of an infected wound.

eye drop: liquid medication administered onto the cornea.

F

factitious disorder (fack-**TISH**-us): a condition in which a person acts as if he or she has a physical or mental illness when he or she is not really sick.

failure to thrive: when someone does not grow as expected due to any number of reasons including malabsorption or malnutrition.

fall risk patient: a person who is at higher risk of falling.

fasciitis (**fas**-ee-**EYE**-tis): inflammation of a fascia.

fasciotomy (**fash**-ee-**OT**-oh-mee): a surgical incision through a fascia to relieve tension or pressure.

fasting blood sugar: a blood test to measure the glucose levels after the patient has not eaten for 8 to 12 hours.

fat embolus (**EM**-boh-lus): the release of fat cells from yellow bone marrow into the bloodstream when a long bone is fractured.

febrile seizure: a tonic–clonic seizure that occurs in infants and young children in response to a fever.

fecal microbiota transplantation: the transplant of stool from a healthy donor, used to restore gut bacteria.

fecal incontinence (in-**KON**-tih-nents): the inability to control the excretion of feces.

fetal alcohol syndrome: condition characterized by growth abnormalities, intellectual disability, brain damage, and socialization difficulties, caused by the mother's consumption of alcohol during pregnancy.

fetal ultrasound: a noninvasive procedure used to image and evaluate fetal development during pregnancy.

fever: a body temperature of 100°F or higher.

fibrillation (**fih**-brih-**LAY**-shun): a potentially life-threatening fast, irregular heartbeat.

fibroadenoma (**figh**-broh-**ad**-eh-**NOH**-mah): a round, rubbery, firm mass that arises from excess growth of glandular and connective tissue in the breast.

fibrocystic breast disease (**figh**-broh-**SIS**-tick): the presence of fibrous tissue and benign cysts in the breasts.

fibroids: benign tumors composed of muscle and fibrous tissue that occurs in the wall of the uterus.

fibromyalgia (**figh**-broh-my-**AL**-jee-ah): a debilitating chronic condition characterized by fatigue; muscle, joint, or bone pain; and a wide range of other symptoms.

filling: the restoration of a decaying tooth by removing the damaged area and replacing it with material to fill it in.

first trimester screening: testing performed between 11 and 13 weeks of pregnancy that involves an ultrasound and a blood test.

fissure (**FISH**-ur): a groove or crack-like sore of the skin; also normal folds in the contours of the brain.
fistula (**FIS**-tyou-lah): an abnormal passage between two internal organs or leading from an organ to the surface of the body.
flat head syndrome: flattening on the back or side of an infant's head.
flatulence (**FLAT**-you-lens): passage of gas out of the body through the rectum.
floaters: particles of cellular debris that float in the vitreous fluid and cast shadows on the retina.
fluid restriction: a limit on the amount of water and other liquids a person drinks per day.
fluorescein angiography (**flew**-oh-**RES**-ee-in **an**-jee-**OG**-rah-fee): a photographic study of the blood vessels in the back of the eye following the intravenous injection of a fluorescein dye as a contrast medium.
fluorescein staining (**flew**-oh-**RES**-ee-in): the application of a fluorescent dye to the surface of the eye via eye drops or a strip applicator.
fluoroscopy (**floo**-or-**OS**-koh-pee): the visualization of body parts in motion by projecting x-ray images on a luminous fluorescent screen.
focal seizure: a seizure involving one part of the brain, which may involve absence seizure-like symptoms and repetitive muscle movements.
Foley catheter: the most common type of indwelling urinary catheter.
folliculitis (foh-**lick**-you-**LYE**-tis): inflammation of the hair follicles.
food allergy: an immune system reaction that occurs after eating a certain food.
food-borne and waterborne transmission: disease transmission caused by eating or drinking contaminated food or water that has not been properly treated to remove contamination or kill pathogens that are present.
formulary (**FOR**-myoo-**layr**-ee): a list of prescription drugs covered by a specific health care plan.
fracture: a broken bone.
fructosamine test (fruck-**TOHS**-ah-meen): a blood test that measures average glucose levels over the past three weeks.
functional disorder: a condition that produces symptoms for which no disease or other organic cause can be identified.
functional endoscopic sinus surgery: a procedure performed using an endoscope in which chronic sinusitis is treated by enlarging the opening between the nose and sinus.
functional MRI: an imaging study that detects changes in blood flow in the brain when the patient is asked to perform a specific task.
functional neurologic disorders: disorders characterized by neurologic symptoms without a physical cause.
fungus (**FUNG**-gus): a simple parasitic organism.
furuncles (**FYOU**-rung-kulz): large, tender, swollen areas caused by a staphylococcal infection around hair follicles or sebaceous glands.

G

galactorrhea (gah-**lack**-toh-**REE**-ah): the production of breast milk in women who are not breastfeeding.
gallstone: a hard deposit that forms in the gallbladder and bile ducts.
Gamma knife surgery: a type of radiation treatment for brain tumors.
ganglion cyst: a benign, fluid-filled lump that occurs most commonly on the outer surface of the wrist.
gangrene (**GANG**-green): tissue death caused by a loss of circulation to the affected tissues.
gastralgia (gas-**TRAL**-jee-ah): pain in the stomach.
gastritis (gas-**TRY**-tis): inflammation of the stomach lining.
gastroduodenostomy (**gas**-troh-**dew**-oh-deh-**NOS**-toh-mee): the establishment of an anastomosis between the upper portion of the stomach and the duodenum.
gastrodynia (**gas**-troh-**DIN**-ee-ah): pain in the stomach.
gastroenteritis (**gas**-troh-en-ter-**EYE**-tis): inflammation of the mucous membrane lining the stomach and intestines.
gastroesophageal reflux disease (gas-troh-eh-**sof**-ah-**JEE**-al **REE**-flucks): the upward flow of acid from the stomach into the esophagus.
gastrointestinal bleeding: loss of blood from the digestive tract.
gastroparesis (**gas**-troh-pah-**REE**-sis): a condition in which gastric motility slows down, causing delayed gastric emptying.
gastrosis (gas-**TROH**-sis): any disease of the stomach.
gastrostomy tube (gas-**TROS**-toh-mee): a surgically placed feeding tube from the exterior of the body directly into the stomach.
general anesthesia: a state of deep sedation where the patient is unresponsive even to painful stimuli.
generalized anxiety disorder: a mental condition characterized by chronic, excessive worrying.

gender dysphoria (**JEN**-der dis-**FOR**-ee-ah): a condition where a person's sex at birth does not match the gender with which they currently identify, causing significant amounts of stress.

genetic disorder: a pathological condition caused by an absent or defective gene.

genital herpes (**HER**-peez): a sexually transmitted disease caused by the herpes simplex virus (HSV) type 1 or 2.

genital warts: small growths in the genital or anal area caused by genital herpes.

genome testing: whole genome screening to identify genetic variants that increase the risk of certain diseases.

germ cell tumor: a tumor in the sperm-producing cells or egg-producing cells, usually in the testicles or ovaries.

gestational diabetes mellitus (jes-**TAY**-shun-al **dye**-ah-**BEE**-teez **MEL**-ih-tus): the form of diabetes that occurs during some pregnancies.

gestational hypertension: high blood pressure that sometimes develops after 20 weeks of pregnancy.

giardiasis (gee-are-**DIE**-uh-sis): a diarrheal disease caused by the parasite giardia.

gigantism (jigh-**GAN**-tiz-em): abnormal growth of the entire body caused by excessive secretion of growth hormone before puberty.

gingivectomy (**jin**-jih-**VECK**-toh-mee): surgical removal of diseased gingival tissue.

gingivitis (**jin**-jih-**VYE**-tis): inflammation of the gums; the earliest stage of periodontal disease.

glaucoma (glaw-**KOH**-mah): a group of diseases characterized by increased intraocular pressure that causes damage to the optic nerve and retinal nerve fibers.

glioblastoma: a type of fast-growing, malignant brain tumor that forms from glial cells.

glomerular filtration rate: a blood test to check how well the kidneys are filtering blood.

glomerulonephritis (gloh-**mer**-you-loh-neh-**FRY**-tis): a type of nephritis caused by inflammation of the glomeruli.

glucose tolerance test: an oral test used to diagnose gestational diabetes during pregnancy, and sometimes to screen for type 2 diabetes.

gluten intolerance: a response to gluten involving digestive distress but not causing the intestinal tissue damage of celiac disease.

glycosuria (**glye**-koh-**SOO**-ree-ah): the presence of glucose in the urine.

goiter (**GOI**-ter): an abnormal, benign enlargement of the thyroid gland.

gonorrhea (**gon**-oh-**REE**-ah): a highly contagious sexually transmitted disease caused by the bacterium *Neisseria gonorrhoeae.*

gout (**GOWT**): a type of arthritis characterized by deposits of urate crystals in the joints.

granulation tissue: the tissue that normally forms during the healing of a wound that will become the scar tissue.

granuloma (**gran**-you-**LOH**-mah): a localized area of inflammation, usually in the lungs.

Graves' disease (**GRAYVZ**): an autoimmune disorder in which the immune system stimulates the thyroid to make excessive amounts of thyroid hormone.

greenstick fracture: a type of fracture in which the bone is bent and only partially broken.

group B strep test: a vaginal and rectal swab test during the third trimester of pregnancy.

group therapy: mental health treatment where people with similar issues meet with counselors for support and to learn coping skills.

growth factors: medications given to encourage, or stimulate, the growth of bone marrow.

guided imagery: a type of treatment in which a patient follows verbal prompts to envision a peaceful location and distance him- or herself from current pain or stress.

Guillain-Barré syndrome (gee-**YAHN**-bah-**RAY**): inflammation of the myelin sheath of peripheral nerves, characterized by rapidly worsening muscle weakness that may lead to temporary paralysis.

gynecomastia (**guy**-neh-koh-**MAS**-tee-ah): the condition of excessive mammary development in the male.

H

halitosis (hal-ih-**TOH**-sis): an unpleasant odor coming from the mouth.

hallucination (hah-**loo**-sih-**NAY**-shun): a sensory perception experienced in the absence of external stimulation.

hallux valgus (**HAL**-ucks **VAL**-guss): an abnormal enlargement of the joint at the base of the great toe.

hamstring injury: a strain or tear on any of the three hamstring muscles that straighten the hip and bend the knee.

hand, foot, and mouth disease: a mild viral infection common in children under 5 years of age characterized by sores in the mouth and throat and a rash on the hands and feet.

hard-tissue sarcoma: cancer arising from bone or cartilage.
Hashimoto's disease (hah-shee-**MOH**-tohz): an autoimmune disease in which the body's own antibodies attack and destroy the cells of the thyroid gland.
hearing aid: an electronic device worn to correct a hearing loss.
hearing test: part of newborn screening done prior to a baby being discharged home from the hospital.
heart block: a congenital or acquired arrhythmia caused by the electrical signal moving through the heart being partially or completely blocked from reaching the ventricles.
heart block, first-degree: slowed electrical conduction between the atria and ventricles.
heart block, second-degree: partial block in electrical conduction between the atria and ventricles.
heart block, third-degree: complete block in electrical conduction between the atria and ventricles.
heart failure: a chronic condition in which the heart is unable to pump out all of the blood it receives.
heart function test: part of newborn screening that uses a pulse oximeter to screen for congenital heart defects.
heart murmur: an abnormal blowing or clicking sound heard when listening to the heart or neighboring large blood vessels.
heart transplant: surgery to replace a person's heart with a healthy heart from an organ donor.
heart valve disease: a condition that prevents one or more heart valves from opening and closing properly.
heart valve regurgitation: a condition where a heart valve does not close tightly, allowing blood to leak back through the opening.
heart valve replacement: surgery to replace a heart valve.
heart valve stenosis: a condition where flaps of a heart valve become stiff, thickened, or fused together, limiting the amount of blood that can pass through.
heat rash: an intensely itchy rash caused by blockage of the sweat glands by bacteria and dead cells.
heat stroke: a medical emergency caused by prolonged exposure to high temperatures.
heel spur: a calcium deposit in the plantar fascia near its attachment to the heel.
HELLP syndrome: a pregnancy complication characterized by hemolysis, elevated liver enzymes, and low platelet count.
hemangioma (hee-**man**-jee-**OH**-mah): a benign tumor made up of newly formed blood vessels.
hemarthrosis (**hem**-ar-**THROH**-sis): blood within a joint.
hematemesis (**hee**-mah-**TEM**-eh-sis): the vomiting of blood.
hematochezia (hee-**mat**-oh-**KEE**-zee-uh): the presence of bright red blood in the stool.
hematocrit (hee-**MAT**-oh-krit): a blood test that measures the percentage by volume of red blood cells in a whole blood sample.
hematoma (**hee**-mah-**TOH**-mah): a swelling of clotted blood trapped in the tissues.
hematopoietic stem cell transplant (hee-**mat**-oh-poy-**EH**-tic): a treatment for cancer in which healthy transplanted stem cells are introduced into the bone marrow via the bloodstream.
hematospermia (**hee**-mah-toh-**SPER**-mee-ah): the presence of blood in the semen.
hematuria (**hee**-mah-**TOO**-ree-ah): the presence of blood in the urine.
hemianopia (**hem**-ee-ah-**NOH**-pee-ah): blindness in one half of the visual field.
hemiparesis (**hem**-ee-pah-**REE**-sis): slight paralysis or weakness affecting one side of the body.
hemiplegia (**hem**-ee-**PLEE**-jee-ah): total paralysis affecting only one side of the body.
Hemoccult® test (**HEE**-moh-kult): a laboratory test for hidden blood in the stool.
hemochromatosis (**hee**-moh-**kroh**-mah-**TOH**-sis): a genetic disorder in which the intestines absorb too much iron.
hemodialysis (**hee**-moh-dye-**AL**-ih-sis): a process by which waste products are filtered directly from the patient's blood.
hemoglobin A1c: a blood test that measures the average blood glucose level over the previous three to four months.
hemolytic anemia (**hee**-moh-**LIT**-ick ah-**NEE**-mee-ah): condition characterized by an inadequate number of circulating red blood cells due to their premature destruction by the spleen.
hemophilia (**hee**-moh-**FILL**-ee-ah): a hereditary bleeding disorder in which a blood-clotting factor is missing.
hemoptysis (hee-**MOP**-tih-sis): expectoration of blood or blood-stained sputum.
hemorrhage (**HEM**-or-idj): the loss of a large amount of blood in a short time.
hemorrhagic stroke (**hem**-oh-**RAJ**-ick): damage to the brain that occurs when a blood vessel in the brain leaks.
hemorrhoidectomy (**hem**-oh-roid-**ECK**-toh-mee): surgical removal of hemorrhoids.

hemorrhoids (**HEM**-oh-roids): a condition that occurs when a cluster of enlarged veins, muscles, and tissues slip near or through the anal opening.

hemostasis (**hee**-moh-**STAY**-sis): to stop or control bleeding.

hemothorax (**hee**-moh-**THOH**-racks): a collection of blood in the pleural cavity.

hematocrit test (hee-**MAT**-oh-krit): measures the percentage of the blood that is made up of red blood cells.

heparin (**HEP**-ah-rin): a common anticoagulant administered by injection or in an IV solution.

hepatectomy (**hep**-ah-**TECK**-toh-mee): surgical removal of all or part of the liver.

hepatic encephalopathy (en-**sef**-ah-**LOP**-ah-thee): altered level of consciousness caused by elevated blood ammonia levels.

hepatitis (**hep**-ah-**TYE**-tis): inflammation of the liver. Hepatitis A and hepatitis B are protected against by HepA and HepB vaccine.

hepatoblastoma: rare type of pediatric liver cancer.

hepatomegaly (**hep**-ah-toh-**MEG**-ah-lee): abnormal enlargement of the liver.

herbal supplement: a dietary supplement containing one or more substances derived from plants.

hereditary cancer syndrome: a known genetic mutation that is linked with an increased cancer risk.

hereditary spherocytosis (**sfee**-roh-sigh-**TOH**-sis): a genetic disorder that causes the red blood cells to be spherical rather than flat.

hernia (**HER**-nee-ah): the protrusion of a part or structure through the tissues normally containing it.

herniated disk (**HER**-nee-**ayt**-ed): the breaking apart of an intervertebral disk that results in pressure on spinal nerve roots.

herpes zoster (**HER**-peez **ZOS**-ter): an acute viral infection characterized by painful skin eruptions that follow the underlying route of an inflamed nerve, also known as shingles.

hertz: a measure of sound frequency that determines how high or low a pitch is.

hiatal hernia (high-**AY**-tal **HER**-nee-ah): the protrusion of part of the stomach through an opening in the diaphragm.

hirsutism (**HER**-soot-izm): excessive bodily and facial hair in women, usually occurring in a male pattern.

hoarding disorder: a mental illness characterized by the overaccumulation of belongings in a way that interferes with daily living.

Hodgkin's lymphoma (**HODJ**-kinz lim-**FOH**-mah): a cancer of the lymphatic system distinguished by the presence of lymphocytes known as Reed-Sternberg cells.

holistic (**hoe-LISS**-tick): a treatment approach that takes into consideration the whole body and its environment, including the mind, body, and spirit.

Holter monitor: a portable electrocardiograph worn by an ambulatory patient to continuously monitor the heart rates and rhythms over a 24- to 48-hour period or longer.

home blood glucose monitoring: test performed by the patient using a drop of blood to measure the current blood glucose level.

homeopathy (**hoh**-mee-**OP**-ah-thee): a treatment system involving the use of substances diluted a thousand-fold in water or alcohol to treat symptoms and diseases.

homeostasis (**hoh**-mee-oh-**STAY**-sis): the processes through which the body maintains a constant internal environment.

hordeolum (hor-**DEE**-oh-lum): a pus-filled lesion on the eyelid resulting from an infection in a sebaceous gland.

horizontal recumbent position: a position in which the patient is lying on the back face up.

hormone receptor-positive cancer: cancer with receptors for specific types of hormones.

hormone replacement therapy: the use of the female hormones estrogen and progesterone to replace those the body no longer produces during and after perimenopause.

hormone therapy: the use of hormones in medical treatment.

hospital-acquired pneumonia: pneumonia contracted during a hospital stay, when a patient's immune system is impaired.

human growth hormone: a synthetic version of the growth hormone that is administered to stimulate growth when the natural supply of growth hormone is insufficient for normal development.

human immunodeficiency virus (HIV): an infection transmitted through exposure to body fluids that damages or kills the T cells of the immune system.

human papillomavirus: a virus that causes genital warts and cervical cancer.

Huntington's disease: a genetic disorder that causes nerve degeneration with symptoms that most often appear in midlife.

hydrocele (**HIGH**-droh-seel): a fluid-filled sac in the scrotum along the spermatic cord leading from the testicles.

hydrocephalus (high-droh-**SEF**-ah-lus): a condition in which excess cerebrospinal fluid accumulates within the ventricles of the brain.

hydronephrosis (**high**-droh-neh-**FROH**-sis): the dilation of one or both kidneys.

hydroureter (**high**-droh-**YOUR**-eh-ter): the distention of the ureter with urine that cannot flow because the ureter is blocked.

hyperbaric oxygen therapy (**high**-per-**BARE**-ik): use of inhaled oxygen in a special chamber with increased air pressure to promote healing and fight infection.

hypercalcemia (**high**-per-kal-**SEE**-mee-ah): abnormally high concentrations of calcium circulating in the blood.

hypercapnia (**high**-per-**KAP**-nee-ah): abnormal buildup of carbon dioxide in the blood.

hypercoagulable state: this occurs when the blood has an increased tendency to form blood clots

hyperemesis (**high**-per-**EM**-eh-sis): extreme, persistent vomiting that can cause dehydration.

hyperemesis gravidarum (**high**-per-**EM**-ih-sis **grav**-ih-**DAHR**-um): excessive vomiting during pregnancy.

hyperesthesia (**high**-per-es-**THEE**-zee-ah): a condition of abnormal and excessive sensitivity to touch, pain, or other sensory stimuli.

hyperglycemia (**high**-per-glye-**SEE**-mee-ah): an abnormally high concentration of glucose in the blood.

hypergonadism (**high**-per-**GOH**-nad-izm): the excessive secretion of hormones by the sex glands.

hyperhidrosis (**high**-per-high-**DROH**-sis): a condition of excessive sweating in one area or over the whole body.

hyperinsulinism (**high**-per-**IN**-suh-lin-izm): a condition of excessive secretion of insulin in the bloodstream.

hyperkinesia (**high**-per-kye-**NEE**-zee-ah): abnormally increased muscle function or activity.

hyperlipidemia (**high**-per-**lip**-ih-**DEE**-mee-ah): the general term used to describe elevated levels of cholesterol and other fatty substances in the blood.

hyperopia (**high**-per-**OH**-pee-ah): a vision defect in which light rays focus beyond the retina; also known as farsightedness.

hyperparathyroidism (**high**-per-**par**-ah-**THIGH**-roid-izm): the overproduction of the parathyroid hormone that causes hypercalcemia.

hyperpituitarism (**high**-per-pih-**TOO**-ih-tah-rizm): the excess secretion of growth hormone that causes acromegaly and gigantism.

hyperplasia (**high**-per-**PLAY**-zhee-ah): an increase in the number of cells in a tissue or organ.

hyperpnea (**high**-perp-**NEE**-ah): breathing that is deeper and more rapid than is normal at rest.

hyperproteinuria (**high**-per-**proh**-tee-in-**YOU**-ree-ah): the presence of abnormally high concentrations of protein in the urine.

hypertension: the elevation of arterial blood pressure to a level that is likely to cause damage to the cardiovascular system.

hyperthermia (**high**-per-**THER**-mee-ah): an extremely high body temperature.

hyperthyroidism (**high**-per-**THIGH**-roid-izm): the overproduction of thyroid hormones.

hypertrophy (high-**PER**-troh-fee): a general increase in the bulk of a body part or organ due to an increase in the size, but not the number, of cells in the tissues.

hyperventilation (**high**-per-**ven**-tih-**LAY**-shun): an abnormally rapid rate of deep respiration that is usually associated with anxiety.

hypnosis: a type of therapy in which a patient is placed in a susceptible state and then given suggestions directed toward their treatment goal.

hypnotherapy: the use of hypnosis to produce an altered state of focused attention in which the patient may be more willing to believe and act on suggestions.

hypnotic: medication that depresses the central nervous system and usually produces sleep.

hypocalcemia (**high**-poh-kal-**SEE**-mee-ah): a condition characterized by abnormally low levels of calcium in the blood.

hypoglycemia (**high**-poh-glye-**SEE**-mee-ah): an abnormally low concentration of glucose in the blood.

hypogonadism (**high**-poh-**GOH**-nad-izm): the condition of deficient secretion of hormones by the sex glands.

hypomenorrhea (**high**-poh-men-oh-**REE**-ah): an unusually small amount of menstrual flow during a shortened regular menstrual period.

hypoparathyroidism (**high**-poh-**par**-ah-**THIGH**-roid-izm): a condition caused by an insufficient or absent secretion of parathyroid hormone.

hypoperfusion (**high**-poh-per-**FYOU**-zhun): a deficiency of blood passing through an organ or body part.

hypophysectomy (high-**pof**-ih-**SECK**-toh-mee): surgical removal of the pituitary gland.

hypopituitarism: a condition in which the pituitary gland does not produce enough growth hormone.

hypoplasia (**high**-poh-**PLAY**-zhee-ah): the underdevelopment of an organ or tissue, usually due to a deficiency in the number of cells.

hypopnea (**high**-poh-**NEE**-ah): shallow or slow respiration.

hypoproteinemia (**high**-poh-**proh**-tee-in-**EE**-mee-ah): the presence of abnormally low concentrations of protein in the blood.

hypospadias (**high**-poh-**SPAY**-dee-as): the congenital abnormality of the urethral opening. In the male the urethral opening is on the underside of the penis; in the female the urethra opens into the vagina.

hypotension (**high**-poh-**TEN**-shun): lower than normal arterial blood pressure.

hypothermia (**high**-poh-**THER**-mee-ah): an abnormally low body temperature.

hypothyroidism (**high**-poh-**THIGH**-roid-izm): a condition caused by a deficiency of thyroid secretion.

hypotonia (**high**-poh-**TOH**-nee-ah): a condition in which there is diminished tone of the skeletal muscles.

hypoxemia (**high**-pock-**SEE**-mee-ah): a condition of having deficient oxygen levels in the blood.

hypoxia (high-**POCK**-see-ah): the condition of having deficient oxygen levels in the body tissues and organs.

hysterectomy (**hiss**-teh-**RECK**-toh-mee): surgical removal of the uterus.

hysterosalpingography (**hiss**-ter-oh-**sal**-pin-**GOG**-rah-fee): an x-ray examination of the uterus and fallopian tubes.

hysteroscopy (**hiss**-ter-**OSS**-koh-pee): the direct visual examination of the interior of the uterus and fallopian tubes.

I

iatrogenic illness (eye-**at**-roh-**JEN**-ick): an unfavorable response due to prescribed medical treatment.

ichthyosis (**ick**-thee-**OH**-sis): a group of hereditary disorders characterized by dry, thickened, and scaly skin.

idiopathic disease (**id**-ee-oh-**PATH**-ick): any disease without a known cause.

idiosyncratic reaction (**id**-ee-oh-sin-**KRAT**-ick): an unexpected reaction to a drug that is peculiar to the individual.

ileal conduit (**ill**-ee-al **KON**-doo-it): use of a small piece of intestine to convey urine to the ureters and to a stoma in the abdomen.

ileectomy (**ill**-ee-**ECK**-toh-mee): surgical removal of the ileum.

ileostomy (**ill**-ee-**OS**-toh-mee): surgical creation of an artificial excretory opening between the ileum and the outside of the abdominal wall.

ileus (**ILL**-ee-us): partial or complete blockage of the small and/or large intestine.

iliotibial band syndrome (**ill**-ee-oh-**TIB**-ee-al): an overuse injury caused by this band of connective tissue rubbing against bone, often in the area of the knee.

illicit drug: a controlled substance without known medical benefit, or any illegally obtained drug.

illness anxiety disorder: psychiatric disorder characterized by recurring anxiety and excessive worry that a physical illness may be present.

immobilization: the act of holding, suturing, or fastening a bone in a fixed position with strapping or a cast.

immunity: the state of being resistant to a specific disease.

immunodeficiency disorder (**im**-you-noh-deh-**FISH**-en-see): a condition that occurs when immune system response is compromised.

immunoglobulins (**im**-you-noh-**GLOB**-you-lins): antibodies that bind with specific antigens in the antigen- antibody response.

immunosenescence (ih-**myoo**-noh-seh-**NEH**-sens): the gradual, natural decline of the immune system as a result of aging.

immunosuppressant (**im**-you-noh-soo-**PRES**-ant): a medication that prevents or reduces the body's normal immune response.

immunosuppression (**im**-you-noh-sup-**PRESH**-un): treatment to repress or interfere with the ability of the immune system to respond to stimulation by antigens.

immunotherapy (ih-**myoo**-noh-**THEH**-rah-pee): a disease treatment that involves either stimulating or repressing the immune response.

impacted cerumen: an accumulation of earwax that forms a solid mass by adhering to the walls of the external auditory canal.

impetigo (**im**-peh-**TYE**-goh): a highly contagious bacterial skin infection characterized by isolated pustules that become crusted and rupture.

impingement syndrome (im-**PINJ**-ment): inflammation of tendons that get caught in the narrow space between the bones within the shoulder joint.

implantable cardioverter defibrillator (**KAR**-dee-oh-**ver**-ter dee-**fib**-rih-**LAY**-ter): a double-action pacemaker that regulates the heartbeat and acts as an automatic defibrillator.

implantable loop recorder: a subcutaneous device implanted beneath the skin of the chest to continuously monitor heart rhythm for up to three years.

implantation bleeding: light vaginal bleeding that sometimes occurs 10 to 14 days after conception.

impulse control disorders: a group of psychiatric disorders characterized by failure to resist an impulse despite potential negative consequences.

incision: a cut made with a surgical instrument.

incomplete fracture: a fracture in which the bone does not break into two separate pieces.

incontinence (in-**KON**-tih-nents): the inability to control the excretion of urine and/or feces.

indirect contact transmission: refers to situations in which a susceptible person is infected by contact with a contaminated surface.

indwelling catheter: a urinary catheter that remains inside the body for a prolonged time based on need.

infection (in-**FECK**-shun): invasion of the body by a pathogenic organism.

infectious disease (in-**FECK**-shus): an illness caused by living pathogenic organisms such as bacteria and viruses.

infectious mononucleosis (**mon**-oh-**new**-klee-**OH**-sis): an infection caused by the Epstein-Barr virus that is characterized by fever, sore throat, and enlarged lymph nodes.

infectious myringitis (**mir**-in-**JIGH**-tis): a contagious inflammation that causes painful blisters on the eardrum.

infective endocarditis: inflammation of the lining or valves of the heart caused by bacteria in the bloodstream.

infertility: the inability of a couple to achieve pregnancy after one year of regular, unprotected intercourse, or the inability of a woman to carry a pregnancy to a live birth.

infestation: the dwelling of microscopic parasites on external surface tissue.

infiltrating ductal carcinoma (in-**FILL**-tray-ting **DUK**-tal): breast cancer that starts in the milk duct, breaks through the wall of that duct, and invades the fatty breast tissue.

inflamm-aging (**in**-flah-**MAY**-jing): ongoing, low-grade, age-related systemic inflammation without apparent cause.

inflammation (**in**-flah-**MAY**-shun): a localized response to an injury or to the destruction of tissues.

inflammatory bowel disease: the general name for diseases that cause inflammation and swelling in the intestines.

inflammatory breast cancer: a rare but aggressive form of breast cancer.

influenza (**in**-flew-**EN**-zah): a highly contagious viral respiratory infection that occurs in seasonal epidemics.

inguinal hernia (**ING**-gwih-nal **HER**-nee-ah): the protrusion of a small loop of bowel through a weak place in the lower abdominal wall or groin.

inhalation administration: the administration of medication in the form of vapor and gases taken in through the nose or mouth and absorbed into the bloodstream through the lungs.

inpatient: level of mental health care which may be voluntary or involuntary depending on the condition of the patient; also any in-hospital medical care.

insomnia: the prolonged or abnormal inability to sleep.

insulinoma (**in**-suh-lin-**OH**-mah): a benign tumor of the pancreas that causes hypoglycemia by secreting additional insulin.

integrative medicine: a health care model based on both allopathic and alternative medicine.

intellectual disability: significant below-average intellectual and adaptive functioning present from birth or early infancy.

intermittent catheter: a urinary catheter inserted as needed to drain urine from the bladder, and then removed.

intermittent claudication (**klaw**-dih-**KAY**-shun): pain in the leg muscles that occurs during exercise and is relieved by rest.

internal fixation: fracture treatment in which pins or a plate are placed directly into the bone to hold the broken pieces in place.

interstitial cystitis (**in**-ter-**STISH**-al sis-**TYE**-tis): chronic inflammation within the walls of the bladder.

interstitial lung diseases: a group of diseases that cause inflammation and scarring of the alveoli and their supporting structures.

intertrigo (**in**-ter-**TRYE**-goh): dermatitis caused by the friction of skin rubbing together in skin folds.

interventional radiology: the use of radiographic imaging to guide a procedure or confirm placement of an inserted object.

intestinal obstruction: partial or complete blockage of the small and/or large intestine caused by a physical obstruction.

intracranial pressure: the amount of pressure inside the skull.

intradermal injection: the administration of medication by injection into the middle layers of the skin.

intramuscular injection: the administration of medication by injection directly into muscle tissue.

intraocular lens: a surgically implanted replacement for a natural lens that has been removed.

intraoral radiography: the placement of dental x-ray film within the mouth with the camera positioned next to the cheek.

intrathecal administration (**in**-trah-**THEE**-kahl): injection of medication directly into the cerebrospinal fluid.

intrauterine device (IUD): a form of long-term birth control inserted through the cervix into the uterus to prevent pregnancy.

intravenous contrast medium (in-trah-VEE-nus): contrast medium injected into a vein to make the flow of blood through blood vessels and organs visible.

intravenous fluids: fluids administered into a vein to combat the effects of dehydration.

intravenous injection: the administration of medication by injection directly into a vein.

intravenous pyelogram: a set of x-ray images of the kidneys, ureters, and bladder.

in vitro fertilization: a procedure in which mature ova are removed from the mother to be fertilized.

involutional ectropion (eck-**TROH**-pee-on): the eversion of the edge of an eyelid.

ionizing radiation (EYE-oh-nye-zing ray-dee-AY-shun): radiation present in medical imaging procedures that can increase cancer risk after repeated exposure.

iritis (eye-**RYE**-tis): inflammation of the uvea primarily affecting structures in the front of the eye.

iron-deficiency anemia: a decrease in the red cells of the blood that is caused by too little iron.

irrigation and debridement: a procedure using pressurized fluid to clean out wound debris.

irritable bowel syndrome: a common condition of unknown cause with symptoms that can include intermittent cramping, abdominal pain, bloating, constipation, and/or diarrhea.

ischemia (iss-**KEE**-mee-ah): a condition in which there is an insufficient supply of oxygen in the tissues due to restricted blood flow to a part of the body.

ischemic colitis (iss-**KEE**-mick koh-**LYE**-tis): a condition that occurs when part of the large intestine is partially or completely deprived of blood.

ischemic stroke: brain damage that occurs when the flow of blood to the brain is blocked by the narrowing or blockage of an artery.

isolette: an apparatus for maintaining a controlled environment for a premature or ill newborn.

J

jaundice (JAWN-dis): a yellow discoloration of the skin, mucous membranes, and eyes.

juvenile idiopathic arthritis: an autoimmune disorder affecting children aged 16 years or younger, with symptoms that include stiffness, pain, joint swelling, skin rash, fever, slowed growth, and fatigue.

K

Kaposi's sarcoma (KAP-oh-seez sar-KOH-mah): a cancer that causes patches of abnormal tissue to grow under the skin or on mucous membranes.

Kawasaki disease: form of vasculitis caused by inflammation of the blood vessels; most common in children.

Kegel exercises: a series of pelvic muscle exercises used to strengthen the muscles of the pelvic floor.

keloid (KEE-loid): an abnormally raised or thickened scar that expands beyond the boundaries of the original incision.

keratitis (ker-ah-TYE-tis): inflammation of the cornea.

keratoconus (ker-**uh**-toh-**KOH**-nus): a condition in which the cornea becomes irregular and cone shaped.

keratosis (kerr-ah-TOH-sis): any skin growth, such as a wart or a callus, in which there is overgrowth and thickening of the skin.

ketonuria (kee-toh-NEW-ree-ah): the presence of ketones in the urine.

ketosis (kee-**TOH**-sis): a normal metabolic process that helps the body utilize stored fat when other sources of energy are lacking.

kinesiology (kih-**NEES**-ee-**ol**-oh-jee): the study of body movements and physical activity.

knee–chest position: position in which the patient is lying face down with the hips bent so that the knees and chest rest on the examination table.

koilonychia (**koy**-loh-**NICK**-ee-ah): a malformation of the nails in which the outer surface is concave or scooped out like the bowl of a spoon.

KUB (kidney–ureter–bladder): an x-ray study to detect bowel obstructions and nephroliths.

kyphosis (kye-**FOH**-sis): an abnormal increase in the outward curvature of the thoracic spine as viewed from the side.

L

labor induction: the stimulation of uterine contractions before labor begins on its own.

labyrinthectomy (lab-ih-rin-THECK-toh-mee): surgical removal of all or a portion of the labyrinth of the ear.

labyrinthitis (lab-ih-rin-THIGH-tis): inflammation of the labyrinth that can result in vertigo and deafness.

laceration (lass-er-AY-shun): a torn or jagged wound or an accidental cut.

lactose intolerance: the inability to digest dairy products due to the absence of the enzyme lactase.

laminectomy (**lam**-ih-**NECK**-toh-mee): surgical removal of a lamina from a vertebra.

laparoscopic adrenalectomy (**lap**-ah-roh-**SKOP**-ick ah-**dree**-nal-**ECK**-toh-mee): a minimally invasive procedure to surgically remove one or both adrenal glands.

laparoscopy (**lap**-ah-**ROS**-koh-pee): visual examination of the interior of the abdomen with the use of a laparoscope.

laryngitis (**lahr**-in-**JIGH**-tis): inflammation of the larynx.

laryngoscopy (**lah**-ring-**GOS**-koh-pee): the visual examination of the larynx and vocal cords using a laryngoscope.

laryngospasm (lah-**RING**-goh-spazm): the sudden spasmodic closure of the larynx.

laryngotomy (**lah**-ring-**OT**-oh-mee): a surgical incision into the larynx.

laser: an acronym for **L**ight **A**mplification by **S**timulated **E**mission of **R**adiation, used to treat skin conditions and other disorders of the body.

laser angioplasty (**AN**-jee-oh-**plas**-tee): a procedure to remove plaque from an artery using beams of light from a laser on the end of a catheter.

laser iridotomy (**ir**-ih-**DOT**-oh-mee): a procedure using a focused beam of light to create a hole in the iris of the eye.

laser photocoagulation (**foh**-toh-koh-**ag**-you-**LAY**-shun): the use of lasers to treat diabetic retinopathy and macular degeneration by sealing leaking or damaged blood vessels.

laser trabeculoplasty (trah-**BECK**-you-loh-**plas**-tee): treatment of open-angle glaucoma by creating openings in the trabecular meshwork to allow fluid to drain properly.

LASIK (**L**aser-**A**ssisted in **SI**tu **K**eratomileusis): treatment of vision conditions that are caused by the shape of the cornea.

latent autoimmune diabetes in adults: a condition in which type 1 diabetes develops in adults.

laxative: medication or food given to stimulate bowel movements.

learning disabilities: disorders found in children of normal intelligence who have difficulties in learning specific skills such as processing language or grasping mathematical concepts.

lesion (**LEE**-zhun): a pathologic change of tissue due to disease or injury.

lethargy (**LETH**-ar-jee): a lowered level of consciousness marked by listlessness, drowsiness, and apathy.

leukemia (loo-**KEE**-mee-ah): a type of cancer characterized by a progressive increase in the number of abnormal leukocytes found in blood-forming tissues, other organs, and in the circulating blood.

leukopenia (**loo**-koh-**PEE**-nee-ah): a decrease in the number of white blood cells circulating in the blood.

leukoplakia (**loo**-koh-**PLAY**-kee-ah): an abnormal white, usually benign lesion that develops inside the mouth in response to chronic irritation.

leukorrhea (**loo**-koh-**REE**-ah): a profuse whitish mucus discharge from the uterus and vagina.

levels of consciousness: terms used to describe the measurement of response to arousal and stimulus.

lichen sclerosus (**LYE**-ken skleh-**ROH**-sus): a progressive inflammatory skin disease that can occur in postmenopausal women.

lipectomy (lih-**PECK**-toh-mee): surgical removal of fat from beneath the skin.

lipedema (lip-eh-**DEE**-mah): a chronic abnormal condition characterized by the accumulation of fat and fluid in the tissues just under the skin of the hips and legs.

lipid panel: a blood test that measures the amounts of total cholesterol, high-density lipoprotein, low-density lipoprotein, and triglycerides.

lipoma (lih-**POH**-mah): a benign, slow-growing fatty tumor located between the skin and the muscle layer.

lipoprotein panel blood test: measures the average levels of cholesterol and triglycerides.

liposuction (**LIP**-oh-**suck**-shun *or* **LYE**-poh-suck-shun): surgical removal of fat beneath the skin with the aid of suction.

lithotomy (lih-**THOT**-oh-mee): surgical incision for the removal of a stone from the bladder.

lithotomy position: an examination position in which the patient is lying on the back with the feet and legs raised and supported in stirrups.

liver transplant: a procedure to replace a liver in a patient whose liver has failed for a reason other than liver cancer.

loading dose: an initial, higher dose of medication given to achieve therapeutic levels when a patient starts on a medication.

lobar pneumonia: a type of pneumonia that affects larger areas of the lungs, often including one or more sections, or lobes, of a lung.

lobectomy (loh-**BECK**-toh-mee): surgical removal of a lobe of an organ.

localized allergic response: redness, itching, and burning where the skin has come into contact with an allergen.

long QT syndrome: a heart rhythm disorder that can cause fast, chaotic, and potentially dangerous arrhythmias.

lordosis (lor-**DOH**-sis): an abnormal increase in the forward curvature of the lumbar spine.

lower GI bleed: blood loss from below the jejunum to the rectum, most frequently from the colon.

lower GI series: radiographic study to examine the lower digestive system using a barium enema to make these structures visible.

lumbago (lum-**BAY**-goh): pain in the lumbar region of the spine.

lumbar puncture: the process of obtaining a sample of cerebrospinal fluid by inserting a needle into the subarachnoid space of the lumbar region to withdraw fluid.

lumbar radiculopathy: nerve pain in the lower back.

lumpectomy: surgical removal of only the cancerous tissue with the surrounding margin of normal tissue.

lung cancer: a condition in which cancer cells form in the tissues of the lung.

Lyme disease (**LIME**): a bacterial infection caused by the spirochete *Borrelia burgdorferi*.

lymphadenitis (lim-**fad**-eh-**NIGH**-tis): inflammation of the lymph nodes.

lymphadenopathy (lim-**fad**-eh-**NOP**-ah-thee): any disease process affecting a lymph node or nodes.

lymphangioma (lim-**fan**-jee-**OH**-mah): a benign tumor formed by an abnormal collection of lymphatic vessels.

lymphedema (**lim**-feh-**DEE**-mah): swelling of the tissues due to an abnormal accumulation of lymph fluid within the tissues.

lymph node dissection: a surgical procedure in which all of the lymph nodes in a major group are removed to determine or slow the spread of cancer.

lymphocytic (lim-foh-**SIT**-ic): referring to lymphocytes.

lymphoma (lim-**FOH**-mah): a general term applied to malignancies affecting lymphoid tissues.

lymphoscintigraphy (**lim**-foh-sin-**TIH**-grah-fee): a diagnostic test that is performed to detect damage or malformations of the lymphatic vessels.

M

macular degeneration (**MACK**-you-lar): a gradually progressive condition in which the macula at the center of the retina is damaged, resulting in the loss of central vision.

macular stains: flat, red, irregularly shaped birthmarks.

macule (**MACK**-youl): a discolored, flat spot on the skin that is less than 1 cm in diameter.

magnetic resonance angiography: a specialized MRI study using a contrast medium to locate problems with blood vessels throughout the body.

magnetic resonance imaging: an imaging technique that uses a combination of radio waves and a strong magnetic field to create signals that are sent to a computer and converted into images of any plane through the body.

maintenance dose: the regular dose of medication given on an ongoing basis to maintain therapeutic levels.

malabsorption (**mal**-ab-**SORP**-shun): a condition in which the small intestine cannot absorb nutrients from the food that passes through it.

malaise (mah-**LAYZ**): a feeling of general discomfort, often the first indication of an infection or disease.

malaria (mah-**LAY**-ree-ah): a disease caused by a parasite that lives in certain mosquitoes and is transferred to humans by the bite of an infected mosquito.

male hypogonadism (**high**-poh-**GOH**-nad-izm): the condition of deficient secretion of hormones by the gonads.

malignant (mah-**LIG**-nant): becoming progressively worse and life-threatening.

malignant ascites: an accumulation of fluid and cancer cells in the abdomen that causes swelling, shortness of breath, and fatigue.

malignant melanoma (mel-ah-**NOH**-mah): a type of skin cancer that occurs in the melanocytes.

malignant pleural effusion: an accumulation of fluid and cancer cells between the outer layer of the lung and chest wall that causes shortness of breath.

malignant tumor: a cancerous growth of body tissue creating a mass.

malingering (mah-**LING**-ger-ing): a condition characterized by the intentional creation of false or grossly exaggerated physical or psychological symptoms.

malnutrition: a lack of proper food or nutrients in the body due to a shortage of food, poor eating habits, or the inability of the body to digest, absorb, and distribute these nutrients.

malocclusion: any deviation from the normal positioning of the upper teeth against the lower teeth.

mammography (mam-**OG**-rah-fee): an x-ray examination of the breast to detect the presence of tumors or precancerous cells.

mammoplasty (**MAM**-oh-**plas**-tee): a cosmetic operation on the breasts.

mania: mood highs, sometimes including a feeling of intense happiness and excitement.

manic behavior: an abnormally elevated, expansive, or irritable mood, including increased energy and activity, severe insomnia, poor judgment, and inappropriate social behavior.

manual disimpaction: physical removal of stool from the rectal vault with a gloved finger.

marriage and family therapy: therapy involving two or more members of a family who learn to work through issues, cope with trauma, or improve communication and relationships with one another.

mastalgia (mass-**TAL**-jee-ah): pain or tenderness in the breast.

mastectomy (mas-**TECK**-toh-mee): surgical removal of the entire breast and nipple.

mastitis (mas-**TYE**-tis): a breast infection that is caused by bacteria that enter the mammary glands, most frequently during breastfeeding.

mastoidectomy (**mas**-toy-**DECK**-toh-mee): surgical removal of part of the mastoid process.

mastoiditis (**mas**-toy-**DYE**-tis): inflammation of any part of the mastoid bone.

mastopexy (**MAS**-toh-**peck**-see): surgery to affix sagging breasts in a more elevated position.

maxillofacial surgery (mack-**sill**-oh-**FAY**-shul): specialized surgery of the face and jaws to correct deformities, treat diseases, and repair injuries.

measles: an acute, highly contagious infection transmitted by respiratory droplets of the rubeola virus.

meatotomy (**mee**-ah-**TOT**-oh-mee): a surgical incision made in the urethral meatus to enlarge the opening.

mechanical fall: a fall that occurs when a person slips, trips, or loses their balance.

medication regimen: a course of treatment involving taking certain medications on a regular basis as instructed.

megaloblastic anemia (**MEG**-ah-loh-**blas**-tick ah-**NEE**-mee-ah): a blood disorder characterized by anemia in which red blood cells are larger than normal.

melasma (meh-**LAZ**-ma): a darkening of patches of the skin on the forehead, cheeks, and neck that sometimes occurs during pregnancy.

melena (meh-**LEE**-nah): the passage of black, tarry, and foul-smelling stools.

Ménière's disease (men-**YEHRS**): a rare chronic disorder in which the amount of fluid in the inner ear increases intermittently, causing vertigo, fluctuating hearing loss, and tinnitus.

meningioma (meh-**nin**-jee-**OH**-mah): a common, slow-growing, and usually benign tumor of the meninges.

meningitis (**men**-in-**JIGH**-tis): inflammation of the meninges of the brain and spinal cord.

meningocele (meh-**NING**-goh-**seel**): the congenital herniation of the meninges through a defect in the skull or spinal column.

meningococcal disease (meh-**ning**-goh-**KOK**-al): characterized by sudden onset of fever, headache, stiff neck, dark purple rash; prevented by MenACWY and MenB vaccine.

menorrhagia: an excessive amount of menstrual flow.

metrorrhagia (**met**-roh-**RAY**-jee-ah): irregular uterine bleeding outside of the menstrual periods.

metabolic syndrome: common medical condition characterized by hypertension, hyperlipidemia, and obesity.

metastasis (meh-**TAS**-tah-sis): the new cancer site that results from the spreading process; also the processes by which cancer is spread.

metastasize (meh-**TAS**-tah-sighz): to spread from one place to another, as in cancer.

metered-dose inhaler: a medical device that administers a specific amount of a medication such as a bronchodilator in aerosol form.

methicillin-resistant *Staphylococcus aureus*: one of several types of bacteria that are now resistant to most antibiotics.

migraine headache (**MY**-grayn): a headache characterized by throbbing pain on one side of the head and sometimes preceded by a warning aura.

mild cognitive impairment: decline from normal mental function characterized by short-term memory loss.

mindfulness meditation: treatment for stress focused on maintaining a calm, constant awareness and acceptance of thoughts and emotions.

mineral: a dietary supplement containing one or more substances which are beneficial for humans.

minimally invasive coronary artery bypass: a bypass procedure performed with the aid of a fiber-optic camera through small openings between the ribs.

miosis (mye-**OH**-sis): the contraction of the pupil.

mitral valve regurgitation: the backward leaking of blood that occurs when the mitral valve does not close tightly.

modified radical mastectomy: surgical removal of the entire breast and nipple, as well as axillary lymph nodes under the adjacent arm.

modified Rankin scale: an assessment tool to measure level of disability after a stroke.

Mohs surgery (**MOZE**): used to treat various types of skin cancer by removing layers of cancerous tissue until a healthy margin is achieved.
molar pregnancy: a rare and serious condition caused by the abnormal division of the fertilized egg.
molecular breast imaging: a nuclear medicine technique using gamma radiation to detect potential tumors in particularly dense breast tissue.
molluscum contagiosum (moh-**LUSS**-kum kon-**TAYJ**-eeh-**oh**-sum): a viral infection that causes small, raised lesions.
monaural testing (mon-**AW**-rahl): hearing testing that involves one ear.
monoclonal antibodies (**maw**-noh-**KLOH**-null **AN**-tih-**bod**-eez): molecules designed to locate and attack specific proteins on cancer cells.
mood stabilizer: medication used to treat mood instability and bipolar disorders.
morgue: a refrigerated area in the hospital where cadavers are kept temporarily.
Morton's neuroma: a condition in which pain on the ball of the foot is caused by a swollen, inflamed nerve, usually between the third and fourth toes.
multiparous (mul-**TIP**-ah-rus): a woman who has given birth two or more times.
multiple myeloma (**my**-eh-**LOH**-mah): a type of cancer that occurs in the blood-making cells of the bone marrow.
multiple sclerosis (skleh-**ROH**-sis): a progressive autoimmune disorder characterized by inflammation that causes demyelination of the myelin sheath.
mumps: an acute viral infection characterized by the swelling of the parotid glands.
muscle biopsy (**BYE**-op-see): diagnostic procedure including removal of a plug of tissue with a biopsy needle for examination.
muscle relaxant: medication administered to relax certain muscles and to relieve the stiffness, pain, and discomfort caused by strains, sprains, or other muscle injuries.
muscle tone: the state of balanced muscle tension that makes normal posture, coordination, and movement possible.
muscular dystrophy (**DIS**-troh-fee): a group of more than 30 genetic diseases that are characterized by progressive weakness and degeneration of the skeletal muscles without affecting the nervous system.
myalgia (my-**AL**-jee-ah): tenderness or pain in the muscles.
myasthenia gravis (**my**-as-**THEE**-nee-ah **GRAH**-vis): a chronic autoimmune disease that affects the neuromuscular junction and produces weakness of voluntary muscles.
mycoplasma pneumonia: a milder but longer-lasting form of pneumonia caused by the bacteria *Mycoplasma pneumoniae*.
mycosis (my-**KOH**-sis): any abnormal condition or disease caused by a fungus.
mydriasis (mih-**DRY**-ah-sis): the dilation of the pupil.
mydriatic drops (**mid**-ree-**AT**-ick): medication placed into the eyes to produce temporary paralysis, forcing the pupils to remain dilated even in the presence of bright light.
myelitis (**my**-eh-**LYE**-tis): inflammation of the spinal cord; inflammation of bone marrow.
myelodysplastic syndrome (**my**-eh-loh-dis-**PLAS**-tick **SIN**-drohm): a type of cancer in which there is insufficient production of one or more types of blood cells due to dysfunction of the bone marrow.
myelography (**my**-eh-**LOG**-rah-fee): a radiographic study of the spinal cord after the injection of a contrast medium through a lumbar puncture.
myeloid (**MY**-eh-loyd): relating to the bone marrow.
myelopathy (my-eh-**LOP**-ah-thee): any pathologic change or disease in the spinal cord.
myelosis (**my**-eh-**LOH**-sis): a tumor of the spinal cord.
myocardial infarction (**my**-oh-**KAR**-dee-al in-**FARK**-shun): the occlusion of one or more coronary arteries caused by plaque buildup.
myocarditis (**my**-oh-kar-**DYE**-tis): inflammation of the myocardium.
myoclonus (**my**-oh-**KLOH**-nus *or* my-**OK**-luh-nus): the quick, involuntary jerking of a muscle or group of muscles.
myofascial pain syndrome: a chronic pain disorder that affects muscles and fascia throughout the body.
myofascial release (**my**-oh-**FASH**-ee-ahl): a specialized soft-tissue manipulation technique used to ease the pain of conditions such as fibromyalgia.
myoma (my-**OH**-mah): a benign tumor made up of muscle tissue.
myomectomy (**my**-oh-**MECK**-toh-mee): surgical removal of uterine fibroids.
myoparesis (**my**-oh-**PAR**-eh-sis): weakness or slight muscular paralysis.
myopathy (my-**OP**-ah-thee): any pathologic change or disease of muscle tissue.
myopia (my-**OH**-pee-ah): a defect in which light rays focus in front of the retina; also known as nearsightedness.

myoplasty (**MY**-oh-**plas**-tee): surgical repair of a muscle.
myorrhaphy (my-**OR**-ah-fee): surgical suturing of a muscle.
myosarcoma (**my**-oh-sahr-**KOH**-mah): a malignant tumor derived from muscle tissue.
myotomy (my-**OT**-oh-mee): a surgical incision into a muscle.
myringotomy (**mir**-in-**GOT**-oh-mee): a small surgical incision in the eardrum to relieve pressure from excess pus or fluid or to create an opening for the placement of ear tubes.
myxedema (**mick**-seh-**DEE**-mah): a severe form of adult hypothyroidism caused by extreme deficiency of thyroid secretion.

N

narcissistic personality disorder: a pattern of extreme preoccupation with the self and complete lack of empathy for others.
narcolepsy (**NAR**-koh-**lep**-see): a sleep disorder consisting of sudden and uncontrollable brief episodes of falling asleep during the day.
nasogastric intubation (**nay**-zoh-**GAS**-trick **in**-too-**BAY**-shun): the placement of a tube through the nose and into the stomach for feeding or suction.
National Institutes of Health Stroke Scale: an examination tool for measuring the severity of neurological deficit after a stroke.
natural childbirth: using relaxation, alternate birthing positions, and/or breathing techniques to make the mother comfortable during an unmedicated birth.
natural immunity: disease resistance without administration of an antigen or exposure to disease, either present at birth or passed on from mother to child through breast milk.
naturopathy (**nay**-cher-**AH**-pah-thee): a form of alternative medicine emphasizing the healing power of nature and support of the body's own healing ability.
nausea (**NAW**-see-ah): the urge to vomit.
nebulizer (**NEB**-you-lye-zer): an electronic device that pumps air or oxygen through a liquid medicine to turn it into a mist that is inhaled via a face mask or mouthpiece.
necrotizing fasciitis (**NECK**-roh-**tiz**-ing **fas**-ee-**EYE**-tis): a rare, severe infection caused by group A strep bacteria.
needlestick injury: an accidental puncture wound caused by a used hypodermic needle, potentially transmitting an infection.
neoadjuvant therapy (**nee**-oh-**AD**-jeh-vant): systemic treatment used to reduce cancer size before surgery.
neoplasm (**NEE**-oh-plazm): an abnormal growth of body tissue in which the multiplication of cells is uncontrolled, abnormal, rapid, and progressive; also known as a tumor.
nephritis (neh-**FRY**-tis): inflammation of the kidney or kidneys.
nephrolith (**NEF**-roh-lith): a stone located in the kidney.
nephrolithiasis (**nef**-roh-lih-**THIGH**-ah-sis): the presence of stones in the kidney.
nephrolysis (neh-**FROL**-ih-sis): surgical freeing of a kidney from adhesions.
nephropathy (neh-**FROP**-ah-thee): any disease of the kidney.
nephrostomy (neh-**FROS**-toh-mee): the placement of a catheter to maintain an opening between the pelvis of one or both kidneys to the exterior of the body.
nephrotic syndrome (neh-**FROT**-ick): a group of conditions in which excessive amounts of protein are lost in the urine.
neural tube defects: congenital anomaly where the spinal canal fails to close completely.
neuritis (new-**RYE**-tis): inflammation of a nerve accompanied by pain and sometimes loss of function.
neurodegenerative disease (**new**-roh-deh-**JEN**-er-ah-tiv): an umbrella term for disorders in which there is a progressive loss of the structure or functions of neurons.
neurodevelopmental disorders: disorders with childhood onset which are characterized by a disturbance in the central nervous system.
neurogenic bladder (new-roh-**JEN**-ick): a urinary problem caused by interference with the normal nerve pathways associated with urination.
neuromuscular-blocking drug: medication that causes temporary paralysis by blocking the transmission of nerve stimuli to the muscles.
neuromuscular therapy: a form of massage that uses soft-tissue manipulation focusing on applying pressure to trigger points to treat injuries and alleviate pain.
neuroplasty (**NEW**-roh-**plas**-tee): surgical repair of a nerve or nerves.
neurorrhaphy (new-**ROR**-ah-fee): surgically suturing together the ends of a severed nerve.
neurotomy (new-**ROT**-oh-mee): surgical division or dissection of a nerve.
neutropenia (**new**-troh-**PEE**-nee-ah): the presence of abnormally few of the white blood cells called neutrophils.

nevus (**NEE**-vus): a small, dark skin growth that develops from melanocytes in the skin.

newborn screening: tests conducted 24–48 hours after birth including a blood test for sickle cell anemia and other genetic, hormone-related, and metabolic conditions.

nitroglycerin (**nye**-troh-**GLIH**-seh-rin): a medication with antihypertensive properties that works by dilating the veins, reducing the workload of the heart.

nitrous oxide: an inhalation analgesic.

nocturia (nock-**TOO**-ree-ah): frequent and excessive urination during the night.

nocturnal enuresis (nock-**TER**-nal **en**-you-**REE**-sis): urinary incontinence during sleep.

nodule: a solid, raised skin lesion that is larger than 0.5 cm in diameter and deeper than a papule.

noise-induced hearing loss: nerve deafness caused by exposure to extremely loud noises.

nonalcoholic fatty liver disease: the accumulation of fat in the liver of people who drink little or no alcohol.

nonalcoholic steatohepatitis: a more serious form of *nonalcoholic fatty liver disease*, consisting of fatty accumulations plus liver-damaging inflammation.

non-Hodgkin's lymphoma (non-**HODJ**-kinz lim-**FOH**-mah): the term used to describe all lymphomas *other than* Hodgkin's lymphoma.

non-small cell lung cancer: the most common type of lung cancer.

nonsteroidal anti-inflammatory drugs: medications administered to control pain by reducing inflammation and swelling.

normal cell growth: the regular process in which cells divide and fulfill a standard life span according to the needs of the body.

nosocomial infection (**nos**-oh-**KOH**-mee-al): a disease acquired in a hospital or clinical setting.

nuclear imaging: the use of radiopharmaceuticals for diagnostic purposes.

nuclear medicine: the use of radiopharmaceuticals for diagnostic or treatment purposes.

nuclear scan: a diagnostic procedure that uses nuclear medicine technology to gather information about the structure and function of organs or body systems.

nullipara (nuh-**LIP**-ah-rah): a woman who has never borne a viable child.

nyctalopia (**nick**-tah-**LOH**-pee-ah): a condition in which an individual with normal daytime vision has difficulty seeing at night.

nystagmus (nis-**TAG**-mus): an involuntary, constant, rhythmic movement of the eyeball.

O

obesity (oh-**BEE**-sih-tee): an excessive accumulation of fat in the body.

oblique fracture: a fracture that occurs at an angle across the bone.

obsessive-compulsive disorder: a mental condition characterized by obsessions and/or compulsions.

occupational therapy: activities to promote recovery and rehabilitation in order to assist patients in performing the activities of daily living.

ocular prosthesis: a replacement for an eyeball that is either congenitally missing or has been surgically removed.

oligohydramnios (**al**-ih-go-hy-**DRAM**-nee-os): a condition in which there is less amniotic fluid than normal.

oligomenorrhea (**ol**-ih-goh-**men**-oh-**REE**-ah): light or infrequent menstruation in a woman with previously normal periods.

oligospermia (**ol**-ih-goh-**SPER**-mee-ah): a sperm count of below 15 million/ml.

oliguria (**ol**-ih-**GOO**-ree-ah): scanty urination.

oncogene (**ON**-koh-jeen): a mutated gene causing the cell to function abnormally.

onychia (oh-**NICK**-ee-ah): inflammation of the bed of the nail.

onychocryptosis (**on**-ih-koh-krip-**TOH**-sis): ingrown toenail.

onycholysis (**on**-ih-koh-**LYE**-sis): the separation of the nail plate from the nail bed.

onychomycosis (**on**-ih-koh-my-**KOH**-sis): a fungal infection of the nail.

oophorectomy (**oh**-ahf-oh-**RECK**-toh-mee): surgical removal of one or both ovaries.

open-angle glaucoma: the most common form of glaucoma.

open fracture: a fracture in which the bone is broken and there is an open wound in the skin.

ophthalmoscope (ahf-**THAL**-moh-skope): an instrument used to examine the interior of the eye.

ophthalmoscopy (**ahf**-thal-**MOS**-koh-pee): the visual examination of the fundus of the eye with ophthalmoscope.

opioid (**OH**-pee-oyd): a controlled substance available by prescription only to relieve severe pain.

opportunistic infection (**op**-ur-too-**NIHS**-tick): infection caused by a pathogen that does not normally produce an illness in healthy humans.

oppositional defiant disorder: a psychiatric disorder characterized by a child or adolescent's persistent angry, uncooperative, and disruptive behavior directed toward authority figures, disrupting daily activities.

oral administration: medication taken by mouth to be absorbed through the walls of the stomach or small intestine.

oral glucose tolerance test (**GLOO**-kohs): a test performed most commonly to diagnose gestational diabetes.

oral or maxillofacial surgeon (mack-**sill**-oh-**FAY**-shul): a physician specializing in surgery of the face and jaws to correct deformities, treat diseases, and repair injuries.

oral rehydration therapy: treatment in which a solution of electrolytes is administered in a liquid preparation to counteract dehydration.

oral thrush: a fungal infection in the mouth caused by the fungus *Candida albicans*.

orbitotomy (**or**-bih-**TOT**-oh-mee): surgical incision into the orbit.

orchiectomy (**or**-kee-**ECK**-toh-mee): surgical removal of one or both testicles.

orchiopexy (**or**-kee-oh-**PECK**-see): the repair of an undescended testicle.

orchitis (or-**KYE**-tis): inflammation of one or both testicles.

organ donation: the process through which a person volunteers to have their organs removed and transplanted into another person.

organic disorder (or-**GAN**-ick): a disorder that produces symptoms caused by detectable physical changes in the body.

orientation: the awareness of different aspects of one's environment.

orthostatic hypotension (**or**-thoh-**STAT**-ick **high**-poh-**TEN**-shun): low blood pressure that occurs upon standing up.

orthotic (or-**THOT**-ick): a mechanical appliance, such as a leg brace or splint, that is specially designed to control, correct, or compensate for impaired limb function.

osteitis (**oss**-tee-**EYE**-tis): inflammation of a bone.

osteoarthritis (**oss**-tee-oh-ar-**THRIGH**-tis): the type of arthritis most commonly associated with aging.

osteochondroma (**oss**-tee-oh-kon-**DROH**-mah): a benign bony projection covered with cartilage.

osteomalacia (**oss**-tee-oh-mah-**LAY**-shee-ah): abnormal softening of bones in adults.

osteomyelitis (**oss**-tee-oh-**my**-eh-**LYE**-tis): inflammation of the bone marrow and adjacent bone.

osteopathic manipulative therapy: mechanical spinal adjustment used in conjunction with conventional medical therapies by an osteopath.

osteopenia (**oss**-tee-oh-**PEE**-nee-ah): thinner-than-average bone density.

osteophytes (**OSS**-tee-oh-**fites**): bony growths also known as bone spurs.

osteoporosis (**oss**-tee-oh-poh-**ROH**-sis): a marked loss of bone density and an increase in bone porosity that is frequently associated with aging.

osteoporotic hip fracture (**oss**-tee-oh-pah-**ROT**-ick): a fracture of a hip weakened by osteoporosis that can occur spontaneously or as the result of a fall.

osteosarcoma (**oss**-tee-oh-sar-**KOH**-mah): a hard-tissue sarcoma that usually involves the upper shaft of long bones, pelvis, or knee.

osteotomy (**oss**-tee-**OT**-oh-mee): surgical cutting and reshaping of a bone.

ostomy (**OSS**-toh-mee): a surgical procedure to create an artificial opening between an organ and the body surface.

otalgia (oh-**TAL**-gee-ah): pain in the ear.

otitis (oh-**TYE**-tis): inflammation of the ear.

otitis media (**MEE**-dee-ah): inflammation of the middle ear.

otomycosis (**oh**-toh-my-**KOH**-sis): a fungal infection of the external auditory canal.

otoplasty (**OH**-toh-**plas**-tee): surgical repair, restoration, or alteration of the pinna of the ear.

otopyorrhea (**oh**-toh-**pye**-oh-**REE**-ah): the flow of pus from the ear.

otorrhagia (**oh**-toh-**RAY**-jee-ah): bleeding from the ear.

otorrhea (**oh**-toh-**REE**-ah): any discharge from the ear.

otosclerosis (**oh**-toh-skleh-**ROH**-sis): ankylosis of the bones of the middle ear resulting in a conductive hearing loss.

otoscope (**OH**-toh-skope): an instrument used to visually examine the external ear canal and tympanic membrane.

outpatient: level of mental health care or other medical treatment performed in an office setting or via telehealth using a video platform.

ovarian cancer: cancer that originates within the cells of the ovaries.

ovarian cysts: fluid-filled sacs in, or on the surface of, an ovary.

overactive bladder: a condition that occurs when the muscles of the bladder contract involuntarily even when the bladder is not full.

overdose: the accidental or deliberate ingestion of more medication than has been prescribed or is safe.

overflow incontinence: continuous leaking from the bladder either because it is full or because it does not empty completely.

over-the-counter drug: medication that can be purchased without a prescription.

overuse injuries: injuries that occur when minor tissue injuries have not been given time to heal.

overuse tendinitis (**ten**-dih-**NIGH**-tis): inflammation of tendons caused by excessive or unusual use of a joint.

P

pacemaker: battery-powered device with connections leading into the heart to regulate the heartbeat.

Paget's disease (**PAJ**-its): a chronic bone disease of unknown cause, characterized by abnormal breakdown of bone tissue followed by abnormal bone formation.

palatoplasty (**PAL**-ah-toh-**plas**-tee): surgical repair of a cleft palate or lip.

palliative (**PAL**-ee-**ay**-tiv): a substance that eases the pain or severity of a disease but does not cure it.

palpation (pal-**PAY**-shun): an examination technique in which the examiner's hands are used to feel the texture, size, consistency, and location of certain body parts.

palpation of the breast: an examination performed by a trained health care provider to check the texture, size, and consistency of the breast.

palpitation (**pal**-pih-**TAY**-shun): a pounding or racing heart with or without irregularity in rhythm.

pancreatectomy (**pan**-kree-ah-**TECK**-toh-mee): surgical removal of all or part of the pancreas.

pancreatitis (**pan**-kree-ah-**TYE**-tis): inflammation of the pancreas.

pancytopenia (**pan**-sight-oh-**PEE**-nee-ah): a condition characterized by lower-than-normal quantities of red blood cells.

pandemic (pan-**DEM**-ick): an outbreak of a disease occurring over a large geographic area, sometimes even worldwide.

panic attack: an unexpected, sudden experience of fear in the absence of danger, accompanied by physical symptoms such as shortness of breath and palpitations.

panic disorder: a condition characterized by having more than one panic attack, resulting in persistent fear of these attacks.

panoramic radiograph: a dental x-ray showing all of the structures in both dental arches in a single film.

papilledema (**pap**-ill-eh-**DEE**-mah): swelling and inflammation of the optic nerve at the point of entrance into the eye through the optic disk.

papilloma (**pap**-ih-**LOH**-mah): a benign, superficial, wart-like growth on the epithelial tissue or elsewhere in the body, such as in the bladder.

Pap smear: an exfoliative biopsy of the cervix.

papule (**PAP**-youl): a small, raised red lesion on the skin that is less than 0.5 cm in diameter.

paradoxical reaction: the result of medical treatment that yields the exact opposite of normally expected results.

paralysis (pah-**RAL**-ih-sis): the loss of sensation and voluntary muscle movements in a muscle through disease or injury to its nerve supply.

paralytic (**pair**-ah-**LIH**-tik): a drug that relaxes all muscles.

paranoia (**pair**-ah-**NOY**-ah): intense anxiety caused by persistent suspicion and mistrust of someone or something.

paraphilic disorders (pahr-ah-**FIL**-ick): psychiatric disorders characterized by altered sexual fantasies, urges, or behaviors.

paraplegia (**par**-ah-**PLEE**-jee-ah): paralysis of both legs and the lower part of the body.

parasite (**PAR**-ah-sight): a plant or animal that lives on or within another living organism at the expense of that organism.

parasomnia: general term for several categories of sleep disorders that occur while falling asleep, during sleep, or while waking from sleep.

parathyroidectomy (**par**-ah-**thigh**-roi-**DECK**-toh-mee): surgical removal of one or more of the parathyroid glands.

parenteral administration (pah-**REN**-ter-al): the administration of medication by a manner other than through the digestive tract.

parenteral nutrition: a specialized solution administered intravenously to patients who cannot or should not get their nutrition through eating.

paresthesia (**par**-es-**THEE**-zee-ah): a burning or prickling sensation that is usually felt in the hands, arms, legs, or feet.

Parkinson's disease: a chronic, degenerative central nervous system disorder characterized by fine muscle tremors, rigidity, and a slow or shuffling gait.

paronychia (**par**-oh-**NICK**-ee-ah): an infection of the skin fold around a nail.

partial colectomy: surgical removal of part of the colon.

partial hysterectomy: surgical procedure in which the uterus is removed and the cervix left in place.

partial knee replacement: a procedure in which only part of the knee is replaced.
partial remission (ree-**MIH**-shun): reduction of cancer in response to treatment.
pathogen (**PATH**-oh-jen): a microorganism that causes a disease in humans.
pathologic fracture: a fracture that occurs when a weakened bone breaks under normal strain.
peak flow meter: a handheld device used to measure how quickly a person with asthma can expel air.
pediculosis (pee-**dick**-you-**LOH**-sis): an infestation with lice.
pediculosis capitis: an infestation with head lice.
pelvic inflammatory disease: any inflammation of the female reproductive organs not associated with surgery or pregnancy.
peptic ulcer disease (**UL**-ser): a disease characterized by sores that affect the mucous membranes of the digestive system.
percussion (per-**KUSH**-un): a diagnostic procedure to determine the density of a body area that uses the sound produced by tapping the surface with the fingers.
percutaneous diskectomy (**per**-kyou-**TAY**-nee-us dis-**KECK**-toh-mee): a procedure to treat a herniated intervertebral disk.
percutaneous nephrolithotomy (**per**-kyou-**TAY**-nee-us **nef**-roh-lih-**THOT**-oh-mee): surgical removal of a kidney stone through a small incision in the back.
percutaneous vertebroplasty (**per**-kyou-**TAY**-nee-us **VER**-tee-broh-**plas**-tee): treatment of osteoporosis-related compression fractures by injecting bone cement to stabilize compression fractures within the spinal column.
perfusion (per-**FYOU**-zuhn): the flow of blood through an organ.
pericardiocentesis (**pehr**-ih-**kar**-dee-oh-sen-**TEE**-sis): the puncture of the pericardial sac for the purpose of removing fluid.
pericarditis (**pehr**-ih-kar-**DYE**-tis): inflammation of the pericardium.
periodontal disease: inflammation of the tissues that surround and support the teeth.
periorbital edema (**pehr**-ee-**OR**-bih-tal eh-**DEE**-mah): swelling of the tissues surrounding the eye or eyes.
periostitis (**pehr**-ee-oss-**TYE**-tis): inflammation of the periosteum.
peripartum onset depression: a mood disorder characterized by feelings of sadness and the loss of pleasure in normal activities that can occur shortly after giving birth.
peripheral artery disease: atherosclerosis of the arteries supplying blood to parts of the body other than the heart or brain.
peripheral edema: swelling in the legs.
peripheral neuropathy (new-**ROP**-ah-thee): a disorder of the peripheral nerves that carry information to and from the brain and spinal cord, producing pain, loss of sensation, and inability to control muscles.
peripheral vascular disease: disorders of blood vessels outside the heart and brain.
peritoneal dialysis (**pehr**-ih-toh-**NEE**-al dye-**AL**-ih-sis): dialysis in which the lining of the peritoneal cavity acts as a filter to remove waste from the blood.
peritonitis (**pehr**-ih-toh-**NIGH**-tis): inflammation of the peritoneum.
pernicious anemia (per-**NISH**-us ah-**NEE**-mee-ah): anemia caused by a lack of a protein that helps the body absorb vitamin B_{12} from the gastrointestinal tract.
PERRLA: an acronym for a standard eye test meaning **P**upils **E**qual, **R**ound, **R**eactive to **L**ight, and **A**ccommodation.
persistent depressive disorder: low-grade chronic depression present on a majority of days for two or more years.
persistent vegetative state: a type of coma in which the patient exhibits alternating sleep and wake cycles; however, the individual is unconscious even when appearing to be awake.
personality disorder: a chronic pattern of inner experience and behavior that causes serious problems with relationships and work.
pertussis (per-**TUS**-is): a contagious bacterial infection of the upper respiratory tract that is characterized by recurrent bouts of a paroxysmal cough.
pessary (**PESS**-ah-ree): a soft, flexible device that fits into the vagina to support its internal structure.
petechiae (pee-**TEE**-kee-ee): very small pinpoint hemorrhages on the skin less than 2 mm in diameter.
Peyronie's disease (pay-roh-**NEEZ**): a form of sexual dysfunction in which the penis is bent or curved during erection.
phacoemulsification (**fack**-koh-ee-**mul**-sih-fih-**KAY**-shun): the use of ultrasonic vibration to shatter and remove the lens clouded by a cataract.
pharyngitis (far-in-**JIGH**-tis): inflammation of the pharynx.
phenylketonuria (**fen**-il-**kee**-toh-**NEW**-ree-ah): a genetic disorder in which an essential digestive enzyme is missing.

phimosis (figh-**MOH**-sis): narrowing of the opening of the foreskin so that it cannot be retracted to expose the glans penis.
phlebitis (fleh-**BYE**-tis): inflammation of a vein.
phlebotomy (fleh-**BOT**-oh-mee): the puncture of a vein for the purpose of drawing blood.
phlegm (**FLEM**): thick mucus secreted by the tissues lining the respiratory passages.
phobia (**FOH**-bee-ah): a persistent irrational fear of a specific thing or situation strong enough to cause significant distress, interfere with functioning, and lead to avoidance of whatever causes this reaction.
phosphodiesterase inhibitor (**foss**-foh-dye-**AS**-ter-ace): medication used to treat erectile dysfunction.
photodynamic therapy (**foh**-toh-dye-**NAH**-mik): a technique used to treat damaged and precancerous skin, as well as various types of cancer.
photophobia (**foh**-toh-**FOH**-bee-ah): excessive sensitivity to light.
photopsia (foh-**TOP**-see-ah): presence of what appear to be flashes of light.
photorefractive keratectomy (**foh**-toh-reh-**FRAK**-tiv **ker**-ah-**TEK**-toh-mee): eye surgery in which the outer layer of cornea is removed before a laser is used to change the shape of a deep corneal layer.
phototherapy: the use of natural or artificial light to treat skin conditions such as vitiligo and eczema.
physical therapy: treatment to prevent disability or to restore function through the use of exercise, heat, massage, or other techniques.
PICC line: peripherally inserted central catheter used when patients need IV therapy for more than seven days.
pigmented birthmarks: irregularities in skin color, such as moles.
pinealoma (pin-ee-ah-**LOH**-mah): a tumor of the pineal gland.
pinworm: infection caused by parasitic worms in the intestines.
pituitary adenoma (**ad**-eh-**NOH**-mah): a slow-growing, benign tumor of the pituitary gland that may or may not cause excess hormone secretion.
placebo (plah-**SEE**-boh): an inactive substance that is given for its suggestive effects.
placenta accreta (ah-**KREE**-tah): when the placenta attaches itself too deeply into the uterine wall.
placenta previa (plah-**SEN**-tah **PREE**-vee-ah): abnormal implantation of the placenta in the lower portion of the uterus.
plantar fasciitis (**PLAN**-tar **fas**-ee-**EYE**-tis): inflammation of the plantar fascia causing foot or heel pain when walking or running.
plaque (**PLACK**): a fatty deposit within the blood vessels; also a soft buildup of bacterial debris on the exterior of the teeth; also a scaly, solid, raised area of closely spaced papules on the skin.
plasmapheresis (**plaz**-mah-feh-**REE**-sis): the removal of blood plasma by drawing blood and then separating the blood into its cellular elements.
platelet count: a blood test that measures the number of platelets in a specified amount of blood.
platelet transfusion: used to treat patients with a low platelet count or poor platelet function.
platelet-rich plasma therapy: a treatment that uses injections of the patient's own platelets to support wound, muscle, and joint healing.
play therapy: targeted therapy for children where coping and communication skills are gained through the use of play with a trained therapist.
pleural effusion (eh-**FEW**-zhun): excess accumulation of fluid in the pleural space that prevents the lung from fully expanding.
pleurisy (**PLOOR**-ih-see): inflammation of the pleura.
pleurodynia (**ploor**-oh-**DIN**-ee-ah): sharp chest pain that occurs when inflamed pleural membranes rub against each other.
pneumatic retinopexy (**RET**-ih-noh-**peck**-see): surgery to reattach the detached area in a retinal detachment using a gas bubble to hold pressure on the retina.
pneumoconiosis (**new**-moh-**koh**-nee-**OH**-sis): any fibrosis of the lung tissues caused by dust in the lungs after prolonged environmental or occupational contact.
pneumocystis pneumonia (**new**-moh-**SIS**-tis new-**MOH**-nee-ah): pneumonia caused by an opportunistic infection with the fungus *Pneumocystis jirovecii*.
pneumonectomy (**new**-moh-**NECK**-toh-mee): surgical removal of all or part of a lung.
pneumonia (new-**MOH**-nee-ah): a serious infection or inflammation of the lungs in which the alveoli and air passages fill with pus and other liquid.
pneumothorax (**new**-moh-**THOR**-racks): the accumulation of air in the pleural space resulting in a pressure imbalance that causes the lung to fully or partially collapse.
polio (**POH**-lee-oh): a highly contagious viral infection of the brainstem and spinal cord that sometimes leads to paralysis.
polycystic kidney disease (**pol**-ee-**SIS**-tick): a genetic disorder characterized by the growth of numerous fluid-filled cysts in the kidneys.
polycystic ovary syndrome (**pol**-ee-**SIS**-tick): a condition characterized by an imbalance of reproductive hormones.

polycythemia (**pol**-ee-sy-**THEE**-mee-ah): a condition which causes the bone marrow to produce too many erythrocytes.

polydipsia (**pol**-ee-**DIP**-see-ah): excessive thirst.

polymenorrhea (**pol**-ee-**men**-oh-**REE**-ah): abnormally frequent menstruation.

polymyalgia rheumatica (**pol**-ee-my-**AL**-jee-ah roo-**MA**-tih-kah): an inflammatory disorder of the muscles and joints characterized by pain and stiffness.

polymyositis (**pol**-ee-**my**-oh-**SIGH**-tis): muscle disease characterized by the simultaneous inflammation and weakening of voluntary muscles in many parts of the body.

polyp (**POL**-ip): a mushroom-like growth from the surface of a mucous membrane.

polypectomy: surgical removal of a polyp.

polyphagia (**pol**-ee-**FAY**-jee-ah): excessive hunger.

polysomnography (**pol**-ee-som-**NOG**-rah-fee): the diagnostic measurement of physiological activity during sleep.

polyuria (**pol**-ee-**YOU**-ree-ah): excessive urination.

port-wine stain: a flat vascular birthmark made up of dilated blood capillaries.

positron emission tomography (**PAW**-zih-tron ee-**MIH**-shun tuh-**MAW**-gruh-fee): an imaging technique that combines computed tomography with radionuclide tracers to produce enhanced images of selected body organs or areas.

postmenopausal labial fusion: a severe version of vaginal atrophy in which the labia minora fuse together.

postmenopause: the period of life after experiencing menopause.

postpartum depression: a mood disorder characterized by sadness and loss of pleasure in normal activities that can occur shortly after giving birth (see *peripartum onset depression*).

posttraumatic stress disorder: the development of characteristic symptoms after a major traumatic event.

pre-active dying: the first stage of the dying process.

prediabetes: a condition in which the blood glucose level is higher than normal but not high enough to be classified as type 2 diabetes.

preeclampsia (**pree**-ee-**KLAMP**-see-ah): a complication of pregnancy characterized by hypertension, edema, and proteinuria.

pregnancy test: a diagnostic test to determine if a woman is pregnant.

premature ejaculation: a condition in which the male reaches climax too soon, usually before or shortly after penetration.

premature infant: an infant born before the 37th week of gestation.

premature menopause: a condition in which the ovaries cease functioning before age 40.

premature rupture of membranes: when the amniotic sac ruptures before the 37th week of pregnancy.

premenstrual dysphoric disorder: a condition associated with severe emotional and physical problems linked to the menstrual cycle.

premenstrual syndrome: a group of symptoms experienced by some women within the two-week period before menstruation.

prenatal genetic testing: screening test for some genetic diseases done during pregnancy.

presbycusis (**pres**-beh-**KOO**-sis): a gradual sensorineural hearing loss that occurs as the body ages.

presbyopia (**pres**-bee-**OH**-pee-ah): condition of common changes in the eyes that occur with aging.

prescription: a written order from a licensed medical professional specifying a medication or product to be dispensed to a patient.

prescription drug: medication that can legally be dispensed only by a pharmacist with an order from a licensed prescriber.

pressure ulcer: an open ulcerated wound that is caused by prolonged pressure on an area of skin over a bony prominence.

preterm labor: when regular contractions begin as the result of the opening of the cervix after the 20th week and before the 37th week of a pregnancy.

priapism (**PRYE**-ah-**piz**-em): a painful erection that lasts four hours or more but is not accompanied by sexual excitement.

primary bone cancer: a relatively rare type of malignant tumor that originates in a bone.

primary ovarian insufficiency: when the ovaries stop functioning normally before the age of 40.

primigravida (**prye**-mih-**GRAV**-ih-dah): a woman during her first pregnancy.

primipara (prye-**MIP**-ah-rah): a woman who has borne one viable child.

probiotics (**pro**-bye-**AH**-tics): living microorganisms with a role in aiding digestion and protecting the body from harmful bacteria.

prolactinoma (proh-**lack**-tih-**NOH**-mah): a benign tumor of the pituitary gland that causes it to produce too much prolactin.

proliferative inflammatory atrophy: a potentially precancerous change to prostate cells.

prone position: a position in which the patient lies face down on the abdomen.

prophylaxis (**proh**-fih-**LACK**-sis): treatment, such as vaccination, intended to prevent a disease or stop it from spreading.

prostaglandin analog: eye drops used to treat glaucoma.

prostate cancer: cancer originating in the prostate.

prostatectomy (**pros**-tah-**TECK**-toh-mee): surgical removal of all or part of the prostate gland.

prostate-specific antigen: a blood test that is used to screen for prostate cancer.

prostatic intraepithelial neoplasia (praw-**STAH**-tik **in**-trah-ep-ih-**THEE**-lee-al **nee**-uh-**PLAY**-zhuh): precancerous change to prostate gland cells.

prostatism (**PROS**-tah-tizm): a disorder resulting from compression or obstruction of the urethra due to benign prostatic hyperplasia.

prostatitis (**pros**-tah-**TYE**-tis): inflammation of the prostate gland.

prosthesis (pros-**THEE**-sis): a substitute for a diseased or missing body part.

proteinuria (**proh**-tee-in-**YOU**-ree-ah): the presence of an abnormal amount of protein in the urine.

prothrombin time (proh-**THROM**-bin): a blood test used to diagnose conditions associated with abnormalities of clotting time and to monitor anticoagulant therapy.

proton pump inhibitor: medication that decreases the amount of acid produced by the stomach.

proto-oncogene (**proh**-toh-**ON**-koh-jeen): a normal gene that controls one of the normal processes such as cell growth, division or death.

pruritus (proo-**RYE**-tus): itching.

pruritus vulvae (**VUL**-vee): severe itching of the external female genitalia.

psoriasis (soh-**RYE**-uh-sis): a common skin disorder characterized by flare-ups in which red papules covered with silvery scales occur on the elbows, knees, scalp, back, or buttocks.

psoriatic arthritis: an inflammatory form of arthritis developed by about 20% of all people with psoriasis.

psychoanalysis (**sigh**-koh-ah-**NAL**-ih-sis): therapy based on the idea that mental disorders have underlying causes stemming from childhood and can only be overcome by gaining insight into one's feelings and patterns of behavior.

psychopharmacology (**sigh**-koh-farm-uh-**COL**-oh-gee): drug therapy for mental disorders.

psychosis (sigh-**KOH**-sis): a disrupted thought pattern that makes it difficult for a person to distinguish what is real and what is not.

psychotherapy: supportive talk therapy to treat mental illnesses by providing insights into a person's thoughts, emotions, and behaviors.

psychotic disorder (sigh-**KOT**-ick): a condition characterized by the loss of contact with reality and deterioration of normal social functioning.

psychotropic drug (**sigh**-koh-**TROP**-pick): medication that acts primarily on the central nervous system, where it produces temporary changes affecting the mind, emotions, and behavior.

ptosis (**TOH**-sis): drooping of the upper eyelid that is usually due to muscle weakness or paralysis.

pubic lice: small parasites that can be transmitted during sexual contact.

pulmonary edema (eh-**DEE**-mah): an accumulation of fluid in the lung tissues.

pulmonary embolism (**EM**-boh-lizm): the sudden blockage of a pulmonary artery by foreign matter or by an embolus that has formed in the leg or pelvic region.

pulmonary fibrosis (figh-**BROH**-sis): the progressive formation of scar tissue in the lung, resulting in decreased lung capacity and increased difficulty in breathing.

pulmonary function tests: a group of tests that measure volume and flow of air by utilizing a spirometer.

pulse oximeter (ock-**SIM**-eh-ter): an external monitor that measures the oxygen saturation level in the blood.

purpura (**PUR**-pew-rah): multiple purple discolorations on the skin caused by bleeding underneath the skin.

purulent (**PYOU**-roo-lent): producing or containing pus.

pustule (**PUS**-tyoul): a small, circumscribed lesion containing pus.

pyelitis: inflammation of the renal pelvis.

pyelonephritis (**pye**-eh-loh-neh-**FRY**-tis): inflammation of the renal pelvis and kidney.

pyelotomy (**pye**-eh-**LOT**-oh-mee): a surgical incision into the renal pelvis.

pyoderma (**pye**-oh-**DER**-mah): any acute, inflammatory, pus-forming bacterial skin infection such as impetigo.

pyonephrosis (**pye**-oh-nef-**ROH**-sis): suppuration of the kidney.

pyosalpinx (**pye**-oh-**SAL**-pinks): an accumulation of pus in the fallopian tube.

pyothorax (**pye**-oh-**THOH**-racks): the presence of pus in the pleural cavity between the layers of pleural membrane.

pyrosis (pye-**ROH**-sis): a burning sensation caused by the return of acidic stomach contents into the esophagus.

pyuria (pye-**YOU**-ree-ah): the presence of pus in the urine.

Q

Qi Gong (**CHEE**-gong): a Chinese system of movement, breathing techniques, and meditation.

quadriplegia (**kwad**-rih-**PLEE**-jee-ah): paralysis of all four extremities.

R

rabies (**RAY**-beez): an acute viral infection transmitted to humans by the bite or saliva of an infected animal.

radial keratotomy (**ker**-ah-**TOT**-oh-mee): a surgical procedure to treat myopia.

radiation therapy: the treatment of cancers through the use of x-rays.

radical hysterectomy: surgical removal of the uterus, ligaments, cervix, and a portion of the vagina.

radiculitis (rah-**dick**-you-**LYE**-tis): inflammation of the root of a spinal nerve that causes pain and numbness radiating down the affected limb.

radiculopathy: a condition caused by the compression of a nerve in the spine; also called a pinched nerve.

radioactive iodine treatment: oral administration of radioactive iodine to destroy thyroid cells.

radioactive iodine uptake test: test using radioactive iodine administered orally to measure thyroid function.

radiofrequency ablation: a minimally invasive procedure that relieves chronic nerve pain by burning part of the nerves, preventing the transmission of pain signals.

radiographic positioning: the description of the placement of the patient's body based on the part closest to the x-ray film.

radiographic projection: the description of the x-ray beam's path through the patient's body.

radiology (**ray**-dee-**OL**-oh-jee): the use of radiant energy and radioactive substances in medicine for diagnosis and treatment.

radiolucent (**ray**-dee-oh-**LOO**-sent): a substance that allows x-rays to pass through and appears black or dark gray on the resulting film.

radiopaque (**ray**-dee-oh-**PAYK**): a substance that does not allow x-rays to pass through and appears white or light gray on the resulting film.

radiopharmaceuticals: drugs containing radioactive materials that produce radiation.

rales (**RAHLZ**): abnormal crackle-like lung sounds heard while breathing in.

range-of-motion testing: a diagnostic procedure to evaluate joint mobility and muscle strength.

Raynaud's disease (ray-**NOHZ**): a peripheral arterial occlusive disease in which intermittent attacks are triggered by cold or stress.

rectal administration: the insertion of medication into the rectum as either suppositories or liquid solutions.

rectocele (**RECK**-toh-seel): a bulging of the front wall of the rectum into the vagina.

recumbent (ree-**KUM**-bent): any position in which the patient is lying down.

recurrent urinary tract infection: cystitis that occurs two or more times in six months or three or more times a year.

red blood cell count: a blood test that is performed to determine the number of erythrocytes in the blood.

refraction test: an examination procedure to determine an eye's refractive error so that the best corrective lenses can be prescribed.

refractive disorder: a focusing problem caused when the lens and cornea do not bend light so that it focuses properly on the retina.

regurgitation (ree-**gur**-jih-**TAY**-shun): the return of swallowed food into the mouth.

Reiki (**RAY**-kee): a technique in which the practitioner transfers healing energy by means of visualization or gentle touch.

remission (ree-**MIH**-shun): complete or partial end of cancer signs and symptoms for at least one month.

renal cell carcinoma: the most common form of kidney cancer in adults.

renal colic (**REE**-nal **KOLL**-ick): acute pain in the kidney area that is caused by blockage during the passage of a kidney stone.

renal failure: the inability of one or both of the kidneys to perform their functions.

renal transplantation: the grafting of a donor kidney into the body to replace the recipient's failed kidneys.

repetitive stress disorders: a variety of muscular conditions that result from repeated motions performed in the course of normal activities.

respiratory arrest: the absence of breathing, either with apnea or agonal respirations.

respiratory distress syndrome: a breathing disorder in an infant caused by underdeveloped lungs.

respiratory failure: a condition in which the level of oxygen in the blood becomes dangerously low or the level of carbon dioxide becomes dangerously high.

respiratory syncytial virus (sin-**SIH**-shul): a common, highly contagious virus spread by respiratory droplets.

restenosis (reh-steh-**NOH**-sis): the condition when an artery that has been opened by angioplasty closes again.

restless legs syndrome: a neurological disorder characterized by uncomfortable feelings in the legs, producing a strong urge to move them.

retinal detachment: the separation of all of the light-sensitive retina from the choroid.

retinal tear: the separation of some of the light-sensitive retina from the choroid.

retinitis pigmentosa (**ret**-ih-**NIGH**-tis pig-men-**TOH**-sah): a progressive degeneration of the retina that affects night and peripheral vision.

retinoblastoma: a type of eye cancer caused by the abnormal growth of retinal cells.

retinoids (**RET**-ih-noydz): a class of chemical compounds derived from vitamin A that are used in skin care and treatment.

retinopathy (**ret**-ih-**NOP**-ah-thee): any disease of the retina.

retrograde ejaculation: when an orgasm results in semen flowing backward into the bladder instead of out through the penis.

retrograde pyelogram: an x-ray of the urinary system taken after a contrast medium has been placed in the urethra and caused to flow upward through the urinary tract.

reversal agent: a drug that immediately reverses the effect of another drug, used in the case of overdose.

revision surgery: the replacement of a worn or failed implant.

Reye's syndrome: a potentially serious or deadly disorder in children characterized by vomiting and confusion, sometimes following a viral illness for which the child was treated with aspirin.

rhabdomyolysis (**rab**-doh-my-**AHL**-eh-sis): a syndrome that can result from muscle injury in which the death of muscle fibers releases their contents into the bloodstream.

rheumatoid arthritis (**ROO**-mah-toyd ar-**THRIGH**-tis): a chronic autoimmune disorder in which the joints and some organs of other body systems are attacked.

rhinophyma (**rye**-noh-**FIGH**-muh): hyperplasia of the tissues of the nose.

rhinorrhea (**rye**-noh-**REE**-ah): the watery flow of mucus from the nose.

rhonchi (**RONG**-kye): a coarse, rattling sound somewhat like snoring, usually caused by secretions in the bronchial airways.

rhytidectomy (**rit**-ih-**DECK**-toh-mee): surgical removal of excess skin and fat from the face to eliminate wrinkles.

rickets (**RICK**-ets): a deficiency disease occurring in children involving defective bone growth due to vitamin D deficiency.

rickettsia (rih-**KET**-see-ah): a small bacterium that lives in lice, fleas, ticks, and mites.

root canal: a procedure in which diseased or damaged pulp in the root canal is removed in order to save the tooth.

Rorschach test: a way to assess a person's personality and emotional functioning by analyzing their interpretation of inkblot images.

rosacea (roh-**ZAY**-shee-ah): a chronic skin condition of unknown cause that produces tiny red pimples and enlarged blood vessels.

roseola: a viral illness common in infants, characterized by a high fever followed by a rash.

rotator cuff tear: a partial or complete tear in the rotator cuff that occurs as the irritated tendon weakens, or as the result of a fall or injury.

rotavirus: characterized by diarrhea, fever, vomiting; protected against by RV vaccine.

rubella (roo-**BELL**-ah): a viral infection characterized by a low-grade fever, swollen glands, inflamed eyes, and a fine, pink rash.

ruptured spleen: a medical emergency that occurs when the covering of the spleen is torn.

S

sacrocolpopexy (sa-kroh-**KOL**-poh-**peck**-see): surgical fixation of a prolapsed vagina to a surrounding structure such as the sacrum.

salmonellosis (**sal**-moh-nel-**LOH**-sis): an infectious disease transmitted by feces, either through direct contact or by eating contaminated raw or undercooked food.

salpingectomy (**sal**-pin-**JECK**-toh-mee): surgical removal of one or both fallopian tubes.

salpingitis (**sal**-pin-**JIGH**-tis): inflammation of a fallopian tube.

salpingo-oophorectomy (sal-**ping**-goh oh-**ahf**-oh-**RECK**-toh-mee): surgical removal of a fallopian tube and ovary.

sarcoma (sar-**KOH**-mah): a malignant tumor that arises from connective tissues.

sarcopenia (**sar**-koh-**PEE**-nee-ah): the loss of muscle mass, strength, and function that comes with aging.

scabies (**SKAY**-beez): a skin infection caused by an infestation of itch mites.

scales: flakes or dry patches made up of excess dead epidermal cells.

Schilling test (**SHILL**-ing): a urine test used to evaluate vitamin B_{12} absorption.

schizoaffective disorder: a psychiatric disorder combining schizophrenia symptoms with bipolar or depressive disorder symptoms.

schizophrenia (**skit**-soh-**FREE**-nee-ah): a psychotic disorder characterized by withdrawal from reality, illogical patterns of thinking, delusions, and hallucinations.

sciatica (sigh-**AT**-ih-kah): inflammation of the sciatic nerve that results in pain, burning, and tingling along the course of the affected nerve.

scleral buckle (**SKLER**-al): a silicone band or sponge used to repair a detached retina.

scleritis (skleh-**RYE**-tis): inflammation of the sclera of the eye.

scleroderma (**sklehr**-oh-**DER**-mah): an autoimmune disorder in which the connective tissues become thickened and hardened, causing the skin to become hard and swollen.

sclerotherapy (**sklehr**-oh-**THER**-ah-pee): treatment of spider veins by injecting a saline sclerosing solution into the vein.

scoliosis (**skoh**-lee-**OH**-sis): an abnormal lateral curvature of the spine.

scotoma (skoh-**TOH**-mah): an abnormal area of diminished vision surrounded by an area of normal vision.

screening tools: validated assessment questionnaires for diagnosing certain mental illnesses and psychiatric disorders.

seasonal affective disorder: a bout of depression associated with the decrease in hours of daylight during winter months.

seborrheic dermatitis (**seb**-oh-**REE**-ick **der**-mah-**TYE**-tis): inflammation resulting from overactivity of the sebaceous glands that causes scaling and itching of the upper layers of the skin or scalp.

seborrheic keratosis (**seb**-oh-**REE**-ick **kerr**-ah-**TOH**-sis): a benign skin growth that has a waxy or "pasted-on" look.

secondary bone cancer: tumors that have metastasized to bones from other organs such as the breasts and lungs.

sedation: the use of sedative medication to induce a calm, relaxed state in order to perform a medical procedure.

sedative: a medication that relaxes the body by suppressing neurotransmitters in the central nervous system.

seizure (**SEE**-zhur): a sudden surge of electrical activity in the brain that affects how a person feels or acts for a short time.

selective mutism (**MEW**-tizm): an anxiety disorder where a child who is capable of speech is unable to speak or communicate.

self-harm: harming oneself intentionally, can vary greatly in severity.

senile emphysema (**SEE**-nye-ahl **em**-fih-**SEE**-mah): age-related change in lung tissue that causes an increase in alveoli size without alveolar wall destruction.

sensorineural hearing loss: hearing loss that develops when the auditory nerve or hair cells in the inner ear are damaged.

sentinel node biopsy: biopsy of the first lymph node to come into contact with cancer cells.

septoplasty (**SEP**-toh-**plas**-tee): surgical repair of parts of the nasal septum.

sepsis (**SEP**-sis): an infection that results from bacteria or other infectious organisms entering the bloodstream.

serum bilirubin test: a blood test that measures the ability of the liver to take up, process, and secrete bilirubin into the bile.

severe combined immunodeficiency: an inherited condition in which immune system abnormalities cause an increased susceptibility to infection and failure to thrive as a result.

severe obesity: the condition of having a body mass index value greater than 40.

sexual dysfunctions: conditions which prevent a person from experiencing satisfaction from sexual activity.

sexually transmitted diseases: infections caused by either a bacteria or a virus transmitted through sexual intercourse or other genital contact.

sexually transmitted infections: potentially contagious infections from exposure to a sexually transmitted disease.

shaken baby syndrome: syndrome that results from a child being violently shaken by someone.

shigellosis (shig-eh-**LOH**-sis): a bacterial infection caused by *shigella*, which can cause diarrhea and fever.

shin splint: pain caused by the muscle tearing away from the tibia.

short stature: condition resulting from the failure of the bones of the limbs to grow to an appropriate length compared to the size of the head and trunk.

sickle cell anemia: a genetic disorder that causes abnormal hemoglobin, resulting in red blood cells that assume an abnormal sickle shape.

side effect: a secondary response that accompanies the principal response for which a drug was taken.

sigmoidoscopy (**sig**-moi-**DOS**-koh-pee): the endoscopic examination of the interior of the rectum, sigmoid colon, and possibly a portion of the descending colon.

sign: objective evidence of disease, such as a fever.

silicosis (**sill**-ih-**KOH**-sis): a form of pneumoconiosis caused by inhaling silica dust.

Sims' position: an examination position in which the patient is lying on the left side with the right knee and thigh drawn up with the left arm placed along the back.

single photon emission computed tomography: a type of nuclear imaging test that produces 3D computer-reconstructed images showing perfusion through tissues and organs.

singultus (sing-**GUL**-tus): myoclonus of the diaphragm that causes the characteristic hiccup sound with each spasm.

sinusitis (**sigh**-nuh-**SIGH**-tis): an inflammation of the sinuses.

skin cancer: a malignant growth on the skin, which can have many causes, including repeated severe sunburns or long-term exposure to the sun.

skin grafts: the replacement of damaged skin with healthy tissue taken from a donor site on the patient's body.

skin tags: small, flesh-colored or light-brown polyps that hang from the skin's surface by fine stalks.

skin tear: a shear injury where a flap of epidermis is pulled away from the underlying tissue.

sleep apnea (**AP**-nee-ah): a potentially serious disorder in which breathing repeatedly stops during sleep for long enough periods to cause a measurable decrease in blood oxygen levels.

sleep deprivation: a sufficient lack of restorative sleep over a cumulative period so as to cause physical or psychiatric symptoms and affect routine performance or tasks.

sleep hyperhidrosis: the occurrence of hyperhidrosis during sleep.

slit-lamp ophthalmoscopy (**ahf**-thal-**MOS**-koh-pee): a diagnostic procedure in which a narrow beam of light is focused to permit the ophthalmologist to examine the structures at the front of the eye including the cornea, iris, and lens.

small bowel obstruction: partial or complete blockage of the small intestine.

small cell lung cancer: fast-growing lung cancer that occurs most often in smokers.

smoke inhalation: chemical damage and burns to the lungs caused by breathing in hot smoke containing products of combustion.

Snellen chart: printed chart used to measure visual acuity.

social anxiety disorder: excessive fear of social situations in which the person fears negative evaluation by others or embarrassing himself or herself in front of others.

soft-tissue sarcoma: cancer of the muscle, fat, blood vessels, or other supporting tissues.

somatic symptom disorder (soh-**MAT**-ick): characterized by physical complaints or concerns about one's body that are out of proportion to any physical findings or disease.

somnambulism (som-**NAM**-byou-lizm): the condition of walking or performing some other activity without awakening.

sonogram: the image created by ultrasonography, also known as an ultrasound.

spasm: a sudden, involuntary contraction of one or more muscles.

speculum (**SPECK**-you-lum): an instrument used to enlarge the opening of any canal or cavity to facilitate inspection of its interior.

sperm count: the testing of freshly ejaculated semen to determine the volume plus the number, shape, size, and motility of the sperm.

spina bifida (**SPY**-nah **BIF**-ih-dah): a congenital defect that occurs during early pregnancy in which the spinal canal fails to close completely around the spinal cord.

spinal anesthesia: regional anesthesia produced by injecting medication into the subarachnoid space.

spinal block: an injection given into the fluid surrounding the spinal cord during labor and delivery.

spinal cord injury: paralysis resulting from damage to the spinal cord that prevents nerve impulses from being transmitted below the level of the injury.

spinal fusion: a technique to immobilize part of the spine by joining together two or more vertebrae.

spinal stenosis: a narrowing of the spaces within the spine.

spiral fracture: a fracture in which the bone has been twisted apart.

spirochetes (**SPY**-roh-keets): long, slender, spiral-shaped bacteria that have flexible walls and are capable of movement.

spirometer (spih-**ROM**-eh-ter): a recording device that measures the amount of air inhaled or exhaled (volume) and the length of time required for each breath.

splenomegaly (**splee**-noh-**MEG**-ah-lee): an abnormal enlargement of the spleen.

spondylolisthesis (**spon**-dih-loh-liss-**THEE**-sis): the forward slipping movement of the body of one of the lower lumbar vertebrae on the vertebra below it.

spondylosis (**spon**-dih-**LOH**-sis): a degenerative disorder that can cause the loss of normal spinal structure and function.

sprain: an injury to a joint, such as ankle, knee, or wrist, that usually involves a wrenched or torn ligament.

sputum (**SPYOU**-tum): phlegm ejected through the mouth that can be examined for diagnostic purposes.

sputum culture and sensitivity: a diagnostic test in which a sputum sample is monitored for bacterial growth and antibiotic sensitivity.

sputum cytology: a procedure in which a sample of mucus is coughed up and examined under a microscope to detect cancer cells.

squamous cell carcinoma (**SKWAY**-mus): a malignant tumor of the squamous cells of the epithelium.

staging: the process of classifying tumors by how far the disease has progressed, the potential for its responding to therapy, and the patient's prognosis.

stapedectomy (**stay**-peh-**DECK**-toh-mee): surgical removal of the stapes bone and the insertion of a prosthetic device that conducts sound vibrations to the inner ear.

staphylococci (**staf**-ih-loh-**KOCK**-sigh): a group of about 30 species of bacteria that form irregular groups or clusters resembling grapes.

staphylococcus aureus (**staf**-ih-loh-**KOCK**-us **OR**-ee-us): a form of staphylococcus that often infects wounds and causes serious problems such as toxic shock syndrome.

stasis dermatitis (**STAY**-sis **der**-mah-**TYE**-tis): lower extremity inflammation caused by chronic venous insufficiency and venous stasis.

steatorrhea (**stee**-at-oh-**REE**-ah): the presence of excess fat in the stool.

stem cell transplant: cancer treatment in which abnormal bone marrow is destroyed and replaced with new stem cells.

stent: a wire-mesh tube that is implanted in a coronary artery to provide support to the arterial wall.

stereotactic radiosurgery: treatment using a three-dimensional coordinate system to accurately find small tumors within the body and deliver radiation to them while minimizing damage to the surrounding tissue.

sterilization: any procedure rendering an individual incapable of reproduction.

stethoscope (**STETH**-oh-skope): an instrument used to listen to sounds within the body.

stillbirth: the birth of a fetus that died before or during delivery.

stimulant: a substance that works by increasing activity in certain areas of the brain to increase concentration and wakefulness.

stomatitis (**stoh**-mah-**TYE**-tis): inflammation of the mucosa of the mouth.

stone: an abnormal mineral deposit that has formed within the body.

stool analysis: the examination of the physical and chemical properties of stool to determine the presence of abnormal elements.

stool tests: specimens of feces that are examined for content and characteristics.

strabismus (strah-**BIZ**-mus): a disorder in which the eyes point in different directions or are not aligned correctly because the eye muscles are unable to focus together.

strain: an injury to the body of a muscle or the attachment of a tendon.

strangulated hernia: a condition that occurs when a portion of the small intestine is constricted inside a hernia and the blood supply to the intestine is cut off.

strep throat: a sore throat caused by bacteria group A streptococci.

streptococci (**strep**-toh-**KOCK**-sigh): bacteria that form a chain.

stress fracture: a small crack in a bone that often develops from chronic, excessive impact.

stress incontinence: the inability to control the voiding of urine under physical stress such as running, sneezing, laughing, or coughing.

stress test: the use of electrocardiography to assess cardiovascular health and function during and after stress such as exercise on a treadmill.

stricture: an abnormal narrowing of a bodily passage such as the esophagus resulting from scar tissue or other damage.

stridor (**STRYE**-dor): an abnormal, high-pitched, musical breathing sound caused by a blockage in the throat or larynx.

stupor (**STOO**-per): an unresponsive state from which a person can be aroused only briefly despite vigorous, repeated attempts.

subconjunctival hemorrhage: bleeding between the conjunctiva and the sclera.

subcutaneous injection (**sub**-kyoo-**TAY**-nee-yus): the administration of medication by injection into the fatty layer just below the skin.

sublingual administration (sub-**LING**-gwal): the placement of medication under the tongue, where it is allowed to dissolve slowly.

subluxation (**sub**-luck-**SAY**-shun): the partial displacement of a bone from its joint.

substance abuse: the addictive use of tobacco, alcohol, medications, or illegal drugs.

sudden infant death syndrome: the sudden and unexplainable death of an apparently healthy sleeping infant between the ages of 1 month to 1 year.

suicide: the intentional taking of one's own life.

sulfonylurea (sull-**fah**-nee-**LOU**-ree-ah): diabetes medication that increases the amount of insulin released by the pancreas.

supplemental oxygen: oxygen administered when the patient is unable to maintain an adequate blood oxygen saturation level from breathing normal air.

suppository (suh-**PAW**-zih-toh-ree): medication in a semisolid form that is placed in the rectum, vagina, or urethra.

suppuration (**sup**-you-**RAY**-shun): the formation of pus.

suprapubic catheterization (**soo**-prah-**PYOU**-bick): the placement of a urinary catheter into the bladder through a small incision made through the abdominal wall.

supraventricular tachycardia (**soo**-prah-ven-**TRICK**-you-lar tack-ee-**KAR**-dee-ah): an episode of irregular heart rhythm that begins and ends abruptly during which there are very rapid and regular heartbeats that originate at or above the AV node.

surgical biopsy (**BYE**-op-see): surgical removal of a small piece of tissue for examination to confirm a diagnosis.

swallow evaluation: an assessment to evaluate a patient's ability to swallow safely after a stroke.

symptom (**SIMP**-tum): subjective evidence of a disease, such as pain or a headache.

synchronized cardioversion: an intervention for restoring normal heart rhythm using a timed, lower voltage electrical shock than defibrillation in a non-emergency situation.

syncope (**SIN**-koh-pee): the brief loss of consciousness caused by the decreased flow of blood to the brain.

syndrome (**SIN**-drohm): a set of signs and symptoms that occur together as part of a specific disease process.

syndrome of inappropriate antidiuretic hormone: overproduction of the antidiuretic hormone ADH, leading to bloating, water retention, and electrolyte imbalance.

synergism (**SIN**-er-jizm): the interaction of two drugs taken together that enhances the effectiveness of both.

synovectomy (sin-oh-**VECK**-toh-mee): surgical removal of a synovial membrane from a joint.

synovitis (sin-oh-**VYE**-tiss): inflammation of the synovial membrane that results in swelling and pain of the affected joint.

synthetic immunoglobulins: a post-exposure preventive measure against certain viruses including rabies and some types of hepatitis.

synthetic interferon: medication administered to treat multiple sclerosis, hepatitis C, and some cancers.

syphilis (**SIF**-ih-lis): a sexually transmitted disease that is caused by the bacterium *Treponema pallidum*.

syringe (suh-**RINJ**): a plastic tube used to measure and administer liquid medication.

systemic lupus erythematosus: an autoimmune disorder characterized by a red, scaly rash on the face and upper trunk that also attacks the connective tissue in other body systems.

systemic reaction (sis-**TEH**-mik): a severe, systemic response to an allergen.

systole (**SIS**-toh-lee): the period of contraction that the ventricles undergo while pumping blood into the aorta and the pulmonary artery.

T

tablet: an object containing medication in solid form, designed to be swallowed or dissolved in the mouth.

tachycardia (**tack**-ee-**KAR**-dee-ah): an abnormally rapid resting heartbeat usually at a rate of more than 100 beats per minute.

tachypnea (**tack**-ihp-**NEE**-ah): an abnormally rapid rate of respiration, usually more than 20 breaths per minute.

targeted therapy: a form of anti-cancer drug therapy that uses drugs or other substances to identify and attack specific cancer cells without harming normal cells.

tarsorrhaphy (tahr-**SOR**-ah-fee): the partial or complete suturing together of the upper and lower eyelids.

teletherapy (**tel**-eh-**THER**-ah-pee): precisely targeted radiation therapy administered at a distance from the body.

temporal arteritis (**TEM**-poh-**ral ar**-teh-**RYE**-tis): inflammation of the temporal arteries that can cause headache, visual impairment, or other symptoms.

tendinitis (**ten**-dih-**NIGH**-itis): inflammation of the tendons caused by excessive or unusual use of the joint.

tendinopathy: general term for irritation or degeneration of a tendon in any joint.

tendinosis: a chronic condition characterized by pain due to repetitive overuse or an injury that has not healed.

tenodesis (ten-**ODD**-eh-sis): surgical suturing of the end of a tendon to bone.

tenolysis (ten-**OL**-ih-sis): the release of a tendon from adhesions.

tenorrhaphy (ten-**OR**-ah-fee): surgical suturing of a tendon.

tenosynovitis (**ten**-oh-**sin**-oh-**VYE**-tis): inflammation of the sheath around a tendon.

tenotomy (ten-**OT**-ah-mee): surgical cutting of a tendon to provide release or allow lengthening.

terminal agitation: a form of delirium that occurs at end of life.

testicular cancer: cancer that originates in the testicles.

testicular self-examination: a self-help step in early detection of testicular cancer by detecting lumps, swelling, or changes in the skin of the scrotum.

testicular torsion: the twisting of the spermatic cord leading into the testicle, causing sharp pain in the scrotum.

tetanus (**TET**-ah-nus): an acute and potentially fatal infection of the central nervous system caused by a toxin produced by the tetanus bacteria.

thalamotomy (**thal**-ah-**MOT**-oh-mee): a surgical incision into the thalamus.

thalassemia (thal-ah-**SEE**-mee-ah): an inherited blood disorder that causes mild or severe anemia due to reduced hemoglobin and fewer red blood cells than normal.

thallium stress test (**THAL**-ee-um): nuclear imaging test performed to evaluate blood flow to the heart during exercise.

therapeutic dose: the amount of medication necessary to achieve the desired outcome.

therapeutic level: a blood test to determine if there is a sufficient quantity of a medication in the blood to achieve the desired outcome.

therapeutic massage: the use of touch and pressure to relieve pain.

therapeutic plasma exchange: plasmapheresis in which the patient's own blood is circulated through a device that removes the disease-causing antibodies and replaces them with healthy donor plasma and/or a plasma substitute.

therapeutic ultrasound: the use of high-frequency sound waves to treat muscle injuries by generating heat deep within muscle tissue.

thoracentesis (**thoh**-rah-sen-**TEE**-sis): surgical puncture of the chest wall with a needle to obtain fluid from the pleural cavity.

thoracotomy (**thoh**-rah-**KOT**-toh-mee): a surgical incision into the chest walls to open the pleural cavity for biopsy or treatment.

thrombocytopenia (**throm**-boh-**sigh**-toh-**PEE**-nee-ah): a condition in which there is an abnormally small number of platelets circulating in the blood.

thrombocytosis (**throm**-boh-sigh-**TOH**-sis): an abnormal increase in the number of platelets in the circulating blood.

thrombolytic (**throm**-boh-**LIT**-ick): medication that dissolves or causes a thrombus to break up.

thrombosis (throm-**BOH**-sis): the abnormal condition of having a thrombus.

thrombotic occlusion (throm-**BOT**-ick ah-**KLOO**-zhun): the blocking of an artery by a thrombus.

thrombus (**THROM**-bus): a blood clot attached to the interior wall of an artery or vein.

thymectomy (thigh-**MECK**-toh-mee): surgical removal of the thymus gland.

thyroid carcinoma: cancer of the thyroid gland.

thyroid replacement therapy: use of synthetic thyroid hormones to replace lost thyroid function.

thyroid scan: a specialized nuclear scan to evaluate thyroid function.

thyroid-stimulating hormone assay: a blood test to measure the circulating blood level of thyroid-stimulating hormone.

thyroid storm: a relatively rare, life-threatening condition caused by exaggerated hyperthyroidism.

tinea (**TIN**-ee-ah): a fungal infection that can grow on the skin, hair, or nails.

tinnitus (tih-**NIGH**-tus): a condition of ringing, buzzing, or roaring sound in one or both ears.

tissue plasminogen activator (plaz-**MIN**-oh-jen): a thrombolytic medication administered to some patients having a heart attack or stroke to dissolve damaging blood clots.

TNM staging: cancer staging system based on size of tumor, lymph node involvement, and presence of metastases.

tolerance: acquired unresponsiveness to a specific antigen or decline in effective response to a drug usually due to repeated use.

tomography (toh-**MOG**-rah-fee): the imaging of cross-sections of a part of the body.

tomotherapy: combination of tomography with radiation therapy to precisely target tumors.

tonic–clonic seizure: a type of seizure involving the whole body.

tonometry (toh-**NOM**-eh-tree): the measurement of intraocular pressure.

tonsillectomy (**ton**-sih-**LECK**-toh-mee): surgical removal of the tonsils.

tonsillitis (**ton**-sih-**LYE**-tis): inflammation of the tonsils.

topical analgesic: medication applied to the skin to relieve pain.

topical application: medication in liquid or ointment form rubbed into the skin on the area to be treated.

topical corticosteroid: topical medication used to reduce inflammation.

topical hemostatic agents: products designed to promote rapid blood coagulation in the event of a traumatic wound.

topical retinoid: topical medication used to treat acne.

torticollis (**tor**-tih-**KOL**-is): a stiff neck due to spasmodic contraction of the neck muscles that pull the head toward the affected side.

total hemoglobin test: a blood test that measures the amount of hemoglobin found in whole blood.

total hip replacement: surgery performed to restore a damaged hip to full function by removing the head of the femur and replacing it with a metal ball.

total hysterectomy: surgical removal of the uterus and cervix, either through the vagina or laparoscopically through the abdomen.

total knee replacement: surgical placement of an artificial joint during which all parts of the knee are replaced.

total protein test: measures the proteins albumin and globulin in the blood.

Tourette's disorder: physical and/or verbal uncontrollable "tics" such as shrugging shoulders, blinking eyes, or yelling offensive words.

toxic shock syndrome: an infection caused by an overgrowth of the bacteria *Staphylococcus aureus*.

toxicity (**TOCK**-sih-seh-tee): the presence of a harmful level of a drug in the body, either by overdose or slowed removal of the drug from the body.

toxoplasmosis (**tock**-soh-plaz-**MOH**-sis): a disease caused by a parasite most commonly transmitted from pets to humans by contact with contaminated feces.

tracheostomy (**tray**-kee-**OS**-toh-mee): surgical creation of a stoma into the trachea in order to insert a tube to facilitate breathing.

tracheotomy (**tray**-kee-**OT**-oh-mee): an emergency procedure in which an incision is made into the trachea to gain access to the airway below a blockage.

traction: a pulling force exerted on a limb in a distal direction in an effort to return the bone or joint to normal alignment.

traditional Chinese medicine: a system of ancient Chinese medicinal treatments, including acupuncture, to prevent, diagnose, and treat disease.

transcatheter aortic valve replacement: a procedure in which the existing aortic valve is left in place and a replacement valve is inserted via a catheter.

transcranial magnetic stimulation: brief, powerful electromagnetic pulses used to alter electrical pathways in the brain.

transcutaneous electronic nerve stimulation: a method of pain control achieved by wearing a device that delivers small electrical impulses to the nerve endings through the skin.

transdermal (tranz-**DUR**-mahl): the administration of medication through the unbroken skin so that it is absorbed continuously to produce a systemic effect.

transesophageal echocardiography (**trans**-eh-**sof**-ah-**JEE**-al **eck**-oh-**kar**-dee-**OG**-rah-fee): an ultrasonic imaging technique that is performed from inside the esophagus to evaluate heart structures.

transfusion reaction: a serious and potentially fatal complication of a blood transfusion in which a severe immune response occurs because the patient's blood and the donated blood do not match.

transgender(trans-**JEN**-der): a person whose gender identity does not match their sex assigned at birth.

transient ischemic attack (iss-**KEE**-mick): a temporary interruption in the blood supply to the brain.

transurethral prostatectomy: the removal of excess tissue from an enlarged prostate gland with the use of a resectoscope.

transvaginal ultrasound (**trans**-**VAJ**-ih-nal): a diagnostic test utilizing ultrasound to image the uterus and ovaries.

transverse fracture: a fracture that occurs straight across the bone.

trauma (**TRAW**-mah): wound or injury.

traumatic brain injury: a blow to the head or a penetrating head injury that damages the brain.

tremor: a repetitive, involuntary muscle movement usually involving the hands, arms, head, or face.

triage (tree-**AHZH**): the medical screening of patients to determine their relative priority of need and the proper place of treatment.

trichomoniasis (**trick**-oh-moh-**NYE**-ah-sis): a sexually transmitted infection caused by the parasite *Trichomonas vaginalis.*

trichomycosis axillaris (**try**-koh-my-**KOH**-sis **ak**-sih-**LAH**-ris): superficial bacterial infection of the hair shafts in areas with extensive sweat glands such as the armpits.

trigeminal neuralgia (try-**JEM**-ih-nal new-**RAL**-jee-ah): inflammation of the fifth cranial nerve characterized by sudden, intense, brief attacks of sharp pain on one side of the face.

trigger finger: the painful and progressive restriction of movement caused by inflammation of a tendon's synovial sheath.

triple-negative breast cancer: breast cancer without receptors for estrogen or progesterone, and low levels of HER2.

triple-positive breast cancer: breast cancer with receptors for estrogen and progesterone, and high levels of HER2.

trismus (**TRIZ**-mus): any restriction to the opening of the mouth caused by trauma, surgery, or radiation associated with the treatment of oral cancer.

tubal ligation: a surgical sterilization procedure in which the fallopian tubes are sealed or cut to prevent sperm from reaching a mature ovum.

tuberculin skin testing: a screening test for tuberculosis in which the skin of the arm is injected with a harmless antigen extracted from the TB bacteria.

tuberculosis (too-**ber**-kew-**LOH**-sis): an infectious disease caused by *Mycobacterium tuberculosis* that usually attacks the lungs.

tumor: an abnormal growth of body tissue creating a mass; also known as a neoplasm.

tympanometry (**tim**-pah-**NOM**-eh-tree): the use of air pressure in the ear canal to test for disorders of the middle ear.

tympanoplasty (**tim**-pah-noh-**PLAS**-tee): surgical correction of a hole in the eardrum, either to cure chronic inflammation or to restore function.

type 1 diabetes: an autoimmune insulin deficiency disorder caused by the destruction of pancreatic islet beta cells.

type 2 diabetes: an insulin resistance disorder in which, although insulin is being produced, the body does not use it effectively.

U

ulcer (**UL**-ser): an open lesion of the skin or mucous membrane resulting in tissue loss around the edges.

ulcerative colitis (**UL**-ser-**ay**-tiv koh-**LYE**-tis): a chronic condition of unknown cause in which repeated episodes of inflammation in the rectum and large intestine cause ulcers and irritation.

ultrasonic bone density testing: a screening test for osteoporosis or other conditions that cause a loss of bone mass.

ultrasonography (**ul**-trah-son-**OG**-rah-fee): the imaging of deep body structures by recording the echoes of sound wave pulses that are above the range of human hearing; also known as ultrasound.

umbilical cord blood: blood that remains in the umbilical cord and placenta after a baby is delivered, a potential source of cells for hematopoietic stem cell transplants.

umbilical hernia: the protrusion of intestine in the area of the belly button, specifically the umbilical ring.

unconscious: a state of being unaware and unable to respond to any stimuli including pain.

upper GI bleed: blood loss from the esophagus, stomach, or duodenum.

upper GI series: radiographic study to examine the upper digestive system using a barium swallow to make these structures visible.

upper respiratory infection: a term used to describe the common cold.

uremia (you-**REE**-mee-ah): a toxic condition in which urea and other waste products normally excreted in the urine are retained in the blood.

ureteral obstruction: blockage of one or both ureters.

ureterectomy (**you**-reh-ter-**ECK**-toh-mee): surgical removal of a ureter.

ureterolith (you-**REE**-ter-oh-**lith**): a stone located anywhere along the ureter.

ureterorrhagia (you-**ree**-ter-oh-**RAY**-jee-ah): the discharge of blood from the ureter.

ureteroscopy (you-**reet**-eh-**ROS**-koh-pee): a treatment for a stone lodged in the ureter.

urethral catheterization: the insertion of a tube through the urethra and into the bladder.

urethritis (**you**-reh-**THRIGH**-tis): inflammation of the urethra.

urethroplasty (you-**REE**-throh-**plas**-tee): surgical repair of the walls of the urethra.

urethrorrhagia (you-**ree**-throh-**RAY**-jee-ah): bleeding from the urethra.

urethrorrhea (you-**ree**-throh-**REE**-ah): abnormal discharge from the urethra.

urethrostenosis (you-**ree**-throh-steh-**NOH**-sis): narrowing of the urethra.

urethrotomy (**you**-reh-**THROT**-oh-mee): a surgical incision into the urethra.

urinalysis (**you**-rih-**NAL**-ih-sis): the examination of urine to determine the presence of abnormal elements.

urinary catheterization (**kath**-eh-ter-eye-**ZAY**-shun): the insertion of a tube into the bladder in order to obtain a sterile specimen, drain urine, or inject medication.

urinary hesitancy: difficulty in starting a urinary stream.
urinary incontinence: the inability to control the voiding of urine.
urinary retention: the inability to completely empty the bladder when attempting to urinate.
urinary tract infection: an infection involving the structures of the urinary system that usually begins in the bladder.
urinary tract obstruction: a blockage that prevents the flow of urine in one part of the urinary tract.
urine culture and sensitivity test: a urine test to identify the cause of a urinary tract infection and determine which antibiotic will be the most effective treatment.
urosepsis (you-roh-**SEP**-sis): a life-threatening systemic bacterial infection that can occur when a urinary tract infection spreads to the kidneys.
urticaria (**ur**-tih-**KARE**-ee-ah): itchy wheals on the skin caused by an allergic reaction.
uterine prolapse (proh-**LAPS**): the condition in which the uterus slides from its normal position in the pelvic cavity and sags into the vagina.
uveitis (**you**-vee-**EYE**-tis): inflammation of the uvea causing swelling and irritation.

V

vaginal atrophy: thinning, drying, and inflammation of the vaginal walls caused by hormonal changes.
vaginal candidiasis (**kan**-dih-**DYE**-ah-sis): a vaginal infection caused by *Candida albicans*.
vaginismus (**VAJ**-ih-**nihz**-mis): an involuntary spasm of the pelvic floor muscles that close off the vagina.
vaginitis (**vaj**-ih-**NIGH**-tis): inflammation of the lining of the vagina.
valvular stenosis (steh-**NOH**-sis): a condition in which there is narrowing, stiffening, thickening, or blockage of one or more valves of the heart.
valvuloplasty (**VAL**-view-loh-**plas**-tee): surgical repair of a heart valve.
varicella (**var**-ih-**SEL**-ah): a highly contagious infection caused by the herpes virus *Varicella zoster*; also known as chickenpox.
varicocele (**VAR**-ih-koh-**seel**): a knot of varicose veins in one side of the scrotum.
varicocelectomy (**var**-ih-koh-sih-**LECK**-toh-mee): the removal of a portion of an enlarged vein to relieve a varicocele.
varicose veins (**VAR**-ih-kohs **VAYNS**): abnormally swollen veins usually occurring in the superficial veins of the legs.
vascular birthmarks: birthmarks caused by blood vessels close to the skin's surface.
vascular dementia: a form of dementia caused by a restriction of blood to the brain.
vasculitis (**vas**-kyou-**LYE**-tis): inflammation of a blood vessel.
vasectomy (vah-**SECK**-toh-mee): the male sterilization procedure in which a small portion of the vas deferens is surgically blocked or cut.
vasoconstrictor (**vas**-oh-kon-**STRICK**-tor): medication that causes blood vessels to narrow.
vasodilator (vas-oh-dye-**LAYT**-or): medication that causes blood vessels to expand.
vasovasostomy (**vay**-soh-vah-**ZOS**-toh-mee): a procedure performed as an attempt to restore fertility to a vasectomized male.
vector-borne transmission: the spread of certain disease due to the bite of a vector (insects or animals that are capable of transmitting a disease).
venipuncture: the puncturing of a vein for the purpose of drawing blood.
venography (vee-**NOG**-rah-fee): a radiographic test that provides an image of specific veins after a contrast dye is injected.
venous stasis (**VEE**-nus **STAY**-sis): a condition of sluggish venous blood flow in the lower extremities.
venous thromboembolism: a blood clot that originates in a vein.
venous ulcer: an irregular open pit in the skin of the lower extremities caused by venous stasis.
ventilator: a mechanical device for artificial respiration that is used to replace or supplement the patient's natural breathing function.
ventricular assist device: an implanted mechanical pump that helps the heart circulate blood.
ventricular fibrillation (ven-**TRICK**-you-lar **fih**-brih-**LAY**-shun): rapid, irregular, and useless contractions of the ventricles.
ventricular septal defect: a congenital heart defect characterized by a hole between the two ventricles of the heart.
ventricular tachycardia (ven-**TRICK**-you-lar **tack**-ee-**KAR**-dee-ah): a very rapid heartbeat that begins within the ventricles.
verrucae (veh-**ROO**-kee): small, hard skin lesions caused by the human papillomavirus.
vertigo (**VER**-tih-goh): a sense of whirling, dizziness, and the loss of balance, often combined with nausea and vomiting.

vesicle (**VES**-ih-kul): a small blister, less than 0.5 cm in diameter, containing watery fluid.

vesicoureteral reflux (**veh**-sih-ko-you-**REE**-teh-ral): the backward flow of urine into the ureters from the bladder.

vesicovaginal fistula (**ves**-ih-koh-**VAJ**-ih-nahl **FIS**-tyou-lah): an abnormal opening between the bladder and vagina.

vestibular rehabilitation therapy (ves-**TIB**-you-lar): a form of physical therapy designed to treat a variety of balance disorders.

video-assisted thoracic surgery: the use of a thoracoscope to view the inside of the pleural cavity through very small incisions.

viral (**VYE**-ral): pertaining to a virus.

viral pneumonia: pneumonia caused by one of several different types of viruses.

viruses (**VYE**-rus-ez): very small infectious agents that live only by invading other cells.

visual acuity (ah-**KYOU**-ih-tee): the ability to distinguish object details and shape at a distance.

visual field testing: a diagnostic test to determine losses in peripheral vision.

viscosupplementation: a treatment using injections of hyaluronic acid in the knee to increase the joint's viscous fluid, providing temporary relief from arthritis pain.

vitamin: a dietary supplement containing one or more substances that are beneficial for humans.

vitiligo (**vit**-ih-**LYE**-goh): a skin condition resulting from the destruction of melanocytes due to unknown causes, resulting in irregular patches of white skin.

vitrectomy (vih-**TRECK**-toh-mee): the removal of the vitreous humor in the eye and its replacement with a saline solution.

voiding cystourethrography (**sis**-toh-you-ree-**THROG**-rah-fee): a diagnostic procedure in which fluoroscopy is used to examine the flow of urine from the bladder and through the urethra.

volvulus (**VOL**-view-lus): twisting of the intestine on itself, causing an obstruction.

Von Willebrand disease (von **VIL**-eh-brond): a genetic bleeding disorder caused by a clotting protein called the von Willebrand factor.

vulvitis (vul-**VYE**-tis): inflammation of the vulva.

vulvodynia (vul-voh-**DIN**-ee-ah): a painful syndrome of unknown cause characterized by chronic burning, dyspareunia, itching, or stinging irritation of the vulva.

W

weaning (**WEE**-ning): the gradual process of decreasing the work of breathing done by a ventilator, to measure whether a person can breathe spontaneously; also the process of discontinuing breastfeeding.

Weber and Rinne tests: hearing tests that use a tuning fork to distinguish between conductive and sensorineural hearing losses.

wedge resection: a surgery in which a small, wedge-shaped piece of cancerous lung tissue is removed, along with a margin of healthy tissue around the cancer.

wellness: actively working toward a state of being in good physical and mental health.

West Nile virus: a virus that causes flu-like symptoms; transmitted to humans by mosquito bites.

wheal (**WHEEL**): a small bump on the skin that itches.

white blood cell count: a blood test to determine the number of leukocytes in the blood.

white blood cell differential: a blood test to determine what percentage of the total white blood cell count is composed of each of the five types of leukocytes.

Wilms tumor (**VILMZ**): a rare type of malignant tumor of the kidney that occurs in young children.

work of breathing: the amount of energy required to inhale and exhale.

X

xeroderma (zee-roh-**DER**-mah): excessively dry skin.

xerophthalmia (**zeer**-ahf-**THAL**-mee-ah): drying of eye surfaces, including the conjunctiva.

xerostomia (**zeer**-oh-**STOH**-mee-ah): the lack of adequate saliva due to diminished secretions by the salivary glands.

x-ray: the image produced by the use of radiant energy to visualize conditions such as bone fractures; also known as a radiograph.

x-ray imaging: the use of x-radiation to visualize hard-tissue internal structures, also known as radiography.

Y

yeast: a type of fungus.

Z

Zika virus (**ZEE**-kah): a virus spread to humans by the bite of an infected mosquito; can cause fever, rash, and birth defects.

Index

C

D

E

I

M

N

Q

R

S

T

U

W

X

Y

Z